S0-EJQ-693

BONE TUMORS: DIAGNOSIS AND TREATMENT

BONE TUMORS

DIAGNOSIS AND TREATMENT

JOSEPH M. MIRRA, M.D.

Associate Professor
Division of Surgical Pathology
University of California, Los Angeles, California
Los Angeles, California

Chapters Written By

RICHARD H. GOLD, M.D.

Professor of Radiology and Chief of Radiology
University of California, Los Angeles, School of Medicine
Los Angeles, California

RALPH C. MARCOVE, M.D.

Clinical Associate Professor of Orthopaedics
Cornell University College of Medicine;
Associate Surgeon, Memorial Sloan-Kettering Institute
and The Hospital for Special Surgery;
Chief, Bone Tumor Service
Hospital for Joint Diseases
New York, New York

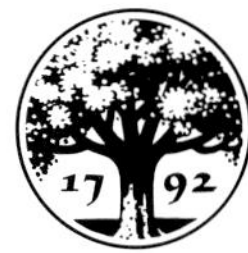

J. B. Lippincott Company
Philadelphia · Toronto

ISBN 0-397-50428-4
Library of Congress Catalog Card Number 80-21537
Printed in the United States of America
1 3 5 6 4 2

Library of Congress Cataloging in Publication Data

Mirra, Joseph M.
Bone tumors, diagnosis and treatment.

Includes index.
1. Bones—Tumors. I. Gold, Richard H., joint author.
II. Marcove, Ralph C., joint author. III. Title.
RC280.B6M57 616.9′92′71 [80-21537]
ISBN 0-397-50428-4

This book I dedicate to my son, Theodore; my mother, Irene; brothers, John and Jan; Aunts, Adeline and Melina; Uncles, Theodore and Tony; and my close friends, Doctor Lloyd Siegel and Carmen Landry.

PREFACE

The intended purpose of this book is to present an integrated clinical, radiologic, and pathologic approach dealing with the diagnosis and principles of treatment of the tumors of bone. Since it is diagnosis that determines therapy, the correct diagnosis is mandatory. There is little room for error or the results will often be diastrous to the patient. Tumors of the mesenchyme are extremely treacherous in that benign lesions can be easily confused with malignant, and the reverse. Stress fractures must be recognized as such, enchondroma of long bones differentiated from chondrosarcoma, "invasive" pigmented villonodular synovitis from a spindle cell sarcoma, traumatic periostitis from periosteal osteosarcoma, osteoblastoma from osteosarcoma, and desmoid tumors from fibrosarcoma. By careful clinical and radiologic correlation, the problems associated with slide diagnosis and the distinction between a benign and malignant tumor can be greatly facilitated. For this reason, this text places great stress upon clinical, radiologic, and pathologic correlation. "Slide readings" alone are to be condemned except in the most obvious cases, which are the minority. Radiographic correlation is vital to bone tumor diagnosis. Correctly interpreted they supply the diagnostician with considerable information about the actual or probable biologic behavior of the lesion in question. Analysis of the radiograph may be the main feature that protects the diagnostician from mistaking a "stress" fracture for an osteosarcoma. A complete rind of reactive bone sclerosis around a lesion almost always signifies benignancy. The diagnosis of a "sclerosing" osteosarcoma with minimal cytologic atypia is often given away by the radiograph because of its massive size, metaphyseal location, infiltrating and coalescing "cumulus-cloud" fluffs of bone production, soft-tissue mass, and ominous periosteal reactions, including the so-called Codman's triangle. Correlation of the radiographic, gross, and microscopic features of individual cases supplies one with an enormous understanding applicable to future case diagnosis. Few of the bone tumors present with a pathognomonic or "classic" radiographic or histologic pattern. Tumors of bone are characterized by considerable variation. For these reasons the text covers, as much as is feasible, the full range of radiographic and histologic patterns an individual tumor may assume, particularly those which, if the pattern is not well known, could lead to diagnostic confusion. The most common or "classic" features are clearly defined first and less common patterns are presented thereafter. Any significant stray from the general or usual range for a contemplated tumor diagnosis should be an immediate danger signal that the presumptive diagnosis may be in error. Therefore, by knowing the full range of manifestations an individual tumor may assume, the diagnostician is alerted to the dangers of including it or excluding it from his list of differential possibilities.

Other factors dealt with in depth in this text include the danger of biopsying from the wrong site, when tissue should be submitted to surgical pathology fresh for tumor imprints or electron microscopy, and when to use superior fixatives such as Zenker's. In order to firmly classify some of the lesions, it may be essential to observe what is occurring at the edge of the tumor with the host bone. This may be all that clearly separates a small "sclerosing" osteosarcoma from an osteoblastoma, for example. This, of course, implies that such an area was sampled by the surgeon. From the text it should become obvious when rebiopsy may be indicated for fresh tissue or from the advancing edge of the lesion. It is also of increasing importance to determine margins because amputation for malignant tumors is rapidly giving way to en-bloc resections in many of the major institutions. How should such specimens be dissected? Does the degree of tumor necrosis caused by preoperative chemo- and radiotherapy influence possible recurrence or survival? The methods of dissection are treated in Chapter 2 and the importance of striving for answers to these questions are also dealt with in the text. Chapter 2 is devoted to the techniques necessary to a vigorous assessment of a bone tumor pathology workup. The techniques of imprints, specimen radiography, slicing the bone, decalcification, embedding, and photography are covered.

The chapter organization of the tumors per se in this text is based upon nine principal histologic features that includes the following tissues or cells: lamellar bone, osteoid and woven bone, cartilage, myxoid, spindle cells, giant cell, round cells and histiocytes, and cystic, vascular, and epithelial cells. Each tumor can be considered to contain one or more of these nine basic histologic components. The bone tumor chapters (7 through 14) and the tables of differential diagnosis (Chap. 6) are based upon this format. Therefore, if an individual tumor can have more than one of the above nine components, it will appear in multiple chapters and tables. The reader must be made aware that if a tumor can contain histologic components A B C . . . , these components may be found in any proportion in an individual case and that any component or combination of components A B C . . . may dominate an individual slide field or the entire lesion. Without this knowledge dominant components not ordinarily considered in the "mind's eye" of the diagnostician as being "typical" of a particular case in study may lead to diagnostic confusion. For example, an osteosarcoma may be dominated by spindle cells, osteoclasts, or cartilage. This may result in erroneous diagnoses of fibrosarcoma, giant cell tumor, or chondrosarcoma. However, by using the differential diagnostic tables of Chapter 6 for spindle cells, giant cell, or cartilage components, the osteosarcoma will always be found to be one of those tumors that enter into the differential diagnosis. In other words, the possibility that a spindle cell, giant cell, or cartilage-predominant tumor could be an osteosarcoma would not be left to chance. In standard bone tumor texts one will not ordinarily find the osteosarcoma in those chapters dealing with fibrous, cartilage, or giant cell tumors. The osteosarcoma will also be mentioned in each of these chapters and the reader referred to the appropriate pages and illustrations to help evaluate this possibility. Therefore, an attempt is made to protect the reader against not knowing which chapter to use in order to help with the diagnosis of a particular case, because this would presuppose a knowledge that the diagnostician may not yet command.

To give another example: under which chapter should "invasive" pigmented villonodular synovitis be included? It can be dominated by the following components: spindle cells, giant cells, round cells, or histiocytes and slitlike spaces. If one is confronted with one or more of these components and one is not aware of this unusual secondary bone tumor, most books will not force the reader to consider this possibility unless the entire book is read with great care. Quite often this lesion is mistaken for a sarcoma by pathologists in whom the diagnosis of PVNS is not made prior to or during biopsy by the radiologist or surgeon. With the system employed in this book the reader must consider "invasive" PVNS if he uses the differential tables of Chapter 6 applicable to spindle cells, giant cells, round cells, or slitlike spaces.

The last chapter in this book is devoted to techniques and principles of treatment applicable primarily to the malignant tumors of bone. Dr. Marcove is one of the world's outstanding bone tumor surgeons and has pioneered the use of cryosurgery to the treatment of benign and malignant bone tumors. The specific details of his method are illustrated and discussed in great depth. The newer chemotherapies and radiotherapy are turning the tables on the malignant bone sarcoma survival statistics. Drs. Marcove and Rosen of Memorial Hospital are at the forefront of their respective fields of surgery and chemotherapy.

ACKNOWLEDGMENTS

The author wishes to acknowledge MedCom Products for the use of many illustrations and some text from their slide and sound teaching sets on Orthopedic Diseases by Joseph Mirra, Peter Bullough, and Robert Freiberger. I also thank J. B. Lippincott Company and Dr. Walter Coulson for their permission to use some of the illustrations that appear in chapters I have written for the book entitled *Surgical Pathology* edited by Walter Coulson.

I also wish to acknowledge the innumerable physicians who have sent me fascinating case material over the years, Ms. Mary Jane Thias, who helped me with Chapter 2, Mrs. Rosalyn Siegel, a close friend, who gave editorial assistance; my secretary, Ms. Mirna Flores, who spent many arduous hours typing the manuscript and who was always a pleasure to work with; and to Mr. Stuart Freeman, Editor-in-Chief of J. B. Lippincott Company; Lewis Reines, former Editor-in Chief of J. B. Lippincott Company; and Ms. Marilyn Fenichel, Copy Editor, Medical Books, for their patience, time, effort, and generosity in preparing the manuscript for publication.

Finally, I give my deepest thanks to those physicians who have always given freely of their time to consult and educate me in the principles of diagnostic pathology, radiology, and surgery. These outstanding and inspiring teachers to whom I owe all includes: Drs. Ralph Marcove, Peter Bullough, Robert Freiberger, Elias Theros, Richard Gold, Robert Mellors, Henry Jaffe, David Dahlin, Lent Johnson, Valentine Yermakov, Gordon Henniger, George Bernard, and Donald Morton.

CONTENTS

BONE TUMORS: DIAGNOSIS AND TREATMENT

INTRODUCTION: DIAGNOSTIC GOALS AND COMMENTS TO THE PATHOLOGIST, RADIOLOGIST, AND ORTHOPAEDIC SURGEON

1

PURPOSE

The ultimate goal of this book is to improve the skills of the reader in diagnosing tumors of the bone and understanding the principles involved in treating them.

Diagnosis determines treatment. Unless the diagnosis is correct, the patient may suffer irreparable consequences. The mesenchymal tissues (bone, soft tissue, and hematopoietic system) are the most treacherous to diagnose precisely because of the tremendous variability of histologic patterns. Hyperplastic, reparative, and pseudoanaplastic lesions are easily mistaken for malignant neoplasms, while lethal malignancies with low-grade anaplasia may initially be confused with benign tumors. Unless one is aware of how inordinately common these pitfalls are, the urgency to correlate all of the available clinical, laboratory and radiographic data may not be fully appreciated. There is no justification for a pathologic diagnosis based solely on a slide "reading" alone or in conjunction with only a tenous presumptive clinical diagnosis on a pathology sheet. This is especially true when tumors of the bone are concerned.

COMMENTS TO THE PATHOLOGIST

Manner in Which This Text Should be Used to Aid Diagnosis

The responsibility for the final diagnosis rests with the pathologist. This text is, therefore, geared to him.

The pathologist should first examine the slide material carefully and then obtain the facts of the case. All of the pertinent clinical, laboratory and radiologic data must be accumulated and reviewed and correlated to the pathologic information. The novice in bone tumor diagnosis should obtain the consultative services of a radiologist who can point out the pertinent bits of radiologic information. Hereafter, the term *bits of information* will be referred to simply as "bits." The pathologist should inquire about the radiologic features of the tumor in question: Is it bordered by sclerosis? Is Codman's triangle visible? Is the pattern of bone destruction centered in the epiphysis, metaphysis, diaphysis? He should learn which features imply a benign lesion and which a malignancy, and should obtain from the radiologist a list of possible differential diagnoses. If the radiologist is quite sure of a particular diagnosis and states that the case is a "classic" this or that, this information will, of course, be extremely valuable and influential in helping the pathologist arrive at a final decision. The pathologist should, nevertheless, be aware that a small percentage of "classic" radiologic diagnoses may be in error. After obtaining the radiologic bits and the presumptive radiologic diagnoses, the pathologist should take the radiographs back to his office and restudy the slides. A list of the main histologic bits or features should be written down. At this point, the book will become extremely useful, because it is organized on the basis of cell types and/or the matrices they may produce.

Broad categories have been chosen by which to group the tumors, such as woven-bone- and cartilage-producing, lesions containing giant cells, round cells, and others. The reader should consult Chapter 6, which contains differential diagnostic tables based upon principal histologic features, the localization of the tumor within a bone, and the type of bone in which the tumor is found (e.g., long bones, skull, spine). On the right-hand side of the tables are the page and figure references that pertain to each of the possibilities. More details about using the tables, with a few examples, are given in the introduction to Chapter 6.

If the accumulated bits are gathered correctly, one should be able to use the tables to make up a list of most of the possible tumors the lesion in question could be. This is not to imply that the tables are fail-safe, but they should be a great aid in obtaining a reasonable differential diagnosis for approximately 95 per cent of the tumors of bone the pathologist will see. The appropriate lesion or lesions may not, however, be identified if the information gathering is in error. Absolutely crucial to the use of the tables is the proper categorization of the cells and tissues present. Small foci of cartilage or osteoid, if not recognized as such, will severely reduce, if not nullify, the usefulness of the tables and obscure the proper diagnosis.

Diagnosis depends upon accurate classification of the tumor in question by appropriate pathologic techniques, which may include imprints, special stains, specimen radiographs, and electron microscopy. The reader is referred to Chapters 2 and 5 for a detailed discussion of the classification of the tumors of bone and the specific pathologic methods recommended in the workup of biopsy, frozen section, en-bloc, and amputation specimens.

Processes Involved in Diagnostic Decision-Making

A few words about the thought processes used in achieving a diagnosis is now appropriate. Basically, in reviewing the slide material and the clinical, radiologic, or other pertinent data, we accumulate bits of vital information. Each bit for any particular tumor can be represented by a statistical probability. For example, suppose that among a series of 100 osteosarcomas, only one is smaller than 2 cm. in maximum size. If we are confronted with an unknown tumor that is only 4 mm. in size, we can safely say, from this one bit of information, that the chance that the tumor is an osteosarcoma is less than 1 per cent. Based upon our personal experience and information in books or papers we consult, we should attempt to put these bits into perspective. This is done by first formulating a differential diagnosis list and then striving, by accumulating more bits or researching more extensively those we have, to arrive at a single (and, we hope, correct) diagnosis. If one's confidence limit approaches 100 per cent, the probability that the diagnosis is correct obviously improves. As one's confidence limit falls, so does the probability of a correct diagnosis. It would be wise, therefore, to seek consultative advice on all cases in which the level of confidence is not high. The level of confidence should, of course, depend on knowledge and experience. For example, let us assume that two pathologists review exactly the same slide material, and radiographs and possess the same clinical information. One pathologist may be able to accumulate only five bits of relevant information, while the other may accumulate not only those five but 25 others as well. Armed with only five bits the first pathologist is in trouble, because many types of bone tumors will almost certainly have those five bits in common. His differential list should be a long one. His final diagnosis will, therefore, be in grave danger of being in error. If his confidence limit is high for a particular diagnosis that is based upon only a few bits, it is not knowledge that supports the diagnosis. On the other hand, 30 bits of information are usually more than enough to favor one diagnosis above all others, and it will likely be correct. Although the reader may at first have been able to collect only a few bits on a particular tumor, by using the text and isolating the diagnostic possibilities based upon those bits, it should become obvious what additional bits are necessary to establish accuracy in diagnosis. Not only should the reader accumulate bits but an individual bit must be related to a "ball park figure" of probability for a particular diagnosis he entertains in his differential list of possibilities. In this manner one will quickly learn how to use the odds to help isolate the best diagnosis.

For example, let us assume that the reader is in possession of only the following "bits": the lesion arises in the metaphysis of a long bone and produces cartilage. This is enough information to obtain a differential diagnostic list from Table 6–3; from this point, he can then gather additional information by referring to those text pages and illustrations from the right-hand side of the table that pertains to each lesion so culled. Or suppose a lesion contains masses of benign osteoclast-like giant cells and oval to spindly stromal cells and the pathologist is entertaining, among others, the diagnosis of a low-grade neoplastic giant cell tumor. Suppose, however, that another of his bits is that the lesion is centered in the diaphysis. If he used the text, he will find that only very rarely is this tumor centered in the diaphysis.

Among over 500 reported cases of neoplastic giant cell tumor, only a few have been reported as arising from this region of a bone. The probability that the lesion in question is a neoplastic giant cell tumor is less than 2 per cent. By accumulating other bits of clinical and radiologic information, as will be made clear in the text, such as the serum calcium and phosphorous, the reader will probably learn that the lesion in question is in reality a giant cell tumor of hyperparathyroidism.

One actual case example will serve to illustrate further the way in which bits placed in proper perspective can be used to arrive at a correct final diagnosis. All of the pertinent bits are italicized.

A *14-year-old boy* was referred to UCLA with a diagnosis of *osteosarcoma* of the right *distal humerus.* Only one slide and this meager history were provided. Review of the slide showed a lesion that produced abundant *osteoid* and *woven* bone. The *osteoblasts* were plump and *exuberant* but contained few *mirror-image mitoses* and *no signs* of *unequivocal* or *frank anaplasia. Osteoclasts* were numerous. The *stroma* was *richly vascular.* Based upon this review, the diagnosis of osteosarcoma was certainly possible, since approximately 20 per cent of osteosarcomas may not show unequivocal anaplasia. But, other lesions, such as the osteoid osteoma, osteoblastoma, and fracture callus, may show similar findings or bits. At this point, it is necessary to accumulate more clinical and radiologic bits. Therefore, a history was taken which included the following information: The patient had had progressively increasing *pain* in this site for over $1\frac{1}{2}$ *years,* with *joint effusion* developing a few days prior to surgical intervention. Because of the effusion and lack of diagnosis, a biopsy of the joint was performed. At operation the *synovium* was *reddish* and *hyperplastic* and an *incidental 3-mm., round, reddish lesion* was seen on the *bone cortex*. The lesion was contained within the joint capsule at the border of the host *metaphyseal cortical bone* and the articular cartilage. This lesion was curetted and sent for diagnosis. It was on the cortical lesion that the diagnosis of osteosarcoma was made. The *synovium showed nonspecific chronic synovitis.* Far fewer than 1 per cent of all osteosarcomas present with as great as a $1\frac{1}{2}$-year history of symptoms and less than 1 per cent are associated with synovitis. The incidence of osteosarcoma with this combination of unusual features is one in 10,000 or less. Therefore, the diagnosis of osteosarcoma is statistically highly improbable. The only lesion that fits every parameter mentioned is the osteoid osteoma with resultant "irritative" synovitis. Thus, the diagnosis was changed, with confidence, to osteoid osteoma. The patient is doing very well after a 2-year follow-up. All symptoms have been relieved and there is no evidence of a residual lesion on radiograph or of metastases.

The reader could have reached these same conclusions by consulting Table 6–2, on woven-bone- and osteoid-producing lesions and Table 6-5, on giant cells (osteoclasts). The lesions that would have been considered—those showing metaphyseal involvement of a long bone with these two principal histologic features—would have included the osteoid osteoma (common), osteoblastoma (common), fibrous dysplasia (common), hyperparathyroidism (common), Paget's disease (uncommon), solitary and aneurysmal bone cysts (common), low-grade neoplastic giant cell tumor (rare), osteogenic sarcoma (common), and metastases with "reactive" bone (uncommon). The patient's age and histologic bits eliminate Paget's disease and metastasis from contention. Reference to the pages and figures of each of the other entities from the right side would have shown that only the *osteoid osteoma* fits all of the observed bits well.

To summarize, the *osteoid osteoma* is a *roundish, red lesion, less than 1 to 2 cm. in size,* characterized by *progressive pain* of *months* to *years duration,* and histologically by an *exuberance* of *osteoblasts, osteoid, woven bone, osteoclasts,* and *prominent vascularity.* When it is located near a joint cavity, it causes *synovitis* and *effusion.* Many cases are located in a *juxtacortical metaphyseal* position. It is entirely *benign* and needs only a curettage or small en-bloc excision for cure.

Bits of information may, therefore, be assigned a certain weight based upon their probability. Bits in the 1 or 99 per cent range of probability are obviously much more important in the final decision-making process than those in the 10 to 90 per cent range. For example, let us assume that a patient is 35 years of age. This bit would not weigh heavily against a diagnosis of osteoid osteoma, if that were one of the diagnoses under consideration, because 10 per cent of patients with this disease are in this age group. However, if the patient were age 65, this diagnosis would be highly improbable ($<1\%$). Such statistical information relating to age can be obtained in the text from the age incidence tables given for each tumor.

Certain bits are so crucial they can literally nullify all others, no matter what the others' possibilities are. For example, suppose a lesion were centered in the epiphysis and was 1.5 cm. in size. The chances of this being an osteosarcoma from these bits is only .01 per cent (1% of osteosarcomas arise in the epiphysis x 1 per cent of osteosarcomas are less than 2 cm. in size).

However, if the lesion is shown unequivocally by microscopic examination to be composed of frankly anaplastic cells that produce osteoid and woven bone and are rich in atypical mitoses, the diagnosis is osteosarcoma, no matter how improbable the other features.

Bits of information usually take precedence in the following order: histologic, radiologic, historical, and laboratory. The importance of the correct categorization of the most subjective of these various types of bits, namely, the histologic, is obvious. The example of the pathologist who confused the exuberant osteoblastic hyperplasia of an osteoid osteoma with an osteosarcoma is a prime example of what could occur if radiologic information is reviewed inadequately and when exuberant mesenchymal reactions are confused with anaplasia. This reemphasizes the need for the correlation of the more objective bits of clinical and radiologic information we have at our disposal with the histologic ones. The radiographic bits represent a built-in system of checks and balances to help protect us from the potentially illusory world of the microscope. The microscope is a potent diagnostic tool, but one must be aware of its limitations, particularly in regard to the complex histologic processes associated with the tumors of the mesenchyme.

Seeking Consultative Advice

If the pathologist has any doubts about his presumed diagnosis, it is advisable for him to seek consultative advice from an experienced bone tumor pathologist. The responsibility of the bone tumor "expert" is to provide a firm and accurate diagnosis and to suggest possible therapy, if this is requested. If he has any reservations about the diagnosis or treatment, this will usually appear in his letter of consultation. A bone tumor consultant has seen several thousand such cases. Because of this vast experience, his accuracy rate is generally high, at least as far as determining whether the tumor is benign or malignant. If several bone tumor experts are consulted, the range of identical diagnosis will fall. The most common differences of opinion among experts are fibrosarcoma versus malignant fibrous histiocytoma, malignant fibrous histiocytoma versus osteogenic sarcoma or malignant giant-cell tumor, mesenchymal chondrosarcoma versus osteogenic sarcoma, pigmented villonodular synovitis versus benign histiocytoma or reparative giant cell granuloma. In all of these instances the diagnosis does not alter biologic behavior and treatment significantly. However, in some cases there will be serious disagreements about whether the tumor is benign or malignant. In my experience the most common examples have been the distinction of osteoblastoma from osteosarcoma, enchondroma from low-grade chondrosarcoma, osteoblastoma from giant cell tumor with woven-bone production, and traumatic reparative lesions from sarcoma. Fortunately, these serious differences in judgment are not common.

In order to aid the bone tumor consultant, the consultees have certain responsibilities to fulfill. Whenever a consultation is requested, the pathologist should send all of the pertinent clinical, laboratory, slide material and radiographs on the case. As a courtesy, copies of the slides and radiographs should be included. This will enable the consultant to keep permanent records and to review the material again, should the need arise. The pathologist should consider the consultant's opinion by comparing it with other opinions and by noting unexpected changes in the status of the patient. For example, in any case diagnosed as benign in which a massive recurrence, metastasis or lethal outcome occurs, the consultant should receive the pertinent history, slides, or autopsy material on which his original diagnosis was based. In some cases benign lesions can transform to malignancies; if this occurs, it will not negate the original diagnosis. In other cases the course of the patient and slide material may show that the original interpretation was in error. The consultant must be made aware of any errors in judgment in order to minimize the possibility of similar mistakes occurring in the future. Bone tumor diagnosis is an extremely difficult task, even for the experts; the responsibilities are great and the risks to the patient, if the diagnosis is in error, are enormous. The future of bone tumor diagnosis depends upon a close cooperative effort between the consultees and consultants. If pertinent follow-up information on the patients is not supplied to the consultants, then errors is diagnosis of similar case material could be compounded many times over.

COMMENTS TO THE RADIOLOGIST

Radiological interpretation is greatly facilitated if the radiologist has a sound understanding of the gross and microscopic pathology of each bone tumor. The manner in which a particular tumor spreads through the bone, the matrices they may produce, the degree of bone destruction, and the reactions of the host bone tissues determine the radiologic patterns. Each tumor often has a "classic" pattern and a range of less typical patterns. The radiologist should not merely memorize radiological tumor patterns; he should first review the illustrations that show the gross features of a lesion and then correlate specimen radiographs (if provided) with the standard radiographic illustrations.

The histologic illustrations that show the various types of calcifications and matrix production and low-power microscopic illustrations of each tumor should also be reviewed. Particular attention should be given to the growth of the tumor. Does it grow in lobules, is it diffusely infiltrative; are the margins of the tumor sharply circumscribed or ill-defined? Does the lesion produce woven bone or lamellar bone? Can these two types of bone be distinguished radiologically? Do malignant lesions produce lamellar bone? Is the tumor characterized by calcifications? What are the radiological signs of a benign versus malignant cartilage tumor? How do these signs correlate with behavior, gross features, other characteristics? These are the kinds of questions the radiologist must ask and attempt to answer from the illustrations and text.

The lesions in this text that the radiologist would most benefit from reading include the osteoid osteoma, osteoblastoma, fibrous dysplasia, Paget's disease, osteosarcoma, enchondroma, chondroblastoma, nonossifying fibroma, chondrosarcoma, chondrosarcoma with fibrosarcomatous transformation, giant cell tumor, hyperparathyroidism and sarcoma arising from bone infarcts. These lesions have very distinct radiographic features when correlated with their gross and microscopic appearances.

COMMENTS TO THE ORTHOPAEDIC SURGEON

The orthopaedist is entrusted with the care and treatment of the patient with the bone tumor. He depends upon the radiologist and pathologist for diagnosis. The care and treatment of the purely benign lesions are generally well understood and this book will add little new information. However, the low-grade malignant tumors (giant cell tumor, chordoma, adamantinoma, parosteal osteosarcoma) and the high-grade malignancies pose numerous problems in treatment. Should the surgeon elect to perform an en-bloc excision, cryosurgery, amputation, radiation, radiation and chemotherapy followed by en-bloc excision, or other methods? We have entrusted Dr. Marcove to write a chapter on these various therapeutic modalities, their techniques, and the manner in which a specific modality is arrived at for the treatment of a specific tumor in a specific location. Knowledge of the variations of the extent of spread, determination of whether the tumor has broken through the bone or not, evaluation of the grade of malignancy and its location, and the age of the patient are all important factors in determining the mode of therapy.

In my experience, the most common errors the orthopaedist makes in treating bone tumors are as follows:

1. Inadequate biopsy material, upon which diagnosis and therapy depend.
2. The meager or inadequate use of the powerful therapeutic techniques of cryosurgery or en-bloc excision, particularly for low-grade malignancies such as the giant cell tumor and low-grade chondrosarcomas.

INADEQUATE BIOPSY. Unless the surgeon and pathologist are aware of the difficulties attendant with particular bone tumors, inadequate biopsies may be performed. Some tumors pose very difficult to impossible diagnostic problems if only formalin-fixed needle or curettage specimens are obtained. Any tumor suspected of being a "round cell" tumor should be sent to the pathologist fresh, not fixed in formalin. The pathologist will be greatly aided in his diagnosis by preparing fresh tumor imprints for cytology and special stains. Fresh tumor can also be fixed in glutaraldehyde for electron microscopic studies, which are especially helpful in differentiating Ewing's tumor from reticulum cell sarcoma and metastatic melanoma from carcinoma.

In other tumors, observing the junction of the tumor with the host bone may be very important in diagnosis. A wedge biopsy of the tumor-host bone interface can provide vital information in distinguishing an exuberant osteoblastoma from an osteosarcoma or a low-grade anaplastic osteosarcoma from an osteoblastoma. Similarly, a small biopsy of a low-grade chondrosarcoma may be mistaken for an enchondroma; more generous amounts of tissue would be much more informative. In dealing with a cartilage tumor by radiograph, the surgeon should always attempt to obtain biopsy material from the most lytic or "fuzzy" areas. The homogeneous stippled calcified areas of a cartilage tumor, on the other hand, usually show the smallest degree of malignancy and may represent an area of enchondroma, while lytic or "fuzzy" areas of calcification often represent that portion of the formerly benign lesion that underwent malignant transformation.

MEAGER OR INADEQUATE USE OF CRYOSURGERY AND EN-BLOC RESECTION. Cryosurgery and en-bloc resection are remarkable techniques for the cure of low-grade neoplastic giant cell tumor and low-grade chondrosarcomas. With cryosurgery, the patients's host bone is retained, morbidity is low, and eventual function is usually excellent. But lack of technical "know-how" and full knowledge of the extent of the tumor in the bone can lead to an inadequately treated zone, recurrence, and potential amputation. Both procedures are excellent and vital techniques that should be at the disposal of any surgeon who treats bone tumors, but proper education about how to use them is a prerequisite. The orthopaedic surgeon interested in treating bone tumors should seek the necessary knowledge and training from a skilled individual or from a medical center proficient in their use.

The actual area of bone a malignant tumor involves is often from 1 to 5 cm. beyond that ordinarily visible by standard radiographs. This is particularly true of the chondrosarcoma, fibrosarcoma, and the round cell malignancies. Any case in which local extirpation is contemplated (cryosurgery versus en-bloc excision), the surgeon must make every attempt to determine safe margins. If any viable tumor is left behind or is cut through at the time of resection, the results will be limb- and life-threatening. Consultation with experienced radiologists and pathologists may be necessary to reduce this error to a minimum. Tomography, computerized bone scans, and the newer techniques of EMI and computerized axial tomography (CAT) scanning will delineate the actual extent of the tumor much more accurately than ordinary radiographs.

The "best shot" at controlling a malignant bone tumor in which local surgery is deemed feasible is at the time of the first procedure. Thereafter, the risks of amputation become much more insurmountable. "Second looks" a few months following the initial procedure may be used to see whether there is any local recurrence before they become clinically obvious. Waiting until recurrence is clincially obvious may preclude treatment short of amputation. The bone tumors in which en-bloc resection and/or cryosurgery play the greatest role include the neoplastic giant cell tumor, Grade I to low Grade II chondrosarcoma, borderline-malignant enchondroma of long bones, parosteal osteosarcoma, adamantinoma, and the chordoma.

PATHOLOGICAL TECHNIQUES AND WORKUP OF SPECIMENS

2

Because bone is a calcified tissue, specialized procedures and equipment are required to obtain slab sections for good, gross visualization of the tumor, specimen radiographs, and histologic studies. The technical procedures and equipment we use in our laboratory will be described in this chapter.

The two pieces of equipment that we find indispensable to the workup of bone tumors are a large, butcher-type band saw and x-ray apparatus. The band saw permits the physician to obtain 2- to 3-mm. slabs of the tumor and surrounding tissues, from which a gross description, closeness of tumor to margins, photographs, radiographs, and sections are obtained. The techniques described herein are neither difficult nor excessively time consuming.

PURPOSES OF THE PATHOLOGICAL WORKUP OF BONE TUMORS

Biopsy and Small Excision Specimens

The purpose of needle and open biopsies of bone tumors is to achieve a specific and firm diagnosis. To do this, great care must be exercised to preserve cytologic detail. In order to obtain the maximum amount of information from the biopsy, it is best to obtain fresh tumor tissue as often as possible. A portion of the fresh tissue should be used to prepare imprints (see p. 10) and a portion for possible electron microscopic studies. The remainder of the tissue should be divided and placed into Zenker's and 10 per cent neutral buffered formalin. Zenker's is a much better preservative for cytologic detail than is formalin. But, before the tissue is placed into these solutions, at least one of the prepared imprints should be stained with hematoxylin-eosin (H and E) to check its quality, and the imprints should be repeated until high quality is obtained. Several unstained imprints should also be reserved for special stains, if desired, after the permanent sections have been reviewed.

If the tissue has been sent to pathology in formalin, imprints cannot be prepared, but a small portion could be placed in glutaraldehyde for possible electron microscopy (EM) studies, particularly if the routine histologic sections are equivocal.

Small excisions are almost always performed for benign bone tumors such as the osteoid osteoma. If the osteoid osteoma is buried in a mass of thick, reactive host bone, the specimen should be radiographed prior to sectioning to identify its exact location.

Large En-Bloc Resection or Amputation Specimens

Large en-bloc resections that include muscle and fascial planes and amputation specimens are usually performed for malignant tumors. The section below lists minimal objectives that must be met.

SPECIFIC DIAGNOSIS. A biopsy represents but a small portion of the tumor. En-bloc and amputation specimens offer the entire lesion to the pathologist; he can obtain significant additional information from these specimens. The biopsy diagnosis can be either verified or amended. It may be found that the malignant tumor has arisen from a formerly benign lesion. Fresh tissue that may not have been available at biopsy can be obtained for imprint analysis and ultramicroscopic studies, particularly if there were any doubts about the precise classification of the tumor.

CLOSENESS OF TUMOR TO MARGINS. Another essential aspect of the workup is to define the adequacy of margins. In order to achieve complete visualization of the tumor and its proximity to margins, the bone and surrounding soft tissues should be sliced into 2- to 3-mm. slabs using a band saw. (See below for the technical details.) The margins of amputation specimens are almost always free of tumor. A single section of the proximal bone margin and one or two from the proximal soft tissues should be sufficient. However, because of the insidious nature and manner of spread of sarcomas, en-bloc resections require numerous sections to ensure the adequacy of the margins. Visualization of entire 2- to 3-mm. slabs will greatly aid in determining from where the most appropriate sections should be obtained. Usually if the tumor is a few millimeters beneath a fascial plane, sections from the tumor's margins do not show microscopic penetration through the fascia. But, if a sarcoma is within 1 cm. or less from a nonfascial plane such as a muscle, fat, or joint margin, the sections from these areas are much more likely to show microscopic infiltration to the margin. I have observed that in two of 13 cases of osteosarcoma in which en-bloc resections were performed through the joint closest to the tumor, that tumor was found to have spread to the joint margin. The tumors were metaphyseal and had broken through the bone at this site. Although the margins appeared to be 1 to 1.5 cm. away from the joint by gross observation, microscopic analysis showed that the tumor extended to the synovial tissue. The presence of viable tumor in margins requires either a more extensive en-bloc resection or amputation.

After analyzing many osteosarcomas, it is my opinion that if en-bloc resection is to be performed to save the limb and the tumor is metaphyseal and has broken through the cortex, the safest procedure is to remove the contiguous joint and bone. From the past experience of others, it was learned that if a sarcoma is close to a joint, the amputation should be well above that joint in order to minimize recurrence. For example, if an osteosarcoma involves the proximal tibial metaphysis, the amputation should be well above the region of the distal femoral metaphysis; that is, an above-knee amputation. But if an osteosarcoma involves the distal femoral metaphysis, either a disarticulation at the proximal femoral head area or transection through the upper femoral shaft many centimeters from the tumor might be performed, depending upon the assessed degree of extension of the tumor up the shaft, the type of sarcoma in question, and the judgment of the surgeon. The same rules should be applied to en-bloc resections of sarcomas that have breached the metaphyseal cortex, since malignant tumors located only short distances from a joint have, in our experience, a significant chance of having spread to the joint tissues. Transected, tumor-contaminated joint tissues can be expected to eventually nullify the essential purpose of en-bloc resection: life as well as limb salvage.

EFFECT OF PREOPERATIVE THERAPY ON THE TUMOR. Several institutions now employ various chemo- and/or radiotherapeutic regimens in the treatment of soft-tissue and bone sarcomas. At our institution, on an experimental basis, en-bloc resection is being performed for limb salvage. Previously the treatment would have been amputation or radiation, or both. The pathologist should evaluate the effect of these therapies upon the tumor. One way to do this is to measure the degree of tumor necrosis by estimating the per cent of necrosis from numerous tissue sections. This can be done by placing tumors in one of five categories, depending on the degree of necrosis of tumor. The categories we use are: 0 to 24 per cent, 25 to 49 per cent, 50 to 74 per cent, 75 to 99 per cent and 100 per cent. Whether or not the degree of tumor necrosis has a direct correlation to survival or an inverse correlation to recurrence remains to be seen. Therefore, depending on the results of such studies, the pathological assessment of tumor necrosis might prove to be useful for monitoring the effectiveness of the various chemoradiotherapeutic regimens. It could also be used to modify or alter dosages in order to achieve maximal tumor necrosis for a particular combination of drugs.

LYMPH NODE AND/OR VASCULAR INVASION. Not uncommonly there is microscopic evidence of vascular invasion by the sarcoma. Metastasis to regional lymph nodes from primary bone sarcomas is an unusual to rare phenomenon. Nevertheless, these tissues should be examined, because their relationship to survival has not yet been adequately studied.

APPARATUS USED IN BONE TUMOR WORKUP

Band Saw

In order to visualize the specimen adequately and to prepare tissue for photography, specimen radiographs, and tissue sections, the bone or limb should be cut into 2- to 3-mm. serial slabs with a rugged band saw. For our purposes we find that a Butcher-

Boy Band Saw Model #B-14, 5.7 amps; 220 volts with a 1.5 horse power (h.p.) motor, excellent for obtaining slab sections with a minimum of bone dust. We have found a fine-tooth blade (Lenox Meat Master blades, 112 inches long by 5/8 inches wide, Gage .020, teeth 10) better than coarse tooth blades. Rebuilt machines can be purchased for a considerably lower price than unused models. Before cutting the bone, the plane of section that will offer the greatest information should be determined by reviewing the patient radiographs.

We have found that soft tissues are likely to be pulled into the machine or stripped from the bone; if this occurs, important margin relationships will be destroyed. In addition, tumors that are soft such as the giant cell tumor may be decimated by the saw. These hazards to proper workup can be eliminated by freezing the specimen overnight or over the weekend. In this manner perfect slabs of soft tissues, tumor, and bone can be achieved with no distortion of bone architecture or destruction of soft-tissue margins. Rapid freezing leads to minimal cytologic distortion. It is our policy, however, to obtain some fresh tumor tissue first (before freezing) for imprint analysis and to fix some fresh tissue in Zenker's for better cytologic detail, and in glutaraldehyde, for possible electron microscopic studies. In order to get to the tumor as rapidly as possible without marring the specimen with numerous scalpel cuts, a preoperative radiograph for orientation is essential. If the tumor has broken through the bone, a sample of the lesion is easily obtained. If it is still confined to bone, a hammer and chisel may be necessary to obtain a portion of fresh tumor tissue. The remainder of the specimen is then rapidly frozen at $-20°F$ or colder.

After slicing the frozen specimen into 2- to 3-mm. slabs, a slurry will cover the surface and obscure gross examination. The slabs should be washed with a stream of cool water and a fine-bristle bottle brush until the colors and landmarks are brilliantly outlined. The surface should then be dried briefly with a paper towel or tissues. The slabs can then be photographed and radiographed and appropriate tissue sections can be made. The bone-tissue sections can be trimmed to cassette size with the aid of the band saw. All of the sections taken should, of course, be properly labelled and placed into cassettes or paper bags. If the tissue sections contain bone, they must first be decalcified. A drawing of at least one specimen slab is essential (see Fig. 2–3).

This drawing should be used to indicate from what portion of the bone each section was taken. Margin surfaces should be inked. Otherwise it would be extremely difficult to state which margin or margins were involved or from which portions additional sections should be obtained if some questions arise after reviewing the case. This drawing, when related to the specimen radiographs and photographs, also greatly aids in identifying which color or consistency of the tumor typifies a particular microscopic tissue, such as cartilage, bone, or other. This kind of information is particularly useful in arriving at an understanding of the processes involved in the growth of an individual tumor or group of tumors and in isolating benign precursor lesions, from which the tumor may have arisen.

Radiographic Apparatus

Specimen radiographs of the slabs can be obtained by either bringing the specimens to the department of radiology or by purchasing a modestly priced radiographic instrument suited to this purpose. We have found the Hewlett Packard, Faxitron Model #43805 with fine-grain film such as Dupont Cronex Lo-Dose Mammography, 8 x 11, to be suitable for obtaining high-quality specimen radiographs. Since the cost of obtaining developing apparatus is quite expensive, the film can be brought to the radiology department, where it can be developed inexpensively.

We have found that for bone specimens of 3 mm. thickness, a kilovoltage of approximately 20 for 2 minutes at a setting of "I" (intermediate) is good for bone definition and a kilovoltage of 15 for 3 minutes at a setting of "L" (light) is good for definition of the soft tissues and tumors that do not produce a bony matrix. These figures will vary according to the thickness of the cut, the matrices the tumor produces, the kind of film used, and the specific details for which the pathologist is looking. But, after some experimentation with the kilovoltages, exposure time and setting, high-quality specimen radiographs can be achieved for each case.

Specimen radiographs are useful for defining the biology of the tumor with respect to its destruction of the bone and its manner of spread, for defining the periosteal reactions induced by the tumor, locating nidi of osteoid osteomata, and for revealing certain aspects that may be missed by gross observation alone. For example, specimen radiographs can help to identify enchondromatous tissue associated with a chondrosarcoma (see Fig. 8–49) or help to identify a bone infarct that may be associated with a bone sarcoma (see Fig. 9–45). It is also extremely useful to correlate the histological features with the patient radiographs. In this manner a greater appreciation of the *in vivo* patient radiographs can be achieved. This can be useful to the understanding of not only the case in question but of future cases, where the correlation of biopsy material to the radiographs may be crucial. In essence, the greater the pathologist's understanding of radiographic, gross, and histologic features of a particular case, the greater his diagnostic acumen will become.

Photographic Setup

Photographic records are useful for teaching and presenting information at conferences, and for reviewing the slide and specimen radiographic material. Not uncommonly, the photographs may settle a question not answerable by referring only to the gross description.

In our laboratory we use a Nikon photomic FTN camera with a 55 mm. Micro-Nikkor-P Auto. f/3.5 lens with or without the M2 extension ring. Without the extension ring, reproduction ratios of 1:2 can be obtained. With the ring, reproduction rates from 1:2 to 1:1 are possible. The light source must be balanced to the color film used; otherwise the pictures will be too blue or too yellow. Fluorescent lights are not recommended, because their color intensity varies significantly from bulb to bulb. Any color daylight film can be used. Color balance can be achieved by using 250W, 120V, 3,200°K incandescent lights with 82A and 80B wratten filters screwed over the Mikro-Nikkor lens.

In order to achieve the greatest photographic depth two incandescent lights on each side should be placed at approximately 45 degrees to the specimen table.

Sledge Microtome

A sledge microtome can obtain larger section than can an ordinary microtome. We use a Leitz sledge microtome model #1400 with sturdy knife holder and profile "D" knives to obtain sections up to 2 in. square. Large sections are useful in helping to determine how the tumor spreads through the bone, its relation to the periosteum and the adequacy of the margins, in identifying benign tumors, from which a particular malignancy may have arisen and correlating gross, specimen radiographic, and histologic features.

TECHNICAL PROCEDURES

Imprints

High-quality imprints are extremely useful in distinguishing one round cell tumor from another. A diagnosis of metastatic neuroblastoma, lymphoma, Ewing's sarcoma, osteomyelitis, eosinophilic granuloma, Gaucher's disease, and others can usually be resolved by using cytologic imprints with standard-tissue sections. The tissue sections are crucial for studying the patterns the tumor cells may be associated with, such as rosette structures (neuroblastoma and Ewing's sarcoma), nesting or glands (carcinoma), but the imprint cannot be surpassed for showing nuclear and cytoplasmic detail.

Obtaining high-quality imprints depends upon several factors. If any are not performed properly, the result may be so poor that it would be of no benefit to diagnosis. These factors include the manner in which the tissue is imprinted to the slides, the quality of the stains, the amount of time the cells are stained with the hematoxylin, eosin or other stains, how firmly the tumor cells are entrapped in stroma, and the degree of necrosis in the sample being imprinted.

The technique of obtaining one or more high-quality imprints is as follows:

1. Set aside several glass slides. The slides should be clean but they need not be scrupulously cleaned.
2. Remove a sample of what appears to be the most viable tumor area. The sample size can be as small as 1 mm. but 3 to 4 mm. is preferable.
3. Pick up this portion with forceps.
4. If there is excess blood or tissue juices on the surface, touch the tissue lightly to tissue paper or a towel to remove excess tissue fluids, which can interfere with cytologic detail.
5. Gently press the tissue to the slide. Do *not* smear it; smearing will rupture cells. If the specimen is not pressed with a reasonable but gentle force, sufficient numbers of cells may not be removed. Approximately 10 to 20 presses should be made per slide. This procedure should be performed in no longer than 20 seconds, since air drying can lead to severe cytologic artifacts. The best imprints are those in which one attains a single monolayer of cells. If excessive fluid is still seen on the surface, the slide(s) should be discarded until a single monolayer of cells is produced. A single monolayer will appear as a fine "vapor" when the slide is turned at an angle for observation. This "vaporlike" deposit of cells will dry in about 15 to 20 seconds. If excess fluid is present, drying will take 30 or more seconds. Experiment and note how long drying takes in various fresh tumors used in surgical pathology for the purpose of perfecting this technique.
6. After the 15 to 20 monolayers of cells are deposited on the slide (time: 20 seconds or less), the slide must be immersed immediately in a fixative for 20 to 30 seconds. The fixative can be either 70 per cent alcohol or a proportion of 10 ml. of 10 per cent formalin to 90 ml. of 70

per cent alcohol. These fixatives are as good as "pap" fixatives, consisting of 50 per cent ether and alcohol, but they do not have their explosive hazards or noxious fumes.

7. One of the imprint slides should be stained with H and E, in the same manner as is done when performing a frozen section. Then the slide(s) should be taken to a microsope. If the cells appear smeared, then either the tissue was pressed too hard to the slide or a smearing motion was used instead of a simple press. If the nuclei are not well stained, the usual problem is that the slide was not placed in hematoxylin long enough. Another slide should be prepared and the length of time in the hematoxylin doubled. If the nuclei are still weakly stained, either the tumor has undergone necrosis in the sample imprinted or the hematoxylin is old and should be changed (the usual problem). If the cytoplasm is pale, the slide should be placed in eosin for a longer period. If the cytoplasm is too pink, leave it in eosin for a shorter time or wash it more thoroughly in 95 per cent alcohol. In order to see nucleoli in Hodgkin's disease or the eosinophilic granules in eosinophilic granuloma, the slide should be placed in the eosin for at least 3 minutes.
8. If an insufficient or meager number of cells are removed, the tumor cells may be entrapped in fibrosis or other dense matrices. Another sample of the tissue should then be removed and 10 to 20 deep cuts made with a new scalpel blade. This procedure usually frees a sufficient number of cells for analysis. This procedure will not work on tumors that produce heavy quantities of fibrous or cartilagenous matrix; the imprint technique should be abandoned in such instances. For the vast majority of tumors, however, sufficient numbers of cells can be obtained.
9. When it is ascertained that excellent cytologic detail has been obtained, the procedure should be repeated on several slides and each slide should be placed in a fixative. After 30 seconds the slides may be removed, air dryed, and used later for special stains, as is necessary.
10. If the tumor is between the interstices of spongy bone, a portion of the cancellous bone should be pressed with greater force against the slide, or portions of the involved marrow can be removed by scalpel and imprinted as explained in Step 5. If these procedures do not work well, a portion of the bone specimen should be scarified by a scalpel, as explained in Step 8.

Special stains may be performed on the post-fixed, air-dried slides. Particularly useful are para-aminosalicylic acid (PAS) stains with and without diastase, including Wright's or Giemsa stain for the "round cell" tumors of bone. Mucin stains should be used for probable carcinomas and melanin stains, for potential metastatic melanomas. Other special stains for enzymes can be used for lymphoma and leukemia identification and classification.

A skilled pathologist can prepare and stain imprints in about 4 minutes. They serve as a potent adjunct to frozen sections and are of inestimable value when coordinated with the permanent sections. It is extremely frustrating to receive a paraffin-embedded specimen with such severe fixation and other processing artifacts that the only reasonable diagnosis is "round cell tumor" of bone. High-quality imprints prepared beforehand protect against this all too common happenstance and the possible need for rebiopsy. This procedure could, of course, be applied to any organ system seen in surgical pathology to aid diagnosis. It is particularly useful in the analysis and classification of lymph node neoplasms.

Decalcification and Post-Fixation of Specimens

Leave the bone sections in the fixative overnight. The next day, after a brief washing in tap water, transfer the specimen in distilled water to a large volume of 10 per cent nitric acid. During the day, agitate the specimen four to five times for a short period of time in order to dislodge air bubbles that cling to the specimen. About 2- to 3-mm. thick specimens should remain in the nitric acid for 3 days at room temperature. Overdecalcification must be avoided or there will be severe loss of cytologic detail. The specimen should be considered properly decalcified when the specimen floats to the surface or bends on slight pressure. The beginner should use the faxitron radiographic apparatus, which measures whether all the calcium has been removed, to learn when decalcification is optimal.

The specimen is then washed in running tap water for 8 hours to remove all traces of acid. At this point they are post-fixed in sulfosalicylic acid (SSA) fixative (100 ml. of 28% SSA, 110 ml. of 40% formaldehyde and 900 ml. distilled water) overnight.

Dehydration, Embedding, and Sectioning

The specimens can be dehydrated and embedded using Peterfi's double-embedding technique (explained in standard histology textbooks). The dou-

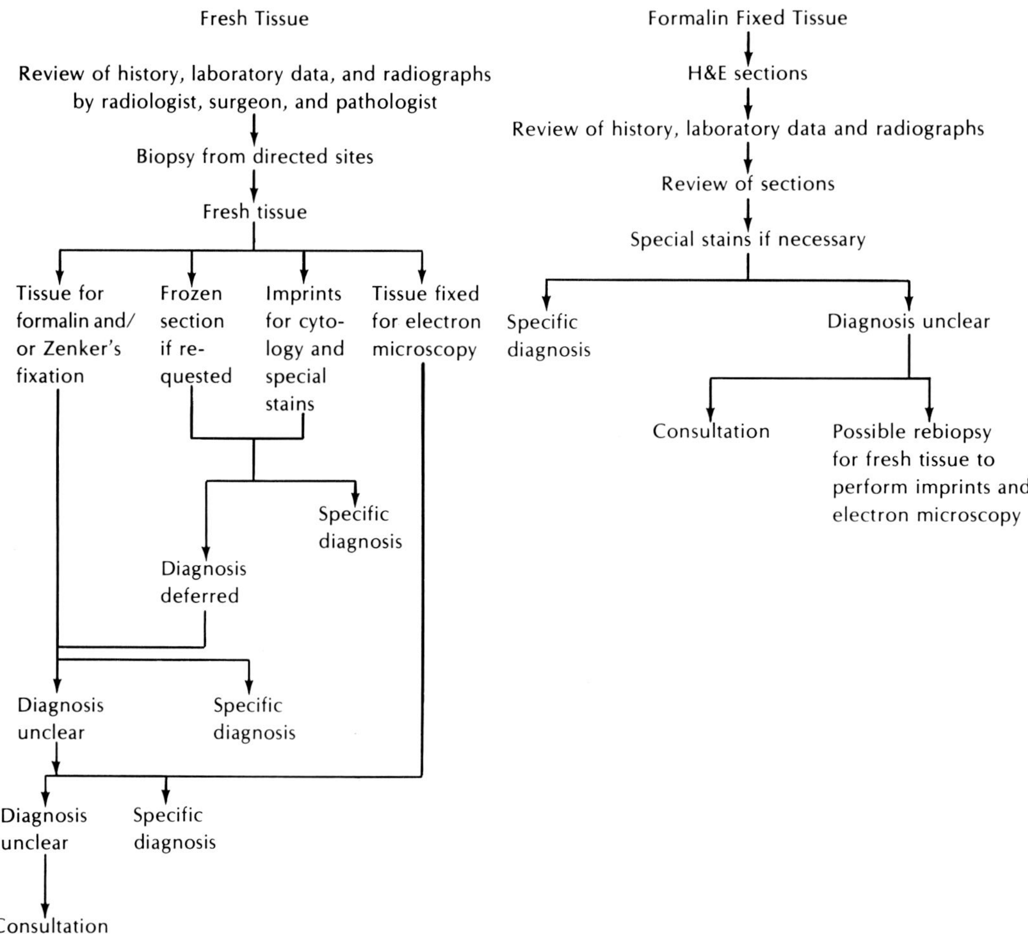

FIG. 2-1. Suggested steps in the diagnosis of an individual bone tumor comparing fresh tissue with formalin fixed tissue.

ble-embedding technique uses paraffin and celloidin. The specimens can be embedded using paper boxes or aluminum foil cups. They should be at least 5 mm. larger than the specimen to be embedded in length, height, and width.

After embedding, the specimens should be hardened in a refrigerator for approximately 1 hour. The blocks are then cut to size and affixed to wooden- or fiber-block supports, with a large margin of paraffin facing the blade.

For routine-size sections, a standard rotary microtome may be used. In order to obtain larger (2 x 2 in.) sections, our laboratory employs the Leitz sledge microtome with a sturdy knife holder and a "D" profile blade. Slice the specimen into a 8- to 10-micron thick ribbon and place it on a board. Place a dropper full of distilled water on a 2-inch slide coated with egg albumin and glycerin fixative. Cut the desired or best section from the ribbon and place it on the distilled water on the slide. Make many cuts in the paraffin surrounding the section to relieve the tension caused by compression of the wax during sectioning. Often most of the paraffin must be cut from around the tissue section in order to allow the section to expand after heating. Then place the slide with the section on a warming table, where the remaining wrinkles are pulled out with teasing needles. When the section has been completely stretched, pour the water off and place the slide in between folded, dampened paper towels and roll flat with a 4-inch brayer or roller.

After storage in a 60°C oven for several hours or overnight, stain the slides routinely, with a few alterations:

1. Cover the sections with a thin solution of celloidin after removing from the second absolute

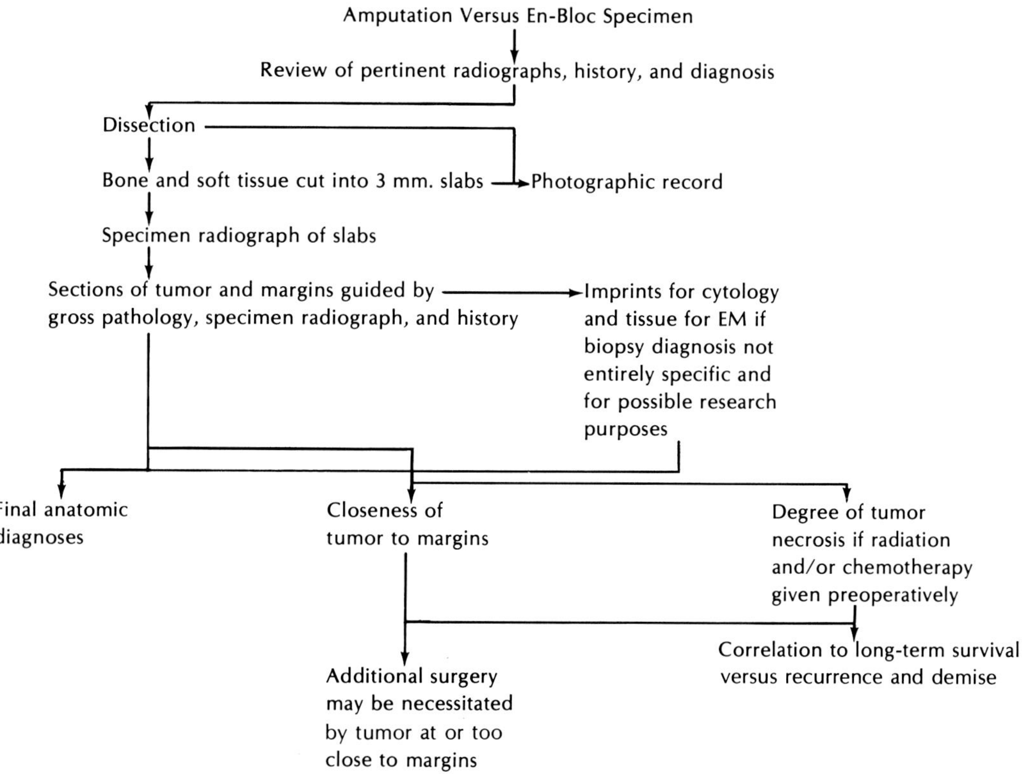
Amputation Versus En-Bloc Specimen
Review of pertinent radiographs, history, and diagnosis
Dissection
Bone and soft tissue cut into 3 mm. slabs
Photographic record
Specimen radiograph of slabs
Sections of tumor and margins guided by gross pathology, specimen radiograph, and history
Imprints for cytology and tissue for EM if biopsy diagnosis not entirely specific and for possible research purposes
Final anatomic diagnoses
Closeness of tumor to margins
Degree of tumor necrosis if radiation and/or chemotherapy given preoperatively
Correlation to long-term survival versus recurrence and demise
Additional surgery may be necessitated by tumor at or too close to margins

FIG. 2-2. Suggested steps in the workup of amputation or en-bloc resection specimens.

alcohol rinse. The celloidin hardens in 80 per cent alcohol after it dries for 2 minutes.
2. Stain the slides for 15 minutes in Harris' hematoxylin.
3. Decolorization is short; it occurs after only 1 to 4 dips in weak acid alcohol (0.5%).
4. Wash the slides in running tap water or dilute sodium bicarbonate for a longer time than for usual tissue sections.

Staining

The equipment used for staining is common to all histology laboratories. The special stains that are most useful for bone tumors are PAS, with and without diastase, reticulin, Giemsa, Wright's stain, and mucicarmine. These are standardized procedures and need not be dealt with in this text.

We have found the hematoxylin-phloxine-tartrazine stain to be an excellent connective-tissue stain, particularly useful for tumors of the mesenchyme. The colors obtained for cells and tissues should be as follows:

Collagen: yellow
Osteoid: yellow
Bone: pink
Cartilage: yellow to yellowish pink
Elastic tissue: refractile pink
Muscle: pink
Erythrocytes: magenta
Osteoclasts and histiocytes: pink
Eosinophils: bright pink granules
Nuclei: blue

Also it is a very good cytologic stain, because nuclear features stand out more clearly than with eosin staining. The hue the phloxine-tartrazine stain produces is less intense than the darker and more obscuring hue of eosin.

The phloxine-tartrazine stain is a modification of Lendrum's stain for inclusion bodies.* The Harris' hematoxylin is used as a nuclear stain as above. To use the phloxine-tartrazine stain, follow these steps.

1. Stain the slides 5 minutes or longer in phloxine (0.5%) and calcium chloride (0.5%) in 70 per cent ethanol.
2. Wash them in tap water for 1 minute.

*Lendrum, A. C.: J. Pathol. and Bacteriol., *59:* 339, 1947.

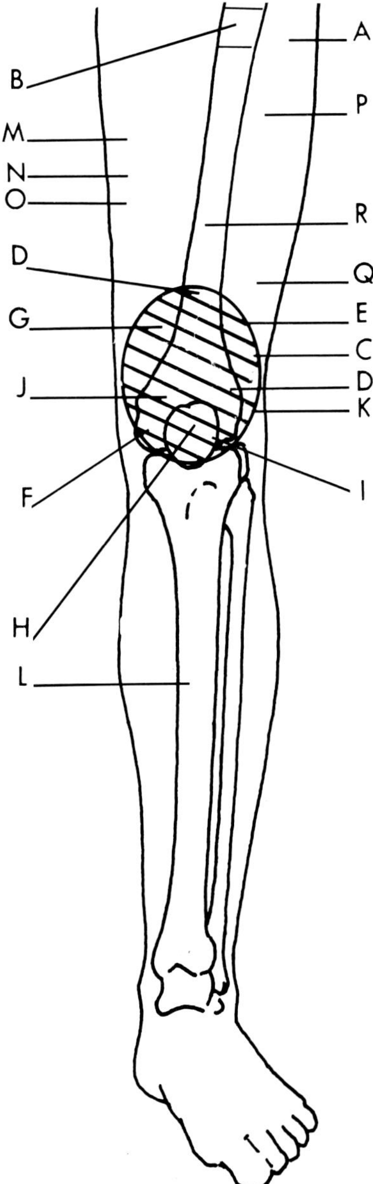

FIG. 2-3. Sample specimen drawing. The tumor is centered in the metaphysis; 10 per cent is cartiliginous and the remainder is fibrous and gritty. It is a soft-tissue mass with probable vascular invasion. The lymph nodes look uninvolved, and 50 per cent of the tumor looks necrotic. The margins look clear of tumor. My overall impression is that the tumor is an osteosarcoma of intramedullary type arising from Paget's disease. (Key: A, B-margins; C, D-soft-tissue extension of femur; E-area of Codman's triangle; F, G, H, I, J, K-sections through tumor; L-tibia section, Paget's disease; M, N, O, P-four lymph nodes; Q-area of probable vascular invasion; R-section of femur, Paget's disease)

3. Rinse in distilled water for 1 minute.
4. Stain and decolorize in a saturated solution of tartrazine NS in ethylene glycol monoethyl ether (cellosolve) for 2 to 4 minutes.
5. Dehydrate quickly through 95 and 100 per cent ethyl alcohol.
6. Clear in xylene.
7. Coverslip.

SUGGESTED WORKUP OF INDIVIDUAL PATIENT MATERIAL FOR CLASSIFICATION (DIAGNOSIS) OR RESEARCH PURPOSES

In most institutions the pathologist usually receives tissue fixed in formalin, rather than fresh biopsy tissue. Imprints and even ultrastructural studies may be critical to establishing particular entities with certainty, particularly for round cell tumors of the bone. Imprints and tissue for electron microscopy require fresh or unfixed tissue. In order to establish a diagnosis, a second procedure may be necessary to obtain fresh tissue. It would be more advantageous if the pathologists educate the clinician to consult with them and a radiologist before they perform the biopsy. Decisions about which areas to biopsy and whether or not fresh tissue would be beneficial to the diagnosis could then be made. Prebiopsy decisions to obtain fresh tissue for imprints and possibly electron microscopy, could protect the patient from less than a fully documented diagnosis and possibly a second operative procedure.

The suggested steps in the workup of biopsy versus en-bloc or amputation specimens to obtain diagnosis and other necessary information are outlined in Figures 2-1 and 2-2.

An unequivocal diagnosis should not be offered at the time of frozen section unless the pathologist is 100 per cent sure of his analysis. Treatment based on less is too dangerous to be acceptable. The same principle applies to diagnosis based on permanent section material. Unless the pathologist is extremely confident of his diagnosis, additional material and/or consultation is strongly suggested. If the pathologist seeks out a consultant, he should supply him with all pertinent clinical and laboratory data and radiographs, in addition to the slide material. A consultant in bone tumors will rarely offer a diagnosis without the pertinent radiographs and other clinical data.

A sample protocol, gross description, and final summary and anatomic and pathologic diagnoses of a hypothetical bone tumor case are given in Figures 2-4, 2-5, 2-6, and 2-7. Figure 2-3 shows a sample specimen drawing.

The kind of specific format that may be used in the workup of en-bloc resection and amputation specimens is as follows:

General information

Patient name ____________

Patient number ____________

Name of prosector ____________

____________ 1. Surgical pathology number
Date of Surgery ____________
Surgeon ____________
Preoperative diagnosis ____________
Preoperative therapy ____________

____________ 2. History ____________

____________ 3. Pertinent laboratory data ____________

____________ 4. Pertinent radiographic data ____________

____________ 5. a) Amputation b) En-bloc excision

____________ 6. LXWXH of tumor in bone

____________ 7. a) Confined to bone b) Broken into soft tissues

____________ 8. Size of tumor in soft tissue (LXHXW)

____________ 9. Tumor centered in epiphysis, metaphysis, diaphysis, and other

____________ 10. Specify which bone or bones are involved

____________ 11. Tumor: soft, firm, rock hard, gritty, cystic, necrotic, hemorrhagic, other (specify)

____________ 12. Tumor shows foci of fibrosis, cartilage, bone, evidence of possible benign bone lesion

____________ 13. Colors: white, pink, red, black, brown, translucent blue, yellow, orange, gray, other (specify)

____________ 14. a) Evidence of vascular invasion b) Nerve involvement

____________ 15. Number of lymph nodes removed

____________ 16. Closest gross distance to margins: 0 mm., 1 to 4 mm., 4 mm. to 1 cm., 1 cm. to 5 cm., > 5 cm.

____________ 17. a) Tissue for electron microscopy submitted, b) Not submitted

____________ 18. Imprints taken or not performed. Stains requested ____________

____________ 19. Photographs, no photographs

____________ 20. Specimen radiographs obtained, not obtained

____________ 21. Special stains ordered on permanent sections: a) PAS with and without diastase, reticulin, phloxine-tartrazine, gram, AFB, Gomori methylanine silver, iron, Fontana for melanin, mucicarmine, other (specify)

FIG. 2-4. Sample protocol for en-bloc resection versus amputation bone tumor specimens.

Received is a right leg that has been amputated in the area of the mid-femur, 25 cm. above the femoral condyles. The leg measures 50 cm. in length. The region above the knee is swollen and measures 40 cm. in circumference. A 3 cm. longitudinal incision with sutures is noted in the lateral aspect of the leg immediately superior to the knee. Review of the patient's radiographs shows a large blastic lesion in the metaphysis that has broken through the cortex in a posterolateral position. The femur and tibia display typical features of severe Paget's disease.

The tumor is approached through the surgical incision. A gritty tumor is encountered with firmer, less gritty areas. Portions of apparently viable tumor are taken and five imprints prepared for H and E and PAS stains. A small sample is fixed in glutaraldehyde for electron microscopy. A portion from this area is submitted in a cassette and labelled EM control. Several sections of fresh tumor are fixed in formalin and Zenker's. The leg is frozen overnight and cut into twelve 2- to 4-mm. slabs. Measurements and other data are listed in the above sheets and the sections taken labelled as per Figure 2-3. The bone of the femur and tibia located away from the tumor has abnormally thick trabeculae and a pumice stonelike appearance consistent with Paget's disease. Sections L and R are taken from nontumor Paget's bone.

FIG. 2-5. Sample gross description.

Sample Diagnoses

Right leg (high above-knee amputation)

- Intramedullary osteogenic sarcoma, distal femoral metaphysis arising in association with Paget's disease
- Soft-tissue extension of tumor
- Tumor thrombus in distal femoral artery
- History of 1 month of preoperative adriamycin and 3600 Rads
- 80 per cent tumor necrosis
- Tumor greater than 5 cm. from proximal margin
- Four lymph nodes removed, all negative for tumor

FIG. 2-7. Final pathologic diagnoses.

Sample Description

Clinical:	20-year history of Paget's disease. Two months history of pain in right knee region. 3600 R and local adriamycin injections given 1 month prior to amputation.
Laboratory:	Markedly elevated serum alkaline phosphatase
Radiologic:	Paget's disease of right femur and tibia
Specimen radiographs:	Paget's and cumulus cloudlike densities of osteosarcoma confirmed in distal femoral metaphysis. Tumor extends through host bone, broken through the cortical metaphysis, resulting in a Codman's triangle.
Gross Pathology:	Typical of bone- and cartilage-producing osteosarcoma, severe Paget's of femur and tibia
Histology:	Mosaic bone pattern of Paget's disease. About 10 per cent of osteosarcoma is cartilage producing. Remainder of tumor produces osteoid-woven bone and focal fibrosarcomatous pattern. Benign osteoclasts permeate the tumor. 80 per cent tumor necrosis (drug and radiotherapy related?)
Imprints:	Consistent with anaplastic osteoblasts.
Special stains:	Phloxine-tartrazine
Electron Microscopy:	Viral-like particles noted in nuclei of the osteoclasts in an area of Paget's disease of bone. None noted in the sarcoma cells.
Other Comments:	Research patient #15 will receive systemic chemotherapy for 1 year. Correlate course to degree of tumor necrosis, margins, vascular involvement, and other data. Tumor grown in athymic nude mice for susceptibility to various chemotherapy and radiotherapy regimens.

FIG. 2-6. Summary of data critical to final diagnoses and for research purposes (optional).

COLOR PLATES

Plate 1

Fracture Repair

A.
First Few Days. The earliest changes in fracture repair are hemorrhage and a proliferation of small spindle cells (H and E, x40).

B.
One to Two Weeks. At about 1 week, the spindle cells may form sarcomalike masses mixed with small capillaries. The cytoplasm is spindly to polygonal. The more polygonal the cell, the more intensely pinkish-blue the cytoplasm. The nuclei are plump and spindly to ovoid. The ovoid nuclei contain a single large nucleolus. Mitoses may be frequent, but they are mirror image. The cells may appear as malignant or more malignant than some fields of osteosarcoma (compare with Plate 5; *A* and *B*).

C.
1 Week. The malignant aura is even further enhanced by the infiltration of sarcomalike spindle cells of the surrounding rounded skeletal muscle fibers trapped in the callus (H and E, x125).

D.
Two to Three Weeks. Osteoid (*x*) is first laid down between 12 and 14 days. Compare the fluffy masses of osteoid and the polygonal rounded cells that produce this specialized collagen matrix to the more longitudinal bundles of collagen separated by spindle shaped fibroblasts in the extreme upper portion of this field (the periosteum). In this illustration, we can also note the gradual transition of the specialized fibroblasts of the periosteum to cells of osteogenic potential in the zone between the quiescent periosteum (upper field) and osteoid production (lower field). The tinctorial qualities of osteoid and collagen are otherwise identical. In contrast, the tinctorial qualities of the other mass (*y*) is within its center darker blue. This signifies the deposition of calcium and the conversion of osteoid to woven bone (H and E, x400).

E.
Three to Four Weeks. Large fluffy masses of osteoid and woven bone become more apparent. Calcification within the osteoid centers has already occurred (*x*), marking the transition from osteoid to primitive woven bone. Plump osteoblasts begin to form a rim around some of the masses; others have a spindly appearance. Well-formed capillaries begin to appear. Some of the large pink round masses surrounded by nuclei at each periphery (*y*) are trapped partially atrophic skeletal muscle fibers. This field still bears a strong resemblance to osteosarcoma (H and E, x250).

F.
Four to Five Weeks. The woven bone masses are remodeled to thinner trabeculae and are lined by a prominent rim or single row of plump osteoblasts. The stroma is composed of a loose fibrous tissue rich in well-formed capillaries. These latter features signify definite maturation to benign bone tissues and should no longer be confused with osteosarcoma by histology alone. There are also some trabeculae of lamellar bone present (*arrow*), also lined by plump osteoblasts. Well-formed lamellar bone cannot be formed in 4 to 5 weeks by callus. Therefore, this tissue must represent host lamellar bone that has been incorporated into the fracture repair site. The plump osteoblasts on the surface of the lamellar bone signify renewed osteocytic activity stimulated by the fracture (H and E, x125).

G.
Five to Six Weeks. Continuation of the maturational process noted in the preceding illustration. Rimming of osteoblasts is still present but the cells have assumed a more spindly configuration, which is a reflection of diminishing activity (H and E, x125).

H.
Six to Eight Weeks. Lamellar bone begins to replace the more primitive woven bone. The intertrabecular stroma is rich in dilated vessels and there is conversion to marrow fat. Osteoblastic rimming is much less prominent (H and E, x40).

I.
Honeymoon Fracture of Rib, 4 Weeks Old. A fracture gap is seen on the extreme left (*short arrow*). The callus tissues are richly vascular and there is prominent woven bone production (*long arrow*) lined by osteoblasts. The woven bone becomes attached to host lamellar bone. High-power examination showed (*X*) that the lamellar bone does not contain nuclei within the lacunar spaces. This is because the vascular supply is interrupted to the lamellar bone a distance of up to 1 cm. or more from the fracture gap (H and E, x10).

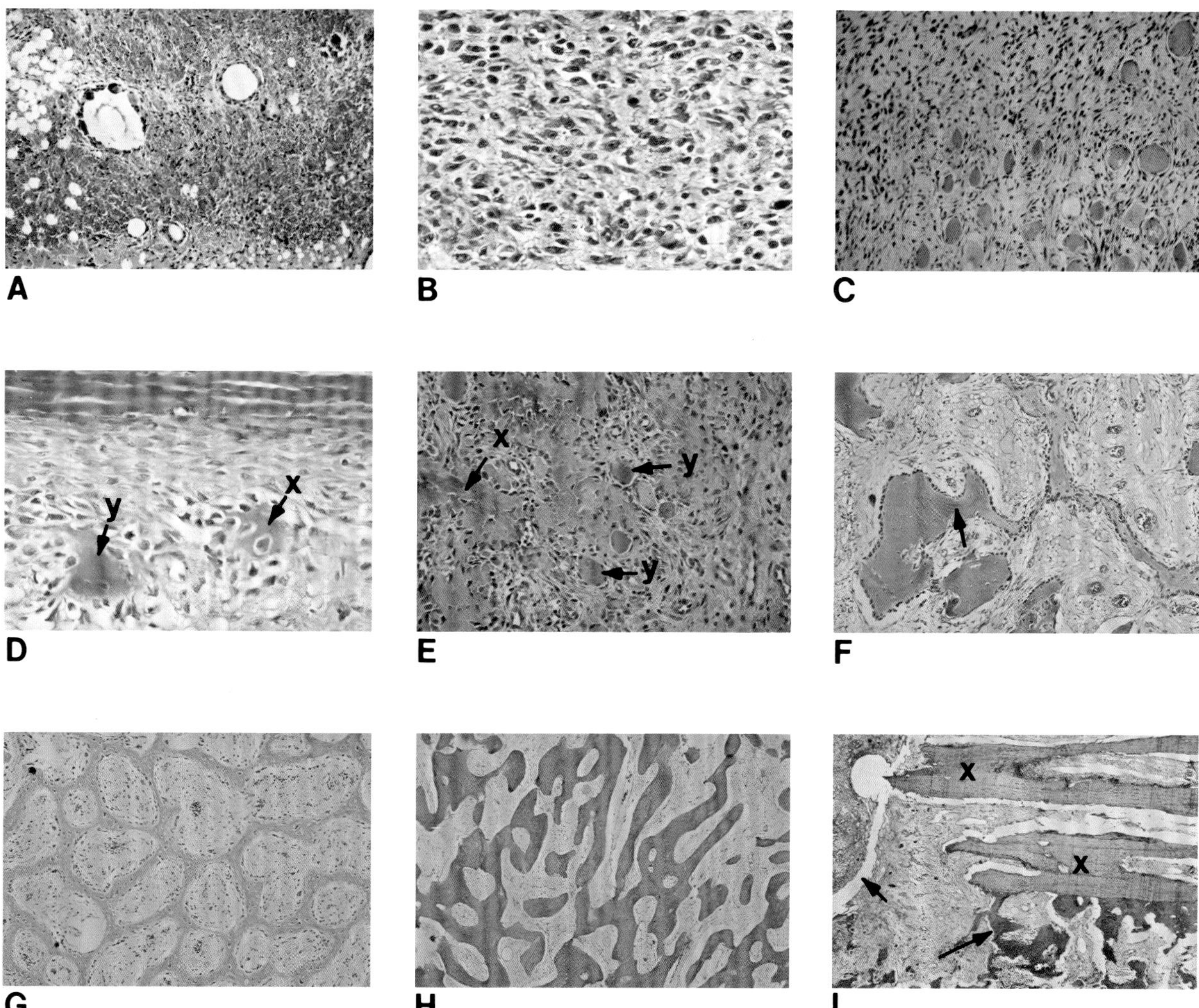

A
B
C
D
y
x
E
x
y
y
F
G
H
I
x
x

Plate 2

Osteoid Osteoma and Osteoblastoma

A.
Osteoid Osteoma. This gross specimen shows a yellowish pink; dense, woven bone 4-mm. nidus (*arrow*) surrounded by a 1-mm. rim of reddish vascular tissue. The surrounding medullary cavity and cortex are densely sclerotic.

B.
Osteoblastoma. This approximately 2-cm. osteoblastoma is characterized by intense vascularity. It is well circumscribed. The surrounding host bone is only minimally sclerotic.

C.
Osteoid Osteoma. This low-power illustration of a small, 2-mm. osteoid osteoma shows its pathognomonic features: A central, round, woven bone nidus (*x*), a fibrovascular zone (*y*) with a diminution in host bone trabeculae, and surrounding reactive bone sclerosis (*z*) (H and E, x10).

D.
Osteoblastoma. The lesion is larger than on osteoid osteoma and tends to have a lobulated outer perimeter. The woven bone of the lesion is well delineated (*arrows*) from the surrounding minimally sclerotic host bone (H and E, x10).

E.
Osteoblastoma or Osteoid Osteoma. If one examines the margins of these lesions on higher power, a sharp delineation between the lesional woven bone, seen to the right of field, and host lamellar bone, seen to the left of field, is observed (*arrows*). Infiltration between host lamellar bone is usually not seen. If infiltration is present, it usually does not extend more than fractions of a millimeter into the host bone (H and E, x40).

F.
Osteoblastoma or Osteoid Osteoma. Lesions in their early, osteoid-rich productive phase are associated with very plump osteoblasts with nuclear features that could easily be confused with osteogenic sarcoma (H and E, x400).

G.
Osteoblastoma or Osteoid Osteoma. Many of these lesions are rich in osteoid and woven bone. The features that aid in determining its benignancy are the prominent focal to diffuse rimming of osteoblasts (in many but not all cases) (*arrows*) and rich fibrovascular stroma. Peppering of osteoclasts is a common feature but may be seen in osteosarcoma as well (H and E, x160).

H.
Osteoblastoma or Osteoid Osteoma. Other lesions may be composed almost entirely of woven bone. The woven bone is generally about as thick as the intertrabecular richly fibrovascular stroma. In this case osteoblasts are still prominently rimming the bone. In other fields or in entire lesions with woven bone production similar to that illustrated, osteoblastic rimming may be minimal to absent. In rare cases dense woven bone can fill almost the entire field, and osteoblastic rimming becomes inconspicuous (H and E, x250).

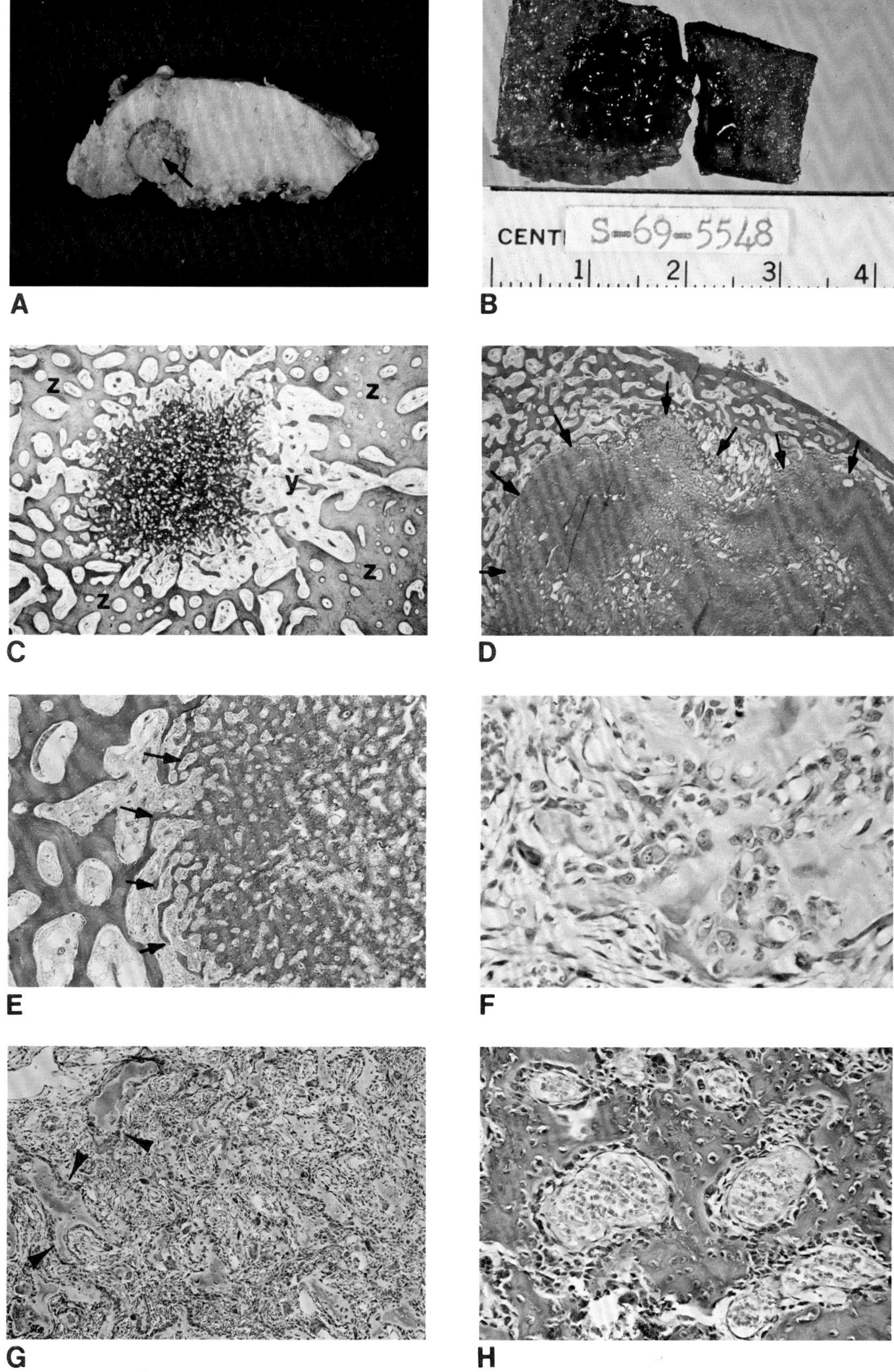
A
B
CENTI
S-69-5548
1 2 3 4
C
z
z
y
z
z
D
E
F
G
H

Plate 3

Osteogenic Sarcoma, Typical Sclerosing Type

Plates 3 through 5 demonstrate the enormous range of histologic patterns and cytologic atypia associated with the osteosarcoma. In general, a single case of osteosarcoma will have one predominant pattern, although on occasion extensive sampling may show multiple tissue patterns. If the predominant pattern is spindle cells, confusion with fibrosarcoma is possible; if histiocyte rich, with malignant fibrous histiocytoma; and if the case shows little cytologic atypia, possible confusion with osteoblastoma and callus. The reverse errors are also possible. The diagnosis of osteosarcoma from biopsy material alone can be made in many instances; however, unless the pathologist is 100 per cent sure of his slide diagnosis expertise, clinicoradiologic correlation in association with careful observation of cytologic features, pattern of spread through the host lamellar bone, and matrix production (as described in Chap. 7), is recommended and should reduce diagnostic error to a minimum.

A.
The lesion is centered in the tibial metaphysis but extends to the articular cartilage. The extension was made easier by the absence of an epiphyseal plate. The lesion is tannish white and is demarcated by a vascular reaction. It has caused small cortical erosions and has resulted in a separation of the periosteum from its cortical attachment (*arrow*).

B.
Close examination reveals that the tumor has permeated through the marrow interstices (*arrow*). The host lamellar bone appears in the area of the tumor as thin, tan-red canal-like structures outlined against the whiter, poorly vascular tumor bone.

C.
The pattern of tumor bone infiltration between the host lamellar bone spicules present in the gross examination is verifiable histologically. It is particularly clear with the use of a phloxine-tartrazine-hematoxylin stain. The host lamellar bone stains an intense pink (*x*). The marrow has been replaced by compact masses of woven bone (*y*) (brownish-purple) and osteoid (*z*) (light yellow-green). These features are virtually pathognomonic of a "sclerosing" osteosarcoma.

D.
Right: Note the wide, long plates of pink residual host bone trabeculae (*x*). The marrow space has been replaced by thinner, smaller, less well-organized islands of pink woven bone (*y*). *Left:* Under polarized light the entrapped host bone is strongly refractile and clearly lamellar. The tumor osteoid and bone is much less refractile and on higher power would show a crisscross or woven rather than lamellar collagen pattern (x40).

E.
This illustration demonstrates the advancing margin of an osteosarcoma under polarized light. The lesion is spreading from the left to the right. The left third of the illustration shows nonpolarized uninvolved marrow fat and trabeculae of host lamellar bone (*x*). The right side shows replacement of the marrow by a polarizable crisscross pattern of tumor osteoid and woven bone (*y*). Note also the trapped host lamellar bone trabeculae (*z*).

F.
Host residual lamellar bone is present in the top and bottom of the field. The remainder of the bluish red trabeculae is woven bone. On high-power examination; the intermingling of lamellar and woven bone give the appearance of callus, except for the fact that instead of fibrovascular or marrow fat spaces between the trabeculae of well formed woven bone, the tissue is almost pure osteoid (*arrows*).

This pattern of dense osteoid abutting plates of well formed woven bone is most common in osteosarcoma of the sclerosing type and exceedingly rare in benign conditions. Although this pattern is usually pathogmononic of osteosarcoma, the extreme nuclear innocence common to fields such as this on highpower examination (Plate 3, *I*) may trap the observer into a diagnosis of benignancy. Correlation with the radiographs, observing whether or not the process infiltrates insidiously between host bone lamellae, and looking assiduously for any areas, no matter how small, for evidence of objective anaplasia or malignant cartilage are some of the necessary prerequisites to diagnose this variant of osteosarcoma with confidence and to prevent confusion with callus or osteoblastoma (x40).

G.
This is a medium-power illustration of the "sclerosing" variant of osteosarcoma. Again, note the entrapped host lamellar bone trabeculae (*x*), the well formed "innocent" tumor woven bone (*y*), and the presence of significantly "ominous" amounts of osteoid (*z*) between the bone trabeculae (x125).

H.
The majority of osteosarcomas in their dense, bone-producing regions do not display atypical cytologic features much greater than that shown in this illustration. However, if the diagnosis of osteosarcoma is made only on the basis of cytologic atypia similar to that shown in this field, then the chances of misdiagnosing callus, osteoblastoma, or osteoid osteoma is a distinct danger, since they may show fields just as cytologically atypical (Plates 2, *F*, and 4, *E, H, I* and Fig. 7-23) (H and E, x300).

I.
It is quite common to find large areas of a sclerosing osteosarcoma with small nuclei of incredible innocence. The denser the degree of bone production, the more "innocent" the nuclei become. The only clue to the probable diagnosis of osteosarcoma from this field is the presence of dense woven bone and intertrabecular spaces completely filled in with masses of osteoid (*arrow*). The final diagnosis in cases such as this will obviously depend on the correlation of other clinical, radiologic, and pathologic data (H and E, x400).

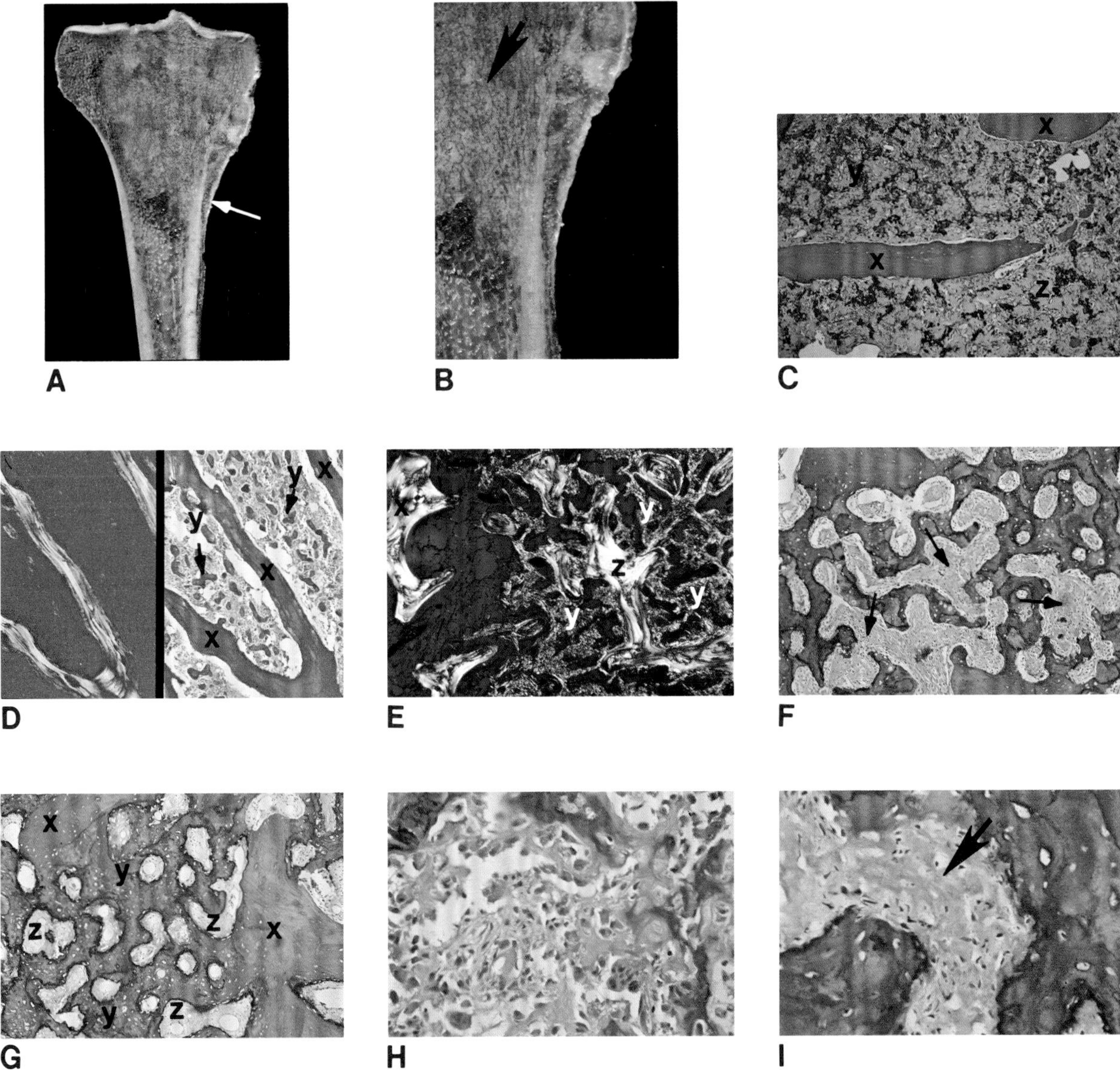
A
B
x
y
x
z
C
y
x
y
x
x
D
x
y
z
y
y
E
F
x
y
z
z
x
y
z
G
H
I

Plate 4

Osteosarcoma and Sarcomalike Areas of Callus and Osteoblastoma

A.
Osteosarcoma. In spite of the "innocence" of the nuclei, the presence of masses and tightly packed "streamers" of osteoid are rarely seen in benign conditions. It is a common pattern of osteosarcoma, however (H and E, x300).

B.
Osteosarcoma. The production of long, tightly knit streamers of closely packed osteoid with little to no intervening fibrovascular tissue and cartilage production (*arrow*) is almost pathognomonic of osteosarcoma. Early callus might be the rare exception (H and E, x40).

C.
Osteosarcoma. In this illustration the presence of tightly knit streamers of osteoid and nuclei with considerable variation in sizes and shapes, staining characteristics, and abnormal chromatin clumping is unequivocal evidence of an anaplastic osseous-productive tumor; by definition, an osteosarcoma (H and E, x400).

D.
Osteosarcoma. This illustration is characterized by a proliferation of cells that are productive of woven bone (*left*) and cellular cartilage (*right*). Although the cells are ominous, they do not meet the rigid specifications of unequivocal anaplasia. Fields such as these should not be diagnosed osteosarcoma without radiologic correlation and additional investigation for fields or patterns that could only be construed as osteosarcoma (H and E, x250).

E.
Callus. This field of a callus shows that the bone and cartilage that may be produced in this condition may be as cytologically ominous as that shown in the previous illustration (H and E, x250). Fields such as these demonstrate that due caution must be used in the interpretation of what is or is not anaplasia. This problem diminishes as the pathologist grows more experienced and learns to differentiate subtler degrees of anaplasia from cytologically "ominous" benign bone-producing tumors and early callus. However, on rare occasion even the experts cannot differentiate an osteoblastoma from an osteosarcoma, or the reverse, by cytologic criteria alone.

F.
Osteosarcoma. If fields of cartilage such as these are seen, then the diagnosis of unequivocal anaplasia is justified. Benign conditions do not produce nuclear features as atypical as those shown here. There is considerable enlargement, variations in size and shape, abnormal chromatin distribution, and multiple small nucleoli. Giant nuclei (*arrow*) such as shown here are not seen in benign cartilage tumors. This voluminous nucleus is at least 35 microns in diameter. Cartilage nuclei of benign lesions rarely exceed 10 to 12 microns and generally have spindly to contracted shapes. One must be aware, however, that benign chondrocytes may shrink from their lacunuae because of artifacts of fixation. The result may be that the observer mistakes the entire shrunken cell for a large nucleus (H and E, x250).

G.
Osteosarcoma. The most ideal areas for the identification of unequivocal anaplasia is in the most cellular or poorest bone-producing areas of the tumor. Note the extreme anaplasia from such an area that includes a quadripolar or nonmirror image atypical mitosis (lower left). At least three mitoses are present. Compare the nuclear features of a few benign osteoclast-like cells that are present (*arrows*) with the surrounding anaplastic cells (H and E, x400).

H.
Callus. This callus was two weeks old and shows a massive proliferation of cells and ominous masses of osteoid production suggestive of an anaplastic tumor. The nuclei are swollen and contain small nucleoli. Since the lesion is from a callus, the cytology would not be typified as anaplasia. However, fields identical to this one may be found in osteosarcoma. This field, therefore, illustrates an example of possible or equivocal anaplasia (in actuality, pseudo-anaplasia). Unequivocal anaplasia is a term that must, of course, be restricted to malignant tumors. The diagnosis of osteosarcoma should never be made in the absence of "objective" anaplasia without radiologic correlation and other histologic patterns that are seen in no other condition (H and E, x250).

I.
Osteoblastoma. The osteoblastoma may show a wild flurry of osteoblasts, small masses of osteoid and woven bone, and moderate vascularity. The osteoblasts are well delineated from one another and contain regular but enlarged nuclei, abundant bluish-pink cytoplasm, and prominent Golgi zones. In spite of the ominous cellularity, this constellation of features, including prominent Golgi zones, is common to osteoblastomas and osteoid osteomas and only rarely seen in osteosarcomas. However, it is not difficult to understand why fields such as these, by "slide reading" alone, could be mistaken for osteosarcoma (H and E, x250).

J.
Osteosarcoma, Giant Cell Predominant. Low-power examination of this lesion mimics a giant cell tumor or perhaps a chondroblastoma. The giant cells probably represent benign, reactive, permeating osteoclasts (H and E, x125).

K.
Osteosarcoma, Giant Cell Predominant. If high-power examination reveals tight masses and streamers of osteoid without osteoblast rimming and stromal cells with unequivocal anaplasia (*arrow*), the diagnosis is osteosarcoma by definition. Some cases of osteosarcoma are dominated by masses of benign osteoclast-like giant cells. These cells are probably benign osteoclasts that permeate numerous benign and malignant tumor of the bone. Much more important to correct diagnosis is a careful analysis of the stromal cells and matrices produced that are found between the osteoclasts. Only in this way is it possible to differentiate the true, ordinary giant cell tumor of epiphyses from other osteoclast-rich benign and malignant tumors (H and E, x300).

L.
Giant Cell or Osteoclastic Sarcoma. *Left:* Huge, massive cells with obviously anaplastic multiple nuclei (x125). *Middle:* The tumor is composed of anaplastic mono- and multinucleated cells. The arrow points to the more definite osteoclast-like appearance of some of the cells (x300). *Right:* Since this tumor is related histogenetically to the ordinary low-grade neoplastic giant cell tumor, it shows features such as histiocytic vacuoles in the cytoplasm (*a*), occasional cells will show the malignant mononuclear stromal cells entering or fusing with the giant cell along its periphery (*b*). In other areas the tumor may show long spindle cells with a storiform pattern, which is an indication of its specialized histiocytic origin (x300).

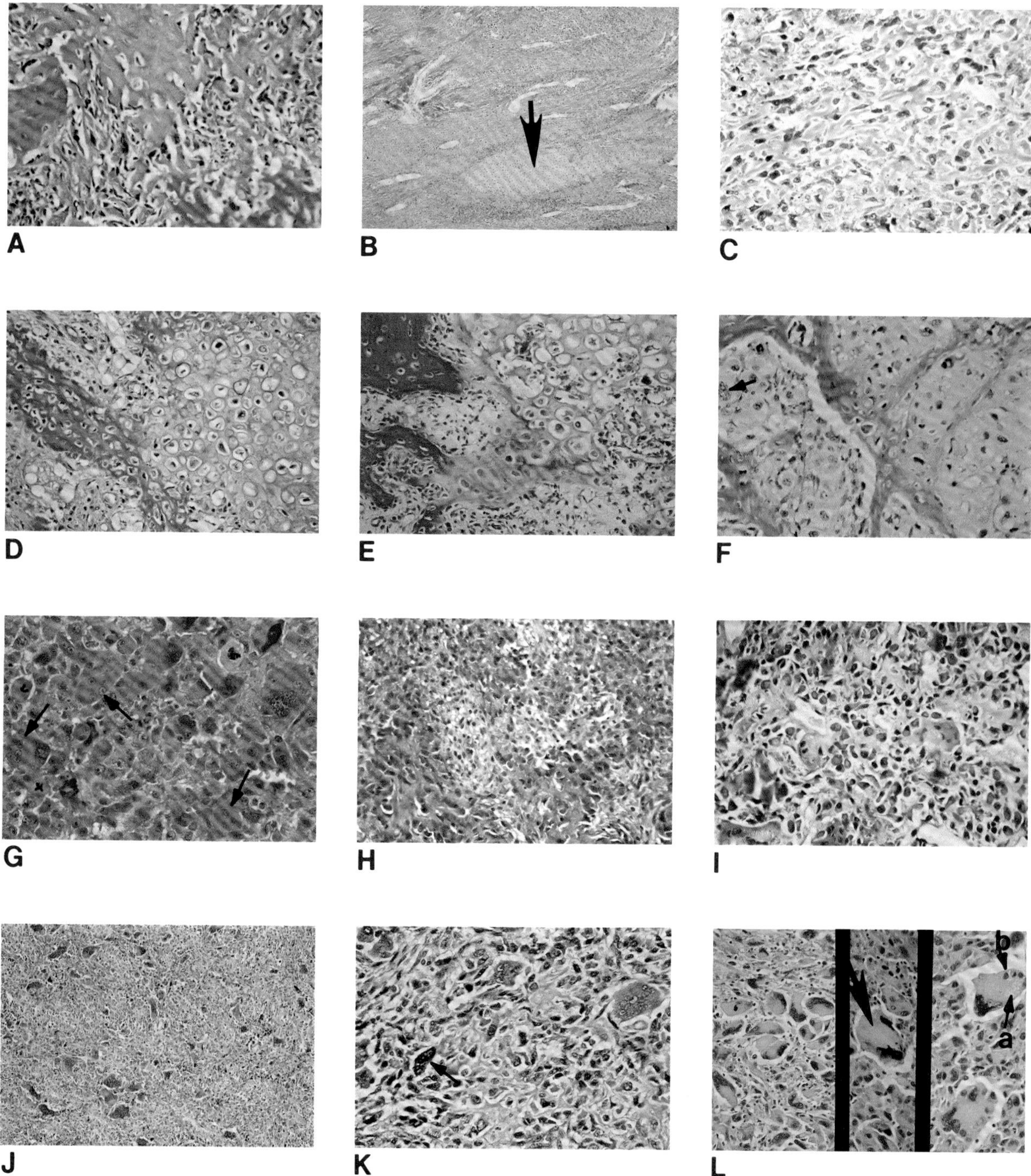
A
B
C
D
E
F
G
H
I
J
K
L
a
b

Plate 5

Osteosarcoma, Less Common Histologic Patterns

A.

Osteosarcoma, Spindle Cell Type. Most fields of this osteosarcoma showed fibrous tissue with remarkable innocence. Only by correlating the radiologic features with the histologic features and finding areas of malignant tumor osteoid and bone production is correct diagnosis possible. Consider, however, the danger of biopsy from such an area with or without radiologic correlation (H and E, x400).

B.

Osteosarcoma, Spindle Cell Type. The cells are spindly and the nuclei are very closely packed. Occasional nuclei show more ominous enlargement. Since the cells are producing very primitive woven bone in this field, the lesion must be a bone-producing tumor. The nuclei are too close together and enlarged to be consistent with fibrous dysplasia. Intense sheets of cells such as these are not seen in osteoid osteoma or osteoblastoma. The only two reasonable possibilities are osteosarcoma or early callus. Although the nuclei of some of the cells are very suggestive of anaplasia, callus certainly must remain in the differential diagnosis (Plate 1, *B*). Therefore, the ultimate diagnosis of osteosarcoma must be established by other criteria. In this case, radiologic features of a large metaphyseal tumor with a soft-tissue mass and Codman's triangles confirmed the slide impression of "fibroblastic" osteosarcoma and ruled out callus (H and E, x400).

C.

Osteosarcoma With Cells Resembling Ewing's Sarcoma. Many of the cells contained small lymphocyte or nuclei similar to those seen in Ewing's tumor. However, the presence of streamers of osteoid and occasional bizarre, enlarged, unequivocally anaplastic nuclei establishes the diagnosis of osteosarcoma. In actuality, this tumor arose from the diaphysis, where this curious mixture of osteosarcoma and cells resembling Ewing's are most commonly found (H and E, x400).

D.

Osteosarcoma, Telangiectatic Type. Low-power examination shows large, cystlike spaces, many of which contain red blood cells (H and E, x40).

E.

Osteosarcoma. Telangiectatic Type. In some cases, the walls of the cysts show masses and streamers of osteoid (*arrow*), an immediate clue to the diagnosis of osteosarcoma. This pattern is rarely seen in simple or aneurysmal bone cysts. Usually the bone deposition in these conditions is composed of larger and fewer number of slivers of osteoid and woven bone (H and E, x125).

F.

Osteosarcoma, Telangiectatic Type. Other cases show proliferations of ominous cells in the stroma surrounding the cystlike vascular spaces. If the degree of anaplasia is not clear-cut, then considerable care must be given to a correlation of all of the pathologic and clinical features. This variant of osteosarcoma is the easiest of all to misdiagnose as a benign tumor (aneurysmal bone cyst) on initial presentation (H and E, x125).

G.

Osteosarcoma Resembling Malignant Fibrous Histiocytoma. The spindle cells in this field are objectively anaplastic. The collagen is arranged in a pinwheel pattern highly suggestive, but by no means diagnostic, of malignant fibrous histiocytoma (MFH). Many sections should be examined to rule out the presence of malignant bone or cartilage production. Realizing that this osteosarcoma variation is possible, the diagnosis of MFH of bone should not be made unequivocally on biopsy tissues alone. In this author's experience, most of the MFH's of bone I have seen were in association with long-standing bone infarcts.

H.

Osteosarcoma, Malignant Fibrous Histiocytoma or Liposarcoma-Like. In occasional osteosarcomas, the cells may become highly active phagocytes. When this occurs, the cytoplasm enlarges and becomes pale, and red globules ("sarcoma bodies") (*arrow*) may be seen in many of the cells. Note the masses of tumor osteoid in the upper and right portions of the field, which proves that the tumor in question is an osteosarcoma (H and E, x250).

I.

Osteosarcoma, MFH or Liposarcoma-Like. Frozen sections of the previous case showed numerous droplets of fat within the tumor cells. Therefore, the presence of fat in the cells of a malignant tumor of bone cannot be used to diagnose MFH or liposarcoma unless great care is taken to eliminate the osteosarcoma from contention (H and E, x250).

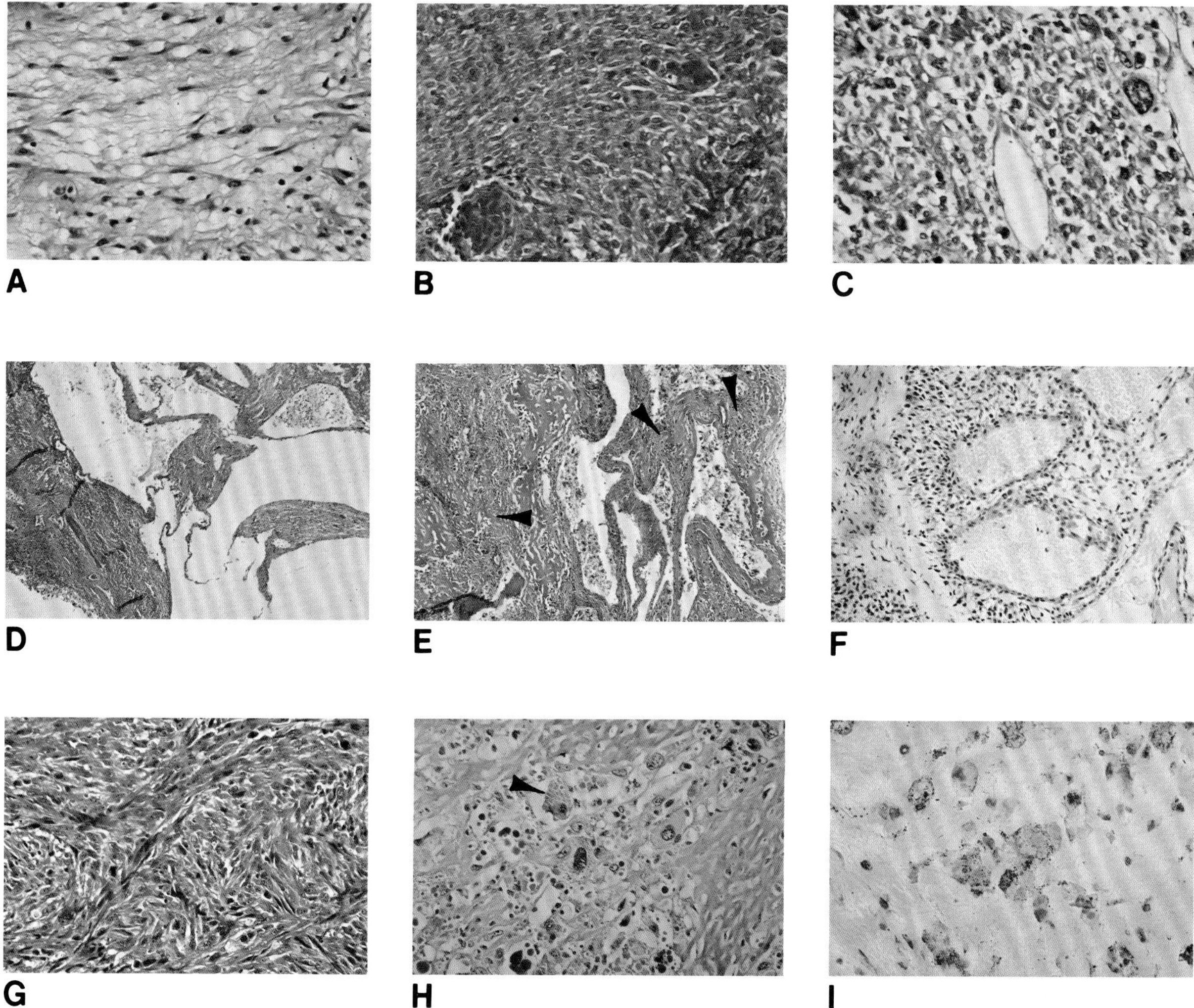

Plate 6

Fibrous Dysplasia, Fibrosarcomatous Transformation of a Low-Grade Chondrosarcoma, Mesenchymal, Chondroblastoma, Chondromyxoid Fibroma, and Chondroblastoma

A.
Fibrous Dysplasia. Note the brown macula with irregular outer contours in the axilla of this patient with fibrous dysplasia. Café au lait spots of neurofibromatosis have less irregular or rounded outer contours.

B.
Fibrous Dysplasia. This disease is characterized by a firm, white, variably gritty tumorlike process that focally destroys bone. An entire bone is rarely involved. The process seemingly "expands" the bone it involves. The bone "expansion" is in reality due to the formation of reactive bone along the periosteal and endosteal surfaces. This gross example is from the sternum.

C.
Fibrosarcomatous Transformation of a Low-Grade Chondrosarcoma That Formed From a Long-Standing Enchondroma. The enchondroma is contained within the distal shaft (*x*). A low-grade chondrosarcoma was identified at (*y*), from which a firm, matrix-free, highly anaplastic and lethal fibrosarcoma (*z*) arose and perforated the cortex. This dedifferentiation or transformation occurs in from 10 to 20 per cent of chondrosarcomas.

D.
Mesenchymal Chondrosarcoma. Typical low-power view that shows variable islands of chondroid or cartilage between which are oval to short spindly cells. The nuclei stain as intensely as those of lymphocytes (x40).

E.
Mesenchymal Chondrosarcoma. Intimate mixture of chondroid to malignant cartilage and monotonous stromal sarcoma cells (x125).

F.
Mesenchymal Chondrosarcoma. In many cases fields that mimic hemangiopericytoma are found.

G.
Chondromyxoid Fibroma. This example shows a florid admixture of spindly fibroma-like cells that are undergoing metaplasia to a primitive chondroid matrix. Mitoses are rare, which helps to distinguish this tumor from the mesenchymal chondrosarcoma (x250).

H.
Chondromyxoid Fibroma. This field demonstrates a bland fibromyxoid area. This benign tumor can contain variable quantities of fibroid, chondroid, and myxoid tissues in virtually any proportion. Note the striking innocence of the nuclei. They are quite similar to the bland nuclei seen in fibrous dysplasia (x250).

I.
Chondromyxoid Fibroma. A field showing a chondrofibroid stroma admixed with vacuolated or myxoid zones. The nuclei are monotonously bland. Mitoses are usually very rare (x300).

J.
Chondroblastoma. Note the swirling masses of chondroid to the left of the field and the intense cellularity and foci of calcification in the remainder of the lesion. It must be remembered that the chondroid of a chondroblastoma rarely occupies more than about 30 per cent of the total lesional tissue.

K.
Chondroblastoma. This field is the most characteristic of the usual areas seen in the chondroblastoma. It contains benign osteoclasts and rounded polygonal cells with distinct cell borders (the chondroblasts). Another highly characteristic feature is as the presence of linear strands of calcified reticulin separating each cell and giving rise to the so-called "chicken-wire" calcifications. More heavy deposits of calcium occur when individual foci of chondroblasts in these foci undergo necrosis, as the next illustration shows (x300).

L.
Chondroblastoma. The "chicken-wire" calcifications have obstructed nutrients to the chondroblasts, resulting in focal cell necrosis and an extensive nodular focus of calcification, as shown here. These foci account for the up to 1-mm. foci of calcifications seen on radiograph. Note that the individual cells are not dissimilar in nuclear and cytoplasmic characteristics to the histiocytes of eosinophilic granuloma. This is not meant to imply any histogenetic relationship but merely to show the ranges of variability these cells may assume. They do not contain large nucleoli, mitoses are usually scarce, and chromatin is usually evenly distributed. These cells must not be mistaken for those of a malignant neoplasm, as they were before Codman defined the lesion as the benign epiphyseal chondromatous giant cell tumor. The constellation of features shown in these three illustrations are virtually pathognomonic of the chondroblastoma.

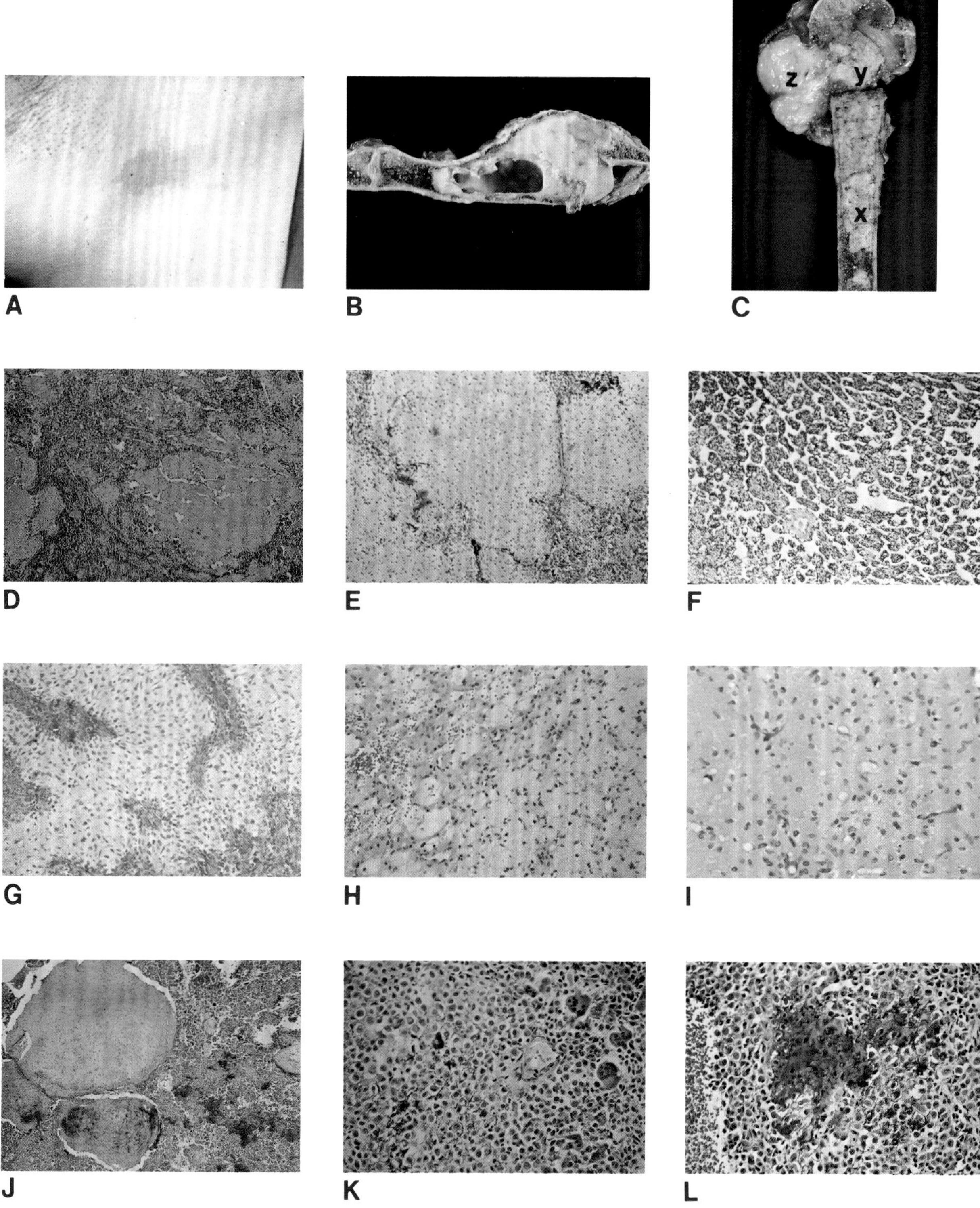
A
B
C
z
y
x
D
E
F
G
H
I
J
K
L

Plate 7

Low-Grade Neoplastic Giant Cell Tumor, Low-Grade Fibrosarcoma, Nonossifying Fibroma, Desmoplastic Fibroma of Bone, Ollier's Disease, Malignant Fibrous Histiocytoma Arising in Bone Infarct, Myeloma, and Reticulum Cell Sarcoma

A.
Low-Grade Neoplastic Giant Cell Tumor. This lesion of a phalanx demonstrates the typical gross features of a giant cell tumor. It is relatively circumscribed, soft, brownish-tan, and may be modified by foci of hemorrhage or necrosis.

B.
Low-Grade Neoplastic Giant Cell Tumor. This tumor was curetted on several occasions. Eventually seeding was noted even under the skin, as shown here (*arrow*). This testifies to the probable low-grade neoplasia of this tumor. The histology of the primary and recurrent lesions did not show sarcomatous transformation. Amputation was performed. Lung metastases did not develop.

C.
Low-Grade Neoplastic Giant Cell Tumor. Another example of the gross appearance of a large, recurrent giant cell tumor of the proximal tibial epiphysis. The lesion is still covered by a thin rim of periosteum on all sides. The lesion was amputated because it was not considered feasible to resect it or treat it with cryosurgery. Histologically, it still conformed to an ordinary giant cell tumor. No malignant transformation was noted and lung transplants or metastases did not develop.

D.
Low-Grade Fibrosarcoma. This low-grade fibrosarcoma involves the distal femur. It was firm and white and modified by hemorrhages and foci of necrosis. The tumor is fairly well circumscribed. More highly anaplastic fibrosarcomas infiltrate the bone extensively and do not show this degree of circumscription.

E.
Nonossifying Fibroma. This is a rare example of a benign nonossifying fibroma *insitu.* It has lobulated outer borders and is whitish to tan to yellow in color. The yellow color is due to accumulations of lipid-laden cells (Mubarak, S.: Am. J. Clin. Pathol., *61*:699, 1974).

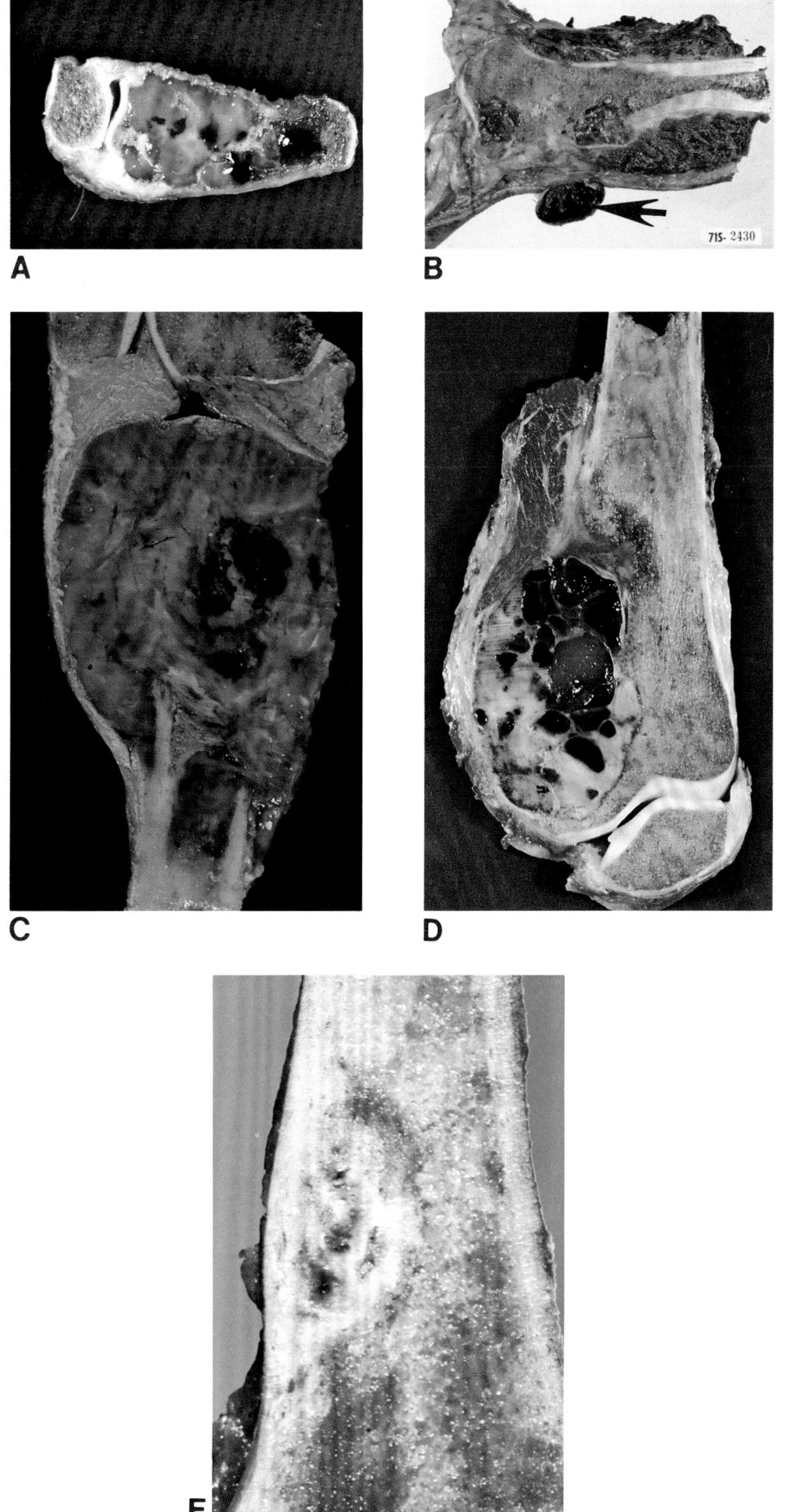
A
B
71S- 2430
C
D
E

Plate 7 (Continued)

Low-Grade Neoplastic Giant Cell Tumor, Low-Grade Fibrosarcoma, Nonossifying Fibroma, Desmoplastic Fibroma of Bone, Ollier's Disease, Malignant Fibrous Histiocytoma Arising in Bone Infarct, Myeloma, and Reticulum Cell Sarcoma

F.
Nonossifying Fibroma. This lesion was removed during a small en-bloc procedure. It is brownish yellow and moderately firm. It sits in an eroded loculated shell of cortical and subcortical bone.

G.
Desmoplastic Fibroma of Bone. This lesion is characterized by thick collagen bundles and sparse, widely set apart, relatively innocuous fibroblastic nuclei. Mitotes should be rare. It must be differentiated from Grade I fibrosarcomas that have metastatic potential. The desmoplastic fibroma is at most a locally aggressive fibroblastic neoplasm. (Milla, J., Bullough, P., and Freiberger, R.: Orthopedic Diseases, Part II. New York, Famous Teachings in Modern Medicine, Med Com Inc., © 1972)

H.
Ollier's Disease. Typical gross appearance of the tibia in a patient with multiple enchondromatosis.

I.
Malignant Fibrous Histiocytoma Arising in Bone Infarct. A malignant fibrous histiocytoma (*z*) is arising in an area of bone infarction (*y*). The fact that the lesion is malignant histiocytic is probably related to the benign histiocytic reaction to the infarct. Large, lipid-laden histiocytes formed distinct orange nodules, an example of which is labelled (*x*). The patient presented with a small tumor due to the fact that it had already eroded the cortex sufficiently to result in an infarction (*arrow*), causing pain, which lead the patient to seek medical attention. This infarct was solitary and may have been caused by an airplane decompression accident 8 years previously. The airliner "flamed out" at approximately 30,000 feet, causing immediate decompression, and it then fell to approximately 15,000 feet before "flame-in." The patient experienced extreme internal ear pain during the episode.

J.
Myeloma. Myeloma deposits are tan to deep reddish and quite soft.

K.
Myeloma. *Left:* In this section of myeloma involving a long bone, several areas of amorphous pink para-amyloid material were noted surrounded by multinucleated giant cells. *Right:* With Congo red and polarized light, the para-amyloid did not polarize. However, amyloid (*arrow*) was noted adjacent to giant cells. This histologic finding implies that perhaps para-amyloid is converted to amyloid post-phagocytosis by the giant cells.

L.
Reticulum Cell Sarcoma. This lesion arose from the os calcis. Note the extension of the soft-tissue component. This is a common accompaniment of the primary reticulum cell sarcoma of bone. It may even lead to joint effusions and be confused with a benign inflammatory monoarticular arthritis.

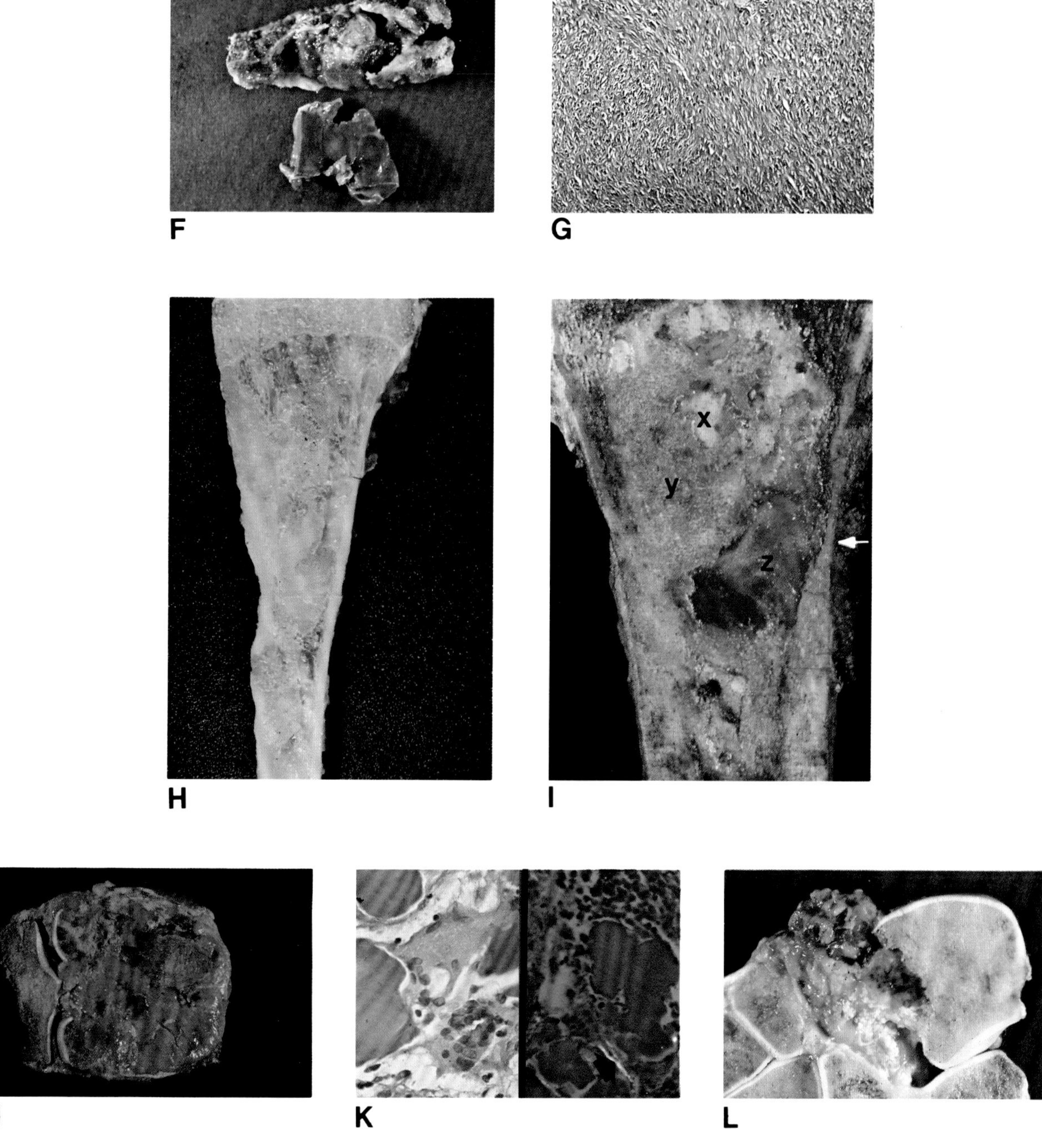
F
G
H
x
y
z
I
J
K
L

Plate 8

Eosinophilic Granuloma (EG), Letterer-Siwe Disease, and Gaucher's Disease

A.
Eosinophilic Granuloma (EG). EG is an extremely cellular lesion in its early phases (x40).

B.
Eosinophilic Granuloma (EG). Note the intimate admixture of fairly large pink mononuclear histiocytes, osteoclast-like giant cells, and smaller eosinophils. These three cell types may be found in any proportion, depending on the area sampled (x400).

C.
Top: In some fields eosinophils may be the predominant cell (x400). *Bottom:* In others the histiocytes may predominate. Note the distinct nuclear cleft in many of the histiocytic nuclei (x400).

D.
Eosinophilic Granuloma (EG). Typical appearance of the histiocytes in the early phase of EG. The nuclei are pleomorphic in size and shape but lack large nucleoli. Large nucleoli should raise the suspicion of Hodgkin's disease. Mitoses may be common in EG but they are mirror image (x1000).

E.
Eosinophilic Granuloma (EG). Imprints of EG show the cytologic features much more clearly. *Left:* The typical nonlipid rich histiocyte. Observe the small to absent nucleoli and even chromatin distribution (x1000). *Right:* A histiocyte that is filling up with lipid (x1000). *Inset:* An eosinophil (x1000). (Mirra, J., Bullough, P., and Freiberger, R.: Orthopedic Diseases, Part III: Histiocytoses and Round Cell Tumors. New York, Famous Teachings in Modern Medicine, Med Com, Inc., © 1973)

F.
Letterer-Siwe Disease. The sella turcica shows distinct orange infiltrates that correspond to large accumulations of lipid-laden histiocytes. The pituitary is seen at top (*arrow*). No histiocytes were seen in the pituitary of this patient and diabetes insipidus was not observed. The cause of the diabetes insipidus in EG is not known but it may be due to extraosseous extension of histiocytes from the bone in this region compressing the posterior pituitary. Patients with diabetes insipidus who come to autopsy should have this area carefully removed and studied in order to determine its pathogenesis. This patient did not have diabetes insipidus.

G.
Gaucher's Disease. This was the actual fresh gross appearance of the femoral head in a patient with Gaucher's disease. It was intensely orange-yellow, a reflection of the histiocytic proliferation. The crack seen beneath the articular cartilage is Waldenströms crescent, a sign of unequivocal avascular necrosis in the area.

H.
Gaucher's Disease. The typical "crumpled paper" appearance of Gaucher histiocytes. It is characteristic but not entirely pathognomonic, as this author has seen a similar appearance in the histiocytes of some Letterer-Siwe patients. If the section is not stained well it is difficult to discern. To see these kerasin-induced filaments, it is best to close the diaphragm as much as possible (x400).

I.
Gaucher's Disease. A large Gaucher cell with a crumpled paper appearance due to the filamentous intracytoplasmic deposits of kerasin (x1000).

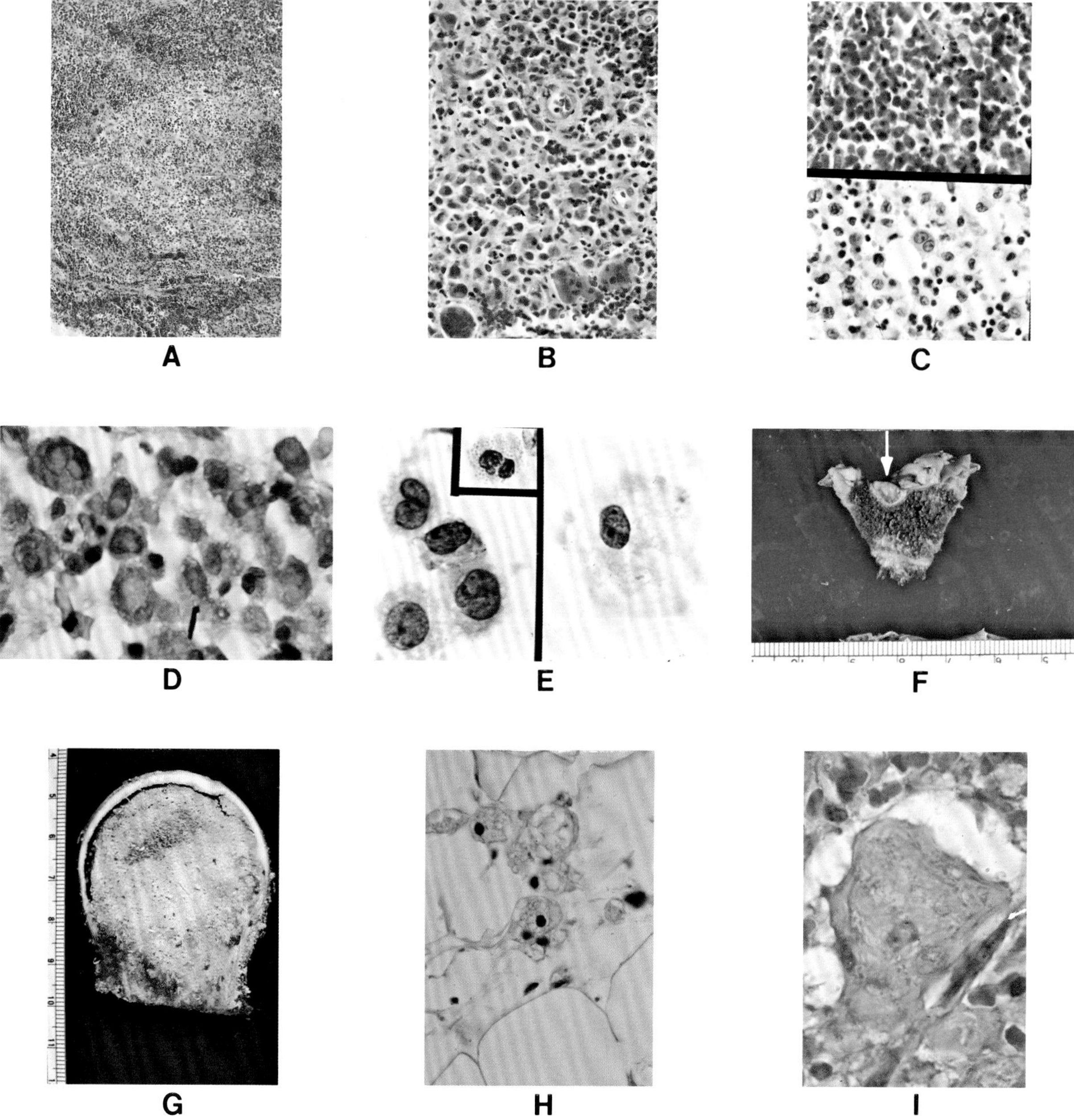
A
B
C
D
E
F
G
H
I

Plate 9

Myeloma, Hodgkin's Disease, and Primary Reticulum Cell Sarcoma of Bone

A.

Myeloma. H and E sections: *Top:* Typical solid sheets of well-differentiated plasma cells typify most myelomas. Double and triple nuclei may abound (x300). *Bottom:* Poorly differentiated myeloma may be confused with other lymphomas, such as histiocytic or poorly differentiated lymphocytic. However, the presence of occasional cells differentiating to plasma cells is key to its recognition as a plasma cell or possibly "immunoblastic" lymphoma (x300).

B.

Imprint. Once again, imprints show cytologic features much more clearly. Note the abundant double nucleated plasmacytes (x1000). (Mirra, J., Bullough, P., and Freiberger, R.: Orthropedic Diseases, eases, Part III: Histio-cytoses and Round Cell Tumors. New York, Famous Teachings in Modern Medicine, Med Com, Inc. © 1973)

C.

Myeloma. Imprint stained with Wright's. Malignant plasmablasts. Note the prominent nucleoli (x1000).

D.

Hodgkin's Disease. *Top:* Hodgkin's disease may affect a bone in a spotty or focal distribution (x40). *Bottom:* In order to rule out Hodgkin's, it is best to search for cellular areas in which large, atypical histiocytes stand out, as in this field (x125).

E.

Hodgkin's Disease. *Top:* Note the presence of benign lymphocytes and atypical histiocytes with very large nucleoli. Nucleoli of this size are not seen in eosinophilic granuloma but are extremely common to Hodgkin's disease. *Bottom left and right:* In order to confirm the suspicion of Hodgkin's, a diligent search for classic cells must be performed. These are two examples of classic bi- and multinucleate Sternberg-Reed cells (x1000).

F.

Hodgkin's Disease. *Top:* Imprint of classic Sternberg-Reed cell (x1000). *Bottom:* Imprint of very atypical histiocytes seen in association with Hodgkin's disease of bone (x1000).

G.

Primary Reticulum Cell Sarcoma of Bone (RCS). *Top:* Note the large size and pleomorphism of the nuclei (x250). *Bottom:* The cells have distinct, rounded cytoplasmic borders. Tapered cytoplasm is not seen. The nuclei show extreme pleomorphism: single, double, multilobulated, and clefted forms. Nucleoli are variable in size and nuclear chromatin is distributed unevenly (x400).

H.

Primary Reticulum Cell Sarcoma of Bone (RCS). Imprints stained with H and E. *Top:* Note the numerous "mulberry" shapes and other signs of nuclear pleomorphism (x400). *Bottom:* Pleomorphic lobulated nuclei with very abnormal chromatin clumping (x1000).

I.

Primary Reticulum Cell Sarcoma of Bone (RCS). Reticulin stain shows each cell surrounded by fibers. The arrow points to a cell encased by the reticulin it produces. This latter sign is quite characteristic of primary RCS. However, good preservation of material and excellent staining is necessary to demonstrate this feature.

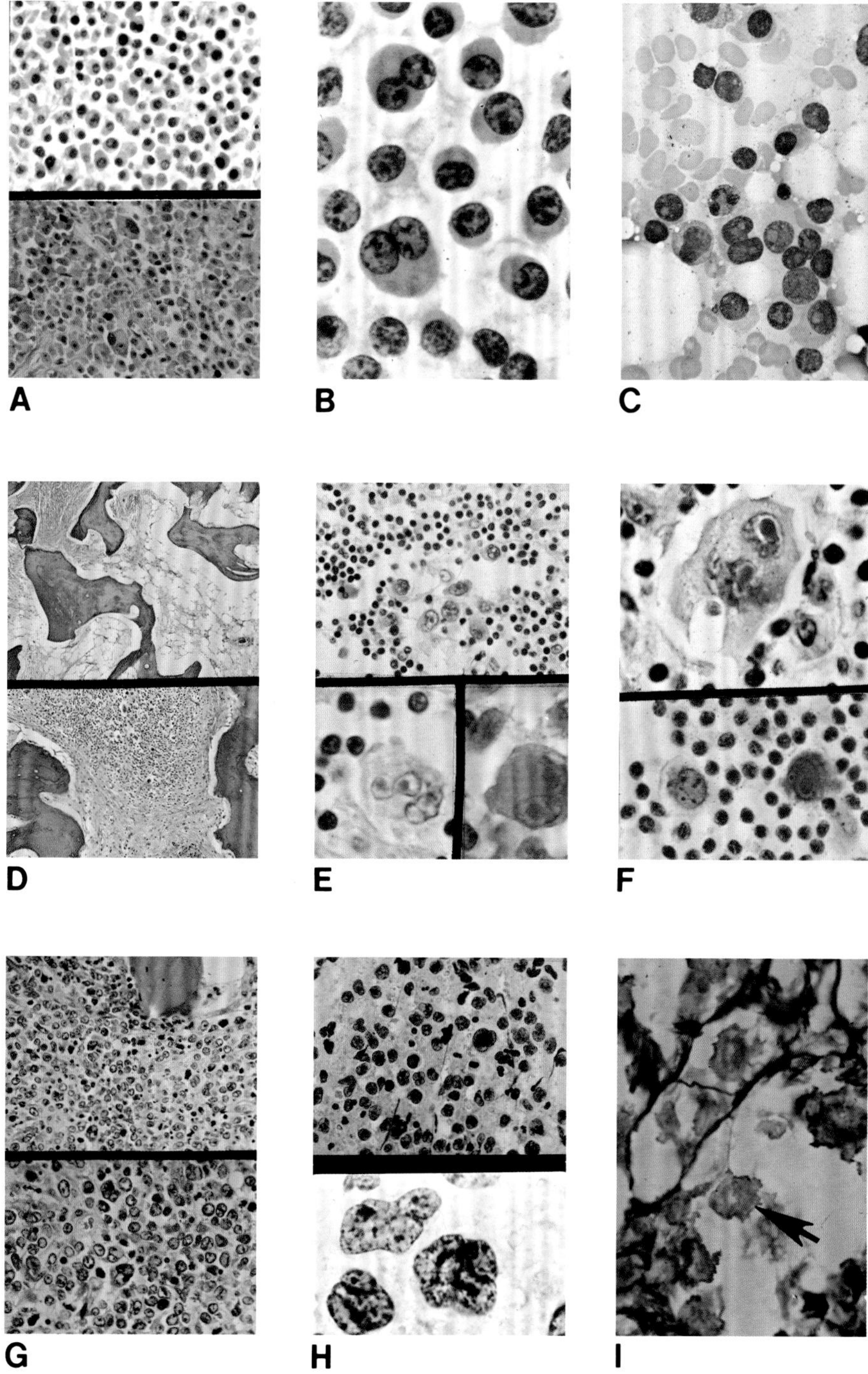
A
B
C
D
E
F
G
H
I

Plate 10

Ewing's Sarcoma, Lymphosarcoma; and Metastatic Neuroblastoma

A.
Ewing's Sarcoma. *Top:* Sheets of cells with pale, round to oval, single, lymphoblast-like nuclei and lacey indistinct cytoplasm characterize this tumor (x250). *Bottom:* The chromatin network is finely dispersed. Nucleoli may be present and are of variable size but usually are small. Mitoses are generally abundant.

B.
Ewing's Sarcoma. *Top:* PAS stain shows intense intracytoplasmic glycogen. *Bottom:* Some sections stained with PAS after diastase digestion. Note the loss of the glycogen staining.

C.
Ewing's Sarcoma. Imprints. The nuclei are roundish and paler staining than well-differentiated lymphocytes. The cytoplasm is pale and minimally to moderately abundant (x1000).

D.
Lymphosarcoma. *Left:* On low-power examination the staining of the nuclei is more intense compared to Ewing's and should suggest a lymphosarcoma. *Right:* The best areas to study to determine whether the cells may be lymphocytic are in those regions where cells are in loosest approximation. The nuclear and cytoplasmic features of this area should be compared and contrasted to Plate 10, *A*, top (x250).

E.
Lymphosarcoma. If the bone specimen is well stained and properly decalcified, the nature of the infiltrate as being of lymphocytic origin should be much easier to appreciate (x250).

F.
Lymphosarcoma. However, imprints of such lesions will be of great help. *Top:* This imprint was from a patient with a presumptive radiographic diagnosis of Ewing's sarcoma. The Wright's stained imprint, however, was read as consistent with poorly differentiated lymphocytic lymphoma. Note the dense blue-staining cytoplasm and lymphoblastic nuclei with very prominent nucleoli (x1000). *Bottom:* In this author's experience such patients presenting with "solitary" lymphoblastic lymphomas of bone generally end up with leukemia within 6 months. This peripheral blood smear is from such a patient (x1000).

G.
Metastatic Neuroblastoma. *Top:* The neuroblastoma to bone is generally a very cellular tumor which, to the casual observer, mimics lymphosarcoma or Ewing's sarcoma on low-power (x125). *Bottom:* Neuroblastoma cells may show distinct or indistinct cytoplasmic borders. The nuclei may resemble well to poorly differentiated lymphocytes or Ewing's nuclei. The principal diagnostic features relate to signs of neural differentiation. These include rosettes (rare in metastases), a fibrillary matrix between tumor cells (not so rare but subtle) and occasional to rare cells with uni- or bipolar extensions. The unipolar extensions give rise to "pear" or "carrot" shaped cells (*arrow*) that are not seen in Ewing's sarcoma or lymphocytic lymphomas.

H.
Metastatic Neuloblastoma. *Top:* A 2-year-old with metastatic neuroblastoma. Autopsy showed extensive bone involvement. The cells here are difficult to distinguish from lymphocytes, although the abundant pink cytoplasm in some cells is a clue to cells of nonlymphocytic origin (x250). *Middle:* However, careful search did reveal some cells with unequal pear-to carrot-shapes (*arrow*) (x400). *Bottom:* Imprint of a neuroblastoma with some "carrot" cells (x400).

I.
Metastatic Neuroblastoma. *Top:* This rosette is from a primary adrenal neuroblastoma. Note the carrot-shaped cells and the central neurofibrillary core. *Second Frame:* Patient with metastatic neuroblastoma. Note the bipolar cytoplasmic extension of the cell in the middle of the illustration that is also consistent with a cell of neural origin. *Third Frame:* Note the long carrot-shaped cell and multinucleation. This kind of cell is never seen in Ewing's sarcoma or lymphocytic lymphoma. This patient also had proven metastatic neuroblastoma. *Bottom:* Imprint of a long, ganglion-like cell in a patient with metastatic neuroblastoma to bone unsuspected until after imprint analysis (x1000).

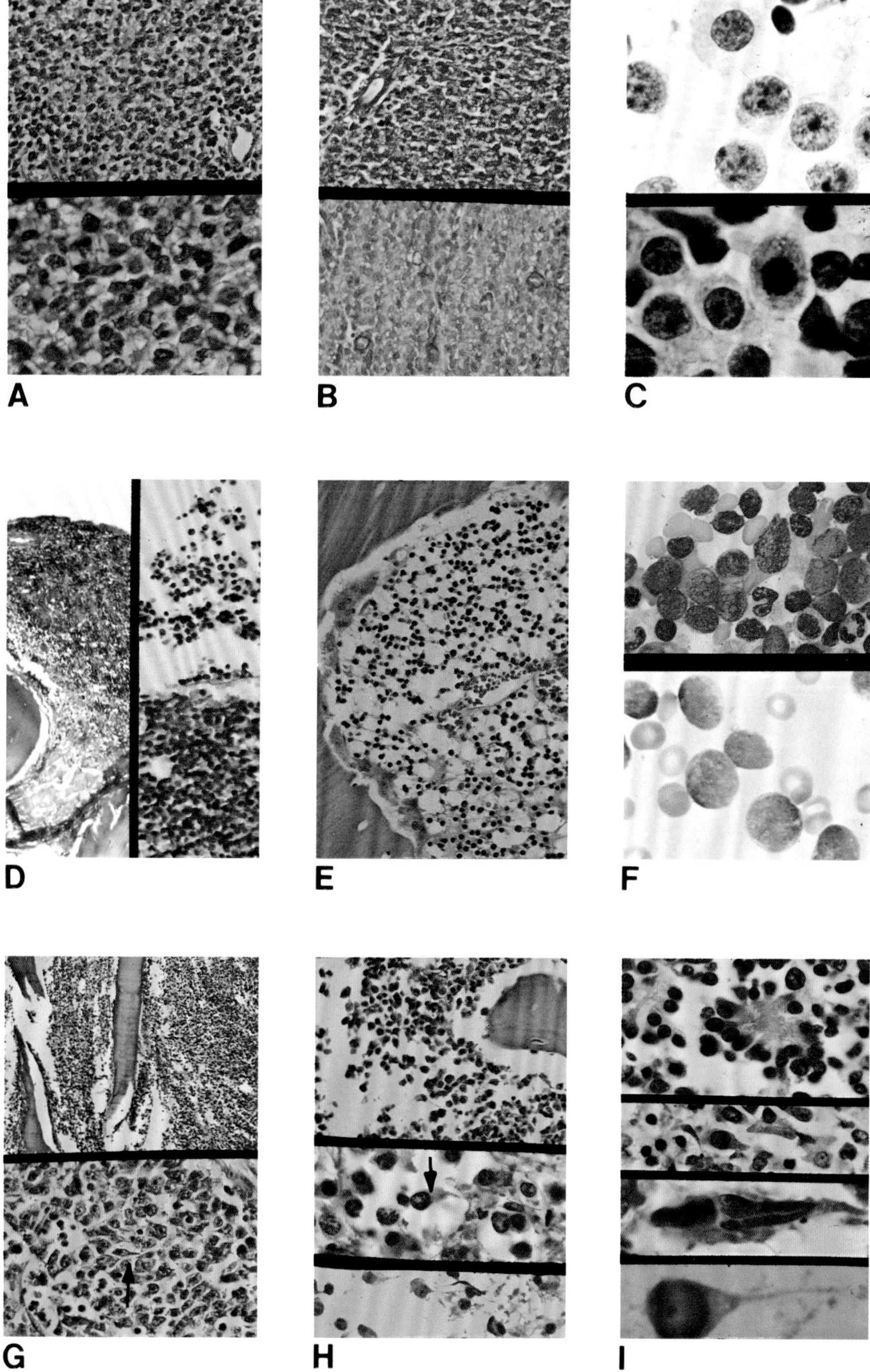
A
B
C
D
E
F
G
H
I

RADIOLOGICAL INTERPRETATION

Richard H. Gold, M.D.

3

INTRODUCTION

Diagnostic radiologists and surgical pathologists share a special kinship. The radiologist is in a sense practicing gross pathology each time he inspects a radiograph, a radionuclide scan, an ultrasonogram, or a computer-assisted transverse tomographic examination. Microscopy plays a discriminatory role in distinguishing a benign primary tumor of bone from a malignant one, but histologic features that may suggest malignancy are sometimes manifested by tumors that neither metastasize nor invade locally; moreover, a single biopsy specimen may not be representative of the most malignant part of a tumor, especially if the tumor has arisen from a benign precursor lesion such as an enchondroma or bone infarct. The radiographic examination may ease the burden of this diagnostic challenge for the pathologist. While frequently not yielding a specific diagnosis, the radiograph may be looked upon as a complementary tool that permits assessment of the relative aggressiveness or indolence of a tumor. An experienced bone pathologist would be loathe to base his diagnosis solely upon histology, preferring instead to correlate histologic features with radiographic ones before coming to a conclusion.[32] It cannot be overemphasized that diagnosis should not depend solely on post-treatment radiographs. Treated lesions can be so altered radiographically to give a false impression of benignancy or malignancy.

THE RADIOLOGICAL APPROACH TO BONE LESIONS

In this chapter I have deliberately avoided a complete review of the radiologic features of *all* bone tumors and tumorlike conditions, which are treated in detail in subsequent chapters. Rather, I have tried to present a logical method of radiologic analysis that should prove helpful in the everyday evaluation of radiographs of any discrete bone disorder that a pathologist is likely to encounter.

Because many bone abnormalities are at first glance radiologically indistinguishable, a logical diagnostic approach using both clinical and laboratory data is mandatory. For every bone lesion, the following disease categories should be considered:

1. Developmental anomalies
2. Trauma
3. Dysplasias and dysostoses
4. Metabolic disease (including dystrophies)
5. Infections and inflammatory processes
6. Tumor and tumorlike conditions
7. Degenerative disease and ischemic necrosis

An orderly sequence of radiologic observation might consist of the following:

1. Soft tissues
2. Periosteal region
3. Cortex
4. Medulla
5. Diaphysis, metaphysis, epiphyseal plate (physis), epiphysis
6. Joint

Most benign and primary malignant bone tumors have favored sites of origin within a bone. Familiarity with these sites may provide a clue to diagnosis. For example, the *chondroblastoma* and *giant cell tumor* are most often centered in the epiphysis. Most *osteosarcomas, chondrosarcomas,* and *fibrosarcomas* are centered in the metaphysis. *Nonossifying fibroma* takes origin at the junction of the metaphysis with the diaphysis (metadiaphyseal). Round cell lesions such as *Ewing's sarcoma, reticulum cell sarcoma,* and *myeloma* usually originate in the diaphysis.

Evaluation of the radiographic appearance of a bone tumor requires an orderly, logical approach.[20] The most important features to consider are: the telltale mineralization of tumor matrix, the site and pattern of bone destruction, and the reactive new bone proliferation. These give the best indications of cellular origin and relative indolence or aggressiveness of the tumor.

Pitfalls to Detection of Early Lesions

Because of its compactness, cortical bone is more resistant to destruction than is cancellous bone. Furthermore, because of the greater radiographic density of cortical bone, even subtle alterations in its structure, such as a nutrient foramen or hairline fracture, are easily seen in radiographs. In contrast, the lattice work of cancellous bone is masked in radiographs by the denser, surrounding cortex. Indeed, close to half or more of the volume of cancellous bone must be destroyed before any change becomes apparent in standard radiographs.[18] In aged persons, generalized loss of bone, particularly of cancellous bone, is a natural process of atrophy that further hinders radiographic detection of primary and metastatic tumor. A malignant tumor of bone may indeed go undetected in standard radiographs until it has become large enough to erode the cortex (Fig. 3-1, *A* and *B*). Malignancies in their early phases may resemble benign bone tumors; the incipient blastic osteosarcoma (Fig. 3-22) may be mistaken for fibrous dysplasia, bone infarct, or osteoblastoma. The incipient lytic osteosarcoma (see Fig. 7-87) can be confused with a bone cyst or giant cell tumor.

Thus, it is easy to see why the *classic* radiographic features of a primary malignant bone tumor usually become manifest only when the local extent of the tumor is far advanced. The classic features that radiologists look for include: cortical destruction with extracortical tumor extension; resultant subperiosteal new bone that is delicate, interrupted, longitudinally lamellated, or perpendicularly spiculated; deposition of an isolated cuff of subperiosteal new bone (Codman's triangle) at the boundary of the neoplasm, where it breaches the cortex; and in osteosarcoma, the cumulus cloudlike mineralization of tumor osteoid.

In contradistinction to a malignant tumor, a benign bone tumor, because of its slow rate of growth, may thin and outwardly displace the cortex, but it rarely breaches the cortex and usually provokes solid or uninterrupted subperiosteal new bone (Fig. 3-2).

Standard tomography (body-section radiography) is more sensitive than standard radiography in indicating the nature and extent of cancellous bone destruction. Tomography permits the site of interest to be subdivided longitudinally into many parallel sections or planes, each only several millimeters thick; a number of radiographs are then made, each with a different section or plane in focus. *Computed tomography,* an elegant variation of standard tomography, is far

FIG. 3-1. Metastasis to tibia from carcinoma of uterine cervix. (*A*) Anteroposterior radiograph reveals a focus of destruction occupying almost the entire width of the shaft. (*B*) Corresponding lateral view reveals endosteal destruction in the posterior cortex. The destruction became visible only when it had extended from the medullary cavity to the cortex (*arrow*), a relatively late event.

FIG. 3-2. Eosinophilic granuloma of femur with radiographic characteristics of a benign tumor: sharp interface with host bone, coarse trabeculation of host bone at margin of tumor, and solid, uninterrupted subperiosteal new bone.

FIG. 3-3. Basic destructive patterns of primary bone tumors according to Lodwick. These patterns correlate with pathologic aggressiveness: (*A*) Geographic pattern implies slow rate of growth. (*B*) Moth-eaten pattern implies intermediate rate. (*C*) Permeative pattern implies a rapid rate. (Lodwick, G.S.: Solitary malignant tumors of bone. The application of predictor variables and diagnosis. Semin. Roentgenol., *1*:293–313, 1966)

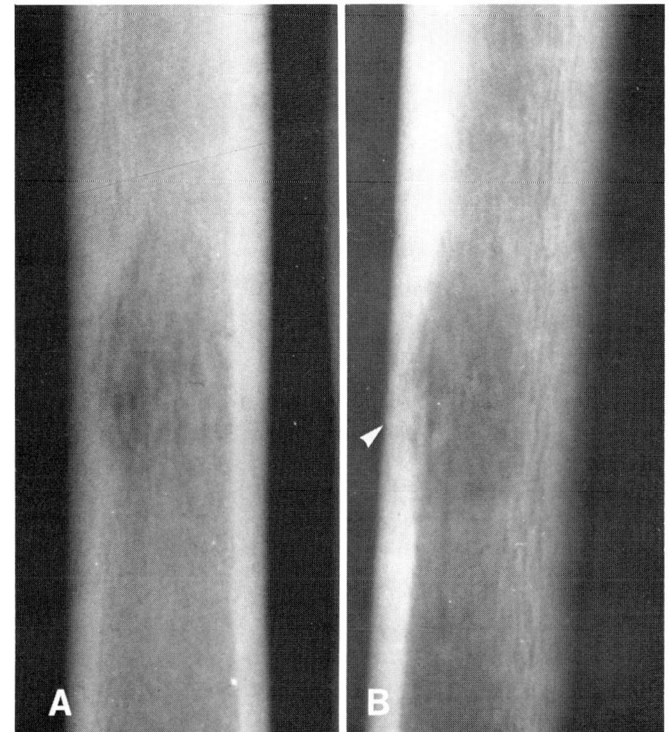

FIG. 3-1

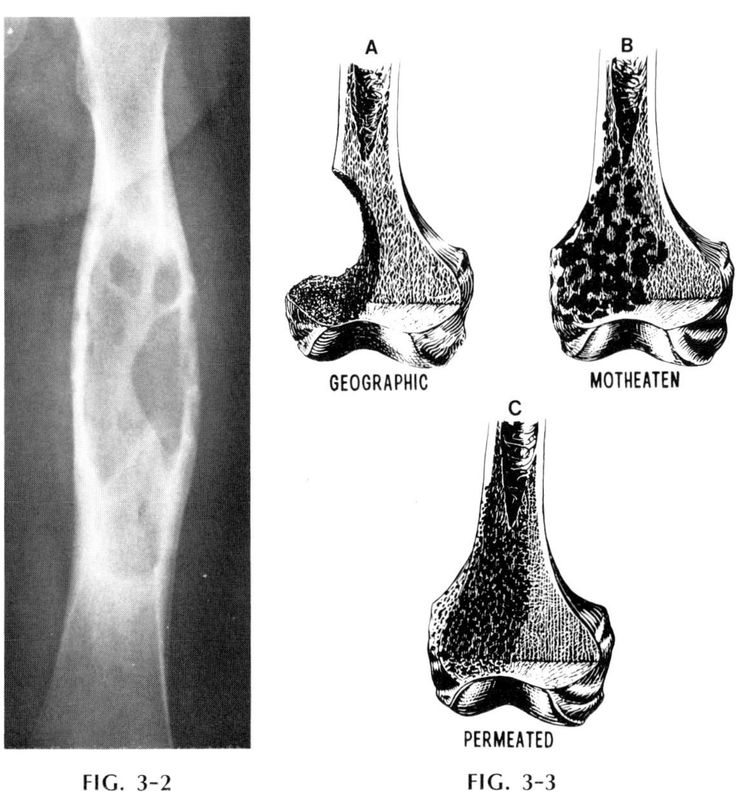

FIG. 3-2

FIG. 3-3

more sensitive than standard tomography in elucidating the intra- and extraosseous extent of bone tumors. Thus, computed tomography may contribute to staging the tumor and to the planning of preoperative and preradiation therapy.

Before an abnormality appears in standard radiographs and even standard tomograms, *radionuclide bone scans and scintigrams* usually reveal an abnormally increased uptake ot radionuclide at the site of a primary or metastatic tumor. Unfortunately, a positive scan is not specific for malignant neoplasm. Radionuclide bone scans must be correlated with radiographs to exclude benign causes of abnormally increased radionuclide activity, notably degenerative joint disease and spondylosis. If benign causes are eliminated and if there are no negative baseline scans, any remaining unexplained focus of increased activity may have to be confirmed by biopsy, especially since it may represent a metastasis.

Pattern of Destruction as an Indicator of Growth Rate

Every bone tumor manifests a radiographic pattern of destruction that can be correlated with its pathologic aggressiveness or indolence (Table 3–1). Lodwick has analyzed the varying patterns and classified them into three basic types: geographic, moth-eaten, and permeative types of destruction (Fig. 3–3).[19]

Geographic destruction is characterized by large, well-defined, greater than 1 cm. holes with a sharply delineated edge (Fig. 3–3, *A*). The key radiographic feature of geographic destruction is a sharp zone of transition between bone that has undergone complete destruction and bone that is completely intact. This pattern implies that the growth rate of the tumor is very slow and has resulted in intimate contact between the true edge of the lesion and the visible margin of destroyed bone. A sclerotic rim at the edge of the process signifies extremely slow growth or quiescence (Fig. 3–4). Slow growing or quiescent lesions exhibiting a geographic pattern may also manifest coarse trabeculation resulting from irregular ridging of the encompassing host bone. Geographic destruction is characteristic of benign or low-grade neoplasms such as the nonossifying fibroma, chondromyxoid fibroma, aneurysmal bone cyst, simple bone cyst, and giant cell tumor (Fig. 3–5).

Moth-eaten destruction is characterized by multiple 2 to 5 mm. holes that have a tendency to coalesce (Fig. 3–3, *B*). The zone of transition of each hole is ill defined. A moth-eaten pattern implies severe cortical

Table 3–1. Classification of Primary Bone Malignancies According to Patterns of Destruction

Tumor	*Peak Age Incidence*	*Location Within Long Bone*	*Periosteal Reaction*	*Matrix Mineralization*
Geographic Destruction				
Chondrosarcoma	40+	Anywhere, central or periosteal	Expanded shell	Cartilage (flocculent and windblown)
Aggressive giant cell tumor (most feature moth-eaten edge and cortical destruction)	25	Epiphyseal-metaphyseal	Nonexistent or expanded shell	—
Some fibrosarcomas (may also manifest moth-eaten pattern)	40+	Metaphysis or diaphysis	Scant and amorphous	—
Moth-Eaten Destruction				
Some fibrosarcomas (may also manifest geographic pattern)	40+	Metaphysis or diaphysis	Scant and amorphous	—
Permeative Destruction				
Ewing's sarcoma	15	Diaphysis	Lamellated and/or spiculated	—
Osteosarcoma	15	Metaphysis (occasionally diaphysis)	Lamellated	Osteoid (cumulus cloud, sunburst)
Reticulum cell sarcoma	40	Diaphysis	Scant and amorphous	—
Sarcoma in Paget's disease	40+	Anywhere	Scant	Not visible in radiograph

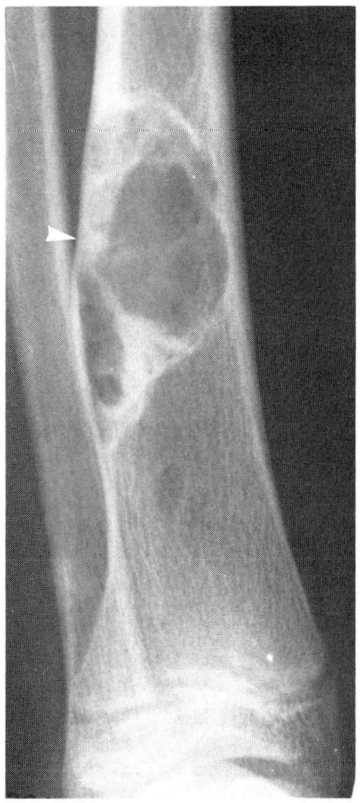

FIG. 3-4

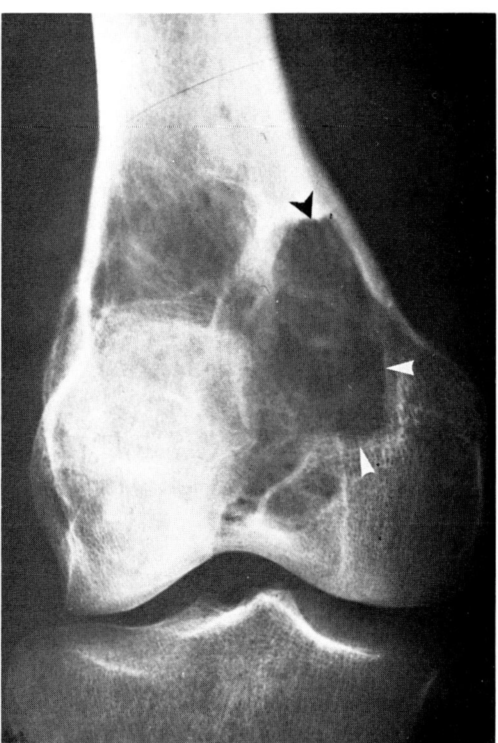

FIG. 3-5

FIG. 3-4. Nonossifying fibroma of tibia. The lesion tends to be eccentric and occupy the metadiaphyseal region. A sclerotic rim at the edge of a focus of geographic destruction implies extremely slow growth or quiescence. Although the cortex has slowly and progressively been outwardly displaced (*arrow*), it has not been breached. The vast majority of lesions with this appearance will be nonossifying fibromas. On rarer occasions a simple bone cyst, monostotic fibrous dysplasia, chondromyxoid fibroma, or an old healed eosinophilic granuloma may be found on biopsy. The probability that a lesion such as shown above would turn out to be malignant post-biopsy would be nearly zero, because of its dense peripheral sclerotic rind.

FIG. 3-5. Giant cell tumor of distal end of femur, resulting in geographic pattern of destruction. The sharp zone of transition (*arrows*) between bone that has undergone complete destruction and bone that is completely intact implies slow growth.

destruction and signifies a moderately aggressive lesion. Moth-eaten destruction is characteristic of some fibrosarcomas.

Permeative destruction is characterized by multiple tiny holes (1 mm. or less) predominating in cortical bone. These holes gradually diminish in size and number from the center of the lesion to its periphery (Fig. 3-3, *C*). Thus, the zone of transition is broad and ill defined. Although the cortex may appear, radiographically, to be almost intact, but with greatly reduced radiodensity, it is, nevertheless extensively involved. A permeative pattern implies that the tumor not only has breached the cortex, but probably has extended throughout most or all of the length of the bone. In short, this pattern of destruction implies great aggressiveness and extensive neoplastic infiltration. Permeative destruction is characteristic of primary reticulum cell sarcoma of bone (Fig. 3-6) and Ewing's sarcoma (Fig. 3-7). Osteosarcoma also manifests permeative destruction, but the pattern is usually obscured by tumor bone. Even permeative destruction, however, is not pathognomonic of malignancy, because osteomyelitis may result in this pattern.

Each of these three aforementioned basic patterns of destruction may occur alone or in combination with one or both of the other patterns (Fig. 3-8). The moth-eaten and permeative patterns signify total penetration of the cortex by the lesion, and it is not critical to distinguish between them. But it is essential to distinguish these two patterns from the geographic pattern in order to make diagnostic and therapeutic decisions. The reason it is so important to make this distinction is that the geographic pattern implies a slow rate of growth; the moth-eaten pattern, an intermediate rate; and the permeative pattern, the most rapid rate of growth. When the observer learns to recognize and understand the implications of each pattern, he may then estimate the growth rate of a bone tumor from a single radiographic examination. Unfortunately, estimating the benignancy or malignancy of certain tumors by these criteria is fraught with risk, especially in the case of giant cell tumors. Moreover, when the physician is considering possible diagnoses of primary bone tumors, he must always bear in mind that the lesion may be metastatic. In patients more than 50 years of age, the incidence of metastatic tumor in bone far exceeds that of primary tumor.

Bubbly Lesions

Certain lesions may exhibit a characteristically bubbly appearance in radiographs. They therefore tend to manifest a geographic pattern of destruction, implying slow growth and usually benignancy.

FIBROUS DYSPLASIA. The fibrous tissue component of this lesion admixed with poorly calcified, primitive, fine trabeculae of new bone creates a characteristic *ground-glass* radiographic appearance. When the proximal femur is involved there may be a characteristic varus deformity and convex-lateral "bending" that is sometimes called a "shepherd's crook." In the intertrochanteric region of the femur the lesion may appear circular with a thick sclerotic rim (Fig. 3-9). Usually the radiographic density of fibrous dysplasia is greater than that of a purely destructive lesion.

ENCHONDROMA. This lesion creates evenly distributed stippled, ringlike or snowflake densities. The calcifications are often the only sign (Fig. 3-10).

EOSINOPHILIC GRANULOMA. The solitary lesion is seldom expansile. The actively progressing lesions usually show no sclerotic rim, and are often associated with a uniform layer of subperiosteal new bone (Fig. 3-2). Incipient lesions may mimic osteomyelitis or sarcoma, particularly Ewing's. Older lesions develop more rounded borders and in the late healing phase develop a rim of sclerosis.

GIANT CELL TUMOR. Rapidly growing (Fig. 3-8) or indolent (Fig. 3-5), this lesion tends to begin in the epiphyseal-metaphyseal region and extends all the way to the subarticular region. This tumor is rarely bordered by sclerosis and does not contain punctate calcifications. These latter signs in a tumor of this region would usually be caused by chondroblastoma.

NONOSSIFYING FIBROMA. This lesion is characterized by its eccentric location between metaphysis and diaphysis and scalloped, thin sclerotic border of reactive host bone (Fig. 3-4).[14]

OSTEOBLASTOMA. This may mimic aneurysmal bone cyst but the osteoblastoma frequently contains radiologically visible mineralizing osteoid (Fig. 3-11).[21,23]

MYELOMA. This so-called solitary plasmacytoma (Fig. 3-12) may appear very expansile and, because it is slow growing, may be surrounded by a thin to thick sclerotic rim of host bone. The lesion may become sclerotic after radiotherapy, or sclerosis may occur when amyloid deposits within the lesion undergo calcification.

FIG. 3-6. Reticulum cell sarcoma of humerus characterized by permeative zone of destruction and absence of subperiosteal new bone. The permeative pattern signifies total penetration of the cortex. A pathologic fracture has occurred (*arrow*).

FIG. 3-7. Ewing's sarcoma: Radiograph of sagitally sectioned amputation specimen. A permeative pattern of destruction and numerous delicate perpendicular spicules of subperiosteal new bone characterize the radiographic changes. The periosteum has been displaced as far as the ulna; chronic pressure has resulted in pressure atrophy (*arrow*). The tumor has infiltrated throughout the length of the radius, a feature typical of the aggressive tumors that produce permeative destruction.

FIG. 3-8. Rapidly growing giant cell tumor of distal end of femur. Although this tumor has basically a geographic destructive pattern, cortical destruction and an indistinct zone of transition (*arrows*) between destroyed and intact bone imply rapid growth. Note its usual extension to the articular cartilage.

FIG. 3-9. Fibrous dysplasia of intertrochanteric region of femur. The thick sclerotic rim implies that the lesion is no longer growing. The radiographic density of the lesion is greater than that of a purely destructive process because the lesion contains fibrous tissue admixed with spicules of immature bone.

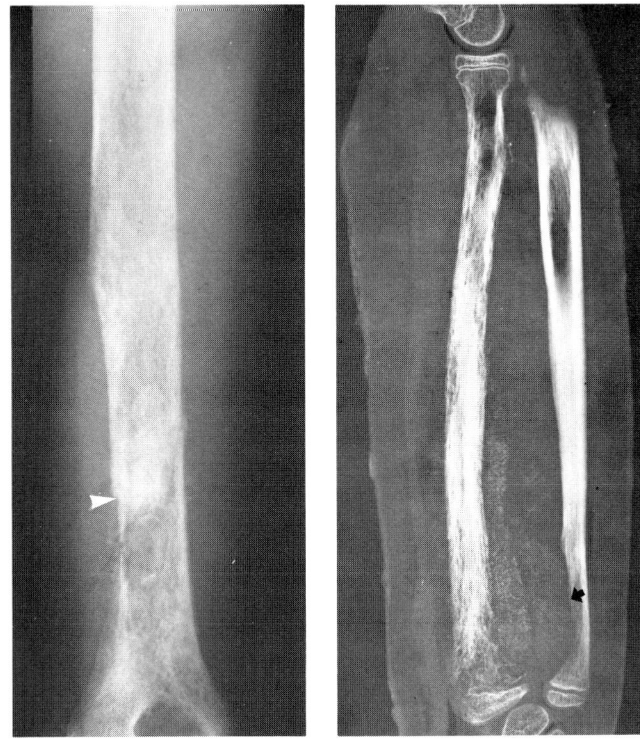

FIG. 3-6

FIG. 3-7

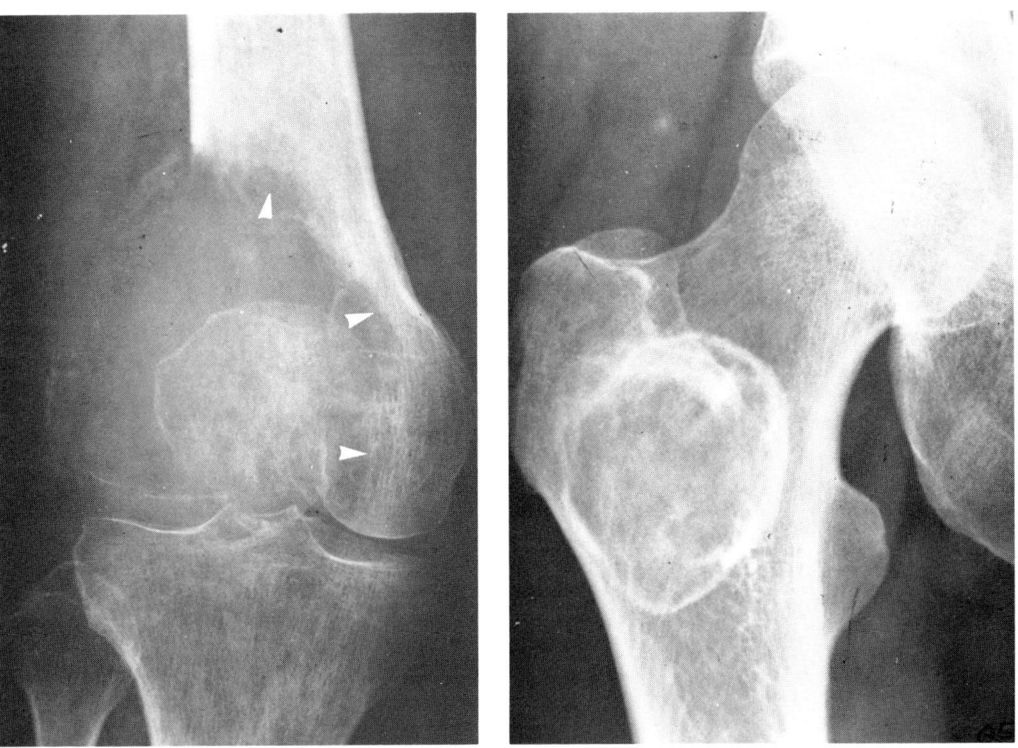

FIG. 3-8

FIG. 3-9

METASTATIC KIDNEY AND THYROID TUMOR. These lesions may be exceedingly bubbly and expansile in appearance (Fig. 3–13).[11]

ANEURYSMAL BONE CYST. This is found anywhere in any bone, is typically eccentric, and looks aneurysmal (Figs. 3–14, 3–15, and 3–26).[5]

ANGIOMA. These multiple lesions are frequently encountered in the bones on both sides of a single joint. Malignant tumors rarely involve contiguous bone ends unless they are metastatic tumors or angiosarcoma. The most common tumorlike lesions that involve contiguous epiphyses are rheumatoid arthritic or osteoarthritic "cysts" (geodes), pigmented villonodular synovitis, gout, or tuberculosis. Most are benign synovial lesions invading bone at the articular cartilage-metaphyseal bone border.

SIMPLE CYST. They are usually unilocular, centrally placed, metaphyseal-diaphyseal, lytic lesions that extend to the epiphyseal plate of young children.[26] As the patient grows older, the lesion may separate from its contact with the epiphyseal plate. They can be bordered by benign host bone sclerosis. On very rare occasion, a "simple bone cyst" may be a telangiectatic osteosarcoma upon histologic examination. Therefore, bone chips should not be taken from the pelvis without a change of instruments, unless the diagnosis is first confirmed pathologically.

HYPERPARATHYROID CYST. A cyst does not heal following parathyroidectomy; brown tumors, however, become calcified after parathyroidectomy.

INFECTION. Brodie's abscess is usually the result of infection with *Staphylococcus aureus* and has a predilection for the distal tibia of a child. *Coccidioidomycosis* tends to affect those regions of the bones with persistent red marrow, that is, the ends of bones and bony protuberances such as tuberosities and trochanters. Look for adjacent soft-tissue edema to suggest inflammation.

Ecchinococcosis. Only 2 per cent of people with visceral disease have bone lesions; these can involve contiguous bones.

CHONDROMYXOID FIBROMA. These lesions are usually encountered in young adults, tend to have a well-defined margin and to affect subcortical areas in the diaphysis of a long bone, to result in irregular cortical displacement, and to sometimes provoke extensive sclerosis over a period of time. The proximal end of the tibia is the most common site to be affected (Fig. 3–16). Unlike other cartilaginous tumors, calcification within this tumor is very rare. Sometimes, chondromyxoid fibromas are locally aggressive and may completely destroy the overlying cortex, thus simulating malignancy.[10]

CHONDROBLASTOMA. This is the only tumor always located in the epiphysis prior to its fusion. Minute, subtle, 1- to 2-mm. calcifications are seen in fewer than half of the cases. If seen, they are quite helpful to radiologic diagnosis. The margin of the lesion may be lobulated as befits its cartilaginous origin (Fig. 3–17). In contrast to the giant cell tumor (GCT) of epiphysis, the chondroblastoma is usually much smaller and often is surrounded by a border of host bone sclerosis.[22] The GCT and chondroblastoma are the two most common primary tumors of epiphyses. Less common is the chondrosarcoma and rarely, enchondroma.

Now string together the first letter of all these lesions. What do you get? "Fegnomasic." What does this word mean? Fegnomashic is an uncontrollable urge to use mnemonic devices.[24]

FIG. 3–10. Enchondroma of femur. The densifications are the only radiographic sign. Radiologic distinction from a bone infarct is difficult. Note that there are no significant focal areas of lysis, cortical thickening, or endosteal scalloping, signs which in all but short tubular bones would point to probable chondrosarcomatous transformation. Enchondromas of the long bones are usually discovered incidentally. Bone pain is an ominous clinical symptom, again in all but the short tubular bones.

FIG. 3–11. Osteoblastoma of fibula. The cortex is outwardly displaced but intact, signifying benignancy. Fluffy, mineralizing osteoid is present within the tumor. However, the radiographic appearance of some osteoblastomas may appear more aggressive and mimic that of an aneurysmal bone cyst or osteosarcoma.

FIG. 3–12. So-called solitary plasmacytoma of vertebra. The lesion originated in the body and extended into a pedicle. Myelography reveals an extradural defect in the column of radiopaque contrast. The thin sclerotic rim at the border of the lesion (*arrows*) signifies extremely slow growth. Nonetheless, almost all solitary plasmacytomas are really precursors of multiple myeloma.

FIG. 3–13. Renal cell carcinoma metastatic to radius. The bubbly appearance and geographic pattern of destruction resemble the features of a benign tumor. It is important to remember, however, that beyond the age of 50, metastatic tumor of bone occurs far more frequently than primary tumor. Bubbly, expansile, radiolucent lesions such as this one are most consistent with renal cell carcinoma, thyroid carcinoma, or myeloma.

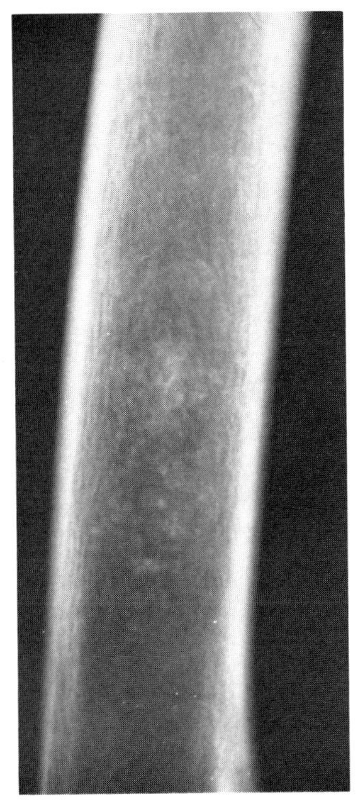

FIG. 3-10

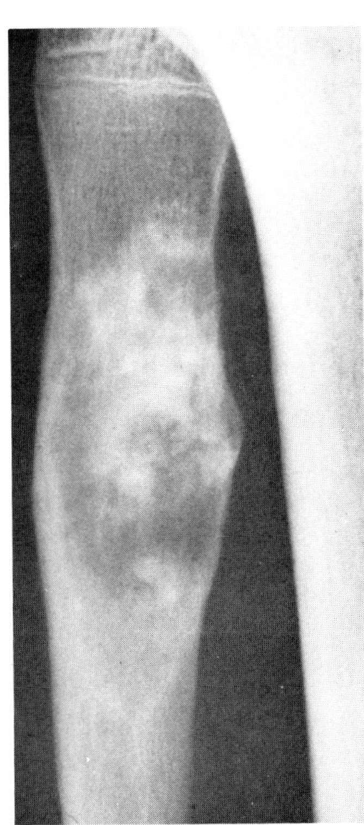

FIG. 3-11

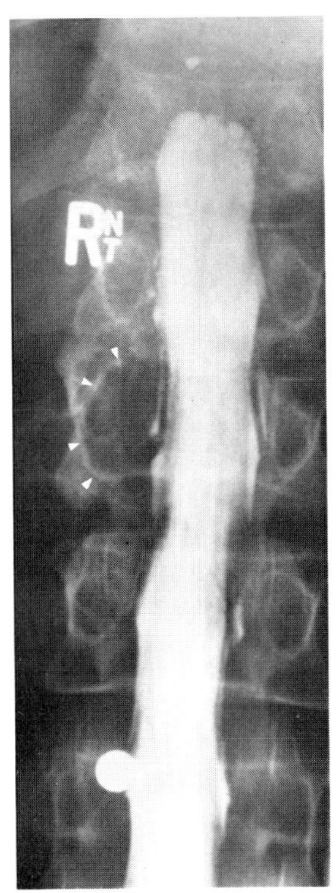

FIG. 3-12

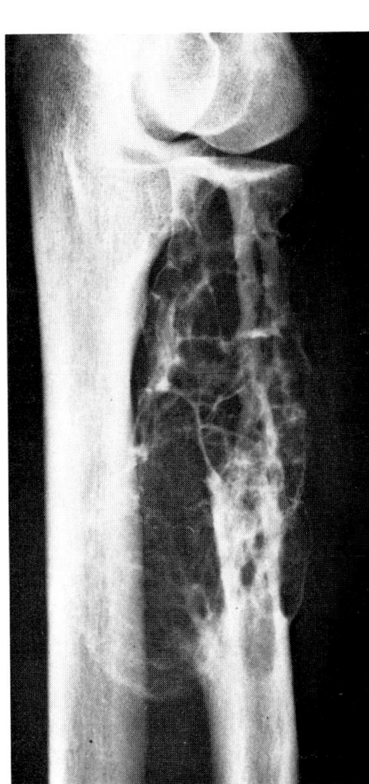

FIG. 3-13

OTHER WAYS TO DIAGNOSE BONE TUMORS

Age of the Patient as an Aid to Diagnosis

While clinical history may have limited value in the diagnosis of bone tumors, the age of the patient is an important consideration. For example, the peak incidence of lytic bone lesions from acute leukemia and neuroblastoma is in the first decade; osteosarcoma and Ewing's sarcoma are most common in the second decade; giant cell tumor is unusual before the third decade; and metastatic tumor and multiple myeloma are the most frequent malignant tumors of bone in patients more than 50 years of age.

Specifically the patient's age can be particularly useful in differentiating Ewing's sarcoma from reticulum cell sarcoma of the flat bones such as the ilium (Fig. 3–18). Both types of sarcoma cause a permeative pattern of destruction, but they may be distinguished in long bones by the extent of periosteal response; Ewing's sarcoma characteristically evokes an extensive, delicately spiculated or lamellated proliferation of subperiosteal new bone, while reticulum cell sarcoma does not. Flat bones, however, unlike long bones, do not have periosteums that have a capacity for vigorous new bone production. Thus, if a tumor occurs in the ilium, which is a flat bone, the fact that no new bone production is taking place makes it difficult to use periosteal response to diagnose a tumor. Ewing's sarcoma seldom occurs beyond the second decade of life, while reticulum cell sarcoma predominates in the third through sixth decades; using this information, the physician may make a logical choice between these two entirely different neoplasms that assume identical radiographic appearances.[20]

Mineralization of the Tumor Matrix

It is possible to recognize the specific type of tumor matrix by its radiologic pattern of mineralization.[8] In general, the greatest degree of mineralization in tumor cartilage or osteoid occurs in the region of greatest maturity, usually the center of the tumor. Since deposits of cartilage have a lobular configuration, calcification within benign tumor cartilage frequently takes the form of rings. These appear as a sheath of mineralized bone at the periphery of lobules of cartilage, but flocculent deposits and sharply defined crystal-like clusters may also be seen (Figs. 3–10 and 3–19). The central predominance of the calcification aids in distinguishing a cartilaginous tumor from a medullary infarct, in which the most heavily calcified portion tends to be at the periphery of the lesion. The pattern of mineralization in tumor osteoid is also variable, depending on the rate of tumor growth. Rapidly growing tumors such as osteosarcoma usually produce fluffy cumulus clouds of poorly differentiated tumor bone with ill defined edges and an unstructured appearance (Figs. 3–20 and 3–22). As the tumor breaks through the cortex it will lift off the periosteum, the result of which can be "sunburst" or "hair-on-end" reactive new bone admixed with cumulus cloud fluffs of tumor bone.

Heterotopic bone formation may occur within soft tissue subsequent to trauma, which may have been recognized or unrecognized. Such ossification—called circumscribed myositis ossificans—may resemble mineralized tumor osteoid in radiographs. The favored site is the quadriceps femoris of the thigh; the next most common site is the brachialis of the upper arm. Bilateral symmetric myositis ossificans of the hips and knees may result from spinal cord trauma or from thermal burns. Myositis (fibrodysplasia) ossificans progressiva is a dysplasia of bone and soft tissue featuring congenitally short thumbs, short great toes, and ossification of the soft tissues; this starts to occur in early childhood and frequently affects the nuchal ligament of the neck first.

Although in the early weeks of the ossification process the central core of circumscribed myositis ossificans may be misinterpreted as soft-tissue osteosarcoma, the overall picture is readily distinguishable pathologically and, later on, radiologically. Maturing

FIG. 3–14. Aneurysmal bone cyst of ulna in boy, age 9. The lesion is typically eccentric and has an aneurysmal appearance.

FIG. 3–15. Aneurysmal bone cyst of ilium in boy, age 14. The cortex has gradually undergone a combination of destruction and reformation, with this expanded, shell-like remnant the end result. The very thin smooth expanded shell (*arrows*) are of great aid in ruling out an osteosarcoma or Ewing's tumor. However, metastatic renal cell, thyroid carcinoma, or myeloma can have a similar radiographic appearance. The patient's age strongly favors aneurysmal bone cyst over the other possibilities, which are usually found in advanced adulthood.

FIG. 3–16. Chondromyxoid fibroma characterized by subcortical location in proximal end of tibia, well-defined margin, and irregular cortical displacement. Unlike other cartilaginous tumors, calcification within chondromyxoid fibroma is rare.

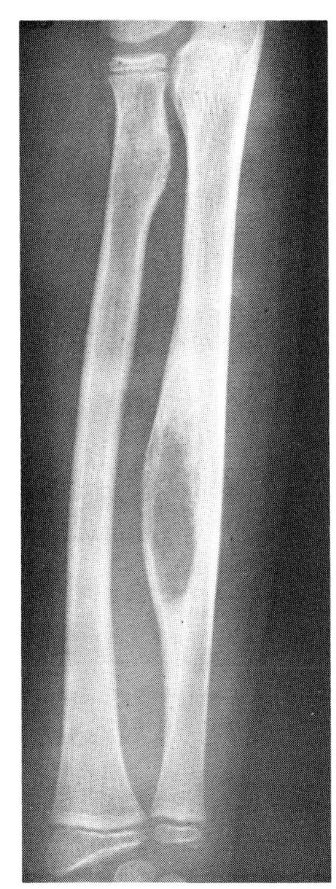

FIG. 3-14

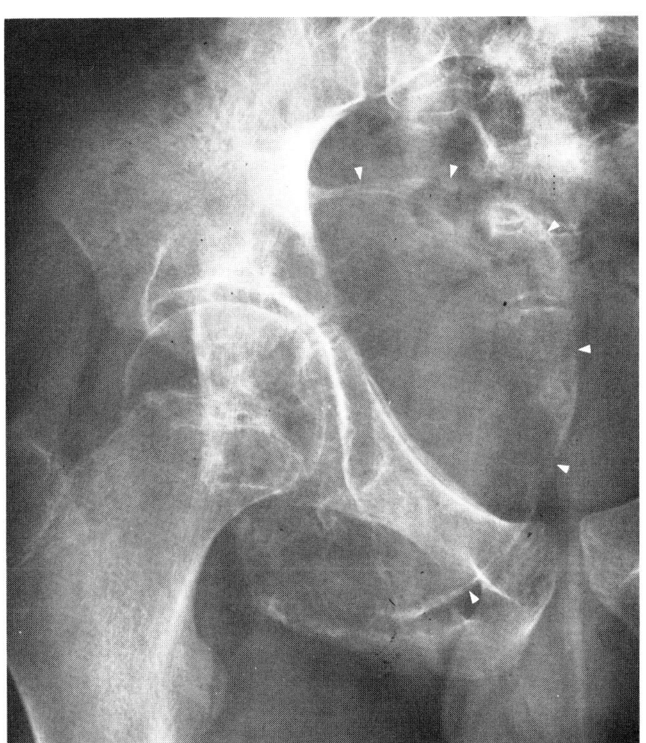

FIG. 3-15

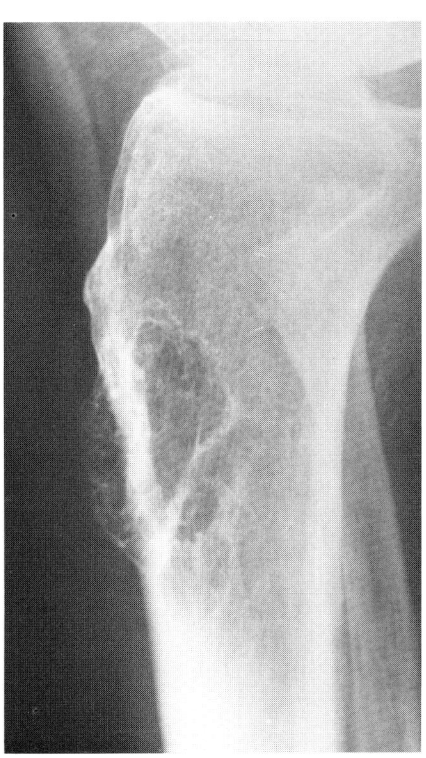

FIG. 3-16

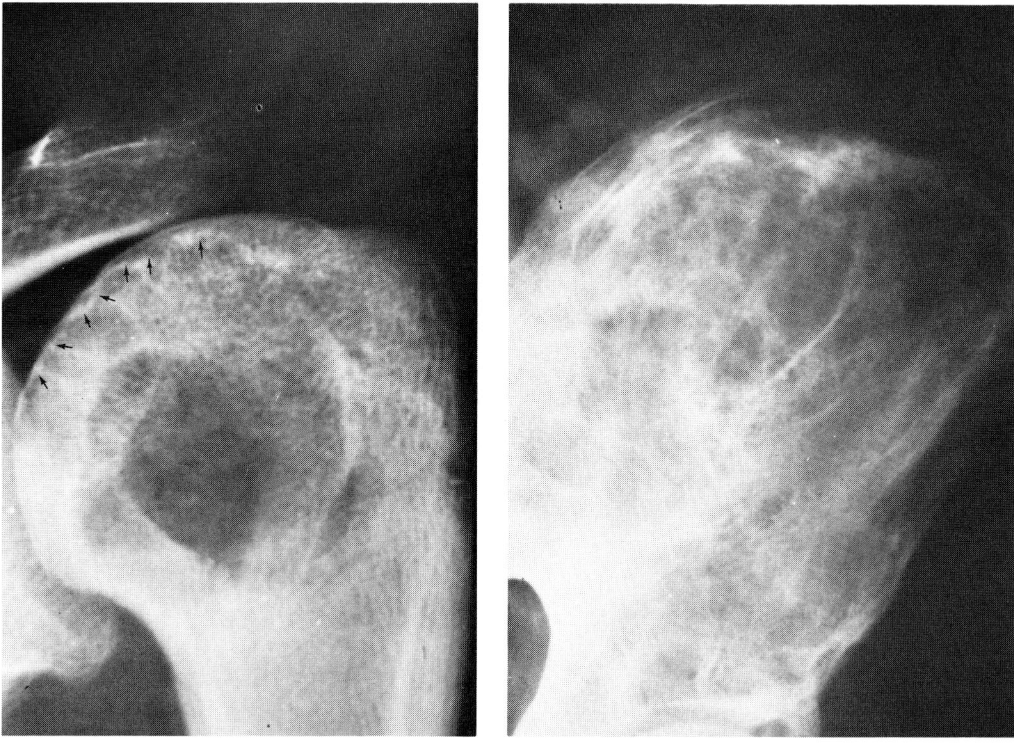

FIG. 3-17 FIG. 3-18

FIG. 3-17. Chondroblastoma of humeral head. This is the only tumor always originating in the unfused epiphysis. The margin is lobulated (*arrows*), as befits its cartilaginous origin. Calcifications, when present, are usually very small and punctate.

FIG. 3-18. Ewing's sarcoma of ilium: Permeative destruction of the ilium of a boy, age 15. The age of this patient with a permeative lesion is a diagnostic clue. Both Ewing's and reticulum cell sarcomas manifest a permeative pattern. In a long bone, Ewing's sarcoma evokes spiculated or lamellated subperiosteal new bone, while reticulum cell sarcoma does not. The periosteum of flat bones, however, does not have a capacity for vigorous production of subperiosteal new bone. The result is a loss of an important distinguishing feature. If we remember that Ewing's sarcoma seldom occurs beyond the second decade, while reticulum cell sarcoma predominates later in life, the age of this patient—15 years—enables us to favor the diagnosis of Ewing's sarcoma.

myositis ossificans exhibits a characteristic "zone" phenomenon—a peripheral zone consisting of a regular arrangement of mature bone, a transitional zone of osteoid tissue, and a central, highly cellular zone containing fibroblasts (preosteoblasts). In soft-tissue osteosarcoma the zone phenomenon is reversed, with new bone production occurring centrally and undifferentiated spindle cells located peripherally.[3] Circumscribed myositis ossificans bone production shows up on radiographs at about three to four weeks from onset of the trauma. By that time the mineralizing part of the lesion has become peripheral, and maturity from poorly differentiated to well-differentiated bone takes place from the periphery inwards (Fig. 3-21).[25] In contrast, the mineralization of osteosarcoma occurs more centrally than peripherally and does not mature from undifferentiated to well-differentiated lamellar bone and marrow fat. In short, the radiographic density of circumscribed myositis ossificans is peripherally oriented, while that of osteosarcoma is centrally oriented.

Periosteal new bone proliferation (post-traumatic periostitis) may accompany myositis ossificans and presumably results from subperiosteal hemorrhage; the new bone rapidly becomes stratified, rather than becoming fluffy or homogeneous, as in osteosarcoma and parosteal osteosarcoma, and eventually becomes smoothly marginated. It stops growing in 9 to 12

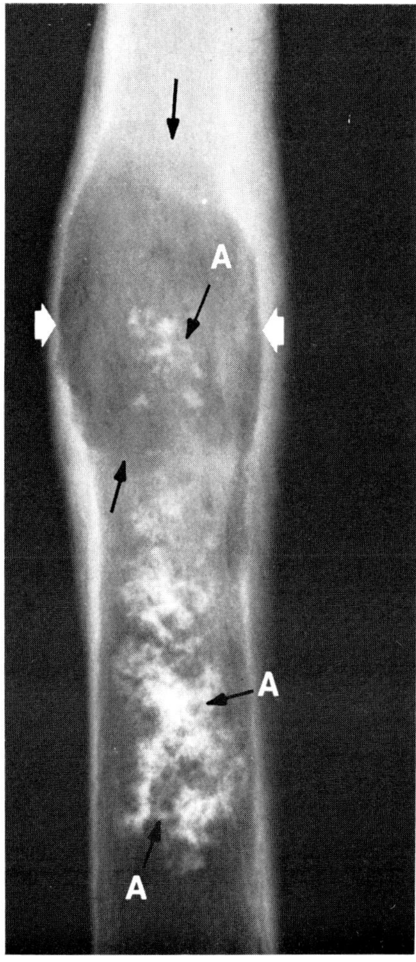

FIG. 3-19. This is one of the most important yet poorly understood radiographic patterns that the radiologist, pathologist, and surgeon must become familiar with. This lesion is one of the most commonly misdiagnosed tumors of bone, because it is not one tumor but at least two. The shaft contains numerous, fairly sharply outlined, flocculent and ringlike mineralization densities, usually always associated with an enchondroma on pathologic examination. Bone infarct is another possibility; however, ringlike or "eggshell" densities (three examples of which are shown in Fig. 3-19, *A*) are not seen in this condition. These "eggshell" densities represent shells of lamellar bone that partially or completely surround or "wall off" islands of radiolucent bland cartilage cores (the enchondroma). Refer to Figures 8-5, 8-6, 8-13, 8-49, and 8-50 for further clarification.

The crucial area is outlined by arrows. This region shows evidence of focal "new growth," which has resulted in and is evidenced by a focal "expansion" of the shaft, cortical ersion, and scalloping, and a large, lytic area signifying malignant transformation to a chondrosarcoma, or even worse, to a chondrosarcoma with fibrosarcomatous transformation. Biopsy must be directed to this region for confirmation of malignancy. Biopsy of the nonexpanded distal shaft ossified and calcified lesion may show only bland enchondromatous tissue with disastrous consequences to the patient, unless the complexities of this radiographic pattern were fully appreciated and biopsy from the area of malignant transformation achieved.

After the initial incomplete diagnosis of enchondroma alone, two circumstances usually occur. The first is massive recurrence within 1 to 5 years, proving the initial diagnosis incomplete or, after thorough curettage of the so-called "enchondroma," the area of malignant change is recognized. However, the wound is usually so contaminated by the extensive curettage for a "benign" tumor that recurrence is to be expected, unless amputation or a massive en-bloc resection, which includes all of the wound tissues, is performed. Another error we have seen on several occasions in regard to this combination of a benign and malignant tumor is to take bone chips from the pelvis in order to pack the curettage cavity without changing instruments, since the surgeon believes he is dealing with a benign tumor. This error will usually lead to an inoperable recurrence in the pelvis, even if the primary tumor could be totally eradicated. It becomes clear, therefore, why recognition of this radiographic pattern is crucial to all concerned.

weeks, as befits its benign origin. After reaching maturity, large masses of myositis ossificans tend to shrink and small ones may disappear completely.

Tumor Size and Potential for Metastasis

In general, the larger a bone tumor, the greater the likelihood that it is malignant. But, assuming a direct relationship between the size of a tumor and its potential for metastasis, while seemingly logical, may at times be erroneous. That tumor size and aggressiveness need not necessarily be interdependent is illustrated by the case of the 13-year-old girl, who complained of intermittent sharp pain in the left thigh for 3 months.[9] Radiographs of the left femur revealed a flocculent, calcific density in the diaphysis of the bone at the junction of the middle and distal thirds (Fig. 3-22). Cortical destruction and subperiosteal new bone proliferation were absent. Tomography confirmed the absence of a fracture line and the lack of cortical destruction. An excision biopsy of the lesion led to a pathologic diagnosis of an osteosarcoma that measured only 2.0 cm. in its greatest dimension. Full-chest tomography immediately following biopsy revealed several small pulmonary metastases that were not visible in the standard preoperative chest radiographs. Death occurred two months after the femoral biopsy.

The classic radiographic features of a primary malignant bone tumor (cortical destruction with extracortical tumor extension, interrupted, lamellated, or finely spiculated subperiosteal new bone) usually become manifest only when the tumor is, locally, far advanced. In a child, therefore, osteosarcoma must be considered whenever fluffy intramedullary densities merge radiographically to form a cumulus-cloud shadow, no matter how small, and even in the absence of other radiographic features of malignancy.

Significance of Soft-Tissue Edema

Situations arise in which it is difficult to decide radiographically and clinically whether a destructive process of bone is inflammatory or neoplastic. In these situations, the *absence* of soft-tissue edema is a valuable clue that the process is not an inflammatory one (Fig. 3-23). Absence of edema is reflected radiographically by a sharp interface between muscle and subcutaneous fat and by well-defined, sharply outlined, fatty septa surrounding the muscle bundles overlying a bone tumor, even though the muscle itself is displaced by the tumor. It should be remembered, however, that some Ewing's sarcomas evoke an inflammatory response with associated soft-tissue edema. Moreover, a massive malignant tumor may, by its pressure, obstruct overlying veins, resulting in edema secondary to venous stasis superimposed upon hypervascularity to the tumor. Thus, the presence of edema is not as specific as its absence in distinguish-

---

FIG. 3-20. Osteosarcoma of femur producing characteristic ill-defined cumulus clouds of tumor bone extending beyond cortex. A Codman's triangle is visible (*arrow*). This triangle and the "sunburst" seen on this radiograph prove, histologically, to be consequent to reactive periosteal new bone stimulated by rapid lift off by the tumor. The cumulus cloud fluffs (*A*) however, represent malignant tumor bone.

FIG. 3-21. Circumscribed myositis ossificans in boy, age 12. He developed painful swelling of the forearm followed by restriction of pronation and supination. One year later a 3-cm. hard, fixed mass between the radius and ulna became evident. It has the radiographic appearance of mature lamellar bone. As characteristic of myositis ossificans, the periphery is the densest and most mature part of the lesion. In contradistinction, mineralization of osteosarcoma is greatest centrally. The very smooth border of this lesion strongly mitigates against soft-tissue osteosarcoma. On rare occasion, however a parosteal osteosarcoma can have round, smooth borders (see Figs. 8-41 and 8-42).

FIG. 3-22. Lethal, 2-cm. osteosarcoma of midfemur in girl, age 13, lateral and anteroposterior views. Although pulmonary metastasis has already occurred, neither cortical destruction nor subperiosteal new bone are present. In a child, osteosarcoma must be considered a prime diagnostic possibility whenever an intramedullary cumulus cloudlike shadow, no matter how small, is present radiographically, even in the absence of classic radiographic criteria of malignancy. This radiographic pattern can also be seen in bone infarct, stress fracture without the usual reactive periosteal callus, or possibly even enchondroma. Great care must be taken in histological assessment (see Figs. 7-43—7-46) to rule out stress fracture, if a biopsy is taken. Osteosarcomas detected at this small size are extremely rare.

FIG. 3-23. Osteosarcoma of femur characterized by subtle cortical destruction (*arrow*), and striking increase in radiographic density resulting from intraosseous deposition of tumor bone. Sharply outlined fatty septa (*arrowheads*) imply that the pathologic process is *not* inflammatory. Another sign of absence of inflammation is a sharp interface between muscle and subcutaneous fat, which is apparent on the original radiograph.

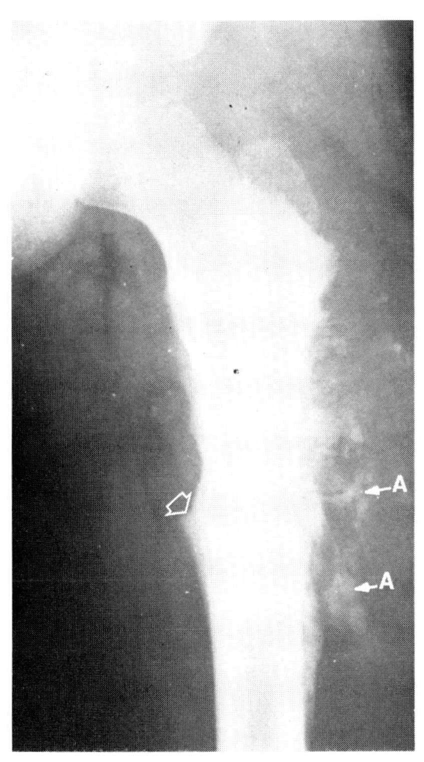

FIG. 3-20

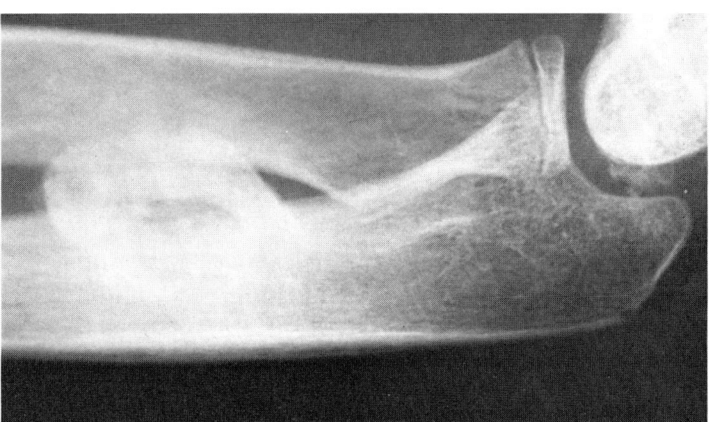

FIG. 3-21

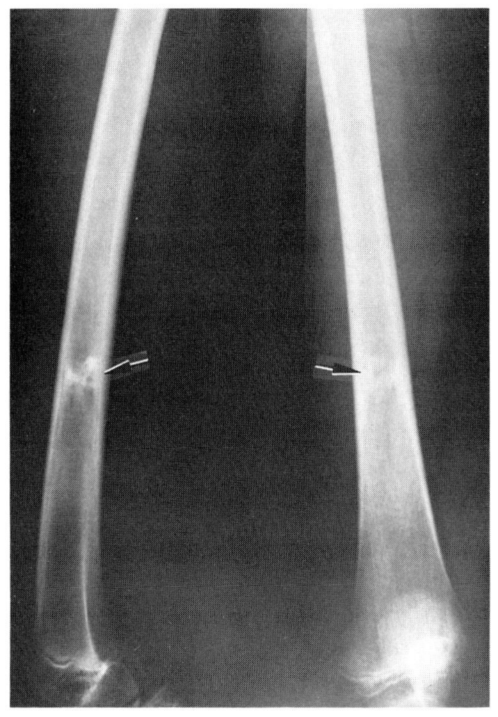

FIG. 3-22

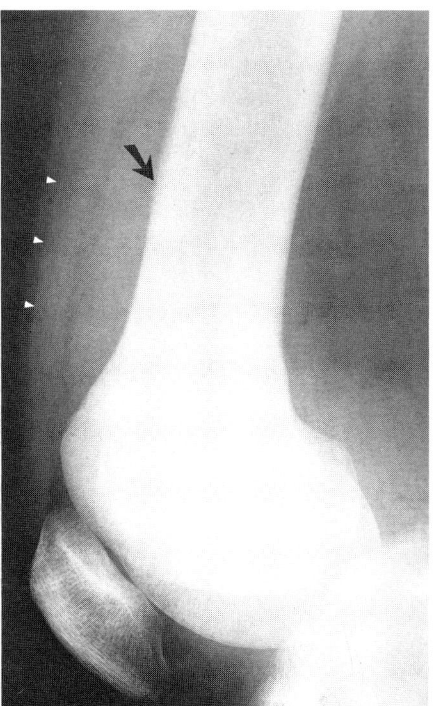

FIG. 3-23

ing between inflammation and tumor. Hyperemia accompanies both inflammatory and malignant neoplastic diseases of bone and results in the enlargement of overlying superficial veins. Since the veins are outlined by a contrasting background of subcutaneous fat, their enlargement may be perceived radiographically.

SIGNIFICANCE OF SUBPERIOSTEAL NEW BONE

Recognition of the benign or malignant origin of subperiosteal new bone is essential in distinguishing a benign lesion from a malignant one.[8] The healthy periosteum, when activated by relatively benign stimuli, produces solid new bone of smooth outline and, when fully developed, of uniform density. These benign stimuli include hyperemia secondary to overlying soft-tissue inflammation, edema caused by venous stasis, subperiosteal hemorrhage, osteomyelitis, eosinophilic granuloma (Fig. 3–2), benign fracture, hypertrophic pulmonary osteoarthropathy (which, however, may be associated with pulmonary or pleural neoplasms), osteoid osteoma, and lipid storage disorders such as Gaucher's disease. The resultant newly formed benign subperiosteal new bone is separated from the underlying cortex by a thin, radiolucent zone. The new bone may be thick or thin and of smooth or irregular contour, depending upon the duration of the process and the intensity and unevenness of the underlying stimulus, but it is always solid and uniform in character. In contrast, subperiosteal new bone that is stimulated by underlying malignant neoplasm is rarely even, uniform, and solid in appearance. It appears delicate and interrupted, typically longitudinally lamellated or perpendicularly spiculated. It should be understood, however, that while these are classic periosteal manifestations of malignancy—particularly osteosarcoma and Ewing's sarcoma—they may occasionally accompany an active, rapidly progressive benign process, such as osteomyelitis or repeated subperiosteal hemorrhage. In the benign processes, however, the spicules of new bone are usually more coarse and the lamellations fewer and thicker than those associated with malignancy.

The characteristic lamellations of subperiosteal new bone in response to Ewing's sarcoma (Fig. 3–24) may disappear centrally where ultrarapid tumor growth destroys the new bone and hinders its further elaboration. The multiplicity of the lamellations probably reflects alternating periods of rapid and slow tumor growth. During a period of slow growth, the periosteum is displaced less rapidly and thus has time to form a layer of new bone, but during rapid growth the periosteum cannot produce an effective encapsulating shell. Instead the tumor penetrates the thin layers of subperiosteal new bone already formed, displacing the periosteum even further peripherally. Unlike the delicate, thin strips of lamellated new bone laid down in response to Ewing's sarcoma, an aggressive benign process such as osteomyelitis tends to manifest thicker layers that may coalesce at various sites along the shaft.

The perpendicular spicules of new bone that may be elaborated by the periosteum in response to Ewing's sarcoma (Fig. 3–7) and osteosarcoma grow along tiny vascular channels between the periosteum and cortex. This type of reaction signifies extremely rapid growth. A shell of new bone appearing at the periphery of the perpendicular spicules implies that the underlying process was once aggressive and rapidly growing but has since become quiescent (Fig. 3–25). Such a response may result from radiation therapy.

A *Codman's triangle* of new bone is an isolated cuff of subperiosteal new bone that may form at the boundary of any mass, benign or malignant, that is rapidly elevating the periosteum. The triangle is found most frequently in association with malignant neoplasm of bone (Figs. 3–20 and 3–24), but it sometimes arises in response to rapid displacement of the periosteum by exudate or blood. The triangle may also result from a rapidly growing aneurysmal bone cyst, osteomyelitis, or trauma (Fig. 3–26).

SPECIFIC RADIOGRAPHIC FEATURES OF MALIGNANT TUMORS OF BONE

MULTIPLE MYELOMA (PLASMA CELL MYELOMA). This tumor of hematopoietic origin is the most common primary malignant tumor of bone. The classic radiographic description of myeloma is that it appears as multitudinous "punched out" holes accompanied by cortical destruction and little or no periosteal reaction. It predominates in those bones in which the red marrow normally persists throughout adulthood (e.g., vertebrae, ribs, skull vault [except for the basiocciput], and pelvis). An equally frequent but less well-appreciated radiographic presentation is a generalized loss of bone density (simulating osteoporosis), with resultant collapse of multiple vertebrae and pathologic fractures of ribs, in the absence of visible, discreet foci of destruction. Occasionally, an expansile focus of myeloma may balloon a segment of

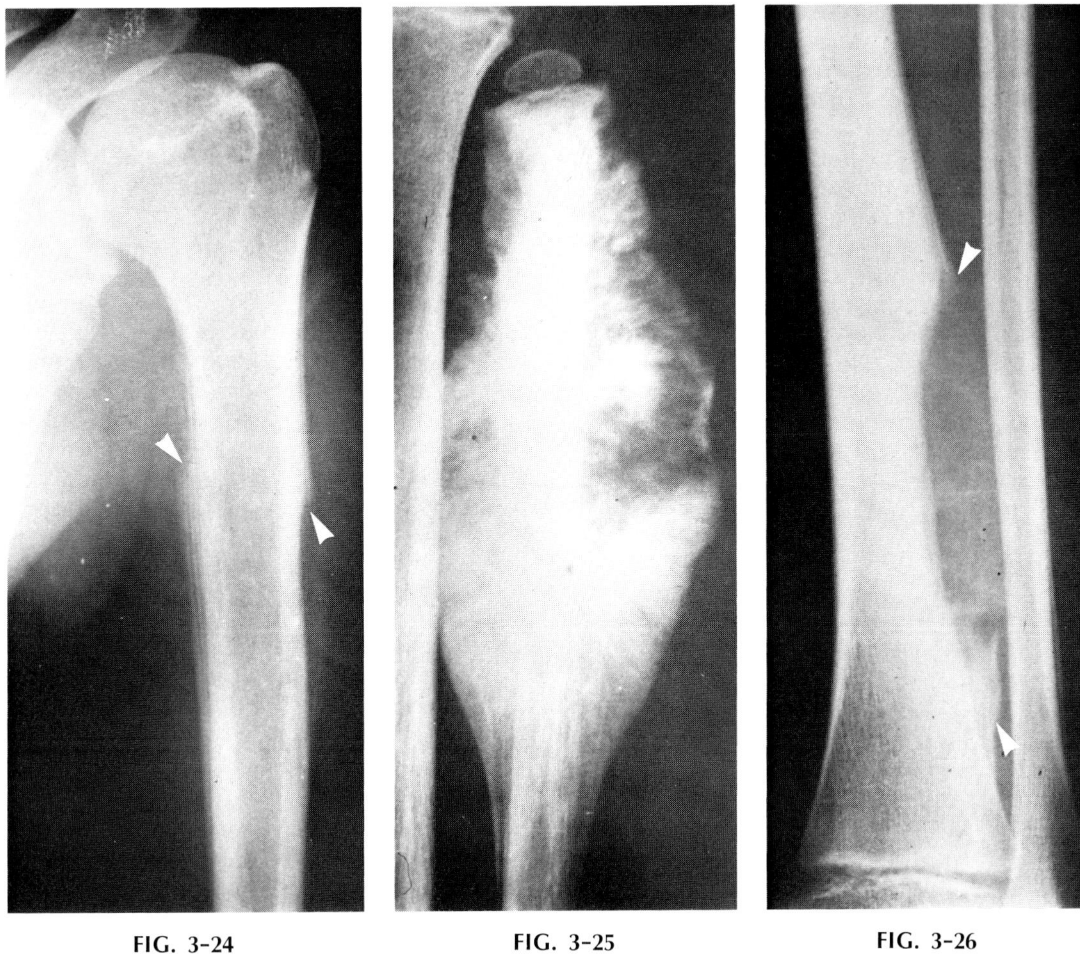

FIG. 3-24 FIG. 3-25 FIG. 3-26

FIG. 3-24. Ewing's sarcoma of humerus. Several layers of subperiosteal new bone disappear in regions where extreme rapidity of tumor growth has destroyed them and hindered their further production. The margins of these ultra-aggressive foci of tumor are marked by subperiosteal Codman's triangles of new bone (*arrows*).

FIG. 3-25. Ewing's sarcoma of fibula following radiation therapy. The peripendicular spicules of subperiosteal new bone have matured, resulting in loss of their delicate character. A shell of new bone has formed at the periphery of the spicules, implying that the process that was formerly aggressive has become quiescent.

FIG. 3-26. Rapidly growing aneurysmal bone cyst. Multiple layers of subperiosteal new bone and Codman's triangles (*arrows*), while most frequently associated with malignancy, may accompany subperiosteal hemorrhage or exudate or, as in this case, a rapidly growing ABC. It is extremely important to realize that incipient, rapidly growing ABC may mimic sarcoma, particularly the lytic osteosarcoma. Great care must be given to the histology of all so-called "lytic osteosarcomas" to rule out exuberant fibro-osteoblastic repair tissue in an ABC (see Fig. 13-50). This is one of the more common errors in bone tumor diagnosis, that is, confusing an ABC for an osteosarcoma. If a thin rim of sclerotic bone is seen peripherally (Fig. 3-15), it almost surely is not an osteosarcoma.

affected bone, frequently a rib. Breaching of the cortex with extraosseous extension of tumor is also a common occurrence.

Myeloma is usually multicentric but may occasionally begin as a solitary destructive focus—so-called solitary plasmacytoma—which eventually disseminates throughout the skeleton. Multiple myeloma is rare before the fifth decade of life; therefore, age is a clue to its diagnosis. Almost all reported cases are entirely osteolytic, but rarely a sclerotic response may occur in association with secondary amyloid deposition within the myeloma lesions. Multiple myeloma may go undetected in radionuclide bone scans because of a lack of affinity of the radionuclide for the myelomatous bone. (Diffuse metastatic disease to bone may also go undetected in bone scans because of the so-called "superscan" effect—diffuse uptake of the radionuclide is so extensive that it prevents appreciation of focal or discrete lesions. In that situation, radionuclide excretion by the kidneys is strikingly diminished because the radionuclide is taken up almost entirely by osseous tissue.) The chief problem in radiologic differential diagnosis lies in distinguishing multiple myeloma from metastatic tumor. Discrete foci of destruction resulting from multiple myeloma are usually very numerous, especially in the skull vault, and, because they are multicentric in origin, they tend to be of similar size, while metastatic lesions tend to be fewer in number and of varying size. Moreover, diffuse metastatic skeletal disease tends to destroy the vertebral pedicles, while multiple myeloma, even when extensive, tends to spare them.

EWING'S SARCOMA (FIGS. 3-7, 3-18, 3-24, AND 3-25). This extremely aggressive and infiltrative tumor is aptly reflected radiographically by a permeative pattern of destruction extending throughout much or all of an affected bone. In long bones, the center of the tumor is usually in the diaphysis. Interrupted, delicately lamellated, or spiculated subperiosteal new bone is frequently an accompanying feature. The peak age incidence is 15 years.

CENTRAL OSTEOSARCOMA (FIGS. 3-20, 3-22, AND 3-23). This tumor manifests the most characteristic radiologic feature of all primary bone tumors—confluent cumulus clouds of mineralized tumor osteoid, sunburst, spiculated, and Codman's triangle periosteal reactions, and unusually, "onion skinning." Striking aggressiveness is implied in radiographs by its permeative destructive pattern, but this pattern is frequently masked by mineralized tumor osteoid. In long bones, the center of the lesion is usually in the metaphysis, but diaphyseal lesions are sometimes encountered. Tumor centered in the epiphysis is rare (1%). Osteosarcoma is the second most common primary malignant tumor of bone; only multiple myeloma occurs more frequently. As with Ewing's sarcoma, the peak age incidence is 15 years. Osteosarcoma may arise occasionally in elderly patients, usually within a focus of Paget's disease of bone. But, the increase in bone density and distortion of bone architecture that results from Paget's disease may make it difficult to recognize, radiologically, the accompanying osteosarcoma. Radionuclide bone scans may reveal extraskeletal metastases of osteosarcoma (including the lungs).

PAROSTEAL OSTEOSARCOMA. This tumor has a peak incidence in the third and fourth decades and presents as a homogeneous, dense lesion arising predominantly in the distal femoral or proximal tibial metaphysis. Classically, a radiolucent zone is present between the tumor and the host bone. This sign may also be seen in traumatic periostitis, however. This zone reflects a space between the tumor mass that overgrows its pedicle and the normal cortex against which it rests. The medullary cavity may be invaded.[7]

PERIOSTEAL OSTEOSARCOMA. This has its peak age incidence falling between those of the central and parosteal types. It is a purely cortical lesion with thickened but intact cortex and without tendencies toward medullary invasion or overgrowth of its base of origin. The matrix is less homogeneous, in comparison to that of parosteal osteosarcoma, and spicules of tumor bone radiate peripherally from the cortex. See pages 538–548 for further discussion.[30]

GIANT CELL TUMOR (FIGS. 3-5, AND 3-8). This tumor arises near the end of a bone, usually at the knee, and predominates in the third decade of life. It is not possible by radiologic analysis to determine which tumors will behave more aggressively. The lesion is always lytic and centered in the epiphysis or metaphysis, but only very rarely in the diaphysis. It almost always extends to the articular cartilage. It does not contain calcifications and is rarely associated with a border of sclerosis. Most lesions appear as a single confluent defect, others have a "bubbly septate," or pseudomultiloculated appearance. These patterns are actually due to variable erosion of the cortex and not to true bony separations within the tumor itself.[12]

FIBROSARCOMA OF BONE. This relatively rare tumor, predominating in patients over the age of 40, usually arises in the shaft or metaphysis of a long bone and results in a geographic or moth-eaten pattern of destruction. Fibrosarcoma may provoke a septated or amorphous shell of subperiosteal new bone, but does not provoke perpendicularly spiculated new bone. Occasionally a fibrosarcoma may burst through the cortex, elevating the periosteum, and envelop a small piece of cortical bone, which then takes on the radiographic appearance of a sequestrum.

CHONDROSARCOMA (FIG. 3-19). This tumor is usually found in patients over the age of 35. It takes two classic radiographic forms: it may appear as a slowly growing central tumor with a geographic destructive pattern expanding a segment of the metaphysis and the adjacent shaft of a long bone;[28] or as a large, eccentric tumor occurring predominantly at the surface of flat bones such as ribs, pelvis, and scapulae and only minimally involving the underlying bone. Both forms of chondrosarcoma frequently manifest typical cartilage matrix calcification, but the absence of this calcification does not exclude the diagnosis. Chondrosarcomas tend to remain relatively circumscribed, unlike Ewing's sarcoma, reticulum-cell sarcoma, and osteosarcoma, which usually infiltrate extensively through the length of the affected bone (whether evident on radiographs or not). Unlike enchondroma, whose multitudinous lobules of cartilage are surrounded by platelike sheaths of lamellar bone that appear radiographically as rings or spheres and whose mineralized matrix is characterized by 1- to 3-mm. punctate calcifications (Fig. 3-10), chondrosarcoma tends to be associated with focal increased radiolucency, extensive cortical scalloping and/or displacement outward, periosteal reaction, soft-tissue mass, or denser, more dispersed and more randomly oriented calcifications with a typical "windblown" appearance. Because cartilage tends to assume a lobular configuration, the border between tumor and host bone may also appear lobulated. Enchondroma is the most common benign tumor of the short tubular bones of hands and feet. The solitary enchondroma of the long and flat bones is a rarely discovered entity. It is usually discovered as an incidental finding on a radiograph taken for some other reason, or after chondrosarcomatous transformation has occurred. Chondrosarcoma, on the other hand, is rare in the short tubular bones, occurring predominantly in the axial skeleton and proximal ends of the femora and humeri. A benign cartilage tumor within the axial skeleton, especially the ribs, pelvis, scapulae, or within the proximal ends of the femora or humeri, is far more likely to undergo transformation into chondrosarcoma or fibrosarcoma than is a benign cartilage tumor located within the more peripheral parts of the skeleton. The onset of pain, an enlarging mass, or a change in radiographic pattern of matrix calcification may signify sarcomatous degeneration within a cartilage tumor that was once benign.

The incidence of chondrosarcoma arising in patients with multiple hereditary cartilage-capped exostoses or multiple enchondromatosis (Ollier's disease) is difficult to ascertain but may be quite high (from 10 to 50%).

PRIMARY RETICULUM CELL SARCOMA OF BONE (FIG. 3-6). This is a rapidly infiltrating tumor occurring predominantly in the long bones of persons age 40 and older. As befits its aggressiveness, the pattern of destruction is permeative and a long segment of bone is usually involved. The periosteal response is typically scant, amorphous, and not spiculated or lamellated. Codman's triangles do not usually occur. When a tumor of bone with pathologic characteristics of reticulum cell sarcoma is discovered concurrently with a known lymph node focus of reticulum cell sarcoma (histiocytic lymphoma), it is usually classified as a *metastasis* from the nodal component. If, on the other hand, a reticulum cell sarcoma of bone occurs in the absence of a nodal focus of tumor elsewhere, it is usually classified as a *primary* tumor of bone. Lymphography, therefore, may play a vital role in classifying reticulum-cell sarcoma that presents in bone. (Lymphography is the radiographic demonstration of the lymphatic system by intralymphatic injection of a radiopaque agent. Applied to the patient with malignant neoplastic disease, lymphography is an aid for staging its extent, a graphic method to observe its progression or regression, and a guide to lymph-node dissection and to accurate placement of fields to be irradiated.) Primary reticulum cell sarcoma of bone is radiosensitive, and long-term survival is not unusual in the localized form of the disease.

SPECIALIZED DIAGNOSTIC TECHNIQUES IN THE EVALUATION OF BONE TUMORS

ARTERIOGRAPHY. Arteriography is gradually being supplanted by computed tomography. Nonetheless, computed tomography is not available universally, and while it is an aid in determining the limits of intraosseous and extraosseous tumor extension, it cannot replace arteriography in accurately mapping the arterial blood supply of a tumor before perfusion chemotherapy.

Selective arteriography cannot replace biopsy, but it is simple to perform, relatively innocuous to the patient, and may serve as a guide to the management of bone tumors.[13,16,31,33,34,37,38] Since most primary malignant bone tumors manifest arteriographic evidence of malignancy, arteriography may complement pathologic studies in differentiating malignant tumors from benign ones. For example, arteriography may

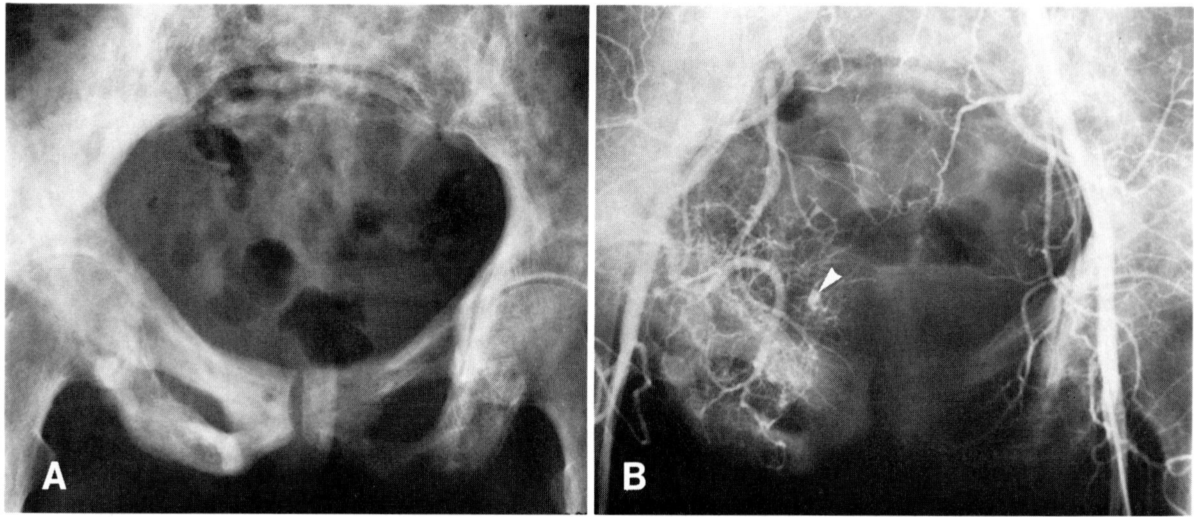

FIG. 3-27. Osteosarcoma arising in focus of Paget's disease. This woman, age 57, complained of pain and swelling in the right suprapubic region. (*A*) Standard radiograph reveals proliferative Paget's disease throughout the pelvis, but no evidence of bone destruction by tumor. (*B*) Aorta-iliac arteriogram discloses a large, vascular tumor arising from the right pubic bone. Numerous, irregularly outlined pelvic vessels that fail to diminish in caliber and that pursue bizarre pathways and a "tumor lake" (*arrow*) signify malignancy.

disclose the onset of malignancy within a long-standing benign cartilaginous tumor or within a focus of Paget's disease (Fig. 3-27) or fibrous dysplasia. Since the area of greatest vascularity often represents the most malignant part of the tumor, arteriography is sometimes helpful in choosing a biopsy site. Arteriography aids in defining the limits of intraosseous and extraosseous tumor extension, limits which are frequently more extensive than those inferred from study of the standard radiographs. Thus, arteriography aids in the planning of surgical or radiotherapeutic treatment, and may also permit accurate mapping of the arterial blood supply of a tumor prior to perfusion chemotherapy.

Disadvantages of arteriography must also be stressed: a normal arteriogram does not exclude malignancy, since some indolent chondrosarcomas, fibrosarcomas and reticulum cell sarcomas may be deceptively innocent in their arteriographic appearance (Fig. 3-28).[33] Neither does arteriography permit differentiation between histologic types of primary malignant tumor, nor between primary and metastatic tumor. Giant cell tumors show great variation in their arteriographic appearance; some rapidly growing tumors are avascular while others that subsequently pursue a benign course show striking hypervascularity, resembling malignancy.[13,16,33] Lastly, serial arteriographic changes do *not* provide a de-

FIG. 3-28. Avascular chondrosarcoma of humerus. The tumor arose in a solitary osteochondroma. (*A*) Standard radiograph reveals tumor matrix mineralized in a punctate and flocculent manner not uncommon in osteochondroma. The main clue to malignant transformation is the presence of ill defined, poorly calcified soft-tissue mass (*arrows*). (*B*) Subtraction image of percutaneous arteriogram. The brachial artery is displaced by the tumor. Although malignant, the tumor is deceptively avascular. (The opacified vessels are clearly seen because the bone and matrix mineralization has been "subtracted" photographically. Subtraction was accomplished by superimposition of the positive arteriographic image (in which bone, matrix mineralization, and opacified vessels appear black) upon a standard negative radiograph exposed immediately prior to the arteriographic injection.

FIG. 3-29. Central osteosarcoma. Comparison of standard film radiograph (*A*), corresponding xeroradiograph (*B*), and xeroarteriogram (*C*). The xeroradiographs provide enhanced detail of bone destruction, tumor matrix mineralization, periosteal reaction, and overlying soft-tissue changes. In the xeroarteriogram, edge enhancement of the borders of small vessels results in exquisite vascular detail.

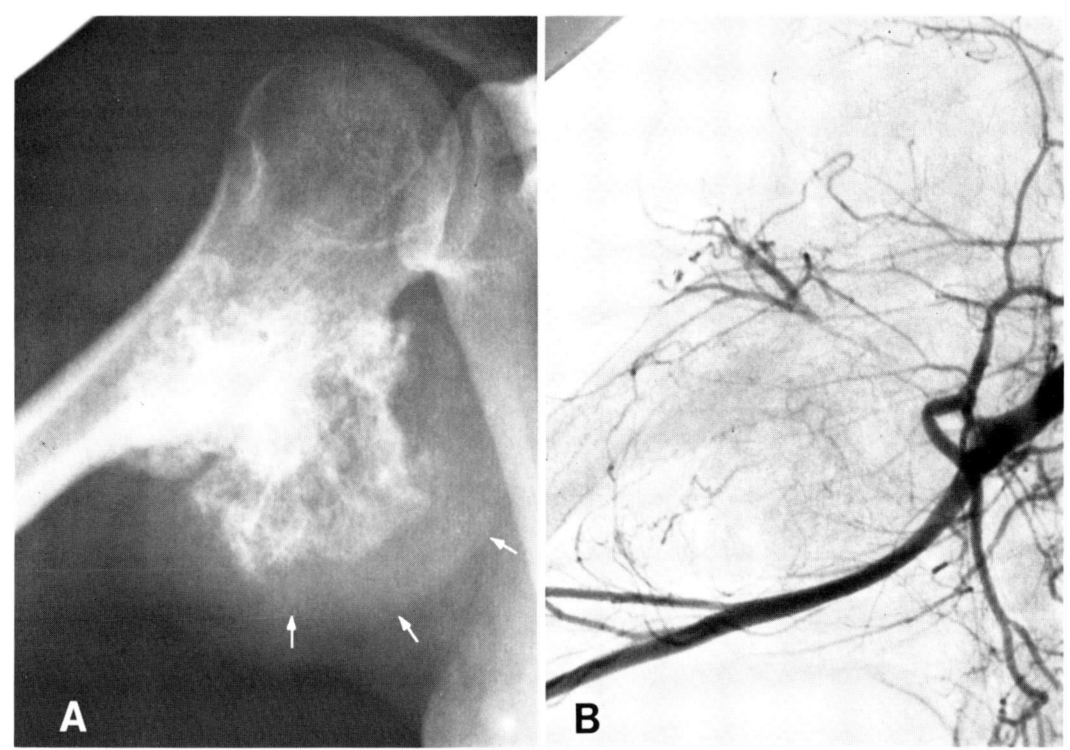

FIG. 3-28

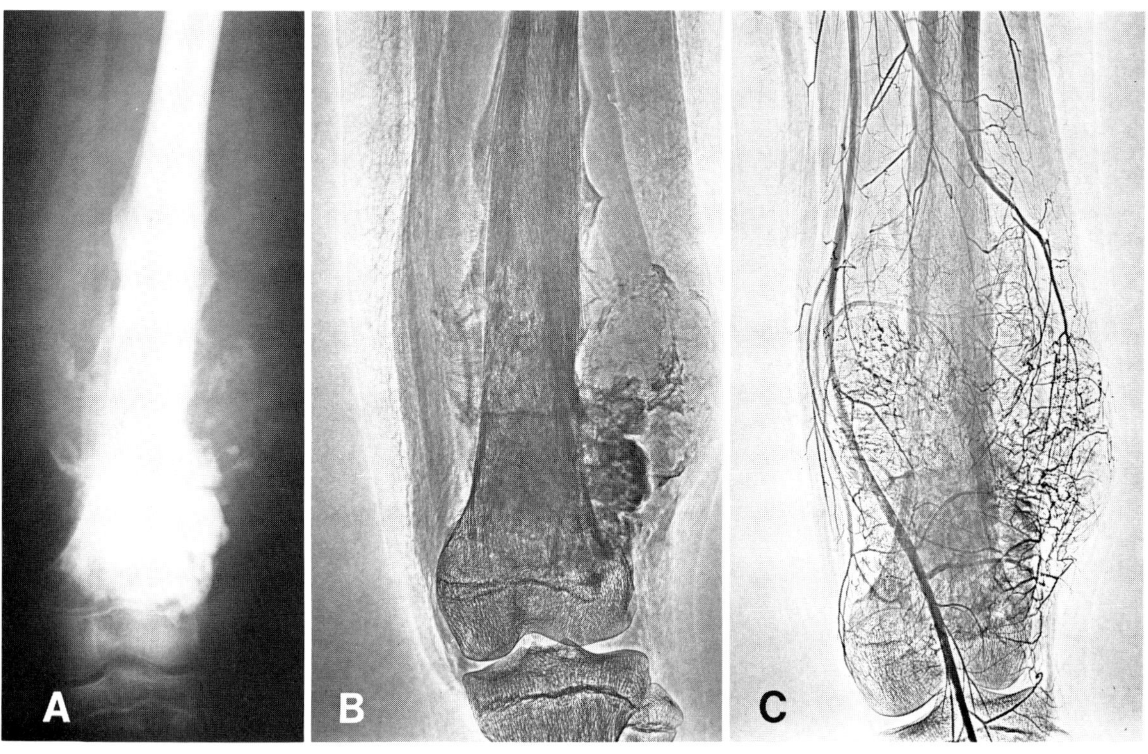

FIG. 3-29

pendable guide to the response of a tumor to radiotherapy.[33]

The most characteristic arteriographic sign of malignancy is the presence of tumor neovascularity.[33] These "tumor vessels" pursue a bizarre, irregular path and because they are in part lined by tumor cells, are ragged in outline and fail to diminish progressively in calibre (in contradistinction to normal or inflammatory vessels). They often terminate in small, scattered "tumor lakes" in which the radiopaque medium pools for a considerable time because the walls of the lakes are inelastic. Arteriovenous shunting is another frequently occurring manifestation of malignancy, but one that may sometimes occur also in benign inflammatory processes such as chronic periostitis and chronic synovitis, including pigmented villonodular synovitis.[17,31] Other arteriographic signs characteristic but not diagnostic of malignancy include: abrupt termination of an otherwise normal artery (possibly a result of local thrombosis or infarction within the tumor), straight veins coursing at right angles to the normal flow of venous return, and a myriad of small vessels encircling the periphery of an area of relative avascularity. The avascular area may be presumed to represent a mass of necrotic tumor, although an abscess or an aneurysmal bone cyst could have a similar appearance. Diffuse staining of tumor by radiopaque medium, while frequently associated with a malignancy, is not diagnostic. It occasionally is encountered in benign diseases, such as benign giant-cell tumors, some aneurysmal bone cysts, chronic periostitis, and chronic synovitis, including pigmented villonodular synovitis.[16,17,31,33]

XERORADIOGRAPHY. In the early 1940s, a photographic process based upon photoelectric rather than photochemical principles was developed. Because the process was a dry one, it was called xerography. In the radiographic counterpart of the process—xeroradiography—the electrostatic image of an object that is interposed in an x-ray beam is recorded upon a thin plate coated with a photoconductor, selenium. The electrostatic image is made visible by applying oppositely charged, blue powder granules to the exposed plate. The blue image is then transferred to paper, thereby becoming a finished xeroradiograph. Xeroradiography is in many ways superior to standard film radiography for evaluating bone tumors (Fig. 3–29, *A* and *B*).[6,35,36] It provides enhanced detail of bone destruction, tumor matrix mineralization, periosteal reaction, and associated soft-tissue changes. Xeroradiographic imaging of arteriograms (Fig. 3–29, *C*) results in edge enhancement of small blood vessels filled with radiopaque medium and reveals them in exquisite detail, far exceeding that recorded in standard film arteriograms and perhaps equal to the detail recorded using special radiographic magnification techniques. Because the xeroradiographic plate is less sensitive than a film-screen combination, the xeroradiographic study must be confined to a relatively thin anatomic part, such as a limb. However, when utilized for evaluation of bone tumor lesions in the limbs, xeroarteriography may complement the routine rapid-sequence film arteriographic examination.[15,27]

COMPUTED TOMOGRAPHY ("CAT SCANNING"). Computed tomography (also known as computerized axial tomography, CAT scanning, computer-assisted tomography, and reconstructed tomography) is a noninvasive process that combines acquisition of information from many different views within a single cross-sectional plane with computation of these data to present a recognizable image. A narrow x-ray beam rotates about that part of the body being examined. The x-rays are either absorbed or unaffected as they pass through a cross-section of various tissues, and the resultant variations are recorded on sensitive detectors moving in parallel and rotating with the x-ray tube. The recorded information is converted to digital form, stored in a computer, and the thousands of data bits reconstructed into an image. The brightness of each portion of the cross-section of any anatomical part in the final image is proportional to the degree to which it absorbs x-rays. Conventional x-ray techniques can reliably detect differences in density of only 5 to 10 per cent, so they can only be used to distinguish tissues of water density from fat and air (more radiolucent) or from calcium and heavy metals (more radiodense). Computed tomography, in contradistinction, may detect density differences as small as 0.5 per cent, resolving anatomic detail heretofore unobtainable with conventional techniques.[1,2] In many selected applications, the intravenous adminis-

FIG. 3-30. Parosteal osteosarcoma originating in sacro-iliac region. (*A*) Standard radiograph shows large mass of mineralized tumor matrix superimposed upon and superior to the left sacro-iliac region. (*B*) Computed tomography discloses huge soft-tissue mass (*white arrows*) and mass of mineralized tumor matrix (*open arrow*) posterior to the fifth lumbar vertebra. The extraosseous extent of the tumor is easily discerned in the CAT scan but is impossible to assess from the standard radiograph.

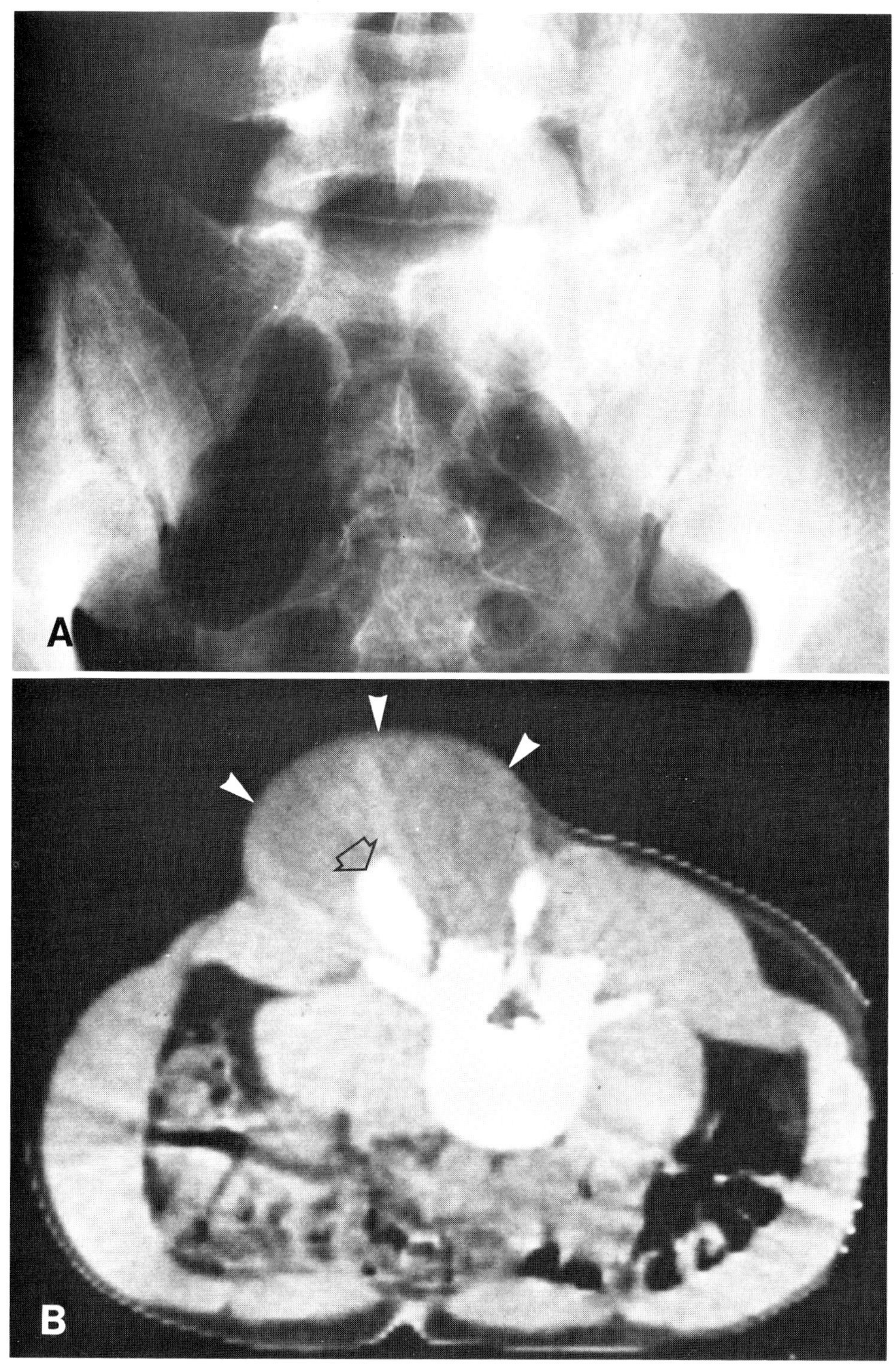

FIG. 3-30

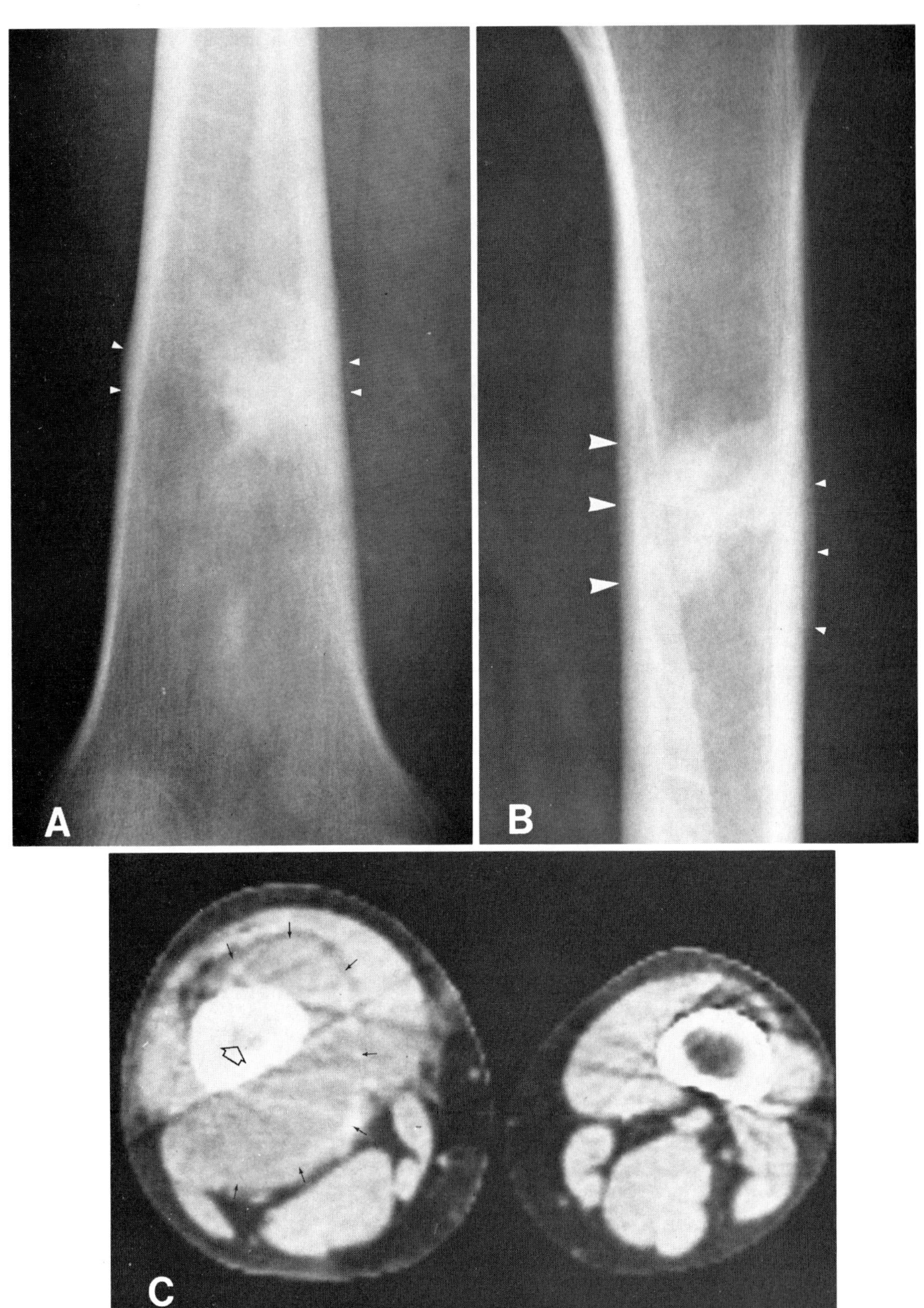

FIG. 3-31

tration of radiopaque contrast agent increases the quantity of information available.

In evaluating skeletal tumors, computed tomography has been effective in determining the extent of disease both in the intra- and extraosseous parts of tumor.[4,29] The extraosseous component of a tumor is far better demonstrated by computed tomography than by conventional radiography. This is because computed tomography can differentiate tissues of only minimally altered density; it is thus very useful in staging, preoperative planning and evaluating whether radiation therapy is needed. Pretreatment assessment is especially useful in areas of complex anatomy such as the pelvis (Fig. 3-30). Thus, computed tomography offers a noninvasive alternative to arteriography in demonstrating the extraosseous extent of disease and is frequently more accurate than arteriography because both vascular and avascular tumors can be readily distinguished from adjacent muscles. Computed tomography is also useful in demonstrating "skip" metastases of osteosarcoma because small foci of intramedullary tumor are of different density than marrow fat. Computed tomography may define intramedullary extension of central as well as cortical osteosarcomas, thereby aiding in the determination of their central, periosteal or parosteal nature (Fig. 3-31). Computed tomography plays no role in the demonstration of zone of transition, which is best reproduced with standard radiography, standard tomography, and xeroradiography.

REFERENCES

1. Abrams, H.L., and McNeil, B.J.: Medical implications of computed tomography ("CAT scanning"). New Engl. J. Med., *298:*255–261, 1978.
2. Abrams, H.L., and McNeil, B.J.: Medical implications of computed tomography ("CAT scanning"). New Engl. J. Med., *298:*310–318, 1978.
3. Ackerman, L.V.: Extraosseous localized non-neoplastic bone and cartilage formation (so-called myositis ossificans). J. Bone Joint Surg., *40-A:*279–298, 1958.
4. Berger, P.E., and Kuhn, J.P.: Computed tomography of tumors of the musculoskeletal system in children. Clinical applications. Radiology, *127:*171–175, 1978.
5. Bonakdarpour, A., Levy, W.M., and Aegerter, E.: Primary and secondary aneurysmal bone cyst: a radiological study of 75 cases. Radiology, *126:*75–83, 1978.
6. Campbell, C.J., Roach, J., and Grisolia, A.: Comparative study of xeroroentgenography and routine roentgenography in the recording of roentgen images of bone specimens. J. Bone Joint Surg., *39A:*577–582, 1957.
7. Edeiken, J., Farrell, C., Ackerman, L.V., and Spjut, H.J.: Parosteal sarcoma. Am. J. Roentgenol. Radium Ther. Nucl. Med., *111:*579–583, 1971.
8. Edeiken, J., Hodes, P.J., and Caplan, L.H.: New bone production and periosteal reaction. Am. J. Roentgenol. Radium Ther. Nucl. Med. *97:*708–718, 1966.
9. Ellman, H., Gold, R.H., and Mirra, J.M.: Roentgenologically "benign" but rapidly lethal diaphyseal osteosarcoma: a case report. J. Bone Joint Surg., *56A:*1267–1269, 1974.
10. Feldman, F., Hecht, H.L., and Johnston, A.D.: Chondromyxoid fibroma of bone. Radiology, *94:*249–260, 1970.
11. Forbes, G.S., McLeod, R.A., and Hattery, R.R.: Radiographic manifestations of bone metastases from renal carcinoma. Am. J. Roentgenol., *129:*61–66, 1977.
12. Goldenberg, R.R., Campbell, C.J., and Bonfiglio, M.: Giant-cell tumor of bone. An analysis of 218 cases. J. Bone Joint Surg., *52A:*619–664, 1970.
13. Herzberg, E.L., and Schreiber, M.H.: Angiography in mass lesions of the extremities. Am. J. Roentgenol. Radium Ther. Nucl. Med., *111:*541–546, 1971.
14. Jaffe, H.L., and Lichtenstein, L.: Non-osteogenic fibroma of bone. Am. J. Pathol., *18:*205–221, 1941.
15. James, P., Baddeley, H., Boag, J.W., *et al.*: Xeroradiography—its use in peripheral contrast medium angiography. Clin. Radiol., *24:*67–71, 1973.
16. Lagergren, C., and Lindbom, A.: Angiography of peripheral tumors. Radiology, *79:*371–377, 1962.
17. Lagergren, C., Lindbom, A., and Soderberg, G.: Hypervascularization in chronic inflammation demonstrated by angiography: Angiographic, histo-pathologic, and microangiographic studies. Acta Radiol., *49:*441–452, 1958.
18. Lodwick, G.S.: Reactive response to local injury in bone. Radiol. Clin. North Amer., *2:*209–219, 1964.
19. ———: Solitary malignant tumors of bone: the application of predictor variables in diagnosis. Semin. Roentgenol., *1:*293–313, 1966.

FIG. 3-31. Central osteosarcoma of the femur with intramedullary and extraosseous extension depicted by CAT scan. Anteroposterior (*A*) and lateral (*B*) standard radiographs reveal an intramedullary cumulus cloudlike formation of mineralized tumor osteoid. Subperiosteal new bone [(*A*, *B*), *small arrows*] and cortical breakthrough by tumor [(*B*), *large arrows*] are subtle. The CAT scan (*C*) discloses massive enlargement of the right thigh, intramedullary involvement by tumor (*open-arrow*) and a large soft-tissue mass consisting of tumor and hemorrhage surrounding the bone and displacing adjacent muscle (*closed arrows*). The abnormalities become even more obvious on comparison of the images of the two limbs.

20. ———: The Bones and Joints: An Atlas of Tumor Radiology. Chicago, Year Book Medical Publishers, 1971.
21. Marsh, B.W., Bonfiglio, M., Brady, L.P., and Enneking, W.F.: Benign osteoblastoma: range of manifestations. J. Bone Joint Surg., *57-A:*1–9, 1975.
22. McLeod, R.A., and Beabout, J.W.: The roentgenographic features of chondroblastoma. Am. J. Roentgenol. Radium Ther. Nucl. Med., *118:*464–471, 1973.
23. McLeod, R.A., Dahlin, D.C., and Beabout, J.W.: The spectrum of osteoblastoma. Am. J. Roentgenol. Radium Ther. Nucl. Med., *126:*321–335, 1976.
24. Meshuga, M.I., and Pazzo, R.U.: Psychopathology of Everyday Obsessions. New York, Academia in Action, 1935.
25. Norman, A., and Dorfman, H.D.: Juxtacortical circumscribed myositis ossificans: evolution and radiographic features. Radiology, *96:*301–306, 1970.
26. Norman, A., and Schiffman, M.: Simple bone cysts: factors of age dependency. Radiology, *124:*779–782, 1977.
27. Parsavand, R.: Infusion angiography using xeroradiography. Radiology, *112:*739–740, 1974.
28. Reiter, F.B., Ackerman, L.V., and Staple, T.W.: Central chondrosarcoma of the appendicular skeleton. Radiology, *105:*525–530, 1972.
29. de Santos, L.A., Goldstein, H.M., Murray, J.A., and Wallace, S.: Computed tomography in the evaluation of musculoskeletal neoplasms. Medical Imaging, *3:*8, 1978.
30. de Santos, *et al.:* The radiographic spectrum of periosteal osteosarcoma. Radiology, *127:*123–129, 1978.
31. Steinbach, H.L.: Angiography of bones and joints. *In* Abrams, H.L. (ed), Angiography. ed. 2, pp. 1299–1321. Boston, Little, Brown, 1971.
32. Stewart, J.R., Dahlin, D.C., and Pugh, D.G.: Pathology and radiology of solitary benign bone tumors. Semin. Roentgenol., *1:*268–292, 1966.
33. Strickland, B.: Value of arteriography in the diagnosis of bone tumors. British Journal of Radiology, *32:*705–713, 1959.
34. Sutton, D.: Percutaneous angiography with special reference to peripheral vessels. British Journal of Radiology, *28:*13–25, 1955.
35. Wolfe, J.N.: Xeroradiography: image content and comparison with film roentgenograms. Am. J. Roentgenol. Radium Ther. Nucl. Med., *117:*690–695, 1973.
36. Wolfe, J.N.: Xeroradiography of the bones, joints and soft tissues. Radiology, *93:*583–587, 1969.
37. Yaghmai, I.: Angiographic features of osteosarcoma. Am. J. Roentgenol., *129:*1073–1081, 1977.
38. Yaghmai, I., *et al.:* Value of arteriography in the diagnosis of benign and malignant bone lesions. Cancer, *27:*1134–1147, 1971.

TUMOR TERMINOLOGY

4

Although most textbooks of pathology define the terms used herein, by no means have these definitions been standardized. A definition must be clear and precise; if they are too broad or vague, they are of little value. A good definition, however, can form a solid foundation to the understanding of classification, diagnosis, behavior, and treatment of bone tumors. Definitions of terms relating to the tumors of bone may be on many levels; principally they are based on histologic and behavioristic qualities. For example, anaplasia may be defined on the basis of its histologic features but its definition should also include the kind of behavior the tumor displays. On a histologic level anaplasia has those cytologic features that are evidence of malignancy. A problem arises when the pathologist discovers a lesion that mimics anaplasia in every regard, but is not malignant. Therefore, unless the tumor is coupled with malignant behavior, it may be nothing more than a pseudoanaplastic benign tumor.

One aspect of pathologic diagnosis is to formulate in our minds definitions of terms; it is another to put these definitions to practical use. Recognition of anaplasia versus pseudoanaplasia will be aided by clarity of definitions and experience, upon which diagnosis depends. But we must always be aware of the limitations of our definitions and the errors in judgment they may lead to if they are not critically applied.

ANAPLASIA-ANAPLASM

ANAPLASIA. Anaplasia is those bizarre cytologic aberrations associated with malignant neoplasms. All anaplastic tumors are malignant but not all malignancies are anaplastic. Pseudoanaplasia refers to those bizarre cytologic aberrations associated with benign tumors.

ANAPLASM. An anaplastic neoplasm is an *anaplasm.* Anaplasia probably occurs because of chromosomal errors, which result in bizarre cytologic alterations and uncontrolled, rapid, life-threatening growth. It is presumed that even if the noxious agent or carcinogen that provoked the anaplastic change is removed, the anaplasm will not be controlled. Anaplastic cells are not normal or embryonal cells, but a type never seen in the normal development of the host. These cells have the ability to destroy local tissues and invade vascular structures, resulting in lethal metastases. Anaplasia may be either of high or low histologic grade. Pseudoanaplasia refers to cytologic aberrations that may be impossible to distinguish from true anaplasia.

SUBJECTIVE ANAPLASIA. The form of low-grade anaplasia that depends heavily upon the experience of the pathologist I will call *minimal or subjective anaplasia.*

OBJECTIVE ANAPLASIA. Extreme anaplasia is universally recognized and is called *frank or objective anaplasia.*

Characteristics of Anaplasia and Anaplasms

Histologically, anaplasia is characterized by:

1. Bizarre changes in the sizes and shapes of nuclei and cytoplasm
2. Increase in the nuclear/cytoplasmic ratio, compared with that of their normal cell counterpart.

3. Abnormalities in chromatin distribution
4. Enlarged single-to-multiple nucleoli
5. Increased mitotic rate
6. Nonmirror image (atypical) mitoses. If a hypothetical mirror were placed in any axis of the mitosis, the image would not identically reflect what actually appears on its other side. Atypical mitoses are due to abnormal bits or clumps of chromosomal material that are distributed differently on one side of the mitotic apparatus as compared to the other. This is one of the most reliable signs of true anaplasia. But, atypical mitoses are not pathognomonic of malignancy. Radiation damage, the application of podophyllin to benign epithelial lesions, and other types of treatment may disturb the normal mitotic apparatus and lead to atypical mitoses and yet not necessarily be associated with a malignant change in the tissue to which these noxious agents have been applied. Atypical mitoses, incuding tripolar type, may rarely be seen in benign tumors such as the atypical fibroxanthoma of skin.
7. Hyperchromatism
8. Loss of polarity. Almost every reparative or benign hyperplastic bone forming tumor will demonstrate, at some time during its course, a well-defined, single layer of plump osteoblasts along the surface of the osteoid or bone it produces (see Fig. 7–14, *A*). This "rimming" of osteoblasts is a sign of polarity seen in benign conditions. Intramedullary osteogenic sarcomas lose this feature and do not assume the degree of polarization as shown in the above illustration.
9. Lack of maturation to benign tissues. Maturation to benign lamellar bone and marrow fat in a bone-producing tumor is an excellent sign of benignancy. Intramedullary osteosarcoma never matures to these benign tissues.

Behavioristically, an anaplasm is a highly malignant tumor. Unless treated it will almost always destroy the host.

Recognition of histologic anaplasia of any grade is extremely important to pathologic diagnosis, but there are some limitations.

Limitations to the Recognition of Anaplasia

Minimal or subjective anaplasia may be almost impossible to differentiate from the exuberant nuclear and cytoplasmic features associated with the growth phases of benign hyperplastic lesions. Even the most experienced cannot separate early fracture callus, or myositis ossificans, from osteosarcoma by cytology alone. Very highly malignant tumors such as the sclerosing osteosarsoma may show cytologic "innocence" to such a degree that objective cytologic evidence of anaplasia is virtually absent. This is the case in perhaps as many as 20 per cent of osteosarcomas or any other sarcoma of bone.

In general, anaplasms are characterized by numerous typical and atypical mitoses, and hyperplastic pseudosarcomas, by frequent but typical mitoses. Hyperplastic lesions show much less variation in size and shape of nuclei and cytoplasm. The nucleus and cytoplasm may, however, be quite plump. Nucleoli, if present, can be variable in size, but usually are solitary.

On rare occasions benign lesions may mimic high-grade cytologic anaplasia in almost every detail. In general these bizarre pseudosarcomas lack mitoses completely, which is the most crucial histological clue indicating its benignancy. But, the atypical fibroxanthoma of skin, an extraosseous lesion, mimics high-grade anaplasia in every respect; it even has numerous atypical mitotic figures. A benign bone tumor with cytologic features mimicking true anaplasia and atypical mitoses has not yet been reported, but in general, whatever rare cytologic variation has been described in nonosseous tissues usually occurs in the bones as well.

The only absolute way to distinguish a pseudosarcoma from a true sarcoma is by its behavior. Pseudosarcomas are not anaplasms. They will eventually stop growing and will not jeopardize the life of the patient, even if left untreated. The opposite is true of sarcomas. In this author's experience, for every 100 sarcomas there are approximately five highly exuberant reparative lesions that are mistaken for low- to moderate-grade anaplastic sarcomas and less than one benign lesion with such bizarre and pleomorphic nuclear features that it is diagnosed as an extremely high-grade sarcoma. (See Figs. 7–47—7–49, Pseudomalignant osteoblastoma). Refer also to sarcoma and pseudosarcoma, which are defined later in this chapter.

DEVELOPMENTAL ERROR LEADING TO TUMOR GROWTH

The process by which a benign tumor forms during fetal or early infantile development as a result of a disturbance in normal growth is defined as a developmental error. Such disturbances result in a faulty mixture of tissue within the organ. This faulty mixture of benign tissues is called a *hamartoma.* These lesions are slow growing and usually do not become clinically evident until early childhood; only rarely do they become evident in infancy or adulthood. The degree of skeletal involvement may vary from a single to multiple bones. A genetic defect will result in multiple developmental disturbances; other causes of the developmental error will usually result in solitary or localized growths. The etiology or pathogenesis of most of these growths is not known. Most have a propensity for eventual malignant transformation if the extent of the disease is great. The malignancy that arises reflects some cellular component of the benign tumorous growth: chondrosarcoma from multiple enchondromatosis, fibro- and osteosarcoma from fibrous dysplasia, chondrosarcoma from osteochondromatosis, and others.

Osteochondromatosis is an example of a genetically transmitted disease with variable penetrance, in which the developmental error (herniation of the lateral margin of the epiphyseal plate) results in multiple, aberrant, cartilage-capped bony protuberances of enchondrally formed bones. Solitary osteochondromas may be due either to very low penetrance of a gene or to other factors. Radiation given to a limb of an infant for treatment of a dermal hemangioma, for example, has resulted in local osteochondroma formation. This, therefore, would be an example, of an iatrogenic-radiation-induced developmental error. Other benign tumorous growths that probably begin in the early period of development include Ollier's disease (multiple enchondromatosis), fibrous dysplasia, osteopoikilosis, and the solitary bone cyst. Malignant transformation may be as high as 50 per cent in severe Ollier's disease, 5 to 10 per cent in extensive fibrous dysplasia, but nearly nil in osteopoikilosis and solitary bone cysts.

DYSPLASIA

Dysplasia is defined as atypical change in the cytology from normal, but it is not as severe a change as anaplasia. In metaplasia the change is from one normal cell type to another. In this text dysplasia will refer to a cytological change and not to skeletal dysplasias. Skeletal dysplasia refers to diseases of bone in which there is an error in bone modeling or maturation (e.g., achondroplasia, metaphyseal dysplasia).

Cytologic dysplasia was first applied to the epidermal tissues, such as the cervix. In dysplasia the nucleus enlarges, the nuclear to cytoplasmic ratio increases, abnormalities in chromatin distribution develop, and changes in organization or polarity occur. Dysplasias may result from chronic inflammation, radiation, or chronic irritation. Dysplasias are capable of regressing if the inciting stimulus is removed. Dysplastic cells are not capable of autonomous growth. But, dysplastic conditions are believed to be precancerous. The most classical benign bone tumorous lesion that is typified by varying degrees of cytologic dysplasia in later years is multiple enchondromatosis. In this condition the degree of dysplasia may be so great that low-grade chondrosarcoma is simulated. Eventually as many as 50 per cent of these patients may go on to develop highly lethal chondrosarcomas. It is also possible to observe dysplasia in long-standing lesions of fibrous dysplasia, in the cartilage cap of multiple osteochondromatosis, Paget's disease, and in the histiocytes of old bone infarcts. All of these lesions may transform to sarcomas. Dysplasia is not noted in osteomas, osteopoikilosis or in the late or healing phases of osteoid osteoma or callus. These latter diseases are almost never associated with sarcomatous transformation.

HYPERPLASIA

Hyperplasia refers to an abnormal increase in benign cells resulting from a known or unknown stimulus. Removal of the stimulus results in reversal of the hyperplasia and attempts by the organ or tissue to restore the normal anatomy. But, if the stimulus is not removed, the growth of the tumorous process may proceed for many years. Such lesions may be mistaken for malignant or neoplastic growths. Although the cells of a hyperplastic process are by definition benign, their nuclei and cytoplasmic characteristics and numbers of mitoses may be sufficiently "ominous" to be confused with malignancy. This is particularly true of the early exuberant developmental stages of any hyperplastic process. Unsuspected hyperplasias of the mesenchyme are the most treacherous of any organ system, because they are hardest to recognize, both clinically and pathologically. Unless the stimulus for the hyperplasia is removed or controlled by the host, they may transform to dysplastic and anaplastic malignant growths. Every benign tumorous process of the bone results from hyperplasia of one or more cellular components. Before pathologists became aware that the brown tumors of hyperparathyroidism were hyperplastic lesions caused by excess parathormone activity, brown tumors were thought of as a relentless neoplasm affecting numerous bones, which led to the eventual demise of the patient. We now know, however, that removing the parathyroid adenoma will result in reversal of the tumorlike lesions and restitution of the bones to normal or nearly normal. This is the classic example of a generalized bone tumorous hyperplasia caused by a known agent. An osteoid osteoma is an example of a benign, sharply localized solitary hyperplasia of osteoblasts activated by an unknown stimulus. Patients with this disease must eventually contain the stimulating agents, whether it is viral or otherwise, because the growth of this tumor is entirely self-limited and will, over the course of many years, disappear and be replaced by normal bone.

Osseous tissue hyperplasia is frequently caused by a stimulus to repair damaged sites, in association with fractures or infection. Unless the pathologist is aware that a fracture accounts for the tremendous proliferation of plump osteoblasts, osteoid, and woven bone seen in a biopsy, he may mistakenly diagnose osteogenic sarcoma. Similarly, osteomyelitis may be mistaken for Ewing's sarcoma because of their similar radiographic features coupled with a poor histologic preparation, in which the lymphocytes and plasma cells may be confused with a round cell sarcoma.

Thus, hyperplastic processes may be confused with malignant tumors, while highly malignant tumors with little cytologic atypia may be confused with hyperplastic processes. The hyperplastic processes most often confused with malignancy include the stress fracture and the osteoblastoma; similarly, cytologically low-grade anaplastic osteosarcomas, chondrosarcomas, and fibrosarcomas may be confused with hyperplastic processes.

NEOPLASIA-NEOPLASM

NEOPLASIA. Neoplasia is an intriguing and perplexing term that has had many definitions, some vague, others less so. The most vague definition is its literal translation, which means new growth. The formation of granulation tissue and of callus are new growths, but they would not be judged neoplastic. These formations obey laws of normal growth and when their purpose is achieved, growth ceases. Hyperplastic tumors also stop growing without jeopardy to the life of the patient, unless the lesion gets so large that it interferes with some vital organ function. A hyperplastic process, therefore, is characterized by controlled growth. Removal of the original stimulus results in regression. The property that distinguishes neoplasia from hyperplasia is ceaseless, autonomous, or uncontrolled growth. The process may have been incited by an offending agent, but unlike hyperplasia, even if the etiologic agent is removed, the process of cell multiplication proceeds. The hallmarks of neoplasia are excessive and uncoordinated growth without a definite limit. The resultant mass of tissue is highly injurious or fatal.

It must be emphasized, however, that autonomy of growth of a neoplastic tumor should not be equated with anarchy. Neoplastic growths depend upon the host for blood supply and nourishment. Their growth may be enhanced, retarded, and even destroyed by hormones, drugs, chemicals, radiation, freezing, heat, infections, host immune defenses, infarction, or other agents. Also the process of neoplasia may, on very rare occasion, spontaneously cease because the cells mature to completely benign tissues. The most classic example of this phenomenon is the transformation of neuroblastoma and its metastases to benign ganglioneuromas. This occurrence has not as yet been proven in any well-known primary bone sarcoma.

NEOPLASM. A neoplasm is a tumor formed by the process known as neoplasia. A neoplasm is, therefore, an abnormal mass of tissue that is unrelenting in growth, unless destroyed therapeutically. It differs from hyperplastic growths in that it persists and progresses throughout the life of the organism, ultimately leading to loss of limb or life. Because of its behavior, a neoplasm as defined here is a malignant tumor. Some tumors, such as leiomyomas, may grow for many years and attain huge size, but eventually growth slows down and ceases altogether. Although the stimulating agent of such tumors is unknown their behavior is that of a hyperplastic growth. The difference between hyperplastic growths is that they consist of normal cells in abundance, while neoplastic growths consist of abnormal cells.

Neoplasms can be divided into two main types:

A *low-grade malignant neoplasm* is a slowly progressive malignant growth. Unless extirpated, it is characterized by numerous local recurrences. In a small percentage of cases metastases may occur, usually many years after the initial discovery. Even with metastasis, the course is much slower and does not portend the same rapidly dismal prognosis as does high-grade or fully malignant neoplasms. Histologically, these tumors show abnormal cells with minimal to equivocal anaplasia. The primary bone tumors that have these properties include low-grade neoplastic giant cell tumor of epiphyses, parosteal osteogenic sarcoma, chordoma, adamantinoma, and Grade I chondrosarcoma. Cure is possible by means of an adequate en-bloc resection or cryosurgery. Extensive lesions may require amputation.

A *high-grade or fully malignant neoplasm* is a tumor characterized by excessively rapid growth, early metastasis, and often a lethal outcome within five years of discovery. These neoplasms usually, but not necessarily, show frank or obvious anaplasia. The fully malignant primary bone tumors are either sarcomas or lymphomas. These include the intramedullary osteogenic sarcoma, high-grade chondrosarcoma and fibrosarcoma, mesenchymal chondrosarcoma, Ewing's tumor, reticulum cell sarcoma, and myeloma.

In this text, there is no such entity as a benign bone neoplasm. Most medical dictionaries and textbooks offer a definition of neoplasia as a continuous growth of cells even if the provoking stimulus is removed. Often neoplasms are then categorized as either benign or malignant. But in my experience, I have seen no benign tumors of bone that are continuously growing neoplasms. Benign lesions, such a fibrous dysplasia, multiple enchondromatosis, and osteochondromatosis do have the capacity to grow for many years, but unless they have undergone a focal malignant transformation, eventually they appear to stop growing or enter a phase where growth is imperceptible. If growth stops or is severely retarded because of as yet unknown host factors, these entities should not, in this author's estimation, be classified as true neoplasms. Those benign tumors of osseous or extraosseous origin that were in the past classified as neoplasms were, traditionally, removed from that category if it were discovered that they were caused by hormonal stimulus, (for example, the giant cell "tumor" or hyperparathyroidism), reparative injury (myositis ossificans), or developmental anomaly (osteochondroma). It is bizarre to classify benign lesions as neoplasms if their provoking stimulus is unknown and to remove them from that category if an etiologic cause of pathogenesis is discovered. Surely if it were discovered that an osteosarcoma were caused by a viral agent, for example, the osteosarcoma would still be a neoplasm. A discovery of a virus may eventually lead to cure or prevention of osteosarcoma, but its simple discovery would not alter its growth activity. A neoplasm, as we have defined it, is always characterized by uncontrolled, relentless, life-endangering growth.

Precise and restricted use of the term neoplasm and accurate categorization of bone tumors into benign lesions or low- or high-grade neoplasms are pivotal to understanding how these various tumors behave; diagnosis and treatment ultimately depend on this understanding. For example, if one categorizes a tumor as benign, it is possible to accept local recurrence, but is it possible to accept such a diagnosis if there are lung metastasis? It is, if the original categorization as a benign tumor was in error; the metastases represent dissemination from a malignant transformation of the original benign primary; or the lung lesions represent benign lung "implants." This phenomenon sometimes occurs with chondroblastomas, although at least 98 per cent of these tumors behave in a completely self-limited or benign fashion. Knowledge of its usual nonneoplastic or nonmalignant behavior lead to the attractive hypothesis that lung lesions no different in appearance from the original chondroblastoma could well represent benign "implants" perhaps due to vigorous curettage rather than to a potentially lethal malignant metastasis. If additional case reports continue to support this particular hypothesis, future chondroblastoma patients with this rare and peculiar phenomenon will be spared unnecessary amputations, excessively large wedge resections of the lung, and possible systemic chemotherapy. If the chondroblastoma were categorized as an unequivocal neoplasm and if lung dissemination were always equated with malignant metastasis, there would have been no chance to conceive or to explore alternative explanations. For additional information about possible benign lung "implants", see Figs. 8-86—8-89, and Table 8-1, Cases 1, 7, 8, and 9. This example illustrates why, in the final analysis, tumors should be categorized based upon their known behavior, which in some cases may take many years to ascertain. Categorization by histology alone is fallible. Entities such as the hemangioendothelioma, hemangiopericytoma, and parosteal osteoma were originally thought to be benign tumors, because they lacked frank anaplasia and were relatively slow growing. Only after study of a number of these patients for many years did it become obvious that lethal metastases were possible and, even then, in only a relatively small proportion of patients, compared with those patients with high-grade anaplasms. Because of their documented behavior, these tumors are now classified correctly as malignant (neoplasms). The hemangioendothelioma and hemangiopericytoma are now usually prefixed by the term *malignant* and the parosteal osteoma is now called the parosteal osteogenic sarcoma. Similarly, numerous lesions that were originally placed into a malignant category because of histologic features confused with anaplasia are now, because of their self-limited behavior, known to be benign. Well-known examples of these benign pseudosarcomas include myositis ossificans (confused with the osteosarcoma), proliferative myo-

Table 4-1. Characteristics of Benign Tumors, Low-Grade; and Fully Malignant Neoplasms of Bone

Benign Tumor	*Low-Grade Malignant Neoplasms*	*Fully Malignant Neoplasms*
	Behavioristic Qualities	
1. Growth slow, eventually ceases of its own accord. It takes a nonlethal course.	1. Growth moderate, but is progressive. Demise may occur 10 to 20 years after initial discovery.	1. Growth rapid. Demise is usually within 5 years.
2. Tendency toward circumscription. Simple excision or curettage usually is curative.	2. Locally invasive. Simple excision or curettage is usually attended by recurrences.	2. Aggressive, destructive, local invasion. Recurrences with simple excision or curettage virtually guaranteed.
3. Adjacent vessels and lymphatics not involved	3. They may invade local lymphatics and blood vessels, usually after one or more recurrences.	3. Early lymphatic and/or blood vessel invasion.
4. Lesion confined to bone	4. They may break out of bone and involve soft tissues late in its course.	4. Breaks out of bone early in its course.
5. Anaplastic transformation, uncommon	5. Anaplastic transformation to highly malignant tumor is possible after several years.	5. Usually gives rise to early, lethal metastases.
6. Does not give rise to lethal metastases. Lung implants are rare.	6. May give rise to lethal metastases late	
	Radiologic Features	
1. Often bordered by zone of reactive host bone sclerosis	1. Rarely bordered by host bone sclerosis	1. Very rarely bordered by sclerosis
2. Almost always confined to bone and covered by at least a thin shell of periosteal new bone	2. Confined to bone in early stages. In late stages, there is invasion of soft tissues.	2. Early invasion of soft tissues by mass.
3. Bland to absent periosteal reactions	3. Bland to absent periosteal reactions	3. Codman's triangles, sunburst, onionskin and other ominous periosteal reactions are usual.
4. Circumscribed	4. Often circumscribed	4. Poorly circumscribed, diffuse to moth-eaten destruction.
	Histologic Features	
1. There is proliferation of exuberant but, nevertheless, nonanaplastic cells.	1. Abnormally exuberant cells with minimal or equivocal anaplasia.	1. Frank anaplasia is the rule. Small percentage show minimal anaplasia.
2. Typical mitoses, usually infrequent.	2. Typical mitoses, moderate in number.	2. Excessive typical and atypical mitotic activity.
3. Lesions tend to abut but usually does not infiltrate extensively between host lamellar bone marrow.	3. Tend to abut but usually does not infiltrate extensively between host lamellar bone marrow.	3. The tumor actively invades the fatty marrow, for considerable distances, leaving residua of host bone lamellae (sign of excessively rapid growth). This is best seen at the margin of the neoplasm with the host bone.

sitis (confused with rhabdomyosarcoma), pseudosarcomatous faciitis (confused with fibrosarcoma), atypical leiomyoma (confused with leiomyosarcoma), Spitz nevus (confused with malignant melanoma), and chondroblastoma and chondromyxoid fibroma (formerly confused with chondrosarcoma). Most of these entities have been delineated only in the last three decades or even more recently. How many other such entities exist? Their isolation will depend upon learning to recognize those tumors with specific histologic patterns that under close examination do not "fit" behavioristically into the malignant neoplastic category into which they were placed.

SARCOMA-PSEUDOSARCOMA

SARCOMA. A sarcoma is a fully malignant neoplasm originating from the connective tissue. The degree of anaplasia varies enormously and the severity of anaplasia does not necessarily correlate with lethality. Intramedullary osteosarcoma and Ewing's sarcoma are highly lethal neoplasms, no matter how minimal the degree of anaplasia. Grade I chondro- and fibrosarcomas of bone have a much longer course and metastasize less frequently than their higher histologic grade counterparts. Even though, by usage, these Grade I tumors are designated sarcomas, they behave like low-grade malignant neoplasms. Metastases almost always occur by means of blood vessels rather than by the lymphatic route. Although primary bone tumors of the hematopoietic system are sometimes called lymphosarcomas, they are more properly classified as lymphomas, since the hematopoietic system is not strictly defined as a connective tissue. The primary sarcomas of bone include the osteosarcoma, chondrosarcoma, fibrosarcoma, reticulum-cell sarcoma (believed to be derived from the connective tissue supporting stromal cells of the hematopoietic system), Ewing's sarcoma, and angiosarcoma. Although smooth muscle and fat are present in bone tissue, the primary leiomyosarcoma and liposarcoma are extremely rare. Since the bone is virtually devoid of myelinated nerves, the neurogenic or Schwannian sarcoma is not believed to occur as a primary tumor of the bone. Neurogenic sarcomas of bone are rare and are usually shown to be in association with a soft-tissue mass, from where they almost surely originated.

PSEUDOSARCOMA. A pseudosarcoma is a benign tumor that, because of its intense cellular exuberance or bizarre cytologic aberrations (pseudoanaplasia), mimics or is capable of being confused with a sarcoma.

The pseudosarcomas are virtually harmless, but because of their bizarre cellular morphology and alarming early, rapid growth behavior, they are often diagnosed as sarcoma. This has disastrous consequences for the patient. There is, however, no group of lesions more exasperating to recognize or more difficult to diagnose than pseudosarcomas. One must begin by asking the question of all lesions in which sarcoma is entertained if it could be a pseudosarcoma. The differentiation between the two often depends on the correlation of the clinical, radiologic and gross appearance with subtle morphologic clues.

HYPERPLASTIC OR REPARATIVE PSEUDOSARCOMAS. In assessing these lesions, this author has come to recognize at least three different forms; each has its own distinctive characteristics. The hyperplastic or reparative pseudosarcomas of bone or adjacent soft tissues include callus ("stress" fracture), myositis ossificans, and traumatic periostitis. These lesions are usually initiated by trauma, which need not necessarily be caused by a direct blow or fall, but may result from overstress of muscles, fascia, or periosteum. For example, stress fracture in a bone may be caused by a direct blunt or torsional injury or it may result from multiple repetitive injuries following abnormal physical exertion. In all probability, such individuals develop microscopic stress fractures, and if these build up in sufficient number before normal processes can repair them, they result in a complete break.

It is well known that exuberant callus can be readily mistaken for osteosarcoma, both radiographically and microscopically. Limbs have been amputated because the clinician and pathologist did not entertain the possibility of pseudosarcoma and never obtained the diagnostically important history that may have pointed to overstress as the cause. As bone is but a calcified form of connective tissue that can be seriously modified by stress, so must uncalcified connective tissues be capable of similar alteration. Tearing of the connective tissues with or without hemorrhaging may well result in reparative pseudotumors. Those lesions characterized by intense hyperplastic activity will morphologically contain masses of exuberant, stimulated mesenchyme with numerous mitoses; it is these features that mimic high-grade cellular sarcoma. But, compared with sarcomas of equivalent cellularity, the pseudosarcoma is typified by mirror-image mitoses. The nuclear and cytoplasmic features of pseudosarcomas, although bizarre, show cytologic clues of benignancy. The cells' cytoplasm and nuclei are much more monotonously "ominous," since most of them have been "turned on," so to speak, by the injury at about the same time. With most sarcomas, the nuclei and cytoplasm differ much more greatly from cell to cell (increased cellular pleomorphism), bizarre giant nuclei are more often seen, and some to many of the mitotic figures are typified by nonmirror images.

As these hyperplastic pseudosarcomatous lesions approach maturity, mitoses become rare to absent and the matrix and cellular morphology, much more organized and bland looking. After these lesions have matured, the chances of diagnosing a high-grade sarcoma are lessened greatly. The problem still remains, however, of differentiating well or minimally anaplastic sarcomas from a maturing pseudosarcoma.

Pseudosarcomas are usually heralded by a sudden burst of growth for the first few weeks, which usually abates within 8 to 10 weeks. They may then actually begin to shrink and on occasion, even disappear completely. This phenomenon has been shown clearly in myositis ossificans. There may be recurrences after a simple excision, but almost always only once in only five to ten per cent of cases. Most recurrences occur in those lesions that have been removed during their early active or immature growth phase. These recurrences are best explained by assuming that an injurious event "triggers" the local mesenchyme into forming a hyperplastic actively mitotic and cellular growth. If the lesion is simply excised before this very active lesion has entered the phase of retardation or cessation of growth and if residual cells remain in the wound, the growth phase may continue through the 8- to 10-week period. In other words, if a reparative pseudosarcoma is incompletely excised before it has had a chance to fully "ripen," a recurrence is possible. If the lesion is removed a second time, it is usually after the period of active growth has passed and recurrence is no longer possible.

It is important, however, to keep the following rule in mind: *Any so-called pseudosarcoma that recurs more than once or shows significant, persistant growth beyond a 12-week period of observation is probably a malignant tumor.* This rule is particularly applicable to soft-tissue and/or periosteal tumors. The above mentioned behavior is extremely rare for true traumatic reparative lesions, unless, of course, the cause of the injury that led to the development of the lesion in the first place is not removed. Most cases of persistently recurrent or "atypical myositis ossificans," which this author has consulted on, have proven to be subtly anaplastic neoplasms, such as osteosarcoma of soft tissue or malignant giant-cell tumor of soft parts with considerable osseous metaplasia. In spite of their cytologic innocence, these tumors eventually metastasized and destroyed the host.

PSEUDOSARCOMA FROM EXOGENOUS AGENTS. Pseudosarcomas may form from exogenous agents, such as ionizing radiation, bleomycin therapy, or others. Pseudosarcomatous fibroblasts sometimes occur in bone lesions treated by radiation.

Irradiation pseudosarcoma is a complex diagnostic problem, because usually the radiation has been given for a malignant epithelial tumor or sarcoma. Quite often, even if the tumor has been destroyed, the radiation-damaged tissue becomes infected easily and results in a mass of tissue impossible to distinguish clinically from necrotic neoplasm. Therefore, the problem on biopsy when confronted with abnormal cells after they have been treated with radiation, is whether they represent neoplastic cells, radiation-damaged benign cells, or both. Even if the original neoplasm were destroyed by the radiotherapy, occasional patients given over 5,000 R may develop a radiation-induced secondary neoplasm (sarcoma or carcinoma). Post-radiation sarcoma generally does not occur until five to seven years after the radiation has been given. Therefore, the problem of distinguishing postradiation fibromatosis from radiation-induced changes in the primary neoplasm from a secondary radiation-induced malignancy is often crucial. But diagnosis of irradiation fibromatosis can be made with reasonable assurance, provided that the following criteria are met:

1. The fibroblasts contain enlarged, bubbly to smudged nuclei, with a minimal amount of mitotic activity.

2. On low-power examination, the fibroblasts do not form a solid tumor mass but occur as a diffuse process in which individual atypical cells are separated from each other by an edematous, highly inflammed and vascular connective tissue.

If there are nests or cohesive sheets of cells with abnormal cytologic features, the diagnosis is much more consistent with recurrent neoplasm or radiation-induced sarcoma.

DEGENERATIVE PSEUDOSARCOMA. The third form of pseudosarcoma appears to be consequent to degenerative, ischemic or other unknown factors that result in extremely bizarre nuclear and cytoplasmic alterations. The main clue to diagnosis is slow to absent growth and usually a benign preoperative or gross diagnosis. The histological diagnosis suggestive of sarcoma usually comes as a surprise to the clinician, since the patient may give a history of a lump of many years duration with very slow to absent growth. The nuclei of degenerative pseudosarcomas are frequently bubbly and show signs, at least focally, of degeneration, including karyorrhexis and smudging of chromatin. Mitotic figures are rare to absent. One must be aware of the fact that karyorrhexis (nuclear destruction) can resemble atypical mitotic figures; care must be taken to carefully evaluate which of the two actually exists. In comparison to the incredibly bizarre shapes and sizes of the nuclei in pseudosarcomas of this type, unequivocal mitotic figures are absent or far less numerous than what would be expected if the tumor were as malignant as it appeared. In order to be more precise, a highly pleomorphic sarcoma usually contains at least one mitosis /10 HPF; in degenerative pseudosarcoma they are either absent or at most 1/40 to 50 HPF.

The most common examples of degenerative pseudosarcomatous changes occur in nonosseous tumors such as leiomyomas, neurilemmomas, and endocrine and soft-tissue tumors, although this author has seen them on two occasions in otherwise innocent bone lesions. One was an osteoblastoma with bizarre pseudosarcomatous cytology*, and the other, a benign chondromyxoid fibroma with bizarre nuclei simulating chondrosarcoma (unpublished observations). The former case was diagnosed osteosarcoma by several pathologists, but the clinician, unable to accept the diagnosis, treated the lesion with a simple en-bloc excision. The five-year course has been entirely benign (see Figures 7-47—7-49). The pseudosarcomatous chondromyxoid fibroma was cured by simple curettage. The point to be made is that although bizarre pseudosarcomatous changes are well recognized in leiomyomas, neurilemmomas, and some endocrine tumors, there is reason to believe that other benign tumors, including those of bone, can be similarly affected. Degenerative pseudosarcomatous cytologic change is probably very rare, perhaps occurring in about 1 per cent of benign tumors. In an extensive retrospective study of 1150† and 600‡ myeomectomies, the incidence of pseudosarcomatous leiomyoma was .96 per cent and .77 per cent, respectively. On the other hand, for every 200 or so primary bone sarcomas, there is one extremely bizarre, falsely anaplastic degenerative pseudosarcoma (noted from personal observations).

TUMOR OF BONE

A bone tumor is any localized osseous mass. As defined in its broad sense, a bone tumor may be either benign or malignant. A tumor may be due to a local inflammatory process, metabolic disorder, developmental error, or any of a host of known or unknown factors. Some authors tend to equate the term *tumor* with neoplastic, malignant, or cancerous growths. In order to reduce confusion, the qualifying adjectives benign, low-grade malignant, or high-grade malignant will be used as often as possible. The terms *tumorlike* or *tumorous* will be used synonymously with benign tumor.

BENIGN TUMOR. A benign tumor is a localized mass that grows by expansion and, given sufficient time, would cease growing. Removal or control of the inciting stimulus should lead to regression. Benign tumors do not endanger the life of the host unless they interfere with the function of a vital organ. Benign tumors do not result in lethal metastases, although iatrogenically induced or chance self-limited distant implants appear to be possible in a very small percentage of cases.

MALIGNANT TUMOR. A malignant tumor is characterized by incessant growth. It invades local tissues and eventually metastasizes. If the tumor is not eradicated, it will progress until it destroys the organism in which it resides. Malignant tumors are either low- or high-grade neoplasms (see Neoplasm).

PRIMARY BONE TUMOR. A primary bone tumor is a mass lesion that arises from one or more cellular components indigenous to the involved bone. They may be either benign or malignant. Benign tumors are often derived from more than one cell type. Malignant tumors are almost always derived from a single-stem cell. If the stem cell is capable of producing more than one type of tissue, various malignant components are possible. For example, the osteosarcoma may be composed of malignant bone as well as of cartilage, since the cell of origin is capable of differentiating in these two directions.

SECONDARY BONE TUMOR. A secondary bone tumor is either due to a malignant metastasis, involvement of a bone by a contiguous benign or malignant tumor of the soft tissues or joint, or by malignant transformation of a formerly benign tumor.

---

*Mirra, J.M., Kendrick, R.A., and Kendrick, R.E.: Pseudomalignant osteoblastoma versus arrested osteosarcoma. Cancer, *37:*2005, 1976.

†Davids, M.A.: Myomectomy: surgical technique and results in a series of 1150 cases. Am. J. Obstet. & Gynecol., *63:*592, 1952.

‡Langstadt, J.R., Javert, C.T.: Sarcoma and Myomectomy. Cancer, *8:*1142, 1955.

CLASSIFICATION OF BONE TUMORS

5

PRINCIPLES OF CLASSIFICATION

Classification forms the basis or system upon which tumors of the bone are diagnosed. The sections that follow identify those principles upon which the classification of bone tumors should be based.

Identification of the Fundamental Cell(s) or Tissue(s) of Origin

Fundamental cells or tissues are those that are produced by the tumor itself; that is, those cells or tissues that are directly related to the origin of the tumor. This definition excludes any host bone cells or tissues that form as a reparative or reactive response to the tumor. In most tumors the blood vessels, osteoclasts, osteoclast-like giant cells, and host reparative bone are not fundamental to the origin of the lesion. For example, osteoclasts are seen in many bone tumors but are of fundamental origin in but a few; namely, the giant cell tumors of hyperparathyroidism, Paget's disease, epiphyses, and the osteoclastic sarcoma. The blood vessels of most tumors merely serve to nourish the lesions and are not of fundamental origin, with the exceptions of the hemangioma and angiosarcoma of bone. Table 5–1 is a classification based upon the fundamental cell(s) and tissue(s) of origin. It is extremely useful to know which cells and tissues can be produced by the tumor per se, and which cannot. By studying this classification, it can be seen, for example, that the osteoid osteoma and the osteoblastoma do not have the inherent capacity to form cartilage. If cartilage is seen, either the tissue forms as a consequence to fracture (of which cartilage is one of the fundamental tissues), or the presumptive diagnosis of these two entities is in error. For example, most so-called osteoblastomas with cartilage production in the absence of a demonstrable fracture often turn out to be subtly anaplastic osteosarcomas.

The second column of Table 5–1 lists the fundamental benign or malignant tissues that must always be present in each of the entities listed to their right. The fundamental tissues include (benign or malignant): bone or osteoid, cartilage or chondroid, fibrous, osteoclastic, vascular, smooth muscle, notochordal, hematopoietic, histiocytic, inflammatory, epithelial, neural, and synovial. Many of these tissues are normally present in the bone; others reach the bone by either metastasis or contiguous spread from the joint or soft tissues. If an entity is being considered, it must contain one or more of the fundamental tissues listed to its left. The diagnosis of osteoblastoma, for example, cannot be made without the production of benign bone by the tumor. One category that requires further explanation is the first, tumors that derive from cells having fibrous, cartilage, and bone-forming potential. The potential to form each is present but only one may be expressed in any given case. By definition, the osteogenic sarcoma must produce malignant bone (or osteoid) in every case. However, malignant fibrous and/or cartilage production may or may not be expressed and is not inherent in

Table 5-1. Classification of Bone Tumors by Fundamental Histogenetic Cell(s) and Tissue(s) of Origin, and by Behavior

Fundamental Precursor Cell(s)	*Fundamental Tissue(s)*	*Benign Lesions*	*Low-Grade Neoplasms*	*Fully Malignant Neoplasms*
Fibro-, osteo-, chondroblast	Bone and/or cartilage and/or fibrous	Callus "Traumatic periostitis"	Parosteal osteosarcoma	Intramedullary osteosarcoma
Osteoblast	Bone	Osteoid osteoma Osteoblastoma Enostosis(es) Osteoma(s)	—	—
Fibro-, osteoblast	Bone, fibrous, and rarely cartilage	Fibrous dysplasia	—	—
Chondroblast	Cartilage	Enchondroma(s) Parosteal chondroma Chondroblastoma Osteochondroma	Chondrosarcoma, Grade I	Chondrosarcoma, Grades II–III
Chondroblast with transformation to fibroblastlike cell or osteoblast	Cartilage and fibrous	—	—	Fibrosarcomatous transformation of low-grade chondrosarcoma
	Cartilage and bone	—	—	Osteosarcomatous transformation of low-grade chondrosarcoma
Fibro-, chondroblast	Chondroid and fibrous	Chondromyxoid fibroma	—	—
Fibroblast	Fibrous	Fibrous cortical defect Nonossifying fibroma	Fibrosarcoma, Grade I	Fibrosarcoma, Grades II–III
		Desmoplastic fibroma*		
Osteoclast	Osteoclastic	Giant cell tumor of hyperparathyroidism and Paget's disease	Giant cell tumor of epiphyses	Osteoclastic sarcoma
Lipoblast	Fat	Lipoma	—	Liposarcoma
Endothelial	Vascular	Hemangioma	Hemangioendothelioma	Angiosarcoma
Perithelial	Specialized vascular	Glomus	Hemangiopericytoma	Pericytic sarcoma ?†
Leiomyal	Smooth muscle	Leiomyoma ?†	Leiomyoblastoma ?†	Leiomyosarcoma
Physaliphorous	Notochordal	Ecchordosis Physaliphora	Chordoma	—
White blood cells, noninflammatory	Hematopoietic	Mastocytosis	Waldenström's macroglobulinemia	Lymphoma Leukemia Myeloma

(*Continued*)

Table 5-1. Classification of Bone Tumors by Fundamental Histogenetic Cell(s) and Tissue(s) of Origin, and by Behavior (Continued)

Fundamental Precursor Cell(s)	*Fundamental Tissue(s)*	*Benign Lesions*	*Low-Grade Neoplasms*	*Fully Malignant Neoplasms*
White blood cells, inflammatory cells and histiocytes	Inflammatory histiocytic	Osteomyelitis Tuberculosis Fungus infections Gout Sarcoidosis Eosinophilic granuloma	—	—
Pure histiocytes	Histiocytic	Gaucher's disease Niemann-Pick disease	—	Reticulum cell sarcoma Malignant fibrous Histiocytoma Hodgkin's disease‡
Epithelial	Epithelium	Epidermal inclusion cyst	Adamantinoma of long limb bones	Carcinoma
Neurocytic	Neural crest and neural	Neurofibroma	—	Neurosarcoma Melanoma Neuroblastoma
Synoviocytic	Synovial	Pigmented nodular synovitis (also histiocytic)	—	—
Uncertain	—	Simple bone cyst Aneurysmal bone cyst	—	Ewing's sarcoma

*Not enough cases of demoplastic fibroma have been accumulated to permit categorization. Some behave with total innocence, others as low-grade neoplasms or "aggressive" benign lesions.

†? Tumors with a potential to be primary in bone but have never been reported as such.

‡Usually associated with benign inflammatory cells and fibrosis. The fundamental cell of origin is, however, either a histiocyte or transformed lymphoblast.

its definition. The parosteal osteosarcoma always expresses woven bone and low-grade malignant fibrosarcoma-like tissue; cartilage production is variable. Callus and traumatic periostitis may express either fibrous tissue with or without bone or with cartilage tissues. In fewer than 2 weeks from the inception of trauma or fracture, the tissues of each of these two entities will consist of only preosteoblastic and/or prechondroblastic spindle cell fibrous-like tissue. Within 2 weeks from inception, bone with or without cartilage begins to appear, while the amount of preosseous spindle cell tissue abates.

In this classification scheme the osteochondroma is defined as being derived from only cartilage precursor cells, yet all osteochondromas are associated with bone production. This seeming contradiction is explained by Virchow and recent experiments that show that the osteochondroma is related to herniation of a portion of the epiphyseal plate cartilage (see Figs. 14-3—14-6). Bone forms as a normal consequence of growth secondary to vascular invasion at the base of the cartilage cap, the same way it occurs in normal endochondral ossification. The bone of an osteochondroma is, therefore, a derivative of the underlying host bone and does not form from the herniated epiphyseal plate cartilage cells per se. Therefore, the bone is not strictly a fundamental tissue of origin, although it does play a prominent role in the secondary phenomena associated with the pathogenesis of the lesion.

If any tissues other than the listed fundamental tissues are present, it may be because:

1. The tissue is consequent to pathologic fracture (e.g., cartilage in fibrous dysplasia). This is not an uncommon phenomenon and can lead to problems in diagnosis.

2. The tissue is secondary to nourishment of the tumor by the host tissues (e.g., vascular tissue). This phenomenon is always present and usually does not obscure diagnosis.
3. The tissue is consequent to reactive host bone production, responding to the local effects of the tumor (e.g., woven-bone production as a response to a metastatic prostatic carcinoma). This is a common phenomenon and can be extremely difficult to distinguish from a fundamental tissue.
4. Tissues are forming as a response to secondary infection, necrosis, or hemorrhage. Generally these tissues include inflammatory and histiocytic cells. They are relatively common responses and may result in diagnostic problems. For example, the massively exuberant histiocytic response to a locally invasive but benign pigmented villonodular synovitis can be mistaken for a histiocytic or other kind of sarcoma.
5. Collision of two histogenetically unrelated tumors. This is an extremely rare occurrence but if it occurs, it will lead to great difficulties in diagnosis. An actual case will serve to illustrate this point. A 30-year-old female presented with a lytic lesion with some calcifications in the femoral metaphysis. Biopsy showed enchondroma and large masses of giant cells and stromal cells identical to a giant cell tumor. Two experts reviewed the case; the first diagnosed it as a neoplastic giant cell tumor with chondromatous metaplasia; the second, as an enchondroma with foci of giant cell reaction. Neither diagnosis is tenable from a histogenetic standpoint. Fundamental osteoclastic lesions cannot produce cartilage, and cartilage-derived cells cannot, themselves, lead to the production of masses of osteoclast-like cells. One year later the patient presented with an epulis (giant cell tumor) of the gum to her dentist. Radiographs showed loss of the lamina dura, forcing the clinician to conclude that the patient had hyperparathyroidism. The serum calcium was markedly elevated and the phosphorus depressed. A large parathyroid adenoma was removed. According to Virchow this phenomenon of two histogenetically unrelated tumors occurring together would be attributed to the propensity for a new pathological process (in this case hyperparathyroidism) to most likely occur in an area of decreased resistance (in this case the region of the enchondroma). In his terminology the enchondroma would represent a *locus minoris resistentiae* to the effects of systemic hyperparathyroidism. All metaphyseal giant cell tumors should be investigated further to rule out hyperparathyroidism (see p. 308). Had a workup been performed at the time of initial presentation, the diagnosis of giant cell tumor due to hyperparathyroidism would have become obvious. Such an example typifies the rare "collision" of two entirely histogenetically unrelated tumors and emphasizes the importance of recognizing the fundamental tissues that are or are not possible for each tumor of bone.
6. The presumed diagnosis is in error.

Classification by Biologic Behavior—Benign, Low-Grade, and Fully Malignant Neoplasms

The tumors of bone must also be classified according to their known biologic behavior. It is upon this separation that therapy obviously depends. Benign lesions are self-limited growths even though they may persist for years. They do not give rise to lethal metastases, and treatment consists of simple procedures. Low-grade neoplasms do not display frank anaplasia but are typified by relentless growth unless they are extirpated. They may give rise to lethal metastases but usually only after one or more recurrences. Nevertheless, 5-year survival rates are high. Treatment generally consists of en-bloc excision or cryosurgery. Fully malignant lesions usually show obvious anaplasia and highly virulent behavior (extremely low 5-year survival rates). Table 5–1 groups the lesions of bone into one of these three biologic modes of behavior.

Identification of the Site of Origin of the Bone Tumor in Question—Primary Versus Secondary

Not only is it important to classify a tumor by its histogenetic type, benignancy versus degree of malignancy, but it is also important to establish whether the tumor is primary or secondary. All three factors determine the treatment to be used. Primary bone tumors arise *de novo* from the affected bone site. Secondary tumors may be of three types: metastatic (by far the most common), spread to the bone by contiguous spread from joint or soft-tissue tumors, and malignant transformation of a preexistent benign bone tumor. Metastatic tumors are treated much differently from tumors that arise from the bone or contiguous tissues. Clinicians usually treat the latter

Table 5-2. Benign Primary and Secondary Tumors of Bone and Their Potential for Malignant Transformation

Benign Tumors	*Primary in Bone*	*Potential to Erode into Bone by Contiguous Joint or Soft-Tissue Tumors*	*Potential to Transform into Highly Malignant Neoplasms*
Fracture callus	Always	None	Extremely rare
Traumatic periostitis	Always	None	None
Enostosis(es)	Always	None	Extremely rare (1 case)
Osteoma(s) of skull	Always	None	None
Osteoid osteoma	Always	None	None
Osteoblastoma	Always	None	Rare to +
Osteochondroma	Always	None	Rare
Osteochondromatosis	Always	None	++
Enchondroma of phalanges	Always	None	Rare
Enchondroma of long bones with clinical symptoms*	Always	None	+++
Enchondromatosis	Always	None	+++
Chondroblastoma	Always	None	Rare
Chondromyxoid fibroma	Always	None	Rare
Monostotic fibrous dysplasia	Always	None	Rare
Polyostotic fibrous dysplasia	Always	None	+
Fibrous cortical defect	Always	None	None
Nonossifying fibroma	Always	None	Extremely rare
Giant cell tumor of hyperparathyroidism and Paget's disease	Always	None	Extremely rare
Bone infarct	Always	None	Rare
Simple bone cyst	Always	None	Extremely rare
Aneurysmal bone cyst	Always	None	None
Lipoma	Always	None	None
Hemangioma	Always	None	None
Eosinophilic granuloma	Always	None	None
Gaucher's disease	Always	None	Rare
Chronic osteomyelitis†	Common	Common	Rare
Tuberculosis and fungus infections†	Common	Common	Rare
Epidermal inclusion cyst	None	Always	None
Pigmented nodular synovitis	None	Always	None
Glomus tumor	None	Always	None
Gout	None	Always	None

Key: extremely rare: <.1% of cases; rare: .1 to 2% of cases; +: 3 to 5% of cases; ++: 6 to 20% of cases; +++: >20% of cases

*In this author's experience the majority of symptomatic solitary enchondromas of the long bones have undergone malignant transformations. There may be, however, many asymptomatic lesions that remain undiscovered and never transform to chondrosarcoma. Those rare enchondromas that are found as incidental findings in patients younger than 40 years of age are usually completely benign.

†For the purposes of this table, primary bone infection will refer to those cases that are consequent to direct vascular dissemination to the bone or to open fractures.

Table 5–3. Fully Malignant Bone Tumors and Their Probability of Being Either Primary or Secondary Neoplasms

		SECONDARY NEOPLASM		
Fully Malignant Neoplasm	*Primary Neoplasm*	*Arose From Benign Lesion Within Bone*	*Metastatic*	*Invaded Bone From Joint or Soft-Tissue Tumor*
Intramedullary osteosarcoma	++	+	Rare (multifocal osteosarcoma may represent metastasis)	Rare
Fibrosarcoma	++	+	+	Rare
Chondrosarcoma	++	+ to ++	Rare	Rare
Fibrosarcomatous or osteosarcomatous transformation of chondrosarcoma	None	+ to ++ (enchondroma)	None	None
Mesenchymal chondrosarcoma	++	None	Rare	Rare to +
Liposarcoma	Rare	None	++	+
Leiomyosarcoma	Rare	None	++	+
Lymphoma	+	None	++	Rare
Hodgkins' disease	+	None	++	Rare
Reticulum cell sarcoma	++	None	++	Rare
Myeloma	++	+	++	None
Malignant fibrous histiocytoma	++	+ to ++	++	Rare
Neurosarcoma	Rare	None	++	++
Neuroblastoma	None	None	+++	None
Angiosarcoma	++	0	+	+
Carcinoma	None	None	++	+

Key: rare = <1% of cases; + = 1 to <20% of cases; ++ = 20 to <100% of cases; +++ = 100% of cases

by local measures to attempt cure. Metastatic tumors, on the other hand, are usually treated symptomatically, with radiation or systemic chemotherapy. Amputation is usually avoided. There is little hope for cure because of the nature of metastatic tumors. These tumors have usually seeded many bone sites, and cure is usually not feasible by surgical procedures. It is extremely important, therefore, to decide whether a malignant spindle cell tumor of the bone represents a primary fibrosarcoma of bone or a metastatic fibrosarcoma, a spindle cell melanoma or undifferentiated carcinoma.

Table 5–2 lists those benign entities of bone that are either primary or erode into the bone by means of contiguous joint or soft-tissue involvement. Table 5–3 lists those fully malignant neoplasms of bone and their relative frequency or probability of being either primary or secondary.

BENIGN LESIONS AND LOW-GRADE MALIGNANT NEOPLASMS AND THEIR PROPENSITY TO TRANSFORM TO FULLY MALIGNANT NEOPLASMS

Many of the benign and low-grade neoplasms have been reported to transform to highly virulent neoplasms. These neoplasms are a subgroup of secondary

Table 5-4. Fully Malignant Neoplasms that may Arise from Benign or Low-Grade Neoplastic Bone Tumors

High-Grade Sarcoma	*Benign or Low-Grade Neoplasms From Which High-Grade Sarcomas May Arise**
Intramedullary osteosarcoma	Paget's disease, radiation osteitis, Fibrous dysplasia, osteochondroma(s), Grade I chondrosarcoma, osteoblastoma, chronic osteomyelitis, osteogenesis imperfecta, bone infarct, osteopoikilosis (1 case)
Chondrosarcoma, Grade II–III	Grade I chondrosarcoma, enchondroma(s), radiation osteitis, Paget's disease, fibrous dysplasia, chondroblastoma, chondromyxoid fibroma
Fibrosarcoma, Grade II–III	Paget's disease, radiation osteitis, giant cell tumor (usually postradiation), chondrosarcoma, fibrous dysplasia, chronic osteomyelitis, nonossifying fibroma
Osteoclastic sarcoma	Paget's disease, giant cell tumor
Malignant fibrous histiocytoma	Bone infarct, chronic osteomyelitis†
Myeloma	Chronic osteomyelitis

*The lesions from which the high-grade sarcomas may arise are listed in approximate order of frequency.

† Most cases have been reported as fibrosarcomas. The illustrations of the majority of reported cases, however, are more consistent with a malignant fibrous histiocytoma. (Personal observations). All of the cases were reported prior to the establishment of MFH as a bone entity.

malignancy. Nevertheless, each is treated the same as its primary malignant counterpart and must be distinguished from metastases. Careful review of history and radiographs and careful dissection and numerous sections are necessary to determine which highly malignant neoplasms arise from benign or less virulent tumors. Such knowledge about the incidence of primary versus secondary malignancies is vital to a more complete understanding of the pathogenesis of the malignant bone tumors. It must be determined, for example, the incidence of malignant transformation of enchondromas of long bones to chondrosarcoma and bone infarcts and fibrous dysplasia to sarcoma. Only in this way will it be possible to determine how closely such patients must be followed, the mode and extent of treatment that should be given to patients with multifocal disease, and how to identify those early signs of malignant transformation to enable the clinician to offer the afflicted patients the best hope of cure. Subtle changes in the radiographic pattern of adult patients with Ollier's disease could lead to a diagnosis of incipient chondrosarcomatous transformation before obvious clinical symptoms develop, at which time salvage of limb or life may be too late.

Table 5–2 lists the known relative incidence of malignant transformation of preexistent benign tumors. Enchondromatosis, osteochondromatosis, and enchondroma of long bones are by far the benign tumors with the highest incidence of malignant change. In this author's estimation these relative incidences, which are based upon reported cases, are probably too low. The more care given to reviewing the past history, radiographs, and thorough dissection of individual cases of malignant tumors, the greater will be the incidence of discovery of these secondary bone sarcomas. Those particular benign entities that should be searched for in dealing with so-called "primary" bone sarcomas are listed in order of frequency in Table 5–4.

DIFFERENTIAL DIAGNOSTIC TABLES AND THEIR USE

6

INTRODUCTION

The diagnosis of bone diseases is difficult, not because the characteristic features of each disease are unknown, but because lesions are rare; therefore, few pathologists can have firsthand experience with the different clinical, radiologic, and pathologic presentations each lesion may assume. The incidence of primary bone tumors is only 1 in 50,000 to 100,000 persons per year. Therefore, in a hospital serving 200,000 people, only two to four primary bone tumors will be seen each year. In spite of their rarity, however, each individual case must be diagnosed accurately if disastrous errors are to be avoided. Osteogenic sarcoma must be differentiated from exuberant callus, the giant cell tumor of hyperparathyroidism from the true neoplastic giant cell tumor, and giant cell tumor with osteoid production from an osteogenic sarcoma with giant cells.

It is beyond the scope of this book to include the very rare congenital malformations and the mucopolysaccharidoses, or the delve into the infectious diseases or diseases of the jawbones in much detail. The lesions presented in depth are those that are most common and those that present the greatest diagnostic difficulties. These include the benign or malignant bone tumors, hamartomatous malformations, hyperparathyroidism, Paget's disease, and traumatic lesions that may be confused with malignancy. A substantial portion of the discussion of individual disease will be devoted to pitfalls in diagnosis, particularly in the differentiation of fracture callus from osteogenic sarcoma, enchondroma from chondrosarcoma, parosteal osteosarcoma from osteochondroma, and neoplastic giant cell tumor from the giant cell tumor of hyperparathyroidism.

The age of the patient, the site of involvement, signs and symptoms, and radiologic and laboratory features are often paramount in establishing a firm diagnosis, since several of the diseases of bone may mimic each other very closely, if not exactly, in one or more parameters. For this reason most of the entities presented in the text will be preceded by a short tabulation of the pertinent clinical, radiological, and pathological diagnostic features. The radiological features of a lesion may be crucial to diagnosis. For instance, in differentiating an enchondroma from a well-differentiated chondrosarcoma or fracture callus from osteogenic sarcoma. The pathologist should make a habit of asking for and reviewing radiographs on all but the most obvious cases, especially when he is asked for a frozen-section diagnosis.

Before formulating a specific diagnosis, one must develop a differential list of possibilities and then proceed to eliminate from this list all but one. Of course, it is also assumed that great care is taken in this elimination process to not only arrive at a final diagnosis but to arrive at the correct one.

The first part of this chapter consists of a series of nine differential tables based upon sites of involvement of the majority of the bone tumors. These are cross-coded with the principal histologic or dominant features of each individual tumor. The tables represent a distillation of the thought processes used by this author in formulating a differential diagnostic list of individual tumors based upon the principal radiologic and histologic data.

ORGANIZATION OF THE TABLES

Main Histologic Components

There are nine tables, each of which is organized on the basis of nine principal tissue or cell types. These are listed at the top of each table. These principal histologic features can be used to characterize the tumors of bone. Some tumors may fit into more than one of these histologic groupings, and in that case a specific tumor may appear in more than one of the tables.

Tumors or Tumorous Lesions of Bone

The particular tumors or tumorous conditions of bone are listed on the left-hand side of the table. They are grouped according to whether they are benign or malignant, and to what degree. (The terms *benign, low-grade,* and *fully malignant* are defined in detail in Chapter 4.)

The tumors are further subdivided according to whether they are solitary or multiple. By solitary, it is meant that only a single bone is, or appears to be, involved at presentation. By multiple, it is meant that more than one bone is involved by an identical process. Virtually every lesion of bone handled in this text can present as truly or apparently solitary, including hyperparathyroidism and Gaucher's disease, which in reality are systemic bone diseases. However, a large, solitary giant cell tumor of hyperparathyroidism or periostitis consequent to an medullary infarct of Gaucher's disease can, upon a single radiograph of the affected painful area, simulate a primary, nonsystemic bone tumor. Therefore, these lesions will be listed as possibly presenting as apparent solitary lesions, even though upon further clinical investigation the systemic nature of the disease process becomes apparent.

Many of the primary benign and malignant bone lesions are always solitary lesions. These are designated by a dash in the multiple column. Some bone tumors are almost always solitary and only rarely multiple. These tumors are designated by the term *rare* in the multiple column.

The advantage of this grouping is that, if more than one bone lesion is found a number of lesions can be virtually eliminated from consideration.

Primary Site of Involvement

The middle portion of the table lists the lesions according to their primary site of involvement, which is either intramedullary or juxtacortical (periosteal). By primary site of involvement is meant the site of origin of the primary bone tumors or the major site of involvement of the secondary tumors (metastatic and those tumors which invade the bone from the surrounding soft tissues or joints). Most primary bone tumors take origin from the medullary substance of the bone. The tumors that arise from the cortex or periosteum are much rarer. Analysis of the radiograph will usually show clearly which side of the table should be used for grouping. A few rules are necessary, however, in certain equivocal cases. When fracture callus is formed the intramedullary portion as well as the juxtacortical and periosteal portions of the bone play an equal role in the genesis of the lesion and, therefore, callus is coded as a intramedullary and juxtacortical lesion.

Periosteal reactions such as "sunburst," "hair-on-end," "onion-skinning," and fine periosteal lines all of which are consequent to an underlying intramedullary bone tumor, should not be considered primary sites of origin and are coded as only primary intramedullary tumors. For example, an intramedullary osteosarcoma that breaks through the cortex and induces a periosteal reaction is listed as an intramedullary osteosarcoma.

On occasion a periosteal tumor may wrap around the bone completely and produce such a thick mantle of periosteal bone that makes it impossible to determine whether the tumor is an intramedullary tumor that has broken out of the bone or a tumor of periosteal origin. Similarly, an intramedullary osteosarcoma may break out of the bone and produce a thick mantel of periosteal bone that obscures its intramedullary origin. In such cases where it cannot be determined what has actually occurred, both sides of the table should be used to formulate a differential list, unless adequate tomograms have been performed to show the true origin of the tumor.

Finally, on occasion a tumor of periosteal origin may grow into the bone, making it difficult to determine its true origin. This often happens with the periosteal chondroma. Also, occasionally a parosteal osteosarcoma may invade the intramedullary substance of the bone. These two possibilities should be kept in mind when faced with a parosteal chondroma that has eroded eccentrically but deeply into the bone; it may be mistaken for a primary intramedullary tumor (indicated by an asterisk on the table). In general, any tumor that appears markedly eccentric should be considered as possibly being of a periosteal or juxtacortical origin.

Type of Bones Involved

Tumors of bone usually have a predilection for certain sites and it is useful to have this information before making a diagnosis. For example, some tumors have a predilection for the skull or jawbones to the exclusion of all others. The tables are subdivided to account for these important differences in distribution. The various categories include the long and short tubular bones of the hands and feet, the flat bones (ribs, pelvis, clavicle, scapula, and sternum), and the spine and skull bones (including jaw). Each tumor is then given a range of known frequency for each of these sites.

Area of Long and/or Short Tubular Bone Involvement

In the tables, the short tubular bones are further subdivided according to whether the epiphyseal, metaphyseal, or diaphyseal areas are involved. It is also particularly useful to define whether the lesion appears to have arisen in the epiphyseal, metaphyseal, or diaphyseal portion of the bone, since many of the tumors tend to occur in certain areas more often than in others. For example, it is extremely useful to know that the chondroblastoma and giant cell tumor almost always involve the epiphyseal or epiphyseal metaphyseal end of the bone. Other tumors, such as the Ewing's sarcoma, are predominantly diaphyseal lesions. In order to determine the predominant site of long-bone involvement, the pathologist should draw an imaginary line through the center of the tumor perpendicular to the long axis of the bone. If the line crosses through the diaphysis then the tumor can be said to be centered in the diaphysis; if the line crosses through the epiphysis, it is epiphyseally centered. The sites of origin are organized primarily by this method. The one exception is a lesion that involves two or three of these areas extensively, making it impossible to identify the area of origin. In such cases, both the epiphyseal and metaphyseal sections of the tables should be consulted. The giant cell tumor is usually centered in the epiphysis or the epiphyseal-metaphyseal region of the bone. The tables will include the giant cell tumor under both these categories. If there is any doubt about which region of the bone is the site of origin, the differential diagnostic tables should be consulted under every likely possibility.

MANNER IN WHICH THE TABLES CAN BE USED

The purpose of the tables is to help formulate a reasonable list of diagnostic possibilities based upon key histologic feature(s), site of origin, and the particular bone involved and to lead him to the appropriate pages and figures in the text that describe each lesion in detail. In general, when trying to diagnose a lesion, the following steps should be taken:

1. Review the slides and list the main diagnostic features: cartilage production, prominent masses of spindle cells, *etc.*
2. Review the radiographs and determine the primary site of origin: intramedullary, juxtacortical (periosteal).
3. Determine the type of bone involved: skull, long bone, *etc.* If a long bone is involved, is the tumor centered in the epiphysis, metaphysis, or diaphysis?
4. Using these data in conjunction with the appropriate tables develop a list of diagnostic possibilities for each table used.
5. The lesions should be further reduced to the appropriate differential list by eliminating all of those entitites that are not common to each of the tables.
6. Refer to the text pages and figures that correspond to those possibilities.
7. Start reading about the most common (+ + +, + +) lesions and end with the most rare (+ or rare).
8. After reading about the differential diagnostic possibilities, determine whether additional information is needed before a firm diagnosis can be made. For example, is it necessary to inquire about possible trauma? Are tomograms necessary? Are serum calcium or phosphorous tests or the results of the white blood or differential blood count needed? Is there a family history of a similar disease?
9. After this additional information has been gathered, decide whether diagnosis is now clear-cut. If not, will additional information be needed? Will special stains need to be ordered or other procedures, such as CAT scans and additional biopsies for imprints and electron microscopy?
10. If, after all of these steps have been taken and additional reading of texts and papers has been done and the diagnosis is still not clear-cut, outside consultation may be necessary.

EXAMPLES

The four examples listed below illustrate how to use the differential diagnostic tables in conjunction with this textbook.

EXAMPLE 1. A dense, rectangular-shaped lesion is noted in the *midiaphysis* of the *tibia* of a 13-year-old boy. Although the periosteum shows some degree of response, the radiographs show conclusively that the lesion also involves the entire width of the medullary bone. This indicates that the primary site of involvement is the intramedullary portion of the diaphysis of a long bone, and it is under this section that is listed in the table. Histologically, the lesion shows three principal components, *osteoid and woven bone, cartilage,* and masses of *spindle cells*. Callus, parosteal osteosarcoma, or intramedullary osteosarcoma all have these features in common, and Tables 6–2, 6–3, and 6–4 could be used to formulate a differential list. The text and figures given on the right-hand side of the table should help the physician determine whether the lesion is a callus due to a stress fracture or a form of osteosarcoma; a significant portion of the text and illustrations are devoted to the differentiation of stress fracture from osteosarcoma. But, unless one has included callus in the differential diagnosis and considered the possibility that a clinically unrecognized stress fracture has occurred, the radiology and histology of the lesion, which was sufficiently alarming, could have led to the erroneous diagnosis of osteosarcoma when in fact the lesion was a stress fracture.

EXAMPLE 2. A 17-year-old female with pain in the knee demonstrates a lytic lesion in the distal *femoral epiphysis*. Histologically, the lesion shows masses of *rounded* to *polygonal* stroma cells, a *chrondroid* or *cartilagelike* matrix, prominent *osteoclast-like giant cells,* a few spindly cells mainly due to scarring, and cholesterol clefts admixed with a few blood vessels. The few spindly cells, vessels, and cholesterol clefts are reactive elements only and do not constitute principal or dominant histologic features. The features that are significant are cartilagelike tissue (Table 6–3) and numerous giant cells (Table 6–5). Although prominent round cells were noted, do not use Table 6–7, which deals with them, because round-cell tumors with bone- or cartilage-matrix production are excluded, as noted at the top of this table. The possibilities, as listed in Table 6–3, include enchondroma, chondroblastoma, callus, chondrosarcoma, and osteosarcoma. The possibilities, as listed in Table 6–5, are osteoid osteoma, osteoblastoma, hyperparathyroidism, Paget's disease, eosinophilic granuloma, simple bone cyst, aneurysmal bone cyst, pigmented synovitis, chondroblastoma, Gaucher's disease, granulomas, sarcoid, giant cell tumor, osteosarcoma, fibrosarcoma, malignant fibrous histiocytoma, osteoclastic sarcoma, Hodgkin's disease, and metastasis. Although this is a long list, by eliminating those tumors that do not appear in both lists, we come down to only two possibilities, the chondroblastoma (common) and the osteosarcoma (rare). In other words, the only two tumors of epiphysis that would be expected to contain numerous osteoclast-like giant cells and cartilage-like- or chondroid-matrix production by the tumor are the chondroblastoma and osteosarcoma. The chondroblastoma is a common tumor; the osteosarcoma, a rare tumor of epiphysis. By referring to the text, it should be possible to determine which of these two tumors the patient actually has. If, by histological examination, unequivocal anaplasia is evident, the diagnosis of osteosarcoma is the likely one. Perhaps, on the first analysis, the physician failed to observe small foci of osteoid produced by malignant stromal cells. After referring to the tables and text, the physician would be alerted to make a more careful search for malignant osteoid or bone.

EXAMPLE 3. A 50-year-old male presents with pain in the leg. The radiographs show a large, lytic intramedullary lesion with spotty calcifications in the *middiaphysis* of the *femur* (long bone). On histologic examination *cartilage* tissue and prominent masses of obviously *malignant spindle cells* are noted. Some of the cartilage appears innocuous, other parts, obviously malignant. The physician then consults Tables 6–3 and 6–4. Although several entities are culled, the only ones appropriate to both categories, with malignant spindle cells and cartilage, are intramedullary osteosarcoma, parosteal osteosarcoma, dedifferentiated chondrosarcoma, and mesenchymal chondrosarcoma. By referring to the text and appropriate figures, the physician should be able to make a specific diagnosis. For example, after reading about each entity, the physician reviews his slides and finds a large focus of chondrosarcoma in apparent "collision" with a fibrosarcoma and, in addition, bland cartilage lobules surrounded by plates of lamellar bone. The diagnosis would therefore be enchondroma of bone with transformation into a chondrosarcoma and further dedifferentiation into a highly malignant fibrosarcoma (chondrosarcoma with fibrosarcomatous dedifferentiation).

EXAMPLE 4. A 6-year-old boy complains of pain in the arm. The diaphysis of the *humerus* (long bone) shows a fine layer of periosteal new bone. Although the shaft shows no definite destruction, it must be assumed that a *medullary* lesion exists. Biopsy of the medulla shows a mass of lymphocyte-like *round cells*.

No matrix is produced by the tumor cells. Table 6–7 is obviously appropriate. After reading about each entity, the physician reviews the slides, but unequivocal site of origin of the cells cannot be distinguished because of overdecalcification of the specimen and crushing of the tumor cells. A rebiopsy is requested and imprints of the tumor show unequivocal "pear"- and "carrot"-shaped cells with occasional multiple nuclei. Vanyl Mandelic Acid studies are ordered, but they are not positive. Electron microscopy of freshly fixed tissue confirms the presence of cells of neural origin. CAT scans of the abdomen reveal a 2 cm. localized nodule in the left adrenal. At laparotomy a small primary neuroblastoma is found and removed. The child is placed on an appropriate chemotherapy regimen.

PROBLEMS IN THE USE OF THE DIFFERENTIAL TABLES

Though there are many advantages to be gained from the use of the differential tables, such as obtaining a reasonable list of diagnostic possibilities in a relatively short period of time and considering possibilities that might otherwise have been overlooked, by no means, should the tables be considered infallible. They are meant to serve merely as a guide to the reader in formulating his diagnosis based on the material on hand and to direct him to most useful portions of the text.

The main stumbling block to the use of the tables is misinterpretation of what is found in the lesion. Many tumors stimulate reactive host bone production; others are infiltrated by benign osteoclasts; and pathologic fracture (callus) may provoke a growth of reparative tissue that has nothing to do with the histogenetic origin of the tumor but which can mislead the investigator into serious errors of diagnosis. Consequently, those obscuring reactive tissues that may appear quite frequently in tumors, presenting serious problems in diagnosis, have been incorporated into the tables where they are most likely to be involved. For example, reparative or reactive woven-bone and osteoid production may be seen in a significant number of neoplastic giant cell tumors; this could lead to a mistaken impression of osteoblastoma or osteogenic sarcoma. In the table of osteoid- and woven-bone-producing lesions, therefore, the giant cell tumor appears in the list of diagnostic possibilities. But not every example of reactive bone production can be adequately incorporated into the tables without rendering them useless. For example, on rare occasions, if a nonossifying fibroma is encountered in its late healing phase, the lesion along its periphery will be in the process of replacement by reparative host bone. In Table 6–2, which lists lesions characterized by osteoid or woven-bone production, nonossifying fibroma is not listed.

Extremely important to diagnosis is the recognition of reactive or reparative host bone, pathologic fracture callus, infiltration of benign osteoclasts into tumors or nonosteoclastic origin, reactive scarring or histiocytic infiltration due to focal hemorrhage or necrosis in a tumor, and the recognition of what constitutes chondroid and osteoid tissues. Without these essential interpretations diagnosis is difficult. In the main text reactive tissues such as chondroid, osteoid, woven and lamellar bone, and giant cells are treated in depth in the introduction to the chapters on bone, cartilage-, and giant-cell-producing tumors in order to reduce diagnostic errors.

Another occurrence that can interfere with the applicability of the differential diagnostic tables is the development of a malignant tumor in a benign lesion. The tables would have to be unreasonably long to account for all of the various combinations and permutations of this occurrence. Unless the two lesions are recognized as separate entities, it is easy to overlook one, usually the benign component. If both lesions are recognized as separate, the principal histologic components of each may be looked up separately to formulate a combined diagnosis, such as osteogenic sarcoma arising in fibrous dysplasia or chondrosarcoma arising from an enchondroma.

Another very rare problem would be when one is confronted by a collision of two histogenetically unrelated tumors (see pp. 55, no. 5).

FEATURES ASSOCIATED WITH TUMORS OF THE BONE THAT ARE USEFUL IN DIFFERENTIAL DIAGNOSES

Specific tumors of bone are associated with a range of clinical and pathologic features. Some features are diagnostic of a particular tumor; other features may typify benignancy or malignancy. For example, an elevated vanyl mandelic acid in association with a metastatic bone tumor is virtually diagnostic of neuroblastoma; a dense border of sclerosis around a circumscribed lesion is a radiologic sign strongly in favor of a benign diagnosis.

In Table 6–10, the left-hand column lists a number of historical, laboratory, radiologic, and pathologic features. The right-hand column lists those tumors or tumorlike conditions that are most often associated

(*Text continues on p. 80.*)

Table 6-1. Lesions Typified by Lamellar Bone Production*

Benign Lesions		Primary Sites of Involvement										Reference in Text	
		Intramedullary						Periosteal or Juxtacortical					
		Long and/or Tubular Bones											
Solitary	*Multiple*	*Diaphyseal*	*Metaphyseal*	*Epiphyseal*	*Flat Bones*	*Spine*	*Skull*	*Long and/or Tubular Bones*	*Flat Bones*	*Spine*	*Skull*	*Pages*	*Figures*
Enostosis	Osteopoikilosis	+	++	++	+	rare	rare	0	0	0	0	85	7-6 to 9
Osteoma	Osteomas	0	0	0	0	0	+++	0	0	0	0	86	7-10, 11, 12
Osteochondroma	Osteochondromatosis	0	0	0	0	0	0	++	++	+	0	521	14-1 to 23; Pl. 3, 4, 5
Callus	Callus	++	rare	rare	+	+	+	++	+	+	+	86	7-13 to 16; Pl. 1, 4
Traumatic periostitis	Traumatic periostitis	0	0	0	0	0	0	++	+	rare	+	550, 560	14-49 to 77
LOW-GRADE MALIGNANT													
Parosteal osteosarcoma, Grade I-II	—	**	**	0	0	0	0	++	rare	rare	0	536	14-37 to 48
FULLY MALIGNANT													
None	None	—	—	—	—	—	—	—	—	—	—	—	

Key: 0 = No cases have been observed or reported; rare = <3% of reported cases; + = uncommon; ++ = common; +++ = exclusive

*On rare occasions, a malignant nonosseous-producing tumor may stimulate reactive host bone, which may develop into lamellar bone. Usually the disparity between the tumor and the reactive bone will not lead to diagnostic difficulties.

**On rare occasions, a tumor with histology identical to the parosteal osteosarcoma may involve the medullary bone extensively and appear to be a primary intramedullary tumor. Usually the bone is woven but foci may show a primitive or fine lamellar bone pattern by polarized microscopy.

Table 6-2. Lesions Which may Contain Prominent Osteoid and/or Woven-Bone Production

BENIGN LESIONS		PRIMARY SITES OF INVOLVEMENT										REFERENCE IN TEXT	
		INTRAMEDULLARY						PERIOSTEAL OR JUXTACORTICAL					
		LONG AND/OR TUBULAR BONES											
Solitary	*Multiple*	*Diaphyseal*	*Metaphyseal*	*Epiphyseal*	*Flat Bones*	*Spine*	*Skull*	*Long and/or Tubular Bones*	*Flat Bones*	*Spine*	*Skull*	*Pages*	*Figures*
Osteoblastoma	—	+	++	rare	+	++	++	rare	rare	rare	rare	108	7–36 to 49; Pl. 2
Osteoid osteoma	—	++	++	rare	+	+	very rare	+	rare	rare	rare	97	7–17 to 35; Pl. 2
Fibrous dysplasia	Fibrous dysplasia	++	++	rare	++	+	++	0	0	0	0	122	7–50 to 71
Hyperparathyroidism*	Hyperparathyroidism	++	++	+	++	+	++	0	0	0	0	308	10–1 to 9
Paget's disease	Paget's disease	++	++	+	++	++	++	0	0	0	0	310	7–61, 10–1 to 19, 10–62 to 70
Callus	Callus	++	rare	rare	+	+	+	++	+	+	+	86, 156	7–13 to 16; Pl. 1, 4
Traumatic periostitis	Traumatic periostitis	0	0	0	0	0	0	++	+	rare	+	550, 560	14–49 to 77
Osteochondroma	Osteochondromatosis	0	0	0	0	0	0	++	++	+	0	521	14–1 to 23
Solitary bone cyst	—	+	++	rare	+	rare	0	0	0	0	0	466	13–6 to 29
Aneurysmal bone cyst	—	+	++	+	+	++	+ (jaw)	**	**	**	** (jaw)	478	13–30 to 50
Giant cell reparative granuloma	—	0	0	0	0	0	+++ (jaw)	0	0	0	0	322	10–23
Giant cell reaction of bone	—	++ (phalanges)	++ (phalanges)	+ (phalanges)	0	0	0	0	0	0	0	322	10–24, 25, 26
Osteoma	Osteomas	0	0	0	0	0	+++	0	0	0	0	86	7–10, 11, 12
"Reactive" bone to other benign lesions	Same	+	+	+	+	+	+	rare	rare	rare	rare	84	—

(*Continued*)

Table 6-2. Lesions that may Contain Prominent Osteoid and/or Woven-Bone Production (Continued)

LOW-GRADE MALIGNANT		PRIMARY SITES OF INVOLVEMENT										REFERENCE IN TEXT	
		INTRAMEDULLARY						PERIOSTEAL OR JUXTACORTICAL					
		LONG AND/OR TUBULAR BOBES											
Solitary	*Multiple*	*Diaphyseal*	*Metaphyseal*	*Epiphyseal*	*Flat Bones*	*Spine*	*Skull*	*Long and/or Tubular Bones*	*Flat Bones*	*Spine*	*Skull*	*Pages*	*Figures*
Parosteal osteosarcoma, Grade I–II	—	**	**	0	0	0	0	++	rare	rare	0	536	14–37 to 48
Low-grade neoplastic giant cell tumor	very rare	very rare	+	++	+	+	rare	0	0	0	0	346, 332	10–43 to 61, 10–77; Pl. *A, B, C*
FULLY MALIGNANT													
Osteosarcoma, intra-medullary type	rare	+	++	rare	+	rare	+	0	0	0	0	138	7–72 to 95, 12–24; Pl. 3, 4, 5
Parosteal osteosarcoma, Grade III	—	0	0	0	0	0	0	++	rare	rare	0	536	—
"Reactive" bone to other malignancies	Same	+	+	+	+	+	+	rare	rare	rare	rare	85, 138	—

Key: 0 = No well documented cases have been observed or reported; rare = <3% of reported cases; + = uncommon; ++ = common; +++ = exclusive

*A systemic bone disease, which may, on occasion, present as an apparent solitary bone tumor.
**Often results in an extensive periosteal "blowout" lesion. However, its primary site of origin appears to be intramedullary in most instances.

Table 6-3. Lesions Containing Cartilage or Cartilage-like Tissue

BENIGN LESIONS		PRIMARY SITES OF INVOLVEMENT										REFERENCE IN TEXT	
		INTRAMEDULLARY						PERIOSTEAL OR JUXTACORTICAL					
		LONG AND/OR TUBULAR BONES											
Solitary	*Multiple*	*Diaphyseal*	*Metaphyseal*	*Epiphyseal*	*Flat Bones*	*Spine*	*Skull*	*Long and/or Tubular Bones*	*Flat Bones*	*Spine*	*Skull*	*Pages*	*Figures*
Enchondroma	Ollier's disease	++	++	+	+	rare	rare (jaw)	0	0	0	0	164, 186, 208	3–19, 8–5 to 17, 8–36 to 45, 8–53 to 65, 14–32 to 34
Parosteal chondroma	Very rare	*	*	0	0	0	0	+++	0	0	0	532	14–24 to 34

Chondroblastoma	—	0	rare	++	+	0	0	0	0	0	0	219	8–71 to 89; Pl. 6, *K, L*
Chondromyxoid fibroma	—	+	++	0	+	+	+	0	0	0	0	234	8–90 to 105, 13–4; Pl. 6, *G, H, I*
Callus	Callus	++	rare	rare	+	+	+	++	+	+	+	164, 86	7–13 to 16; Pl. 1, 4
Traumatic periostitis	Traumatic periostitis	0	0	0	0	0	0	++	+	rare	+	550, 560	14–49 to 77
Osteochondroma	Osteochondromatosis	0	0	0	0	0	0	++	++	+	0	521	14–1 to 23; Pl. 3, 4, 5
Fibrous dysplasia	Fibrous dysplasia	++	++	rare	++	+	++	0	0	0	0	122	7–50 to 71
Aneurysmal bone cyst	—	+	++	+	+	+	+ (jaw)	**	**	**	** (jaw)	234, 488	13–50
LOW-GRADE MALIGNANT													
Parosteal osteosarcoma Grade I–II	—	***	***	0	0	0	0	++	rare	rare	0	536	14–37 to 48
Chordoma	—	0	0	0	0	+++	0	0	0	0	0	243	8–106 to 117
FULLY MALIGNANT													
Chondrosarcoma and its variants	—	++	++	+	++	+	+ (jaw)	rare	rare	rare	0	164, 178, 201, 536	3–19, 8–18 to 52
Osteosarcoma	rare	+	++	rare	+	rare	+	0	0	0	0	152	7–72 to 95, 12–24; Pl. 3, 4, 5
Mesenchymal chondrosarcoma	—	+	+	0	++	rare	++	+	+	+	+	212	8–66 to 70; Pl. 6, *D, E, F*
Parosteal osteosarcoma, Grade III	—	0	0	0	0	0	0	++	rare	rare	0	536	—

Key: 0, No well documented cases have been observed or reported; rare = <3% of reported cases; + = uncommon; ++ = common; +++ = exclusive
*The parosteal chondroma may erode into bone and be mistaken for a primary intramedullary tumor.
**Often results in an extensive periosteal "blowout" lesion. However, its primary site of origin appears to be intramedullary in most instances.
***On rare occasion, a tumor with histology identical to the low-grade parosteal OS may involve the medullary bone extensively and appear to be a primary intramedullary tumor.

Table 6-4. Lesions That may Contain Prominent Masses of Fibrous Tissue or Spindle Cells

Benign Lesions		Primary Sites of Involvement										Reference in Text	
		Intramedullary						Periosteal or Juxtacortical					
		Long and/or Tubular Bones											
Solitary	*Multiple*	*Diaphyseal*	*Metaphyseal*	*Epiphyseal*	*Flat Bones*	*Spine*	*Skull*	*Long and/or Tubular Bones*	*Flat Bones*	*Spine*	*Skull*	*Pages*	*Figures*
Callus	Callus	++	+	rare	+	+	+	++	+	+	+		7–13 to 16; Pl. 1, 4
Traumatic periostitis	Traumatic periostitis	0	0	0	0	0	0	++	+	rare	+		14–49 to 77
Hyperpara-thyroidism	Hyperpara-thyroidism	++	++	+	++	+	++	0	0	0	0		10–1 to 9
Paget's disease	Paget's disease	++	++	+	++	++	++	0	0	0	0		7–61, 10–1 to 19, 10–62 to 70, 13–54
Fibrous dysplasia	Fibrous dysplasia	++	++	rare	++	+	++	0	0	0	0		7–50 to 71
Fibrous cortical defect	Fibrous cortical defect	+	++	0	rare	rare	0	0	0	0	0		9–1 to 21
Nonossifying fibroma	rare	+	++	rare	rare	rare	0	0	0	0	0		9–1 to 21; Pl. 7, *E*, *F*
Desmoplastic fibroma	—	++	++	rare	rare	0	rare (jaw)	++	rare	0	0		9–22 to 30; Pl. 7, *G*
Chondromyxoid fibroma	—	+	++	0	+	rare	0	0	0	0	0		8–90 to 105; Pl. 6, *G*, *H*, *I*
Simple bone cyst	—	++	++	rare	+	rare	0	0	0	0	0		13–6 to 29
Aneurysmal bone cyst	—	+	++	+	+	+	+ (jaw)	**	**	**	** (jaw)		13–30 to 50
Eosinophilic granuloma	Eosinophilic granuloma	++	+	rare	+	++	++	0	0	0	0		10–20 to 22, 11–5 to 24; Pl. 8, *A* to *F*
Pigmented teno-synovitis (PVNS)	PVNS	0	+	++	0	rare	0	0	0	0	0		10–27 to 36
Giant cell rep-arative granuloma	—	0	0	0	0	+++ (jaw)	0	0	0	0	0		10–23
Giant cell reac-tion of bone	—	++ (phalanges)	++ (same)	+ (same)	0	0	0	0	0	0	0		10–24, 25, 26
Osteomyelitis	Osteomyelitis	+	++	++	+	+	rare	0	0	0	0		7–33, 34; 11–1 to 4

LOW-GRADE MALIGNANT													
Low grade neoplastic giant cell tumor	very rare	very rare	+	++	+	+	rare	0	0	0	0	332	10–43 to 61, 10–77; Pl. 7, *A, B, C*
Parosteal osteo-sarcoma, Grades I–II	—	†	†	0	0	0	0	++	rare	rare	0	536	14–37 to 48
Adamantinoma of long bones	unusual (contiguous bone)	++ (usually tibia)	++ (same)	rare (same)	0	0	0	0	0	0	0	440	12–2 to 11
Hemangioendo-thelioma	Hemangioendo-thelioma	+	+	+	+	+	+	0	0	0	0	516	—
Hemangiopericytoma	—	+	+	*	+	*	*	0	0	0	0	509	13–72 to 76
FULLY MALIGNANT													
Fibrosarcoma	very rare	+	++	+	+	rare	+	rare	rare	rare	+	276, 351, 364, 572	9–31 to 40, 10–73 to 80; Pl. 7, *D*
Osteosarcoma, intramedullary	rare	+	++	rare	+	rare	+	0	0	0	0	153	7–72 to 95, 12–24; Pl. 3, 4, 5
Dedifferentiated chondrosarcoma	—	++	+	+	++	rare	0	0	0	0	0	201	8–49 to 52
Mesenchymal chondrosarcoma	—	+	+	0	++	rare	++	+	+	+	+	212	8–66 to 70; Pl. 6, *D, E, F*
Malignant fibrous histiocytoma	—	++	++	+	+	+	+	0	0	0	0	284	9–41 to 56; Pl. 7, *I*
Rare	Hodgkin's disease	++	+	rare	++	++	+	0	0	0	0	276, 406	11–45 to 50; Pl. 9, *D, E, F*
Osteoclastic sarcoma	—	+	++	+	0	0	0	0	0	0	0	356	10–62 to 70; Pl. 4, *L*
Parosteal osteo-sarcoma, Grade III	—			0	0	0	0	++	rare	rare	0	536	—
Angiosarcoma	uncommon	++	++	+	+	+	+	0	0	0	0	516	13–77 to 81
Metastasis	Metastases	++	+	rare	++	++	++	rare	0	0	0	275, 448	8–118, 12–12 to 23

Key: 0, No well documented cases have been observed or reported; rare = <3% of reported cases; + = uncommon; ++ = common; +++ = exclusive

*Possibility of hemangiopericytoma should be considered, though there are only thirteen case reports. I have one case in my collection (clavicle to be reported).
**Often results in an extensive periosteal "blowout" lesion. However, its primary site of origin appears to be intramedullary in most instances.
†Refer to double asterisk comment of Table 6–1.

Table 6-5. Lesions That may Contain Numerous Osteoclasts and/or Giant Cells

BENIGN LESIONS		PRIMARY SITES OF INVOLVEMENT										REFERENCE IN TEXT	
		INTRAMEDULLARY						PERIOSTEAL OR JUXTACORTICAL					
		LONG AND/OR TUBULAR BONES											
Solitary	*Multiple*	*Diaphyseal*	*Metaphyseal*	*Epiphyseal*	*Flat Bones*	*Spine*	*Skull*	*Long and/or Tubular Bones*	*Flat Bones*	*Spine*	*Skull*	*Pages*	*Figures*
Osteoid osteoma	—	++	++	rare	+	+	very rare	+	rare	rare	0	306, 97	7–17 to 35; Pl. 2
Osteoblastoma	—	+	++	rare	+	++	++	rare	rare	rare	rare	306, 108	7–36 to 49; Pl. 2
Hyperpara-thyroidism	Hyperpara-thyroidism	++	++	+	++	+	++	0	0	0	0	308	10–1 to 9
Paget's disease	Paget's disease	++	++	+	++	++	++	0	0	0	0	310	7–61, 10–1 to 19, 10–62 to 70, 13–54
Giant cell reparative granuloma	—	0	0	0	0	0	+++ (jaw)	0	0	0	0	322, 258	10–23
Giant cell reaction of bone	—	++ (phalanges)	++ (same)	+ (same)	0	0	0	0	0	0	0	322	10–24, 25, 26
Eosinophilic granuloma	Eosinophilic granuloma	++	+	rare	+	++	++	0	0	0	0	320, 376	10–20 to 22, 11–5 to 24; Pl. 8, *A–F*
Nonossifying fibroma	rare	+	++	rare	rare	rare	0	0	0	0	0	258	9–1 to 21; Pl. 7, *E, F*
Simple bone cyst	—	+	++	rare	+	rare	0	0	0	0	0	462	13–6 to 29
Aneurysmal bone cyst	—	+	++	+	+	++	+ (jaw)	*	*	*	* (jaw)	478	13–30 to 50
Pigmented synovitis (PVNS)	PVNS	0	+	++	0	rare	0	0	0	0	0	322	10–27 to 36
Chondroblastoma	—	0	rare	++	+	0	0	0	0	0	0	219	8–71 to 89; Pl. 6, *K, L*
Gaucher's disease	Gaucher's disease	++	++	++	+	+	+	0	0	0	0	392	11–24 to 34; Pl. 8, *G, H, I*

Granulomatous infections	Granulomatous infections	+ +	+ +	+ +	+	+ +	rare	0	0	0	0	332	—
Sarcoidosis	Sarcoidosis	+ + (usually phalanges)	+ + (usually phalanges)	rare (usually phalanges)	rare	+	+	0	0	0	0	332	10–40 to 42
LOW-GRADE MALIGNANT													
Low-grade neoplastic giant-cell tumor	very rare	very rare	+	+ +	+	+	rare	0	0	0	0	332	10–43 to 61, 10–77; Pl. 7, *A, B, C*
Chordoma	—	0	0	0	0	+ + +	0	0	0	0	0	243	8–106 to 117
FULLY MALIGNANT													
Osteosarcoma intramedullary	rare	+	+ +	rare	+	rare	+	0	0	0	0	153, 351, 362	7–72 to 95, 12–24; Pl. 3, 4, 5
Fibrosarcoma	—	+	+ +	+	+	rare	+	rare	rare	rare	rare	351, 364	9–31 to 40, 10–73 to 80; Pl. 7, *D*
Malignant fibrous histiocytoma	—	+ +	+ +	+	+	+	+	0	0	0	0	284	9–41 to 56; Pl. 7, *I*
Osteoclastic sarcoma	—	+	+ +	+	0	0	0	0	0	0	0	356	10–62 to 70; Pl. 4, *L*
Rare	Hodgkin's disease	+ +	+	rare	+ +	+ +	+	0	0	0	0	406	11–45 to 50; Pl. 9, *D, E, F*
Metastasis	Metastases	+ +	+	rare	+ +	+ +	+ +	rare	0	0	0	305, 368	8–118, 12–12 to 23

Key: 0 = No well documented cases have been observed or reported; rare = <3% of reported cases; + = uncommon; + + = common; + + + = exclusive

*Often results in an extensive periosteal "blowout" lesion. However, its primary site of origin appears to be intramedullary in most instances.

Table 6-6. Lesions That May Contain Myxoid Tissue

BENIGN LESIONS		PRIMARY SITES OF INVOLVEMENT: INTRAMEDULLARY — LONG AND/OR TUBULAR BONES			INTRAMEDULLARY			PERIOSTEAL OR JUXTACORTICAL				REFERENCE IN TEXT	
Solitary	*Multiple*	*Diaphyseal*	*Metaphyseal*	*Epiphyseal*	*Flat Bones*	*Spine*	*Skull*	*Long and/or Tubular Bones*	*Flat Bones*	*Spine*	*Skull*	*Pages*	*Figures*
Chondromyxoid fibroma	—	+	++	0	+	rare	0	0	0	0	0	458, 234	8–90 to 105, 13–4; Pl. 6, *G, H, I*
Myxoma	—	0	0	0	0	0	+++ Jaw and Nasopharynx	0	0	0	0	456	13–1 to 3
LOW-GRADE MALIGNANT													
Chordoma	—	0	0	0	0	+++	0	0	0	0	0	243	8–106 to 117
FULLY MALIGNANT													
Myxoid chondrosarcoma	—	+	++	+	++	rare	rare	+	+	0	rare	186	—
Carcinomatous metastasis	Carcinomatous metastases	++	+	rare	++	++	++	rare	0	0	0	456	—

Key: 0 = No well documented cases have been observed or reported. rare = <3% of reported cases; + = uncommon; ++ = common; +++ = exclusive

Table 6-7. Lesions in Which Sheets of Oval to Round Cells and/or Histiocytes May Predominate to the Exclusion of Bone- or Cartilage-Matrix Production

		PRIMARY SITES OF INVOLVEMENT: INTRAMEDULLARY — LONG AND/OR TUBULAR BONES			INTRAMEDULLARY			PERIOSTEAL OR JUXTACORTICAL				REFERENCE IN TEXT	
Solitary	*Multiple*	*Diaphyseal*	*Metaphyseal*	*Epiphyseal*	*Flat Bones*	*Spine*	*Skull*	*Long and/or Tubular Bones*	*Flat Bones*	*Spine*	*Skull*	*Pages*	*Figures*
Osteomyelitis	Osteomyelitis	+	++	++	+	+	rare	0	0	0	0	373	7–33, 11–1 to 4
Eosinophilic granuloma	Eosinophilic granuloma	++	+	rare	+	++	++	0	0	0	0	376	10–20 to 22, 11–5 to 24; Pl. 8, *A* to *F*
Gaucher's disease	Gaucher's disease	++	++	++	+	+	+	0	0	0	0	392	11–25 to 34; Pl. 8, *G, H, I*
Nonossifying fibroma	Rare	+	++	rare	rare	rare	0	0	0	0	0	258, 382	9–1 to 21; Pl. 7, *E, F*
"Invasive" PVNS	PVNS (contiguous bone)	0	+	++	0	rare	0	0	0	0	0	322	10–27 to 36

LOW-GRADE MALIGNANT													
None	None	—	—	—	—	—	—	—	—	—	—		—
FULLY MALIGNANT													
Solitary myeloma	Multiple myeloma	++	+	+	++	++	++	0	0	0	0	398	11–35 to 43; Pl. 7, *J, K;* 9, *A, B, C*
Rare	Lymphoma, leukemia	+	++	+	+	++	+	0	0	0	0	424	10–71 to 75; Pl. 10, *D, E, F*
Rare	Hodgkin's disease	++	+	rare	++	++	+	0	0	0	0	406	11–45 to 50; Pl. 9, *D, E, F*
Primary Reticulum cell sarcoma	—	++	+	+	+	+	+	0	0	0	0	411	11–51 to 58; Pl. 7, *L;* 9, *G, H, I*
Ewing's sarcoma	Unusual	++	+	rare	++	+	rare	0	0	0	0	419	11–59 to 70; Pl. 10, *A, B, C*
Metastatic neuroblastoma	Metastatic neuroblastoma	++	+	rare	+	++	++	0	0	0	0	428	11–76 to 80; Pl. 10, *G, H, I*
Metastasis	Metastases	++	+	rare	++	++	++	rare	0	0	0	434	8–118, 12–12 to 23
Malignant (Fibrous) histiosarcoma	—	++	++	+	+	+	+	0	0	0	0	290	9–41 to 56; Pl. 7, *I*

Key: 0 = No well documented cases have been observed or reported; rare = <3% of reported cases; + = uncommon; ++ = common; +++ = exclusive

Table 6-8. Lesions that Contain Epithelial or Epithelial-Like Cells

BENIGN LESIONS		PRIMARY SITES OF INVOLVEMENT										REFERENCE IN TEXT	
		INTRAMEDULLARY						PERIOSTEAL OR JUXTACORTICAL					
		LONG AND/OR TUBULAR BONES											
Solitary	*Multiple*	*Diaphyseal*	*Metaphyseal*	*Epiphyseal*	*Flat Bones*	*Spine*	*Skull*	*Long and/or Tubular Bones*	*Flat Bones*	*Spine*	*Skull*	*Pages*	*Figures*
Epidermal inclusion cyst	—	+ (usually phalanges)	++ (usually phalanges)	+ (usually phalanges)	rare	0	+	0	0	0	0	438	12-1
LOW-GRADE MALIGNANT													
Adamantinoma of long bones	Unusual (contiguous bone)	++ (usually tibia)	+ (usually tibia)	rare (usually tibia)	0	0	0	0	0	0	0	440	12-2 to 11
FULLY MALIGNANT													
Osteosarcoma	rare	+	++	rare	+	rare	+	0	0	0	0	454, 138	12-24
Metastasis	Metastases	++	+	rare	++	++	++	rare	0	0	0	448	8-118, 12-12 to 23

Key: 0 = No well documented cases have been observed or reported; rare = <3% of reported cases; + = uncommon; ++ = common; +++ = exclusive

Table 6-9. Lesions With Unicameral Cyst, Large Vascular Spaces, Vascular-Derived Tumors, or Slitlike Spaces

		PRIMARY SITES OF INVOLVEMENT											
		INTRAMEDULLARY						PERIOSTEAL OR JUXTACORTICAL				REFERENCE IN TEXT	
BENIGN LESIONS		LONG AND/OR TUBULAR BONES											
Solitary	*Multiple*	*Diaphyseal*	*Metaphyseal*	*Epiphyseal*	*Flat Bones*	*Spine*	*Skull*	*Long and/or Tubular Bones*	*Flat Bones*	*Spine*	*Skull*	*Pages*	*Figures*
Solitary bone cyst	—	+	++	rare	+	rare	0	0	0	0	0	462	13–6 to 29
Aneurysmal bone cyst	—	+	++	+	+	++	+ (jaw)	*	*	*	* (jaw)	478	13–30 to 50
Hemangioma	Hemangio-matosis	+	+	+	+	++	++	0	0	0	0	492, 504	13–51 to 71
Pigmented synovitis (PVNS)	PVNS (contiguous bone)	0	+	++	0	rare	0	0	0	0	0	322	10–27 to 36
LOW-GRADE MALIGNANT													
Adamantinoma	Unusual (contiguous bone)	++ (usually tibia)	+ (usually tibia)	rare (usually tibia)	0	0	0	0	0	0	0	440	12–2 to 11
Hemangioendo-thelioma	Hemangioendo-thelioma	+	+	+	+	+	+	0	0	0	0	516	—
Hemangio-pericytoma	—	+	+	rare	+	+	+	0	0	0	0	509	13–72 to 76
FULLY MALIGNANT													
Angiosarcoma	uncommon	++	++	+	+	+	+	0	0	0	0	516	13–77 to 81
Telangiectatic osteosarcoma	—	+	++	rare	+	+	+	0	0	0	0	154	Pl. 5, *D, E, F*
Mesenchymal chondrosarcoma	—	+	+	0	++	rare	++	+	+	+	+	212	8–66 to 70; Pl. 6, *D, E, F*

Key: 0 = No well documented cases have been observed or reported; rare = <3% of reported cases; + = uncommon; ++ = common; +++ = exclusive

*Often results in an extensive periosteal "blowout" lesion. However, its primary site of origin appears to be intramedullary in most instances.

Table 6-10. Checklist of Historical and Physical Findings, Laboratory, Radiologic, and Histologic

Clinical and Pathologic Features	*Probable Tumors or Tumorous Entities*
History and Physical Examination	
Age (Years)	
0–2	Many lesions but considerable or peak incidence for: fracture (battered-child syndrome), osteomyelitis, Caffey's disease, Letterer-Siwe disease, metastatic neuroblastoma
2–20	Many lesions but considerable or peak incidence for: fracture ("stress," battered-child, and congenital-insensitivity-to-pain syndrome), childhood leukemias and lymphomas, intramedullary osteosarcoma, osteochondroma(s), Ewing's sarcoma, metastatic neuroblastoma, osteomyelitis, nonossifying fibroma, simple bone cyst, osteoid osteoma, fibrous dysplasia, osteoblastoma, aneurysmal bone cyst, Ollier's disease, chondroblastoma, Gaucher's disease, unifocal and multifocal eosinophilic granuloma, myositis ossificans and traumatic periostitis, chondromyxoid fibroma, cortical irregularity syndrome, pigmented villonodular synovitis, mesenchymal chondrosarcoma, hemangiomatosis
20–40	Many lesions but considerable or peak incidence for: lymphoma and leukemia, giant cell tumor of epiphyses, hyperparathyroidism, Hodgkin's disease, reticulum cell sarcoma of bone, enchondroma, metastatic melanoma, parosteal osteosarcoma, mesenchymal chondrosarcoma, adamantinoma, hemangioma
40+	Many lesions but considerable or peak incidence for: metastatic carcinoma, adult leukemias and lymphomas, myeloma, Paget's sarcoma, chondrosarcoma, fibrosarcoma, fibro- and osteosarcomatous transformation of chondrosarcoma, chordoma, malignant fibrous histiocytoma (MFH), MFH arising in bone infarcts, angiosarcoma, primary reticulum-cell sarcoma of bone, parosteal osteosarcoma
Pain	Nonspecific symptom of almost every bone tumor
Pain greatly relieved by aspirin	Usually indicative of osteoid osteoma or osteoblastoma (less commonly)
Severe trauma	Fracture, myositits ossificans, and traumatic periostitis
Repetitive trauma	Stress fracture
Family history of bone disease	Osteochondroma(s), neurofibromatosis, Paget's disease, Gaucher's disease, osteopoikilosis, Hodgkin's disease (very rare)
History of benign bone disease for many years	Paget's disease, osteomyelitis, osteochondroma(s), fibrous dysplasia, simple bone cyst, nonossifying fibroma, Gaucher's disease, hyperparathyroidism, osteoblastoma, chondroblastoma, chondromyxoid fibroma
Fever	Osteomylitis, Hodgkin's disease, Ewing's sarcoma, eosinophilic granuloma, Gaucher's disease with bone infarction
Renal stones, renal failure, ulcer, fatigue, constipation, abdominal pain, nausea, vomiting, polyuria, polydypsia	1° and 2° hyperparathyroidism
Polyuria	Hyperparathyroidism, eosinophilic granuloma (Letterer-Siwe and Hand-Schüller-Christian disease)
Exophthalmos	Orbital tumor such as embryonal rhabdomyosarcoma, neuroblastoma, mesenchymal chondrosarcoma, and Letterer-Siwe and Hand-Schüller-Christian disease

Features and the Most Common Bone Tumors or Tumorous Processes With Which They are Associated

Clinical and Pathologic Features	*Probable Tumors or Tumorous Entities*
History and Physical Examination	
Skin infiltrates	Letterer-Siwe disease, lymphomas, metastases
Brown skin macules	Neurofibromatosis, fibrous dysplasia, multiple non-ossifying fibroma syndrome
Precocious puberty	Fibrous dysplasia
Hemorrhagic diatheses	Leukemia, amyloidosis, Gaucher's disease
Skin and soft-tissue hemangiomas, including phleboliths	Skeletal hemangiomatosis, Maffucci's syndrome
Lymphadenopathy	Carcinoma, lymphoma–leukemia, Hodgkin's disease, melanoma, Letterer-Siwe and Hand-Schüller-Christian disease, metastatic sarcoma
Hepatomegaly	Carcinoma, melanoma, lymphoma–leukemia, Gaucher's disease, Letterer-Siwe and Hand-Schüller-Christian disease, metastatic sarcoma
Splenomegaly	Lymphoma–leukemia, Gaucher's disease, Letter-Siwe and Hand-Schüller-Christian disease, melanoma, metastatic sarcoma
Laboratory Features	
↑ Alkaline phosphatase	Metastases, Paget's disease, osteosarcoma, myeloma, Paget's sarcoma, leukemia
↑ Acid phosphatase	Carcinoma of prostate, Gaucher's disease
↑ Serum calcium	Myeloma, primary (1°) and secondary (2°) hyperparathyroidism, metastases
↓ Serum phosphorous	Primary hyperparathyroidism, hypophosphatemic osteomalacia secondary to benign soft-tissue tumor (sclerosing hemangioma)
↑ Serum phosphorous	Secondary hyperparathyroidism
Anemia	Leukemia, carcinoma, myeloma, Hodgkin's disease, Ewing's sarcoma, Gaucher's disease, Letterer-Siwe and Hand-Schüller-Christian disease
Leukocytosis	Leukemia–lymphoma, osteomyelitis, Ewing's sarcoma, Gaucher's disease
↑ Vanyl mandelic acid	Neuroblastoma
Monoclonal spike on electrophoresis	Myeloma, Waldenström's macroglobulinemia
Radiologic Features	
Solitary bone lesion	Most 1° bone tumors, less common in metastatic carcinoma, melanoma, neuroblastoma
Multiple bone lesions	Metastases, multiple fibrous cortical defects, lymphoma–leukemia, Paget's disease, Ollier's disease, osteochondromas, fibrous dysplasia, Ewing's sarcoma, neuroblastoma, hyperparathyroidism, multifocal osteosarcoma, eosinophilic granuloma (all types), Gaucher's disease, osteopoikilosis, bone infarcts, giant cell tumor (very rare), fibrosarcoma (very rare), hemangiomatosis, angiosarcoma, nonossifying fibromas
Predominantly blastic	Metastases (prostate and breast), osteosarcoma, osteoblastoma, parosteal osteosarcoma, bone infarcts
Purely lytic	Metastases, many 1° bone tumors, myeloma, hyperparathyroidism
Mixed lytic and blastic	Metastases, lymphoma–leukemia, osteomyelitis, Paget's, osteosarcoma, fibrous dysplasia, chondrosarcoma, osteoblastoma, bone infarct, Hodgkin's disease
Solitary lytic of epiphysis	Giant cell tumor, chondroblastoma, chondrosarcoma, osteomyelitis, pigmented villonodular synovitis, rheumatoid arthritis, tuberculosis, gout, enchondroma (rare), osteosarcoma (very rare), coccidiodomycosis (rare)

(Continued)

Table 6-10. Checklist of Historical and Physical Findings, Laboratory, Radiologic, and Histologic Features and the Most Common Bone Tumors or Tumorous Processes With Which They are Associated (Continued)

Clinical and Pathologic Features	*Probable Tumors or Tumorous Entities*
Radiologic Features	
Lytic lesions of two contiguous epiphyses	Rheumatoid arthritis, tuberculosis, gout, pigmented villonodular synovitis, coccidiodomycosis, angiosarcoma
Expansive lytic and/or "blowout" lesions	Fibrous dysplasia, hyperparathyroidism, giant cell tumor, chondrosarcoma, aneurysmal bone cyst, myeloma, metastases, (kidney, thyroid), osteoblastoma
Cystic lytic lesion, tibial shaft	Fibrous dysplasia, adamantinoma, simple bone cyst, metastases
Cystic lytic lesions of tibia and fibula or radius and ulna of one limb with no other affected bone	Adamantinoma, invasive soft tissue tumor such as aggressive fibromatosis
Lytic lesion sacrum	Chordoma, giant cell tumor, metastases, chondrosarcoma, sclerosing lipoma (very rare), neurilemmoma (very rare)
"Cumulus" cloud fluffs	Incipient osteosarcoma, osteosarcoma, fibrous dysplasia, osteoblastoma, stress fracture
"Ground-glass" appearance	Fibrous dysplasia, ostoblastoma, osteosarcoma
Thickened trabeculae along lines of stress	Osteoporosis, Paget's disease, hemangioma, hemangiomatosis
Spotty calcifications	Enchondroma, bone infarct, chondrosarcoma, chondroblastoma, osteochondroma
Spotty calcifications and prominent area of lysis	Chondrosarcoma arising in enchondroma, sarcoma arising in bone infarct, fibrosarcomatous and osteosarcomatous transformation of chondrosarcoma
Punched-out lytic holes in multiple bones	Myeloma, metastasis, Gaucher's disease, neuroblastoma, hyperparathyroidism, all forms of multifocal eosinophilic granuloma
Metaphyseal bands of radiolucency	Leukemia, chronic debilitating disease, such as Letterer-Siwe disease, malnutrition, and others.
Codman's triangle(s)	Osteosarcoma, malignant 1° and 2° bone tumors, osteomyelitis, aneurysmal bone cyst
"Sunburst" periosteal reactions	Osteosarcoma, hemangioma of skull, carcinoma of prostate, other carcinomas (rare)
"Onion skinning"	Ewing's sarcoma, osteomyelitis, osteosarcoma, Gaucher's disease, eosinophilic granuloma, acute bone infarcts
Bone "expansion"	Usually benign lesions such as aneurysmal bone cyst, osteoblastoma, fibrous dysplasia, Ollier's disease. Renal and thyroid carcinoma, myeloma, chondrosarcoma, *not* osteosarcoma or untreated Ewing's sarcoma
Border of sclerosis around lesion	Benign lesions, malignant tumors arising in benign
Moth-eaten to permeative destruction	1° and 2° malignant bone tumors, osteomyelitis, eosinophilic granuloma, metastases, reticulum-cell sarcoma
Cortical erosion with soft-tissue mass	Usually malignant 1° or 2° bone tumors, infections, giant-cell tumor, aneurysmal bone cyst, chondromyxoid fibroma, parosteal malignancies, parosteal chondroma, eosinophilic granuloma (rare), chondroblastoma (rare)
Erosion of distal phalangeal tufts, medial scalloping of metaphyses, loss of lamina dura, cortical erosion canals	Hyperparathyroidism

Table 6-10. Checklist of Historical and Physical Findings, Laboratory, Radiologic, and Histologic Features and the Most Common Bone Tumors or Tumorous Processes With Which They are Associated (Continued)

Clinical and Pathologic Features	*Probable Tumors or Tumorous Entities*
Histological Features	
Lesions characterized by:	
Lamellar bone	Refer to Table 6-1.
Osteoid and woven bone	Refer to Table 6-2.
Cartilage	Refer to Table 6-3.
Spindle cells	Refer to Table 6-4.
Giant cells	Refer to Table 6-5.
Myxoid tissue	Refer to Table 6-6.
Round cells and/or histiocytes	Refer to Table 6-7.
Epithelial cells	Refer to Table 6-8.
Cyst, cyst-like, and vascular spaces	Refer to Table 6-9.
Diffuse infiltration or involvement of marrow between host bone trabeculae	Possible in all high-grade malignant tumors, Paget's disease, osteomyelitis, hyperparathyroidism, Gaucher's disease, eosinophilic granuloma, fracture healing
Cartilage lobules surrounded by cuffs of host lamellar bone	Enchondroma
Dead fat, dystrophic calcification	Bone infarct (malignant fibrous histiocytoma, fibro- and osteosarcoma arising in bone infarcts)
Prominent osteoblastic rimming	Usually in benign conditions or reactive bone formation to benign or malignant tumors. On rare occasion reported in parosteal osteosarcoma
"Pear"- or "carrot" -shaped cells in a round-cell tumor of bone	Neuroblastoma, metastatic oat cell carcinoma
Glycogen within the cytoplasm of a round cell tumor	Ewing's sarcoma (most cases), neuroblastoma (some), lymphoma (some), osteomyelitis (some). *Not* seen in reticulum-cell sarcoma
Reticulin around each tumor cell	Reticulum cell sarcoma, malignant fibrous histiocytoma (on occasion), glomus tumor, chondroblastoma, hemangiopericytoma, metastatic leiomyosarcoma, and endolymphatic stromal myosis of uterus (both very rare)
Fat in tumor cells	Malignant fibrous histiocytoma, liposarcoma, metastatic hypernephroma, osteosarcoma (rare), other sarcomas (rare)
Malignant tumor seen in association with benign precursor lesions	Paget's disease, Ollier's disease, enchondroma, radiation osteitis, giant cell tumor, osteochondromas, fibrous dysplasia, osteoblastoma, chondroblastoma, nonossifying fibroma, bone infarct, osteopoikilosis (very rare)
Acinar pattern	Carcinoma
Mucin production	Carcinoma, chordoma
Melanin pigment	Melanoma
Light polarizable crystals	Gout, pseudogout
Histiocytes with "crumpled paper" appearance	Gaucher's disease

(Continued)

Table 6-10. Checklist of Historical and Physical Findings, Laboratory, Radiologic, and Histologic Features and the Most Common Bone Tumors or Tumorous Processes With Which They are Associated (Continued)

Clinical and Pathologic Features	*Probable Tumors or Tumorous Entities*
Histological Features	
Physaliphorous cells	Chordoma
Cholesterol clefts	Usually benign tumors such as nonossifying fibroma, chondroblastoma, eosinophilic granuloma, pigmented villonodular synovitis, giant cell tumor of tendon sheath, bone infarct
Vascular invasion	Fully malignant lesions, giant-cell tumor
Lymph node involvement	Fully malignant 1° and 2° bone tumors (particularly lymphomas, melanomas, and carcinomas), the histiocytoses (particularly Letterer-Siwe and Hand-Schüller-Christian disease), infections (bacterial, fungus, and tuberculous), sarcoidosis

with each feature. This table represents a condensation of those features and tumors discussed in the text and is especially helpful in the formulation of a reasonable differential or specific diagnosis. The left-hand column can be used by the reader as a checklist to help ensure that certain features which may be of importance to diagnosis have not been inadvertantly left out of the data-gathering process. Obviously, the table cannot list every feature or variation for each tumor. The diseases in the right-hand column are listed in order of approximate frequency. The feature of multiple bone lesions by itself is, on a purely statistical basis, associated more commonly with metastasis than with multiple enchondromatosis or polyostotic fibrous dysplasia, for example. Although one would never diagnose metastatic disease simply on the basis of multiple bone lesions, one should certainly entertain such a diagnosis when formulating a differential list.

INTRAOSSEOUS TUMORS THAT PRODUCE OSTEOID, WOVEN, AND/OR LAMELLAR BONE

7

INTRODUCTION

This chapter deals with those bone tumors (nonperiosteal in origin) that are involved in the production of osteoid, woven, and/or lamellar bone. There are two hamartomatous processes characterized by only an abnormal proliferation of bone. This bone is predominantly lamellar and there are no stromal abnormalities. The two entities are the bone island or enostosis (solitary and multiple forms) and the osteoma of skull. The primary intraosseous bone tumors characterized by the production of osteoid and/or woven bone, in every instance, include three benign tumors—the osteoid osteoma, osteoblastoma, and fibrous dysplasia—and one malignant tumor, the osteosarcoma. These lesions also coexist with an abnormal proliferation of intertrabecular or stromal elements, compared to that found in normal adult bone. Variable quantities of osteoid and woven bone may be seen in the cyst walls of the aneurysmal bone cyst and the simple bone cyst, the giant cell tumor of hyperparathyroidism, the neoplastic epiphyseal giant cell tumor, and even within the cartilagenous lobules of the chondrosarcoma. But, this chapter will discuss only those conditions in which bone production is crucial to diagnosis. This includes those benign and malignant tumors in which the presence of bone is not usually encountered; but when these tissues are seen in considerable quantity may result in an incorrect diagnosis. Also treated are those benign bone productive lesions, such as unsuspected stress fracture, in which the ominous nature of the cellular proliferation may suggest an osteogenic sarcoma.

An example of a low-grade malignant tumor that may contain significant quantities of osteoid and woven bone is the giant cell tumor. It is not well known, but up to 40 per cent of these tumors contain foci of osteoid and woven bone.[3] In some cases these tissues appear at the margin of the advancing tumor and represent reactive host bone. In some cases, however, these tissues are buried deep in the lesional tissue and may give the impression that they are an integral part of the neoplastic process. Because of this little known fact, serious errors in diagnosis have been made, such as mistaking the giant cell tumor for an osteoblastoma, or more disastrously, an osteogenic sarcoma with "prominent giant cell reaction."

There is no area in the field of bone tumor pathology more fraught with the dangers of serious misdiagnosis than the lesions covered in this chapter.

Essential to interpretation of bone-producing tumors is a basic comprehension of the normal processes of bone development and fracture repair. The skeleton is composed of fat, vascular, neural, hematopoietic, and fibrous tissue, cartilage, and bone matrix and the cells that produce them and maintain their structural vitality.

The bone or *osseous tissue* of our skeleton is composed of four basic components:

1. Collagen fibers
2. Cement substance (mucopolysaccharides or proteoglycans)
3. Mineral (hydroxyapatite)

(Text continues on p. 84.)

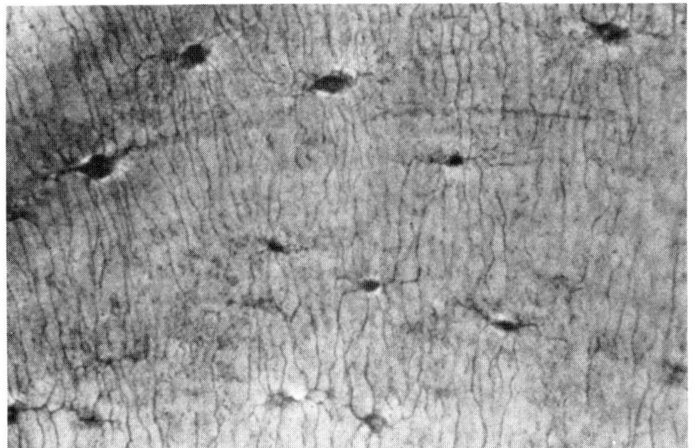

FIG. 7-1

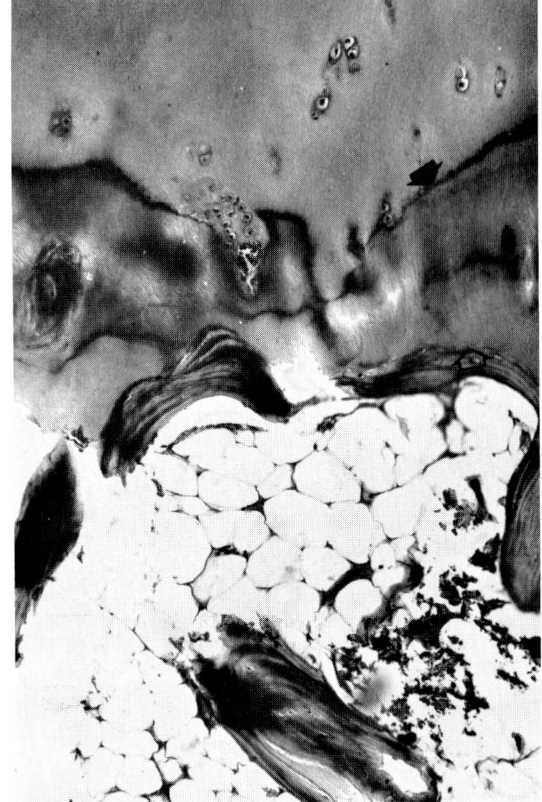

FIG. 7-2

Types of Bone and Calcified Cartilage

FIG. 7-1. Osteocyte canaliculi. Osteocytes maintain their viability in a heavily calcified tissue by means of cytoplasmic extensions from one cell to another (picrothionine stain).

FIG. 7-2. Tidemark of articular cartilage. Chondrocytes do not possess cytoplasmic extensions from cell to cell, so that when trapped in heavily calcified tissues, they undergo necrosis. The chondrocytes in the articular cartilage (upper part) show viable nuclei. There is an absence of chondrocytic nuclei in the calcified tidemark zone (delineated by open and closed arrows), where the subchondral bone and calcified cartilage enmesh (X100).

FIG. 7-3. Lamellar bone, single trabecula. (*A*) Ordinary light. (*B*) Polarized light (X300).

FIG. 7-4. Osteoid, woven, and lamellar bone. (*A*) Osteoid is lightly stained and contrasts sharply with the more hematoxyphilic bone tissues. (*B*) shows the same field under polarized light. Note that the osteoid and woven bone contains collagen in a "basket weave" or "crisscross" pattern and contrasts sharply to the lamellar pattern seen in mature bone. The osteoid and woven bone is being produced by an osteosarcoma. The lamellar bone is a trapped host bone spicule (X250).

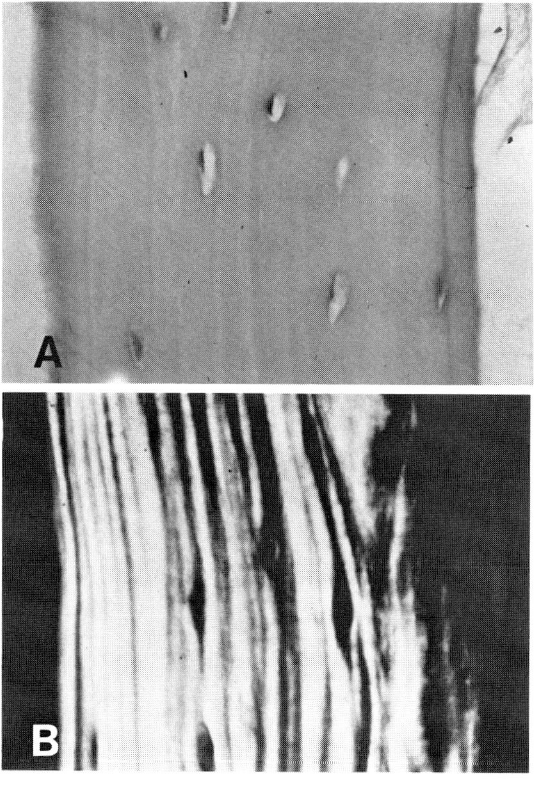

FIG. 7-3

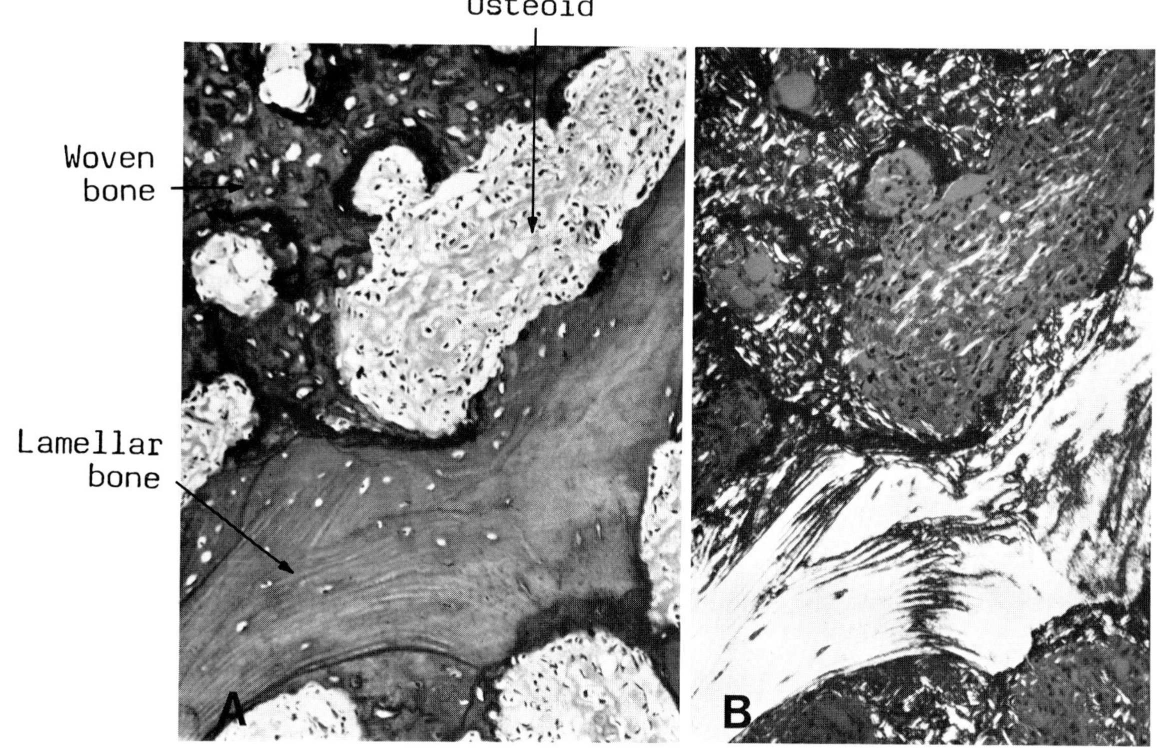

FIG. 7-4

4. Osteoblasts and osteocytes

All of the matrix as it is first laid down by osteoblasts is unmineralized and by definition *osteoid.* During the active phase of bone deposition the *osteoblasts* (bone-forming cells) are plump with conspicuous nuclei, deeply staining eosinophilic cytoplasm, and often have a prominent golgi zone and distinct cell borders; in the inactive phase of bone deposition they are flattened with an oval to spindly nucleus and light pink cytoplasm. This is not to imply that the flattened osteoblast is also inactive but rather that it has entered a phase where its unique role as a producer of osteoid is no longer its task. Its other physiologic functions, including mineral homeostasis, may be quite active. As soon as the osteoblast becomes trapped or surrounded on all sides by the matrix it produced, it is defined as an *osteocyte.* The osteocytes maintain communications one to another through fine cytoplasmic extensions known as *canaliculi.* Normally, it is not possible to see these canaliculi with ordinary hematoxylin and eosin (H and E) staining, but they stand out brilliantly with the use of picrothionine staining (Fig. 7–1). The function of the canaliculi is to pass nutrients from the surface to the more deeply situated cells. This unique adaptation permits the osteocytes to live in densely calcified tissue, where other cells could not survive, since highly calcified tissues do not permit sufficient nutrients needed for cell life to pass this barrier. (Chondrocytes, for example, do not possess this structural adaptation of canaliculi.) After cartilage undergoes significant calcification, the cells become necrotic. Under normal physiologic conditions, this occurs in the vacuolating or calcifying zone of the growing epiphyseal plate and at the calcified junction of the articular cartilage known as the "tidemark" zone (Fig. 7–2). This zone abuts on and joins to the underlying subchondral bone trabeculae.

The mineralized matrix is organized into either *cortical compact bone* or *intramedullary trabecular (spongy or cancellous) bone.* Irrespective of whether the bone is arranged into trabeculae or into cortical bone, it is evident on microscopic examination using polarized light that there are two distinct types of bone tissue. In one, the collagen fibers are arranged in definite layers or lamellae. This bone is the predominant type present in the normal adult human skeleton and is referred to as *lamellar bone.* The collagen lamellae lie parallel to the long axis of the trabecula; this can be seen on routine H and E section (Fig. 7–3, *A*) but more dramatically, with polarized light (Fig. 7–3, *B*). Note on the polarized illustration that individual lamellae are bright, while alternate lamellae are dark (extinguished). The explanation for this finding is that collagen fibers have an oriented periodicity with the capability of rotating polarized light. Those fibers that run perpendicular to the plane of polarized light will appear refractile or bright; those that run parallel to the plane of polarized light will appear dark. If the lamellae of an individual trabecula could be dissected, it would be apparent that each lamella is analogous to a sheet of paper in which all of the collagen fibers run in one direction. The same is true of the adjacent lamella or sheet, with the exception that each runs at a right angle to the adjacent one. Therefore, when one sheet is polarized, it will polarize opposite to its adjacent sheet. The reason that the collagen fiber orientation appears as a line rather than a sheet in Figures 7–3 and 7–4 is due, of course, to the fact that our view is basically two dimensional, since our section is only 7 μ thick. If this book were held on its end, the edges of the pages would assume a linear configuration when viewed from a biplanar system. Our ordinary light microscopic view of the world of tissues is similarly two dimensional.

The function of this unique arrangement of collagen fibers is that it greatly adds to the strength of the bone under compressive load and shear forces. In mature cortical bone, the collagen lamellae are arranged in concentric rings or tubes around vascular spaces, the so-called *haversian systems.*

The second type of bone is called *woven bone* (fiber or nonlamellar). Phylogenetically, it is the older or more primitive type of osseous tissue. The woven, "basket-weave," or "crisscross" pattern of collagen, though appreciable on H and E section with transmitted light (Fig. 7–4, *A*), is much clearer with polarized light (Fig. 7–4, *B*). This bone has much less strength, compared with lamellar bone. The bone of our skeleton begins as the woven type. Within the first few years of childhood, it is gradually replaced by lamellar bone. Woven bone usually forms within 3 weeks from inception of an osteoblastic process, such as callus or myositis ossificans. It takes many weeks before lamellar bone is produced from the inception of the newly stimulated osteoblastic process. Mature lamellar bone and marrow fat is seen in the normal adult skeleton and begins to emerge from callus after approximately 7 or more weeks from inception. Fully mature lamellar bone is strongly birefringent by polarized light. Less mature or immature lamellar bone is characterized by less intense birefringence, thinner lamellae, and often a greater degree of undulation of each lamella. Fully mature lamellar bone is seen in the normal adult bone, the enostoses, osteoma of skull, and the late healing phases of callus, myositis ossificans, and traumatic periostitis, among others.

Woven bone is seen in the fetal skeleton, osteogenesis imperfecta, early callus, myositis ossificans and traumatic periostitis, the nidus of the osteoid osteoma, the lesional tissue of osteoblastoma, fibrous dysplasia, Paget's disease, osteosarcoma, as a "reactive" process to many other benign and malignant tumors, or in any lesion in which bone is being produced rapidly. Immature lamellar bone can be seen at some stage of development of most benign bone productive tumors and occasionally, in malignant bone productive tumor areas. The usual exceptions to these rules include the osteoid osteoma, osteoblastoma, and fibrous dysplasia. Although they are benign woven bone producing tumors, rarely are they seen in association with lamellar bone production by the tumor tissues themselves. The irritative effects of these benign tumors may, however, cause the surrounding host bone or periosteum to produce abnormal quantities of bone, including the lamellar type. In unusual instances, the intramedullary osteosarcoma is associated with lamellar bone production within the tumor itself. Less than fully mature lamellar bone may rarely be seen as a component of the lesional tissue in very dense bone productive osteosarcoma, the so-called "sclerosing" osteosarcoma. The presence, therefore, of lamellar bone production by the tumor tissues themselves is usually, but not necessarily, a sign of benignancy. A surer sign of benignancy, rarely violated, is the following: if it can be ascertained that the tumor tissues themselves are maturing to lamellar bone and marrow fat, the lesion is benign. The usual tumorous processes in which this occurs include callus, myositis ossificans, and traumatic periostitis. Note that all three are trauma-related processes of the mesenchyme.

On the other hand, it should be reemphasized that although the maturation of bone to the mature lamellar type and marrow fat is almost always an indication of benignancy, the absence of this finding within the substance of a lesion does not mean that it is malignant. For example, in the first few weeks of myositis ossificans, callus, and traumatic periostitis, and even in the late phases of fibrous dysplasia, osteoid osteoma, and osteoblastoma, there may not be any development of these recognizably mature, benign osseous tissues.

Rare exceptions to the general rule that maturation to lamellar bone and marrow fat signifies benignancy include the following examples. (1) The association of a slow-growing malignant tumor with "reactive" induction of trapped or surrounding host bone or soft-tissue mesenchyme to form lamellar bone and marrow fat. (2) The subsequent malignant transformation of a benign osseous productive lesion that had matured into lamellar bone and marrow fat. For example, there are at least two recorded instances of sarcomatous transformation of myositis ossificans left in-situ for 45 years in one case[1] and the other, after 16 years.[2]

BENIGN TUMORS OR TUMORLIKE PROCESSES

SOLITARY ENOSTOSIS (BONE ISLAND)

An enostosis is a completely benign, indolent, asymptomatic, roundish, lesion between 2 mm. and 2 cm. in size located in the medullary canal. It is composed of mature lamellar bone frequently containing haversian systems, thereby resembling an "island" of misplaced cortical bone (Figs. 7-6 and 7-7). Under normal circumstances a bone island would not be seen in surgical pathology, because it is a completely innocent and asymptomatic lesion. But, if there is pain originating from the local soft tissues, joint space, or other bone lesion and radiographs are taken, an enostosis will appear as a "spot" in the bone (Fig. 7-5). This "spot" could be mistaken for a solitary metastasis or an osteoid osteoma, prompting biopsy or excision.

If the microscopic features of an enostosis (Figs. 7-6 and 7-7) are examined more closely, it becomes apparent that the surrounding bone spicules blend imperceptibly into the enostosis. The surrounding host bone shows no evidence of reactive sclerosis, as would be expected in an osteoid osteoma. If a radiograph (Fig. 7-5) of a bone island is examined we see, as in the microscopic section, that the host bone spicules blend into the dense enostotic mass along its periphery and that the surrounding host bone is perfectly normal in appearance. No other lesion has these radiographic features. If the standard radiographs do not show the peripheral blending into the lesion clearly, tomograms or bone scans should resolve the difficulty. A reactive lesion such as a metastasis will appear "hot" on scan; an enostosis, however, is a quiescent lesion and should appear very similar to the surrounding normal bone.

OSTEOPOIKILOSIS (MULTIPLE ENOSTOSES OR "SPOTTED BONE" DISEASE)

This is a rare hereditary (autosomal dominant) benign disorder characterized radiologically and histologically by multiple lesions, each of which is indistinguishable from the solitary enostosis (Figs. 7–8 and 7–9). The lesions are asymptomatic. The condition may also be associated with multiple osteochondromatosis and a tendency to keloid formation.

Osteoma of Skull

Bony excrescences of the skull are comparatively rare. They are seen in relation to the nasal sinuses and to the vault of the skull (Fig. 7–10). Most examples of this entity are solitary. If the lesion is on the vault of the skull, there are usually no symptoms and it is removed for cosmetic reasons alone. If the lesion is arising in a bone adjacent to a paranasal sinus, symptoms related to sinusitis may occur. Involvement of the orbit may lead to proptosis and blurring of vision.

Microscopically, these lesions are usually composed of condensed masses of mature lamellar bone, although variable quantities of woven bone may be admixed (Figs. 7–11 and 7–12). The stroma may either be fat or fibrofatty, with variable amounts of vascular and hematopoietic elements.

Gardner and Richards described an autosomal dominant condition (Gardner's syndrome) characterized by the association of multiple osteomas of the skull and mandible. If the long bones are involved, they show irregular cortical thickening resembling the "candle-wax drippings" of melorheostosis. Other lesions include multiple sebaceous cysts, desmoid tumors, skin fibromas, and colonic polyposis. The gene defects have variable expressivity, since not all of the components of the syndrome are present in every affected individual.

Predominantly Woven Bone and Osteoid-Producing Tumors

The remaining benign bone-producing tumors are characterized by osteoid and woven-bone production. These conditions include stress fracture, osteoid osteoma, osteoblastoma, and fibrous dysplasia. Although stress fracture may proceed to lamellar bone production in its phase of resolution, lamellar bone is rarely, if ever, seen before 7 weeks from its inception. Lamellar bone production is rarely, if ever, seen within the lesional fissures of osteoid osteoma, osteoblastoma, or fibrous dysplasia.

Stress Fracture

Importance

Stress or fatigue fractures may result in pain and striking radiologic and pathologic features which, if unrecognized by the clinician and/or pathologist, can and have resulted in the diagnoses of osteogenic or other sarcoma.

Pathogenesis

Todd, *et al*[9]., in a study of arthritic femoral heads, showed by stereomicroscopy, dissection, and tetracycline labeling that individual trabeculae may fracture. Each trabecular fracture in turn may produce its own individual globular accretion of callus (Fig. 7–13). These elegant anatomical studies suggest that the usual fractures of bone as we normally see them, and their repair tissues, is but a gross reflection of the processes which may occur in an individual unit of bone, namely a single trabecula. Since isolated trabecula may undergo the same processes of fracture and callus repair as does the entire bone, it is possible that every day we may be experiencing microfractures without radiological evidence or clinical symptomatology. If a bone is subjected over a short period of time to repetitive stresses, to which it is unaccustomed, it is reasonable to assume that individual trabecular fractures occur, and that if their number

(*Text continues on p. 91.*)

Solitary Enostosis

FIG. 7–5. Note the gradual blending of the surrounding host trabecular bone (*arrows*) into the dense, irregularly outlined enostosis. This feature, in addition of the lack of reactive bone surrounding the lesion, is characteristic of the enostosis.

FIG. 7–6. Trabeculae of the host bone blend into the bone island (H and E, X10).

FIG. 7–7. On high power, the lesion is composed of compact lamellar bone with haversian systems resembling misplaced cortical bone (H and E, partial polarized light, X40).

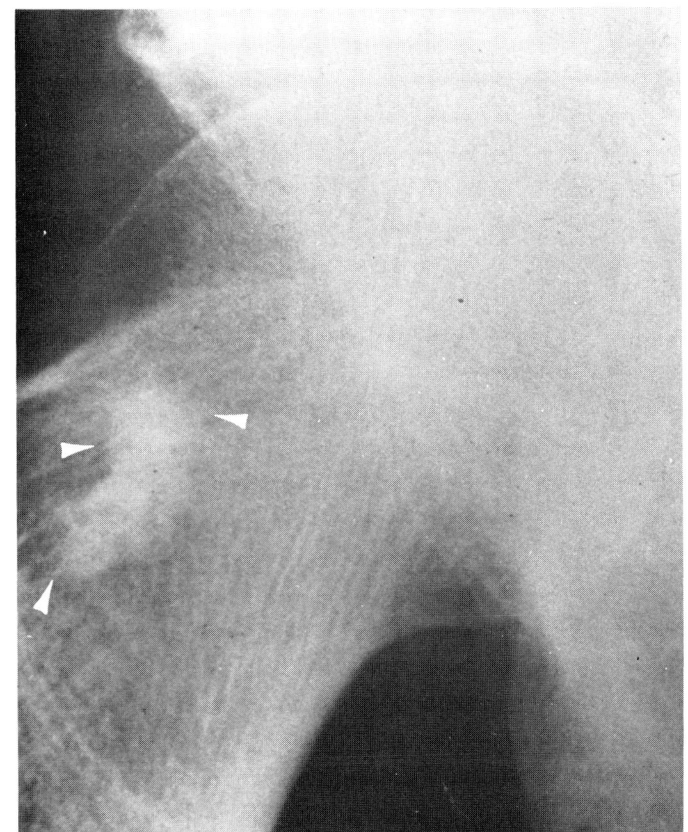

FIG. 7-5

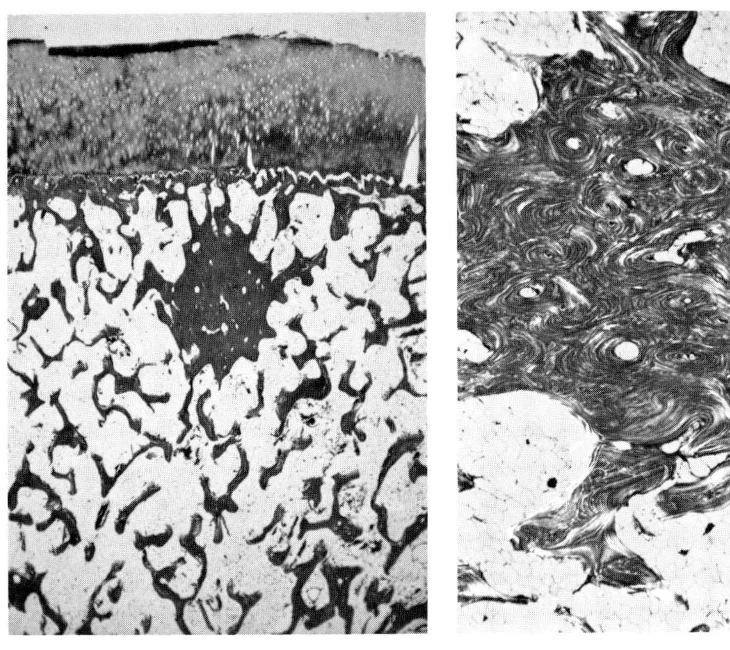

FIG. 7-6

FIG. 7-7

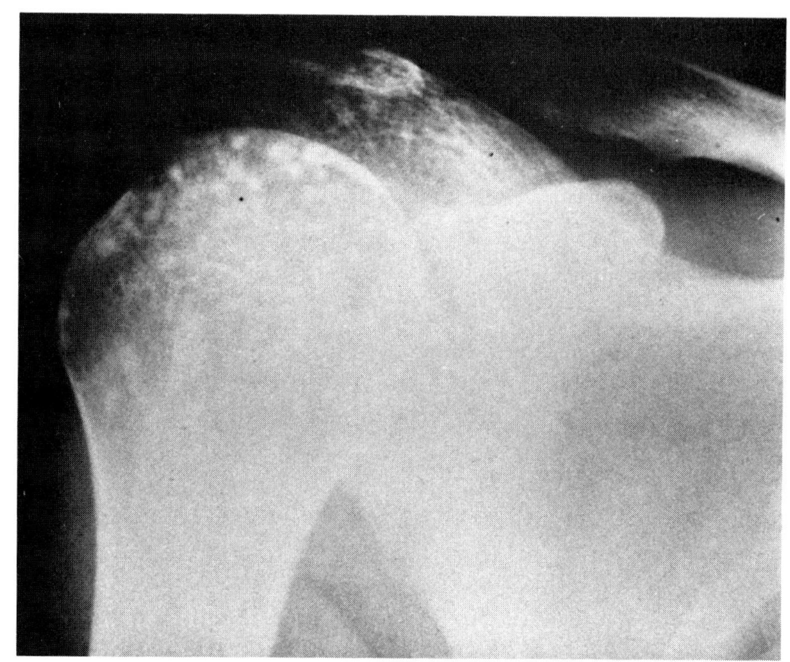

FIG. 7-8

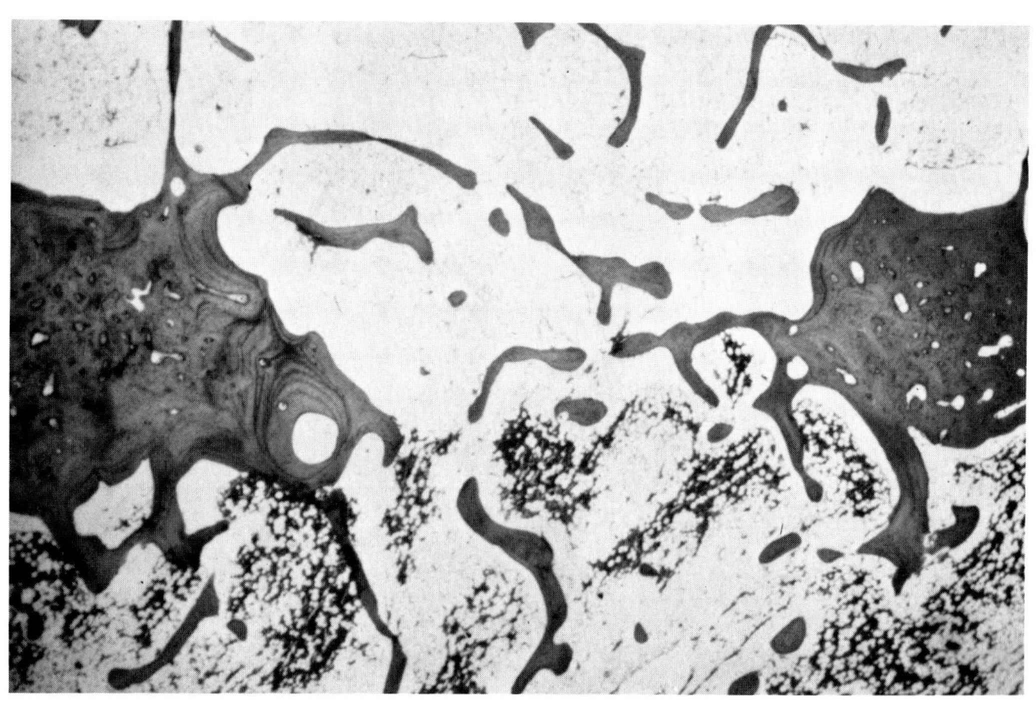

FIG. 7-9

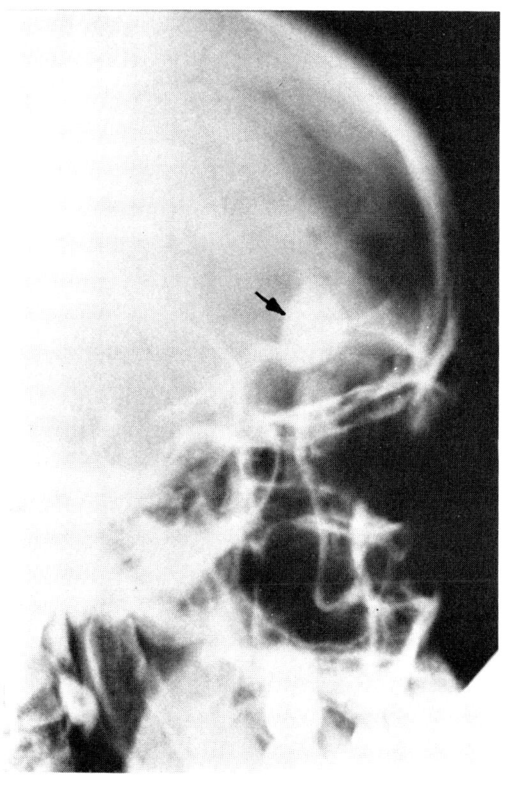

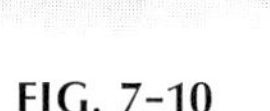

FIG. 7-10

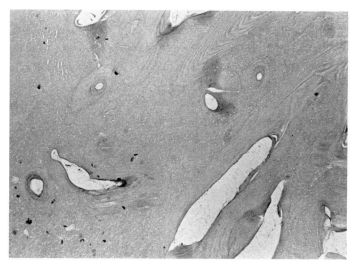

FIG. 7-11

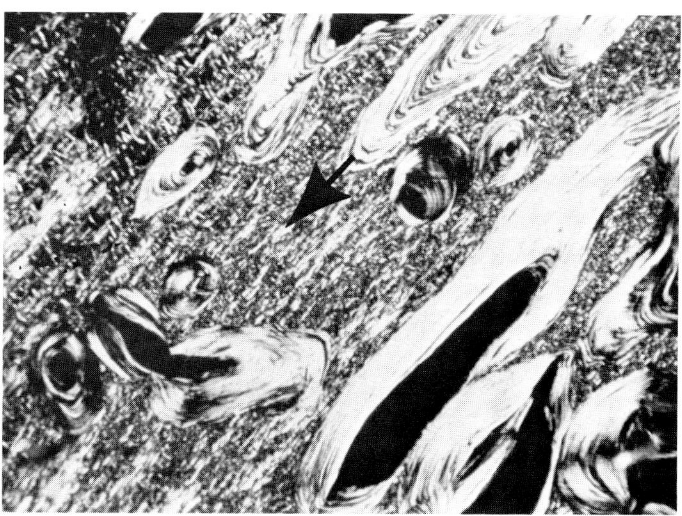

FIG. 7-12

Multiple Enostoses (Osteopoikilosis)

FIG. 7-8. Multiple bone islands characterize osteopoikilosis.

FIG. 7-9. Except for their multiplicity, the bone islands of osteopoikilosis are indistinguishable from the solitary enostosis (H and E, X20).

Osteoma of Skull

FIG. 7-10. The osteoma of the skull is dense and well circumscribed (*arrow*).

FIG. 7-11. The osteoma is composed of dense, benign bone (H and E, X40).

FIG. 7-12. Polarized light shows a mixture of lamellar and woven bone (*arrow*) and haversian systems.

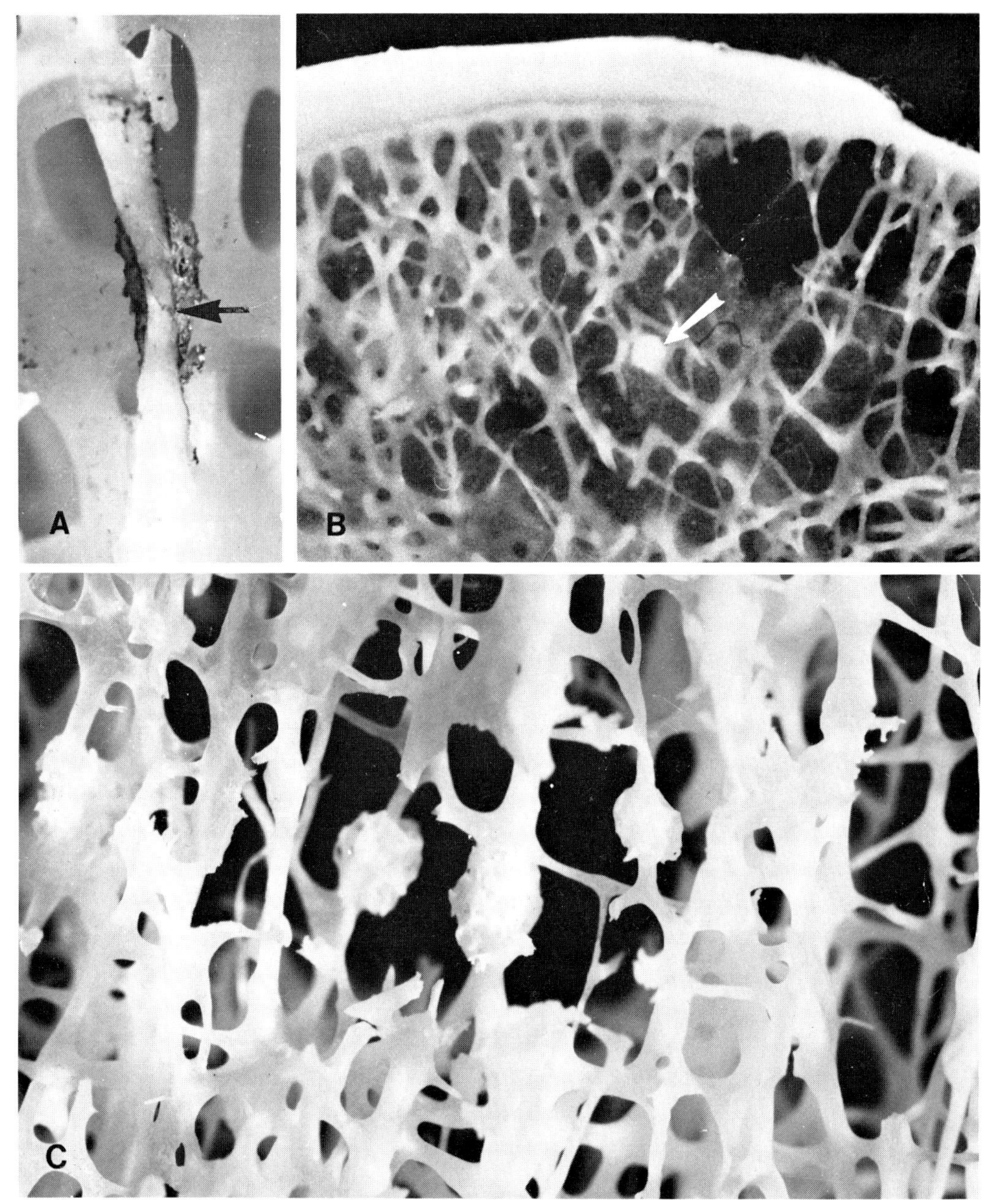

FIG. 7-13

Isolated Trabecular Fractures

FIG. 7-13. (*A*) Fracture line of a trabecula (*arrow*) after removal of a portion of the surrounding callus and India ink impregnation. (*B*) Gross photograph of macerated femoral head showing an individual trabecular callus (*arrow*). (*C*) Several callosities are shown in this high-power illustration of a macerated specimen of a femoral head. (Todd, R., Freeman, M., and Pirie, C.: J. Bone Joint Surg., *54B:* 723, 1972)

exceeds a certain limit, gross fatigue fracture will result (the so-called stress fracture).

Sites of Involvement

Stress fractures most frequently occur in the bones of normal patients who have undertaken strenuous activities to which they are unaccustomed. Usually they occur in the second or third metatarsal ("march" or "soldiers" fracture) or tibia and fibula (from jumping or long distance running).[8] Rare sites include the obturator ring (from repeated stooping), lower ribs (from chronic coughing), first rib (from carrying heavy pack), middle ribs ("Honeymoon" fracture), cervicodorsal spinous processes ("clay shovelers" fracture and golf players), ulna (from handling a pitchfork), calcaneus and metatarsal sesamoids (prolonged standing), and lamina fracture of lower lumbar spine, also known as spondyolysis (may be seen in $33\frac{1}{3}$ per cent of teenage Judo athletes).

Of course, fracture may also occur in abnormal bones consequent to stresses that normal bones would probably withstand. Those primary bone diseases most prone to stress fracture include osteogenesis imperfecta, osteoporosis, osteopetrosis, fibrous dysplasia, Paget's disease and, of course, all malignancies.

Radiological Features

Symptomatic stress fractures are usually only a hairline crack in the bone, where the fracture ends remain opposed without deviation. The patient experiences pain in the affected region and if standard radiographs are taken at this time there may be no evidence of a fracture line unless tomograms are ordered. However, if the patient presents to a physician 3 or more weeks after the fracture, striking bony proliferation of the periosteum and often the shaft of the bone is present. The lesion in the metatarsal shown in Fig. 7–15 would be easily recognized by the medical community as periosteal stress fracture callus, even though the shaft does not yet show a striking increase in radiodensity or a clear-cut fracture line.

On occasion, however, the exuberance of stress fracture that occurs in the midshaft of the tibia may suggest a malignant tumor (Fig. 7–16). If the radiograph of the midshaft shows characteristic features of a stress fracture, namely a horizontal or rectangular shape zone of sclerosis, (this suggests that there is a central fracture line), a biopsy need not be performed if the following measures are taken: an athletic or stressful history is obtained, tomograms taken to show a fracture line, and radiographs repeated to show the resolution of the process. The tomogram should be taken to show an obvious crack (Fig. 7–16, *right*) if not evident on the standard film.

Eccentric or concentric periosteal new bone is usually seen in association with stress fracture. If it is absent and tomograms show no fracture line, the blastic lesion of the shaft may well represent another condition, possibly the osteosarcoma. Compare Figure 7–16 with Figure 7–43, *A*, which shows a small, fluffy blastic mass in the midshaft of the femur. Note that it shows no periosteal new bone and the tomogram shows no fracture line (Fig. 7–41, *B*). Biopsy was considered necessary to establish a diagnosis since the lesion did not conform to the expected features of the usual stress fracture. The tumor was indeed an osteogenic sarcoma (see p. 116 and Figs. 7–43 to 7–46) and the patient died $2\frac{1}{2}$ months later with massive pulmonary metastases.

Unusually, a stress fracture will show neither a fracture line on tomogram nor periosteal new bone. Such cases may show only a rectangular or more irregular cumulus cloud blastic focus on radiograph. Since these cases cannot be adequately delineated from other lesions, including the osteosarcoma, it is incumbent upon the judgment of the involved clinicians, based upon their assessment of the patient's history and careful scrutiny of the radiologic findings, to elect for immediate biopsy or to follow the lesion with serial radiographs, to ensure its benignancy. If the lesion shows gradual resolution within weeks to months it is safe to assume that it was an unusual stress fracture that presented with less than diagnostic radiographic features.

In summary, the radiologic components of a typical stress fracture 3 or more weeks old are:

1. A horizontal, linear, or rectangular bony sclerotic process, usually within the diaphysis (rarely, metaphysis) and generally no more than 3 cm. in length. Incipient osteosarcomas are generally more than 4 to 5 cm. in length at initial presentation.
2. Fluffy, concentric, or eccentric periosteal new bone in most cases.
3. A fracture line evident on tomogram. However, the fracture line may no longer be present if callus completely bridges the fracture gap.

In contrast, fluffy, confluent "cumulus cloudlike" densities evident within the medulla, with or without the production of periosteal new bone, and the absence of a fracture line, along with clinical symptoms, could represent a process such as osteosarcoma, osteoblastoma, cartilage tumor, or bone infarct.

(*Text continues on p. 94.*)

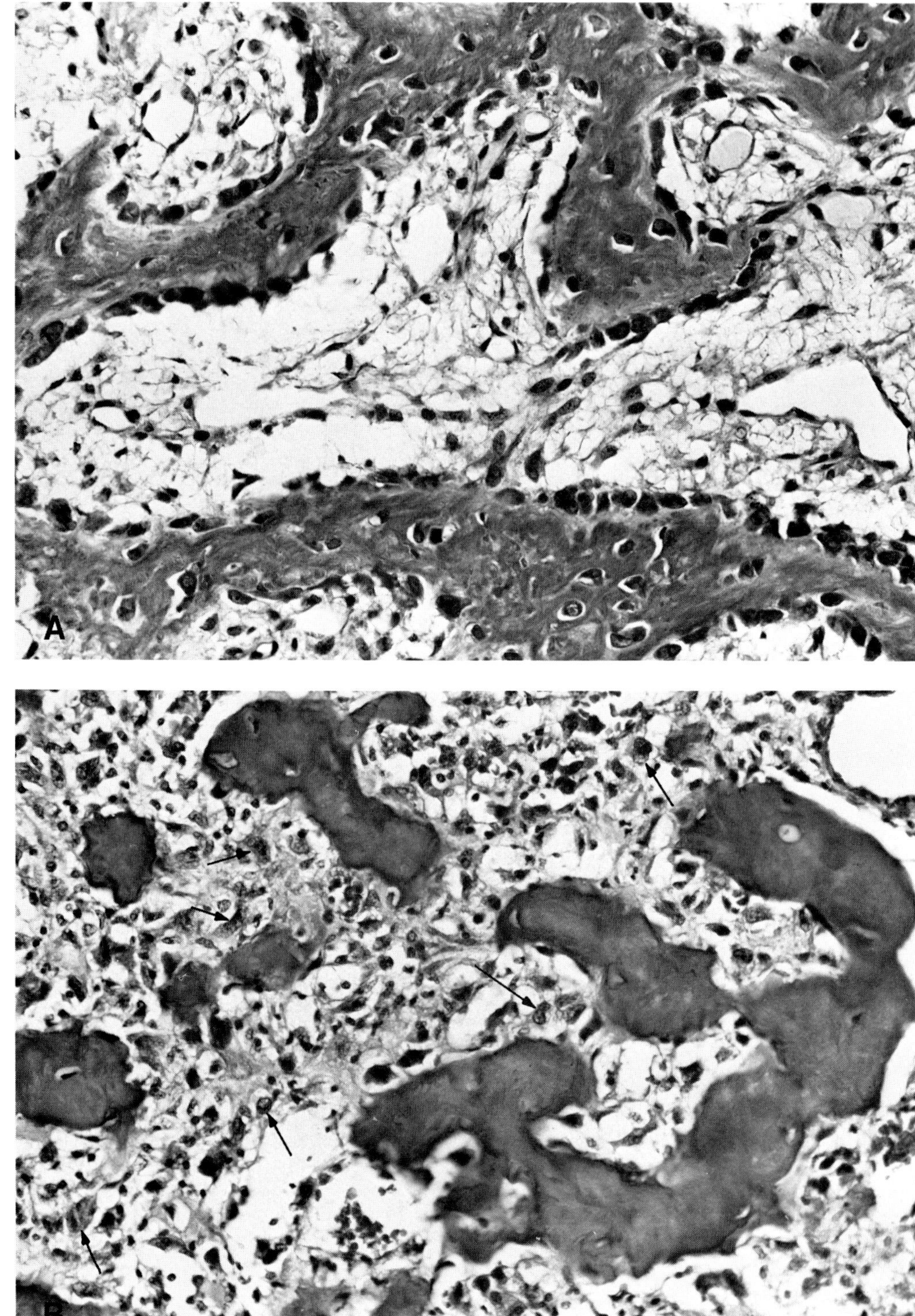

FIG. 7-14

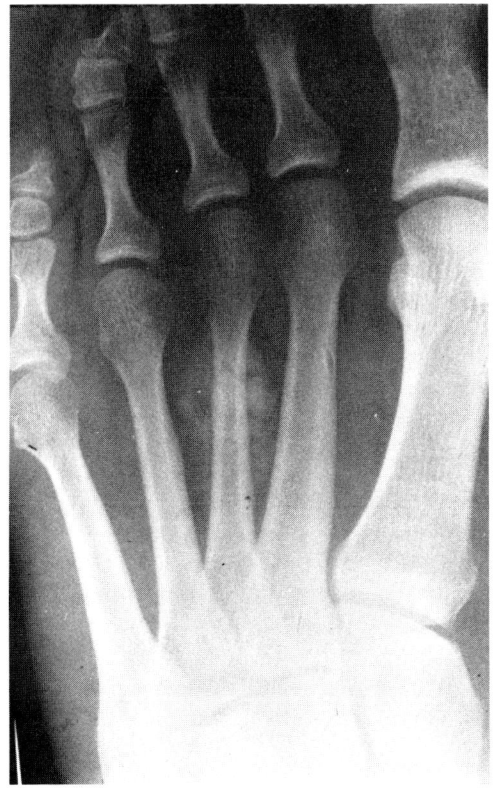

FIG. 7-15

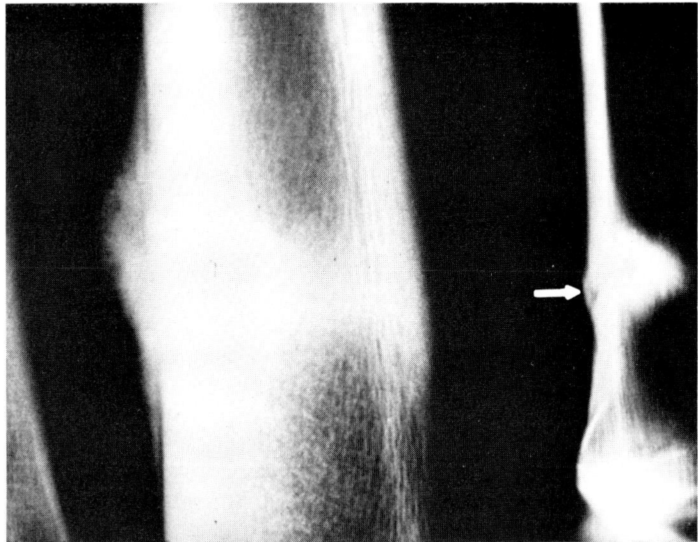

FIG. 7-16

Benign Versus Malignant Bone

FIG. 7-14. (*A*) Benign, prominent osteoblastic rimming of 4- to 5-week-old callus. Note the extreme prominence of the one to two layers of osteoblasts lining the woven bone they are producing. The nuclei are plump but regular in size and shape or are "in phase" with one another. Quite often they may show prominent Golgi zones when highly activated. The intertrabecular tissues are being converted to early fatty marrow. The stroma is hypocellular. (*B*) Woven bone production of an osteosarcoma for comparison. Prominent "in phase" osteoblastic rimming is not present even though the woven bone is quite mature looking. Note well the following: the irregularities in size and shape of the osteoblast nuclei (*arrows*); the absence of conversion to fatty marrow despite the relative maturity of the woven bone; the stroma packed with atypical cells; and the irregular size and shape of the blood vessels and the fact that they are difficult to see compared to the vessels in callus 4 to 5 weeks old showing a similar degree of woven bone maturity (H and E, X250).

Stress Fracture

FIG. 7-15. This so-called "march" or "soldiers" fracture shows periosteal fluffs of new bone in the midmetatarsal. The fracture line is not visible on this ordinary film.

FIG. 7-16. (*Left*) This radiograph of the midtibia shows the pseudomalignant aura a stress fracture may assume. The periosteal new bone is abundant. A clue to its nature is the horizontal or linear nature of the bone production in the midshaft. (*Right*) Tomographic demonstration of the fracture seen most clearly in the cortex (*arrow*), although it was also demonstrable in the medulla in the original films. The fracture probably did not extend through the entire cortex, which would explain the unusual eccentric nature of the periosteal new bone.

Histopathology of Callus Compared and Contrasted to Other Conditions, Especially the Osteosarcoma

By studying the pathologic features of fracture repair, we can observe the full gamut of bone production, from the most primitive preosseous and osseous tissues to the most highly organized or mature tissues. A thorough study of callus in its various phases of development will also lead to a greater comprehension and recognition of the tissues associated with other bone-producing tumors. The discussion that follows describes the morphological and cytologic features of fracture repair tissues, at different stages of maturation. The purpose of this discussion is primarily to help the pathologist distinguish callus tissues from sarcomatous tissues were a stress fracture to be biopsied unknowingly.

FIRST WEEK. During the first few days the tissues are replete with hemorrhage, foci of necrosis, and tissue debris. This is followed by granulation tissue, macrophages to remove the debris, and spindly cells, haphazardly arranged with very ominous pseudoanaplastic cytologic features (preosteoblasts and prechondroblasts). These cells are at first embedded in a loose edematous stroma, which imparts a tissue culturelike appearance. This primitive tissue is diffusely infiltrative, dissecting through muscle, fascia, periosteum, and bone marrow, as would a malignant tumor. (Plate 1, *A*).

SECOND TO THIRD WEEK. Most of the features of the first week are still present; however, the spindly cells noticeably increase in density, losing to some extent their tissue-culture (fasciitis-like) appearance and assuming a more solid spindle-cell fibrosarcoma-like pattern (Plate 1, *B*). The nuclei are hyperchromatic and there may be small-to-modest size single nucleoli. The cytoplasm is dark pinkish-blue and tapered to elongated. Typical mitoses may be frequent. Skeletal muscle bundles, if present on the biopsy, will also show spindle-cell infiltration (Plate 1, *C*), further contributing to the aura of "malignant" invasion. If we compare the spindle cells of early callus (Plate 1, *B*) to those seen in some examples of less anaplastic-appearing osteosarcoma (Plate 5, *A* and *B*), if anything, the callus appears more cellularly ominous. In fact, it may be virtually impossible, as the plates attempt to show, to differentiate early callus from some types of osteosarcoma by histology alone, reemphasizing the need for clinical, radiologic, and pathologic correlation of all spindle-cell, osteoid- and woven-bone-producing tumors.

At approximately 12 to 14 days after the fracture occurs, the spindly cells focally become plump, rounded, or polygonal and prove their preosseous histogenetic origin by the production of primitive osteoid and/or cartilage. Plate 1, *D*, shows a very early phase of osteoid (*arrow*) and contrasts it to primitive woven bone. One difficulty often confronting the pathologist is the differentiation of osteoid (a specialized form of collagen produced by osteoblasts) from collagen (a matrix produced by fibroblasts). Fibroblastic collagen is laid down in a longitudinal direction, is distinctly fibrillar, and the cells that produce the matrix maintain a flattened to spindly shape. Osteoid, on the other hand, tends to be laid down in amorphous masses (Plate 1, *D*), although in osteosarcoma there is a tendency to form tightly knit osteoid streamers (Plate 4, *B* and *C*), the latter resembling fibroblastic collagen more closely. But one of the most distinctive features of osteoid is that the cells that produce it tend to assume the shape of osteoblasts and osteocytes; namely, polygonal to rounded cells which become trapped in their own matrix (Plate 1, *D*, *arrow*). Although these features typify osteoid, its ultimate identification rests upon its conversion to woven bone. This conversion is marked by the deposition of calcium within its central matrix portion and the trapping of polygonal cells within the bone matrix (by definition osteocytes) and of other polygonal cells (osteoblasts) along its outer perimeter (Plate 1, *E*). It generally takes several days before calcium is visibly deposited within the newly formed osteoid. The calcified osteoid areas (by definition woven bone) appear bluish-pink, compared to uncalcified osteoid, which is pink, because calcium is hematoxyphilic (Plate 1, *E*). However, if the tissues are subjected to overdecalcification, all of the calcium may be leached from the tissues and the woven bone may appear tinctorially no different from osteoid, thereby, obscuring their separation.

An osteoblast is probably an evolutionary form of the fibroblast, perhaps explaining why it is not always possible to distinguish osteoid from collagen on tissue section. Even more specialized procedures such as electron microscopy and chemical analysis may fail at this task. We know, for example, that the periosteum has a collagenous appearance and cells that resemble ordinary fibroblasts. But, if the periosteum is stimulated by fracture or tumor, it will transform to an osteoinductive tissue (Plate 1, *D*). This attests to the very close relationship between what we define as collagen and its precursor cell, the fibroblast, and osteoid and its precursor cell, the osteoblast. Nevertheless, we must still attempt to differentiate osteoid from collagen on tissue section, and most importantly, malignant osteoid and collagen production from benign and reactive osteoid and collagenous tumorous proliferations, since diagnosis depends upon these distinctions.

During the first 3 weeks from inception of fracture callus, myositis ossificans, or any benign bone-producing lesion, the cellular proliferation may be so exuberant that it mimics sarcoma. But there may be subtle histologic clues that suggest benignancy. Very close examination of nuclear features and mitotic figures are important.

In general, callus which is 3 to 4 or more weeks old, is typified by cells that appear to be "in phase" with one another at any local site, although they may appear to be in a different "phase" of maturation at a contiguous site. By similar phase of maturation, it is meant that the nuclear and cytoplasmic features appear similar from cell to cell, even if individual nuclei are ominously plump or spindly shaped (Fig. 7–14, *A*). The cells and their nuclei are regularly ominous. In most sarcomas, areas usually can be found in which the cell shapes and their nuclei are irregularly ominous (Fig. 7–14, *B*). With anaplasia the cells in any high-power field appear to be in different phases of maturation; some nuclei are large, others small; there are extensive variations in shape, chromatin clumping, and size of the nucleoli (Plate 4, *G*).

Among mitotic figures, there are important differences between benign exuberant lesions and sarcomas. Although mitoses may be numerous in early callus, they all are mirror images (typical mitoses). With sarcomas, bizarre or atypical mitotic figures appear that are not mirror images. This results from defects in either the chromosomal or spindle apparatus that are rarely, if ever, seen in benign bone tumors.

THIRD TO FIFTH WEEK. By the third to fifth week callus maturation begins to show histologic changes that approach objective histologic benignancy.

During the third to fourth week calcium is seen, under the light microscope, to be deposited within the osteoid. In these early weeks the woven bone is oriented in an irregular pattern (Plate 1, *E*). Although a similar pattern of osteoid and bone deposition that is shown in Plates 3, *F* and *G*, can also be seen in osteosarcomas, changes in the osteoblasts and stroma occur that are rare in osteosarcoma and common in benign conditions such as callus. Those changes that suggest benignancy are prominent osteoblastic rimming and the early conversion of the stroma to a loose, bland, fibrous to fibrofatty tissue rich in prominent blood vessels (Fig. 7–14, *A*). Conversion of the stromal tissues of an osteosarcoma to fatty marrow does not occur (Fig. 7–14, *B*).

PROMINANT, ORDERLY RIMMING OF OSTEOBLASTS. Plate 1, *E* shows masses of osteoid and early woven bone, trapped skeletal muscle, and a stroma beginning to develop prominent capillaries in a $3\frac{1}{2}$-week-old callus. Some of the osteoblasts (*arrow*) show a continuous and orderly alignment along the osteoid and bone matrix, a feature that could be defined as early osteoblastic rimming. Rimming of the osteoblast is occasionally seen in osteosarcoma tumor bone (personal observations) but is not as prominent, continuous, or orderly as that shown in this illustration.

By the fourth week of callus formation, the degree of osteoblast rimming in some foci is exquisitely prominent (Fig. 7–14, *A;* Plate 1, *F*). The osteoblasts are plump, the cytoplasm a deep pinkish blue, and the cells stand out sharply from each other and the surrounding stroma. Golgi zones may be prominent. The nuclei are enlarged, fairly regular in size and shape, and may contain a single prominent nucleolus. In essence, the nuclear and cytoplasmic features suggest that the osteoblasts that line a trabecular surface are "in phase" with each other. The plumper the cell, the greater the tendency for it to lie perpendicularly to its surface of matrix production, while the more spindly cells assume a more horizontal configuration. If one observes five to 10 contiguous osteoblasts, there are only slight variations in the angles of the long axes of the cells to the underlying matrix. In osteosarcoma, the osteoblasts, if they rim the bone at all, show a greater degree of disorganization, typified by a more random distribution of the axis of each cell in relation to the underlying bone matrix and greater nuclear and cytoplasmic variation from cell to cell. I have not seen a focus of intramedullary osteosarcoma bone with osteoblastic rimming having the degree of orderly prominence shown in Plate 1, *F*, and Fig. 7–14, *A*. The only exception to this rule are areas along the advancing margin of osteosarcoma that may stimulate the host bone or periosteum to produce reparative osteoid and woven bone with prominent osteoblast rimming. This is, however, merely a benign reparative host tissue response to the advancing tumor. Therefore although I use unequivocal prominent, orderly osteoblastic rimming as a sign of benign bone production, this feature must be used in context and does not, in itself, mean that the entire lesion in question is necessarily benign.

Focal to diffuse prominent, orderly rimming of osteoblasts may be seen in many other benign conditions: osteoid osteoma, osteoblastoma, Paget's disease, rickets, hyperparathyroidism, and osteogenesis imperfecta. The one benign condition in which osteoblastic rimming is rarely prominent is fibrous dysplasia. In this peculiar disease, bone appears to be produced by fibroblastic cells (so-called fibro-osseous metaplasia). Typical osteoblasts are rare. However, its radiologic features and bland, stromal fibrous tissue should easily distinguish this condition from osteosarcoma.

In most osteosarcoma tissues, there is not even the slightest hint of "rimming" (Fig. 7–14, *B*). In general the malignant osteoblasts are much more randomly distributed (Plate 3, *F, G, H,* and *I,* and Plate 4, *A, B, C,* and *D*) and do not align or rim the osteoid and bone they produce in a continuous fashion. In some cases there is only a suggestion of rimming not unlike that seen in the very early weeks of callus (Plate 1, *E*).

"Benign" rimming as shown in Plate 1, *F* and Fig. 7–14, *A,* is seen in active bone growth areas. As callus matures or enters its phase of less active growth, distinctive benign plump osteoblastic rimming may disappear or may only be present in small focal areas. However, when this occurs there are other signs of benignancy, such as maturation to lamellar bone and marrow fat. This latter feature will also eventually occur in myositis ossificans, traumatic periostitis, and the healing phases of rickets and hyperparathyroidism. Within the lesional tissues themselves of osteoid osteoma and osteoblastoma, some very exuberant to quiescent examples may show absence of osteoblastic rimming and of mature lamellar bone and marrow fat. They always contain areas of osteoid and/or woven bone. These characteristics are difficult to distinguish from a sclerosing osteogenic sarcoma by microscopy alone. Other features, which will be discussed later in this chapter, will distinguish these two benign entities from even subtly anaplastic osteosarcomas.

With these complexities in mind, the principle of benign osteoblastic "rimming" can be useful in the diagnosis of equivocal or problem cases. The pathologist can be more confident that the lesion in question is benign if foci of benign rimming are seen in the curettage or biopsy tissues of an osteoid- and woven-bone producing lesion. It must be ascertained by microscopic analysis of the entire slide material that these foci are representative of the tumor and are not merely benign osseous tissues of the host bone or periosteum induced by the tumor. Again, it cannot be overemphasized that the absence of orderly osteoblast rimming does not rule out a benign condition and its presence does not necessarily preclude an associated malignancy. Its presence or absence must be properly interpreted to be useful. Admittedly, this requires experience, which the novice in bone tumors can attain by diligent observation of all active bone-productive lesions.

MATURATION TO A BLAND FIBROVASCULAR STROMA. Between the fourth and fifth weeks the cellular and spindly stroma of callus undergoes maturation to a more hypocellular fibrous but highly vascular tissue with many fewer mitoses (Plate 1, *F* and *G*, Fig. 7–14, *A*). These features, in addition to the prominent osteoblastic rimming, should no longer be confused with malignancy solely by histologic criteria. On the other hand, the stroma between the woven-bone production of a sclerosing (intense osteoid and bone-producing) osteosarcoma is composed of dense masses of osteoid and/or rounded to spindly cells with sparse vessels (Plate 3, *F* and *G,* Fig. 7–14, *B*). Those osteosarcomas with a prominent vascular stroma are usually associated with a prominent cellular stromal proliferation (Plate 5, *F*) and lack the bland, hypocellular, fibrovascular stroma as shown in fairly mature callus 4 to 6 weeks old.

FIVE WEEKS OR MORE. After 5 or more weeks the bone of callus (Plate 1, *H*) is arranged into an even more benign-looking pattern. Immature lamellar bone begins to make its appearance (Plate 1, *H* (*arrow*)), and the stroma is composed of loose fibrous tissue and early fat, with or without hematopoiesis. The lamellar bone is first deposited along the outside perimeter of the woven bone scaffolding. Note that in this phase of callus maturation, the osteoblasts show flattened rimming or are inconspicuous; both are signs of less intense bone production, which would be expected as callus approaches complete healing. Even though the osteoblastic rimming may no longer be prominent, its conversion to fat and lamellar bone takes precedence in the evaluation of benignancy.

CARTILAGE IN CALLUS. Cartilage may be present in almost all stages of fracture repair, except for the preosseous phase (first 2 weeks). The cartilage of callus may pass through stages of marked hypercellularity (Plate 4, *E*) and be virtually indistinguishable from low-grade anaplastic, Grade I chondrosarcoma, or Grade I chondrosarcomatous tissue in an osteosarcoma (Plate 4, *D*). Grade I chondrosarcomas are in effect clinical and pathologic diagnoses that cannot be determined by merely reading a slide. But, callus cartilage does not display the cytologic atypia seen in unequivocal chondrosarcomas, such as Grades II–III objective anaplasia (Plate 4, *F,* and Figs. 8–23, 8–24, 8–44, and 8–47), which are diagnosable by histology alone.

Differential Diagnosis

Osteosarcoma Versus Fracture—A Case Example

This section will conclude with a case that emphasizes why it is important to diagnosis to recognize the features we have just described. A young woman was sent to our hospital for further possible treatment after removal of an "osteosarcoma" of the rib. On low-power examination (Plate 1, *I*) the lesion showed a fracture line, host lamellar bone, and an infiltrate of woven bone which, in places, abuts the lamellar bone. High-power examination showed nonviable lamellar bone adjacent to the fracture line, woven bone, a loose fibrovascular stroma, and foci of prominent osteoblastic rimming. These features suggested callus in a rib fracture; this discrepancy in diagnosis prompted a critical review of history and radiographs. The radiograph showed an obvious fracture line that did not necessarily rule out osteosarcoma, because pathologic fracture may occur in osteosarcoma as well. Although the woven-bone infiltrate between the lamellar bone and spicules is seen in osteosarcoma (Plate 3, *G*) it can also be seen in callus. The presence of blandish fibrovascular tissue and prominent osteoblastic rimming and the lack of unequivocal or objective anaplasia was much more in keeping with a callus of approximately 4 weeks duration. In reviewing the chart, no history of trauma was mentioned. However, in questioning the patient and asking her specifically if she remembered a traumatic episode about 1 month previously, she offered the following crucial clinical information. She was married 4 weeks before the rib resection, and during her honeymoon experienced a painful episode in her rib cage during a vigorous embrace. This information clinched the diagnosis as nothing more than the so-called "honeymoon" fracture. She is perfectly well years later. This case illustrates, quite well the need for critical cytologic and tissue pattern evaluation, to always question the diagnosis of sarcoma without the unequivocal features of anaplasia, and to review the radiographs and to obtain further history, if necessary.

Massive Hyperplastic Callus

It is important to be aware that a bone or bones severely modified by a benign disease process such as osteogenesis imperfecta[6,7] may develop repeated fractures so ominous in their total radiologic and pathologic presentation that osteosarcoma is simulated. These massive hyperplastic calluses are extremely difficult diagnostic problems. Fortunately, they are extremely rare. The main clue to their diagnosis is an underlying primary benign bone disease that has resulted over the course of years in tremendous loss of bone substance. Pathologically, the lesional tissues may contain masses of osteoid, woven bone, fibrous tissue, and hyperplastic cartilage. Unequivocal anaplasia is not seen. However, differentiating it from a low-grade anaplastic sclerosing osteosarcoma that arose from a chronic benign disease process of bone requires considerable expertise. Cases in which the diagnosis of massive callus is entertained but in which there is doubt require consultative advice.

Osteoid Osteoma

Capsule Summary

Incidence. Some 2.6 per cent of excised primary bone tumors.

Age. Most patients are children to young adults. The youngest reported patient was 8 months old.[16]

Clinical Features. Pain worst at night, greatly relieved by aspirin, may cause limp, muscle atrophy, painful scoliosis; synovitis and bone growth abnormalities if located intracapsularly or near a growing epiphyseal plate.

Radiologic Features. Radiolucent to dense radioopaque central nidus, lucent collar and variable degrees of host and periosteal sclerosis.

Gross Pathology. Cherry-red to bony yellow-white nidus.

Histopathology. Osteoid and/or woven bone, osteoclasts, fibrovascular stroma. Cartilage is never produced.

Course. Benign

Treatment. Local excision. Symptoms immediately relieved.

Definition. An osteoid osteoma (OO) is a distinctive, totally benign entity characterized by a smaller than 2 cm. nidus of osteoid and/or woven bone and one that evokes considerable pain and often "reactive" sclerosis of the surrounding host bone. It usually affects children or young adults. The OO is probably not a true neoplastic condition as we have defined it in this text, since those cases that have not been treated may resolve either completely or by a residue of sclerosis with loss of the nidus.[10,27]

Importance. The pain the lesion provokes before a radiograph is performed may be mistaken for a neurotic symptom and remain untreated for months or years before the diagnosis is made and excision instituted. The signs and symptoms may mimic neurogenic and muscular dystrophies and idiopathic scoliosis and its radiographic features may be confused with osteomyelitis, Ewing's tumor, and eosinophilic granuloma. If the lesion is located near a joint, pain, effusion, and reactive inflammation may mimic an infectious synovitis. Attention to high-power microscopic fields alone can result in confusion with osteogenic sarcoma.

Diagnostic Radiologic Features

In most instances a definitive diagnosis of osteoid osteoma is possible from routine radiographs in conjunction with tomography. The constellation of char-

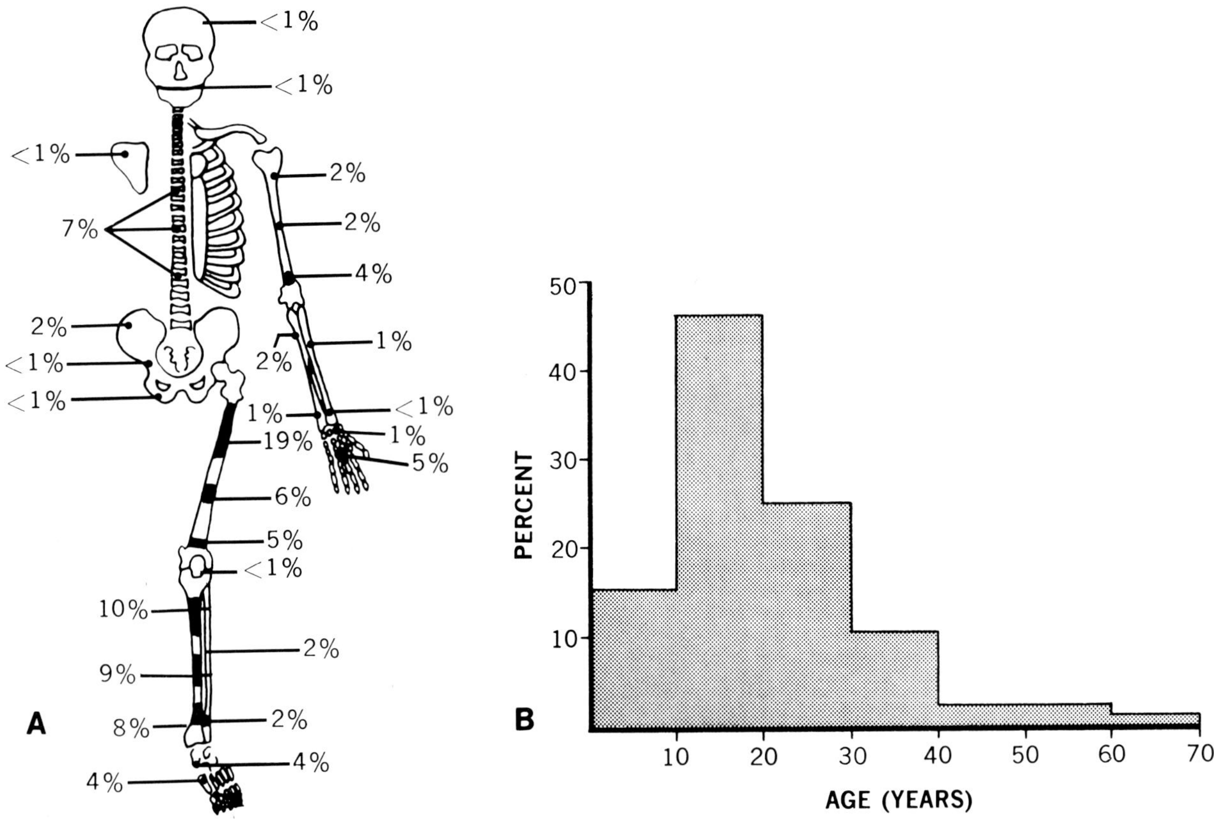

FIG. 7-17. (*A*) Osteoid osteoma Frequency of areas of involvement in 448 patients. Male: female incidence, 2.5:1. (*B*) age distribution of patients with osteoid osteoma. The lesion seldom occurs after the age of 40. (Mirra, J., Bullough, P., and Freiberger, R.: Orthopedic Diseases, Part I: Bone Tumors. New York, Famous Teachings in Modern Medicine, MedCom, Inc., © 1971)

acteristic radiographic features are (Figs. 7–18 and 7–19):

1. A central spherical to oval bony density usually less than 1 cm. in diameter (the *nidus*).
2. A thin (1 to 3 mm.) collar of lucency surrounding the nidus.
3. Variable degree of increased *homogeneous* host bone and/or periosteal density, which surrounds the nidus.

The main difficulty in radiologic diagnosis is that the OO often causes such dense sclerosis in surrounding host bone that the nidus is totally obscured on routine radiographs. Unless the diagnosis is considered and penetrating tomograms ordered, the OO may be confused with other entities. Those cases that present with less usual symptoms and radiologic appearances will be discussed following the pathological description of the process.

Gross Pathology

LOCALIZATION OF THE NIDUS. The first and most important step in the pathologic diagnosis of an OO is to find the nidus. This may not be a simple task, as the nidus can be as small as 1 to 2 mm. in size and buried deeply in a mass of sclerotic reactive host bone. If the nidus is not readily appreciated upon gross examination of the removed bone or its fragments, the specimen should be taken to the radiology department and penetrated adequately, since diagnosis and proper treatment are absolutely dependent upon its demonstration. If the bone is adequately penetrated by specimen radiography and the nidus not seen, then either the lesion was not surgically removed or the presumptive diagnosis was in error. The nidus on the specimen radiograph will appear as either a spherical, ovoid or elliptical, or lucent or dense mass (Fig. 7–19). Its radiographic density will depend, of course, on the ratio of osteoid to woven bone present in the nidus.

GROSS APPEARANCE OF THE NIDUS AND SURROUNDING BONE. The diagnostic features of an osteoid osteoma are to be found in its nidus and the reactions the tumor provokes in the surrounding host bone. The nidus of an osteoid osteoma is a spherical, less than 1 cm., osseous tissue (Figs. 7–19 and 7–20, Plate 2, *A*) usually surrounded by a circular 1 to 3 mm. zone of decreased bone trabeculae. On microscopic examination (Plate 2, *C*), this latter zone corresponds to bland, loose, fibrovascular tissue in which bone trabeculae are markedly attenuated. Less commonly, the nidus may assume an ovoid to elliptical shape (Fig. 7–30, *B*). The nidus is usually found endosteally, near the cortex (Figs. 7–28 and 7–29), deep within the cortex (Plate 2, *A*) or in the superficial aspect of the cortex, which is easily visible from the periosteal surface by either the surgeon, at the time of operation, or by the pathologist, at gross examination (Fig. 7–20). Ordinarily, the resected bone specimen must be cut for gross observation of the nidus.

The color of the nidus varies from deep red to yellow-white, and its texture, from soft to extremely dense, depending on the degree of vascularity and bone deposition. Those lesions which are deep red are rich in blood vessels and osteoid but poor in woven bone. Those which are hard and yellow-white (Plate 2, *A*) are rich in dense woven bone and contain fewer vessels.

An OO nidus is usually less than 1 cm. in its greatest dimension and is rarely more than 2 cm. If ever they are larger than 2 cm., differentiating it from an osteoblastoma may be impossible by microscopic analysis alone. This author tends to agree with Dr. Jaffe[19] that the osteoid osteoma is a distinctive clinicopathologic entity. However, some authors believe the osteoblastoma is but a "giant osteoid osteoma"[30] or an OO is but a circumscribed osteoblastoma. To this day the problem is unresolved; but in general, the OO is characterized by more severe pain, marked irritative effects on surrounding bone and soft tissues, marked relief from aspirin, and a size smaller than 1 cm.

Osteoblastomas, on the other hand, are usually less pain provoking, less irritative, tend to expand the bone in a fusiform fashion, are generally over 3 cm. in size, and have a different overall skeletal distribution (Figs. 7–17 and 7–36). However, by microscopic examination alone (eliminating size) the two are virtually indistinguishable and illustrations for one could serve for the other.

Histopathology

LOW-POWER EXAMINATION. An osteoid osteoma nidus always contains either osteoid or woven bone in variable proportions. On low-power examination an OO nidus is sharply delineated from the surrounding host bone (Figs. 7–21, 7–22, and 7–29 and Plate 2, *C*). The nidus is most often surrounded by a 1 to 3 mm. zone of loose fibrovascular tissue (Plate 2, *C*). *Osteoid osteomas and osteoblastomas both have lesional tissue that is composed of osteoid and/or woven bone and rarely contain residue of host lamellar bone.* This can best be seen with polarized light. The woven bone of an OO nidus or osteoblastoma may abut host lamellar bone or fuse with it along its edge but rarely does it insinuate itself between the lamellar bone marrow by more than fractions of a millimeter (Plate 2, *C* and *E*). *In contrast, the woven bone and osteoid of osteosarcoma can be seen to infiltrate host lamellar bone marrow for many millimeters to centimeters along its advancing edges, and in callus, in the vicinity of its central fracture zone* (Plates 1, *I* and 3, *B–F*). However, if random sections or biopsies are not taken through these areas of osteosarcoma or callus, this crucial histological difference may not be appreciated. If on excisional biopsy or curettage, osteoid and woven bone is found to infiltrate between host lamellar bone for any significant distance, this feature can be used to virtually eliminate OO and osteoblastoma from diagnostic contention. Since OO and osteoblastoma may at times not be easily distinguished by cytologic criteria alone from some osteosarcomas, these extremely important, fundamental histologic differences in pattern, if observed, can facilitate their crucial separation (personal observation).

In general, benign tumors of any tissue remain confined or circumscribed. On the other hand, malignant tumors are typified by relentless infiltration of the surrounding tissues. Since the marrow is a soft tissue, a malignant tumor would obviously infiltrate through it much more easily than it would through bone matrix. It is first the normal marrow that is replaced along the advancing edge of most highly malignant bone sarcomas. Only after many days to weeks may the entrapped host bone be resorbed. The virtual absence of significant lesional osteoid and woven bone infiltration between host bone trabeculae in OO and osteoblastoma is perhaps a reflection of their slower, more circumscribed benign growth. In essence, the OO and osteoblastoma replace the host bone along a fairly sharp or solid "wall" of osteoclastic destruction, while osteogenic sarcoma advances along a "permeative front" before host bone destruction by osteoclasts is completed. This crucial difference cannot be overemphasized and must be learned by the reader.

HIGH-POWER EXAMINATION. The osteoid osteoma and osteoblastoma are virtually indistinguishable on high-power examination. In general, OO is smaller than 2 cm. in maximal dimension, and osteoblastoma, greater than 2 cm. In some cases, however, there is an overlap in size and clinical and radiologic correlation may become necessary for more accurate classification. The discussion below includes a description of the OO under high-power examination, the osteoblastoma, and those features that differentiate these two tumors from osteosarcoma.

The OO and osteoblastoma always contain osteoid and/or woven bone. Some are rich in osteoid (Figs. 7–23 and 7–25, Plate 2, *F*), others contain a mixture of osteoid and woven bone (Fig. 7–24), while others are composed predominantly of dense woven bone (Fig. 7–26). Since osteosarcomas also have a similar variation of these identical tissues, these features alone cannot serve to differentiate these lesions. Osteosarcomas, we are led to believe from textbooks, are obviously anaplastic and OO and osteoblastoma obviously benign cytologically. Unfortunately, there is some degree of cytologic overlap and their distinction is not always simple. In this author's experience, 20 to 30 per cent of biopsies from osteosarcomas show cytologic features not easily distinguishable from exuberant benign bony proliferative diseases, including the OO and osteoblastoma. On the other hand, these latter two lesions may show a wild flurry of plump to spindly osteoblasts with ominously large nuclei, particularly in the osteoid-rich areas (Fig. 7–23; Plate 2, *F*) and actually look more "malignant" than some sclerosing or highly bone-producing osteosarcomas (Plate 3, *I*). Fortunately, the radiographic appearance of most sclerosing osteosarcomas leaves no doubt of the diagnosis, in spite of the innocuous cytologic features some may show.

Almost every case of OO, even those with the most ominous histologic appearance, is easily distinguishable from an osteosarcoma on the basis of its single nidus and size (smaller than 2 cm.). Only very rare osteosarcomas ($< 1\%$) ever present in the size range of 2 cm. and if so, as radiologic, "cumulus cloud" fluffs and not as a single nidus (Fig. 7–43). Thus it is extremely important that radiographs be reviewed. If, by some fluke, only curetted specimens are obtained and radiographs not reviewed and the only history given to the pathologist is bone tumor, the trap is set for the diagnosis of osteosarcoma. Let us consider the following actual case. A 14-year-old boy had a history of pain of $1\frac{1}{2}$ years duration of the elbow. Eventually he developed joint effusion. Radiography showed a joint effusion and a small, 2 mm. "hole" in the distal humeral cortex in close proximity to the articular cartilage. At operation there was synovitis and a reddish nodule protruding from the bone cortex, which was curetted. The lesion was identical to that shown in Plate 2, *G*. The pathologist was so startled by this appearance that he diagnosed osteosarcoma and the patient was referred to UCLA for amputation. Review of the slide material suggested OO or osteoblastoma based upon focal prominent osteoblastic rimming and other histologic principles discussed in this section. Radiographs were reviewed with the patient's history, which absolutely confirmed our tentative slide diagnosis of a benign bone-producing lesion, namely, the osteoid osteoma.

Sites of Involvement

No bone is totally exempt from possible involvement, although only one case has been reported in the vault of the skull.[23] The diaphyses and metaphyses are involved most commonly.[10] The nidus is usually located near to or in the bone cortex and on occasion, intra- or subperiosteally. In rare instances

Osteoid Osteoma

FIG. 7–18. This radiograph shows the pathognomonic features of an osteoid osteoma; these features are: (*a*) A round, central nidus smaller than 2 cm. in dimension; (*b*) a 1- to 2-mm. peripheral zone of lucency; and (*c*) dense, reactive surrounding host bone sclerosis.

FIG. 7–19. (*A*) Specimen radiograph, nidus (*1*) rim of lucency (*2*) and reactive host bone sclerosis (*3*). (*B*) Macerated specimen showing the same features.

FIG. 7–20. This osteoid osteoma was located in the outer portion of the cortex and was easily visualized by gross inspection. It is round, gritty, and surrounded by a reddish rim of vascular tissue.

FIG. 7–21. Sharp delineation of the round nidus (*arrow*) from the surrounding dense host lamellar bone (H and E, X10).

FIG. 7–22. The nidus is sharply delineated (*arrow*). The host bone cortex is sclerotic (H and E, X10).

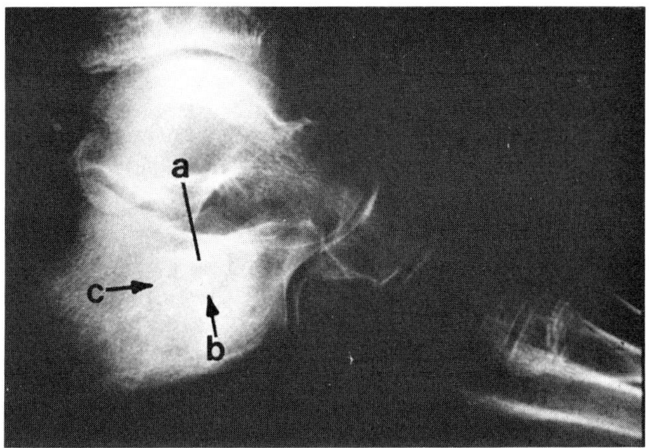

FIG. 7-18

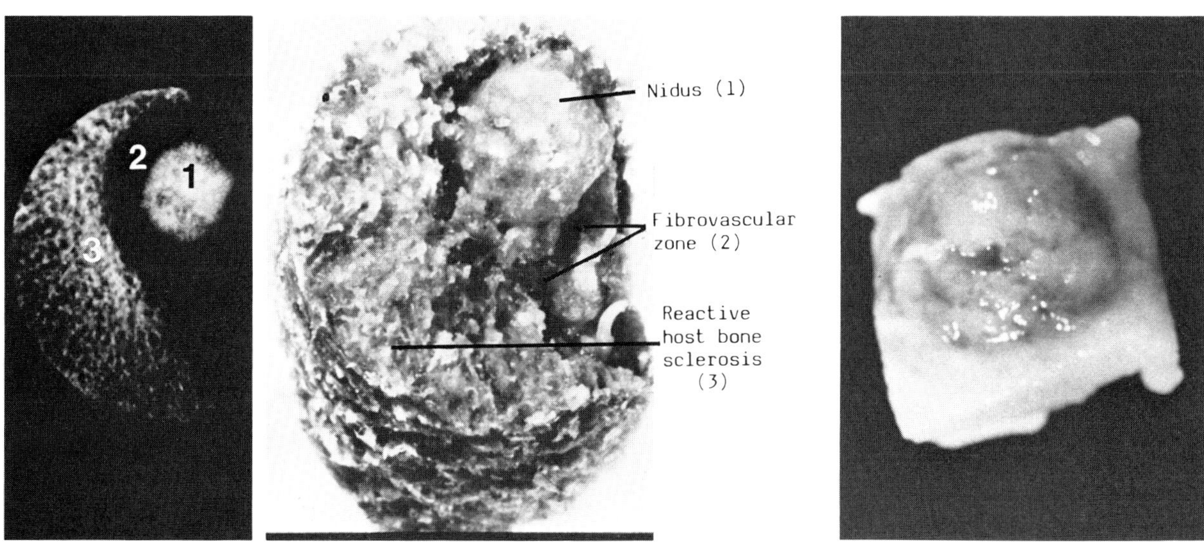

FIG. 7-19

FIG. 7-20

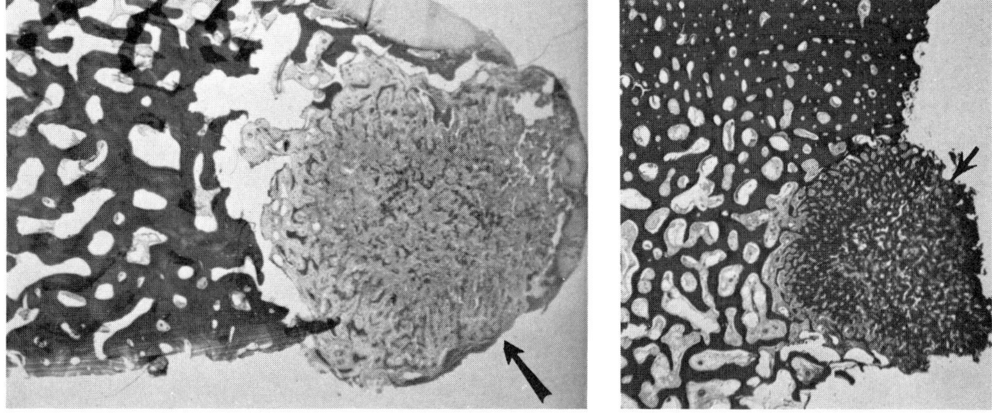

FIG. 7-21

FIG. 7-22

multiple nidi within the same bone have been reported.[12]

Clinical and Radiographic Characteristics of the OO

PAIN. The pain is often slowly progressive, frequently disturbs sleep, and in more than half the cases, is greatly relieved by increasing doses of aspirin. Exquisite point tenderness can be illicited if the nidus is located at the bone surface. Symptoms are usually present 6 months to 2 years before diagnosis.

SWELLING AND REDNESS. Superficial lesions may result in swelling and redness, in combination with pain and mimic osteomyelitis. However, radiographic examination should alert the clinician to the actual diagnosis (Figs. 7–27 and 7–28).

REACTIVE BONE SCLEROSIS. Perhaps the most common and confusing radiographic change is dense reactive host bone and/or periosteal sclerosis, both of which may totally mask the nidus by ordinary radiographic penetration, which is usually inadequate (Fig. 7–30 *A*). Unlike osteomyelitis or malignant bone tumors, which usually result in patchy areas of sclerosis and lysis and irregular patterns of periosteal new bone such as "sunburst," Codman's triangles, and "onion-skinning" reactions, the OO will result in a homogeneous intraosseous, and periosteal new bone. In long bones (Fig. 7–30, *A*) the sclerosis is usually eccentric, homogeneous, and circumscribed and the periosteal new bone has very smooth convexly oriented borders, which are also homogeneous in their density. This is in contrast to the less homogeneous and irregularly bordered pattern of intramedullary and periosteal densification in a case of osteomyelitis, in which a central niduslike structure is in reality a sequestrum, or dead bone fragment (Fig. 7-33).

Unless high penetrating tomograms are taken the dense bone sclerosis may obscure the nidus and be mistaken for osteomyelitis or a malignancy. The value of tomography in any painful, solitary lesion of bone showing smooth-bordered homogeneous sclerosis cannot be overestimated (Fig. 7–30, *B*). A biopsy of a clinically unrecognized OO will almost certainly miss the small nidus and probably result in an erroneous clinical and pathologic diagnosis of osteomyelitis, since the irritated surrounding sclerotic host bone usually shows mild reactive chronic inflammation and fibrosis.

In one reported case,[17] the reactive sclerosis associated with an OO extended across an intervertebral disc to involve the adjacent vertebral body as well, a most curious and unique finding. Radioactive scanning may help locate the nidus and be useful as a guide to selecting more specialized tomographic procedures.[11,14]

JOINT EFFUSION. If the OO is located in an intracapsular position, the lesion may result in severe impairment of joint function, reactive synovitis, and effusion. *There is no periosteum in the intracapsular portion of the bone, so that reactive periostitis is not seen when the nidus is located in this position.*

MUSCULAR SYSTEM AND SCOLIOSIS. Focal muscular atrophy may occur. If the OO is in a spinal bone, the lesion usually results in muscular spasm with resultant curvature of the spine (Fig. 7–31, *A*). The spine will not be rotated, as is the case in most forms of true scoliosis, but will merely be curved. Therefore, all young patients presenting with a painful two-dimensional curvature of the spine should receive tomograms to attempt to delineate a possible OO nidus. The nidus should be in the center of the curve and on the concave side, since it is the muscles on this side that are closest to the nidus and have undergone the greatest spasm (Fig. 7–31). Excision of the nidus dramatically relieves the pain and the curvature abates in a few weeks time.

ABNORMALITIES IN BONE GROWTH. In rare instances, if the nidus is located near a growing epiphysis, there may be acceleration of bone growth.[15,22]

Differential Diagnosis

OSTEOBLASTOMA. On high-power examination, an osteoblastoma is virtually indistinguishable from an OO. On low-power examination, it is greater than

Histology of Osteoid Osteoma or Osteoblastoma

FIG. 7–23. Osteoid osteoma or osteoblastoma, on high-power examination, may show fields replete with osteoid and a wild flurry of ominously plump osteoblasts virtually indistinguishable from some osteosarcomas, if attention is paid to only high-power histology (H and E, X400).

FIG. 7–24. The features that help in distinguishing fields such as these from osteosarcoma are the following: Thick, irregularly serrated osteoid and woven bone trabeculae; prominent rimming of osteoblasts along the osteoid and bony seams; and intense vascularity associated with a peppering of osteoclasts (H and E, X125).

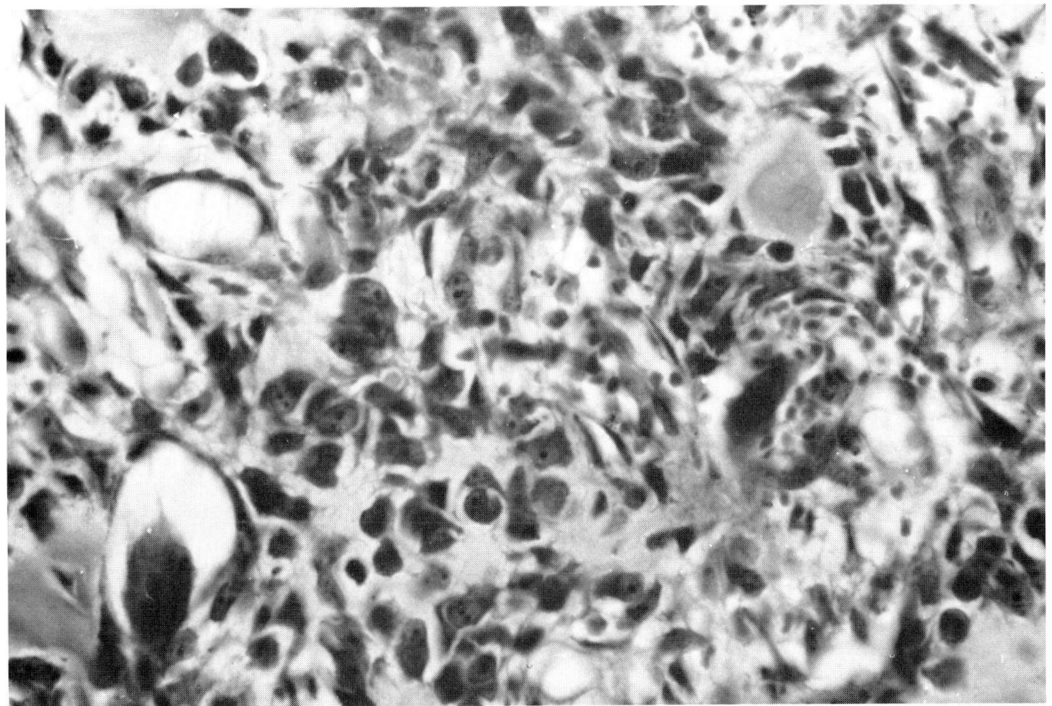

FIG. 7-23

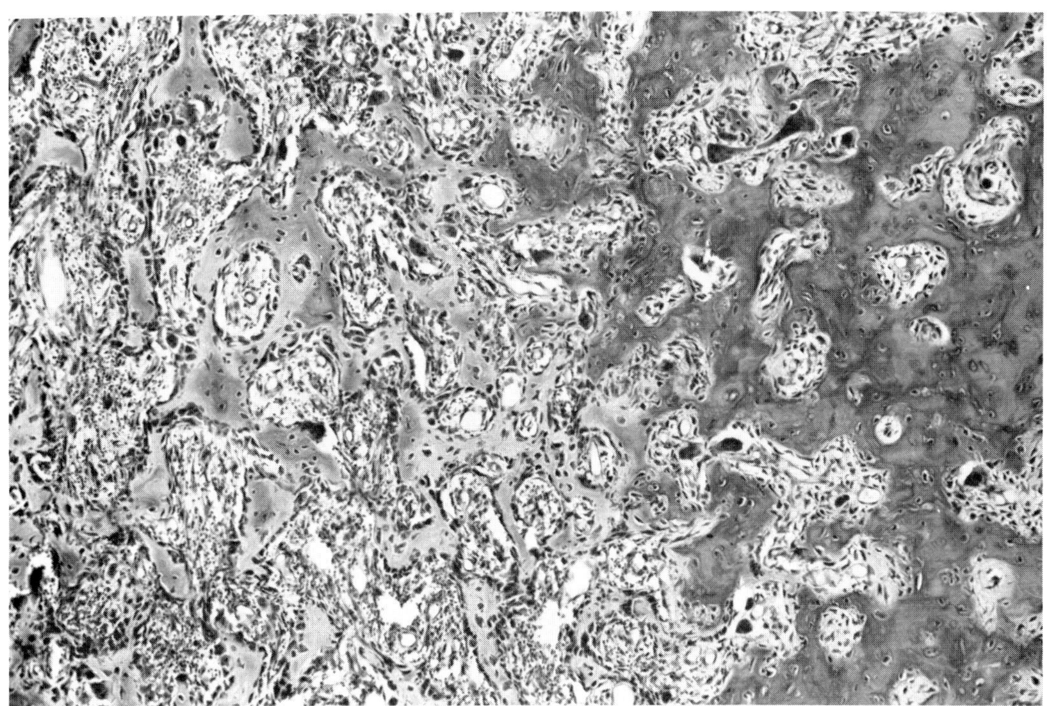

FIG. 7-24

2 cm. in diameter. With curetted tissue, these distinctions are lost, so that it is necessary to correlate the specimen with radiographs. Osteoblastomas (Figs. 7-37–7-41) are fairly large lesions (2–10 cm.) that tend to "expand" the bone, do not have a small nidus, (small is considered 2 cm.), and generally cause no more than a thin border of reactive sclerosis.

OSTEOSARCOMA. Osteosarcomas with minimal anaplasia may be most difficult to distinguish from osteoid osteomas or osteoblastomas from a high-power field alone. In almost every instance the radiological and size differences are so great that confusion with OO is not possible. In my experience, there has been only one case of a 2 cm. osteosarcoma[92] that could have been confused with a benign OO (See p. 116 and Figs. 7-43–7-46 for a more complete discussion). In these cases, the principle aids to diagnosis were "fluffs" or "cumulus cloudlike" densities by radiograph, cartilage production with atypical cytologic features, and the absence of the usual radiological signs of stress fracture. These features all point to either the osteosarcoma or unusual stress fracture (see p. 91).

SOLITARY ENOSTOSIS. This does not cause pain or reactive surrounding host bone sclerosis and is composed of lamellar bone, in contrast to the osteoid and woven bone of OO.

OSTEOMYELITIS. In general osteomyelitis results in bone sclerosis mixed with patchy areas of lucency and more irregular, usually concentric periosteal new bone, as compared with that of the OO. On rare occasions osteomyelitis may closely simulate OO (Fig. 7-33). In actuality the central nidus in osteomyelitis is a fragment of dead bone termed the sequestrum. This fragment is more irregular in shape than the well-defined nidus of OO. The lucent "collar" is usually wider than that seen in OO and represents pus and resorbed bone. Figure 7-34 shows a small intracortical collection of pus that simulated OO on radiograph. On rare occasions the nidus of an OO may be quite long or elliptical and thus more closely resemble a sequestrum (Fig. 7-30, *B*).

BRODIE'S ABSCESS (FOCAL CHRONIC OSTEOMYELITIS). Brodie's abscess is a focal collection of inflammation or pus in which the host bone has encapsulated the lesion by dense fibrous tissue and bone. The central area is lucent. The lucent area is usually larger than 2 cm. although smaller lesions may be radiologically indistinguishable from a OO with lucent nidi. The Brodie's abscess is rare, compared with the OO. Biopsy or aspirate examination clearly distinguishes these two lesions.

EWING'S TUMOR. Ewing's tumor will not show a nidus on tomograms. Biopsy, imprints, and special stains are diagnostic.

EOSINOPHILIC GRANULOMA. Small lesions may mimic OO with a lucent nidus. Biopsy is a diagnostic mixture of benign histiocytes and eosinophils.

METASTASIS. On very rare occasions a small intracortical metastasis mimics OO (Fig. 7-35). Biopsy is diagnostic.

Course and Treatment

The lesion is completely benign. There are no recorded instances of malignant degeneration. Simple excision suffices. However, since the lesion is quite small and may be located in poorly accessible areas, its complete removal may be a difficult task. Exact localization, by tomography, bone scan or insertion of a needle into the lesion by fluroscopy may greatly facilitate its removal. If the lesion is not totally removed, the remaining portion of the nidus may result in a re-exacerbation of symptoms.

Although, the vast majority of OO's are removed surgically, there are a few cases reported of spontaneous healing.[13,21,27] I know one radiologist who followed by means of serial radiography his osteoid osteoma of femur for 10 years before all trace of it disappeared. However, he had to live with significant pain requiring up to 14 to 16 aspirin tablets per day for 4 of those 10 years.

(*Text continues on p. 108.*)

Histology of Osteoid Osteoma or Osteoblastoma

FIG. 7-25. Prominent rimming of osteoblasts, a feature almost always signifying a focus of benign osteoid or bone production, in spite of the plumpness of the cells (H and E, X400).

FIG. 7-26. While some of these lesions are rich in osteoid, others are replete with dense woven bone. This is such an example. Note the thickness of the trabeculae, the serrated borders, and the prominence of capillaries and osteoclasts. Rimming of osteoblasts in this field is inconspicuous to minimal. This latter feature is usually reduced in those cases with dense woven bone and probably signifies a reduction in its growth activity (H and E, X125).

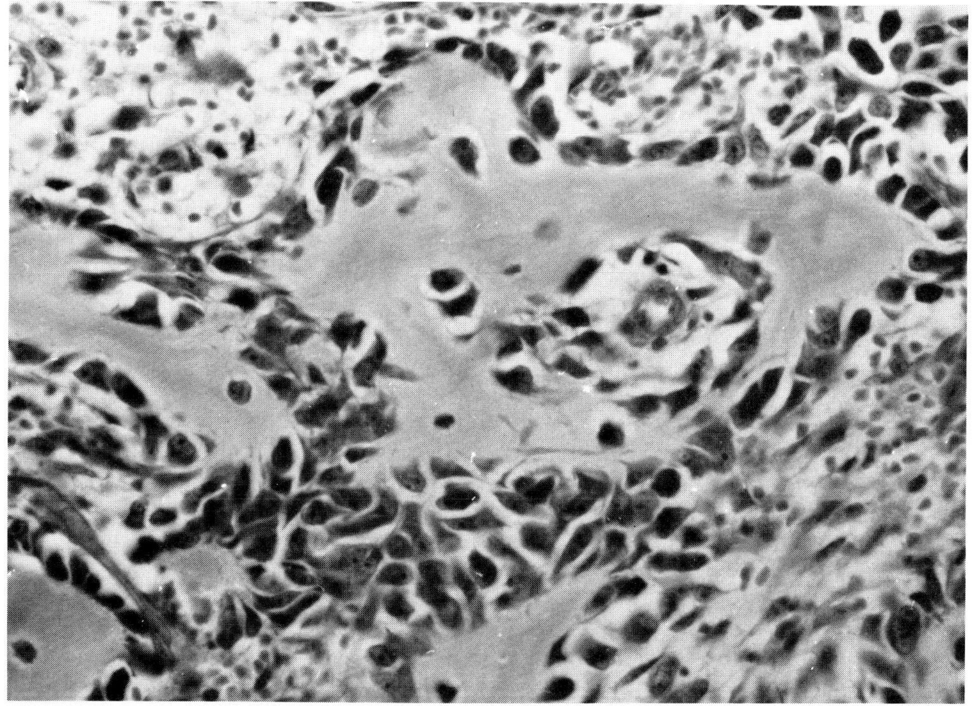

FIG. 7-25

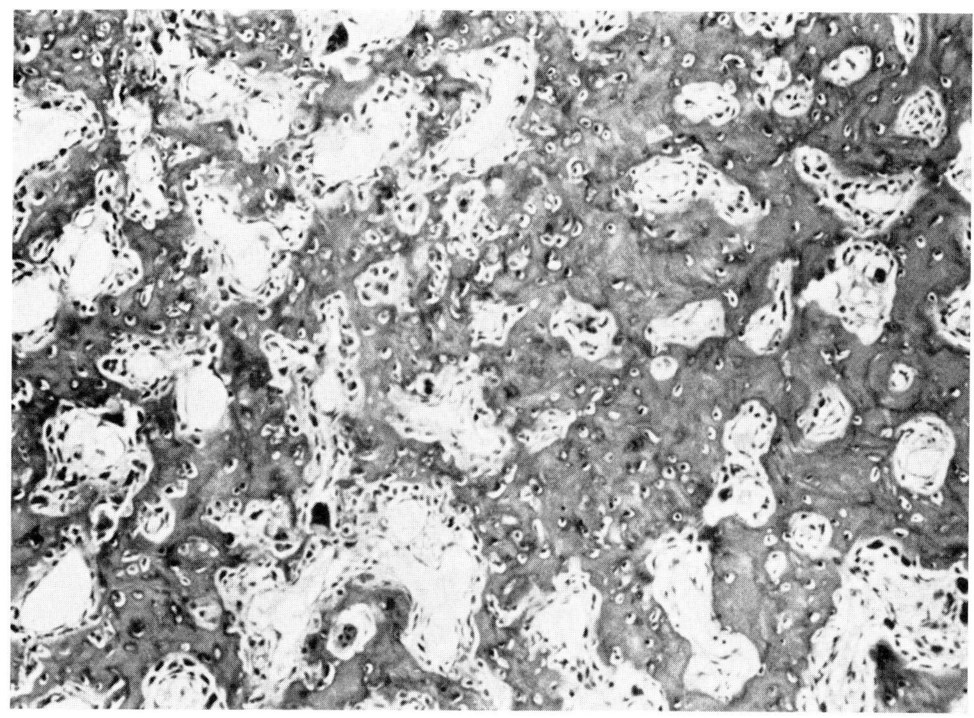

FIG. 7-26

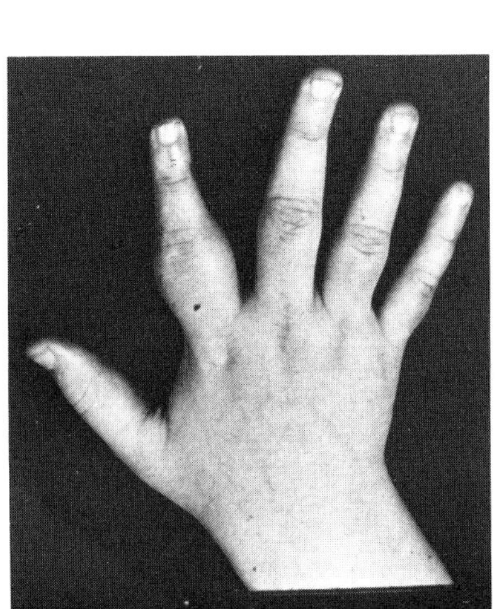

FIG. 7-27

FIG. 7-28

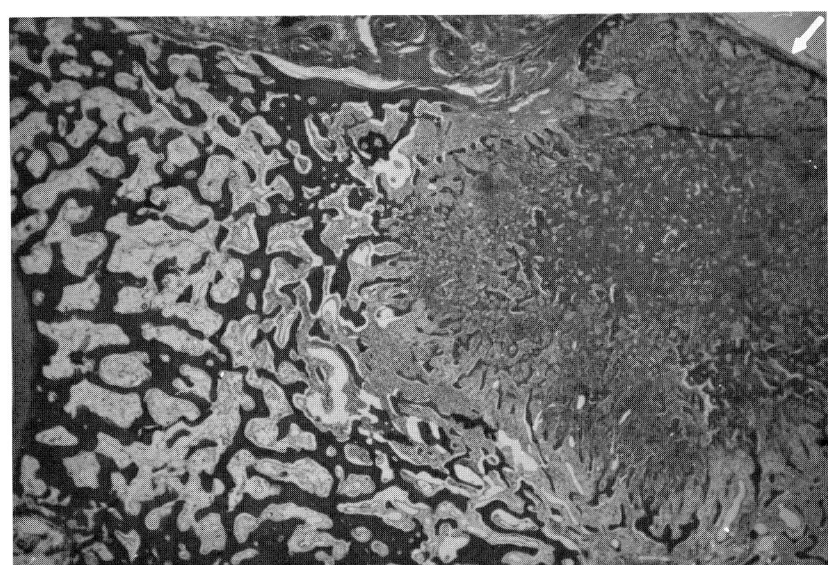

FIG. 7-29

Osteoid Osteoma

FIG. 7-27. The marked tenderness, swelling, and redness of the second digit clinically resembles osteomyelitis.

FIG. 7-28. Radiographs, however, clearly show that the irritation of the soft tissues was consequent to an intracortical osteoid osteoma.

FIG. 7-29. Intramedullary to intracortical osteoid osteoma of a phalanx. As in other lesions of this type, the lesional bone is clearly delineated from host lamellar bone. The portion of the lesion that extends beyond the normal confines of the bone is covered by a thin shell of periosteal new bone (*arrow*).

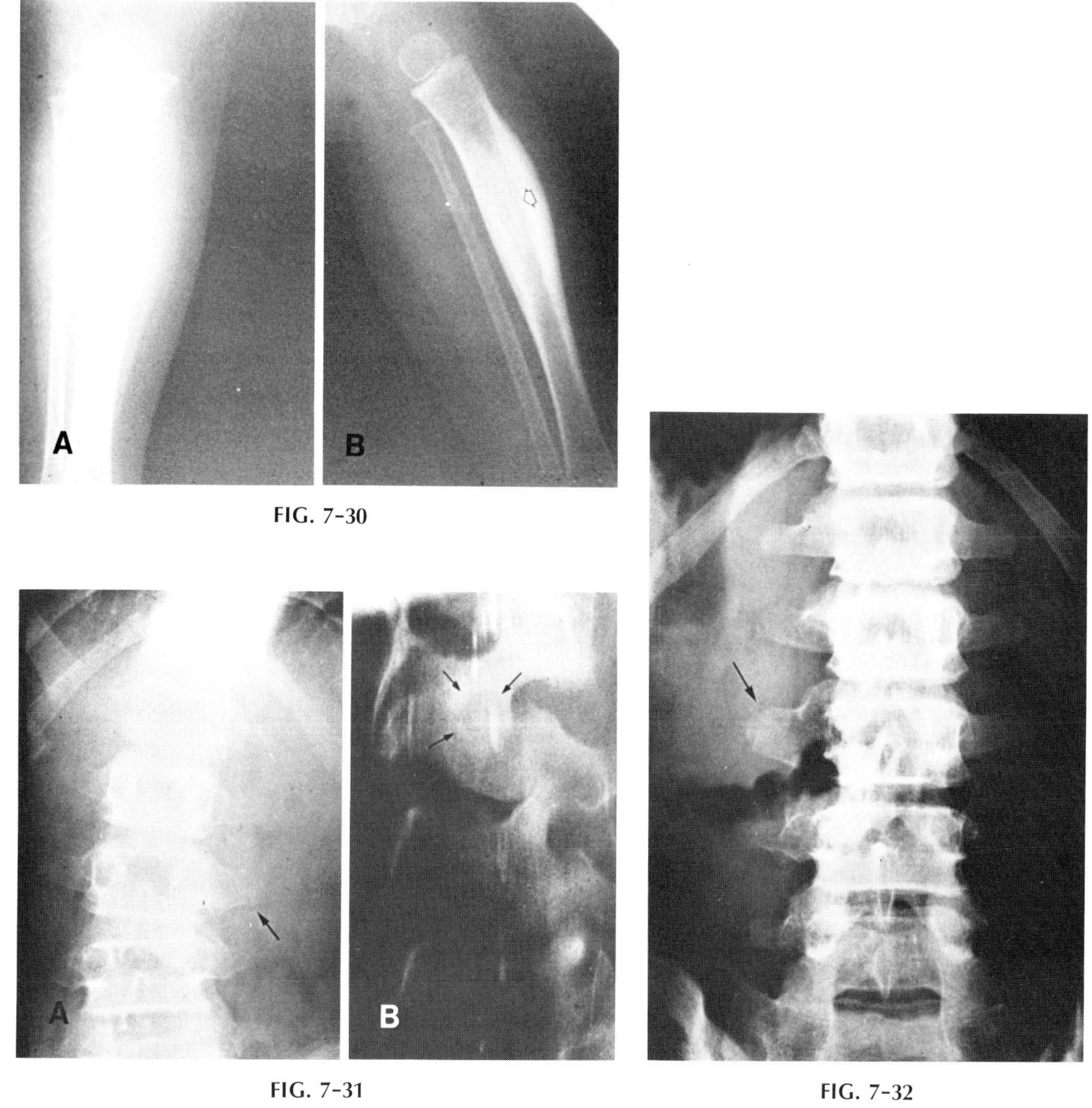

FIG. 7-30

FIG. 7-31

FIG. 7-32

Osteoid Osteoma

FIG. 7-30. This osteoid osteoma (OO) arose in the tibia of an 18-month-old boy. It is characterized by massive homogeneous density and smooth periosteal sclerosis. Lesions such as these are commonly seen in association with OO. Penetrating tomograms are crucial to diagnosis (*B*). In contrast to most OOs, this nidus is distinctly more elongated in the longitudinal axis. It is of interest to note that two similar long elliptical nidi are described by Norman, *et. al.*[22] in two very young patients (16 months and 2 years old). Long elliptical nidi are not seen in patients with closed epiphyses. This would imply that the shape of an OO nidus can be affected by bone growth. The younger the patient and the closer the lesion to an area of rapid growth, the longer the nidus appears to be. Unless the full extent of these long elliptical nidi are removed entirely, treatment will be inadequate and pain is likely to recur.

FIG. 7-31. (*A*) Patient presented with back pain. Radiograph revealed a curve in the lumbar spine. There is an increase in size in the transverse process, which is in the center of the convex portion of the curve. This is a clue to the presence of an OO, and tomograms should be concentrated at this spot (*arrow*). (*B*) Tomogram clearly outlines the OO (*arrows*).

FIG. 7-32. Several weeks post-resection, the spine is no longer functionally scoliotic. The transverse process that had contained the nidus is still enlarged, however (*arrow*).

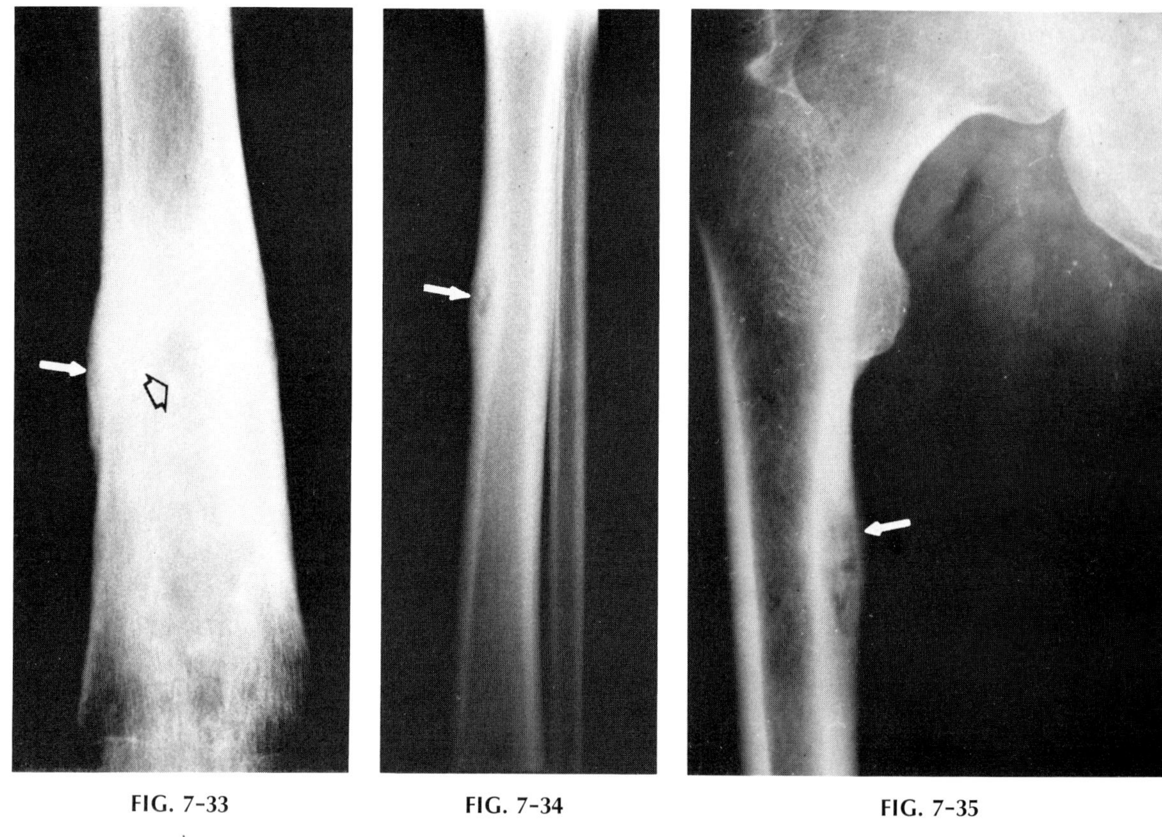

FIG. 7-33 FIG. 7-34 FIG. 7-35

Lesions Mimicking Osteoid Osteoma

FIG. 7-33. Osteomyelitis. A central mass of two dead bone slivers (sequestrum) (*black arrow*). The sequestrum may resemble an OO nidus. The uneven to undulating periosteal new bone (*white arrow*) and the uneven distribution of reactive bone sclerosis and irregular lucencies some distance from the "nidus" is almost never seen in osteoid osteoma, but is a frequent accompaniment of osteomyelitis.

FIG. 7-34. Pus was found in this small intracortical abscess (*arrow*) that otherwise simulated an osteoid osteoma (OO) almost exactly, except perhaps for the fact that the niduslike area has an ill-defined or shaggy contour. Such osteomyelitis lesions that so closely resemble OO are rare in comparison to the incidence of true osteoid osteomas with this appearance.

FIG. 7-35. Metastatic renal cell carcinoma. On very rare occasions, a metastatic tumor may bear some resemblance to an OO. In contrast to OO, however, there is concentric layering of the periosteum adjacent to the lesion (*arrow*). Secondly, instead of a clear-cut round nidus, the intracortical lesion has a shaggy or ill-defined contour.

Osteoblastoma

Capsule Summary

Incidence. Some 0.5 per cent biopsied bone tumors.

Age. Peak incidence, persons 10 to 20 years old. Over 80 per cent of patients are younger than 30 year old.

Clinical Features. Pain, swelling, rarely gross fracture. Neurological symptoms, functional scoliosis, and muscle atrophy, if the spine is involved.

Radiologic Features. The tumor's growth usually results in fusiform expansion. The affected bone is covered by a thin rim of periosteal new bone. Ominous periosteal reactions are uncommon; on rare occasion may mimic osteosarcoma or osteomyelitis. Center of lesion is variable: it is either lucent, mixed lucent and blastic, or predominantly blastic. Usually has a mixed pattern and tends to affect diaphyses and metaphyses of long bones and the posterior arch, when the spine is involved. Tomograms should show sharp circumscription of the lesions' borders. Vertebral bodies are rarely affected.

Gross Pathology. Red, if highly vascular; gritty and more yellowish if there is considerable bone production. It is larger than 2 cm. and well circumscribed. Outer contours may be lobular.

Histopathology. There are usually lobulated outer borders. Infiltration of surrounding host lamellar bone either does not occur or is minimal (less than 1 mm. of the intertrabecular marrow). Usually, there is no lamellar bone trapped in the lesional area. The absence of demonstrable infiltration by the lesional tissue between lamellar bone marrow is helpful in differentiating the osteoblastoma from the osteosarcoma. Cartilage has not been reported in association with the osteoblastoma and unequivocal anaplasia is, of course, not present. High-power features are identical to that of the osteoid osteoma.

Course. Benign. Recurrences are very uncommon. When there are recurrences an osteosarcoma mistaken for osteoblastoma or malignant transformation of osteoblastoma must be considered and ruled out.

Treatment. Curettage and packing with bone chips.

General Features

DEFINITION. The osteoblastoma is a rare, benign, usually larger than 2 cm. circumscribed lesion composed principally of osteoid and woven bone. Its histologic features are almost identical to that of the osteoid osteoma, a fact which prompted Dr. Dahlin to call it the "giant osteoid osteoma." However, differences in the severity of pain, the sites of involvement (See Figs. 7-17 and 7-36), radiographic features, gross and low-power microscopic features are sufficiently distinctive, some authors believe, to justify labeling them as different entities. On occasion their features overlap and distinguishing between them is not possible.

IMPORTANCE. The greatest problem for the pathologist is not distinguishing osteoblastoma from osteoid osteoma but distinguishing the osteoblastoma from intramedullary osteosarcoma. The consequences of incorrect diagnosis are, of course, disastrous. Even the most highly qualified experts will admit to errors of this kind on occasion. The usual story is that of a patient with a blastic or lytic and blastic lesion confined to the bone that is diagnosed as "osteoblastoma" but who will return in several months to at most 2 years with massive bone destruction, a soft-tissue mass, and metastases. Similarly it is probable that some osteosarcoma "cures" include cases of osteoblastoma.

The other entity that is confused with osteoblastoma is the giant cell tumor with prominent osteoid and woven-bone production. This entity is discussed later, in the differential diagnosis section. It is important to separate these two lesions, because giant cell tumor acts like a low-grade malignant neoplasm, while the osteoblastoma is almost always controlled by simple curettage or if more "aggressive" (very large size or recurrence), by en-bloc excision or, in this authors opinion, by cryosurgery.

INCIDENCE. The osteoblastoma represents approximately 0.5 per cent of biopsied primary bone tumors. Osteoid osteomas are five times as common and osteosarcomas, 38 times as common.

Sites of Involvement

The osteoblastoma generally involves the metaphyses or diaphyses of the long bones. Approximately 42 per cent of osteoblastomas involve the spine and sacrum, while only 7 per cent of osteoid osteomas involve these areas. Approximately 3 per cent involve the skull bones and mandible, in contrast to the osteoid osteoma, in which less than 1 per cent (only 1 reported case) involved these bones. Osteoblastomas are centered in the medullary portions of the shaft, while osteoid osteomas tend to be located near to or in the cortex or subperiosteally. Osteogenic sarcoma is similar to osteoblastoma in that it is usually centered in the deep medullary substance, most commonly involving the metaphysis of the bones around the knee, proximal humerus, and skull. Osteosarcoma is rare in the spine (3%). However, since osteosarcoma is 38 times as common, the *actual* number of osteosarcomas of the spine compared to osteoblastoma will be approximately equal.

Clinical Features

Pain or discomfort are the prominent complaints in most cases.[40] Symptoms are usually present for a few months to a year. The pain is usually not severe and only occasional cases are relieved dramatically by aspirin. In one rare instance I have seen of a 7-year-old boy with an osteoblastoma of the femur (Fig. 7-42), the lesion, in a period of 2 years, resulted in loss of appetite, severe cachexia, high output cardiomegaly, reversal of albumin-globulin ratio, systemic periostosis, leg edema, and chronic fever.[42] We attributed these unusual symptoms to an inappropriate and overwhelming host immune response to the tumor. Massive numbers of plasma cells were seen at the edge of the lesion.

Tenderness over the tumor is the most consistent physical finding. If located near a joint, there may be some loss of motion or a limp.

Those lesions that arise near to, or in the spine, may result in muscle spasm and functional scoliosis, muscle or sensory deficits, and, in up to 50 to 60 per cent of cases, abnormal tendon reflexes.[40]

Radiographic Features

Osteoblastoma usually results in a uniform fusiform expansion of the bone (Figs. 7-37–7-40). Even if it extends into the soft tissues, it is usually always covered by a thin rim of periosteal new bone (Figs. 7-38–7-40).[42] The borders of the lesion appear well delineated from the surrounding host bone and often there is a thin rim of reactive intramedullary bone sclerosis. The lesional center may be variably blastic and stippled densities may be seen (Fig. 7-39). Rarely, the lesional center is almost completely lucent (Fig. 7-41). Most lesions are about 4 to 6 cm. in size, although their range is 2 to 10 cm. Ominous periosteal new bone and Codman's triangles are rarely seen. If seen, such cases will be difficult to distinguish from osteosarcoma or osteomyelitis. Some cases may show extensive prominent reactive host bone and smooth periosteal sclerosis, similar to that seen in the osteoid osteoma (OO). An OO is characterized by a spherical to ovoid nidus, a lucent collar, and much more commonly than osteoblastoma, a severe extensive reactive bone sclerosis and thick but smooth periosteal reactive sclerosis.

An osteosarcoma is usually characterized by poorly delineated borders, ominous periosteal reactions, including Codman's triangles, and a soft-tissue mass not delineated by a thin shell of bone. In rare cases of small or incipient osteosarcomas, however, the radiographic features may be virtually identical to that of osteoblastoma. Rarely, if ever, does the osteosarcoma result in smooth bone "expansion." On very rare occasions the osteoblastoma may mimic the usual osteosarcoma radiologically. Only careful microscopic assessment for anaplasia and/or cartilage and a wedge biopsy, which includes the edge of the lesion as it abuts the host bone, will distinguish the two.

In the long bones, osteoblastomas are most often centered in the diaphysis or metaphysis. Extension to the epiphyseal region is most common in the short tubular bones of the hands or feet. The lesion does not, however, cross a growing epiphyseal plate. Osteoblastomas of the spine usually arise from only the posterior elements and rarely extend into the vertebral body. The most common destructive *primary* bone tumor of the vertebral body is the giant cell tumor. Although, hemangiomas of the vertebral bodies are perhaps the most common malformation of vertebral bodies, they tend to result in accentuation of the vertical bony trabeculae.

On occasion, osteoblastomas may grow quite rapidly as evidenced by serial x-ray studies, so that this feature may not be very useful in distinguishing the osteoblastoma from the osteosarcoma. However, if a small osteosarcoma is considered benign radiographically (Fig. 7-85, *A*) and a biopsy is not taken, or if it is and called benign, within a few weeks to months the error will become startlingly obvious (Fig. 7-85, *B*). In essence, rapidly growing osteoblastomas usually remain confined by at least a rim of periosteal new bone, which is usually fine or thin, while small osteosarcomas will soon erode into the soft tissues and present with a soft-tissue mass not covered by a fine, smooth, concentric rim of periosteal new bone.

Gross Pathology

Osteoblastomas range in size from 2 to 10 cm. Since they contain woven bone, they are variably gritty. Their color is usually a deep red to reddish brown or pink (Plate 2, *B*), a reflection of their intense vascularity. Lesions with less vascularity are usually yellowish and harder, because they contain greater amounts of bone than the intensely red lesions. If a lesion is removed intact, it is well circumscribed (Plate 2, *B*, Fig. 7-42, *A* and *B*) and surrounded by a shell of cortical bone or thickened periosteum. If the cortex is focally destroyed and a soft-tissue mass is observed, it is much more likely to be a malignant tumor, because benign osteoblastomas almost never have this feature. Osteoblastomas may erode the cortex and "bulge" the bone in a concentric or fusiform fashion and be covered by a fine to thick (rare) shell of periosteal new bone. This latter feature is particularly common in osteoblastomas that arise in small bones or confined sites such as metacarpal bones (Fig. 7-38) or transverse or spinous processes of the vertebral column (Fig. 7-40). This feature is also commonly seen in association with the aneurysmal bone cyst and fibrous dysplasia.

Histopathology

If one examines a number of osteoblastomas and osteoid osteomas, it becomes apparent that on medium- to high-power examination, it may be impossible to clearly distinguish one from the other. Some osteoblastomas will show very prominent plump osteoblasts, osteoid, woven bone, vascularity and osteoclasts; others may show thickened masses of woven bone with a diminution in vascularity, osteoclasts, and flattened osteoblasts. The same is true of the OO.

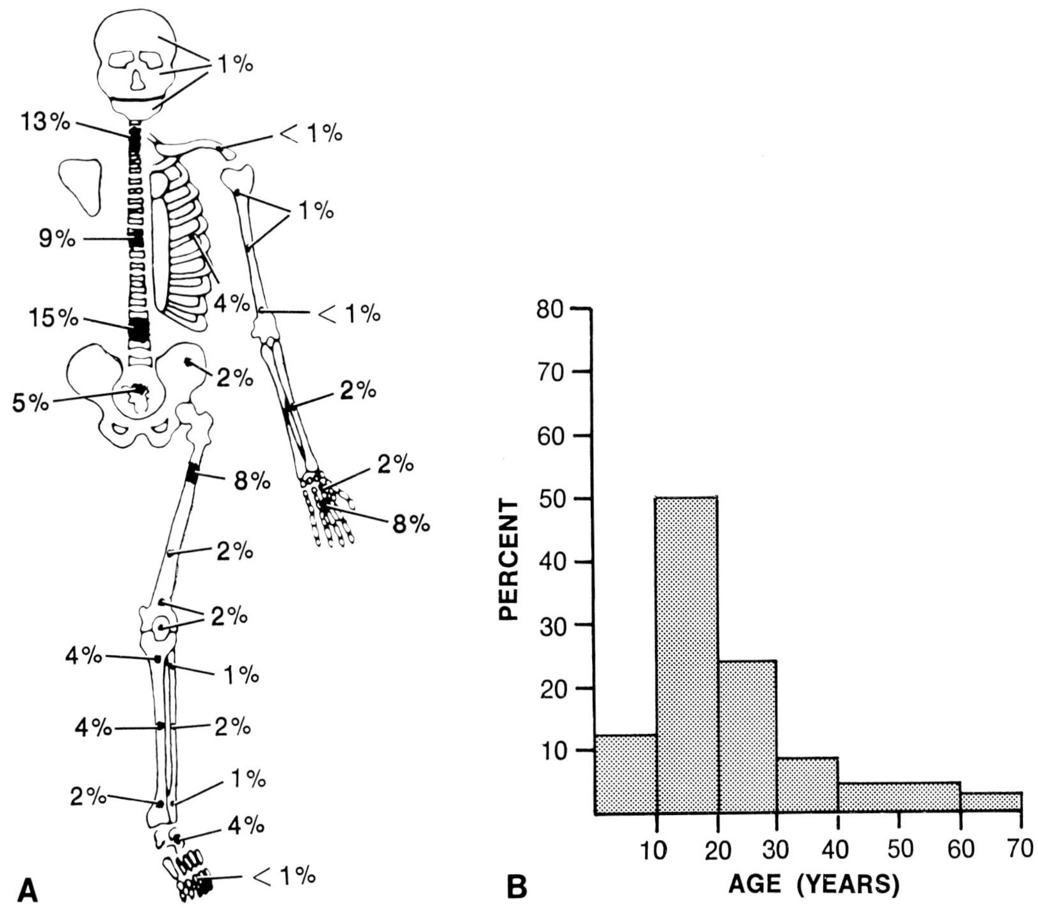

FIG. 7-36. (*A*) Frequency of areas of involvement in 144 patients. This rare lesion accounts for only 0.5 per cent of all primary bone tumors. Male: female incidence, 2:1. (*B*) The graph shows age distribution of patients with osteoblastoma. (Mirra, J., Bullough, P., and Freiberger, R.: Orthopedic Diseases, Part I: Bone Tumors. New York, Famous Teachings in Modern Medicine, MedCom, Inc., © 1967)

In some regions, osteoblastomas may show prominant sheets of osteoblasts (up to 10 cells thick). This is usually not seen in OO. In general, osteoid osteomas are removed intact; their size (less than 1 cm.) and round shape permit easy distinction from osteoblastomas, which are usually removed as curetted specimens. If an osteoblastoma is removed intact, it is distinguishable from the O.O. by its greater size and a lobulated outer perimeter (Plate 2, *D*).

Distinguishing Microscopic Features of Osteoid Osteoma and Osteoblastoma: Differentiation from Osteosarcoma

In most texts, it is emphasized that osteoblastoma can be distinguished from osteosarcoma because the osteoblastoma lacks anaplasia. Unfortunately, the distinctly active plump hyperplastic cells of an osteoblastoma can be interpreted as anaplasia by those unfamiliar with this lesion. The second common assumption is that almost every osteosarcoma has so many features of anaplasia that confusion with other entities should be negligible. But, I have seen at least five cases that were diagnosed as osteoblastoma by experts in which there were massive recurrence, metastases, and death within 1 to 4 years of initial diagnosis, proving that in reality they were osteosarcomas from inception.

In my experience, I have seen approximately 150 osteosarcomas, 30 osteoid osteomas, and seven osteoblastomas. Between 20 to 30 per cent of biopsy tissues from these osteosarcomas, in my opinion, did not contain sufficient atypia to be objectively diagnosed by most pathologists as osteosarcoma by cytologic criteria alone. In approximately, 90 per cent of these cases, the radiograph showed clear-cut sarcomatous features. However, in some instances the radiographic features of osteoblastoma and osteosarcoma may overlap, and when combined with only minimal cytologic anaplasia with respect to the osteosarcoma or marked cellular exuberance or atypia with respect to the osteoblastoma, the trap is set for error.

Also my studies of osteosarcoma have shown that the degree of cytologic atypia or anaplasia is independent of radiographic appearance. Small osteosarcomas that have not yet broken through the cortex may look highly anaplastic, while large, obviously malignant lesions may show minimal cytologic evidence of anaplasia. According to these observations, to calculate the incidence of osteosarcomas by combining "bland" radiographic features with less than objective anaplasia, we should multiply 10 per cent (incidence of incipient osteosarcomas with initial benign radiographic appearance) by 20 per cent (incidence with less than unequivocal anaplasia). The result is 2 per cent, which means that 2 per cent of osteosarcomas may show a combination of "benign" radiologic and "innocent" histologic features. This figure therefore represents the approximate percentage of osteosarcomas that could pass for an osteoblastoma. Let us assume we are confronted with 100 cases that are either osteosarcomas or osteoblastomas. Among these 100 cases, we should, on an incidence basis, have approximately 97 osteosarcomas and two to three true, benign osteoblastomas, since the incidence of osteosarcomas to osteoblastoma is about 38 to one. However, based upon the above observations, approximately two of the 97 osteosarcoma cases have a combination of deceptively innocent radiological and pathological features that could pass for osteoblastoma. This calculation is quite similar to my actual experience. I have seen seven osteoblastomas with benign long-term follow-up, 150 osteosarcomas, and five cases of "osteoblastomas," which killed the patients 1 to 4 years after diagnosis, proving that these osteoblastomas were in fact osteosarcomas. However, in my review of these five "osteoblastoma" cases, there were certain histologic features that were present that distinguish these two tumors.

These histologic aids are as follows:

1. *Osteoblastomas do not produce cartilage.* In four of the five osteosarcomas originally diagnosed as osteoblastomas, there were small but definite focal islands of hyalin cartilage. The cartilage was cellular but in most cases lacked objective anaplasia. The islands of cartilage should be studied; if it is Grade II to III chondrosarcoma (Plate 10, *F*), it is virtually diagnostic of osteosarcoma.

Cartilage production, then, is an important feature in attempting to differentiate an osteoblastoma from osteosarcoma. However, one must be aware that it may be possible for osteoblastoma to induce a pathologic fracture, a component of which can be cartilage. Therefore, the cartilage and radiographs must be reviewed to rule out callus. If no fracture is present, then the possibility that the tumor may be an osteogenic sarcoma must be considered, because this is the most common bone-producing tumor, that comes to biopsy and is also associated with cartilage production. If an unsuspected "stress" fracture is the actual cause of the lesion, then extra care must be taken to avoid confusing it with either an osteoblastoma or with an OS.

Another possible exception to this criterion of cartilage production relates to a unique case reported by Zabski, *et al.*[48] They observed a benign lesion which arose in a rib of a 21-year-old female that had a peculiar combination of osteoblastoma and chondro-

---

Osteoblastoma

FIG. 7-37. One of the spinous processes (*arrow*) is "expanded" and covered by a thin rim of periosteal bone.

FIG. 7-38. Most osteoblastomas show this smooth concentric "expansion" and are covered by a thin rim of bone. A thin collar or rim of periosteal sclerosis (*arrow*) testifies to its benign nature.

FIG. 7-39. The distal end of the clavicle is "expanded" and covered by a rim of bone. There are spots of densification within the lesion, which distinguishes this lesion from an aneurysmal bone cyst. A cartilage tumor would, however, have to enter into the differential diagnosis.

FIG. 7-40. Smooth-bordered expansion of a transverse process (*arrow*) of a cervical vertebrae in addition to increased density within the lesion characterized this osteoblastoma.

FIG. 7-41. In this example of a biopsy-proven osteoblastoma, the unusual features are the lack of expansion, small size, and lucent center. The lesion is surrounded by a subtle, but definite, border of benign sclerosis.

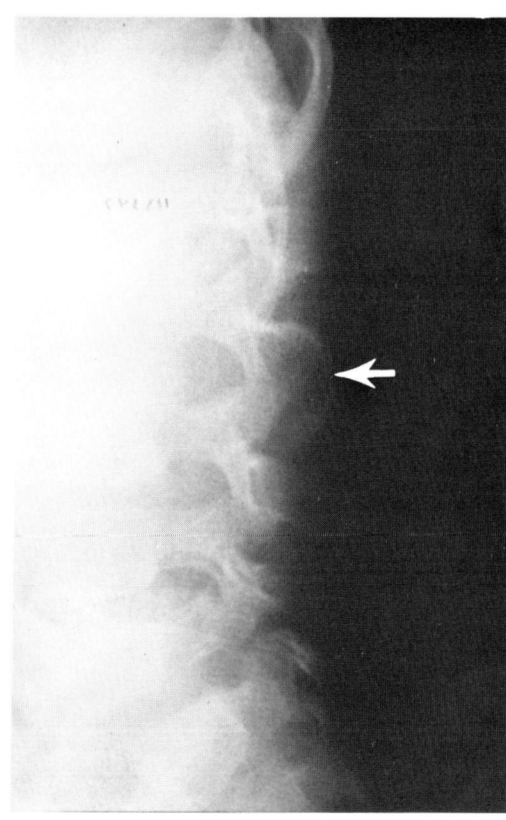

FIG. 7-37

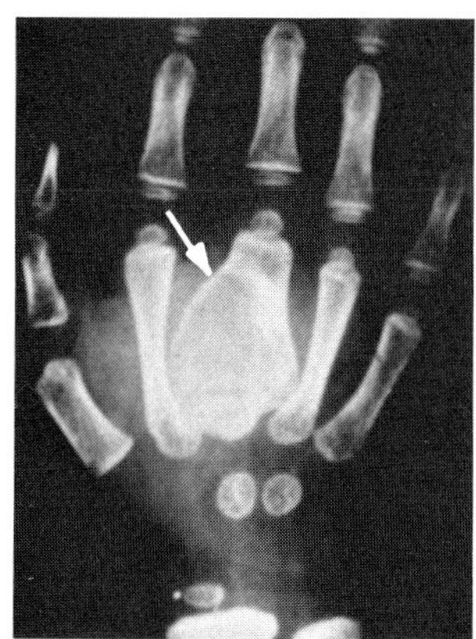

FIG. 7-38

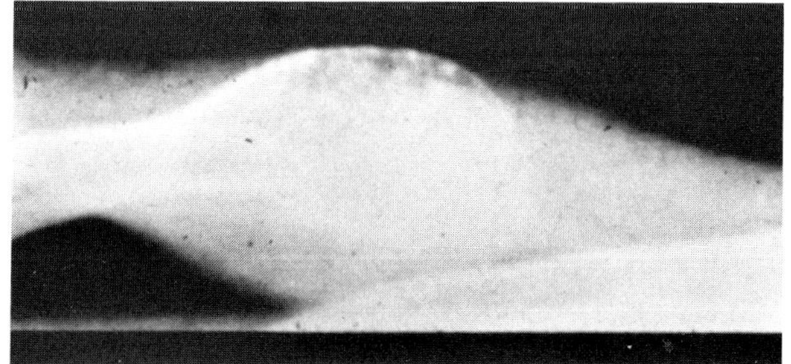

FIG. 7-39

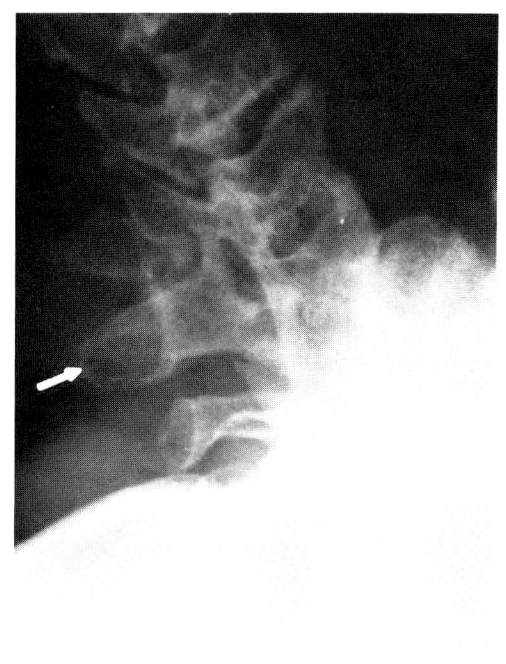

FIG. 7-40

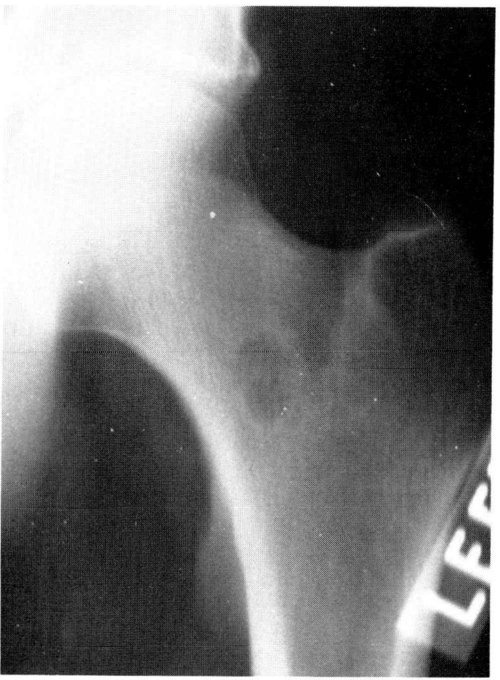

FIG. 7-41

blastoma features, which prompted their diagnosis of an osteochondroblastoma. Even so, this unique case had evidence of cartilage production different from that seen in osteosarcoma. In osteosarcoma, the cartilage production is usually pure hyaline. In this case, foci of rounded to polygonal chondroblasts maturing to hyaline cartilage indistinguishable from a chondroblastoma were seen.

2. A second important histologic aid in differentiating an osteoblastoma from a minimally anaplastic osteosarcoma is related to the pattern of osteoid and woven-bone deposition. *Most osteoblastomas produce thick trabeculae of osteoid and woven bone with irregular serrated borders (Plate 2, G and H). The stroma is usually as wide as the trabeculae are thick and contain numerous prominent capillary vessels and osteoclasts.* Although *osteosarcomas* may produce bone of this type, *they usually produce focal or extensive areas of compact osteoid or poorly calcified woven bone with a "tightly-knit" or "streamer" pattern (Plate 4, A, B, and C), with a paucity of prominent vessels.* In these areas osteoclasts are usually absent and the nuclei are quite small and deceptively innocent looking (Plate 3, *H* and *I*). Yet, osteosarcoma composed entirely of this compact osteoid and woven-bone pattern with small osteoblastic and osteocytic nuclei may behave in as virulent a fashion as their high-grade anaplastic counterparts. This author has seen this pattern of osteoid and woven bone in numerous osteogenic sarcomas. But, this is not an infallible aide, as this pattern of tightly knit streamers of osteoid tissue was also present in one indisputable osteoid osteoma (personal observation) and in a focus of a small femoral lesion of an adult male of an osteoblastoma with benign long term follow-up studies despite simple curettage (x-ray of this patient shown in Fig. 7–41). Nevertheless, this pattern of masses of ominous closely knit streamers of collagen, in my experience, is seen in a ratio of 25 osteosarcomas per 1 benign lesion.

3. *Search for infiltration of tumor cells, osteoid, or woven bone between host lamellar bone marrow.* Another feature that has been observed by this author in a small sample of intact osteoblastomas and numerous intact osteoid osteomas that for this observer helps to distinguish these lesions is that in the two benign conditions, the lesional osteoid and woven bone (seen most clearly with polarized light) is quite sharply delineated from the surrounding host lamellar bone (Plate 2, *C* and *E*, Fig. 7–42). In almost every instance of OO and osteoblastoma the host lamellar bone is totally absent or replaced in the lesional area. Small portions of host lamellar bone and marrow may, however, be trapped between the lobulated margins of the osteoblastoma. Even so, careful scrutiny demonstrates a distinct "front" of osteoblastomatous tissue that abuts host lamellar bone and marrow fat. Infiltration of the marrow, even in these trapped portions of host bone, by tumor cells is not seen. In contrast, intact specimens of osteosarcoma show that the neoplasm in virtually all instances infiltrates the marrow, i.e., insinuates itself millimeters to centimeters between the host lamellar bone at its advancing edges (Plate 3, *B* and *C*). This feature shows up much clearer with polarized light (Plate 3, *E*). In the deep zones of osteosarcoma, however, the host lamellar bone may be completely replaced. Therefore, to use this pattern as a diagnostic aide, intact specimens or biopsies of the marginal zone of lesion with host bone should be obtained. In reviewing the literature on osteoblastoma, this author has seen only one reference to the clear separation of osteoblastoma woven bone from host bone.[30] Since this finding may ultimately prove to be of great value in distinguishing equivocal cases of osteoblastomas from osteosarcomas, the following surgical procedure is suggested: *In assessing a possible osteoblastoma, the surgeon should submit for pathological examination not merely curettage specimens in which the margins of*

Osteoblastoma

FIG. 7-42. (*A*) Rare gross example of an intact osteoblastoma. Note its sharp circumscription (*arrows*). It caused massive cortical and periosteal new bone deposition (*a*), which mimicked osteomyelitis or osteosarcoma on radiograph and obscured its true diagnosis. (*B*) This illustration corresponds to a low-power histologic composite of the upper two slides shown in the previous illustration. Again note its sharp circumscription (**A**, *black arrows*) and lack of infiltration between the marrow of the host lamellar bone, which would occur in an osteosarcoma. Note also the massive cortical periosteal new bone reaction **(*B*)** and the osteporotic but lesion-free medulla **(C).** (*C*) Two coalescent lobules of woven bone production of another osteoblastoma removed intact. Note its distinct front or line of separation or absence of marrow invasion between host bone lamellae along its margins (*arrows*). Osteoblastomas tend to have this lobulated appearance in comparison to the more exquisite spherical shape of osteoid osteomas but lack the multiple invasive nodular foci of tumor bone between host marrow seen along its advancing peripheral margins in osteosarcoma (H and E, X 10).

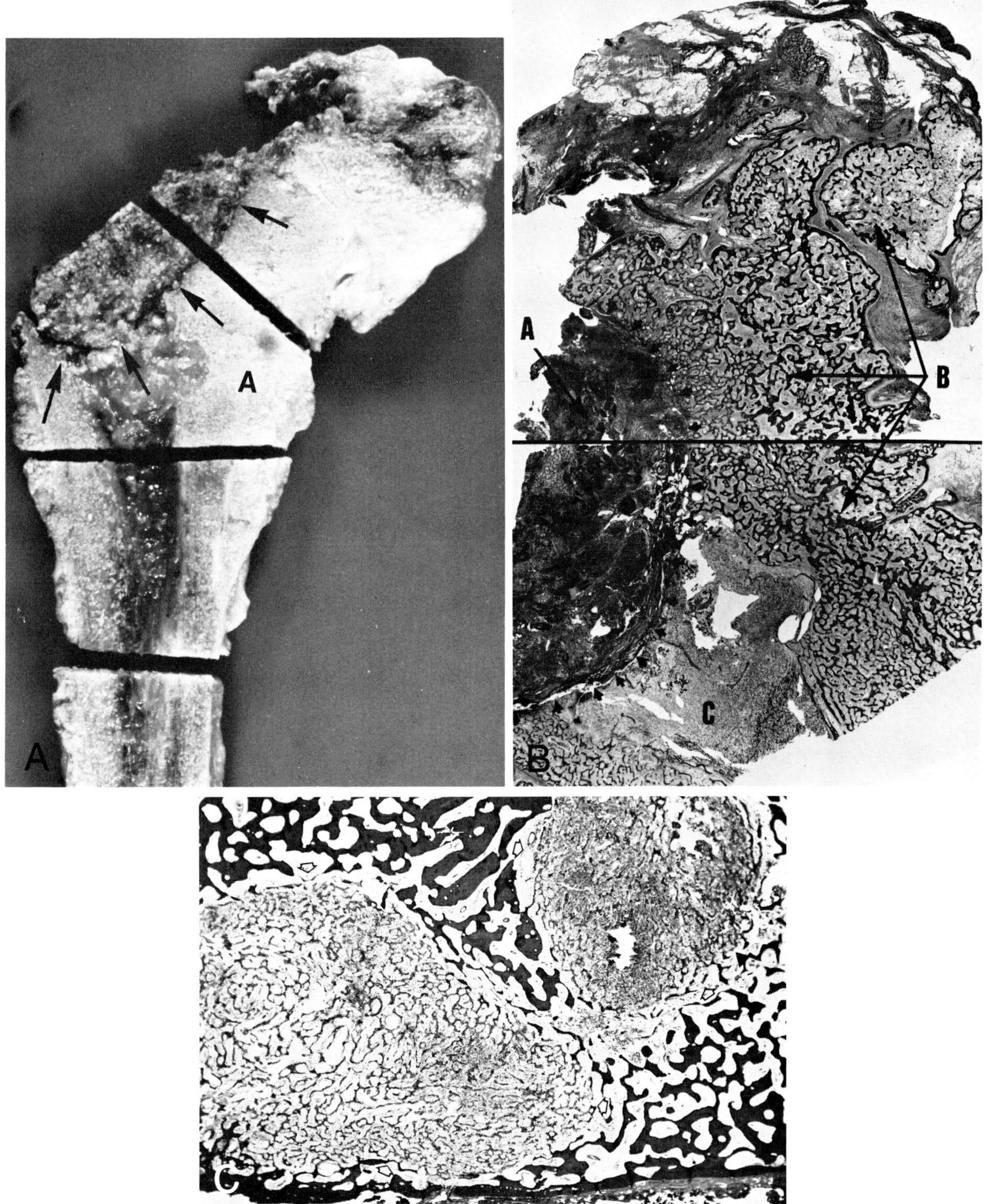

FIG. 7-42

the lesion are destroyed but an intact wedge that includes a margin of lesion with host bone.

But, when the pathologist receives a curettage or small biopsy specimen showing predominantly osteoid and woven bone production, he should still search for the pattern of lamellar bone infiltration by these tissues. Its absence does not rule out osteosarcoma, since in the deeper portions of this lesion the lamellar bone may be totally resorbed. Its presence could, however, signify osteosarcoma (most likely), stress fracture, or possibly fibrous dysplasia.

4. *Search for prominent rimming of osteoblasts.* Prominent rimming of osteoblasts can be found in osteoblastoma and OO and rarely in areas of malignant tumor bone production (see p. 95, Fig. 7–25, Plate 2, *G* and *H*). Prominent well-defined, and well-oriented osteoblastic rimming is not seen in all osteoblastomas and OO's, nor may it be seen throughout the lesion. Usually the rimming is prominent in only small foci, most often at the peripheral aspect of the tumor tissues. Benign osteoblastic rimming may be seen in osteosarcoma, at the advancing edge of the tumor with normal host bone or periosteum; the rimming representing a reactive response of benign tissues to the infiltrating tumor. Therefore, this feature must be used in context and requires interpretation and experience before it can be properly used as a diagnostic aid.

5. *Search for presence or absence of unequivocal anaplasia.* In osteoblastoma and OO, there is an absence of unequivocal anaplasia. There may be, however, such a wild flurry of cellular proliferation that it may be mistaken for anaplasia (Fig. 7–23, Plate 2, *F*). By objective anaplasia it is meant bizarre sizes and shapes of nuclei, abnormal chromatin distribution, variation in nucleolar size, and frequent typical and nonmirror image mitoses (Plate 4, *G*). Approximately 80 per cent of biopsied osteosarcomas will show these latter features in one field or other. The smaller the sample size and the more sclerosing or densely bone-producing the osteosarcoma, the greater is the chance of not finding objective anaplasia.

In addition to the wild flurry of cells seen in osteoblastoma, it appears possible that on extremely rare occasions this lesion may undergo degenerative changes, which result in bizarre nuclei that may mimic high-grade anaplasia. The principle histologic distinguishing feature is the total absence of mitosis. A case with this peculiar microscopic presentation is discussed later in this section (see pp. 120 and Figs. 7–47–7–49).

Osteoblastoma Versus Osteosarcoma—A Case Example

A specific case example[93] will illustrate more clearly how these five histologic aids help distinguish osteoblastoma from osteosarcoma.

The patient, a 12-year-old white female cheerleader, complained of intermittant pain in the thigh of 3 months duration. A specific episode of trauma or of scuba diving was denied. Physical examination was unremarkable. Radiographs only showed a single bone lesion. It was a small (less than 2.5 cm.) and had fluffy "cumulus cloudlike" density, and was located in the femoral diaphysis (Fig. 7–43, *A*). Cortical bone destruction was not present and periosteal new bone was absent. Tomography showed no fracture line (Fig. 7–44, *right*). The lesion, therefore, was not representative of the usual stress fracture since evidence of a fracture line and, as importantly, periosteal new bone, was absent as well.

Based upon the radiological appearance, possible diagnoses uncluded bone infarct, enchondroma, osteoblastoma, osteosarcoma, and unusual stress fracture. Osteoid osteoma was not feasible because a nidus was not present and there was not significant diffuse reactive sclerosis or smooth-bordered periosteal new bone. Radiographs did not show punctate calcifications of 1 to 2 mm.; this helped to rule out the diagnosis of enchondroma.

The presence of coalescing "cumulus cloudlike" fluffs of bone is suggestive of incipient osteogenic sarcoma (see also Fig. 7–85) and for this reason, in spite of the seemingly benign radiographic appearance, biopsy was performed.

The biopsy revealed a predominance of compacted masses of osteoid and woven bone with little intervening stroma, a paucity of blood vessels and osteoclasts and seemingly innocent cytologic features (Fig. 7–44). Only occasional mirror-image mitoses were found. In addition to this tissue were several small islands of hyalin cartilage with cellularity and focal nuclear atypia severe enough to suggest chondrosarcoma tissue to those with enough experience with cartilage productive tumors (Fig. 7–45). Osteoid and woven bone were found infiltrating between lamellar bone (Fig. 7-46). Benign osteoblastic rimming was not seen.

Let us now consider these features and the manner in which we can arrive at a specific diagnosis by elimination. Bone infarct is ruled out by the absence of masses of dead bone and fat and the absence of dystrophic calcification and fibrosis. Osteoid osteoma and osteoblastoma are ruled out by the presence of cartilage islands. Enchondroma and chondrosarcoma are eliminated by the presence of osteoid and woven bone production directly from an undifferentiated (noncartilagenous) stroma and "stress" fracture was eliminated by the absence of a fracture line and periosteal callus on radiographic analysis, and most importantly; by cartilage atypia, which in this author's experience, exceeded the bounds of callus cartilage. Osteoid and woven bone may form by metaplastic activity on the surface or within cartilage lobules and still be acceptable as a primary cartilage tumor. However, if tumor osteoid and bone forms from a noncartilagenous stroma, by definition the tumor in question cannot be a primary cartilage tumor. Therefore, by process of elimination all benign and primary cartilagenous tumor possibilities are excluded in this case. The only lesion to explain all of the features, including the pattern of infiltration between lamellar bone and the absence of benign osteoblastic rimming, is an osteogenic sarcoma with minimal atypia of the tumor bone and subtle low-grade chondrosarcoma.

Based upon this diagnosis and further consultation with Drs. Lichtenstein and Dahlin, an amputation was to be performed, provided that lung metastases were not present. Unfortunately, tomograms of the chest taken but one week after biopsy showed several 1 to 2 cm. cannonball metastases, in spite of the radiological and histological innocence of this osteosarcoma. The patient died of massive pulmonary metastases $2\frac{1}{2}$ months after initial biopsy.

A summary of the differential features of osteoblastomas and osteosarcomas is presented in Table 7–1.

Differential Diagnoses

OSTEOSARCOMA. Approximately 10 per cent of osteosarcomas may show radiologic features that may suggest osteoblastoma and 2 per cent may show radiographic and microscopic features of comparative "innocence" that could be confused with osteoblastoma. These figures can, of course, be either higher or lower, depending on the experience of the diagnosticians involved. The differential radiologic and histologic features of this overlapping group has been dealt with in detail in the preceding section. A more in-depth discussion of the great variety of radiographic and microscopic presentations an osteosarcoma may assume are treated later in this chapter.

OSTEOID OSTEOMA. The distinction between OO and osteoblastoma has been discussed previously (see pp. 99, 100, and 102).

GIANT CELL TUMOR WITH OSTEOID AND WOVEN-BONE PRODUCTION. Approximately 40 per cent of giant cell tumors (GCT) produce some degree of woven bone. This author has seen at least three cases in which 50 per cent of the lesional tissue or more had this feature. In one case, this feature resulted in an erroneous diagnosis of osteosarcoma, and in two, an erroneous diagnosis of osteoblastoma.

The distinction is of importance, because a neoplastic GCT is a low-grade neoplasm best treated by total eradication, such as by freezing or en-bloc resection; osteosarcoma, however, should be treated by radical methods and osteoblastoma, by simple curettage and packing with bone chips.

The distinction between a neoplastic GCT and one with associated bone production is discussed in detail in the section on osteosarcoma. The distinction between osteosarcoma and GCT with bone production is more difficult than the distinction between GCT and osteoblastoma, because osteosarcomas may produce areas replete with numerous osteoclast-like giant cells and stromal cells, which, on cursory examination, may resemble those of a GCT. An osteoblastoma, on the other hand, does not produce areas solidly packed with giant cells and stromal cells, as seen in the classic GCT (see Figs. 10–52 to 10–54). In osteoblastoma and OO, true osteoclasts merely pepper the osteoid and woven bone that is produced (Plate 2, *G*, Fig. 7–24). In other words, these are not solid areas composed purely of giant cells and stromal cells without intervening bone and osteoid. In GCT there may be areas that resemble osteoblastoma, but in osteoblastoma there will be no significant areas which resemble the nonbone-containing areas of a GCT.

HYPERPARATHYROIDISM. On rare occasions the brown tumor of hyperparathyroidism may present as a solitary focus of bone involvement. Since this hormone-induced tumor may appear virtually identical on histologic examination to the true neoplastic GCT, it is conceivable that it could be mistaken for an osteoblastoma. It is good practice to recommend at least 3 serum calciums and phosphorus for all patients with GCT-like areas, whether or not there is associated new bone production, particularly if the lesion is in a nonepiphyseal site. The vast majority of neoplastic giant cell tumors are centered in the epiphyseal-metaphyseal region; the GCT of hyper-

(*Text continues on p. 120.*)

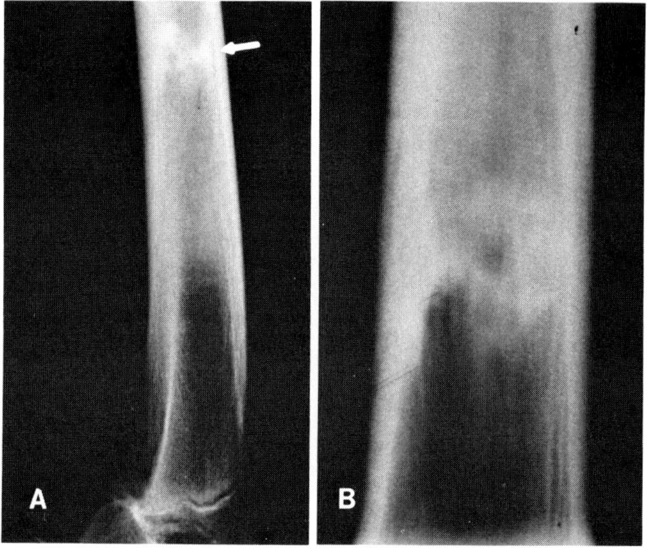

FIG. 7-43

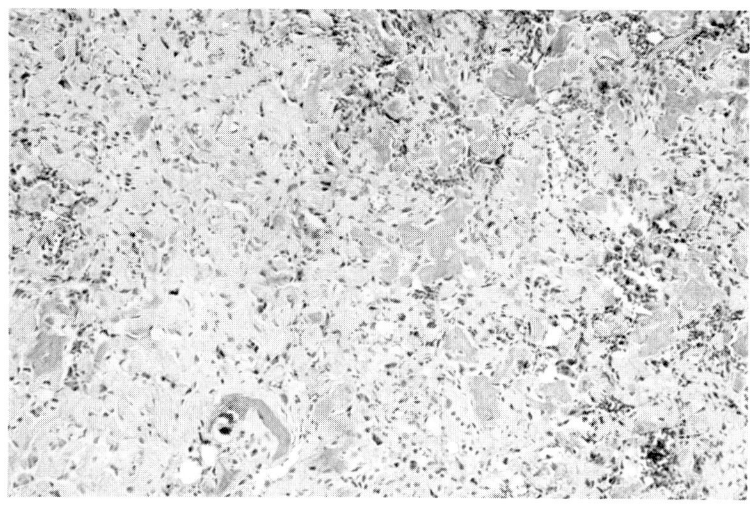

FIG. 7-44

Incipient Blastic Osteosarcoma

FIG. 7-43. (*A*) Small intramedullary fluffs (*arrow*) in the middiaphysis of the femur ("cumulus cloud" like appearance). (*B*) Tomograms failed to reveal a fracture line. Absence of periosteal bone of any kind is also not in support of a diagnosis of the usual stress fracture. In rare cases of stress fracture the above features can be simulated, however, Clinicopathologic correlation is essential to differentiation.

FIG. 7-44. Biopsy of this lesion revealed focal masses of osteoid and woven bone that were tightly packed. The nuclei are innocent in appearance. There is no benign rimming of osteoblasts. The stroma is not rich in dilated capillaries (H and E, X125).

FIG. 7-45. Other fields were composed of a cellular cartilage suggestive of either a very cellular enchondroma or Grade I chondrosarcoma (H and E, X125). Cartilage is not present in osteoblastoma unless associated with pathologic fracture.

FIG. 7-46. Other fields showed host lamellar bone (*black arrows*) between which there was infiltration by a woven bone and osteoid-forming (*white arrow*) tumor (H and E, X40). All of these features combined make the diagnosis of osteosarcoma inevitable, in spite of the bland radiograph and pathological features. This case represents the smallest osteosarcoma yet reported.[93]

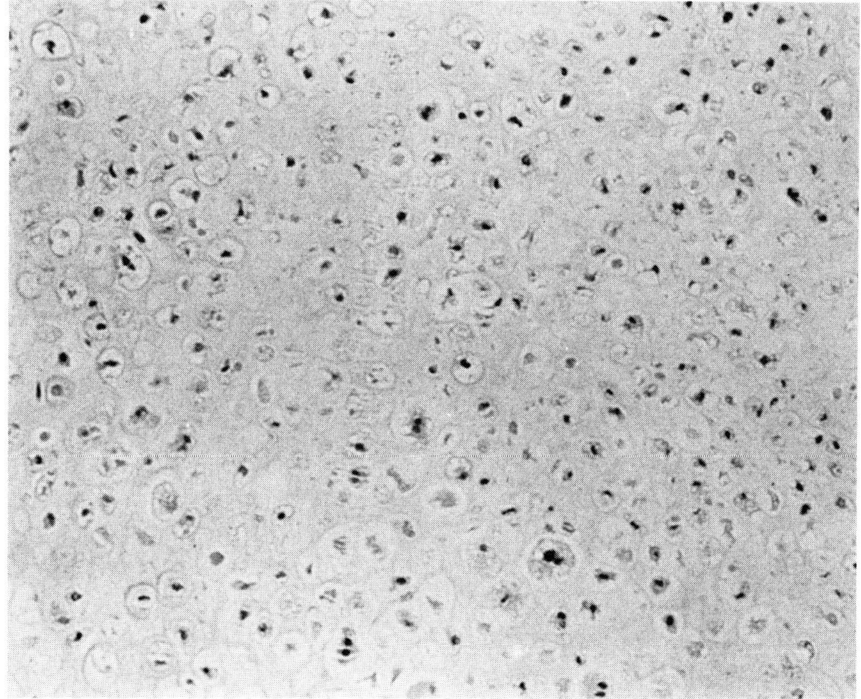

FIG. 7-45

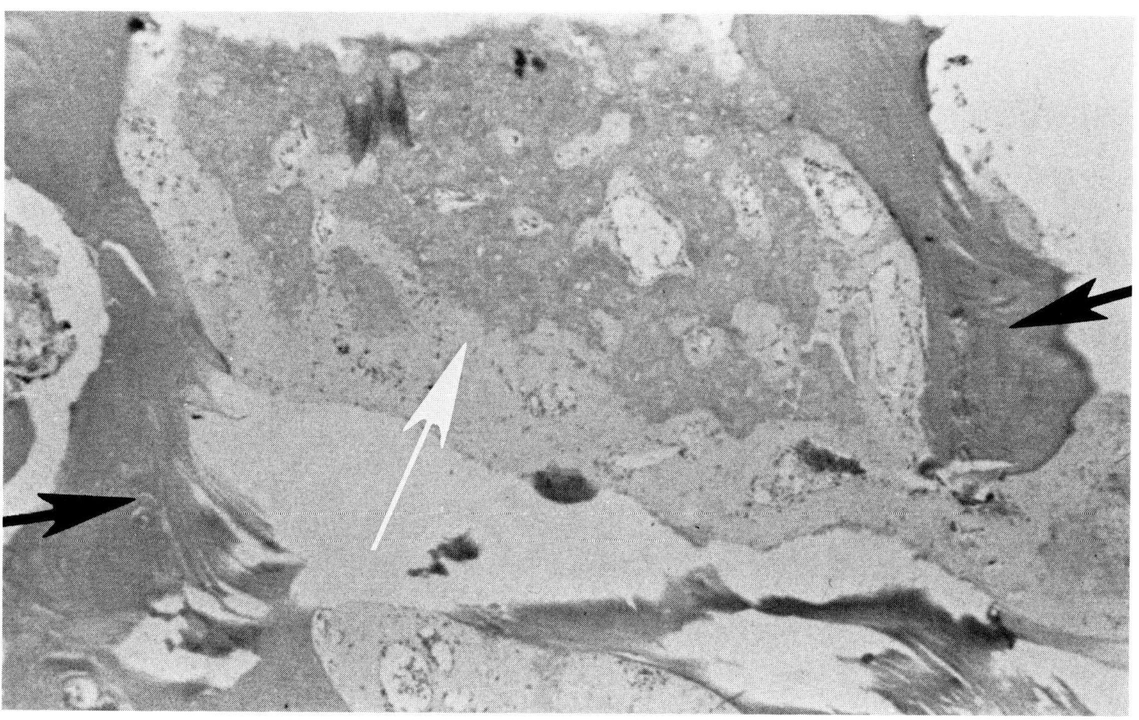

FIG. 7-46

Table 7-1. Differential Features of Osteoblastoma and Osteosarcoma

Radiographic	*Osteoblastoma*	*Osteosarcoma*
1. Confined to bone	Usual	10%
2. Tends to "expand" bone evenly and covered by thin rim of periosteal new bone	Common	Rare, if ever
3. Focal or eccentric cortical destruction	Rare	Common
4. Soft-tissue mass without rim of periosteal bone	Rare	Common
5. Cumulus cloudlike fluffs	Possible	Common
6. Ominous periosteal new bone	Rare	Common
Morphologic		
1. Islands of hyalin cartilage with absence of pathologic fracture by radiograph	Absent, or at least not yet reported	Common
2. Osteoid and/or woven bone infiltration between host lamellar bone marrow at the lesion-host bone interface	Absent*	Almost always, particularly at margins of tumor growth
3. Thick, irregularly serrated osteoid and woven-bone trabeculae with prominent vascular stroma and osteoclasts	Usual	Unusual
4. Prominent focal benign rimming of osteoblasts	Fairly common	Absent†
5. Compact masses and "streamers" of osteoid with little intervening fibrovascular stroma	Unusual	Common
6. Marked "ominous" cellularity	Common	Common
7. Objective anaplasia (must include atypical mitotic figures)	Absent	Common (80% of cases)
8. Bizarre nuclei with abscence of mitoses	Very rare‡	Absent‡
Behavior		
1. Recurrences (assuming the absence of radiation therapy, chemotherapy or amputation).	Rare	Common
2. Metastases	Rare§	85% in less than 2 years without chemotherapy

*This feature has been seen in the limited number of osteoblastomas removed intact that this author has reviewed. More cases will have to be reported before this feature can be used with security.
†Benign rimming of osteoblasts may be seen in host bone or periosteal sites reactive to osteosarcoma, but is not present in the tumor bone, per se.
‡Refer to description of pseudomalignant osteoblastoma versus arrested osteosarcoma (see below).
§About 3% of cases 5 years or more after curettage may transform to a rapidly growing sarcoma which may destroy the patient by local growth or metastases.

parathyroidism is uncommonly centered in this portion of the bone.

PSEUDOMALIGNANT OSTEOBLASTOMA VERSUS ARRESTED OSTEOSARCOMA. A few years ago this author was consulted on a most unusual case for which he could find no adequate explanation unless certain assumptions were made; namely, that the lesion in question was either an osteoblastoma with bizarre pseudomalignant cytologic features or an osteosarcoma that had spontaneously arrested in growth.

In March of 1970, a 17-year-old Negro male injured his leg and immediate radiographs showed an expansile cyst-like lesion of the fibula with a smooth border of periosteal new bone and absence of soft-tissue mass. Even though it looked benign radiographically, a biopsy was requested, but it was refused by the parents. Some 15 months later, it remained virtually unchanged by radiograph (Fig. 7-47). Permission for biopsy was given at this time. On low-power microscopic examination (Fig. 7-48), the lesion consisted of thick woven bone and osteoid with irregularly serrated borders, peppered by osteoclasts and rich in a vascular stroma. On high-power examination, the nuclei were bizarre (Fig. 7–49) and the cells were a mixture of bizarre mononuclear osteoblasts and osteoclasts. By usual criteria, these cells were anaplastic and the lesion was diagnosed as an osteosarcoma. Because of the benign radiological and behavioral characteristics, the surgeon elected to only en-bloc resect the fibula, in spite of the pathologic diagnosis. In reviewing numerous slides from this case, I found evidence of significant nuclear karyorrhexis, cytoplasmic degeneration, and nucleolar and chromatin smudging. Not a single mitotic figure was observed, nor evidence of cartilage formation. The patient is alive and well 8 years later, in spite of biopsy, curettage, and simple en-bloc resection. Since this lesion showed virtually no change in size after 15 months of radiologic follow-up and had an absence of: mitoses, cartilage, infiltration between lamellar bone trabeculae, and tight streamers of osteoid (behavior and histology extremely unusual for any ordinary osteosarcoma), the conclusion I came to was that the lesion either represented an osteoblastoma with pseudomalignant nuclear features due perhaps to degenerative changes or an osteosarcoma with a spontaneous arrest in growth. It is well known, for example, that certain other nonmalignant lesions may show very disturbing nuclear features that may mimic anaplasia in such a way that occurs in endocrine tumors, neural tumors, and leiomyomas of the uterus. On the other hand, it is also known that on very rare occasions malignant tumors may spontaneously arrest in growth or mature to benign tissues. There are at least 176 well-recorded cases of this phenomenon.[94]

I sent this case to Dr. Dahlin, who concurred with the diagnosis of pseudomalignant osteoblastoma and commented that he has seen two similar cases (observations to be published).

Although I have seen pseudomalignant cytologic changes in tissues other than bone in a number of instances, including radiation pseudosarcoma, neurilemmomas, endocrine tumors, and others, I have seen this phenomenon in only one other bone case. This lesion was a small trabeculated expansile lesion of a toe. Curettage showed a chondromyxoid fibroma, but the individual nuclei of some cells were so large that a Grade II to III chondrosarcoma was simulated. There were no mitoses, and long term follow-up showed no evidence of recurrence or metastases. Based upon my experience, therefore, I suspect that bizarre pseudomalignant cytologic changes may occur in approximately 0.1 to 0.5 per cent of benign bone lesions. This figure correlates well with the incidence of pseudosarcomatous changes in incidental leiomyomas of the uterus, which has been recorded to be approximately .5 to 1 per cent of cases.[33] Therefore, in very rare cases, benign bone tumors may show microscopic features that, by ordinary histological criteria, would be deemed anaplastic.

Recognition of these rare benign histologically pseudomalignant entities and their true incidence in bone will depend upon keeping an open mind and searching for these cases with completely benign radiologic and clinical features in association with bizarre nuclei but showing an absence of mitoses (most important feature), nuclear and cytoplasmic degeneration and tissue patterns otherwise in keeping with a well-known benign lesion. Obviously, bizarre pseudosarcomas of bone exist and need to be recognized and reported.

Course and Treatment

In approximately 90 to 95 per cent of osteoblastomas in which curettage or local excision is performed, total cure is achieved.[40] Portions of bone with osteoblastoma that can be sacrificed without harm to the patient, such as ribs or fibula, are best treated by excision. But up to 40 per cent of all lesions involve the posterior elements of the spine; these areas are sometimes inaccessible to simple curettage and these are perhaps best treated by radiotherapy. Unfortunately, the literature is lax on reports stating what the most appropriate dosage should be. If radiation is considered necessary, the radiotherapists must obviously strive to define the lowest dose which will effect cure, since the dangers of myelitis and sarcomatous degeneration after many years have to be considered particularly when dosages of 4500 R. or more are used.

Marsh[40], in his 1975 article, indicated that he has had good results with radiation dosages between 1000 and 5500 R. Of 14 patients who received immediate postoperative irradiation, two had recurrences many years later and one of these patients succumbed to the complications of massive local recurrence without metastasis. Unequivocal anaplasia was not seen in the recurrence specimen, although the behavioral characteristics certainly suggested malignant transformations. In one of 13 spinal osteoblastomas where patients did not receive radiation, recurrence leading to paraplagia occurred 7 months later. This complication was treated by laminectomy and 5000 R.

Only two patients with osteoblastoma were treated

by radiation in nonspinal sites. One of these two cases had a recurrence 21 months after 2800 R. had been given. The patient was well 7 years after en-bloc resection of the femoral shaft. The investigators state: "Most, if not all of the lesions of the spine must have been incompletely removed by curettement. Since the incidence of recurrence was no greater in lesions which could be thoroughly curetted, we surmised that incomplete curettage can effect a cure in a high percentage of patients."[40]

Recurrences beyond two years of initial operation are very uncommon (about 5%). In those cases with rapid, massive, local recurrence and metastases within two years from initial treatment, the tumor in question was almost certainly an osteosarcoma from the start. *Most cases of osteoblastoma that recur after 5 or more years from initial biopsy diagnosis lead to the demise of the patient and signify malignant transformation.* At least five such cases are described by Mayer,[41] Stutch, *et al.*,[41] Seki, *et al.*,[45] Lichtenstein,[39] and Marsh.[40] Relentless massive local recurrences and metastasis in three cases were seen in association with variable degrees of atypia and anaplasia. We should not necessarily conclude from these facts that even some cases of osteoblastoma are malignant from inception, but more likely (in this author's opinion), that some are capable of transforming into osteosarcoma many years later and that others are probably osteosarcomas mistaken for the osteoblastoma. Malignant transformation certainly occurs in other benign lesions: fibrous dysplasia can transform into fibro- and osteosarcoma; enchondroma into chondrosarcoma; and bone infarct reparative tissues to sarcoma. We never call any of these benign precursor lesions malignant; this would be a misnomer. Similarly the term *malignant osteoblastoma,* which is used occasionally, is a serious misnomer. The fact that we cannot always distinguish an osteosarcoma from osteoblastoma by our present level of histologic expertise is certainly no justification for use of this term.

Schajowicz[43] has reported eight cases of a locally aggressive tumor which he has called "malignant osteoblastoma." Radiologically, none of the lesions had the classical appearance of osteosarcoma. Most cases were characterized by lysis with expansion and thinning of the cortex. Some lesions were epiphyseal and resemble giant cell tumor. The histologic features were those of osteoblastoma but suggestive of malignancy. The lesions were highly cellular and showed more ominous cytologic features than ordinary osteoblastomas. Multinucleated giant cells were always present and in some cases resembled giant cell tumor. Mitoses were generally abundant and atypical mitoses, rare to absent. Cartilage was never seen. Four of the cases were characterized by local recurrences from 6 months to 2 years later. In no instance was death directly related to the tumor, nor was metastasis noted. Unfortunately, I could not tell from the article whether some of the cases presented were giant cell tumors with foci of abundant bone production, benign osteoblastomas with more than usual cytologic atypia (pseudomalignant osteoblastomas), an "aggressive" osteoblastoma such as was shown in Fig. 7–42 *A* and *B*; which I think is the most likely possibility, or truly a distinct entity, as Dr. Schajowicz suggested. The absence of lethal metastases surely throws doubt on the use of the term *malignant.*

Fibrous Dysplasia

Capsule Summary

Incidence. A not uncommon bone disorder.

Age. Infancy to adulthood. Those patients with polyostotic (multiple bone) fibrous dysplasia (FD) are usually

---

Pseudomalignant Osteoblastoma

FIG. 7–47. Within the shaft of the fibula, a mixed lytic and blastic lesion has focally "expanded" the bone and is covered by a thin rim of periosteal new bone. There is no soft-tissue mass. This radiograph, taken 13 months after the first, was virtually unchanged.

FIG. 7–48. On microscopic examination this lesion of the fibula showed thick, irregularly serrated masses of woven bone and a highly vascular stroma peppered with osteoclasts (H and E, X40).

FIG. 7–49. High-power examination of this fibula lesion revealed mononuclear and multinuclear giant cells with bizarre nuclear pleomorphism simulating anaplasia. Not a single mitosis was seen after examination of thousands of cells in which the tissue was well fixed and stained. This tumor represents either a very extremely rare example of an osteosarcoma with growth arrest or, more likely, an osteoblastoma with "degenerative" pseudosarcomatous cytologic changes (H and E, X250).

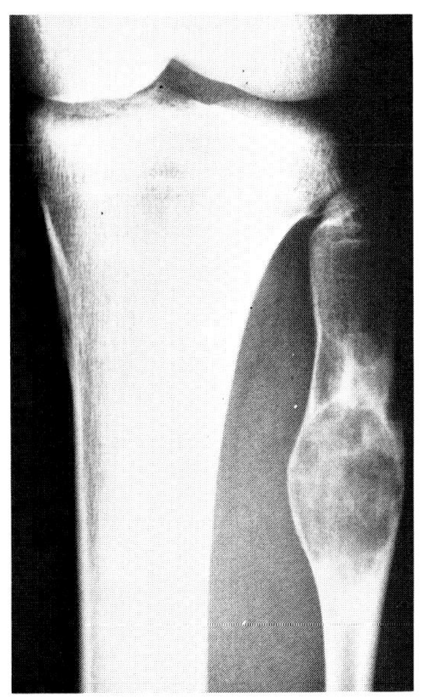

FIG. 7-47

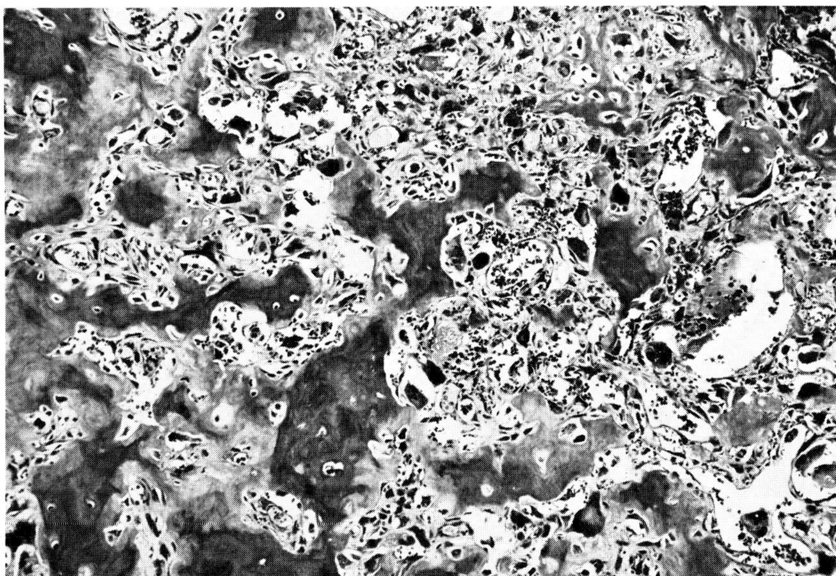

FIG. 7-48

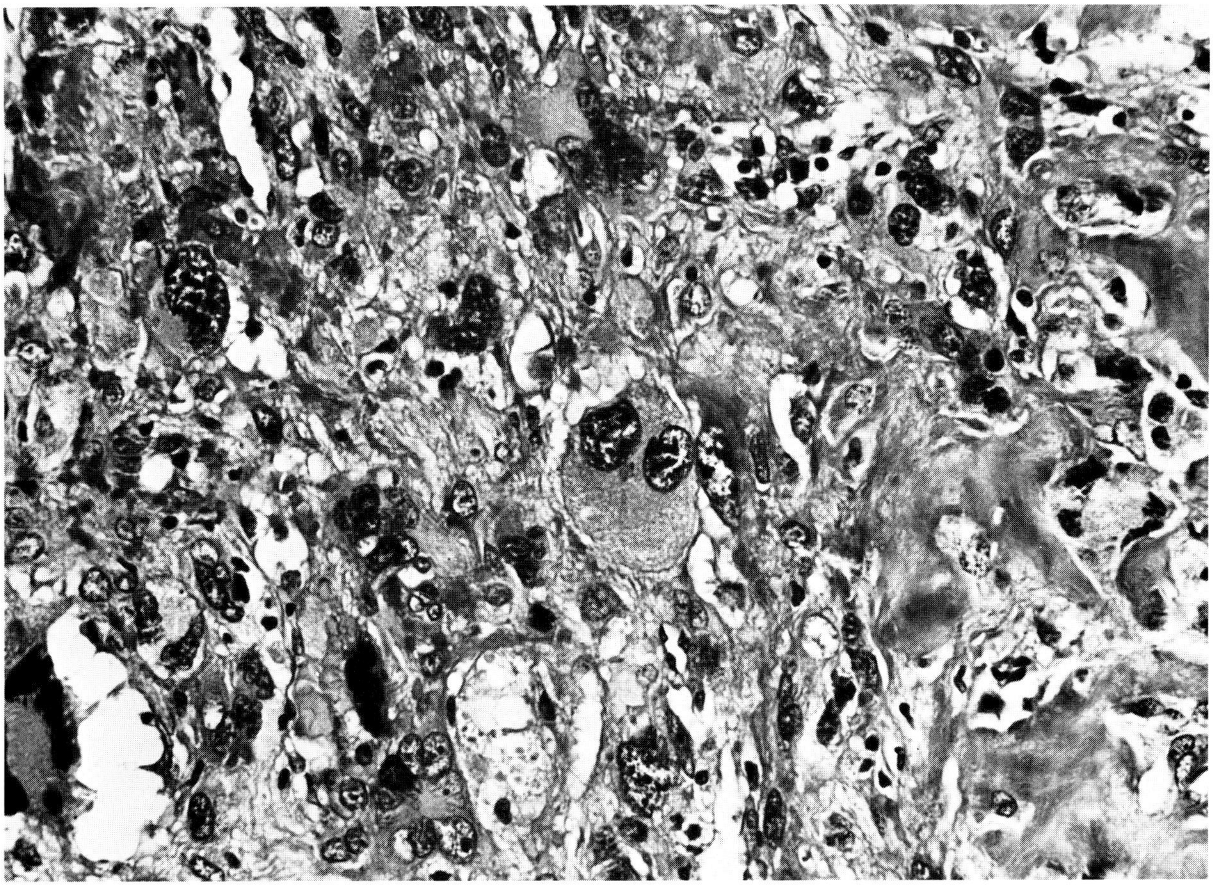

FIG. 7-49

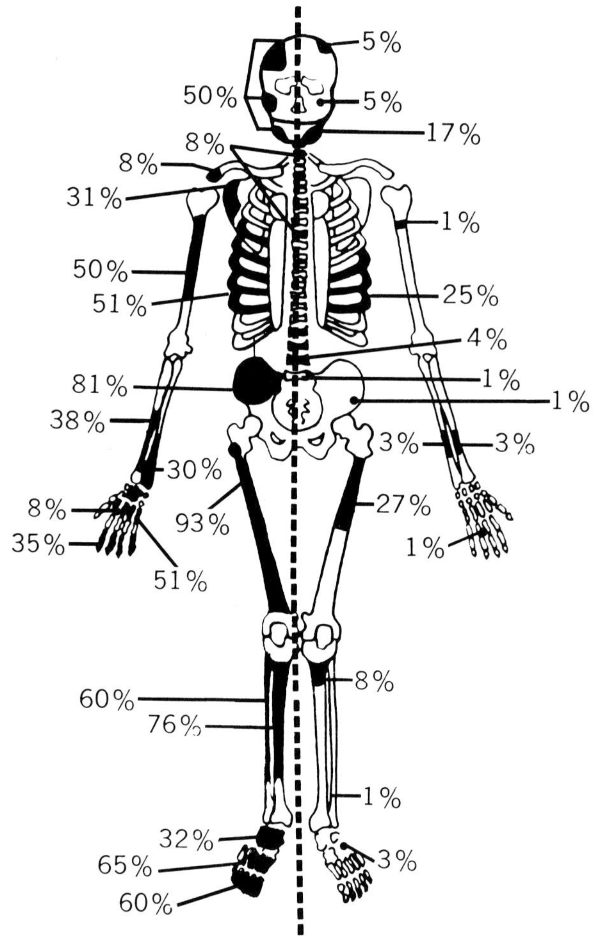

FIG. 7-50. Fibrous dysplasia. Frequency of areas of polyostotic involvement (*left*) in 62 patients and monostotic involvement (*right*) in 64 patients. Male:female incidence, 1:1.5.

discovered much earlier than those with monostotic (single bone) involvement.

Clinical Features. Symptoms vary greatly, depending upon the number of bones involved and the extent of involvement of individual bones.

Monostotic FD. Swelling with or without pain if it is associated with fracture. Cutaneous pigmentation is uncommon. Serum alkaline phosphatase, calcium, and phosphorus are within normal limits.

Polyostotic FD. A limp, swelling, physical deformity, pain due to fractures, and abnormal cutaneous pigmentation are common; precocious puberty and premature skeletal maturation are less common. Hyperthyroidism, diabetes mellitus, myxomas of soft tissue, and increase in serum alkaline phosphatase are unusual associated features.

Radiologic Features. Any bone may be affected. Lesions are usually centered in the metaphysis or diaphysis. Small lesions are often surrounded by sclerosis. Larger lesions may "expand" the bone concentrically or eccentrically, but even these lesions are covered by a fine rim of periosteal bone. They may be lytic, bubbly, or trabeculated, with or without a pathognomonic "ground-glass" appearance.

Gross Pathology. Foci of the host bone become replaced by variably gritty tissue. Often there are small to large areas of cystic degeneration. Extensive bone involvement results in gross deformities consequent to fracture repair and swelling.

Histopathology. The condition is characterized by a benign fibrous tissue matrix from which variable quantities of woven bone are formed by fibroosseous metaplasia. Plump osteoblastic rimming is either absent or confined to small foci only. Cartilage is rarely seen.

Course. Benign, but may be very disabling and deforming if numerous bones are involved. Malignant transformation to a sarcoma is a rare complication.

Treatment. Symptomatic, for pathologic fractures and deformities.

Definition. Fibrous dysplasia is a benign, nonfamilial disorder of the skeleton characterized by a hamartomatous proliferation of fibroosseous tissues. But extraskeletal anomalies may also be found, including precocious puberty, areas of cutaneous pigmentation, hyperthyroidism, and soft-tissue myxomas. Many cases show but a single focus of skeletal involvement (monostotic fibrous dysplasia); others show multiple bone involvement (polyostotic fibrous dysplasia).

Clinical Features

Fibrous dysplasia is not an uncommon primary bone tumor. It is a more common disease of females than of males. Most lesions probably begin in childhood but symptoms usually do not become manifest before late childhood to adolescence.

SKELETAL INVOLVEMENT. The most benign expression of the disease is when only a single bone (monostotic fibrous dysplasia) is affected. These patients probably represent a forme fruste of the more severe form of the disease (polyostotic fibrous dysplasia). When only a single bone is involved, complaints are usually consequent to a fracture or painless swelling. Asymptomatic lesions may be discovered accidentally on radiographic analysis performed for some other reason. Symptoms depend on the size of the lesion and the bone involved. If the upper end of the femur is involved, there often is a limp and mild pain; if a rib or jaw is involved, a painless lump; if the orbit is involved, there may be proptosis.

Large lesions are prone to repeated fractures. Although fracture healing is usually quite good, after many years the bone or bones may become bowed, shortened, and expanded. Involvement of the vertebral bodies, although uncommon, may result in collapse and kyphoscoliosis (Fig. 7–51). Severe rib and spine involvement may result in respiratory difficulties (Fig. 7–52). Patients with the most severe form of polyostotic fibrous dysplasia develop crippling deformities and if the facial bones are involved, bizarre deformity and severe proptosis. A peculiar aspect of the disease is that when multiple bones are involved, the lesions tend to involve one side of the body (Fig. 7–51) much more than the other. Occasionally only a single limb bud may be involved. Ollier's disease (multiple enchondromatosis) may have a similar predisposition to involve one side of the body more than the other. Von Recklinghausen's disease (multiple hereditary osteochondromatosis) tends to be bilaterally symmetrical.

The patient with polyostotic fibrous dysplasia is usually taller than average in childhood because of an advanced skeletal age. However, closure of the epiphyses usually occurs prematurely consequent to precocious puberty and leads to smaller than average adult height.

CUTANEOUS PIGMENTATION. The most common of the nonskeletal abnormalities are patches of abnormal cutaneous brownish-yellow to yellow pigmentation (Plate 6, *A*). The borders of the patches are irregular in contrast to the regular borders of the cafe-au-lait spots of neurofibromatosis. The patches may develop anywhere on the body but they are not necessarily found in the region of affected bones. Careful search of the back or buttocks is essential in patients suspected of having FD, since these sites may be involved to the exclusion of others. Approximately $\frac{1}{3}$ of patients with the polyostotic form have these patches; fewer patients with the monostotic form have them.

PRECOCIOUS PUBERTY. Approximately 20 per cent of female patients with the polyostotic form may present with vaginal bleeding, premature development of the sexual organs, and secondary sex characteristics in childhood, sometimes even before the age of three. Male children may present with enlarged genitals or advanced secondary sex characteristics.

The triad of bone lesions, precocious puberty, and cutaneous pigmentation has been named *Albright's syndrome.* The triad is rare, occurring in only one of every 30 to 40 patients with skeletal lesions.

OTHER ABNORMALITIES. In some patients there may be associated hyperthyroidism, diabetes mellitus, arteriovenous aneurysm, coarctation of the aorta, rudimentary kidney, and single to multiple soft-tissue myxomas. To 1976, 14 cases of benign soft-tissue myxomas in association with FD had been reported.[65] Some 86 per cent of the myxomas developed in patients with the polyostotic form. Some 93 per cent of the myxomas were multiple in origin and were usually located in the areas of severest bone involvement. The right side of the body and lower extremity were most often the sites of origin. Albright's triad was found in six of these patients. One of the patients developed an osteogenic sarcoma at a site of dysplastic involvement. Only one of the 14 patients developed recurrent myxoma. Two excisions were required following a 10-year course. One year following the last operation the patient showed no evidence of recurrence.

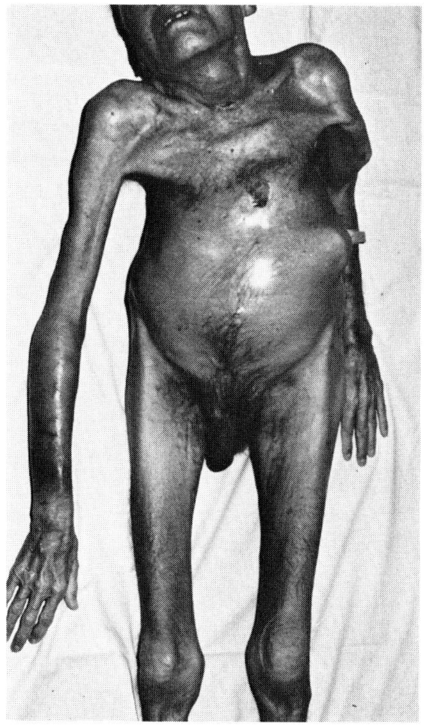

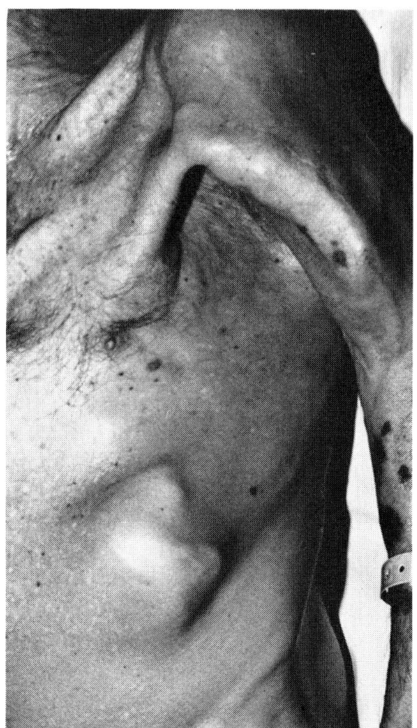

FIG. 7-51 FIG. 7-52

Fibrous Dysplasia

FIG. 7-51. This patient had severe polyostotic F.D. Note the tendency to involve one side of the body. The left arm is deformed and shortened. Involvement of the spine resulted in kyphoscoliosis and respiratory insufficiency.

FIG. 7-52. The arm is deformed consequent to swelling and multiple repeated fractures. Several of the ribs show pronounced swellings due to slow expansive growth of the hamartomatous process.

Histopathology

Since the radiographic and gross features will be much clearer following a description of the histopathology of FD, we will in this instance discuss the histopathologic features first.

HIGH POWER FEATURES. The characteristic microscopic features are the production of a benign fibrous tissue stroma in which spicules of woven bone are formed directly from this stroma. Most cases show very bland fibrocytes with oval to spindly nuclei (Fig. 7–53). The nuclear chromatin is stippled and evenly distributed. Nucleoli are not prominent and mitoses are rare. The nuclei are widely separated from one another, although in occasional cases they are more tightly packed (Fig. 7–54). The stroma has a loose, finely fibrillar quality not unlike that of neural tissues (Fig. 7–53). In unusual cases, as much as 95 to 98 per cent of the lesional tissue may be fibrous. Unless careful search or attention is paid to small islands of metaplastic bone, the diagnosis may not be considered.

Small islands of osteoid that become converted to woven bone appears to form directly from this spindly fibrocytic stroma; they don't appear to pass through a stage of plump osteoblasts characteristic of other benign bone-productive lesions (Figs. 7–53 and 7–54). This apparent direct conversion of fibrous tissue to bone has been referred to as *fibro-osseous metaplasia* and is rarely seen in conditions other than FD. An exception to this rule is the parosteal osteosarcoma.

The osteoid and woven bone produced is rarely lined by plump osteoblasts with abundant bluish-pink cytoplasm, a feature characteristic of most other benign bone productive conditions. An occasional trabeculum may show some plump osteoblastic rimming but this feature should not detract from the diagnosis if careful attention is given to correlating histologic, radiologic, and clinical features.

LOW-POWER FEATURES. The woven bone that is produced tends to, but does not necessarily, assume a characteristic curled configuration with circular "C" and "Y" shapes (Fig. 7–55). In some cases the shapes may not be substantially different from normal bone trabeculae (Fig. 7–56). In most cases the width of the abnormal trabeculae is $\frac{1}{2}$ to $\frac{1}{3}$ the thickness of normal cancellous bone (Fig. 7–58). There is a tremendous variability in the amount of bone produced. In those cases with maximal bone production the ratio of bone to fibrous tissue is about 1 to 1 (Fig. 7–57). Those cases with minimal bone production may show bone to fibrous tissue ratios of 1 to 50 or less (Fig. 7–59). The woven-bone spicules of FD may be discrete and separated from each other by fibrous tissue (Fig. 7–55) or form a contiguous network in which fibrous tissue is separated into islands (Fig. 7–56). These features may vary from field to field or bone to bone. The process rarely, if ever, involves the entire affected bone. Basically, the process is a fibro-osseous hamartoma that replaces the normal host bone. On low-power examination, it can be seen that there is usually a sharp demarcation between the lesional tissue, which is composed of fibrous tissue and woven bone, and adjacent areas of normal host lamellar bone and marrow fat (Fig. 7–56). This usually sharp transition zone is better appreciated by using polarized light in order to differentiate host lamellar bone from the lesional woven bone (Fig. 7–57). This feature is common in most benign tumorous processes. The reverse is true of most malignant tumors. The osteosarcoma and fibrosarcoma, both lesions that should be considered in the differential histologic diagnosis, infiltrate for considerable distances between host bone lamellae at their advancing margins. Therefore, with polarized light examination, these tumors at their margins will show an intimate mixture of neoplastic tissue and host lamellar bone.

OTHER MICROSCOPIC FEATURES. Microscopic features by type of tissue are listed below.

CYSTS. Microscopic and macroscopic areas of cystic degeneration are commonly seen (Fig. 7–69). They may be lined by a delicate fibrous tissue capsule and are frequently associated with small numbers of osteoclasts (giant cells).

MYXOID TISSUE. Small foci of myxoid degeneration of the fibrous stroma is seen occasionally.

GIANT CELLS. Small foci of giant cells are not uncommon and usually are associated with foci of hemorrhage or cystification. They are usually not so pronounced that the lesion would be confused with a giant cell tumor.

HEMORRHAGE, NECROSIS, AND FOAM CELLS. Foci of degeneration, necrosis, and hemorrhage are common. Histiocytes respond to these degenerative foci and eventually may form islands of xanthoma cells.

CARTILAGE. Cartilage does not appear to form from direct metaplasia from the fibrous tissue except on rare occasions. When cartilage is seen, it is usually traced to remnants of a former epiphyseal plate or more commonly, to sites in which fracture has occurred. Recently, this author has seen three very unusual cases of fibrous dysplasia in association with extensive cartilage without evidence of fracture. In one case dysplastic cartilage formed directly from epiphyseal plate and periosteum admixed with and away from areas of fibrous dysplasia. This unusual case mimicked a combination of two disease processes, namely fibrous dysplasia and Ollier's disease.

Gross Pathology

The gross features depend upon the amount of woven bone produced in the lesional fibrous tissue, the degree of degenerative changes (cysts), and the extent of bone involvement. Since the basic proliferating process is fibrous, the tissue will be firm and white (Fig. 7–60, Plate 6, *B*). Most cases produce significant quantities of woven bone so that the tissue will be gritty. A magnifying glass may be necessary to appreciate the very fine spicules of bone produced that are usually in the range of 0.1 mm. in width by 0.5 mm. in length. Normal bone trabeculae are at least 2 to 3 times thicker. It is common to find areas of cystic degeneration. The cysts may range from 1 mm. to several centimeters in size and contain a mucoid serous or serosanguineous fluid (Plate 6, *B*). Areas of cartilage may be seen.

The lesion begins as a fibro-osseous tumorous mass in the intramedullary substance; if growth proceeds, it leads to cortical erosion (Fig. 7–60). Eventually the normal contours of the bone are moderately to severely "expanded" (Plate 6, *B*).

The outer surface of the bone is usually smooth and covered by at least a thin shell of reactive periosteal bone.

Even if the bone is extensively involved there are usually remnants at one or both ends of normal bone (Fig. 7–60). In the regions of the lesional tissue, no normal trabecular architecture can be appreciated either grossly, microscopically, or by radiograph (Figs. 7–60, 7–63). This is in striking contrast to Paget's disease, for example, in which those unfamiliar with the basic pathologic differences may confuse it with FD on the basis of radiographic analysis. Paget's disease of bone is a nontumorous infection-like process (possibly a slow virus disease) that results in a disorganized, continuous modeling and remodeling of the bone architecture. Although, the normal bone architecture is considerably modified by Pagetoid woven bone trabeculae it is not destroyed (Figs. 7–61 and 7–62) by dense, benign, fibro-osseous tissue, as it is in fibrous dysplasia.

Radiologic Features

The radiologic features of FD merely reflect its basic pathologic process and the responses of the host bone to the process. As we have seen, the basic pathologic process is that of a slow-growing hamartomatous mass of fibrous and woven-bone tissues which focally replace the normal host bone. The lesion begins in one (monostotic) or more bones (polyostotic) of the intramedullary space. Some lesions remain confined to the intramedullary area but usually there is slow replacement of the cortex. Those which erode the cortex in a symmetrical fashion lead to concentric "expansion" of the bone, while others may result in focal cortical erosion and protrude into the soft tissue as an eccentric mass. The lesions are always covered by a smooth, thin, rim of reactive, periosteal host bone. As the lesion is slow growing the host intramedullary bone often forms a collar of reactive sclerosis. The volume of normal bone replaced may vary from as little as a cubic centimeter to hundreds of cubic centimeters. Rarely is the entire bone replaced by the hamartomatous process. Advanced cases are characterized by striking deformity of the bone. These features are summarized in a specimen radiograph of a humerus and spine from a case of severe polyostotic involvement (Fig. 7–63).

Fibrous dysplasia is an indolent tumorous growth that replaces the host bone along a well-demarcated, lobulated front. It does not lead to bone replacement by first permeating extensively through the marrow spaces, as is the case in most malignant conditions. Ominous or significant periosteal reactions do not occur unless there has been a fracture in that site or the lesion has undergone transformation to a highly malignant sarcoma. Therefore, FD of bone, unmodified by these latter two conditions, has smooth, rounded, or lobulated contours, no matter how extensive the amount of host bone replaced. If the gross pathology of this disease is briefly reviewed at this time (see Fig. 7–60, Plate 6, *B*), it will be easier to proceed with an analysis and understanding of its radiologic features.

The density of the lesion on radiograph depends upon the degree of woven bone produced and/or the extent to which the overlying cortex has been replaced in order to be able to visualize the degree of woven-bone production within the lesion itself. If the lesion is small, or if it produces little woven bone or if the cortex is not sufficiently destroyed to remove its obscuring effects, it will appear as a lucent mass (Fig. 7–64). If the cortex is thinned or if the bone is "expanded" and only covered by a thin shell of reactive periosteal bone and if the lesion produces significant quantities of the fine-woven bone peculiar to this disease, then a *"ground-glass"* appearance quite characteristic and almost pathognomonic of FD will be appreciated (Figs. 7–65 and 7–67–7–70). However, a ground-glasslike appearance can on occasion be seen in osteoblastoma and osteosarcoma. The fea-

---

Fibrous Dysplasia

FIG. 7–53. FD is characterized by a loose fibrillar fibrous tissue. The fibroblast nuclei are widely spaced, oval to spindly in shape, and have a bland chromatin distribution. Mitoses are rare. Note the association of spicules of primitive woven bone to the right of the field, without prominent osteoblastic rimming (H and E, X400).

FIG. 7–54. Some cases or fields may show a more ominous cellularity, which could be mistaken for a sarcomatous process. Spicules of woven bone are forming from the stroma without the association of prominent osteoblastic rimming, a process known as fibro-osseous metaplasia. Although distinction from an osteosarcoma may be impossible from analysis of isolated fields such as this one, their separation should not be difficult when combined with an analysis of the radiographs and total pathologic picture (H and E, X250).

FIG. 7–55. The shapes that the woven bone spicules assume, in many cases of FD, are quite characteristic of this disease and no other. These shapes consist of circles and "C" and "Y" configurations. Other changes commonly seen in FD and which are seen in this field are evidence of small cystic areas of degeneration and a sprinkling of chronic inflammatory cells (H and E, X40).

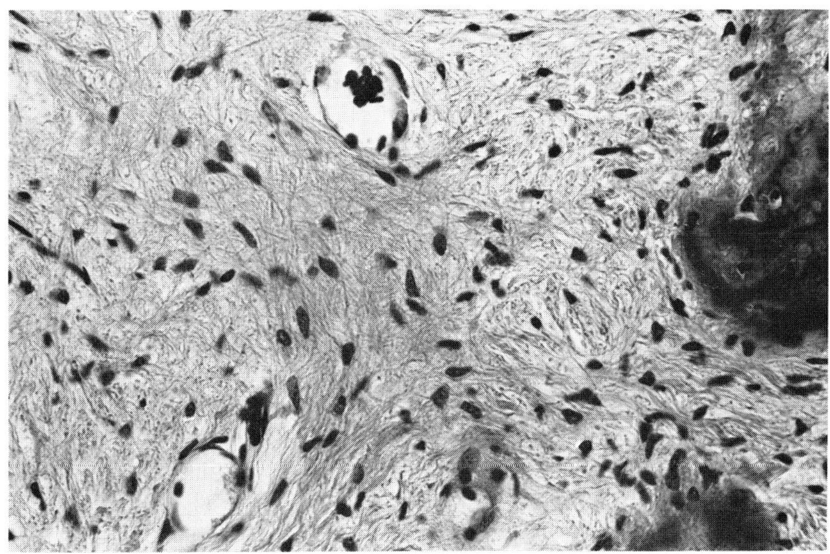

FIG. 7-53

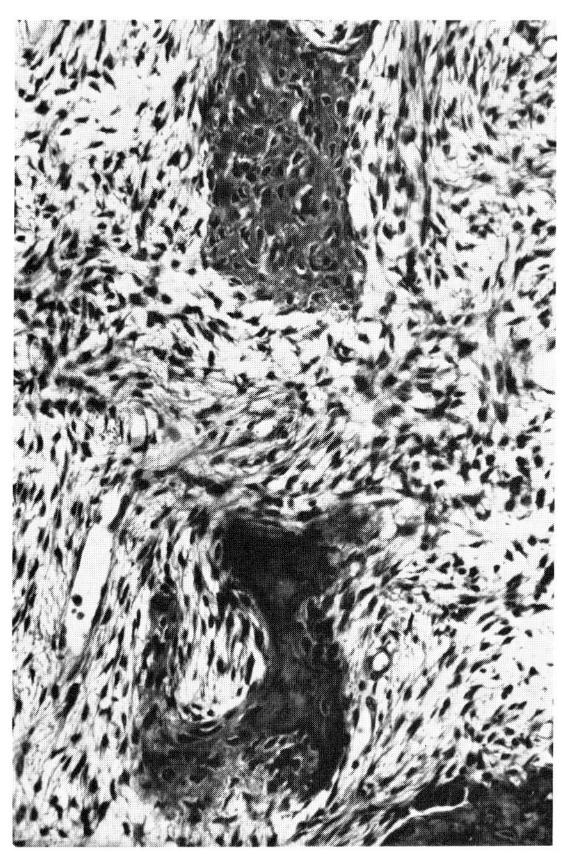

FIG. 7-54

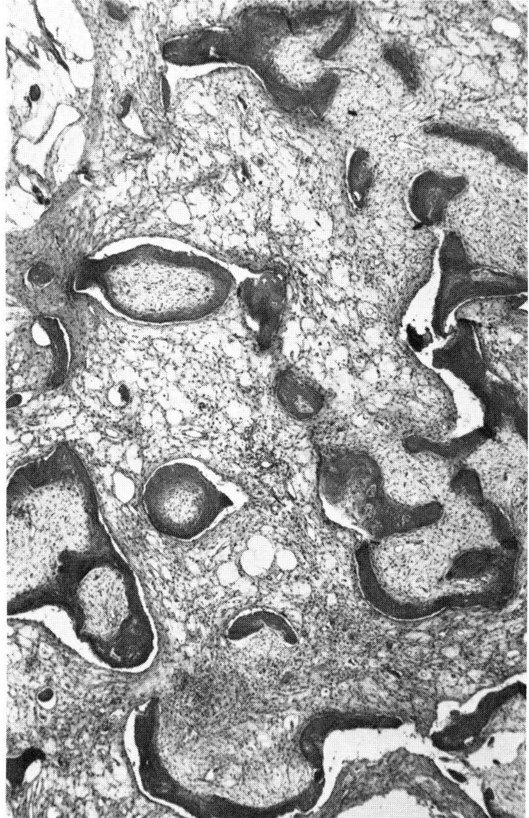

FIG. 7-55

tures of FD are, therefore, those of a slow-growing benign lesion (i.e., the lesion is roundish or lobulated), results in even or eccentric smooth-bordered expansions of the bone, (Figs. 7–65 and 7–66), is always covered by a thin rim of periosteal new bone, and is often surrounded by a border of intramedullary host bone sclerosis.

Fibrous dysplasia may affect any bone. In the long bones the lesions usually begin in the diaphysis or metaphysis. The epiphysis is usually spared, except in the most severe cases. Numerous bones may be involved and may show striking deformities. The range of features FD may assume in the long bones is illustrated in Figures 7–64 to 7–68.

One of the complications of severe involvement is dramatic curvature (Fig. 7–68 and 7–69). The Shepherd's Crook deformity seen most commonly in the femur and tibia could give rise to the mistaken impression that the bones "bent" into this shape. However, bone is a rigid tissue, even those affected by severe bone destroying disease. Changes in shape must be either consequent to remodeling or a result of fracture healing. Fig. 7–69, *D* shows a classic example of a Shepherd's crook deformity consequent to FD. However, serial radiographic studies clearly show its pathogenesis (Fig. 7–69).

Involvement of the flat bones, jaw (Fig. 7–70) and skull (Fig. 7–71) are common. Involvement of the spine (Fig. 7–63) is uncommon. FD affects the skull bones in the following order of frequency: frontal, sphenoid, ethmoid, maxilla, mandible, zygoma, parietal, occipital, and temporal. Increased densities, particularly at the base of the occiput, are quite characteristic of skull lesions in FD. The skull lesions may be either radiodense, radiolucent, or mottled. The increased density at the skull base usually involves the wings of the sphenoid, sella turcica, roof of the orbit, and vertical plate of the frontal bone. Displacement of one orbit, inferiorly and laterally, is a common deformity. Similar lesions may be seen in the frontal or parietal bones, maxilla, and mandible.

FD of the frontal, parietal, or occipital skull has a radiographic appearance rarely seen in other diseases. The lesion will appear irregular in shape, multilocular, and surrounded by a variable border of reactive sclerosis.[62] FD characteristically results in a cystlike expansion of the diploic space with bulging of the outer table. The inner table is virtually unchanged (Fig. 7–71).

The two lesions that may simulate FD of the skull most closely are meningioma and Paget's disease. The so-called en-plaque type of reactive bone sclerosis seen in infiltrative meningioma at the base of the skull is radiologically similar to FD affecting this area. However, there usually are distinctive differences between the two. Meningioma infiltrates the bone and causes reactive sclerosis without causing enlargement of the bones. In FD, the process results in a slow tumorous replacement of the bones with enlargement. Therefore, anterior-posterior views will usually show distinct bone enlargement in the areas of involvement and commonly enlargement of the floor or roof of the orbit with displacement of the eyeball. The exquisitely sharp margination of pure osteolysis of Paget's disease (osteoporosis circumscripta) is not seen in FD. The proliferative bone-producing type of Paget's is usually characterized by bony nodules on the inner aspect of the middle table and marked osteoporosis of the outer table. The inner table is hyperostotic and the outer, atrophic. Bubbly cystlike extrusion of the outer table as seen in a tangential view of FD is not seen in Paget's disease. A most important aid to differential diagnosis of FD versus meningioma or Paget's is the age of the patient. FD patients are usually under 30, while patients with meningioma and Paget's disease are almost always seen in patients over 30.

(*Text continues on p. 134.*)

Fibrous Dysplasia

FIG. 7–56. The hamartomatous process almost never replaces the entire bone. If one examines the edge of the lesion, it can be seen to advance along a broad front. Note the abnormal tissues on one side and normal bone and marrow (*top*) on the other. The process does not extensively infiltrate the marrow elements first, as do malignant processes (H and E, X40).

FIG. 7–57. This polarized light view of the same area shows the clear-cut separation between host lamellar bone (*A*) and the lesional woven bone (*B*).

FIG. 7–58. The spicules of the lesion may fuse to adjacent host lamellar bone (*arrow*) but do not extend for considerable distances between them (H and E, X40).

FIG. 7–59. Some areas of the lesion may show masses of bland fibrous tissue with minimal to absent bone production. It is not unusual to find cysts and foci of giant cells (*arrows*) either within or outside the cysts (H and E, X125).

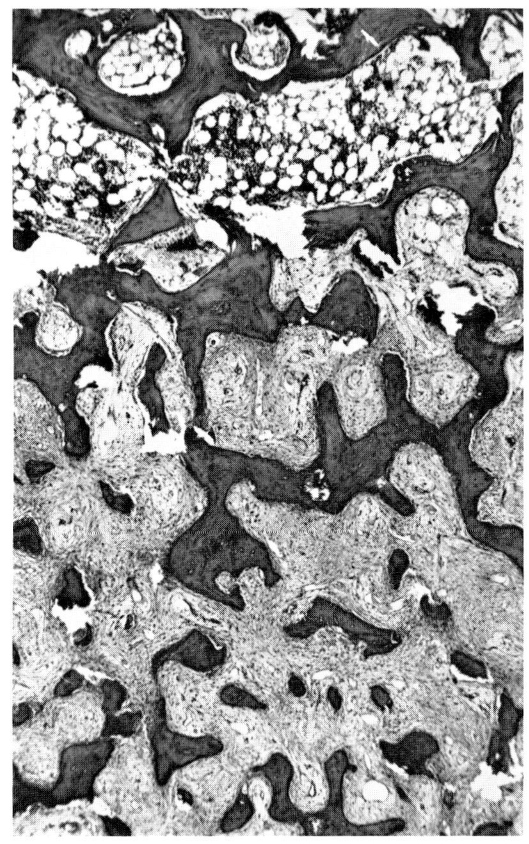

FIG. 7-56

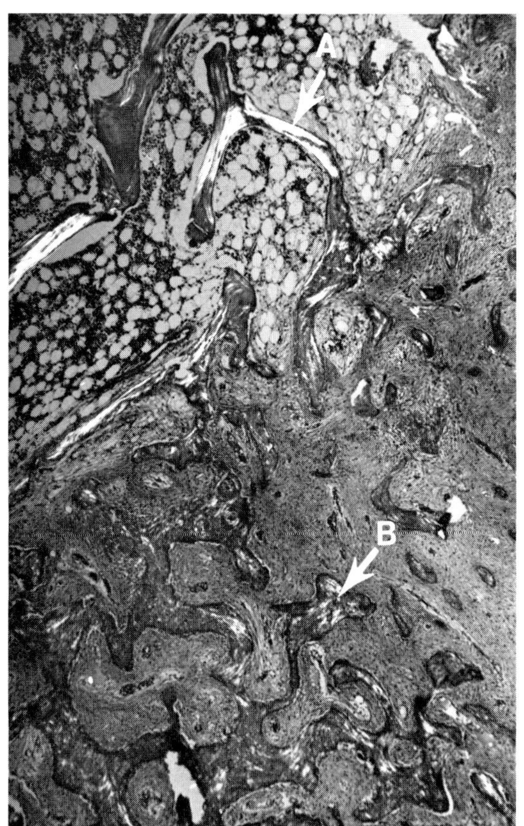

FIG. 7-57

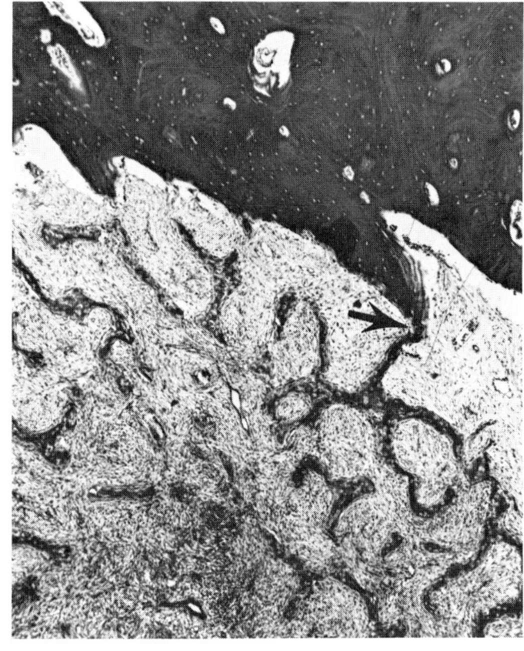

FIG. 7-58

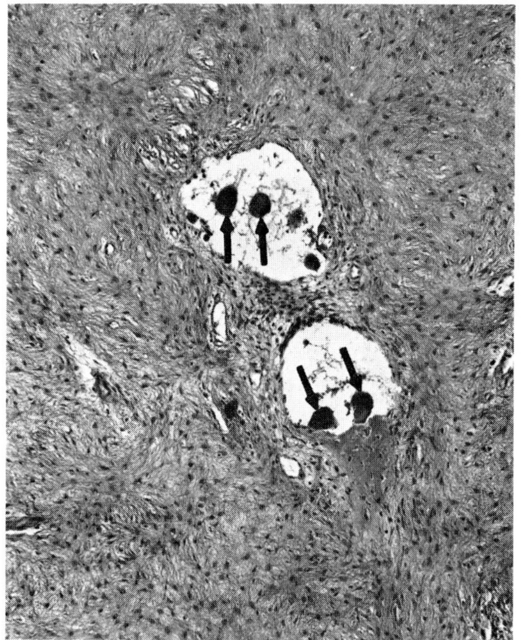

FIG. 7-59

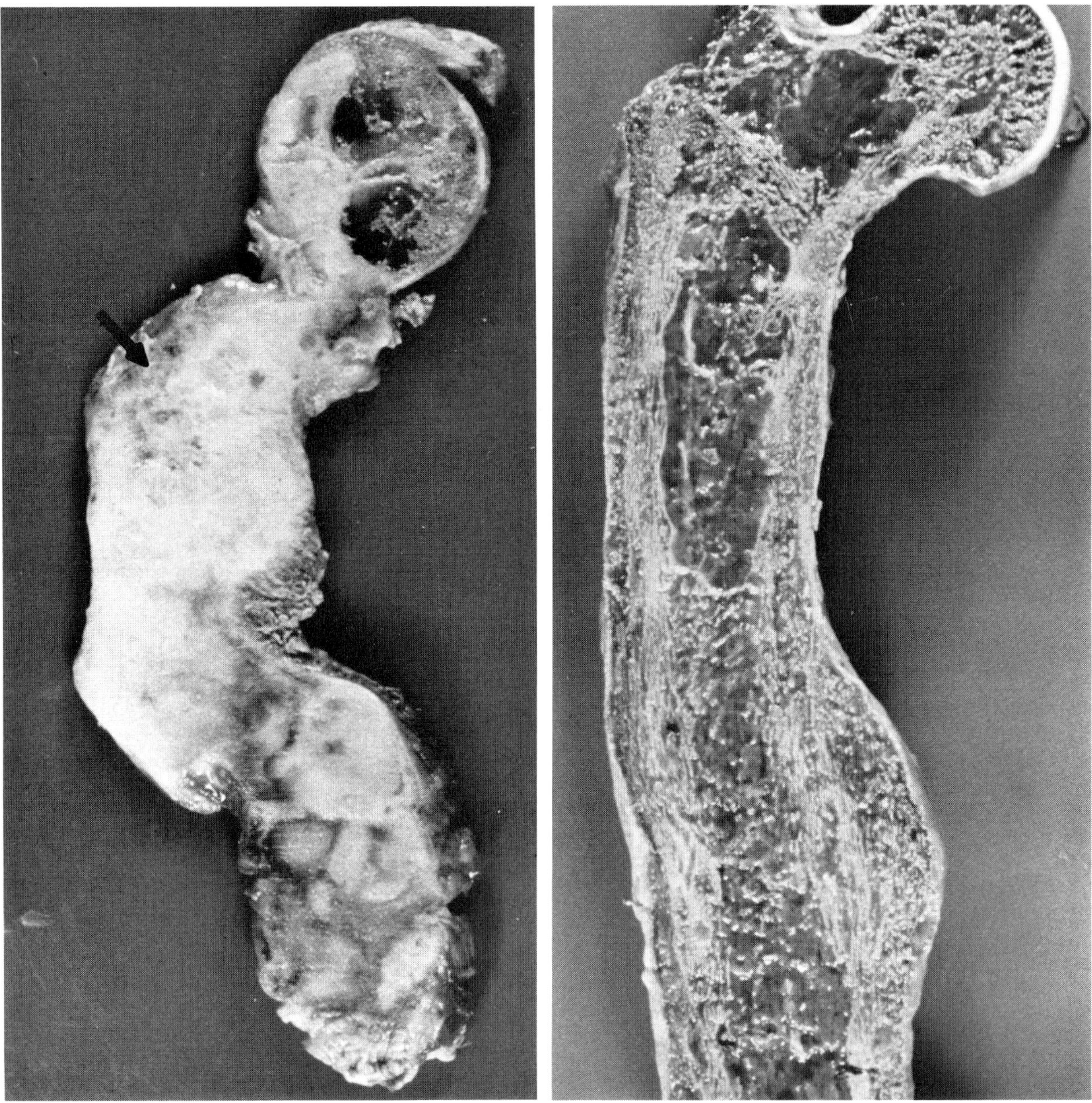

FIG. 7-60 FIG. 7-61

Fibrous Dysplasia Compared to Paget's Disease

FIG. 7-60. The gross features of FD are well illustrated by this case of humeral involvement. The tissue is firm and white and gritty in areas of bone production. Only the proximal epiphyseal end appears uninvolved by the process. The bone is severely deformed due to tumorous swelling. Multiple fractures have resulted in angulated deformities. The edges of the lesion are smooth-bordered and are surrounded by a thin or thick rim of periosteal or cortical bone. Some islands of translucent bluish cartilage (*arrow*) may be seen in former fracture sites. Small foci of cystic degeneration are also present. The reader is urged to compare this specimen to those *in vivo* and to radiologic features from the same patient in order to gain a more complete understanding of the process (see Figs. 7-52, 7-63, and 7-68).

FIG. 7-61. In distinction to FD, Paget's disease of the bone is not characterized by a tumorous replacement. Rather it is typified by an abnormal modeling and remodeling of the host cancellous and cortical bone. Paget's bone has a pumicelike appearance and eventually results in a thickening of the trabeculae, particularly those oriented along the lines of stress. However, as in FD, the bone contour may be similarly widened and deformed.

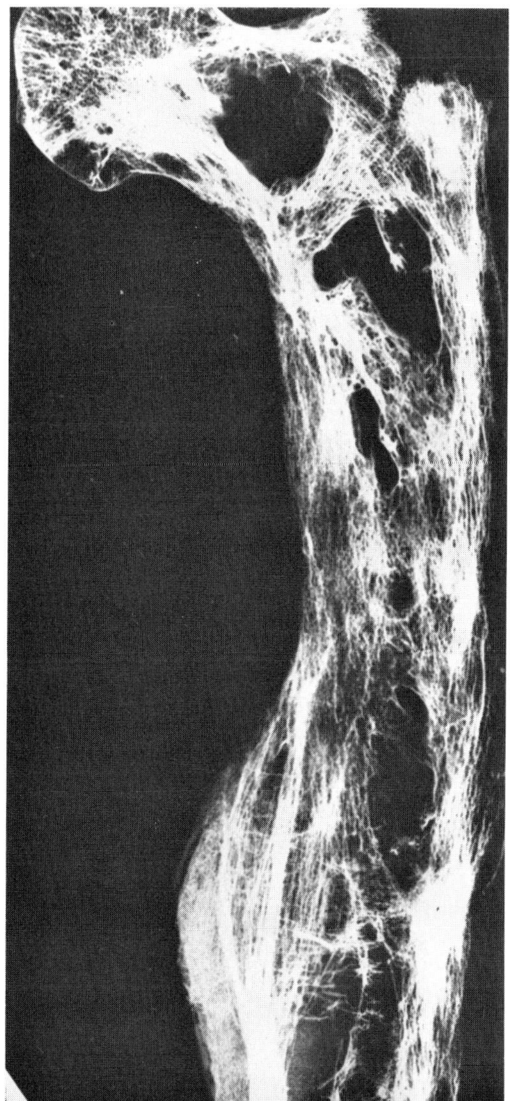

FIG. 7-62

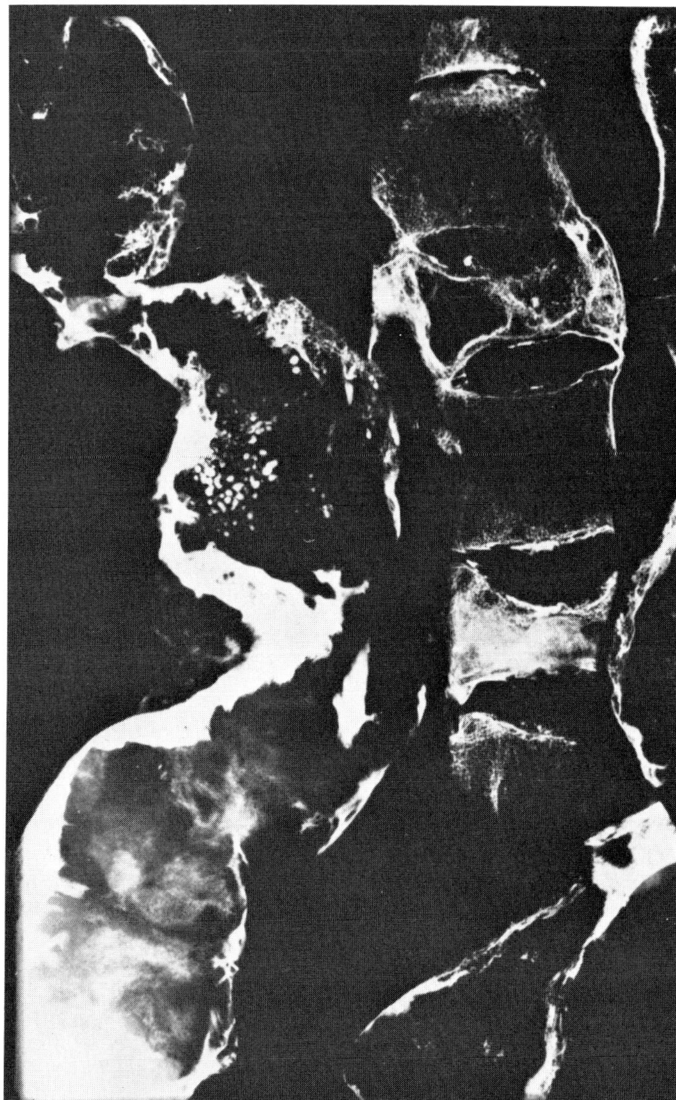

FIG. 7-63

Fibrous Dysplasia Compared to Paget's Disease

FIG. 7-62. Specimen radiograph of the above femur of Paget's disease shows the distortion of the normal bone architecture and thickening of bone trabeculae, particularly those along the lines of stress. Considerable new bone may be formed from the periosteal membrane (lower half of illustration), which results in cortical irregularity and thickening. In contrast, FD results in cortical erosion by the tumorous process and is covered by a rim of periosteal new bone.

FIG. 7-63. Humerus (*left*), spine (*middle*) and sternum (*right*) from patient (Fig. 7-51) with polyostotic FD. Humerus: the only residual bone with fairly normal trabecular contours is confined to the peripheral areas and represents reactive periosteal bone and remnants of cortex. The interior is replaced by a tumorous process. The lower half shows a pathognomonic "ground-glass" appearance due to the deposition of myriads of fine trabeculae of woven bone so characteristic of this disease. The dense, rounded opacities in the upper half represent foci of calcification with cartilage islands in an old fracture area. Spine: Note the tendency to skip bones. Those vertebral bodies affected by the process are undergoing collapse even though some appear denser than normal bone. The density is due to the deposition of woven bone, which is much weaker than lamellar bone, and will not withstand stress as efficiently as will the latter.

Course and Treatment

Fibrous dysplasia is a benign disease that may be slowly progressive for several decades. Treatment of patients with the polyostotic form often requires numerous and complicated orthopaedic procedures in an attempt to reduce deformities and stabilize fractures. The majority of pathologic fractures heal well with conservative therapy. All surgical methods employed should be integrated into a comprehensive orthopaedic program for the prevention of deformities.[58]

Sarcomatous degeneration is an uncommon occurrence. Approximately 50 cases have been reported to date.[59] The most common type is osteogenic sarcoma, although fibrosarcoma (spindle-cell sarcoma) is second in frequency. Chondrosarcomatous transformation is rare. There is a slight predominance of malignant change in patients with the polyostotic form. The actual percent incidence of sarcomatous degeneration in patients with polyostotic disease may be much greater than with the monostotic form, if we assume that a large number of patients with monostotic disease may remain undiscovered because symptoms are absent or mild. Most of the patients have not had radiation therapy prior to the development of the sarcoma.[59] The prognosis is extremely poor.

Differential Diagnosis

SOLITARY BONE CYST WITH FIBRO-OSSEOUS REPAIR TISSUES. If a solitary bone cyst is modified by a cortical infraction (which may not be obvious on radiograph), hemorrhage into the cyst may occur. Eventually, this cyst may become organized by fibro-osseous tissues. A biopsy at this stage may lead to the erroneous conclusion of fibrous dysplasia. This probably is not a serious error since both are benign conditions, and the ultimate treatment may not differ significantly. Since bone cysts are solitary they could only be confused with a monostotic form of FD. If other fibro-osseous bone lesions are noted then the solitary bone cyst can be eliminated from consideration. If a solitary bone cyst had previously been diagnosed by radiograph and biopsy, then the presence of these tissues in a recurrent lesion should not alter the diagnosis. If, however, a solitary bone cyst with fibro-osseous repair presents for the first time, its confusion with monostotic FD is much more probable, though usually the radiological features of a bone cyst are sufficiently distinctive (Figs. 13–11 to 13–17) to prevent this from occurring. However, on surgical exploration of a bone cyst modified by fibro-osseous repair, the amount of solid tissue encountered by the surgeon is generally much less and the amounts of cystic areas much greater than if he had entered a

---

Fibrous Dysplasia

FIG. 7-64. A prime example of monostotic FD of the distal ulna. The lesion is small, lucent, and metaphyseal. Its outer contours are irregular in shape but the reactive surrounding bone sclerosis is a good sign that the lesion in question is benign. Because of the absence of a "ground-glass" appearance, the radiologic diagnosis of FD would not be firm, if entertained at all. Tomograms demonstrated a small cortical infraction, which must have been the cause of symptoms that prompted medical attention, in spite of its small size. Most patients with this disease are discovered in youth to young adulthood. Note the open epiphyses.

FIG. 7-65. This midshaft monostotic lesion show features pathognomonic of FD. The bone is smoothly expanded by a tumorous mass. Its outer rim is covered by a fine layer of periosteal new bone. A "ground glass" appearance is noted.

FIG. 7-66. This patient with polyostotic FD does not show a characteristic "ground-glass" appearance, but does show a trabeculated area of lucency in the shaft and an eccentric trabeculated bubblelike mass covered by a fine rim of periosteal new bone. This constellation of features is usually seen in three diseases: fibrous dysplasia, Gaucher's disease, and aneurysmal bone cyst.

FIG. 7-67. Massive involvement of the humerus by FD. Note the pathognomonic "ground-glass" appearance (*arrow*). Patients with this degree of involvement almost always have polyostotic disease. In the absence of a ground-glass appearance, one would also have to consider multiple enchondromatosis, Gaucher's disease, or severe untreated hyperparathyroidism (rare).

FIG. 7-68. Severe involvement of the humerus and scapula is evident on this radiograph. The characteristic "ground-glass" appearance is noted (*arrows*). Compare this *in vivo* radiograph with the specimen radiograph (Fig. 7–63) and gross specimen (Fig. 7–60).

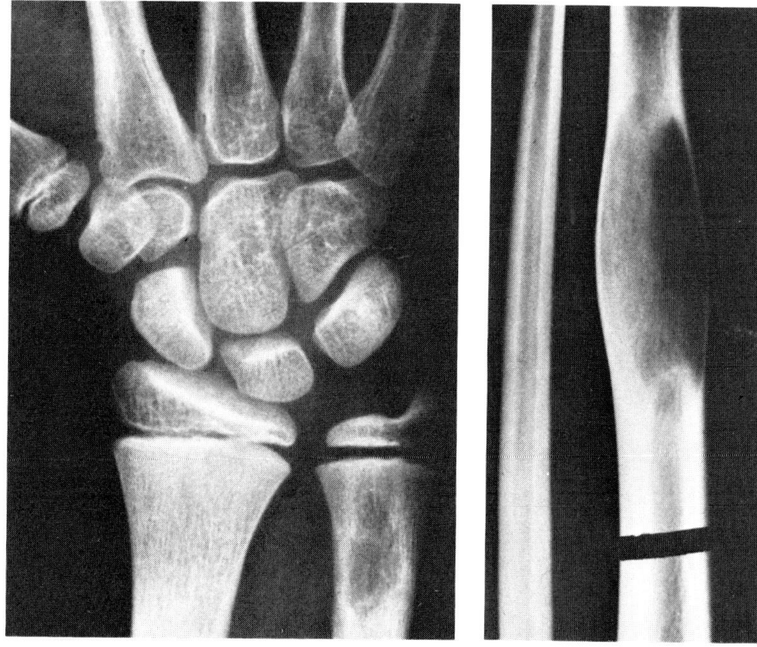

FIG. 7-64

FIG. 7-65

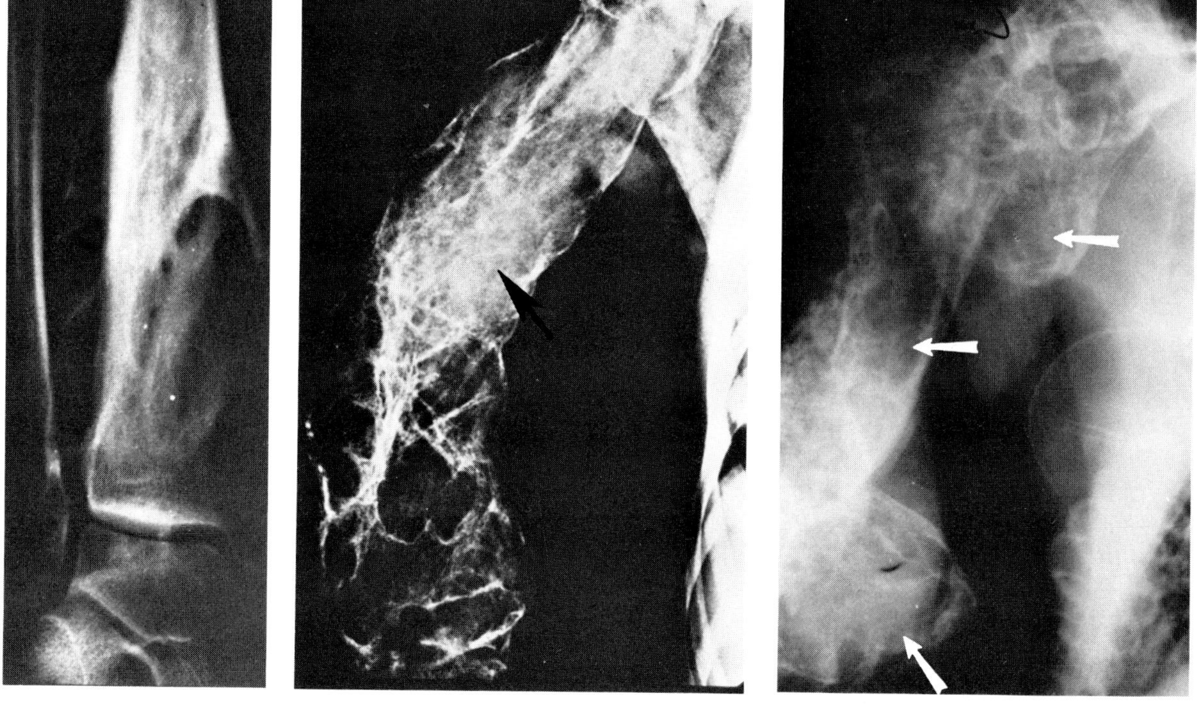

FIG. 7-66

FIG. 7-67

FIG. 7-68

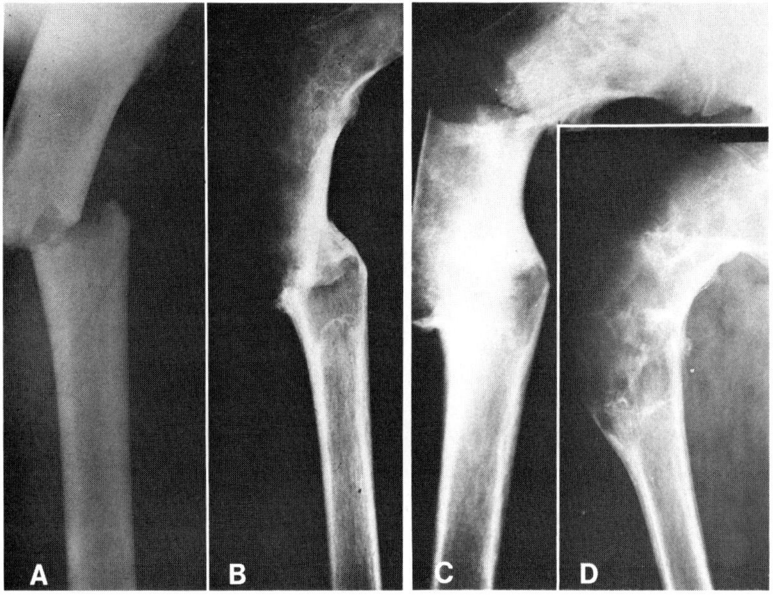

FIG. 7-69

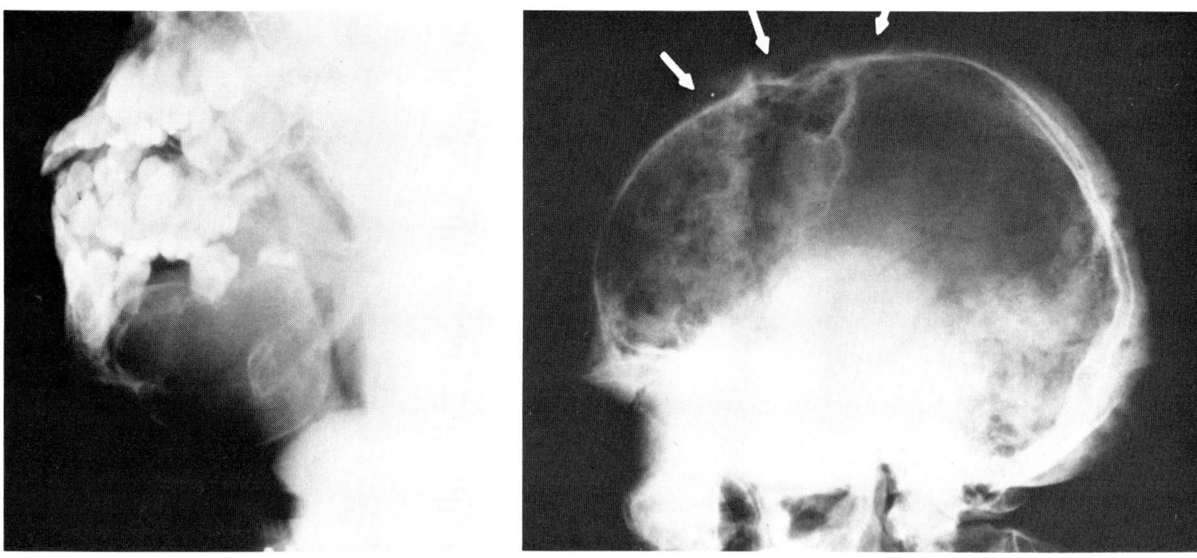

FIG. 7-70

FIG. 7-71

Fibrous Dysplasia

FIG. 7-69. This series of radiographs shows that the so-called Shepherd's Crook deformity (*D*) forms as a result of repeated fractures with repair and is not due to the fact that the bone is bent into that position.

FIG. 7-70. Mandibular involvement is common. Note the characteristic "ground-glass" appearance, bone "expansion," and fine rim of periosteal bone.

FIG. 7-71. Extensive skull involvement. The characteristic features of FD (assuming the "ground-glass" appearance is not plainly seen) are that some of the lesions are bordered by a zone of reactive sclerosis and, furthermore, that there is a cystlike expansion of the diploic space with bulging of the outer table (*arrows*). The inner table is not affected much; in contrast to Paget's disease, in which the inner table is usually thickened, and the outer, atrophic.

fibrous dysplastic lesion. Pathologically, the fibro-osseous repair tissues of a bone cyst contain a more uneven distribution of bone production. The bone may be laid down in more solid masses (Fig. 13–17) and do not have the usual curled "C" and "Y" shapes, as fibrous dysplastic lesions do. Plump osteoblasts lining the bone may be moderately to extensively prominent. In addition, careful search should be made for remnants of remaining cyst lining (Fig. 13–15), the characteristic feature of the simple bone cyst. Also, there may be quantities of hemosiderin pigment, cholesterol crystals, and other signs of necrosis and hemorrhage.

DESMOID (DESMOPLASTIC FIBROMA). This is an extremely rare fibroblastic tumor that may behave as a neoplasm (p. 270 and Figs. 9–22 to 9–30). The tissue (Figs. 9–28 and 9–29) is identical to extra-abdominal desmoids and does not form woven bone.

FIBROSARCOMA. Low-grade anaplastic fibrosarcomas may resemble cellular areas of fibrous dysplasia. However, greater nuclear pleomorphism (Figs. 9–30 and 9–34 to 9–37), increased frequency of mitoses (one mitosis per five HPF's or greater), absence of a rim of sclerosis, more permeative pattern of destruction on radiograph, and infiltration between host lamellar bone trabeculae should separate this malignant entity from FD.

OSTEOSARCOMA. Low-grade anaplastic osteosarcoma may produce relatively innocent fibrous tissue and woven-bone trabeculae not unlike FD. However, these tissues will invade extensively between lamellar bone trabeculae and mitoses are more frequent. Islands of malignant cartilage may be found. It is important to correlate the histologic material with the radiographic material, because the majority of osteosarcomas have virtually pathognomonic radiographic features (p. 139 and Figs. 7–73 to 7–92 and Plates 3 and 4).

OSSIFYING FIBROMA. This entity is discussed in the next section.

Ossifying Fibroma

Although the entity ossifying fibroma is almost always seen in relation to jaw bones, cases have been reported in long bones. Kempson (1966) reported 2 cases in young children. Both involved the tibia. The radiological features were indistinguishable from fibrous dysplasia. The tissues showed a mixture of benign fibrous tissue and fine spicules of woven bone. The pathologic distinction from FD was the fact that the bulk of the bone spicules were rimmed by prominent plump to spindly osteoblasts. This feature is rarely observed in FD and when present only in small foci. The clinically distinctive feature for these authors was that both cases recurred following curettage and involved large areas of the tibia. Such "aggressive" behavior is not to be expected following curettage of FD. The authors suggested wide excision and periosteal stripping combined with bone grafting in dealing with this lesion in the long bones. However, in my estimation this lesion could represent early active fibrous dysplasia in a rapid growth phase in which osteoblastic rimming may be prominent. Whether or not this is a distinct entity remains to be seen. This issue could perhaps be resolved by reviewing biopsy material from infants affected with polyostotic lesions to see if osteoblastic rimming is prominent in its incipient growth phase. If at some later age another biopsy is necessary and the features are typical of fibrous dysplasia because osteoblastic rimming is no longer prominent, then the *ossifying fibroma* of long bones may not be a distinct entity.

Brown Tumor of Hyperparathyroidism

This lesion is characterized by prominence of giant cells, fibrous tissue, areas of hemorrhage, and hemosiderin pigment, and often, small areas of osteoid and woven-bone production. Refer to p. 308 and Figs. 10–1 to 10–9 for a more complete description.

Simple Bone Cyst and Aneurysmal Bone Cysts

Both lesions may be associated with slivers of osteoid and woven bone in their cyst or cystlike walls. Fracture with hemorrhage into a simple bone cyst may lead to the formation of extensive fibroosseous tissues. This could be confused with fibrous dysplasia. These changes are discussed and illustrated in another section. (refer to p. 466 and Fig. 13–17).

LOW-GRADE MALIGNANT INTRAOSSEOUS LESIONS ASSOCIATED WITH OSTEOID AND WOVEN-BONE PRODUCTION

Neoplastic Giant Cell Tumor

Variable degrees of osteoid and woven bone may be produced in up to 40 per cent of GCT's and confusion with osteosarcoma or osteoblastoma is possible. Refer to p. 346 and Fig. 10–59 for a more detailed description.

HIGH-GRADE MALIGNANT INTRAOSSEOUS LESIONS ASSOCIATED WITH "REACTIVE" OSTEOID AND WOVEN-BONE PRODUCTION

Almost any high-grade malignant tumor, whether it is primary or metastatic, can be associated with reactive osteoid and woven-bone production. Metastatic breast carcinoma, for example, can result in massive reactive bone sclerosis. In most every instance the anaplasm can be easily distinguished from the reactive host bone it may stimulate. The reactive bone will commonly show benign features, such as prominent benign osteoblastic rimming.

There is only one primary intraosseous tumor associated with nonreactive malignant bone production—the osteogenic sarcoma.

Intramedullary Osteogenic Sarcoma

The osteosarcoma (OS) that arises from the intramedullary bone is a highly malignant tumor with distinctive radiologic and pathologic characteristics that permit it to be distinguished from the less lethal osteosarcomas of periosteal origin.

The intramedullary osteosarcoma can be either primary or secondary; solitary or multiple. The primary tumor usually affects adolescents or young adults. Secondary osteogenic sarcoma may develop as a complication or radiation therapy for some other lesion, from Paget's disease, fibrous dysplasia, bone infarct (rare), osteochondroma (rare), and osteoblastoma (rare). Most patients with secondary osteosarcoma are over age 40, as it usually takes many years before transformation of a benign precursor lesion to a highly malignant tumor is possible. Most osteosarcomas are solitary lesions, although between 1 and 2 per cent may be multiple. The multiple tumors may present within a short time interval from each other (*synchronous*) or months to years later (*metachronous*).

Primary Intramedullary Osteogenic Sarcoma

Capsule Summary

Incidence. Some 19.5 per cent of all biopsied primary bone tumors. Male:female incidence is 2:1.

Clinical. Painful, rapid growth, and swelling are present and alkaline phosphatase may be elevated.

Radiologic. Usually a metaphyseal sclerotic lesion with considerable periosteal new bone and soft-tissue mass. Unusual to rare features include diaphyseal and epiphyseal primary location, pure lysis, absence of periosteal new bone and soft-tissue mass, "onion skinning" periosteal reactions, similar to Ewing's tumor, small "cumulus-cloud" densities, or rarely, cystlike features mimicking benign conditions such as nonossifying fibroma, aneurysmal bone cyst, chondroblastoma, and giant cell tumor.

Gross. Usually yellowish white with areas of cartilage, hemorrhage and necrosis. Rarely, it is almost entirely hemorrhagic and cystic (telangiectatic osteosarcoma).

Histologic. Usually objective anaplasia with atypical mitoses, osteoid, and woven to immature lamellar bone. However, between 20 and 30 per cent of cases may show equivocal or minimal anaplasia. Many histologic patterns are possible. Patterns may mimic chondrosarcoma, fibrosarcoma, undifferentiated tumors such as Ewing's tumor or melanoma, aneurysmal bone cyst (telangiectatic osteosarcoma), histiosarcoma, and giant cell sarcoma. By definition, this neoplasm must show the presence of malignant stromal cells producing either osteoid or primitive bone.

Course. Usually rapidly fatal. In 15 to 30 per cent of cases, there is a 5-year survival rate with amputation alone.

Treatment. Amputation or combinations of radiotherapy, chemotherapy, and en-bloc excision or amputation.

Definition. An intramedullary osteosarcoma is a highly malignant bone-forming tumor characterized by frankly to subtly anaplastic stromal cells with the evidence of the *direct* formation of osteoid and/or primitive bone by these cells. These tumors may also produce malignant cartilage. If osteoid and/or primitive bone forms from a noncartilagenous malignant stroma, even if the great bulk of the tumor is chondrosarcomatous, it is still, by definition, an osteogenic sarcoma.

Importance. The osteosarcoma (excluding multiple myeloma) is the most common of the histologically verified primary bone tumors, either benign or malignant. The fibrous cortical defect is probably the most common of all bone tumors, but it is rarely biopsied.

The osteogenic sarcoma is extremely variable in its radiological and morphological presentation which may cause diagnostic confusion in trying to identify which sarcoma it may be or even mistaking it for a benign entity. Careful analysis of all osteoid and woven-bone producing-lesions is necessary to avoid drastic errors in diagnosis and therapy.

Clinical Features

More than 85 per cent of patients with primary osteogenic sarcoma present before the age of 30. More than 60 per cent present in the second decade.

The most common presenting complaint is pain, often associated with swelling. At first the pain is slight and intermittent. Within weeks the pain increases in severity and duration and local swelling occurs. Complaints may vary from 1 to 8 months, rarely longer. If pain is present in the area in question for more than 12 months, the diagnosis of primary intramedullary OS must be viewed with extreme

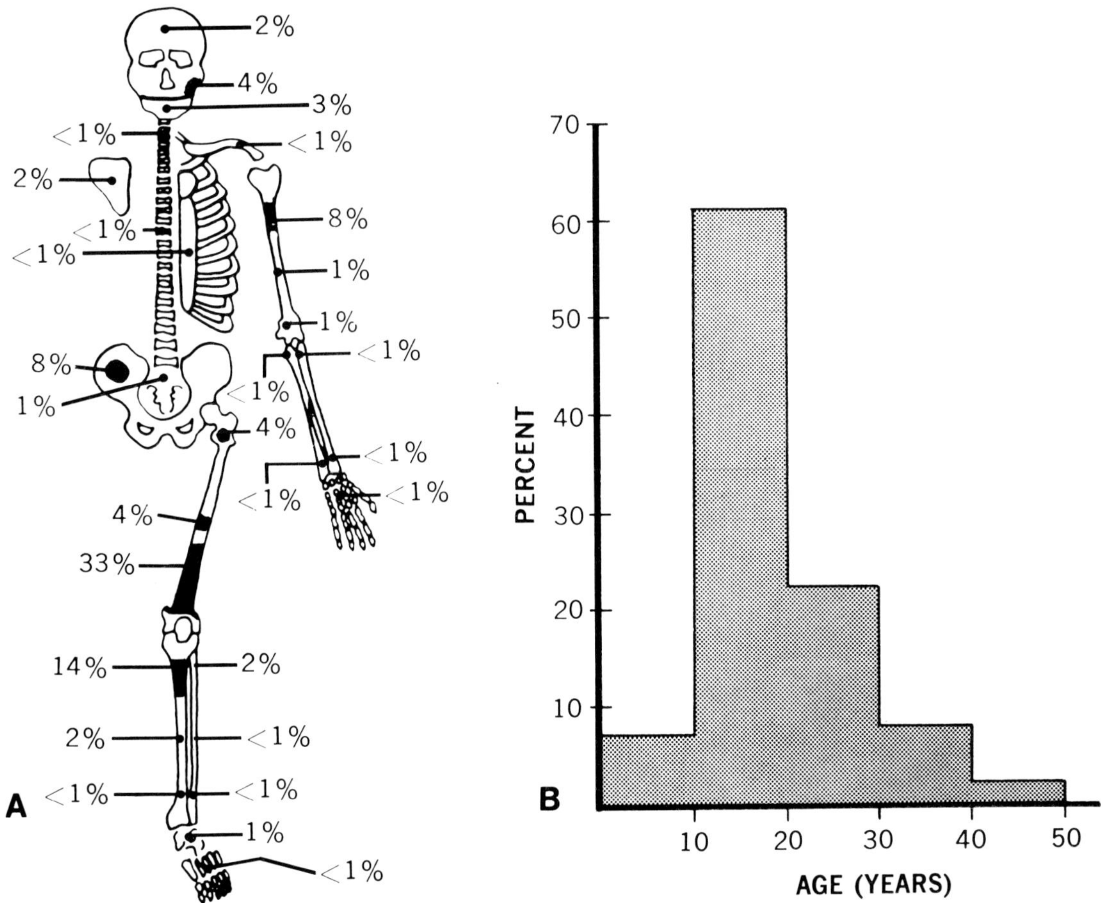

FIG. 7-72. (*A*) Primary osteogenic sarcoma (excluding Paget's sarcoma, postirridation sarcoma, and sarcoma complicating fibrous dysplasia). Frequency of areas of involvement in 854 patients. Male:female incidence, 2:1. (*B*) The graph shows age distribution of patients with primary osteogenic sarcoma (excluding Paget's sarcoma and postirradiation sarcoma).

suspicion, because this is one of the most rapidly growing of all tumors.

The serum alkaline phosphatase is the only helpful laboratory test. But, if it is elevated, it is usually not more than two to three times higher than normal for that age at the time of initial presentation. If, after extirpation of the primary bone tumor, the serum alkaline phosphatase begins to rise, metastases and/or recurrence is to be expected. The gradual rise may precede obvious clinical dissemination by up to several months.

Radiologic Features

INTRODUCTION. In diagnosing OS, radiographic interpretation is often as important, and in some cases permits easier recognition of the tumor than pathological examination alone. An obvious large "sclerosing" (dense, bone-producing) OS by radiographic examination, may present with deceptively "innocent" cytologic features. On the other hand, it is possible that on pathological examination, an obviously anaplastic OS may present with radiological features considered benign.

The radiographic features of an osteosarcoma depend basically on three factors: its degree of tumor bone production; whether it has broken through the bone cortex; and its location within the bone. Several types of periosteal reaction may be seen if the tumor has broken through the cortex.

1. DEGREE OF TUMOR BONE PRODUCTION. The majority (approximately 90 per cent) of osteosarcomas

produce significant degrees of tumor bone visible on radiograph. Those with minimal to absent visible tumor bone production are defined as lytic OS.

2. CORTICAL DESTRUCTION WITH SOFT-TISSUE MASS. Approximately 90 per cent of osteosarcomas have broken through the bone cortex and show a soft-tissue mass on initial presentation.

3. LOCATION WITHIN BONE. Approximately 90 per cent of long-bone osteosarcomas are centered in the metaphysis, 9 per cent in the diaphysis, and 1 per cent in the epiphysis. These figures are summarized in Table 7–2.

The combinations of the three factors (degree of tumor bone, soft tissue mass, location) are virtually independent of each other. From the table, it is possible to estimate the chances of an osteosarcoma having a particular combination of patterns. For example, it can be calculated that the most common pattern an osteosarcoma may assume is a *tumor-bone-producing lesion* with *soft-tissue mass centered in the metaphysis.* From the table below it can be calculated that approximately 75 per cent of OS will present with these three features (90% x 90% x 90%). On the other hand, the most uncommon presentation would be an osteosarcoma centered in the epiphysis that is lytic and confined to bone with no soft-tissue mass. The chances of such an occurrence would be .01% (10% x 10% x 1%). The importance of these calculations to clinical and pathologic diagnosis is that the fewer typical radiographic features a presumed osterosarcoma has, the more attention has to be paid to assessing its histologic features.

An osteosarcoma may, however, assume a tremendous range of radiographic features. In most cases the radiographic features are virtually pathognomonic. This knowledge is of extreme importance, because between 20 and 30 per cent of osteosarcomas are not easily diagnosable from a slide reading alone. Also some benign lesions, such as aneurysmal bone cyst, osteoid osteoma, osteoblastoma, and early callus may have such cellular exuberance that they may be confused with osteosarcoma. The chances for these errors could be reduced by at least 75 per cent simply by radiologic correlation.

Table 7–2. Radiographic Features of Osteosarcoma of Long Bones

Tumor Bone Production		*Cortical Bone Destruction With Soft-Tissue Mass*		*Tumor Centered in*	
Present	90%	Present	90%	Metaphysis	90%
Absent	10%	Absent	10%	Diaphysis	9%
				Epiphysis	1%

Usually, by the time most patients undergo radiographic examination, the tumor has grown to a large size and has broken through the confines of the bone. Even at initial presentation, subclinical or clinical lung metastases are present in more than 80 per cent of patients. This represents the number of patients who eventually manifest lung metastases, even though amputation may be performed only a few days following diagnosis. It is most unfortunate that this tumor is rarely discovered in its early phases of development; that is, when it is small and confined to bone, when the possibility for cure would be at its greatest. A corollary of these unfortunate circumstances is that in most cases of osteosarcoma, the tumor in and of itself does not cause sufficient pain to force the patient to seek medical attention. This would imply that not pain within the tumor per se but consequences of its growth, such as pathologic fracture or local swelling, cause the patient to seek medical attention. At initial presentation, it is not common to note gross fractures by standard radiographs. However, if specimen slices of the resected bone are subjected to gross examination and specimen radiography, it is not unusual to discover small cortical infractions.

TYPICAL AND DIAGNOSTIC RADIOGRAPHIC FEATURES. Most primary intramedullary osteogenic sarcomas take origin in the long bones and the majority of these (approximately 75 per cent) present with features that are virtually diagnostic. At initial presentation, the radiographic features of most cases are advanced and reflect the highly destructive nature of the tumor. The virtually diagnostic radiographic features are listed below (Figs. 7–73–7–76).

1. The lesion is large (greater than 5 cm. in its longest dimension) and is usually centered in the metaphysis, less commonly in the diaphysis, (Fig. 7–76) and rarely in the epiphysis (Fig. 7–87).

2. The lesion arises from the intramedullary bone and breaks through the cortex to form a lobulated (Fig. 7–73) or roundish (Fig. 7–74) eccentric or concentric soft-tissue mass, usually associated with evidence of fluffy tumor bone deposition (Figs. 7–73–7–76). The soft-tissue mass is *not* covered by a fine, smooth, concentric rim of periosteal new bone, which is seen in benign conditions. In fibrous dysplasia or osteoblastoma, for example, the tumorous processes may bulge the bone eccentrically into the region of the soft tissue, but the mass is covered by a thin rim of periosteal bone, testifying to their slow growth (Fig. 7–65). A benign tumor that can give rise to a rapidly growing destructive lesion with a soft

tissuelike extension is the aneurysmal bone cyst (ABC) in its incipient rapid growth phase (Figs. 13-36 to 13-39). It can easily be confused with the lytic type of osteogenic sarcoma. Fortunately, the biopsy usually affords ready distinction. However, in the healing or slow-growth phase of an ABC, exuberant fibro-osseous repair tissues that may even contain chondroid (Fig. 13-50, *B*) may set the trap for a diagnosis of osteosarcoma. This phase is, however, characterized by a radiologic sign of benignancy which the radiologist and pathologist must be aware of. This sign is the deposition of a fine, thin, rim of periosteal new bone surrounding the "soft-tissue mass" (Figs. 13-37 to 13-42). This radiologic sign cannot be overstressed as an aid to distinguish the alarming pseudosarcomatous histologic aura of a healing ABC from an osteosarcoma.

If the OS forms a very dense periosteal collar of bone (Fig. 7-77), its intramedullary origin may be obscured. Such cases are no longer radiologically diagnostic because bone-productive lesions of periosteal origin may appear identical. The differential diagnosis of lesions similar to that illustrated in Figure 7-77 would include parosteal and periosteal osteosarcoma (p. 536 and Figs. 14-38 and 14-40) and benign traumatic periostitis (p. 560). It is extremely important to separate these entities since there are major differences in their behavior and modes of therapy.

3. The periosteum is often stimulated by the rapidly growing tumor to form "ominous" reactive new bone in the form of one or more Codman's triangles (Figs. 7-76, 7-84), "hair-on-end" (Fig. 7-83), "sunburst" patterns (Fig. 7-79), and less commonly "lamellated" or "onion-skin" patterns (Fig. 7-90).

PERIOSTEAL REACTIONS. The *Codman's triangle* (Fig. 7-84) is usually seen in association with malignant tumors such as Ewing's tumor or osteosarcoma and occasionally in benign processes such as osteomyelitis and rapidly expanding aneurysmal bone cyst. Sections through the Codman's triangle itself often do not contain the tumor per se. "Sunburst" and "hair-on-end" periosteal reactions also commonly accompany malignant tumors that have broken through the cortex and rapidly lift up the periosteum. Since they usually are associated with malignant lesions, they can be called "ominous" periosteal reactions. However, even these reactions are by no means pathognomonic of malignancy, since benign lesions can on occasion result in identical patterns. The rare hemangioma of skull bones, for example, is often accompanied by a "sunburst" reaction.

The fact that these "sunburst" and "hair-on-end" patterns in association with osteosarcoma are truly periosteal reactions and not formed by malignant tumor bone per se are substantiated by the following factors (Figs. 7-78-7-82):

1. Similar reactions are associated with tumors that cannot in and of themselves produce bone, such as hemangioma and Ewing's tumor.
2. Similar reactions may be seen at the borders of the periosteum adjacent to, but not yet infiltrated by, tumor.
3. Sections through these regions with or without the presence of tumor show that the oriented spicular patterns of bone deposition seen on radiograph are indeed produced by stimulated periosteal osteoblasts (Figs. 7-80 to 7-82).

ATYPICAL RADIOLOGIC FEATURES. Those osteosarcomas that present in their early or incipient phases and those that produce little or no radiological evidence of tumor bone production (lytic osteosarcomas) will cause radiologic diagnostic confusion. These less than usual or atypical presentations include the following:

INCIPIENT OSTEOSARCOMAS. In a small percentage of cases (approximately 10%) the osteogenic sarcoma may present before it has broken through the cortex. These tumors are in their incipient phase of development and are smaller than the usual osteosarcoma. Osteosarcoma with these unusual presenting features can therefore be easily misconstrued as a benign or at most low-grade malignant tumor on both clinical and radiologic grounds. And, of course, whenever a malignant tumor presents with a "benign" radiologic pattern, the chances of repeating that error after pathological examination is increased as well if the tumor does not show frank or obvious anaplasia.

There are two types of incipient osteosarcomas: the blastic and the lytic.

Incipient Blastic (Cumulus Cloudlike) Osteosarcoma. Incipient blastic osteosarcoma has multiple coalescing, fluffy, whitish masses with rounded contours, imparting a cumulus cloud appearance on radiographic examination (Figs. 7-43 and 7-85, *A*). There is no rim of benign reactive host bone sclerosis or soft-tissue mass. The entire mass is generally 2 to 4 cm. in length. There is no breach of the cortex, because by definition this should no longer be considered "incipient." Although by no means pathognomonic, most cases I have seen with these features were either osteosarcoma or stress fracture. On tomogram the incipient blastic OS does not show a fracture line or significant periosteal reaction, as does the usual stress fracture. If the history and tomograms do not support a diagnosis of stress fracture, a biopsy should be performed. If there is any doubt, a serial radiographic study should be performed. If the lesion shows gradual to rapid increase in size, biopsy is indicated. The pathologist must be made fully aware by the clinician of the radiologic problem of stress fracture versus osteosarcoma diagnosis if biopsy is performed. On the other hand it is incumbent upon the pathologist to review the history and radiographs on any less than frankly unequivocal osteosarcoma diagnosis he is contemplating by slide material alone to rule out a possible stress fracture, which the clinicians may have missed.

Other entities that this type of osteosarcoma may be confused with include the enchondroma, bone infarct, osteoblastoma, and fibrous dysplasia. However, each of these entities usually has distinguishing features on radiographic analysis. The enchondroma usually contains 1 to 3 mm. punctate, ringlike or spheroidal densifications and if broader zones of calcification are seen, they do not have the diffuse homogeneous cumulus cloudlike appearance of the incipient blastic osteosarcoma. The pattern of calcification in bone infarct is more solid and irregular in distribution. Osteoblastomas tend to be more circumscribed, rounder, or less multifocal in appearance. Often they result in smooth bone expansion and commonly are surrounded by a border of reactive host bone sclerosis. In monostotic fibrous dysplasia, the bone deposition is rarely as great as in blastic osteosarcomas, the lytic area may have a more ground-glass appearance, and often the lesion is surrounded by a sclerotic border of reactive bone. The osteosarcoma, on the other hand, has not, to my knowledge, ever resulted in smooth bone "expansion."

A specimen radiograph (Fig. 7–86) of a blastic osteosarcoma shows the pattern of tumor bone deposition characteristic of osteosarcoma more clearly. Small fluffs of woven tumor bone infiltrate between spicules of the normal host lamellar bone in numerous coalescing sites. In the absence of fracture this infiltrative pattern by a woven-bone-producing tumor is virtually pathognomonic of the osteosarcoma, as we have already alluded to in the discussion on osteoblastoma (p. 114 and Fig. 7–42, Plate 2, *B* and *D*), and later in our discussion dealing with the gross and histological features of OS (p. 148 and Plate 3, *A–G*).

In essence, it appears that in incipient phases of blastic osteosarcomas, the tumor begins in a small focus and spreads through marrow to other contiguous foci. As these foci enlarge, the pattern of coalescent homogeneous cumulus cloudlike densities are produced. After the tumor has enlarged significantly and has broken the cortex, the great masses of bone produced may obscure this cumulus cloud bone producing pattern on standard radiographs. However, in 3- to 4-mm. specimen radiographs of slices of even large osteosarcomas, remnants of this pattern are usually maintained (Figs. 7–83 and 7–86).

Incipient Lytic Osteosarcoma. Incipient osteosarcomas with a purely lytic component are from 2 to 4 cm. in size, have not broken through the cortex, and therefore usually have not incited a periosteal new

(*Text continues on p. 146.*)

Osteosarcoma, Typical

FIG. 7–73. Virtually diagnostic features of osteogenic sarcoma (OS). The lesion is metaphyseal, large, has broken through the cortex, is dense or bone producing, results in ominous periosteal reactions ["sunburst" spiculations (*a*) and Codman's triangle (*b*)]. Note also the angulation of the humeral head due to pathologic fracture (*c*).

FIG. 7–74. The pathognomonic features of this case include the presence of a large bone-producing "cumulus cloud" mass arising in the intramedullary portion of the metaphysis and focal penetration of the cortex in association with a roundish bone-productive soft-tissue mass.

FIG. 7–75. Note the virtually diagnostic signs: "cumulus cloud" density (*a*), hazy metaphyseal soft tissue mass (*b*) and two faint Codman's triangles (*c*).

FIG. 7–76. Even though this tumor is centered in the diaphysis, there can be no doubt about the diagnosis. The medulla is involved. The lesion is obviously producing fluffs of tumor bone. There are ominous periosteal reactions including a sunburst reaction and Codman's triangles (*arrows*).

FIG. 7–77. Although this tumor appears similar to Figure 7–76, it cannot be ascertained whether or not the medullary portion of the bone is involved. Therefore, it is not possible without biopsy or penetrating tomograms to rule out a parosteal osteosarcoma or a very unusual periosteal reaction to trauma (traumatic periostitis). In actuality, this lesion proved to be an intramedullary sclerosing OS, breaking out of the bone, wrapping around it and simulating the above two lesions. This patient developed lethal metastases within 1 year.

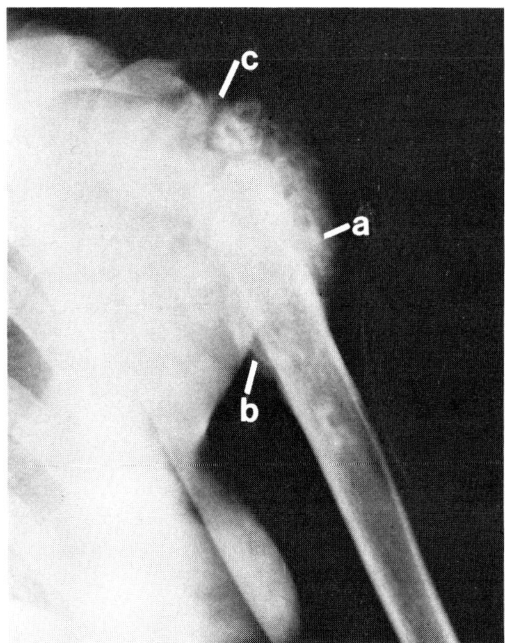

FIG. 7-73

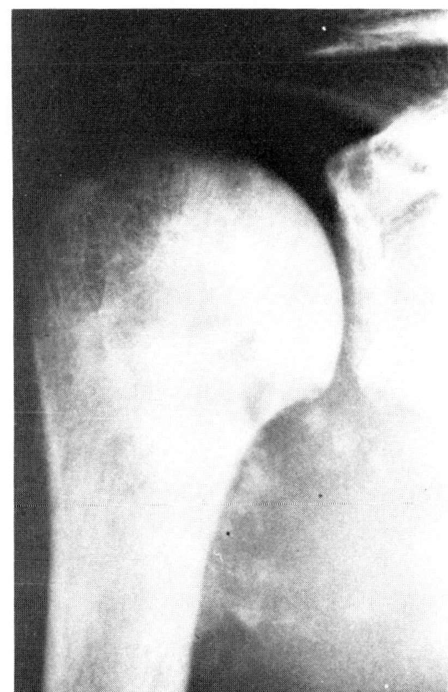

FIG. 7-74

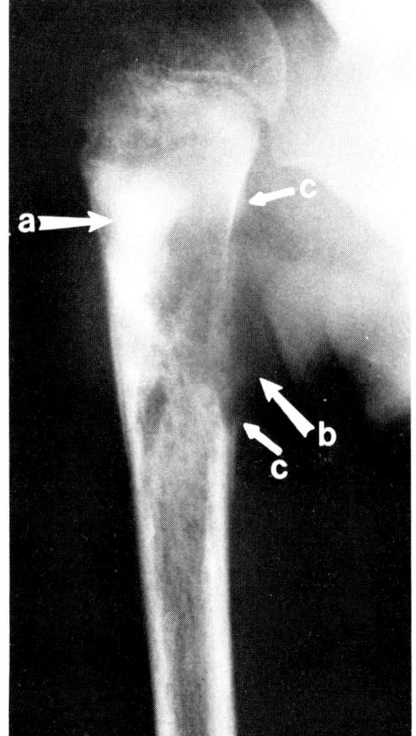

FIG. 7-75

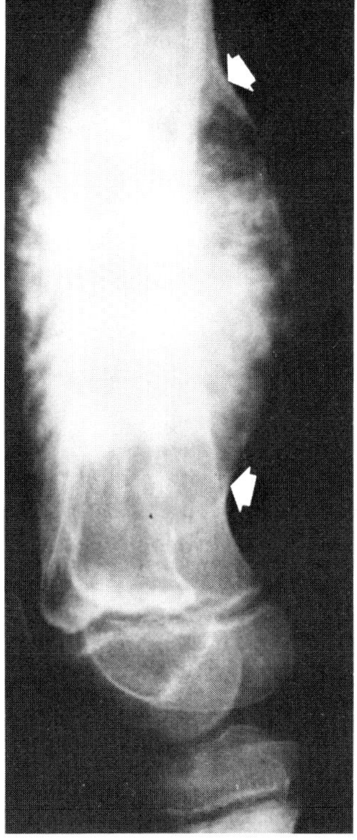

FIG. 7-76

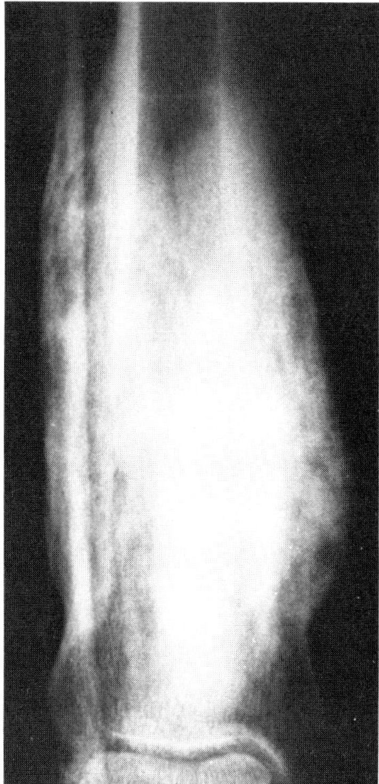

FIG. 7-77

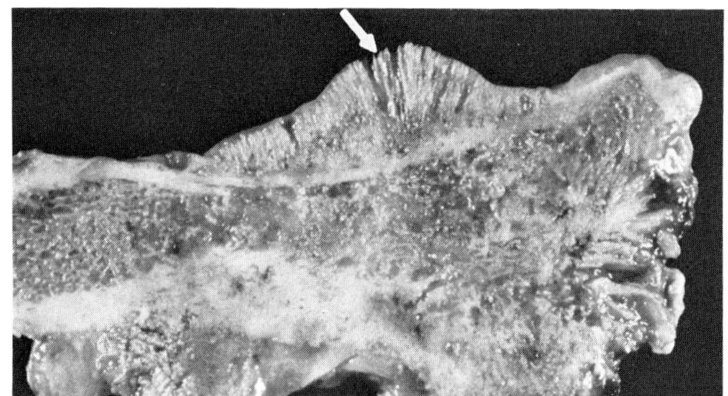

FIG. 7-78

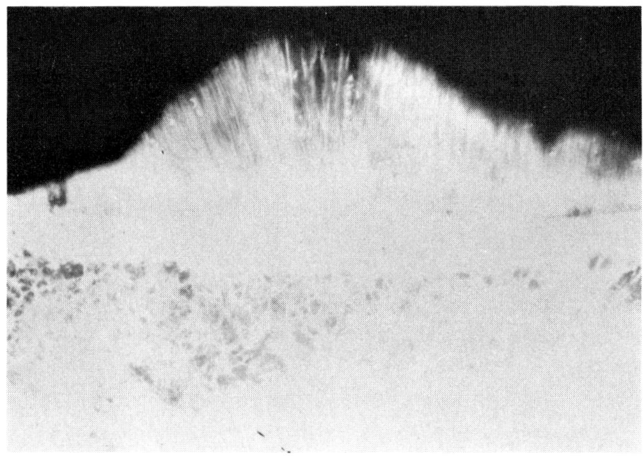

FIG. 7-79

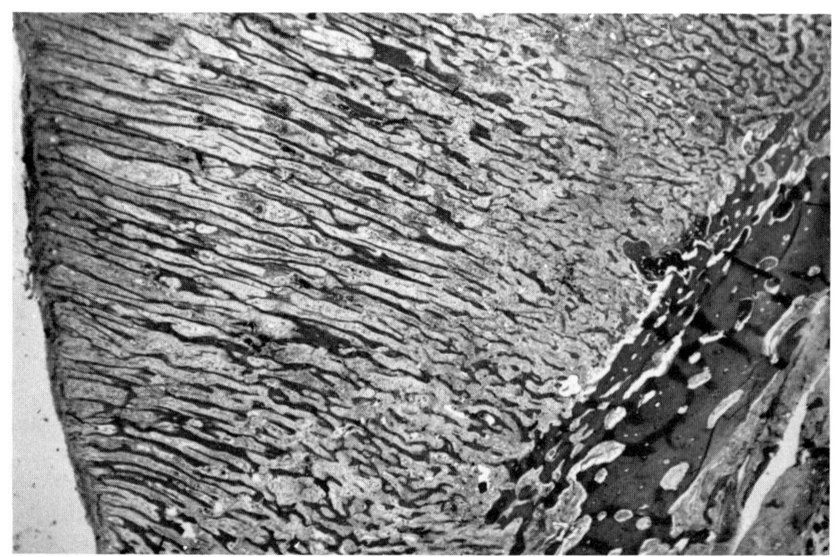

FIG. 7-80

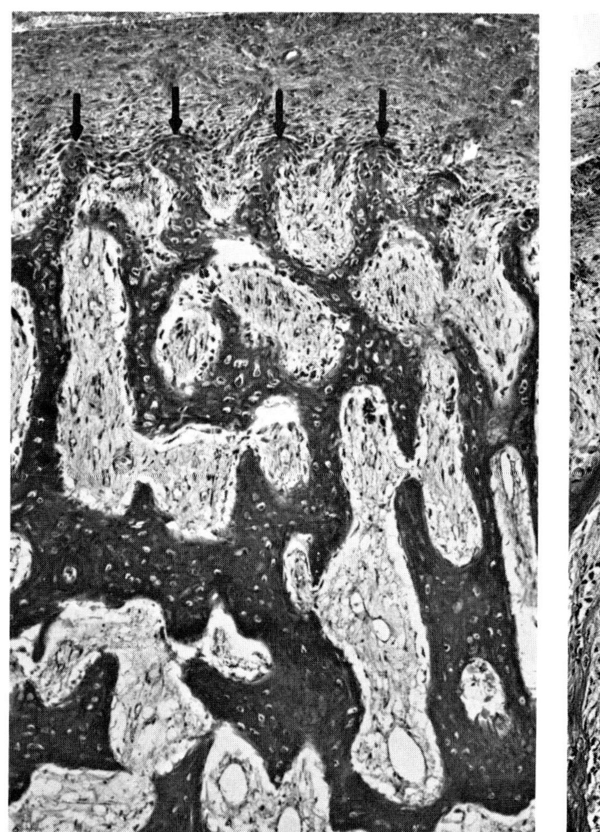

FIG. 7-81

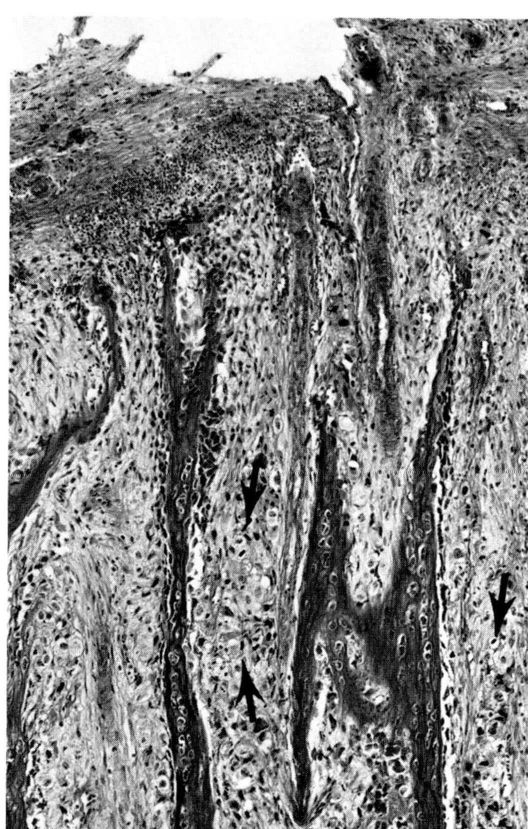

FIG. 7-82

Pathogenesis of Periosteal Reactions in Osteosarcoma

FIG. 7-78. This tumor of the pelvis was a predominantly chondroblastic osteosarcoma. Note the sunburst bone spiculation (*arrow*).

FIG. 7-79. Specimen radiograph of same area.

FIG. 7-80. Note the strikingly oriented pattern of the bone spicules. The right portion of the field represents the bone cortex (H and E, X40).

FIG. 7-81. A section through the margin or Codman's triangle area of the sunburst not yet infiltrated by tumor shows that the bone is being produced by stimulated periosteal osteoblasts (*arrows*). Note the benign osteoblastic rimming of the deeper spicules (H and E, X125).

FIG. 7-82. In the center of the sunburst reaction identical bone spicules can be seen rimmed by benign osteoblasts produced by the outer zone of periosteum. Malignant cartilage is seen between the individual trabeculae (*arrows*). This case clearly demonstrates that the sunburst and other well-oriented patterns of bone seen in association with OS is a reactive periosteal reponse and is not tumor bone, per se. Tumor bone is disoriented, fluffy, or "cumulus cloudlike." However, the periosteal reactive bone is triggered by tumor penetrating the cortex with rapid elevation or intermingling with the periosteal tissue (Figs. 7-78 to 7-82 are from the same case) (H and E, X125).

bone reaction. Their borders are rounded and lack a rim of benign reactive host bone sclerosis. Only a small percentage of osteosarcomas (fewer than 1%) present with these features. The diagnosis of osteosarcoma will almost never be considered by the radiologist or clinician. Other tumors that have similar radiologic presentations are the solitary bone cyst, aneurysmal bone cyst, eosinophilic granuloma or nonossifying fibroma for those located in the metaphyses and diaphyses or giant cell tumor for those extremely rare incipient lytic osteosarcomas centered in the epiphysis (Fig. 7–87). Unfortunately, the only one of the above entities that can be separated from the rare incipient lytic osteosarcoma without biopsy is the nonossifying fibroma (NOF). The NOF is almost always surrounded by a rim of reactive host bone sclerosis that is not seen in osteosarcomas. However, with the exception of the nonossifying fibroma, all of the other entities a lytic osteosarcoma may mimic are subjected to biopsy since their treatment depends upon a definitive pathological diagnosis. Therefore, we should not expect that this, the most "innocent" radiologic form an osteosarcoma may take, will escape pathologic examination even in its incipient phase of development.

ADVANCED LYTIC OSTEOSARCOMAS WITH PERIOSTEAL REACTION AND/OR SOFT-TISSUE MASS. Between 5 and 10 per cent of advanced (nonincipient) osteosarcomas may present as predominantly lytic lesions with "ominous" periosteal reactions (Fig. 7–88, 7–90) with or without soft-tissue mass (Fig. 7–90, 7–91). Although the presence of a large soft-tissue mass is a very important clue to determining whether the bone tumor in question is malignant, the diagnosis of osteosarcoma may not be easily apparent from radiographs. As a good rule of thumb, however, most lytic malignant tumors of the metaphysis in patients under 30 years of age that manifest focal cortical destruction and ominous periosteal new bone (Fig. 7–88) with a large, rounded soft-tissue mass (Fig. 7–89) usually prove to be osteosarcomas on histologic examination. This rule does not apply to lytic tumors with a permeative or "moth-eaten" pattern of bone destruction centered in the diaphysis. Generally, these tumors prove to be Ewing's tumor, fibrosarcoma, or reticulum-cell sarcomas, although on occasion, pathological examination will show osteosarcoma (Figs. 7–90 and 7–91).

There is usually no way to clearly distinguish lytic osteosarcomas from these other lesions on radiological examination without performing a biopsy. However on occasion, the predominantly lytic osteosarcoma may give itself away by producing a small focus of cumulus cloudlike tumor bone within the shaft or in the soft-tissue mass (Fig. 7–91). Since the diagnosis of these lytic osteosarcomas may be quite difficult even with pathologic examination, it is suggested that if any area of cumulus cloudlike densities are observed, no matter how small, that the biopsy include tissue from this region.

Gross Pathology

The gross features of an osteosarcoma depend upon its degree of bone and cartilage production, vascularity, degenerative foci, and extent of involvement. Large lesions (Fig. 7–92) involve the entire width of the intramedullary bone at the affected site and usually have eroded the bone cortex at one or more sites, lifting up the periosteum and extending into the soft tissues as a variable sized lobulated mass. Most osteosarcomas are whitish and gritty to extremely hard depending, of course, on the amount of tumor bone produced. There are frequently foci of

Osteosarcoma

FIG. 7–83. Specimen radiograph of an OS, which shows a "hair-on-end" reactive periosteal bone. The intramedullary portion of the tumor shows characteristic islands of fluffy "cumulus cloudlike" bone infiltrating between host cancellous bone (*arrows*). The tumor has breached the epiphysis and extends to the secondary ossification center. Interference with normal vascular invasion of the epiphyseal plate has led to its widening, compared to the uninvolved distal femoral epiphysis of the opposite femur.

FIG. 7–84. Codman's triangle on specimen radiograph of a 3-mm. slice of bone involved by OS. The bone of the outer part of the triangle can be seen clearly to arise from a layer of periosteum (*a*), which has been lifted from its cortical mooring by the tumor (*b*).

FIG. 7–85. Osteogenic sarcoma, incipient blastic. (*A*) In its incipient phase, before the cortex has been penetrated, most osteosarcomas are typified by coalescing homogeneous fluffs imparting a "cumulous cloud" appearance. If this pseudobenign radiologic pattern is not recognized, biopsy may not be performed until the diagnosis becomes grossly manifest. (*B*) A mere 2 months later, the diagnosis becomes obvious and illustrates the tremendously rapid growth and destructive qualities of this highly malignant tumor.

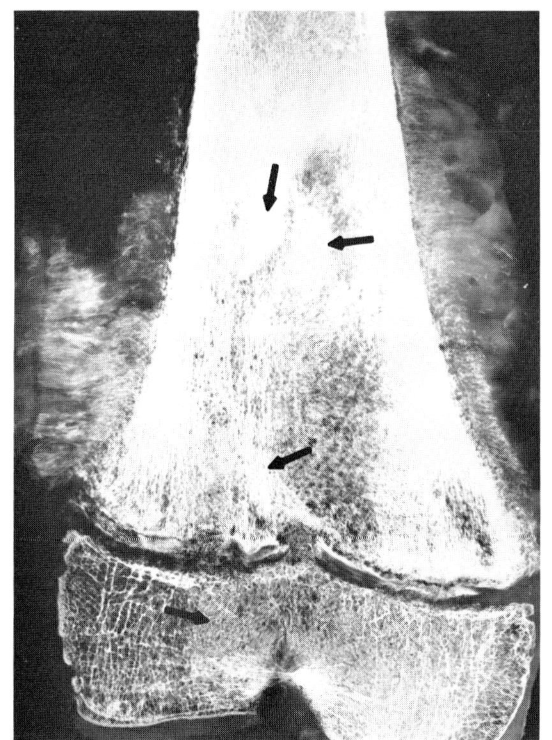

FIG. 7-83

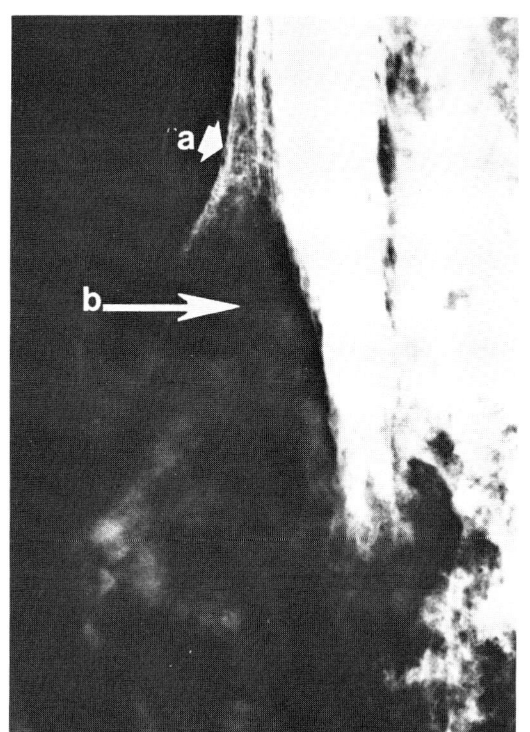

FIG. 7-84

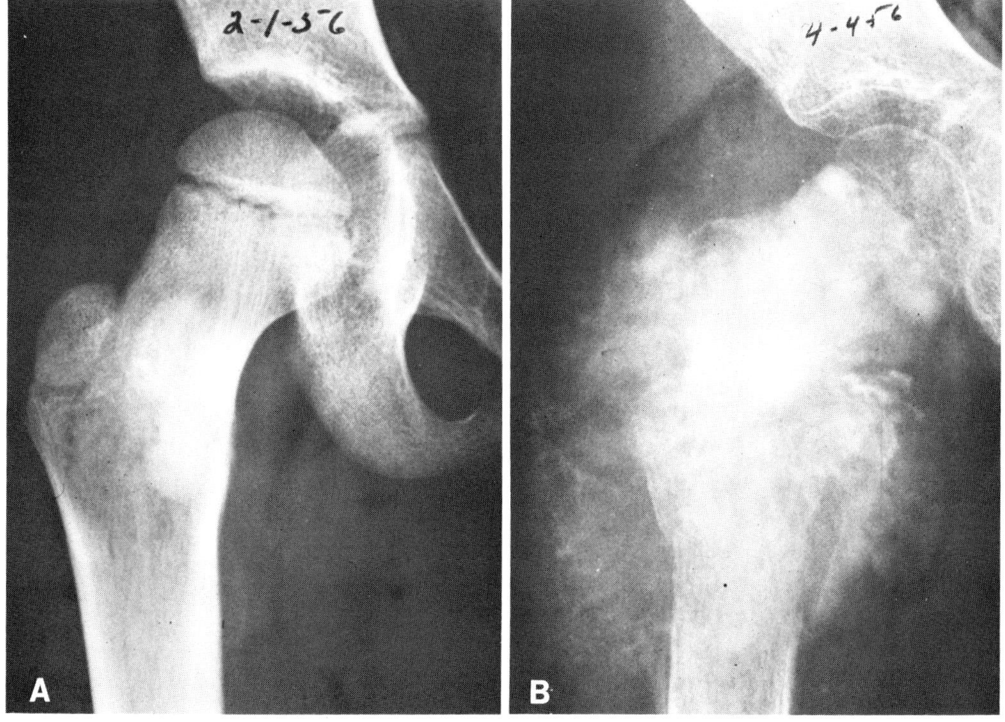

FIG. 7-85

hemorrhage and small to large islands of translucent bluish cartilage. The lesions rarely extend through the medullary canal more than $\frac{1}{3}$ the length of a long bone. If an epiphyseal plate is present, the tumor usually does not destroy it and extend to the secondary ossification center. In some cases, however, the tumor does destroy a small portion of the epiphyseal cartilage and extends to the secondary ossification center at this point.

The osteosarcoma with a predominantly lytic radiographic presentation, on gross examination, is firm (if abundant collagen is produced) to soft and gray to tan. The rare, always lytic, telangiectatic osteosarcoma is soft, hemorrhagic, and cystlike in appearance.

The pattern of tumor infiltration between host bone trabeculae (Plate 3, *A* and *B*) is best appreciated by using a magnifying glass or stereomicroscope and correlating these gross findings with specimen radiographs (Fig. 7–86) and microscopy (Plates 3, *C* and *F*). This is an exercise that should be performed not merely to satisfy academic interest but to gain greater insight into the pattern of infiltration of malignant bone tumors such as the osteosarcoma.

Characteristic Histopathology

The distinguishing feature of the osteosarcoma is the production of osteoid and/or woven bone by unequivocally anaplastic stromal cells (Plate 4, *C* and *K*). By unequivocally anaplastic is meant that the nuclei are bizarre in size and shape, chromatin abnormalities are marked, nucleoli are often prominent, and atypical (nonmirror) image mitotic figures are present. It is usually easiest to observe the most severe degrees of anaplasia in the most cellular areas of an osteosarcoma than in those in which osteoid and/or woven bone production is at a maximum (Plate 4, *G*). Most osteosarcomas will show blatantly obvious fields of anaplasia, even though the degree of anaplasia may vary from field to field. But it is possible to mistake highly exuberant reparative or cellular benign growths for anaplasia. If there is any doubt whether anaplasia truly exists, greater effort must be spent on a thorough analysis of all of the histologic, radiographic, and clinical features. And the more an individual case strays from classic patterns, the greater the care must be given to interpretation.

Most osteosarcomas contain significant quantities of osteoid and/or woven bone. These deposits vary from large thick masses of osteoid (Plate 4, *A*) to a closely "knit" to "streamer" type of osteoid with inconspicuous intervening vessels (Plates 3, *F* and *J*, and 4, *B* and *C*). These patterns of osteoid deposition are rarely seen in benign conditions and are an important aid when considering the diagnosis of osteosarcoma, particularly in the highly bone-producing form of osteosarcoma, where signs of anaplasia are

---

Osteosarcoma

FIG. 7–86. A specimen radiograph that clearly shows the characteristic pattern of coalescing "cumulous cloud" fluffs of OS tumor bone infiltrating through the marrow spaces. Microscopically this pattern is demonstrated by entrapped trabeculae of host lamellar bone (Plate 3*C*, *D*, *E*, *F*, and *G*). This is an extremely important pattern to be aware of because it can be used to differentiate histologically bland osteosarcomas from osteoblastoma. In order to distinguish these two lesions, biopsy should be directed at the margin of the lesion with the normal host bone. Osteosarcoma will show insidious invasion through the marrow spaces along its advancing front; osteoblastomas will be sharply delineated from the surrounding host bone (Fig. 7–42, *A*, *B*, and *C*).

FIG. 7–87. Osteosarcoma, incipient lytic. This is an extremely rare example of an OS that simulated in every detail a giant cell tumor. To our surprise, the lesion demonstrated a Grade III anaplastic osteosarcoma (see Fig. 7–93).

FIG. 7–88. Osteogenic sarcoma that could be confused with a benign process. (*A*) The lesion is metaphyseal and lucent. Unlike nonossifying fibroma, which it resembles most closely, the lesion is *not* surrounded by a border of reactive sclerosis and *has* eroded the cortex (*arrow*), inciting a faint but nevertheless significant periosteal reaction, which cannot be seen in this reproduction. These are features highly suggestive of a malignant process and despite its small size, the most common lesion in this metaphyseal site with these features is OS. However, in rare instances an eosinophilic granuloma or osteomyelitis could present with an identical radiographic pattern. At any rate, biopsy is mandatory. In this case, biopsy showed unequivocal OS. (*B*) The lesion is yellowish-gray and hemorrhagic and there is evidence of light-gray spicules of osteoid production. The cortex and epiphyseal plate are focally destroyed. This would rule out eosinophilic granuloma, because there has never been a reported case that breached a growing epiphyseal plate. Osteomyelitis can be associated with reactive bone and due to lytic enzymes associated with the process, it often leads to destruction of the epiphyseal plate. Biopsy easily distinguishes these three processes. This patient died 2 years later with multiple pulmonary metastases.

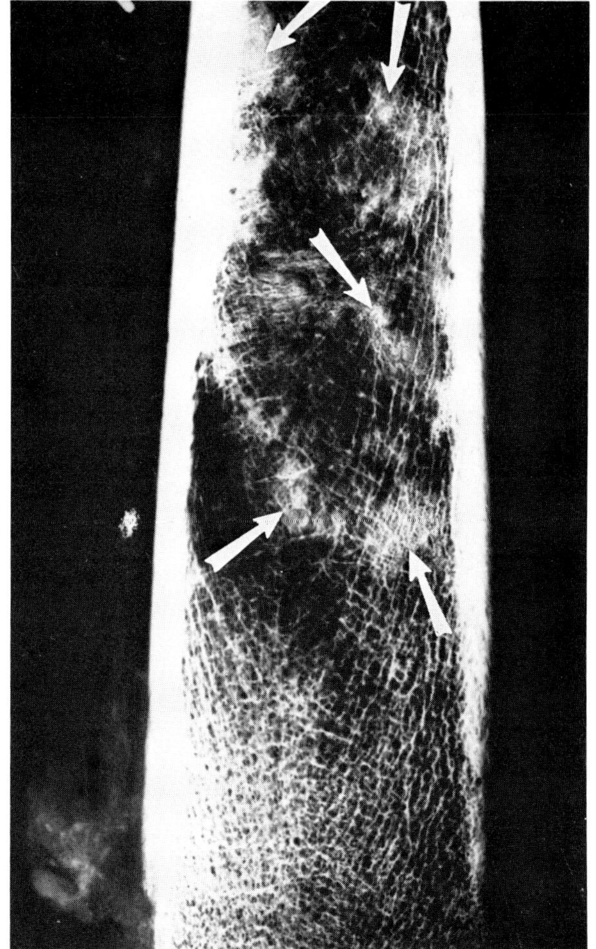

FIG. 7-86

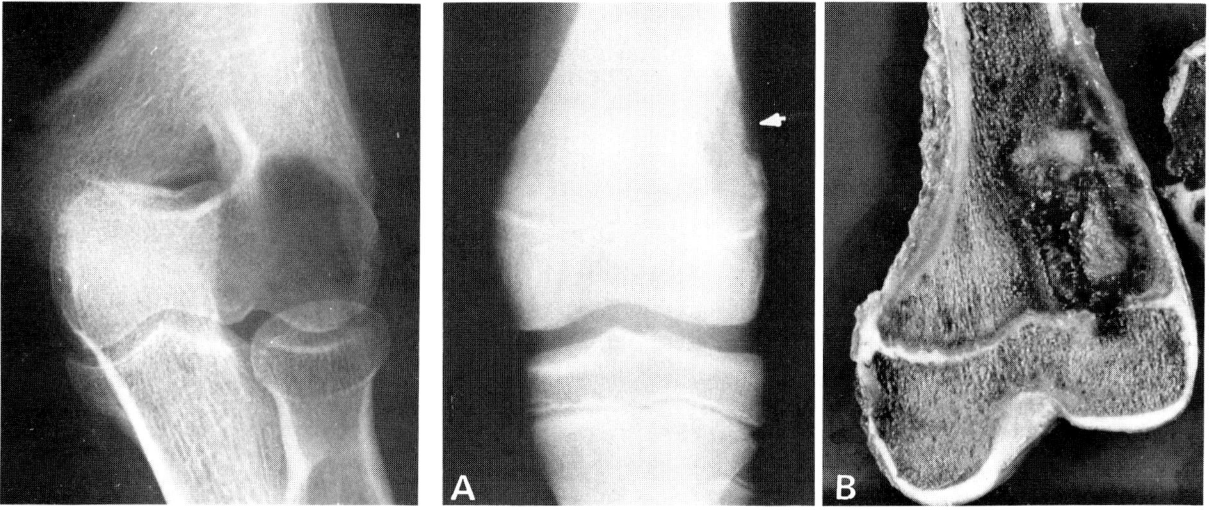

FIG. 7-87

FIG. 7-88

minimal (Plate 3, *I*). The osteosarcoma often produces variable quantities of woven bone (Plate 3, *C–H*) which in and of itself is not diagnostic of the tumor. But, unlike most other lesions there are usually masses of osteoid between the tumor woven bone trabeculae (Plates 3–6 to 3–9). Osteosarcomas do not produce tumor bone lined by a single row of prominent osteoblasts, so-called "benign" rimming (Fig. 7–14, *B*, p. 95).

A very important aid to the diagnosis of osteosarcoma is the presence of cartilage. High-grade chondrosarcoma (Plate 4, *F*) is not uncommonly found in variable amounts and if present, usually simplifies the diagnosis. In order to diagnose osteosarcoma, one must find areas of osteoid and/or woven bone production forming from undifferentiated stromal cells. The presence of woven bone within or surrounding lobules of malignant cartilage (Fig. 8–33) is not diagnostic of osteosarcoma, because bony metaplasia of cartilage tissues is not infrequently seen in association with pure chondrosarcoma.

Variable numbers of benign osteoclasts are often found sprinkled through the lesion (Plate 4, *K*). They represent a reactive element and are not derived from the neoplastic cells, because they do not show anaplasia and because identical cells may be found in numerous unrelated benign and malignant bone tumors.

Other malignant components that may be seen in osteosarcoma in variable proportions include spindle cells, malignant small and large round cells, and malignant giant cells.

Unusual Histologic Features Which Cause Diagnostic Difficulties

There are two main reasons osteosarcoma may be difficult to diagnose from biopsy alone. The first is that not all osteosarcomas are so blatantly anaplastic that they can be recognized easily, and the second, that the nonbone producing components of an osteosarcoma may so dominate the histology that confusion with other malignant entities or even benign conditions is possible. Table 7–3 lists several benign conditions that are confused with osteosarcoma, and vice versa.

From the table, it is apparent that the most difficult lesions to separate from osteosarcoma are callus and conversely, "osteoblastoma" from osteosarcoma.

Histopathologic Variations of Osteosarcoma

SCLEROTIC OR OSTEOID AND WOVEN BONE PREDOMINANT OSTEOSARCOMA (SCLEROTIC OSTEOSARCOMA). It is the densely bone-producing osteosarcoma that is most often confused with benign lesions such as osteoblastoma, osteoid osteoma, or callus. The reason is that the histological features of the cells of osteosarcoma in areas of intense osteoid and woven bone production are small, innocuous or innocent looking (Plates 3, *I*, and 4, *A*). In fact, they may be much more innocuous looking than those in early callus (Plates 1, *B*, and 4, *H*) osteoblastoma, or osteoid osteoma (Fig. 7–23, Plate 4, *I*).

Osteosarcoma

FIG. 7–89. Lytic osteosarcoma, advanced stage. The interior of the bone is trabeculated, not unlike that seen in benign conditions such as Gaucher's disease and fibrous dysplasia (FD) (Fig. 7–66). However, unlike FD there is evidence of ragged cortical destruction and a soft-tissue mass *not* covered by a fine rim of periosteal bone (a sign of slow growth). Therefore, the features are most consistent with a malignant process. Its metaphyseal location favors the diagnosis of a lytic OS, although fibrosarcoma and, rarely, Ewing's sarcoma, and aneurysmal bone cyst (incipient) would also have to be considered in the radiologic differential diagnosis. The gross specimen to the right is from the same case. Note from Figures 7–88 and 7–89 how much more extensive and destructive these lesions are than one would surmise from the standard radiograph.

FIG. 7–90. Lytic osteosarcoma mimicking Ewing's tumor, reticulum cell sarcoma, or fibrosarcoma. In this unusual example of an osteosarcoma, the features are those of a tumor that permeates the bone and is resulting in a moth-eaten pattern of destruction usually seen in other malignant entities or in osteomyelitis. The presence of very fine onion-skinlike lamellae of periosteal new bone (*arrows*) is rarely seen in osteomyelitis.

FIG. 7–91. Osteosarcoma mimicking Ewing's tumor. (*A*) The lesion is in the midshaft and has permeated the cortex and resulted in a fine "hair-on-end" spiculation. In most cases, this pattern is characteristic of Ewing's tumor. Although this tumor has most of the microscopic features of Ewing's, there are small foci of malignant spindle cells producing primitive osteoid and woven bone. (*B*) The diagnosis of OS was suspected on the basis of the fact that the lateral radiograph showed a fluffy mass of irregular densification suggestive of tumor bone (*arrow*).

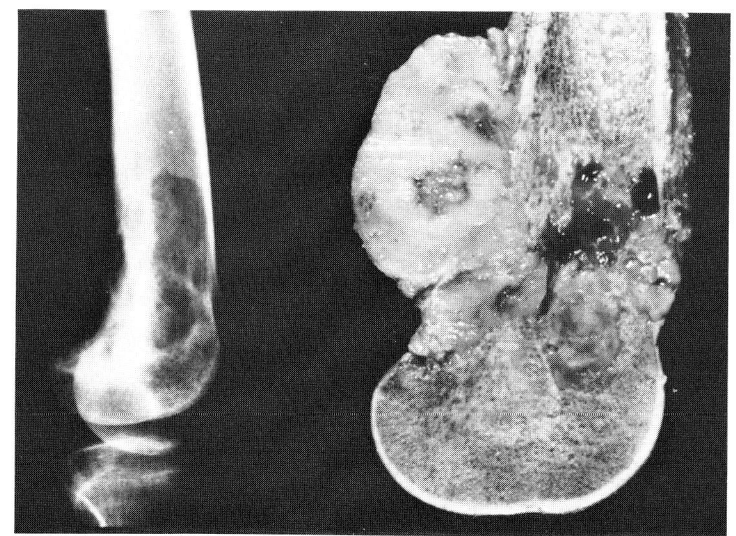

FIG. 7-89

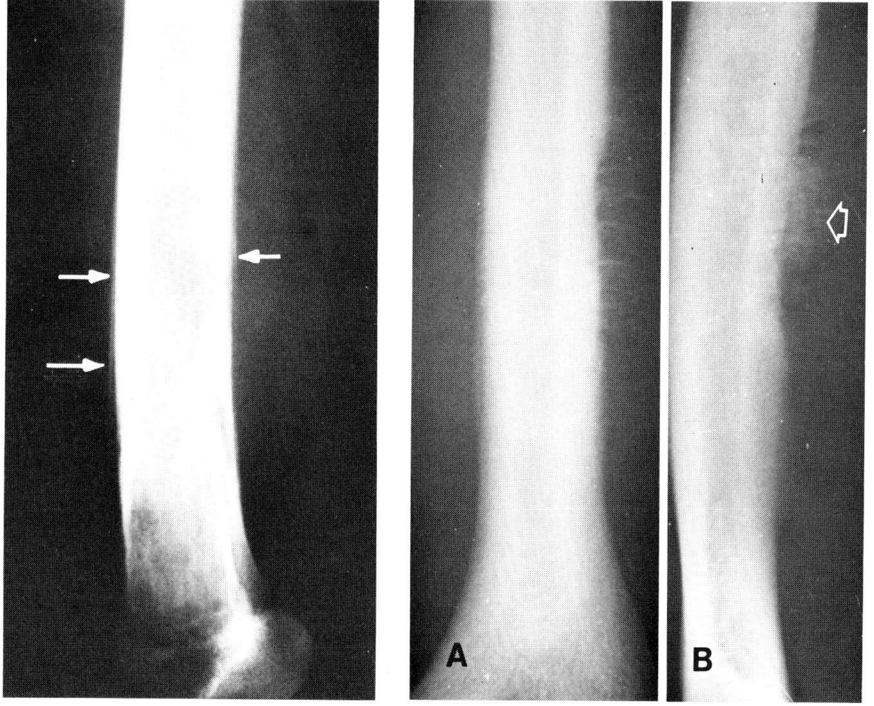

FIG. 7-90

FIG. 7-91

Table 7-3. Incidence of Pathologic Misdiagnosis from 150 Intramedullary Osteosarcomas and 650 other Primary Bone Tumors (Personal Observations)

BENIGN TUMOR DIAGNOSED AS OSTEOSARCOMA			OSTEOSARCOMA INCORRECTLY DIAGNOSED BENIGN		
Correct Diagnosis	*Sites*	*Number of Cases*	*Incorrect Diagnosis*	*Sites*	*Number of Cases*
Stress and "honeymoon" (rib) fracture	Rib, tibia	2	Osteoblastoma	Femur (2), radius, humerus, tibia	5
Atypical hyperplastic callus	Femur	2			
Pseudomalignant osteoblastoma	Fibula	1			
Osteoid osteoma	Humerus	1	Atypical aneurysmal bone cyst*	Femur	1
Giant cell tumor	Sacrum	1			
Aneurysmal bone cyst	Humerus	1			

*In actuality a telangiectatic osteosarcoma.

Also look for pattern of dense woven bone and "streamers" of osteoid between relatively intact host lamellar bone. Sclerotic osteogenic sarcoma always infiltrates the intertrabecular marrow space and replaces it with masses of dense woven bone and foci of tightly knit "streamers" and masses of osteoid. The pattern of tightly knit streamers and masses of osteoid (Plates 3, *D–H*, 4, *A–C*) are in and of themselves highly suggestive of osteosarcoma, since this pattern is rare to benign conditions. The host lamellar bone may be virtually intact and viable. (Use polarized light examination to appreciate this important aid to diagnosis and see Plate 3, *B* and *C*). This infiltration pattern may extend for several millimeters to many centimeters. It is most apparent along the advancing edges of the tumor. But in the more central portions of the tumor, the host lamellar bone may be completely destroyed. Therefore, the absence of this finding on biopsy does not necessarily rule out osteosarcoma. In osteoid osteoma and osteoblastoma the lamellar bone is destroyed at the junctional site of the lesional tissue with the host bone and the pattern of marrow infiltration between host lamellar bone trabeculae is not seen (Plate 2, *B* and *E*). Callus may infiltrate between the bone trabeculae at the site of fracture, but if biopsied after 3 to 4 weeks post-injury, is usually characterized by benign osteoblastic "rimming" (see p. 95 and Plate 1, *F–H*) at the woven bone stage and a loose fibrovascular or early fatty stroma. At the woven bone stage of callus, tightly knit streamers of osteoid admixed with the woven bone spicules are rarely seen. Osteosarcoma tissues never maturate to lamellar bone and marrow fat, as is seen in the later stages of callus.

If any cellular (those with minimal to absent bone producing) areas are seen, they should be closely examined, since it is in these areas that the greatest degree of nuclear anaplasia exists.

Refer to page 116 and Figs. 7–43 to 7–46 for a detailed discussion of these principles using a specific case example.

CARTILAGE PREDOMINANT OS (CHONDROBLASTIC OS). Although obvious malignant cartilage is present in most cases of osteosarcoma, those cases with less than blatant cartilage anaplasia or those with a great preponderance of cartilage may cause diagnostic problems. Those with foci of cartilage with minimal anaplasia (Plate 4, *D*) may not be sufficiently distinctive to separate from hyperplastic callus cartilage (Plate 4, *E*). Correlation with history and radiographic features is crucial. An important rule is to remember that in any bone-producing lesion, if cartilage is present in the lesional tissue, it usually signifies that the cartilage is either secondary to callus or to osteosarcoma. Osteoid osteoma and osteoblastoma do not produce cartilage.

Those cases of osteosarcoma with a predominance of obviously malignant cartilage (Plate 4, *F*) can be mistaken for chondrosarcoma. This error can only be avoided if in all lesions in which the diagnosis of chondrosarcoma is considered a diligent search is made to rule out areas of direct tumor osteoid and woven bone production from malignant stromal cells without their first passing through a stage of cartilage differentiation. One fact is worth while mentioning. In any patient under the age of 30 the presence of chondrosarcomatous tissue in association with a metaphyseal lesion almost always can be proven to be an OS. Proof, of course, depends on examining multiple sections for areas diagnostic of OS.

SPINDLE CELL, FIBROSARCOMA, OR MALIGNANT FIBROUS HISTIOCYTOMA-LIKE OSTEOSARCOMA. Most examples of osteosarcoma will show some fields with prominent spindle cell patterns. Those with minimal or equivocal anaplasia (Plate 5, *A* and *B*) can obviously be mistaken for a benign condition. Fortunately, it is extremely rare for an osteosarcoma to present with a deceptively innocuous spindle cell pattern. Recognition of its true nature will depend upon radiologic correlation and diligent search for areas of obvious anaplasia, foci of tumor bone (Plate 5, *B*), malignant cartilage, and marrow infiltration between lamellar bone trabeculae.

Most cases of osteosarcoma with a predominant spindle cell pattern will be obviously anaplastic and will usually resemble fibrosarcoma. If the bundles of cells are arranged in a pinwheel or "storiform" pattern, its histology may resemble the malignant fibrous histiocytoma (Plate 5, *G*). The only way to differentiate these tumors with certainty is to examine ample sections for the presence or absence of osseous production by the tumor cells.

LARGE CELL PREDOMINANT OSTEOSARCOMA. If an osteosarcoma is characterized by large cells (over 40 microns) with prominent nucleoli, confusion with carcinoma, metastatic melanoma (Plate 4, *G*), primary reticulum cell sarcoma, or liposarcoma is possible (Plate 5, *G–I*). In rare cases, osteosarcoma cells may become highly active phagocytes. When this occurs, the cells may grow to enormous proportions as they distend their cytoplasm with the products of phagocytosis, which may include large red globules (Plate 5, *H*) and even fats (Plate 5, *I*). As a result of conversion to lipids, the cytoplasm becomes pale and if these features predominate, the mistaken diagnosis of a primary malignant fibrous histiocytoma (MFH) or liposarcoma is possible. This author has observed peculiar red bodies (by H and E stains) in the cyto plasm of approximately 3 per cent of osteosarcomas. They can range in size from a few to up to 20 microns in size. They are PAS positive, diastase resistant, and fat positive. Therefore, these bodies are probably composed of glycolipids or glycolipoproteins. I have seen these peculiar products of phagocytosis, which I designate "sarcoma bodies" in three rhabdomyosarcomas, six osteosarcomas, and one MFH of soft tissue. These bodies appear to be breakdown products of erythrophagocytosis (personal observations). Similar bodies have been described in the endodermal sinus tumor (Telium bodies). Carcinomas and melanomas have not, in my experience, been associated with their production.

GIANT CELL PREDOMINANT OSTEOSARCOMA. If benign osteoclast-like giant cells predominate (Plate 4, *J* and *K*), it is possible to confuse it with a giant cell tumor. However, the majority of cases of GCT are epiphyseal lesions. Primary epiphyseal osteosarcoma is very rare. Histologically, the stromal cells between the giant cells of an osteosarcoma usually display signs of objective anaplasia if careful attention is given to them. In addition, the anaplastic stromal cells will, in some fields, be seen to produce tightly knit streamers of osteoid (Plate 4, *K*), a pattern not seen in GCT, although it is possible for the giant cell tumor to produce trabeculae of osteoid and woven bone frequently lined or rimmed by benign osteoblasts (Fig. 10–59). The giant cell predominant osteosarcoma should be differentiated from the giant cell sarcoma of bone (p. 356). This tumor usually arises in Paget's disease and contains no areas of tumor osteoid, woven bone, or cartilage, and most important, the stromal and giant cells are anaplastic (Plate 4, *L*). The prognosis for this tumor is equally dismal, if not worse, than the OS.

SMALL CELL OR ROUND CELL PREDOMINANT OSTEOSARCOMA. On rare occasions an osteosarcoma is characterized by a predominance of small bland-appearing to obviously malignant cells (Plate 5, *C*) and may mimic chondroblastoma, Ewing's tumor, reticulum cell sarcoma, or metastatic tumor. The diagnostic feature of osteosarcoma is that the cells can be found, in foci, to produce osteoid and very primitive woven bone (Plate 5, *C*). In addition, PAS stains of these tumor cells show they are rich in glycogen, as is true of Ewing's tumor. This particular correlation of Ewing-like cells occurring mostly in diaphyseally located osteosarcomas was pointed out to me by Dr. Lee Theros (personal communication), who in turn obtained this interesting observation from Dr. Lent Johnson. These facts are interesting in that they suggest that the Ewing's cells may perhaps be osteogenic precursors, rather than precursors of the hematopoietic system. Dr. Hutter, *et al.*[102] reported 25 cases of a primary bone sarcoma that contained a curious mixture of osteosarcoma, chondrosarcoma, vascular sarcoma-like areas, and fields indistinguishable from Ewing's tumor. They speculated that the histologic variations in these tumors, which they called primitive multipotential sarcoma of bone, depended more on the metabolic field or environment in which the tumor arose than on specific cell or origin. This concept was originally formulated in a very interesting article by Johnson.[105] Basset[88] also emphasized the importance of the cell's environment on its functional activity. He concluded that the cell has a definite genetic determination and that the resources of its environment may influence the products that the cell can synthesize and return to the extracellular milieu. Therefore, if we speculate that Ewing's tumor and osteosarcoma are histogenetically related tumors, we could say that the metabolic influences of the midshaft are usually conducive to the development of undifferentiated stem cells (Ewing's tumor), while the environment of the metaphysis is more conducive to osseous differentiation of these same stem cells. Since these hypothetical factors may not be equally influential with respect to individual cases, we could expect tumor "hybrids," composed of a combination of features characteristic of Ewing's tumor and osteosarcoma, as reported in Hutter's article, and which this author has also seen on occasion. Some of the tumors that appear in Hutter's article, however, are clearly mesenchymal chondrosarcomas and should be excluded from the other cases, since this is now known to be a distinct and separate entity.

VASCULAR OR CYSTLIKE PREDOMINANT OSTEOSARCOMA. (TELANGIECTATIC OSTEOSARCOMA). This is a rare variant of osteosarcoma and the most difficult to diagnose by radiograph and structural features. All of the histologic features of aneurysmal bone cyst (ABC) may be mimicked on low-power examination (Plate 5, *D–F*). On high-power examination, however, careful analysis will reveal cells considerably more pleomorphic than seen in A.B.C. Evidence of anaplasia, nonmirror image mitoses, and quite often, "ominous" tightly knit streamers of osteoid in the cystlike walls become evident upon careful analysis (Plate 5, *E* and *F*). In ABC, osteoid may be present in the bones' walls but usually as a few small slivers and rarely, if ever, as masses of closely packed osteoid. The fibroblastic cells may be exuberant but they do not show objective anaplasia or atypical mitoses.

Differential Diagnosis

The preceding discussion covered most of the benign and malignant entities that can be confused with osteosarcoma, and vice versa. The most common benign lesions that can ever so closely resemble low-grade anaplastic osteosarcoma on a histologic basis are the exuberant bone-producing osteoblastoma (Table 7–1) osteoid osteoma, the exuberant fibro-osseous chondroid reparative lesions of early callus, healing simple bone cyst, and aneurysmal bone cyst. The reader is referred to each entity for an in-depth discussion of each of the features that serve to distinguish them from osteosarcoma. The three benign lesions most treacherous to distinguish from the osteosarcoma are the stress fracture (p. 86), the osteoblastoma (p. 110), and the aneurysmal bone cyst (p. 478) because of their marked radiologic and pathologic similarities in some cases. Nevertheless, there are subtle but definite differences that can be used to distinguish each of these three benign entities from the osteosarcoma. The reader is urged to review each of these three benign entities in detail. The manner in which each of these lesions is differentiated from os is treated in detail in the sections on each of these entities.

Two further entities that may result in an erroneous diagnosis of osteosarcoma are the pseudomalignant osteoblastoma (p. 120 and Figs. 7–47–7–49) and massive atypical hyperplastic callus.

The following conditions are so difficult to separate from osteosarcoma that they also deserve special attention.

Osteosarcoma

FIG. 7-92. The lesion arises from the medullary bone, destroys the cortex, and forms a lobulated soft-tissue mass. The tissue is whitish-yellow, variably gritty, and may show hemorrhagic areas and islands of cartilage (*a*). Note the pathologic fracture (*b*). Also note the "cumulus cloudlike" masses of tumor bone in the midshaft (*c*).

FIG. 7-93. This case corresponds to the incipient lytic OS shown in Fig. 7–87. The tumor is composed of highly anaplastic giant cells and smaller mononuclear cells. Condensations of osteoid are present, some of which are becoming calcified, as shown by the hematoxyphilia (*arrow*). In some fields primitive malignant cartilage was seen (H and E, X250).

FIG. 7-94. The bone was en-bloc resected one month after adriamycin and 3500 R of radiation therapy. The epiphyseal area of involvement of this distal hemerus is clearly seen.

FIG. 7-95. However, examination of multiple sections through this area showed complete replacement by a loose fibrous connective tissue and numerous capillaries. Not a single tumor cell was seen. Similar features of 100 per cent tumor necrosis were seen in two of 12 cases treated in the identical manner (H and E, X125).

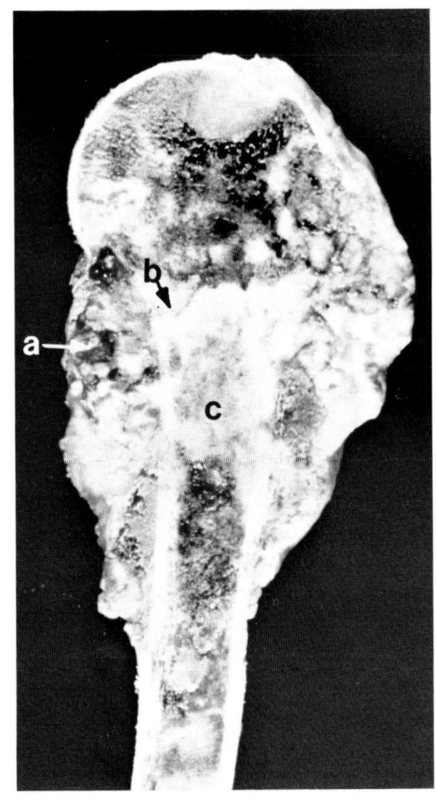

FIG. 7-92

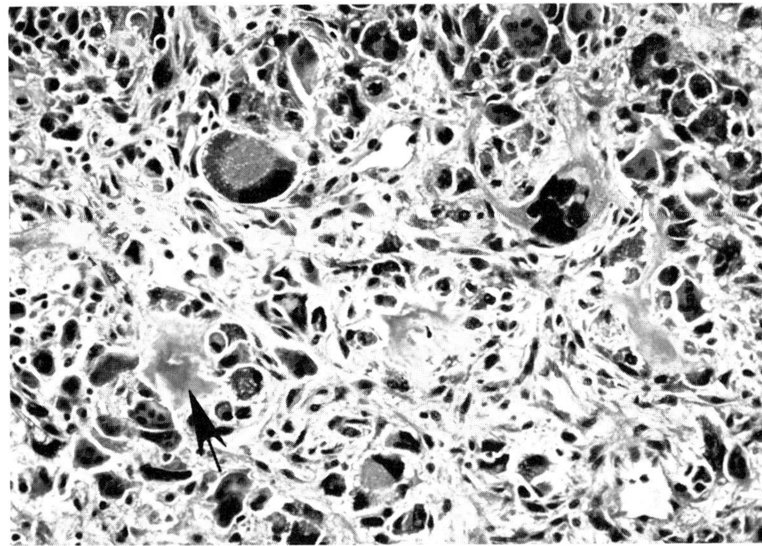

FIG. 7-93

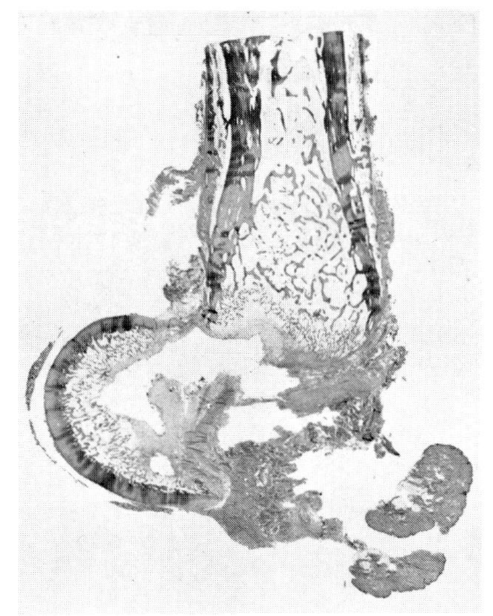

FIG. 7-94

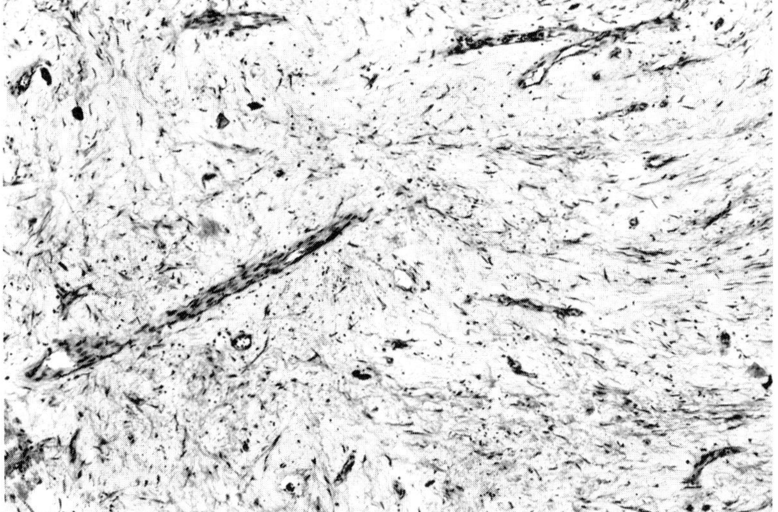

FIG. 7-95

ATYPICAL HYPERPLASTIC CALLUS. Atypical hyperplastic callus may be so extensive in its involvement that osteosarcoma is almost exactly mimicked on radiograph and even by histology, with the only exception being the absence of atypical mitotic figures and bizarre large or obviously anaplastic nuclei. However, the degree of nuclear hyperplastic atypia can fall within the range of some osteosarcomas. What features should make us suspicious of massive hyperplastic callus?

OSTEOGENESIS IMPERFECTA. On rare occasion patients with severe osteogenesis imperfecta may develop massive hyperplastic and atypical callus that mimics osteosarcoma.[87,88,96] Patients with this condition eventually resolve the tumorous callus without amputation. Since some patients with this disease have also developed osteosarcoma,[108] there is obviously a problem distinguishing hyperplastic callus from sarcoma. Crucial to diagnosis are the presence of fracture lines by tomogram in the areas of massive bone formation and the absence of unequivocal anaplasia and bizarre mitotic figures.

ANTECEDENT HISTORY OF BENIGN BONE DESTRUCTIVE LESIONS. On rare occasions large benign lesions that are extensively bone destructive may lead to massive callus similar to those seen in osteogenesis imperfecta. Careful review of history, documentation of a proceding benign lesion, and absence of the typical features of osteosarcoma on biopsy should lead to consideration of this entity. The pathogenesis of this lesion is probably from severe cortical erosion, consequent to the lesional process, repeated fractures, and a peculiar response by the host leading to the production of massive callus.

DOCUMENTATION OF INDOLENT GROWTH. *The vast majority of osteosarcomas become rapidly progressive and present with destructive growths and symptoms in 6 months or less. Any deviation from this pattern of clinical behavior makes the diagnosis extremely suspect.* This deviation in behavior was present in several reported cases of hyperplastic callus complicating osteogenesis imperfecta.

It is extremely rare to find in the literature any fully documented cases of osteosarcoma with indolent growth left in-situ for $1\frac{1}{2}$ years or more before biopsy without metastasis unmasking its true, highly malignant nature. Lindbom[110] mentioned three such cases. The radiology of two cases are presented but no histological illustrations. It is possible that these osteosarcomas (with documented metastasis) may have arisen from prior benign lesions. This certainly may follow in the wake of fibrous dysplasia, Paget's disease, and postirradiation.

In this author's experience *a tumor with radiographic evidence of indolent bony growth of at least $1\frac{1}{2}$ years duration is more likely to be a benign condition mimicking an osteosarcoma than an osteosarcoma.* If an osteosarcoma results from transformation of a formerly benign process, its radiologic and morphological presentation is usually rapidly progressive and unequivocally malignant. Benign massive, tumorous osteosarcoma-like processes are, admittedly, very rare. They require the greatest scrutiny before they can be recognized.

Course and Treatment

The osteogenic sarcoma is one of the most malignant tumors known to man. Its usual course in 80 to 85 per cent of patients is multiple pulmonary metastases and death within 2 years of diagnosis, in spite of amputation and/or preoperative high-dosage irradiation. The marked propensity for lung metastases over other organs has prompted Martini, *et al.*[114] to perform multiple pulmonary-wedge resections in selected patients. The selection depends upon whether the treatment of the primary bone lesion was considered adequate; no evidence of metastases at the time of treatment of the primary tumor; and whether the primary tumor presented in a long bone. Twenty-two such patients were treated by either one or several pulmonary-wedge resections. After 3 years 45 per cent of the patients were alive and well, a significant increase from the usual survival statistics. Most of the patients who succumbed to the disease did so either because of eventual overwhelming lung metastases and/or metastases to other organs, such as brain (two cases) or liver (one case). Their conclusion suggested that 5-year survival rates could be augmented by 5 to 20 per cent by resection of pulmonary metastases, provided that certain criteria were satisfied (p. 589).

More recent developments in the field of tumor chemotherapy and radiation therapy may hold great promise for those persons with sarcoma, even those with the dreaded osteosarcoma. In the last few years, systemic chemotherapy appears to be significantly modifying the usual rapid development of metastases and has resulted in significant increases in survival statistics.[100,105,121]

Currently at UCLA, the divisions of oncology, under Dr. Donald Morton's direction, and orthopedic surgery, under Dr. Harlan Amstutz's direction, have begun a program of treating osteosarcoma patients preoperatively with intraarterial infusion of Adriamycin and 3500 R. One month later, the affected segment of bone, including a margin of healthy tissue, is removed by en-bloc resection and a cadaver allograft or metal prosthesis inserted. The patients are then placed on systemic chemotherapy that includes high dose methotrexate, Citrovorum Rescue Factor, and Adriamycin. At the time of this writing 12 such patients have received this treatment. The average follow-up has been 8 months with only a single case of recurrence and none with metastasis. Pathological examination of the removed tissues has been remarkable in at least two of these cases. These cases showed 100 per cent necrosis of tumor (measured by loss of tumor nuclei). The tumor tissue was either hemorrhagic or necrotic. In one case there was replacement by a bland scar tissue (Figs. 7-87, 7-93-7-95). In the other, only the tumor osteoid, bone, or cartilage matrix remained. In contrast, the surrounding host bone, marrow, cartilage, and soft tissues showed minimal to no loss of nuclei. Although the follow-up time has been short and the number of cases too small to draw definitive conclusions, the effects to date seem to hold promise for the future of sarcoma treatment.

Secondary Intramedullary Osteogenic Sarcoma

More than half of the osteogenic sarcomas that arise after the age of 40 can be shown to follow in the wake of another disease. The two most common antecedent lesions are Paget's disease and postirradiation. Less common antecedent lesions include fibrous dysplasia,[103] low-grade chondrosarcoma (p. 201 and Fig. 8-51), bone infarcts,[117] osteogenesis imperfecta,[108] bone cysts,[108] and osteoblastoma.[41,47]

PAGET'S SARCOMA. Most patients with Paget's sarcoma transformation have polyostotic disease and present over the age 50. The earliest radiographic change signifying malignancy is a small focal area of destruction in the subcortical portion of the bone. The osteosarcoma that arises in association with Paget's disease is similar in histological patterns to the primary intramedullary type. On occasion the sarcomas appear to be pure fibrosarcomas, others giant cell (osteoclastic sarcomas), or chondrosarcomas. All of these tumors show extreme anaplasia and are not difficult to diagnose as malignant. The prognosis is extremely poor; only a few cases have been reported with long-term survival after amputation.[119]

IRRADIATION SARCOMA. The fact that osteosarcoma may complicate radiation therapy and from exposure to radium used in painting luminous watches was first established in 1922 and 1929 by Beck and Martland, respectively.[90,115] The interval between radiation exposure and sarcoma is between 7 and 48 years, with a median of 23 years.[94] In rare cases the interval may be shorter. If radiation is given to a benign or low-grade malignant bone tumor such as the GCT and a highly malignant osteosarcoma develops in just a few months or 1 to 2 years, great care must be given to verify that the original tumor was not an osteosarcoma. An osteosarcoma may also develop in areas that have been radiated for extraskeletal tumors, such as is used to control breast carcinoma and Hodgkin's disease or in patients who had been given radioactive thorium for the treatment of tuberculosis and ankylosing spondylitis.

The shortest duration between radiation and the development of a malignant tumor that I have ever seen was 3 years. This unfortunate 18-year-old developed a highly malignant squamous cell carcinoma of the scalp three years after 7000 rads was given to the same region for a fungus infection. The dosage was meant to be 700 rads but the protective screen to reduce the dosage was inadvertently not placed.

The probability of developing an osteosarcoma is in proportion to dosage. Most cases with external irradiation had dosages over 3000 rads, although cases with as little as 1500 rads have been reported. The percent risk may nevertheless be small since Phillips and Sheline,[118] in a follow-up of 2,300 patients surviving 5 years after radiotherapy for a variety of malignant tumors, found that only two developed radiation osteosarcoma, an incidence of .1 per cent of survivors.

Most of the postradiation-induced sarcomas are similar pathologically to the primary intraosseous osteosarcoma. Less commonly, the tumors are fibrosarcomas, and rarely, chondrosarcoma. The 5-year survival rate of 51 cases was approximately 18 per cent.[123]

Multiple Osteosarcomas of Bone

A small percentage of patients with osteosarcoma appear with multiple skeletal lesions. The lesions may appear *synchronously* while others may appear months to years later and are defined as *metachronous.* Amstutz[86] in a review of the literature of these unusual cases, divided them into three types:

TYPE I. Child-adolescent, multiple and synchronous in type (13 cases). These patients usually present with multiple osteosarcomas in the incipient blastic phase in the metaphyses of long bones. Because of their synchronous nature, radiographic appearance of incipient growth, and location within metaphyses, there is good reason to believe that these cases represent osteosarcomas of multicentric rather than metastatic origin. Lung metastases may or may not be evident at initial presentation. The prognosis for this group is extremely poor; survival was usually less than 1 year following diagnosis.

TYPE II. Adult, low-grade multiple malignancies (3 cases). These three patients were adult women and had multiple synchronous histologically low-grade anaplastic osteosarcoma without evidence of Paget's disease. These lesions were confined to the axial and proximal appendicular skeleton. Their course was more protracted, compared to Type I. Survival ranged from $2\frac{1}{2}$ to 6 years.

TYPE III. Metastatic type (11 cases). These cases arose predominantly in adulthood and were characterized by the development of a single osteosarcoma and a disease-free interval of between 5 and 44 months. After this disease-free interval, one or more skeletal osteosarcomas became manifest; the length of survival from initial symptoms ranged from 7 months to 7 years. The average survival time for males (nine cases) was 19 months and for females (two cases), $6\frac{1}{2}$ years. The patient who has survived 6 years showed no evidence of residual disease after the last follow-up study.

Fitzgerald, *et al.*,[97] reported 12 cases of multiple metachronous osteosarcoma with two long-term survivors. This represented an incidence of 1.5 per cent from the cases of osteosarcoma they observed. The time interval between the development of the first and second osteosarcoma ranged from 5 to 163 months (average, 35 months). Even though the lesions could have represented metastatic disease, it was evident that radiographically, most lesions were metaphyseal and indistinguishable from a new primary sarcoma of bone. Two of the 12 patients were long-term survivors. One patient was alive and well 12 years after the first sarcoma and 7 years after treatment of the fourth sarcoma. They concluded that these patients should not be assumed to have incurable disease and should be treated accordingly.

REFERENCES

Introduction

1. Fine, G. and Stout, A.P.: Osteogenic sarcoma of the extraskeletal soft tissues. Cancer, *9:* 1035, 1956.
2. Pack, G.T. and Braund, R.R.: The development of sarcoma in myositis ossificans. J.A.M.A., *119:*776, 1942.
3. Schuffstall, R.M. and Gregory, J.: Osteoid formation in giant-cell tumors of bone. Am. J. Pathol., *29:* 1123, 1953.

Benign Tumor or Tumorlike Processes

4. Murray, R.O., and Jacobson, H.G.: The Radiology of Skeletal Disorders. pp. 130–137. Baltimore, Williams and Wilkins, 1971.
5. Todd, R.C., Freeman, M.A.R., and Pirie, C.J.: Isolated trabecular fatigue fractures in the femoral head. J. Bone Joint Surg., *54B:*723, 1972.

Osteogenesis Imperfecta

6. Apley, A.G.: Hyperplastic callus in osteogenesis imperfecta. J. Bone Joint Surg., *33B:*591, 1951.
7. Baker, S.L.: Hyperplastic callus simulating sarcoma in two cases of fragilitis ossium. J. Pathol. and Bact., *LVIII:*609, 1946.
8. Fairbank, Sir H.A.T., and Baker, S.L.: Hyperplastic callus formation with or without evidence of a fracture in osteogenesis imperfecta. Br. J. Surg., *36:* 1, 1948.
9. Klenerman, L., and Townsend, A.C.: Osteosarcoma occurring in osteogenesis imperfecta. Report of 2 cases. J. Bone Joint Surg., *49B:*314, 1967.

Osteoid Osteoma

10. Freiberger, R.H., Loitman, B.S., Helpern, M., and Thompson, T.: Osteoid osteoma: a report of 80 cases. Am. J. Roentgenol. Radium Ther. Nucl. Med., *82:* 194, 1959.
11. Gilday, D.L.: Diagnosis of obscure childhood osteoid osteoma with the bone scan. J. Nucl. Med., *15:*494, 1974.
12. Glynn, J.J.: Osteoid osteoma with multicentric nidus. J. Bone Joint Surg., *55A:*855, 1973.
13. Golding, J.S.R.: The natural history of osteoid osteoma with a report of 20 cases. J. Bone Joint Surg., *26B:*218, 1954.
14. Gore, D.R., and Mueller, H.A.: Osteoid-osteoma of the spine with localization aided by 99 MTC-Polyphosphate Bone Scan. Clin. Orthop., *113:* 132, 1975.
15. Guistra, P.E., and Freiberger, R.H.: Severe growth disturbances with osteoid osteoma. Rad., *96:*285, 1970.
16. Habermann, E.T. and Stern, R.E.: Osteoid osteoma of the tibia in an 8 month-old boy. J. Bone Joint Surg., *56A:*633, 1974.
17. Heiman, M.L., Colley, C.J., and Bradford, D.: Osteoid osteoma of vertebral body. Report of a case with extension across intravertebral disc. Clin. Ortho., *118:* 159, 1976.
18. Jaffe, H.L. "Osteoid Osteoma": A benign osteoblastic tumor composed of osteoid and atypical bone. Arch. Surg., *31:*709, 1935.
19. Jaffe, H.L.: Tumors and Tumorous Conditions of the Bones and Joints. pp. 92–106. Philadelphia, Lea & Febiger, 1958.
20. MacLellan, D., and Wilson, F.C.: Osteoid osteoma of the spine. J. Bone Joint Surg., *49A:* 111, 1967.

21. Moberg, E.: The natural course of osteoid osteoma. J. Bone Joint Surg., *33A:* 166, 1951.
22. Norman, A., and Dorfman, H.D.: Osteoid osteoma inducing pronounced overgrowth and deformity of bone. Clin. Ortho., *110:* 233, 1975.
23. Prabhakar, B., Reddy, D., Dayananda, B., and Raghava, R.: Osteoid osteoma of skull. J. Bone Joint Surg., *54B:* 146, 1972.
24. Schulman, L., and Dorfman, H.D.: Nerve fibers in osteoid osteoma. J. Bone Joint Surg., *52A:* 1351, 1970.
25. Sherman, M.S., and McFarland, G., Jr.: Mechanism of pain in osteoid osteomas. South. Med. J., *58:* 163, 1965.
26. Simon, W.H., and Beller, M.L.: Intracapsular epiphyseal osteoid osteoma of the ankle joint. Clin. Orthop., *108:* 200, 1975.
27. Vickers, C.W., Pugh, D.C., and Ivins, J.C.: Osteoid osteoma: a fifteen year follow-up of an untreated patient. J. Bone Joint Surg., *41A:* 357, 1959.

Osteoblastoma

28. Bloom, M.H., and Bryan, R.S.: Benign osteoblastoma of the spine. Clin. Orthop., *65:* 157, 1969.
29. Byers, P.D.: Solitary benign osteoblastic lesions of bone. Osteoid osteoma and benign osteoblastoma. Cancer, *22:* 43, 1968.
30. Dahlin, D.C., and Johnston, E.W.: Giant osteoid osteoma. J. Bone Joint Surg., *36A:* 559, 1954.
31. Dias, L.S., and Frost, H.M.: Osteoblastoma of the spine. Clin. Orthop., *91:* 141, 1973.
32. Dias, L.S. and Frost, H.M.: Osteoid osteoma-osteoblastoma. Cancer, *33:* 1075, 1974.
33. Fechner, R.: Surgical pathology of the reproductive system and breast. Pathol. Annu., *6:* 306–308, 1971.
34. Gibbons, J.M., Jr., and Hammond, G.: Benign osteoblastoma. Lahey Clinic Bull., *13:* 97, 1963.
35. Golding, J.S.R., and Sissons, H.A.: Osteogenic fibroma of bone. A report of 2 cases. J. Bone Joint Surg., *36B:* 428, 1954.
36. Jaffe, H.L. Benign osteoblastoma. Bull. Hosp. Joint Dis., *18:* 141, 1956.
37. Lichtenstein, L.: Benign osteoblastoma. A category of osteoid and bone forming tumors other than classical osteoid osteoma, which may be mistaken for giant cell tumor or osteosarcoma. Cancer, *9:* 1044, 1956.
38. Lichtenstein, L., and Sawyer, W.R.: Benign osteoblastoma. J. Bone Joint Surgery, *46A:* 755, 1964.
39. Lichtenstein, L.: Bone Tumors. ed. 4. St. Louis, C.V. Mosby, 1972.
40. Marsh, B.W., Bonfiglio, M., Brady, L.P., and Enneking, W.F.: Benign osteoblastoma: range of manifestations. J. Bone Joint Surg., *57A:* 1, 1975.
41. Mayer, L.: Malignant degeneration of so-called benign osteoblastoma. Bull. Hosp. Joint Dis., *28:* 4, 1967.
42. Mirra, J.M., *et. al.:* Osteoblastoma associated with severe systemic toxicity syndrome. Am. J. Surg. Pathol, in press.

42a. Mirra, J.M., Kendrick, R.A., and Kendrick, R.E.: Pseudomalignant osteoblastoma versus arrested osteosarcoma. Cancer. *37:* 2005, 1976.
43. Pochaczevsky, R., Yen, Y.M. and Sherman, R.S.: The roentgen appearance of benign osteoblastoma. Rad., *75:* 429, 1960.
44. Schajowicz, F., and Lemos, C.: Osteoid osteoma and osteoblastoma. Acta Orthop. Scand., *41:* 272, 1970.
45. Schajowicz, F.: Malignant osteoblastoma. J. Bone Joint Surg., *58B:* 202, 1976.
46. Seki, T. *et. al.:* Malignant transformation of benign osteoblastoma. J. Bone Joint Surg., *57A:* 424, 1975.
47. Stutch, R.: Osteoblastoma—a benign entity? Ortho. Rev., *4:* 27, 1975.
48. Zabski, Z., Cutler, S., and Yermakov, V.: Osteochondroblastoma—unclassified benign tumor of the rib. Cancer, *36:* 1009, 1975.

Fibrous Dysplasia

49. Albright, F.: Polyostotic fibrous dysplasia: a defense of the entity. J. Clin. Endocrinol. Metab., *7:* 307, 1947.
50. Albright, F., Butler, A.M., Hampton, A.O., and Smith, P.: Syndrome characterized by osteitis fibrosa disseminata, areas of pigmentation and endocrine dysfunction, with precocious puberty in females. New Engl. J. Med., *216:* 727, 1937.
51. Berger, A., and Jaffe, H.L.: Fibrous (fibro-osseous) dysplasia of jawbones. J. Oral Surg., *11:* 3, 1953.
52. Coleman, M.: Osteitis fibrosa disseminata, Brit. J. Surg., *26:* 705, 1939.
53. Coley, B.L., and Stewart, F.W.: Bone sarcoma in polyostotic fibrous dysplasia. Ann. Surg., *121:* 872, 1945.
54. Dabska, M., and Buraczewskin, J.: On malignant transformation in fibrous dysplasia of bone. Oncology, *26:* 369, 1972.
55. Dockerty, M.B., Ghormley, R.K., Kennedy, R.L.J., and Pugh, D.G.: Albright's syndrome (polyostotic fibrous dysplasia with cutaneous pigmentation in both sexes and gonadal dysfunction in females). Arch. Intern. Med., *75:* 357, 1945.
56. Falconer, M.A., Cope, C.L., and Robb-Smith, A.H.T.: Fibrous dysplasia of bone with endocrine disorders and cutaneous pigmentation (Albright's disease). Q. J. Med., *11:* 121, 1942.
57. Gibson, M., and Middlemiss, J.G.: Fibrous dysplasia of bone. Br. J. Radiol., *44:* 1, 1971.
58. Harris, W.H., Dudley, R., and Barry, R.: The natural history of fibrous dysplasia. J. Bone Joint Surg., *44A:* 207, 1962.
59. Huvos, A., Higinbotham, N., and Miller, T.: Bone sarcomas arising in fibrous dysplasia, J. Bone Joint Surg., *54A:* 1047, 1972.
60. Jaffe, H.L.: Fibrous Dysplasia of Bone: A disease entity and specifically not an expression of neurofibromatosis. J. Mt. Sinai Hosp., *12:* 364, 1945.
61. ———: Fibrous dysplasia of bone. Bull. N.Y. Acad. Med., *22:* 588, 1946.

62. Leeds, N., and Seaman, W.B.: Fibrous dysplasia of the skull and its differential diagnosis. Radiology, *78:*570, 1962.
63. Lichtenstein, L.: Polyostotic fibrous dysplasia. Arch. Surg., *36:*874, 1938.
64. Lichtenstein, L., and Jaffe, H.L.: Fibrous dysplasia of bone: a condition affecting one, several or many bones, the graver cases of which may present abnormal pigmentation of skin, premature sexual development, hyperthyroidism or still other extraskeletal abnormalities. Arch. Pathol., *33:*777, 1942.
65. Logan, R.: Recurrent intramuscular myxoma associated with Albright's syndrome. J. Bone Joint Surg., *58A:*565, 1976.
66. McCune, D.J., and Bruch, H.: Osteodystrophia fibrosa: report of a case in which the condition was combined with precocious puberty, pathologic pigmentation of the skin and hyperthyroidism. Am. J. Dis. Child., *54:*806, 1937.
67. Peck, F.B., and Sage, C.V.: Diabetes mellitus associated with Albright's syndrome (osteitis fibrosa disseminata, areas of skin pigmentation, and endocrine dysfunction with precocious puberty in females). Am. J. Med. Sci., *208:*35, 1944.
68. Phemister, D.B., and Grimson, K.S.: Fibrous osteoma of the jaws. Ann. Surg., *105:*564, 1937.
69. Pugh, D.G.: Fibrous dysplasia of the skull: a probable explanation for leontiasis ossea. Radiology, *44:*548, 1945.
70. Rushton, M.A.: Regional osteitis fibrosa affecting the facial bones. Proc. R. Soc. Med., *40:*316, 1947.
71. Schlumberger, H.G.: Fibrous dysplasia of single bones (monostotic fibrous dysplasia). Mil. Surgeon, *99:*504, 1946.
72. ———: Fibrous dysplasia (ossifying fibroma) of the maxillaean mandible. Am. J. Orthod., *32:*579, 1946.
73. Sherman, R.S., and Sternbergh, W.C.A.: The roentgen appearance of ossifying fibroma of bone. Radiology, *50:*595, 1948.
74. Smith, A.G., and Zavaleta, A.: Osteoma, ossifying fibroma, and fibrous dysplasia of facial and cranial bones. Arch. Path., *54:*507, 1952.
75. Snapper, I.: Medical Clinics on Bone Diseases. pp. 157–171. New York, Interscience Publishers, Inc., 1943.
76. Stauffer, H.M., Arbuckle, R.K., and Aegerter, E.E.: Polyostotic fibrous dysplasia with cutaneous pigmentation and congenital arteriovenous aneurysms. J. Bone Joint Surg., *23:*323, 1941.
77. Sterngerg, W.H., and Joseph, V.: Osteodystrophia fibrosa combined with precocious puberty and exophthalmic goiter. Am. J. Dis. Child., *63:*748, 1942.
78. Strassburger, P., Garber, C.Z., and Hallock, H.: Fibrous dysplasia of bone. J. Bone Joint Surg., *33A:*407, 1951.
79. Sutro, C.J.: Osteogenic sarcoma of the tibia in a limb affected with fibrous dysplasia. Bull. Hosp. Joint Dis., *12:*217, 1951.
80. Thannhauser, S.J.: Neurofibromatosis (von Recklinghausen) and osteitis fibrosa cystica localisata et disseminata (von Recklinghausen). Medicine, *23:*105, 1944.
81. Vines, R.H.: Polyostotic fibrous dysplasia. Arch. Dis. in Child., *27:*351, 1952.
82. Windholz, F.: Cranial manifestation of fibrous dysplasia of bone. Am. J. Roentgenol., *58:*51, 1947.
83. With, W.A., Leavitt, D., and Enzinger, F.M.: Multiple intramuscular myxomas, another extraskeletal manifestation of fibrous dysplasia. Cancer, *27:*1167, 1971.
84. Zimmer, J.F., Dahlin, D.C., Pugh, D.G., and Clagett, O.T.: Fibrous dysplasia of bone: an analysis of 15 cases of surgically verified costal fibrous dysplasia. J. Thorac. Cardiovas. Surg., *31:*488, 1956.

Ossifying Fibroma

85. Kempson, R.L.: Ossifying fibroma of the long bones. A light and E-M study. Arch. Pathol., *52:*218, 1966.

Intramedullary Osteogenic Sarcoma

86. Amstutz, H.C.: Multiple osteogenic sarcomata-metastatic or multicentric? Report of 2 cases and review of literature. Cancer, *24:*923, 1969.
87. Apley, A.G.: Hyperplastic callus in osteogenesis imperfecta. J. Bone Joint Surg., *33B:*591, 1951.
88. Baker, S.L.: Hyperplastic callus simulating sarcoma in two cases of fragilitis ossium. J. Pathol. and Bacteriol., *LVIII:*609, 1946.
89. Basset, C.A.L.: Current Concepts of Bone Formation. J. Bone Joint Surg., *44A:*1217, 1962.
90. Beck, A.: Zur Frage des Roëntgensarkoms, zugleich ein Beitrag zur Pathogenese des Sarkoms. Munch. Med. Wochenschr., *69:*623, 1922.
91. Cahan, W.G., *et. al.:* Sarcoma arising in irradiated bone. Report of 11 cases. Cancer, *1:*3, 1948.
92. Coventry, M.B., and Dahlin, D.C.: Osteogenic sarcoma. A critical analysis of 430 cases. J. Bone Joint Surg., *39A:*741, 1957.
93. Ellman, H., Gold, R., and Mirra, J.M.: Roentgenographically "benign" but rapidly lethal diaphyseal osteosarcoma. J. Bone Joint Surg., *56A:*1267, 1974.
94. Evans, R.D.: The effect of skeletally deposited alpha-ray emitters in man. Br. J. Radiol., *39:*881, 1966.
95. Everson, T., and Cole, W.: Spontaneous regression of cancer. A Study and Abstract of Reports in the World Medical Literature and of Personal Communications Concerning Spontaneous Regression of Malignant Diseases. Philadelphia, W.B. Saunders, 1966.
96. Fairbanks, Sir H.A.T., and Baker, S.L.: Hyperplastic callus formation with or without evidence of a fracture in osteogenesis imperfecta. Br. J. Surg., *36:*1, 1948.
97. Fitzgerald, R.H., Dahlin, D.C., and Sim, F.H.: Multi-

ple metachronous osteogenic sarcoma. Report of 12 cases with 2 long term survivors. J. Bone Joint Surg., *55A:*595, 1973.

98. Gerson, B., Dorfman, H., Norman, A., and Mankin, H.: Patterns of localization of strontium[85] in osteosarcoma. J. Bone Joint Surg., *54A:*817, 1972.
99. Haskell, C.M., Eilber, F.R., and Morton, D.L.: Adriamycin (NSC–123127) by arterial infusion. Cancer Chemother. Rep., *6:*187, 1975.
100. Haskell, C.M., Silverstein, M.J., and Rangel, D.M.: Multimodality cancer therapy in man. A pilot study of adriamycin by arterial infusion. Cancer, *33:*1485, 1974.
101. Hatcher, C.H., and Cambell, J.C.: Benign chondroblastoma of bone: its histologic variations and a report of late sarcoma in the site of one. Bull. Hosp. Joint Dis., *12:*411, 1951.
102. Hutter, R.V.P., Foote, F., Francis, K. and Sherman, R.: Primitive multipotential primary sarcoma of bone. Cancer, *19:*1, 1966.
103. Huvos, A.G., Higinbotham, N.L., and Miller, T.R.: Bone sarcomas arising in fibrous dysplasia. J. Bone Joint Surg., *54A:*1047, 1972.
104. Jaffe, H.L.: Intracortical osteogenic sarcoma. Bull. Hosp. Joint Dis., *21:*189, 1960.
105. Jaffe, N., Frei, E., Traggis, D., and Bishop, Y.: Adjuvant methotrexate and citrovorum factor treatment of osteogenic sarcoma. N. Engl. J. Med., *291:*994, 1974.
106. Johnson, L.C.: A general theory of bone tumors. Bull N.Y. Acad. Med., *29:*164, 1953.
107. Johnson, L.L., Vetter, H., and, Putschar, W.G.J.: Sarcomas arising in bone cysts. Virchows Arch. [Pathol. Anat.], *335:*428, 1962.
108. Klenerman, L., Ockenden, B.G. and Townsend, A.C.: Osteosarcoma occurring in osteogenesis imperfecta. J. Bone Joint Surg., *49B:*314, 1967.
109. Klenerman, L., and Townsend, A.C.: Osteosarcoma occurring in osteogenesis imperfecta. Report of 2 cases. J. Bone Joint Surg., *49B:*314, 1967.
110. Lindbom, A., Soderberg, G., and Spjut, H.: Osteosarcoma: a review of 96 cases. Acta. Radiol., *56:*1, 1961.
111. Lowbeer, L.: Multifocal osteosarcomatosis. A rare entity. Bull. Pathol., *9:*52, 1968.
112. Marcove, R.C., *et. al.:* Osteogenic sarcoma under the age of twenty-one. J. Bone Joint Surg., *52A:*411, 1970.
113. Marcove, R., *et. al.:* Osteogenic sarcoma in childhood. N.Y.S. J. Med., *71:*855, 1971.
114. Martini, N., *et. al.:* Multiple pulmonary resections in the treatment of osteogenic sarcoma. Ann. Thorac. Surg., *12:*271, 1971.
115. Martland, H.S.: The occurrence of malignancy in radioactive persons. Cancer, *15:*2435, 1931.
116. McKenna, R.J., Schwinn, C.P., Soong, K.Y. and Higinbotham, N.L.: Sarcomata of the osteogenic series. An analysis of 552 cases. J. Bone Joint Surg., *48A:*1, 1966.
117. Mirra, J.M., *et. al.:* Malignant fibrous histiocytoma and osteosarcoma in association with bone infarcts. J. Bone Joint Surg., *56A:*932, 1974.
118. Phillips, T.L., and Sheline, G.E.: Bone sarcomas following radiation therapy. Rad., *81:*992, 1963.
119. Price C.H.G., and Goldie, W.: Paget's sarcoma of bone: a study of 80 cases. J. Bone Joint Surg., *51B:*205, 1969.
120. Price, C.H.G., and Truscott, D.E.: Multifocal osteogenic sarcoma. J. Bone Joint Surg., *39B:*524, 1957.
121. Rosen, G., Suwan, S., and Kwan, C,: High dose methotrexate with citrovorum factor rescue and adriamycin in childhood osteosarcoma. Cancer, *33:*1151, 1974.
122. ———: Chemotherapy, *en bloc* resection, and prosthetic bone replacement in the treatment of osteogenic sarcoma. Cancer, *37:*1, 1976.
123. Sherman, R.S., and Soong, K.Y.: A roentgen study of osteogenic sarcoma developing in Paget's disease. Rad., *63:*48, 1954.
124. Spjut, H.J., Dorfman, H.D., Fechner, R.E., and Ackerman, L.V.: Atlas of Tumor Pathology. second series, p. 192, 1970.
125. Weinfeld, M. and Dudley, R.: Osteogenic sarcoma. J. Bone Joint Surg., *44A:*269, 1962.

INTRAOSSEOUS CARTILAGE- AND CHONDROID-PRODUCING TUMORS

8

This chapter deals with those benign, low-, and high-grade malignant cartilage or chondroid (cartilage-like) tumors of intraosseous origin. These include callus, enchondroma, chondroblastoma, chondromyxoid fibroma, chordoma, chondrosarcoma, chondrosarcoma with fibrosarcomatous or osteosarcomatous transformation, mesenchymal chondrosarcoma, and osteosarcoma.

Although the enchondroma and the chondroblastoma are classified as benign and the chondrosarcoma as malignant, the line of distinction between benign and malignant may not be as fine as we would hope. How, for example, should we classify those rare unequivocal "benign" chondroblastomas, which demonstrate lung "metastases" no different from the primary lesion? How do we explain the fact that in some cases of chondroblastomatous lung metastases, unremoved nodules may reach a certain maximum size, fill in with bone, and remain static for years? How should cartilage lesions that are cytologically indistinguishable from an enchondroma but which behave with chondrosarcomatous virulence be classified? Are there any parameters by which we can identify these lesions? It is very important that the criteria used to determine whether an enchondroma or chondroblastoma in question is biologically benign or malignant are as refined as possible. Without such care patients will either suffer radical operative procedures they may not need or receive minor surgery, when radical ablation of the tumor was required. At this point, however, our knowledge is not complete and the criteria applied to the diagnosis of these lesions are in need of greater refinement.

DEFINITION OF TERMS

CARTILAGE. Cartilage is composed of chondrocytes and their matrix. The matrix contains collagen and mucopolysaccharides. The mucopolysaccharides impart to cartilage its sheen and slipperiness. Because of the great amount of water cartilage traps in its interstices, it has a high hydrostatic pressure and with that, resistance to compressibility.

Living chondrocytes are necessary to maintain a continuous production of mucopolysaccharides. Collagen imparts to cartilage its tensile strength, the same as it does to bone. Normal articular tissue, epiphyseal plate, enchondroma, mature callus, chondrosarcoma, and osteosarcoma can produce or are characterized by *hyaline cartilage.* It is glistening, translucent, and slippery. On H and E section it is easily recognizable. The matrix is homogeneous, bluish-pink, usually light staining and holds rounded chondrocytes contained within lacunae. Unlike osteocytes, chondrocytes do not possess canaliculi. Therefore, highly calcified cartilage will lead to cellular necrosis. With routine fixation the chondrocyte may shrink away from its lacuna, leaving a pericellular space. Polarization of cartilage demonstrates its collagen fibers. The most mature types of hyaline cartilage such as articular cartilage will demonstrate numerous highly refractile polarizable collagen fibers that are oriented in arcades. Along the surface of the articular cartilage the fibers run parallel to the cartilage, while the fibers below the surface run perpendicular to it (Fig. 8–1). More primitive tumor hyaline cartilage will demonstrate fewer, less light polarizable fibers. If the cartilage loses substantial amounts of its mucopolysaccharides or if mucopolysaccharide production diminishes, the cartilage will have a fibrillar appearance by light microscopy; this type is called *fibrocartilage.* It is seen in degenerative arthritis and it can be present in enchondroma, chondrosarcoma, osteosarcoma, and callus. Still, in these lesions it is easily recognized as cartilage.

Certain other tumors of bone produce a very primitive cartilage or cartilage-like substance; this substance is called *chondroid.* It is important to distinguish chondroid from cartilage, osteoid, collagen, mucoid or myxoid substances. Recognizing chondroid is, or can be, extremely important for the diagnosis of chondroblastoma, chondromyxoid fibroma, osteosarcoma, and mesenchymal chondrosarcoma.

Chondroid may be pink or pinkish blue in color and may contain rounded cells or more polygonal to stellate-shaped cells (Plate 6, *D, E, H,* and *J*). Quite often these cells shrink due to fixation and leave a space on H and E section. I have tried to liberally illustrate those tumors that produce chondroid and where color is essential to their recognition, color plates have been provided. Chordomas may also produce a very primitive chondroid substance, so primitive that its confusion with myxoid chondrosarcoma, mucinous carcinoma, or liposarcoma is possible.

Primitive cartilage or chondroid may be produced in the more anaplastic tumors, including the osteosarcoma, the Grade III chondrosarcoma, and mesenchymal chondrosarcoma. Enchondromas do not produce less than easily recognizable cartilage. Well-differentiated chondrosarcomas and enchondromas produce almost pure hyaline or fibrocartilage. On the other hand, the chondroid-producing tumors rarely produce pure chondroid to the exclusion of other tissue. Rarely does chondroid substance occupy more than 30 per cent of the total lesional tissue of chondroblastoma or 75 per cent of the chondromyxoid fibroma. A significant portion of the tissue of these two tumors is cellular and nonchondroid. This knowledge can be a great diagnostic aid. For example, suppose a 20-year-old girl presents with a rounded lytic lesion of the femoral epiphysis. The radiologists will surely consider either chondroblastoma or giant cell tumor. If biopsy shows 100 per cent fibro- to hyaline cartilage, an incorrect diagnosis of chondroblastoma will be avoided by those who know that chondroblastomas are not composed entirely of pure cartilage. The actual diagnosis in this case must either be an enchondroma or chondrosarcoma. Therefore, not only is the recognition of cartilage and chondroid important to diagnosis, but also the relative proportion of either cartilage or chondroid to other lesional tissues; also an in-depth analysis of the components of the noncartilagenous tissue should be made.

ENCHONDROMA. This is a benign, totally hyaline- or fibrocartilagenous-producing tumor arising in the medullary substance of a bone. Enchondroma may be either *solitary* or *multiple* (*Ollier's disease*).

PAROSTEAL CHONDROMA. Parosteal chondroma is a benign cartilage tumor arising from the periosteum. The vast majority are solitary.

CHONDROSARCOMA is a malignant, pure cartilage-producing neoplasm. Grade II and III chondrosarcomas have objective microscopic anaplasia. Grade I chondrosarcomas do not have unequivocal cytologic anaplasia. The diagnosis of Grade I chondrosarcoma depends heavily upon correlating clinical and pathologic findings.

CENTRAL CHONDROSARCOMA. Those chondrosarcomas which arise from the medulla.

PERIPHERAL CHONDROSARCOMA. Those chondrosarcomas which arise from a juxtacortical (periosteal, intracortical, or intraosteochondromatous) position.

PRIMARY CHONDROSARCOMA. Those chondrosarcomas in which no benign precursor lesion is found. They may be either central or peripheral.

SECONDARY CHONDROSARCOMA. Those chondrosarcomas which arise from a benign lesion. These include focal malignant transformation in an enchondroma, parosteal chondroma, Ollier's disease, osteochondroma(s), chondroblastoma, or chondromyxoid fibroma. These tumors may be either central or peripheral.

CHONDROSARCOMA WITH FIBROSARCOMATOUS OR OSTEOSARCOMATOUS TRANSFORMATION. A highly malignant and often lethal change usually occurring in Grade I to II chondrosarcomas. The transformation occurs in from 10 to 20 per cent of chondrosarcomas. These lesions show a mixture of Grade I to II chondrosarcoma, spindle-cell sarcoma, or osteosarcoma. An enchondromatous lesion may be present. Diagnosis depends on correlating clinical and pathologic findings.

CHONDROMYXOID FIBROMA. A rare, benign lesion composed of variable quantities of chondroid, myxoid, and fibrous tissues.

CHONDROBLASTOMA. A rare, benign lesion characterized by islands of chondroid to cartilage and a stroma composed of chondroblasts, giant cells and "chicken-wire" and spotty calcifications. In contrast to enchondroma and chondrosarcoma, this lesion is never entirely composed of pure cartilage.

CHORDOMA. An uncommon to rare low-grade malignant neoplasm which arises from notochordal rests. It is always seen in association with the distribution of the primitive notochord, that is, in association with the bones or soft tissues of the spine. Most occur in the sacrum or at the base of the skull. It may produce foci of chondroid and, occasionally, easily recognizable cartilage.

MESENCHYMAL CHONDROSARCOMA. A rare, high-grade malignant neoplasm composed of spindly to ovoid primitive mesenchymal stromal cells which produce islands of chondroid or hyaline cartilage. Hemangiopericytoma-like areas are often present. It is never entirely composed of pure cartilage and must be distinguished from the osteosarcoma and chondrosarcoma with fibrosarcomatous transformation.

CALLUS OR FRACTURE REPAIR

Callus forms as a consequence to fracture. Fracture may be due to a blow or torsional injury, excessive internal stress (see stress fractures, p. 86, Figs. 7–13—7–16, and Plates 1, *A–I*, and 4, *E*) or in association with a pathologic process (pathologic fractures). Cartilage in fracture healing almost never forms to the exclusion of other tissues. It is admixed with variable degrees of new bone and/or fibrous tissue. In Chapter 7 we have dealt with the complexities of distinguishing stress fractures from osteosarcoma. There is, however, a similar problem in misinterpreting the intense cellularity of early fracture cartilage with chondrosarcoma. The same clinical, radiologic, and pathologic principles outlined in Chapter 7 would apply to the distinction between the cartilage of injury and chondrosarcoma.

If callus cartilage is consequent to pathologic fracture in a noncartilage-producing tumor, the separation of the two is usually clear-cut. If a fracture is noted on radiograph in association with a primary cartilage-producing tumor, the distinction between callus cartilage and tumor cartilage may be quite difficult. It is wise to ascertain when the fracture took place and if the biopsy was taken from the area of fracture, and to use these facts in an assessment of the tumor in question. Callus cartilage will also be associated with new bone formation, if the fracture is older than 3 weeks. Prominence of osteoblastic rimming and knowledge of the processes of fracture repair will denote the regions of fracture repair and aid in avoiding diagnostic confusion (Plates 1, *A–I*, and 4, *E*). It is worth remembering that one is usually not dealing with callus cartilage unless the radiograph shows either evidence of a recent fracture line by tomograms, an old healed fracture, or some degree of periosteal reaction.

ENCHONDROMA VERSUS CHONDROSARCOMA

Perhaps the most common serious error in bone tumor diagnosis is the failure to distinguish an enchondroma from a low-grade chondrosarcoma. There are several excellent papers which formulate the problem and which attempt to elucidate criteria which would reduce the risk of error. Because the problem of differentiating a chondrosarcoma from an enchondroma is complex and of prime importance, both entities will be discussed as a unit, rather than separately.

Gilmer and colleagues stated the problem succinctly: "The majority of ectopic deposits of cartilage maintain an orderly arrangement, remain quiescent and cause no difficulty. However, they have the potential under some unknown stimulus of becoming invasive and malignant. This potential is certainly greater in ectopic than in normal tissues.

The tendency to rely on histology as a guide to diagnosis, treatment and prognosis can lead to disaster. The most experienced pathologists regularly refer to biologic and clinical data pertinent to a lesion before interpreting the histologic findings. The diagnosis, then, should represent a synthesis of all available data, not just a "reading" of the slides. . .

An ectopic deposit of cartilage which seems to be

Articular Cartilage

FIG. 8-1. Normal hyaline (articular) cartilage. (*A*) The components of normal hyaline cartilage include rounded chondrocytes and a homogenous intercellular matrix that is rich in mucopolysaccharides and collagen. *Note:* In the calcified cartilage region (tidemark zone, arrow), viable chondrocytes are no longer present. (*B*) Polarized light shows the bright, well-oriented collagen fibers of the articular cartilage that are obscured by the mucopolysaccharide component by ordinary light microscopy. Beneath the calcified tidemark zone is polarized subchondral lamellar bone (*arrow*) (x40).

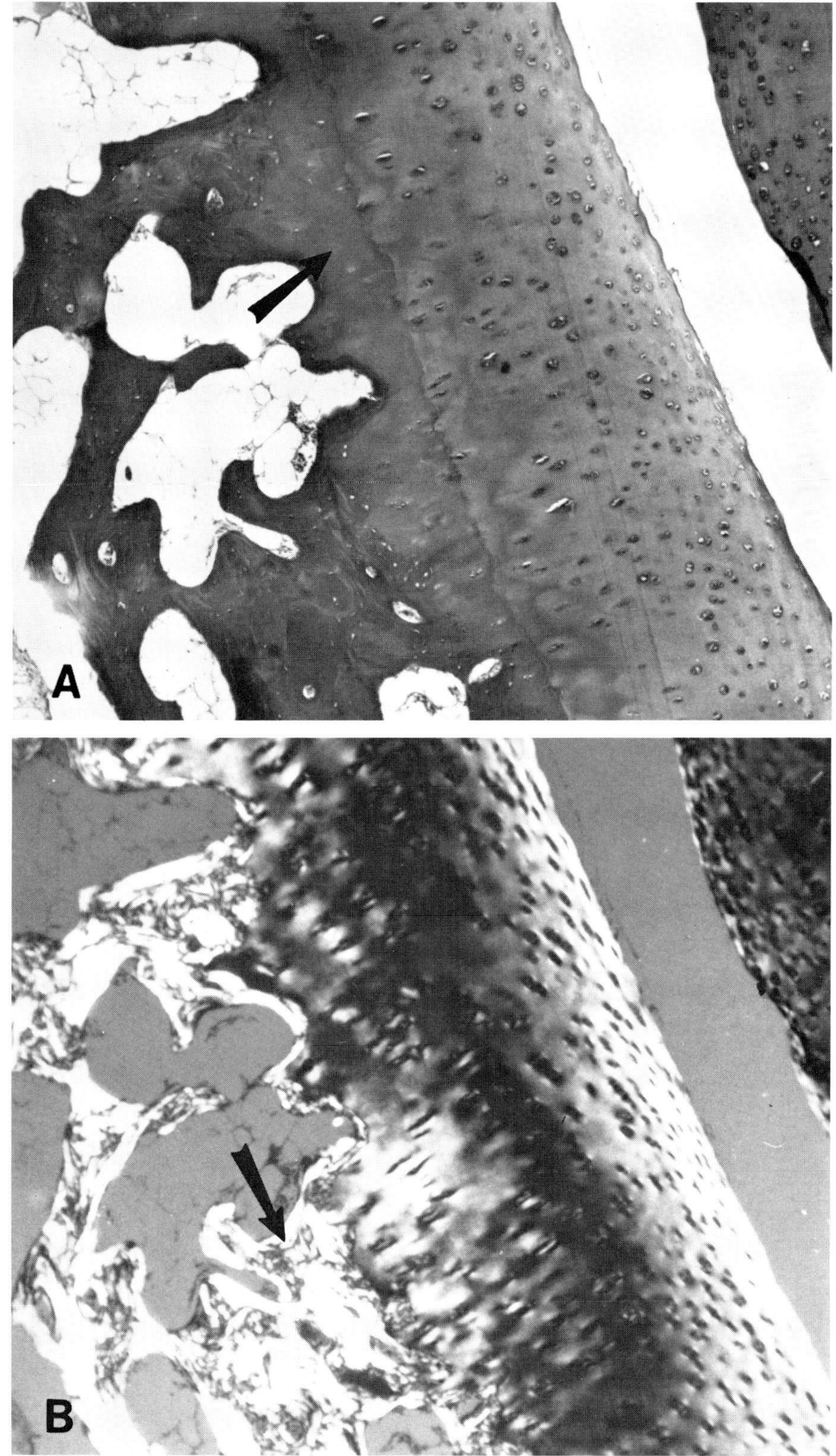

FIG. 8-1

dormant may present within a few months unequivocal evidence of malignancy. A lesion in the metacarpal of a growing child may be biologically benign and yet have histologic features which, considered alone, would warrant the diagnosis of malignancy. Because of its location, it causes no alarm, but the same lesion in an adult femur or humerus becomes ominous.

Probably one of the more common errors on the part of the pathologist is the failure to recognize the more subtle differences which, under certain circumstances, indicate an early or indolent chondrosarcoma. As a consequence, the clinician may be lulled into a false sense of security by the diagnosis of enchondroma, being assured that even if the tumor is malignant, there is time to wait for recurrence, because cartilage tumors as a rule grow slowly. However, even with a report in hand which indicates a fairly active lesion, the clinician influenced by misguided conservatism, is prone to equivocate, when the location alone indicates the urgency of prompt radical surgery. . . Histology and biology do not always parallel."[9]

Coley and Higinbotham addressed themselves not only to the problem of distinguishing enchondroma from chondrosarcoma but to the potential risks of the enchondroma transforming into chondrosarcoma.[3] Both were astute clinicians who obtained very careful follow-up studies on their patients. They were one of the first to note the discrepancy between the pathologic diagnosis of "enchondroma" of long and flat bones and the course of many of their patients, which was clearly that of chondrosarcoma. This prompted them to publish their findings and to make the following observations: "We are convinced that the risk of a benign cartilage tumor undergoing subsequent malignant degeneration is not a negligible one and that the attention of the medical profession should be drawn to it. Pain is the most reliable indication that sarcoma has already developed in a benign cartilage tumor, and it should be emphasized that pain in these cases is much more insidious, less constant, and less severe in the early stages than is the case in osteogenic sarcoma or primary chondrosarcoma. . . When both the clinical symptoms and the roentgenographic features point to chondrosarcomatous degeneration of a benign cartilage tumor then the likelihood becomes even stronger that such is the case. Following this, if a biopsy is performed and a pathologic diagnosis of "benign chondroma" is returned, this diagnosis should be accepted with the greatest reluctance. Many of our cases with such a combination of clinical, radiologic, and microscopic findings have gone on to obvious sarcoma and ultimately the pathologist has demonstrated chondrosarcoma at subsequent operation or biopsy. . . We believe the reasons for this lack of agreement between clinical and roentgenographic findings on the one hand, and microscopic on the other may be two-fold. First in a benign tumor that undergoes malignant change this transformation presumably begins at some one focus which at first may represent only a very small portion of the tumor itself. Therefore, unless biopsy fortuitously includes that area at which malignant change is taking place the pathologist is bound to report chondroma rather than chondrosarcoma. . . The second reason, we believe, lies in the fact that malignant changes in benign cartilage takes place by slow, almost insensible gradations, ranging from frankly benign cartilage through a slight cellular atypism to obviously sarcomatous tissue. . . We have, therefore, reached the conclusion that the diagnosis of chondrosarcomatous degeneration is often justified on the clinical and roentgenographic findings without the support of the histologic confirmation so essential when dealing with most malignant neoplasms. . . Finally, a plea is made for more aggressive treatment of benign tumors of cartilage, for earlier recognition of the tendency to insidious transformation to chondrosarcoma, and for more prompt aggressive surgical treatment once the malignant phase has been recognized." These statements are as true and meaningful today as they were over 30 years ago.

Early Grade I chondrosarcomas arising in enchondromas can be recognized if careful attention is paid to the clinical symptoms, age of the patient, and by obtaining biopsy material from the most "suspicious" areas on radiograph. It is the interpretation of these data and comparison to ordinary enchondromas which are the crucial factors in diagnosis. The main purpose of biopsy should not be to distinguish an enchondroma from a Grade I chondrosarcoma on the basis of cytologic parameters alone, since the two may be virtually indistinguishable. The gradation between cellular enchondromas and Grade I chondrosarcomas are extremely subtle and highly subjective; therefore, reliance upon cytologic differences alone will result in hopeless confusion in formulating a diagnosis.

The purpose of a biopsy should be the following:

1. To establish that the tumor is a pure cartilage-producing tumor, as suspected. Tumors of intramedullary origin, composed entirely of pure cartilage, are either enchondroma or chondrosarcoma. All other cartilage tumors of the medulla contain foci of noncartilage lesional components.

2. To look for patterns of invasion seen only in chondrosarcoma.
3. If objective anaplasia is present, to permit the diagnosis of Grade II to III chondrosarcoma by objective cytologic criteria.
4. To determine whether highly malignant fibrosarcomatous or osteosarcomatous transformation is present in a preexistent cartilage tumor.

The problems of diagnosis of a specific case can be simplified, if we first divide them into three groups; namely, unequivocal enchondroma, chondrosarcoma, and "borderline" lesions. Only after a thorough understanding of unequivocally benign enchondroma, compared with unequivocally malignant chondrosarcoma, is it possible to place the "borderline" lesions into their most appropriate category.

GROUP I. UNEQUIVOCAL ENCHONDROMA

Enchondroma of the Hands and Feet

Clinical Features

Analysis of the skeletal distribution of enchondromas (Fig. 8–2) shows the striking propensity for enchondromas to occur in the bones of the hands and feet (over 55% of cases). We should understand, however, that these figures do not necessarily reflect their true incidence. These figures apply to symptomatic enchondromas and those which have been discovered incidentally and have been subjected to biopsy. Scherer[19] made sections of 1,125 right femurs and found 22 instances of cartilagenous rests. It is reasonable to conclude from these data that enchondromas of the hands and feet are discovered in much greater proportion, compared with other bones, because the small size of the finger bones in relation to the size of the lesion predisposes to pathologic fracture, prompting the patient to seek medical attention. In most cases, lesions of similar or even larger size in the long bones and pelvis would not be expected to have produced symptoms. The importance of the possibility that long bones may harbor many more cartilage rests than come to biopsy is that perhaps many more of the so-called primary intraosseous chondrosarcomas seen are in truth secondary chondrosarcomas. Since the chondrosarcoma may overlap with enchondroma in terms of nuclear atypia, or lack of it, the problem associated with clarifying the actual incidence of secondary chondrosarcoma becomes evident. The only cases in which chondrosarcoma can be determined with absolute assurance to arise from cartilage rests are those cases in which an enchondroma is present on a radiograph for many years before the development of an obvious chondrosarcoma, or in those patients with multiple enchondromatosis who show chondrosarcomatous transformation. Although only six cases of unequivocal solitary enchondromas of the long and flat bones, ranging from 7 to 30 years duration before the onset of chondrosarcoma have been reported,[4] this author suspects that this incidence is much higher than these few cases would appear to support. The reasons for this suspicion will be discussed later.

The enchondroma is the most common bone tumor of the hands and feet. Approximately 98 per cent of the cartilage tumors in these sites behave in a benign fashion, even if the lesion shows "ominous" cellularity and nuclear features, which might lead to a high suspicion of malignancy in other sites.

Chondrosarcoma of the small tubular bones is very rare. This diagnosis is usually reserved for those cases showing frank anaplasia, invasion of the soft tissues, massive recurrence post-curettage, or metastases (an extremely rare occurrence). In general, a hyaline cartilage tumor of the short tubular bones should be considered benign unless proven otherwise. The opposite is true of solitary, pure cartilage-producing tumors of the long and flat bones of adults. In general, these should be considered malignant until proven otherwise.

Of the patients with enchondroma of the hands or feet, 75 per cent have a solitary lesion. The remainder have multiple enchondromas (Ollier's disease). The discussion which follows is concerned with only the solitary enchondroma. The manifestations of Ollier's disease are treated later.

About 66.6 per cent of patients with solitary enchondroma of the hands and feet present with pain consequent to an infraction through the lesion. The remainder of the lesions are discovered incidentally, usually following hand trauma. The patients range in age from 10 to 80 years, with a mean age of 35.[20]

Radiographic Features

On radiograph the lesions are usually centrally placed and, occasionally, slightly eccentric. Most lesions are 1 to 3 cm. in size, although rare giant forms have been described which respond well to local excision.[20] Although the methods of distinguishing these benign "giant" forms from chondrosarcoma were not clearly stated by Takigawa, I will assume that this unusual benign variant had "expanded" the bone but was confined by periosteum and did not

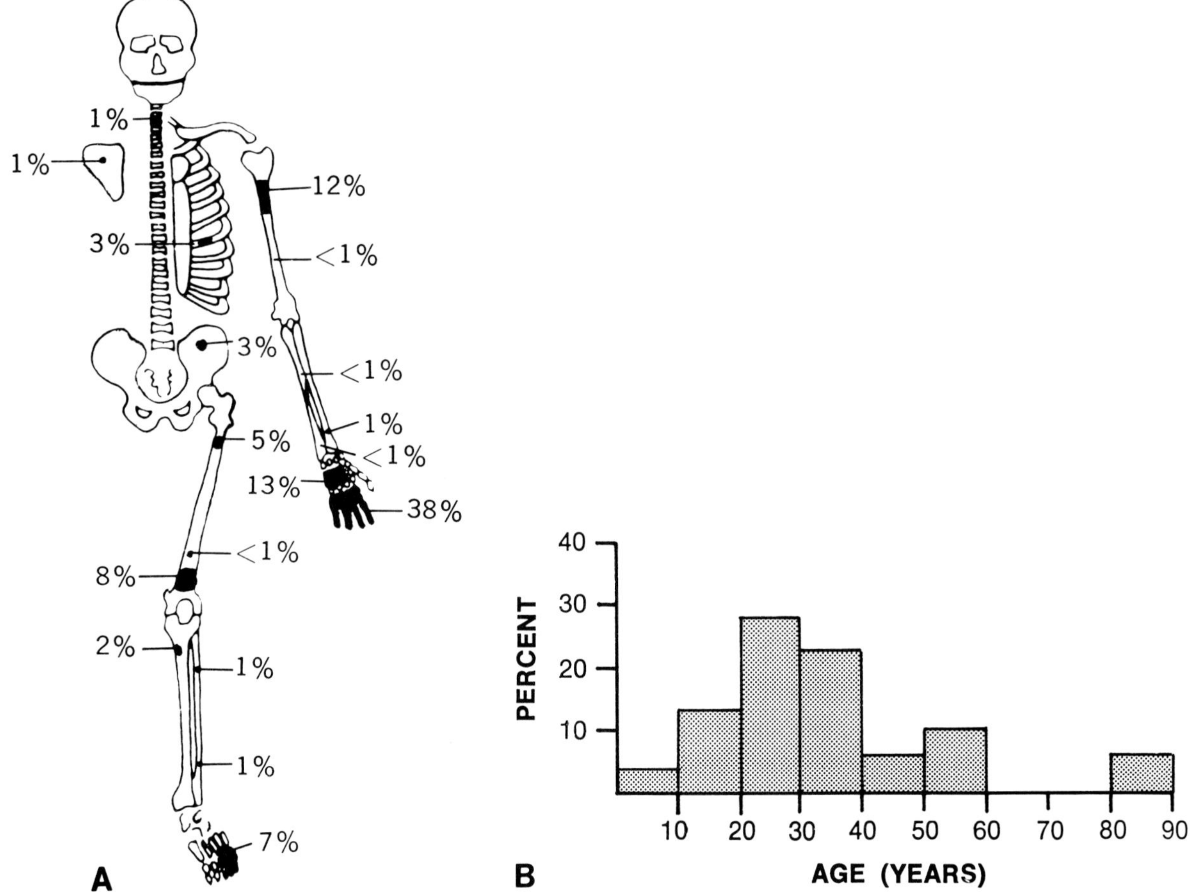

FIG. 8-2. (*A*) Solitary enchondroma. Frequency of areas of involvement in 153 patients. Male:female incidence, 1:1.2. (*B*) Age distribution in patients with solitary enchondroma of the hand (75 cases).[20] Average age: 33 years. Male:female incidence, approximately 1:1. (Mirra, J., Bullough, P., and Freiberger, R.: Orthopedic Diseases, Part II. New York, Famous Teachings in Modern Medicine, MedCom, Inc., © 1972)

show invasion of the soft tissues or joint space and had no signs of objective anaplasia.

Most enchondromas are well circumscribed, lytic, and show diagnostic, stippled, 1- to 3-mm. densities (Fig. 8-3); these characteristics are a great aid in distinguishing them from the other rarer bone tumors of the hands or feet.

Gross Pathology

It is rare to see enchondromas removed intact. The specimen usually consists of numerous small fragments of curettaged, glistening, bluish translucent cartilage and fragments of bone. The calcified cartilage fragments are whitish in color and gritty.

Histopathology

The tissues usually consist of numerous fragments of cartilage and bone, with disruption of the cartilage in relation to the surrounding bone (Fig. 8-4). If larger fragments are submitted, there is an improved chance of viewing the cartilage in relation to the surrounding bone (Figs. 8-5 and 8-6). *Most enchondromas will show focal areas or islands of cartilage surrounded by plates of lamellar to woven-lamellar bone* (Figs. 8–6 and 8–13). The intervening tissues are host bone and marrow fat. A pattern of partial to complete circumferential plates of lamellar to woven-lamellar bone about cartilage lobules signifies slow to absent cartilage growth, as would be expected in a benign lesion (personal observation).

The cartilage is either hyaline or fibrous in type. If the cartilage has become calcified and associated with vascular invasion, bony metaplasia to woven and lamellar bone is possible on the peripheral or central aspects. Heavily calcified enchondromatous tissue tends to form variably stained darker bluish islands (Fig 8–9). The mixture of variably stained islands imparts a mosaic or "jigsaw puzzle" pattern to the cartilage (Fig. 8–11). This pattern is common in enchondromas, particularly those of long bones, and is strongly suggestive of an enchondroma, even if complicated by sarcomatous transformation.

On high-power examination, enchondroma cartilage contains variable degrees of cellularity. In contrast to chondrosarcomas, most enchondromas show a lesser degree of cellularity and more evidence of chondrocyte nesting (Fig. 8–7). These features may also be found in Grade I chondrosarcoma and are, therefore, not pathognomonic. The heavily calcified portions of either enchondroma or chondrosarcoma will show degenerating to fully necrotic chondrocytic cells. The chondrocytes in either enchondroma or chondrosarcoma are usually rounded and sit in lacunae. The cytoplasm tends to shrink away from the lacunus leaving a space around the cell—the lacunar space. In more unusual cases of enchondroma there is fairly marked cellularity and the cytoplasmic features are more ovoid to spindly than rounded (Fig. 8–8). These features are "ominous" in that they mimic a Grade I chondrosarcoma. However, even with features such as is shown in Figure 8–8, if there is no clinical or radiographic evidence to support chondrosarcoma of the bones of the hands or feet, the diagnosis is still most likely to be enchondroma. But a lesion with similar microscopic features in long bones is much more likely to be a low-grade chondrosarcoma.

In essence, there are no objective cytological features which distinguish a cellular enchondroma from a Grade I chondrosarcoma. Diagnosis depends on correlation of clinical, radiologic, and pathologic findings. The only pattern which, in this author's opinion, is diagnostic of an enchondroma by histology alone is the presence of partial to complete circumferential plates of lamellar bone around cartilage lobules. In long bones, however, the association of chondrosarcomatous transformation of an enchondroma is much more likely, compared to benign enchondromas of the hands or feet. Therefore, the presence of enchondromatous tissues does not exclude the possibility of chondrosarcomatous transformation of a portion of the enchondroma.

Course

Recurrences and/or the unequivocal demonstration of malignant transformation of benign cartilage tumors of the hand are extremely rare. Culver, *et. al*[5], however, have presented a chondrosarcoma of a finger in which a small fragment of highly calcified, bland, almost totally acellular cartilage was embedded. They suggested that this radiographic and microscopic remnant most probably represented residua of a formerly benign enchondroma.

Hyalin cartilage tumors of the fingers or toes are to be considered benign enchondromas, unless proven otherwise. In order to diagnose chondrosarcoma there must be soft-tissue or joint invasion, evidence of Grade II to III anaplasia, massive recurrence, or metastases.

Unequivocal Enchondroma of Long and Flat Bones

Definition

In this text, an unequivocal enchondroma of long and flat bones is defined as a pure, cartilage-productive lesion in which the clinical, radiographic, and microscopic features arouse no suspicion of malignancy. What is meant by "arouse no suspicion of malignancy" will be outlined below. Even so, this definition does not exclude an enchondroma in which a small focus of chondrosarcomatous transformation has evaded our diagnostic acumen. Perhaps the only sure evidence that an enchondroma of the long bones is completely benign in all portions is with follow-up studies of 5 or more years, in which the course remains completely benign, following curettage. This would not, however, be a practical consideration of a specific case in which diagnosis and therapy must be immediate.

Clinical Features

INCIDENCE. In striking contrast to the bones of the hands and feet, the ratio of chondrosarcoma to pure, benign enchondroma of the long and flat bones, in this author's experience, is approximately 10 to 1. If we use the figures from Dahlin's textbook[6] of a very large series of patients, the ratio is 6 to 1 (300 primary chondrosarcomas versus 50 solitary enchondromas exclusive of the hands and feet).

AGE. Patients under the age of 15 showing an intramedullary, pure cartilage tumor with innocent histological features is almost always an enchondroma. Malignant cartilage tumors in the young (chondro- and osteosarcomas) show high-grade anaplasia in the majority of cases. Grade I chondrosarcomas begin to make their appearance at about the age of 20. However, the mean age incidence of chondrosarcoma is 47. The age at which enchondroma of the long and flat bones is found in published reports of a small series of 20 patients is 37 years.[3,12,13] The ages of the patients ranged from between 8 and 60 years. Unfortunately, in two-thirds of these patients there were no published 5-year follow-up results. All six of Coley and Higinbotham's reported cases eventually developed chondrosarcoma in between 7 and 30 years. From the available data it is reasonable to state that in dealing with a patient with a "borderline" cartilage lesion, the risk of developing a chondrosarcoma is much greater in a patient over 45 years of age, compared with a patient under the age of 35.

Obviously, there is a great need for publication of series of enchondromas of long and flat bones, with at least 5-year follow-up results. If a malignant lesion develops in less than this time, the case will probably not be acceptable as a secondary chondrosarcoma by some authors. This author suspects that the reason so few enchondromas of long and flat bones are published with long-term follow-ups is that the chances of discovering them incidentally is low and many of the cases have already undergone malignant transformation at initial discovery. When within a couple of years the original diagnosis of a simple enchondroma is seen to be in error, the original diagnosis is often amended to chondrosarcoma. In this author's experience, however, the examination of many enchondromas and chondrosarcomas of long bones has lead him to the conclusion that a significant proportion of so-called "primary" chondrosarcomas have radiographic and histologic evidence of a preceding benign enchondromatous lesion. This lack of unequivocal clinical proof of a preexistent enchondroma in association with most chondrosarcomas may well explain Dahlin's (1956) failure to find a single case from among 212 chondrosarcomas. He states: "chondrosarcoma secondary to proved enchondroma was not encountered in this series." Later in this section, radiologic and histologic features will be presented which, if found in association with a chondrosarcoma, are, in this author's opinion, strong presumptive evidence of a preexistent enchondroma.

SYMPTOMS. If a long bone lesion is discovered as an incidental finding with histologic features of bland cartilage, then it is likely to be totally benign. Such cases are, however, rare. If an "enchondroma" of long or flat bones is discovered because of symptoms directly referable to that area, the index of suspicion of malignancy or malignant transformation must be high. Such lesions must be considered "borderline" on this basis alone. Borderline hyaline cartilage tumors will be discussed later.

Radiologic Features

Those features most consistent with a completely benign enchondroma of the long bones, (one which has not developed a focus of malignancy) should include the following (Figs. 8–10 and 8–36):

1. The lesion contains well-defined punctate, ring-like, spheroidal to short linear densities.
2. Its shape varies from round to polygonal or elliptical.
3. Its size ranges from 1 to 8 cm. in longitudinal direction. Most tumors are 3 to 4 cm. in size.
4. The lesion is confined to the medullary portions of the bone.

(*Text continues on p. 174.*)

Enchondroma of Phalanges

FIG. 8–3. Enchondroma of phalanges. The classical phalangeal enchondroma is represented by a metaphyseal-diaphyseal, well-circumscribed, variably expansile, lytic lesion containing 1- to 3-mm. punctate calcifications. Many present with a small cortical infraction (*arrow*).

FIG. 8–4. Typical curettage specimen of enchondroma consists of numerous disoriented fragments of hyaline cartilage (x40).

FIG. 8–5. If large segments of enchondroma are removed at curettage, lobules of hyaline cartilage surrounded by partial to complete circumferential plates of reactive host lamellar bone may be seen. The intercartilagenous tissue consists of host bone and marrow fat (x40).

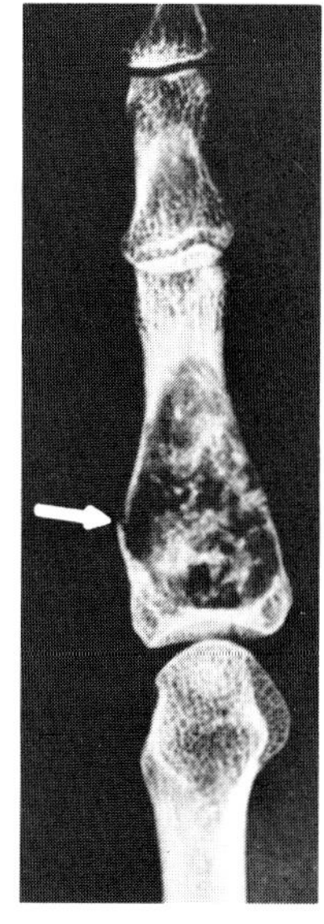

FIG. 8-3

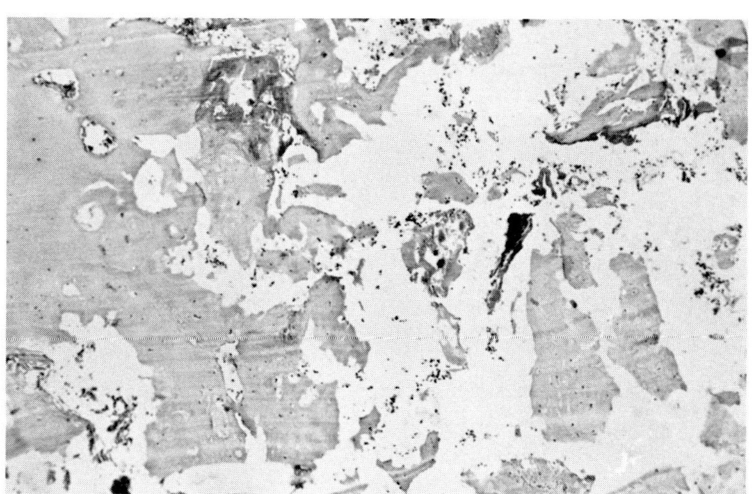

FIG. 8-4

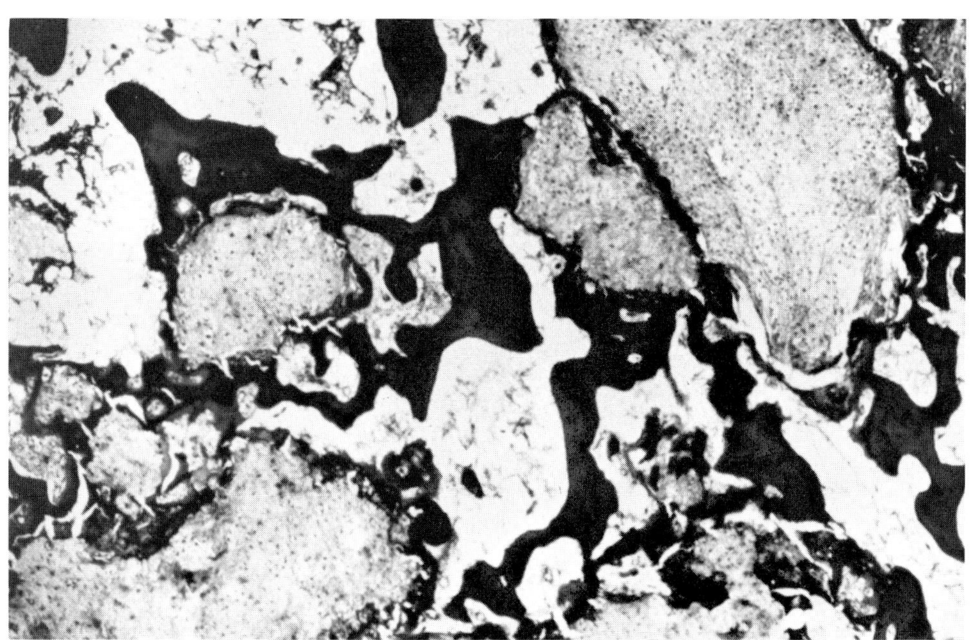

FIG. 8-5

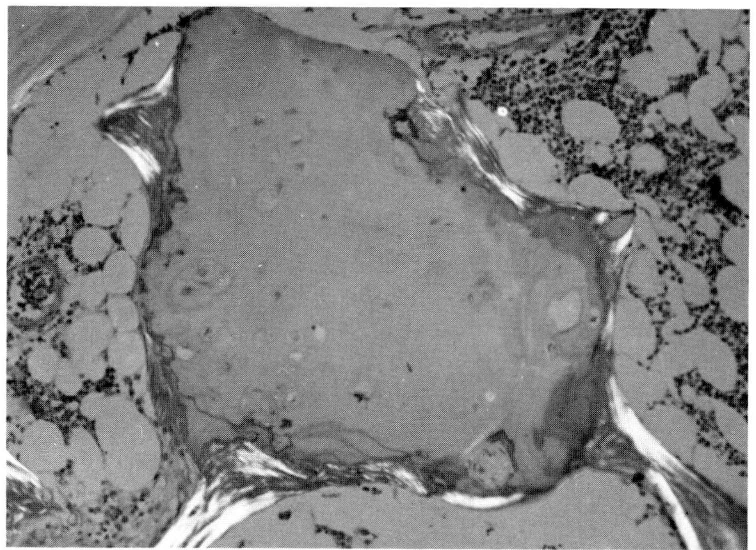

FIG. 8-6

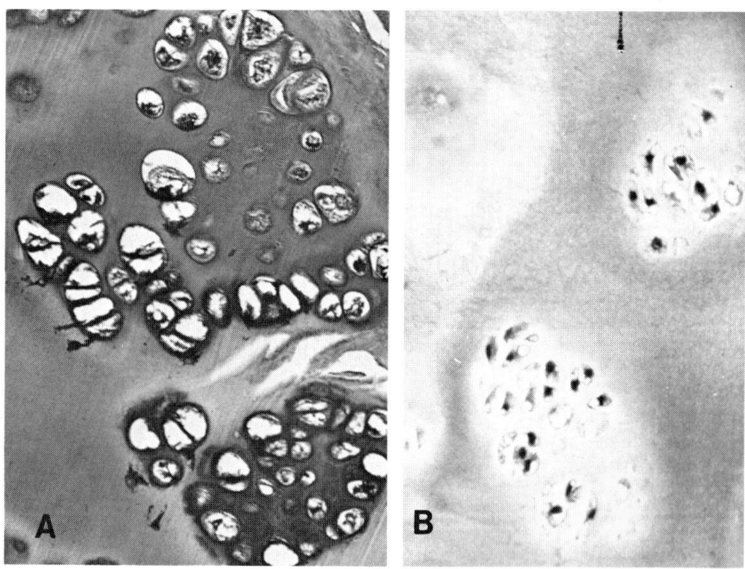

FIG. 8-7

Enchondroma

FIG. 8-6. Polarized light will show that some of the metaplastic bone that encompasses the cartilage is mature lamellar, signifying very slow to absent growth, a sign of benignancy. This type of pericartilagenous ossification accounts for the ringlike, spheroidal densifications seen on radiographic examination (x125).

FIG. 8-7. Note the disposition of chondrocytes into regular islands and the small innocuous nuclei. These two features are common to enchondroma, although such features may occasionally be present in very well differentiated chondrosarcoma (*A*: x125, *B*: x250).

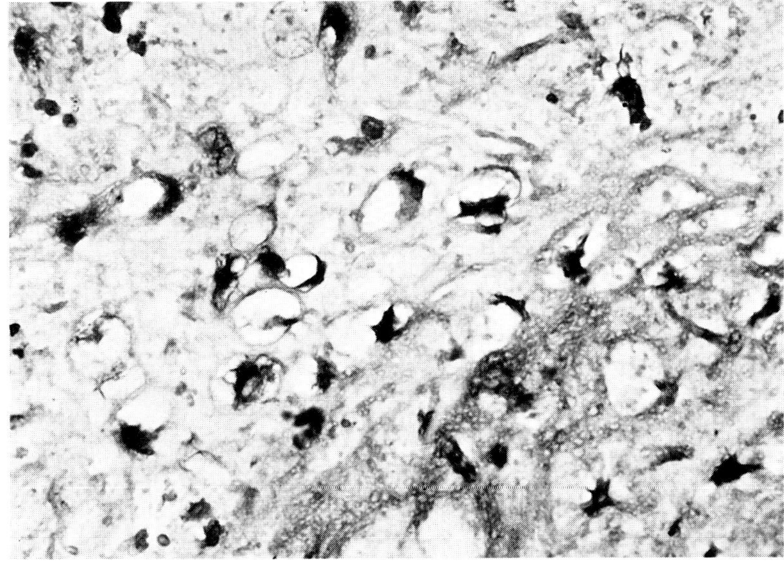

FIG. 8-8

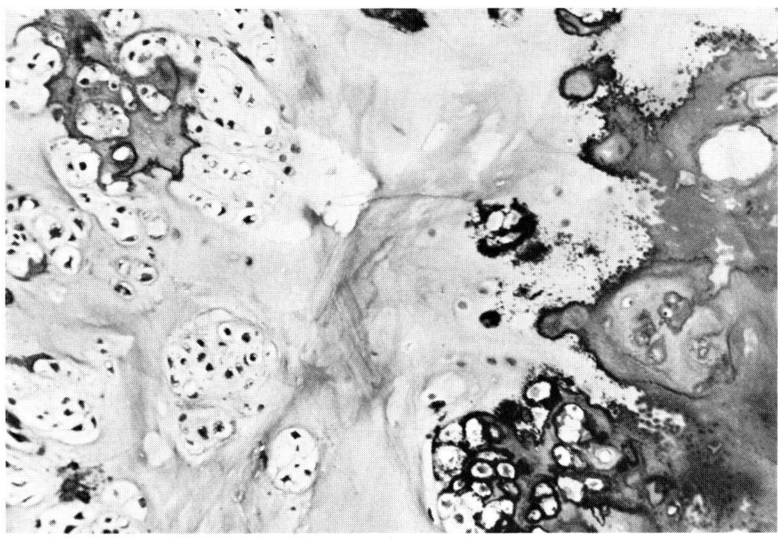

FIG. 8-9

Enchondroma

FIG. 8-8. Atypical features of an enchondroma probably related to fixation artifacts. Note the bubbliness and swelling of nuclei and cytoplasm. Nevertheless, if these are not recognized as artifact, these features could be mistaken for a low-grade chondrosarcoma. Enchondromas even without artifactual changes may show disturbing loss of chondrocyte circumscription into islands and atypical stellate nuclei. Differentiation from chondrosarcoma depends on correlating clinical, radiologic, and pathologic features (x400).

FIG. 8-9. Heavy calcification in a typical enchondroma. Such areas account for the larger, more irregular calcifications seen on radiograph, as compared to the smaller ringlike or spheroidal densifications that correspond to plates of bone that surround some of the cartilage lobules (x125).

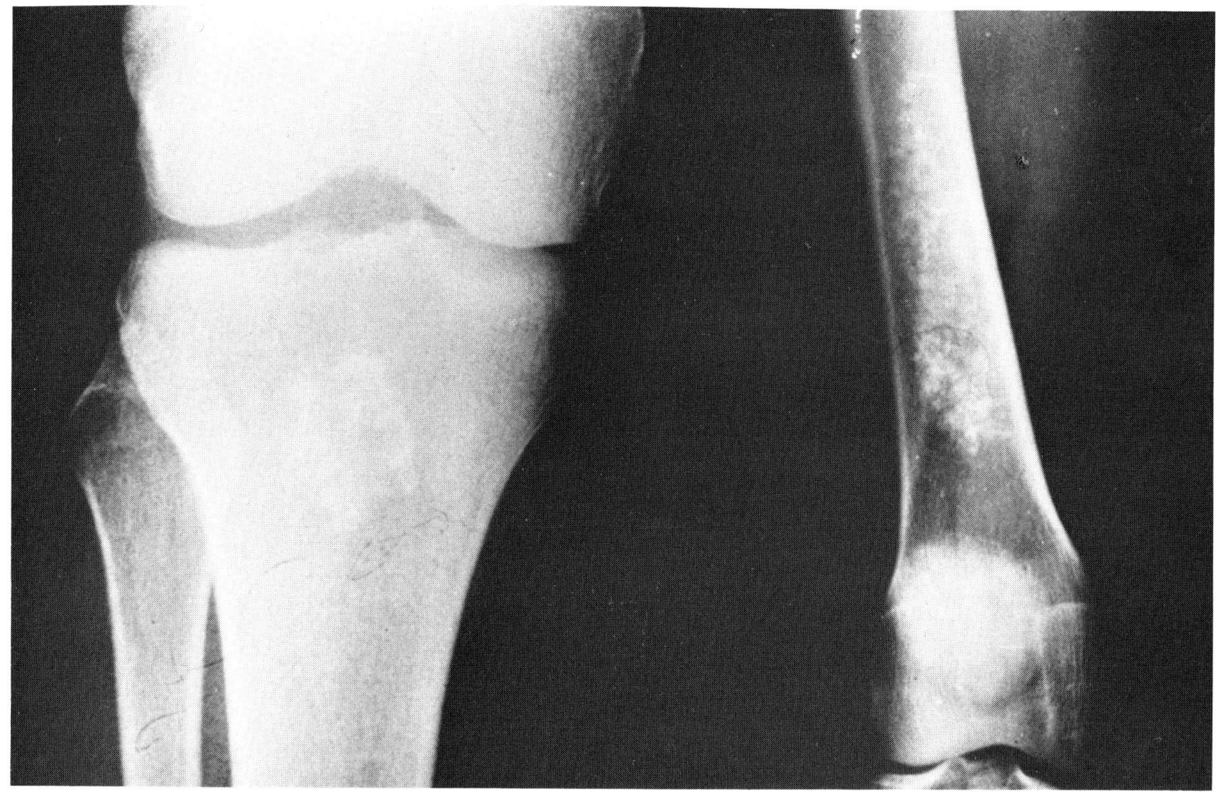

Enchondroma of Long Bones

FIG. 8-10. Unequivocal enchondroma of long bones. *Left and right:* Two examples of benign enchondromas. The lesions are well circumscribed and contain 1- to 3-mm. spheroidal to short, linear calcifications. Note the absence of zones of lysis, scalloping of the cortex, periosteal reactions, and soft-tissue mass. These are ominous signs, usually seen in association with chondrosarcoma or chondrosarcomatous transformation of an enchondroma.

5. The lesion is homogenous with respect to calcification. There are *no* focal areas of lysis significantly different from the homogeneity of the rest of the lesion.
6. There is no evidence of focal cortical erosion, "scalloping" of the cortex, significant cortical thickening or bone "expansion," ("borderline" cartilage tumor group). There must be no significant cortical thickening in association with proliferative periosteal reactions, or soft-tissue mass (malignant cartilage tumor group).

Enchondroma

FIG. 8-11. Calcified areas frequently show a "jigsaw" puzzle pattern of calcification and small nuclei with little cellularity. Note the plates of lamellar bone encompassing the outer portion of the cartilage lobules (*arrows*) (x40).

FIG. 8-12. The finding of metaplastic plates of lamellar bone surrounding cartilage (*arrow*) of a central cartilage-producing tumor is virtually diagnostic of enchondroma. In this example, the cartilage shows total loss of nuclei because it has become completely surrounded by a densely calcified tissue (x125).

FIG. 8-13. In order to fully appreciate this feature of partial to complete encompassing plates of lamellar bone (*arrows*), it may be necessary to use polarized light. Note also the hypocellularity to almost total absence of chondrocyte nuclei, consistent with an "old" enchondroma (x60).

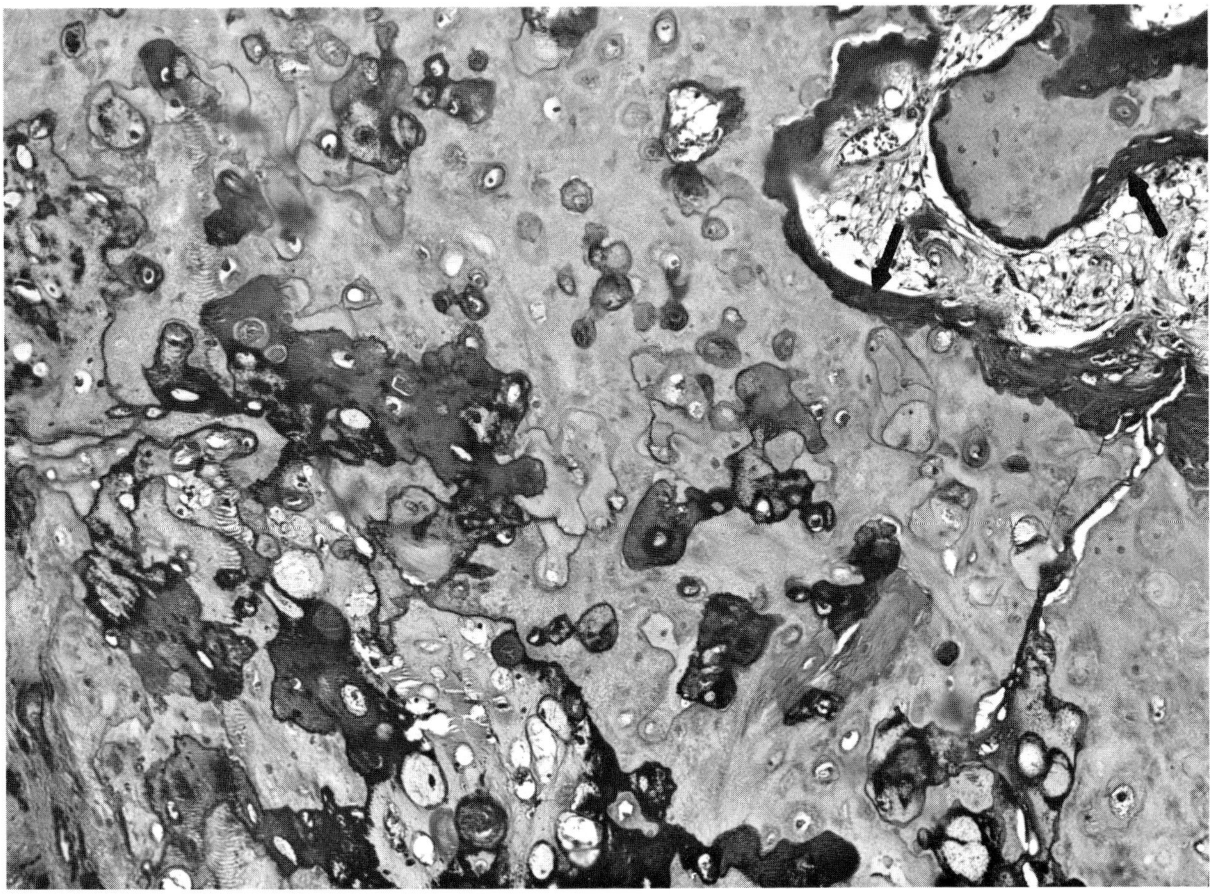

FIG. 8-11

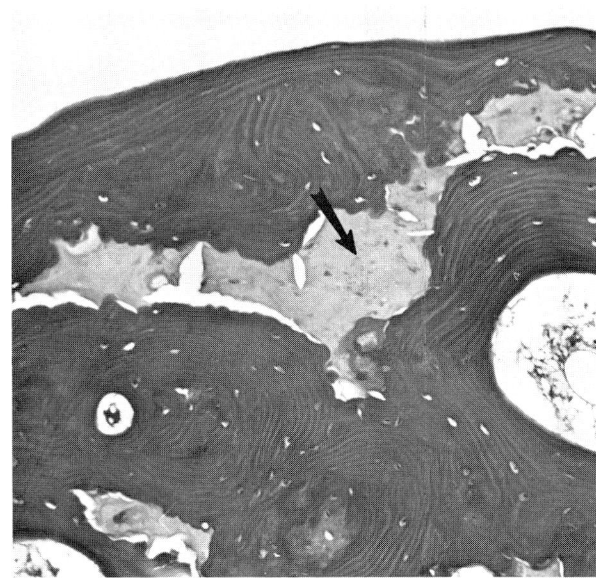

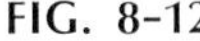

FIG. 8-12

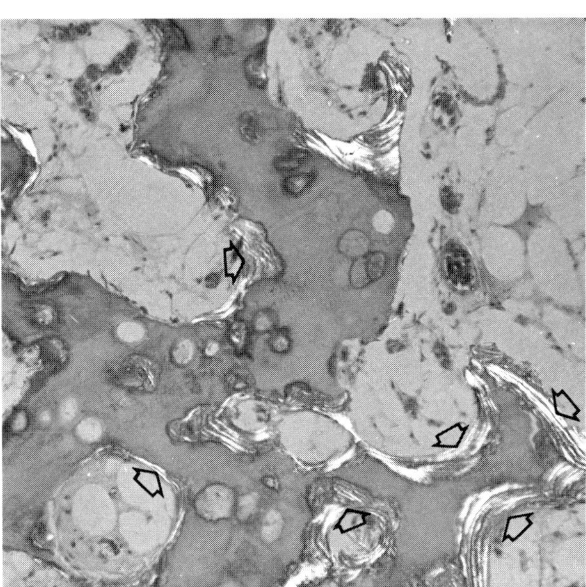

FIG. 8-13

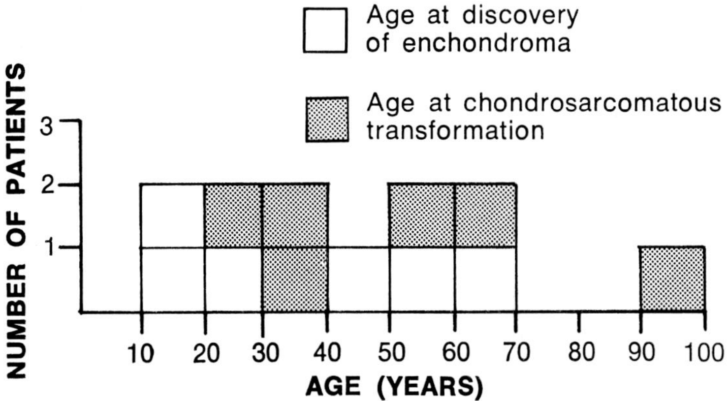

FIG. 8-14. Age distribution of patients with enchondroma of long bones with a follow-up of at least 5 years, compared to their age at chondrosarcomatous degeneration (six cases). Average age of long bone enchondroma patients is 31 years. Average age of chondrosarcomatous transformation is 46 years (Data obtained from Coley, *et al.*).

Gross Pathology

Curettage specimens demonstrate islands of glistening, translucent, bluish cartilage. Using a magnifying glass or stereomicroscope, some to many of the cartilage lobules can be seen to be encompassed by a partial to complete shell of reactive host bone. If the cartilage itself is calcified it will become gritty and appear whitish yellow.

Histopathology

Microscopic examination must show evidence to support slow to absent growth of the cartilage and neither unequivocal anaplasia nor invasion of the marrow fat or soft tissues. In this author's estimation, *the only microscopic feature of unequivocal enchondromatous tissue is the presence of plates of lamellar bone surrounding lobules of cartilage in a partial to complete circumferential manner* (Figs. 8-5, 8-6, 8-12, 8-13, 8-15, 8-49, *C*, and 8-61) (personal observations). But even if unequivocal enchondromatous tissues are seen this does not preclude sarcomatous transformation in a focus of the formerly benign cartilage tissues. The presence of thin to thick plates of fully mature lamellar to woven-lamellar bone signifies extremely slow to absent growth of the cartilage; this is inconsistent with the more rapid growth of chondrosarcoma. This feature is best appreciated using polarized light (Fig. 8-13). It must take many weeks to months for the host to form circumferential plates of lamellar bone by enchondral ossification. Mature lamellar bone does not form as a reactive tissue around chondrosarcoma lobules, because this tumor is characterized by more rapid, unrelenting growth. In contrast, chondrosarcoma may be associated with bone production in and surrounding the cartilage lobules, but it is of the woven bone type (Fig. 8-33). The plates of lamellar bone that surround the cartilage lobules in enchondroma must also be distinguished from remnants of host lamellar bone trapped in an area of chondrosarcomatous invasion. In this instance the trabeculae maintain their normal orientation and are merely trapped in the sarcoma; they do not form in a circumferential manner by enchondral ossification (Figs. 8-26 and 8-27). The absence of lamellar bone around some or many of the cartilage lobules does not rule out enchondroma. If the biopsy is highly fragmented this important pattern may be lost and diagnosis obscured. Its absence only makes the diagnosis of an enchondroma more suspect. The diagnosis of cartilage tumors must always depend heavily upon correlating clinical, radiologic, and pathologic features.

Enchondroma

FIG. 8-15. Cellular enchondroma of rib surrounded by plates of lamellar bone (*arrows*) at its periphery (x10).

FIG. 8-16. Medium-power showing organization of chondrocytes into multiple discrete islands (x40).

FIG. 8-17. High-power examination shows very small, round nuclei, further confirmation that the lesion is an enchondroma (x300).

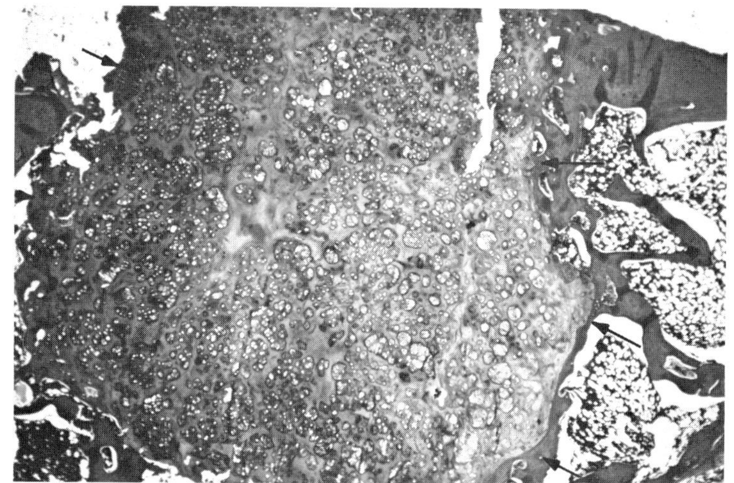

FIG. 8-15

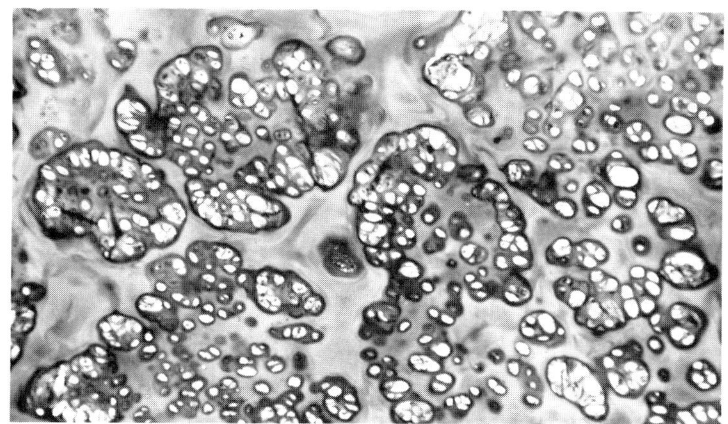

FIG. 8-16

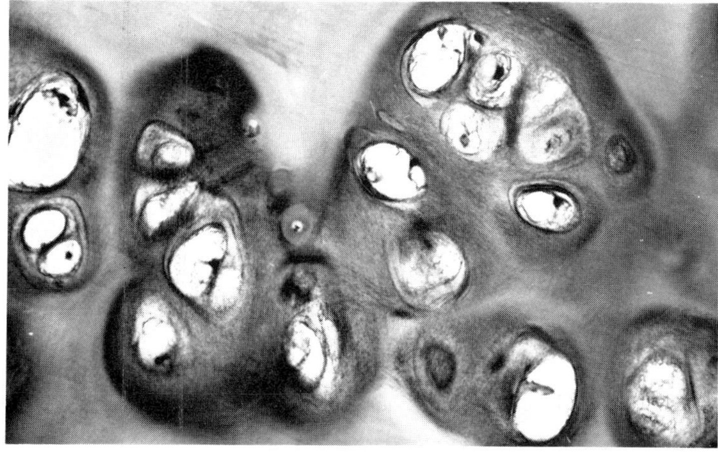

FIG. 8-17

On the other hand, the finding of enchondromatous tissues in association with a malignant cartilage tumor is important to recognize and to report, if we are to obtain a more complete understanding of the potential danger of harboring a sizable enchondroma. It will also enable us to more clearly determine the true ratio of primary to secondary central chondrosarcoma. Among my own cases of chondrosarcoma, I have seen what I consider virtually diagnostic radiologic and histologic areas of enchondroma in approximately 20 per cent of cases.

A second feature seen in enchondromas of the hands, feet, and long bones is the presence of bland islands of heavily calcified cartilage in which distinct blue lines separate one area from another. This feature imparts a "mosaic" or "jigsaw puzzle" pattern to the calcified cartilage lobule (*Fig. 8–11*). Although chondrosarcoma cartilage may undergo various degrees of calcification, this peculiar jigsaw puzzle pattern is unusual to rare unless there was other radiographic or microscopic evidence that supported a preexistent enchondroma (Fig. 8–49, *C, D,* and *E*).

The other histologic features of enchondroma of long bones are similar to those discussed for the hands and feet. These latter features, however, overlap insensibly with Grade I chondrosarcoma.

Certain histologic features must be absent in order to rule out a chondrosarcoma. There must be no areas that show unequivocal anaplasia, infiltration between fat cells (Figs. 8–27 and 8–28), vascular invasion, or soft-tissue mass. Another pattern highly suggestive of enchondroma is the presence of discrete islands of cartilage separated from other islands by zones of normal bone. In chondrosarcoma the masses of cartilage become confluent and replace large areas of the former host bone (Fig. 8–39, *C* and *E*). The islands of chondrosarcoma cartilage in this confluent stage are often separated from one another by thick bands of fibrous connective tissue (Figs. 8–29 and 8–39, *E*). This latter pattern is uncommonly seen in solitary enchondromas of the long and flat bones. However, patients with Ollier's disease may have large confluent islands of cartilage with fibrous tissue bands separating cartilage lobules (Fig. 8–60).

Course and Treatment

If the lesion is truly an enchondroma, it will respond favorably to curettage and packing with bone chips. For long and flat bones, this treatment should be employed for only those pure cartilage tumors deemed unequivocally benign by all of the diagnostic procedures available. However, in any pure cartilage tumor with borderline radiologic and pathologic features (p. 186) the risk of not recognizing a primary or secondary chondrosarcoma by cytologic parameters are great. Simple curettage could result in eventual amputation or loss of life. When such borderline tumors can be very adequately treated by cryosurgery with low morbidity and maintenance of the patient's own bone stock,[16] it does not, in this author's opinion, appear to be worth the risk of employing less comprehensive procedures. The only borderline feature that might not justify cryosurgery is pain in the absence of atypical radiologic and pathologic findings, because the pain may be unrelated to the intraosseous cartilage tumor. For example, a patient with an enchondroma of the femur may develop pain in the knee consequent to trauma, osteoarthritis, or a host of other factors. Radiographs of the knee may inadvertently reveal the enchondroma. Therefore, the symptom of pain without a thorough history as to its possible causes and correlation to the radiologic and pathologic features cannot be used, in and of itself, as a justification for cryosurgery of a long or flat bone pure cartilage-producing lesion.

The only unequivocal evidence of benignancy of a hyaline cartilage lesion of the long and flat bones is complete healing without recurrence (Fig. 8–36). If a lesion recurs in an adult post-curettage and if biopsy shows a recurrent cartilage tumor, the index of suspicion of chondrosarcoma has to be extremely high. Such lesions are probably best treated with freezing or en-bloc resection, even if the lesion shows neither signs of objective anaplasia nor has broken through the cortex.

GROUP II. UNEQUIVOCAL CENTRAL CHONDROSARCOMA

The unequivocal central chondrosarcoma group includes all those cases with objective Grade II to III anaplasia and those cartilage tumors with unequivocal radiographic or clinical evidence of malignant biologic behavior.

Central or intraosseous chondrosarcomas are either primary or secondary. Secondary chondrosarcomas most frequently arise in association with enchondroma(s) and only rarely with chondroblastoma or chondromyxoid fibroma. Most of the reported cases of secondary chondrosarcoma were seen in association with Ollier's disease (multiple enchondromatosis). Those cases of chondrosarcoma arising in chondroblastoma or chondromyxoid fibroma usually occur many years after biopsy and curettage of the formerly benign lesion. If there had been no prior tissue or radiographic diagnosis, these latter two lesions are sufficiently distinctive from ordinary chondrosarcoma to be recognized provided, of course, that the primary benign tumor has not been totally replaced by the sarcoma and sections have been obtained from the benign areas. If the patient has a prior diagnosis of Ollier's disease, any chondrosarcoma that develops is presumed to be secondary, even if histological demonstration of enchondromatous tissue is no longer possible. But, if a chondrosarcoma arises from a solitary enchondroma it is difficult to distinguish the two. There are only a few enchondromas of long and flat bones with a 5-year follow-up prior to the development of a frank chondrosarcoma.[4] Cases will be presented in this section and the section on fibrosarcomatous transformation of primary and secondary chondrosarcomas with radiographic, specimen radiographic, and histologic criteria that support the contention that chondrosarcomatous transformation of clinically "silent" enchondromas are probably not as rare as the literature would lead us to believe.

Clinical Features

Most patients are over 40 years of age. The mean age at presentation of primary chondrosarcoma is 47, compared to those patients with multiple enchondromatosis, who often develop chondrosarcoma in their late 20's or 30's. Patients with solitary enchondromas who develop chondrosarcoma have the same basic age distribution as those with primary chondrosarcomas. The skeletal and age distributions of primary, central and secondary, central and peripheral chondrosarcomas are shown in Figs. 8–40 and 8–48.

The patients present with pain or local swelling. Those patients with secondary chondrosarcomas tend to have noted an insidious increase in pain. In contrast, those patients without evidence of a preexistent benign lesion tend to develop more rapid and severe pain. Occasionally, patients with chondrosarcoma present with pathologic fracture, synovial effusion, or paresthesias.

Radiologic Features

The radiologic features of an unequivocal chondrosarcoma are classical. Most lesions are centered in either the metaphysis or diaphysis. About 10 per cent may begin in the epiphyseal region. The radiographic features of an unequivocal chondrosarcoma are the following:

1. The lesion is large and ill-defined (Figs. 8–18, 8–19, and 8–37, *B*).
2. The contours of the bone are enlarged or "expanded" (Figs. 8–18, 8–19, and 8–37, *B*).
3. The cortex is focally or extensively eroded. The inner cortex may have "scalloped" borders (Fig. 8–19). Other cases may show extensive cortical thickening, a sign of chondrosarcomatous invasion of haversian systems (Fig. 8–18).
4. The interior of the lesion may have circular radiolucencies that represent large lobules of cartilage (Figs. 8–18 and 8–19). These lobules may impart a bubbly appearance (Fig. 8–18).
5. Variably sized calcifications are usually present that have a characteristic "granular," "fuzzy" (Fig. 8–19), and "windblown" appearance (Fig. 8–37, *B*).
6. There is an associated soft-tissue mass and/or periosteal reaction (Figs. 8–18, 8–19, 8–37, *B*).

These are the most important features of unequivocal malignancy in a pure cartilage-producing tumor. Even if there is no unequivocal anaplasia, the presence of these radiographic features must be construed as biologic evidence of malignancy when associated with a central cartilage tumor of the long or flat bones, provided, of course, that these reactions are not merely the callus of pathologic fracture.

Gross Pathology

Grade I to II chondrosarcomas are composed of confluent lobules of glistening, bluish, cartilage (Fig. 8–19, *B*). Foci of calcification or metaplastic ossification are yellowish to white and gritty to hard. The more poorly differentiated chondrosarcomas can be yellowish to gray and can lose their glistening, translucent qualities completely.

Chondrosarcoma often erodes the cortical borders resulting in "scalloping" (Fig. 8–19, *B*). The lesion may infiltrate for many centimeters beyond what is apparent by standard x-ray examination.

Unless the tumor has significant calcifications within it or has significantly eroded the cortex, the full extent of its insidious infiltration into the bone, which can be many centimeters beyond what is apparent on the standard radiograph, will not be appreciated. If an en-bloc excision is to be performed, vigorous efforts to determine the actual extent of

(*Text continues on p. 182.*)

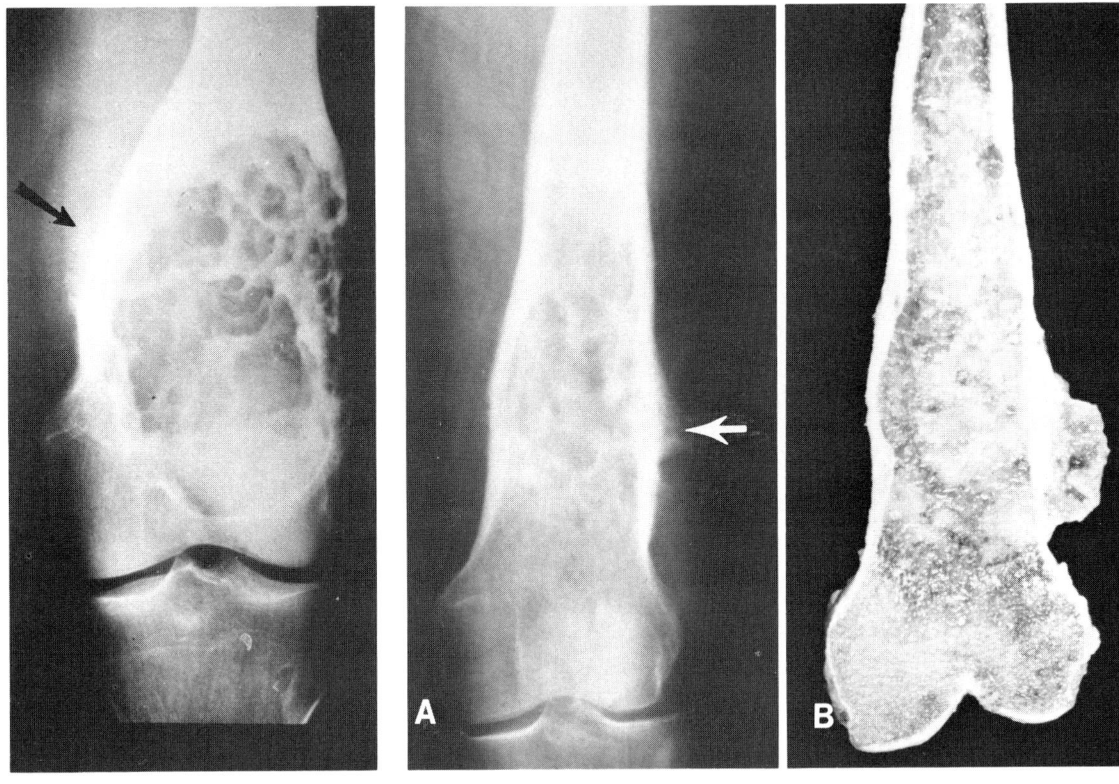

FIG. 8-18

FIG. 8-19

Chondrosarcoma

FIG. 8-18. Unequivocal chondrosarcoma. This radiograph is virtually pathognomonic of chondrosarcoma. The lesion contains rounded lytic lobules, has "expanded" the bone, and has permeated the cortex, resulting in a soft-tissue mass (*arrow*). The thickened "cortex" beneath the mass is the result of reactive periosteal and cortical new bone consequent to permeation of haversian systems by chondrosarcoma.

FIG. 8-19. (*A*) This chondrosarcoma shows a tumor with lobulations, early bone "expansion," periosteal reaction and prominent soft-tissue mass (*arrow*). The "scalloped" contours of the cortex is seen best slightly proximal to the soft-tissue mass. The intraosseous component has a "fuzzy" or "washed-out" appearance, compared to the more distinct calcifications usually associated with enchondroma. From this radiograph, what would you consider the proximal and distal limits of the neoplasm? (*B*) Gross specimen corresponding to previous radiographic lesion. Note that the lesion extends several centimeters proximally and distally from what would be expected from analysis of the standard radiographic films. This feature is common in chondrosarcoma and dictates the necessity for more complete evaluation to determine its true extent of invasion before attempting to cure by en-bloc resection, if that procedure is desirable.

Grade II Chondrosarcomas

FIG. 8-20. Grade II chondrosarcomas. (*A*) There is marked cellularity, hyperchromatism, and pleomorphism of nuclei and cytoplasm. These features are usually diagnostic of a chondrosarcoma when associated with a pure, hyaline, cartilage-producing tumor of long or flat bones. It should be noted, however, that the chondromyxoid fibroma can have similar high-power histology, but this tumor is not a pure hyaline, cartilage-producing tumor (see Fig. 8-103). (*B*) Although the nuclei are rounded, they are moderately enlarged and if several chondrocytes show double nuclei (*arrows*) in a single field, the diagnosis is usually assured of being low-grade chondrosarcoma (both x400).

FIG. 8-21. Low Grade II chondrosarcoma. Although the nesting of chondrocytes resembles enchondroma, occasional nuclei (*arrows*) are too large and plump to be considered benign. This field was selected from the soft-tissue extension of an obvious chondrosarcoma by radiographic analysis (x300).

FIG. 8-22. Grade II chondrosarcoma. Many of the nuclei are large, plump, and hyperchromatic. A highly abnormal cell cluster is seen in this example (*arrow*). Also note the hypercellularity (x400).

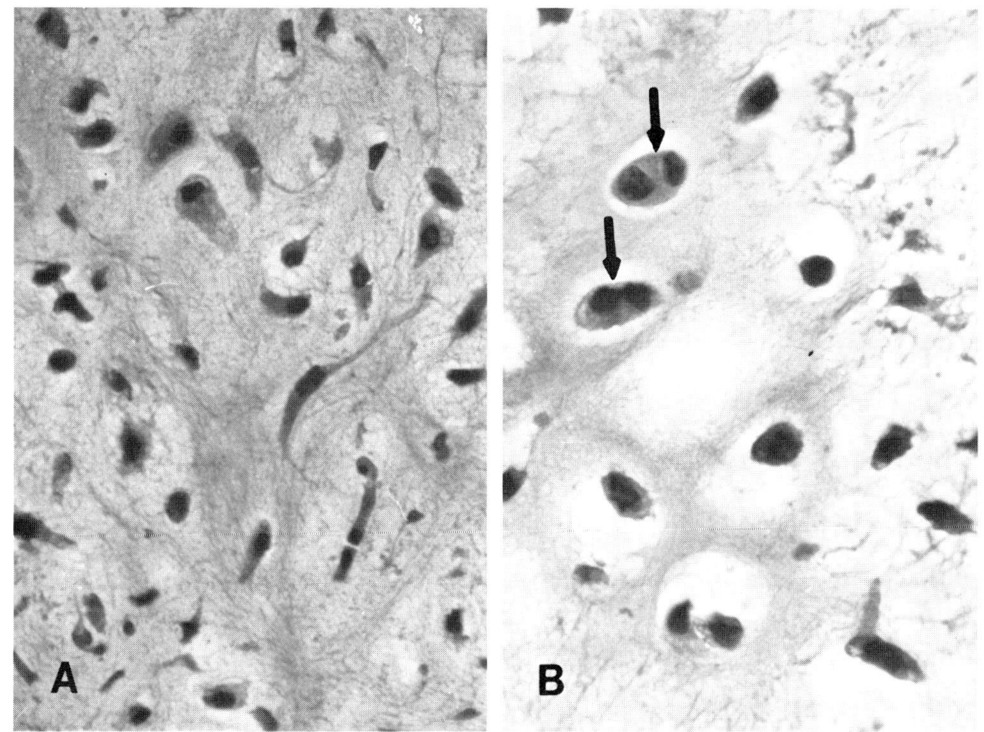

FIG. 8-20

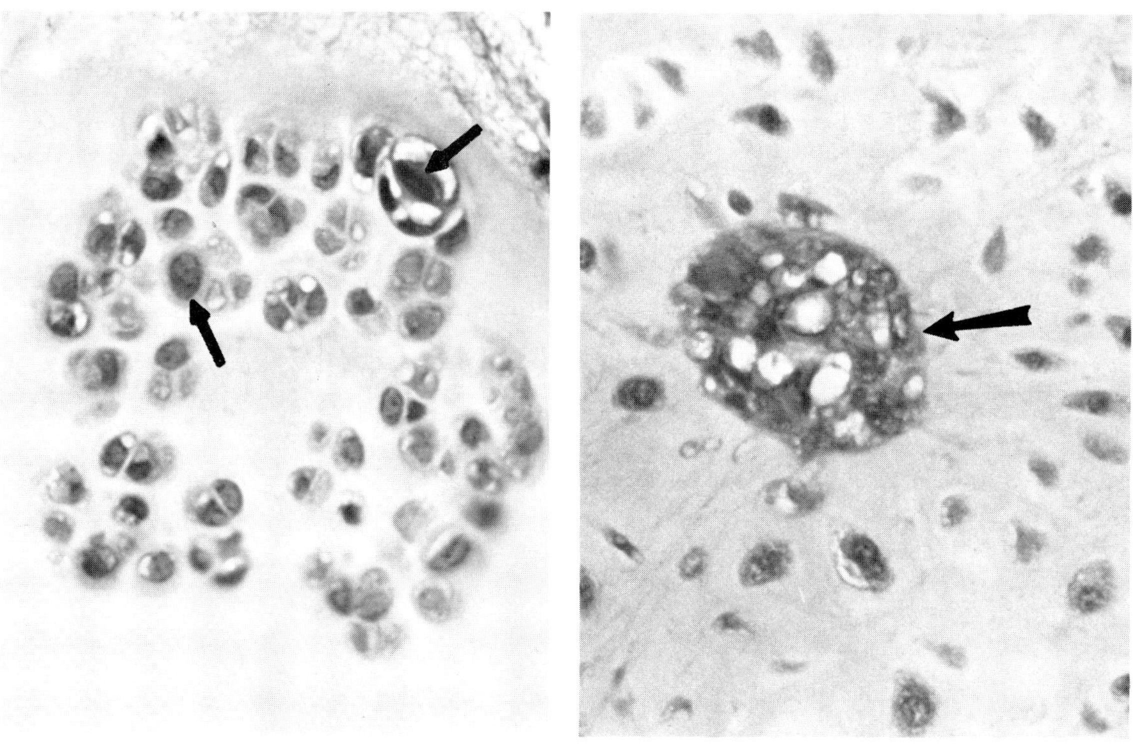

FIG. 8-21

FIG. 8-22

intraosseous penetration by standard tomograms or computed tomography may be necessary to reduce the risks of cutting through tumor.

If the tumor is located near the end of the bone, infiltration into the joint tissues is possible. Crossing of joints by malignant bone tumors is an extremely rare event. However, it is possible for a chondrosarcoma to cross a joint through the ligamentum teres or glenohumeral ligament (personal observations).

HISTOPATHOLOGY

Cytologic Features

Chondrosarcomas are graded by degree of nuclear atypia. Grade I chondrosarcomas overlap cytologically with cellular enchondroma(s) and, in particular, with Ollier's disease. The diagnosis of Grade I chondrosarcoma, therefore, depends on clinical, radiographic, and morphologic patterns, rather than on cytologic characteristics.

Grade II to III chondrosarcomas do, however, show objective features of cytologic anaplasia (Figs. 8–20, 8–24, 8–44, 8–45, *B*, 8–46, and 8–47). In examining for anaplasia, the slides should be scanned on low and medium power. It is best to avoid areas of heavy calcification and to identify and study those regions that show the greatest degree of cellularity, the largest nuclei, and the best preservation of nuclear detail. Nuclei may become entombed in areas of calcification and show considerable enlargement, compared to nuclei in noncalcified areas. Since nuclear size is one of the parameters important in assessing anaplasia, it is wise to avoid heavily calcified areas, which often result in extensive nuclear degeneration and distortion. The features of objective cytologic anaplasia include the following:

1. NUCLEAR FEATURES. Malignant cartilage nuclei are most often plump, round to oval, and occasionally, long and spindly. The most obviously malignant nuclei are roundish and from 11 to 15 microns in diameter. (Figs. 8–21, 8–23, 8–24, and 8–45, *B*). The chromatin pattern is distinct and shows variable degrees of clumping. Avoid nuclei that show smudging of nuclear chromatin, if possible, because these may represent artifactual distortion. In enchondromatous lesions the nuclear chromatin is usually indistinct. Most often, the nuclei are small, in the range of 5 to 8 microns. An extremely important aid in the diagnosis of nuclear malignancy is the presence of prominent pink to red nucleoli measuring 2 to 3 microns. Double and triple nucleoli (not nuclei) are virtually diagnostic of malignancy. In benign cartilage tumors nucleoli are quite tiny and indistinct.

The more malignant the tumor, the greater will be the individual variation in sizes and shapes of the nuclei, nucleoli, chromatin clumping irregularities, and mitotic rate.

Double and triple nuclei within a single cell are important signs of malignancy, provided that fields can be found in which at least three or four such cells can be seen (Figs. 8–20, *B* and 8–46, *A*). Benign cartilage tumors can show occasional double nucleated forms, usually no more than one per single 300x high-power field (HPF) (Fig. 8–43, *arrow*).

Nuclei that are in the average range of 8 to 10 microns are usually indicative of a low-grade chondrosarcoma, atypical enchondroma, or Ollier's disease. If more than five nuclei/300x HPF can be found in the range of 11 microns or more, the diagnosis of chondrosarcoma is extremely probable. Ollier's disease represents the most common exception to this rule. These cases of Ollier's disease with nuclear atypia approaching anaplasia may represent a dysplastic or presarcomatous phase of cytologic changes. These nuclei will not, however, show prominent nucleoli or numerous double and triple nuclear forms. In dealing with cases of Ollier's disease, unless there is atypia at least equivalent to Figures 8–23 and 8–24, the diagnosis of chondrosarcoma should depend on correlating clinical and radiologic features with pathologic patterns of tumor involvement, such as search for soft tissue extension and infiltration of the marrow.

Nuclei that are greater than 20 microns in diameter

Grade II–III Chondrosarcoma

FIG. 8–23. Grade II–III chondrosarcoma. The degree of anaplasia on the left is equivalent to Grade II; that on the right, to a Grade III chondrosarcoma. The diagnosis should reflect the most ominous portions, that is, Grade III chondrosarcoma (x250).

FIG. 8–24. Grade III chondrosarcoma. (*A*) and (*B*): Bizarre sizes and shapes of nuclei and cytoplasm, chromatin clumping irregularities, large and multiple nucleoli, and extreme cellularity. Note the mitosis in metaphase (*arrow*) (both x400).

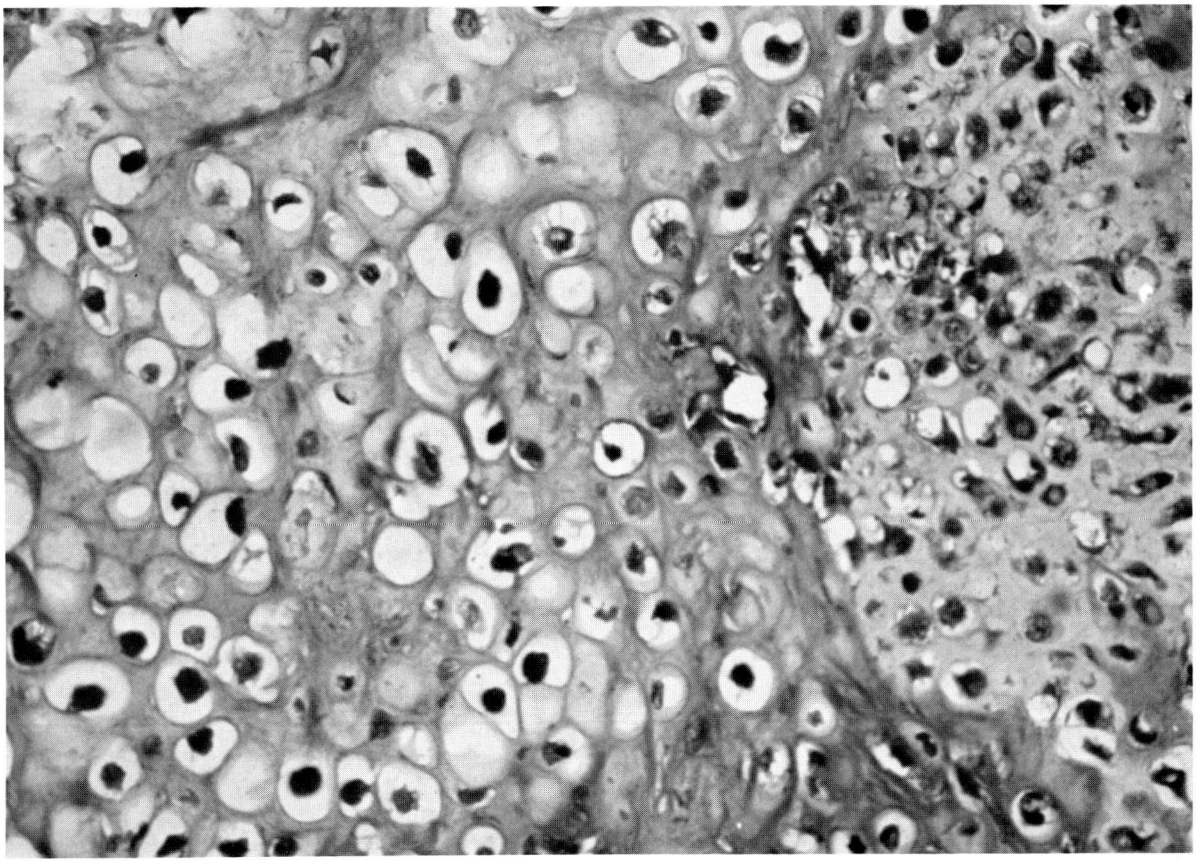

FIG. 8-23

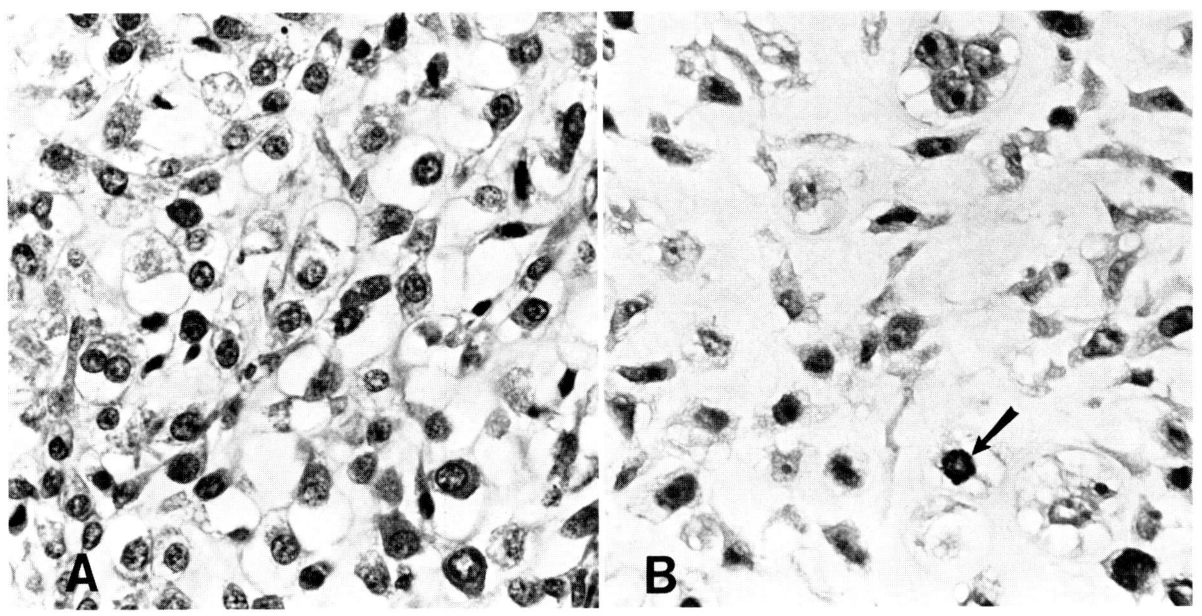

FIG. 8-24

are almost always diagnostic of chondrosarcoma. Very rare exceptions to this rule do occur in certain benign cartilage lesions. Rare cases of synovial chondromatosis may show nuclei in this size range and yet be benign.

2. CYTOPLASMIC CHARACTERISTICS. Cells with prominent cytoplasm showing marked variations in shape are seen in some chondrosarcomas. If cells with long, tapered cytoplasm approaching 30 microns or more are seen, the diagnosis of chondrosarcoma is virtually assured (Fig. 8–20, *A*). Atypical enchondromas may show cells with tapered cytoplasm, but they rarely exceed 15 to 20 microns.

3. MITOSES. Mitoses are rarely, if ever, seen in enchondromas. One mitotic figure per 1 to 2 HPF's is virtually diagnostic of chondrosarcoma provided, of course, that the proliferating cartilage of a callus is ruled out by the appropriate clinical and pathologic parameters.

Cellularity (Viable Nuclei)

Enchondromas generally show between 10 to 40 viable nuclei in one 300x HPF (Figs. 8–41, *A*, 8–42, *A*, and 8–45, *A*). Rare cases of long and flat bone enchondromas will be more cellular and in the range of chondrosarcoma. Chondrosarcomas are usually two to three times more cellular as enchondroma in the range of 40 to 200 viable nuclei per one 300x HPF (Figs. 8–23, 8–24, 8–44, and 8–45, *B*).

Although cellularity cannot be used to diagnose chondrosarcoma with certainty, it is a useful measure, because cases with a low cellularity are usually benign, while the opposite is true of those with a high degree of cellularity. This author uses viable nuclei to measure cellularity since enchondromas may show many cellular spaces without viable nuclei, even in the absence of significant matrix calcification. Therefore, by using viable nuclei rather than cell spaces to determine the parameter of cellularity, it is possible to obtain lower, more biologically significant figures.

Patterns of Tumor Involvement

Patterns of tumor growth and host bone responses to the cartilage may be extremely important to final diagnosis. The following features should be sought.

SIZE OF LOBULES, PERILOBULAR FIBROSIS, AND EXTENT OF BONE REPLACEMENT. Enchondromas usually show small- to moderate-sized lobules of cartilage, usually distinct from one another and separated by a variable amount of normal host bone and marrow (Figs. 8–5, 8–6, 8–13). On the other hand, chondrosarcomas are characterized by incessant growth; the lobules become massive in size, confluent, and may totally replace the host bone in total low-power fields (Figs. 8–30, 8–39, *E*). Between the confluent lobules bands of fibrosis may form (Figs. 8–29, 8–39, *E*). Solitary enchondromas uncommonly show these features. This is not true in Ollier's disease, however.

INFILTRATION BETWEEN HOST BONE TRABECULAE. Chondrosarcoma may infiltrate between host bone trabeculae before the latter can be resorbed or altered by remodeling (Fig. 8–26). This pattern of infiltration is usually seen along the advancing margins of chondrosarcoma and is analogous to the malignant pattern described for osteogenic sarcoma (see Figs. 7–46 and Plates 3, *C* to *G*). In enchondroma the host bone trabeculae are usually resorbed or remodeled in the zones of cartilaginous growth and do not maintain their normal configuration (Figs. 8–5, 8–6, and 8–15). This conforms to what we would expect in a slow growing benign process.

INFILTRATION OF MARROW FAT. Another pattern virtually diagnostic of chondrosarcoma is infiltration and compression of marrow fat by individual cartilage cells along the advancing margins of the tumor (Figs. 8–27, 8–28).

"Borderline" Cartilage Tumor Versus Chondrosarcoma

FIG. 8–25. (*A*) Borderline enchondroma versus Grade I chondrosarcoma by histologic features alone. In actuality the clinical and radiologic features from which this field was taken indicated chondrosarcoma. However, a similar field could have been selected from atypically cellular but clinically benign enchondroma or from patients with Ollier's disease (x250). (*B*) Increased nuclear size and open chromatin network, features of an unequivocal low Grade II chondrosarcoma (x400).

Invasive Patterns of Chondrosarcoma

FIG. 8–26. Chondrosarcoma (*arrow*) infiltrating through the marrow spaces, resulting in entrapment of host lamellar bone spicules. The latter maintain their normal orientation and must be distinguished from the circumferential plates of metaplastic lamellar bone that form around benign cartilage, such as enchondroma (Figs. 8–5, 8–6, and 8–13), parosteal chondroma (Fig. 14–27), and quiescent osteochondroma (Fig. 14–15). Note the normal fatty marrow to the right of the field (x25).

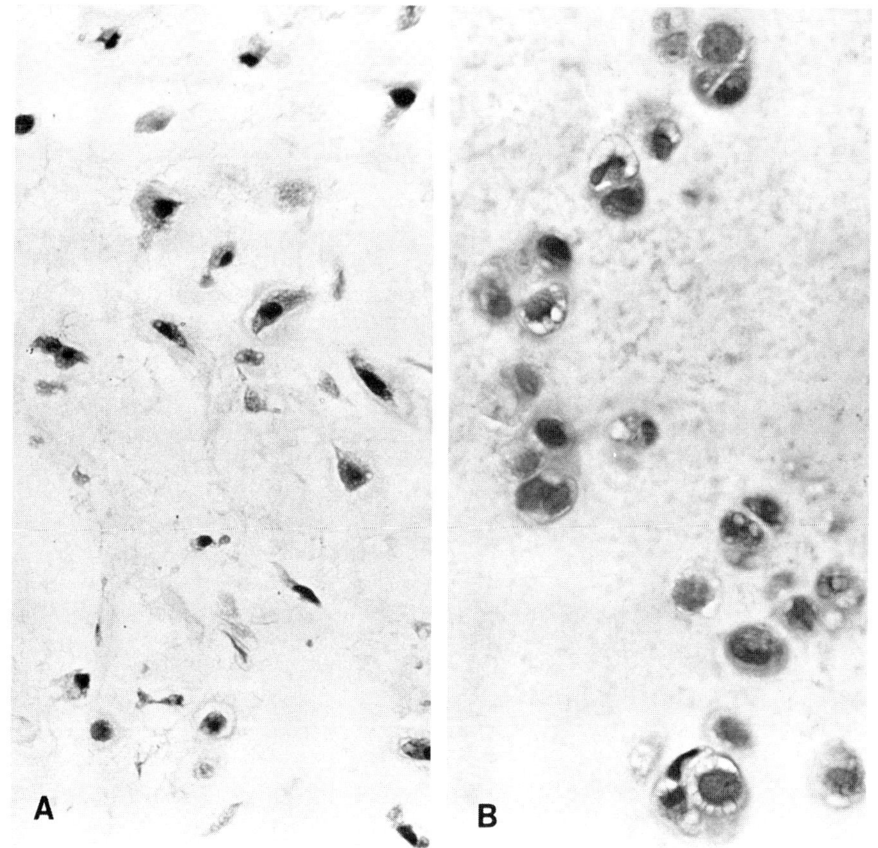

FIG. 8-25

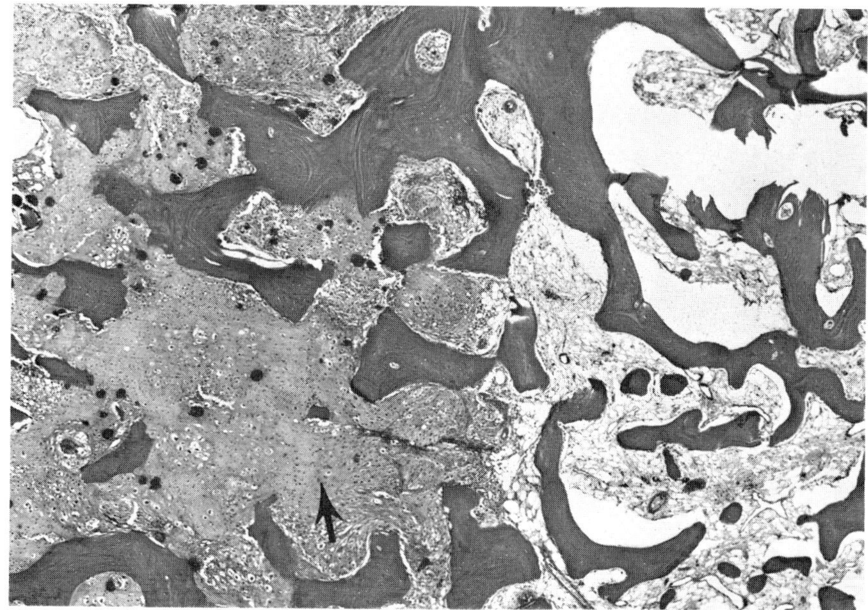
FIG. 8-26

Histopathologic Types of Chondrosarcoma

HYALINE TO FIBRO-MYXOID TYPES. The vast majority of enchondromas show a homogeneous hyaline cartilage matrix with variable degrees of calcification. The low-grade chondrosarcomas may show an identical matrix (Fig. 8–46). However, higher-grade chondrosarcomas will often show focal to extensive and bubbly to myxoid to fibrillar matrix changes or loss of the general homogeneity common to pure hyaline cartilage (Figs. 8–24 and 8–44).

On the other hand, chondroblastomas and chondromyxoid fibromas generally produce a primitive chondroid matrix and little, if any, pure hyaline cartilage. The amount of chondroid and cartilage tissue, in chondromyxoid fibroma and chondroblastoma rarely exceeds more than 75 per cent or 50 per cent, respectively, of the total lesional tissue. In enchondroma and pure chondrosarcoma, between 95 and 100 per cent of the lesional tissue is cartilagenous, if we exclude osseous metaplasia.

CLEAR CELL TYPE. Unni, *et al.*,[21] have described a clear-cell type of chondrosarcoma in 16 patients. This type has distinctive clinical, radiologic, and pathologic features and should be differentiated from the more ordinary type of chondrosarcoma. Their patients ranged in age from 19 to 61 years (average age, 39). Most cases were osteolytic, expansile lesions, most often affecting an end of the femur and humerus, and most often not showing a soft-tissue mass at initial presentation. The tumor is characterized by distinct lobularity both grossly and microscopically and the presence of cells with strikingly clear cytoplasm (Fig. 8–35, *A*). Foci of ordinary chondrosarcoma could be seen in some cases. Other features included foci of osseous metaplasia (Fig. 8–34), minimal to moderate nuclear atypia, fine lines of calcification between tumor cells, osteoclast-like giant cells, and small chondroblastoma-like cells (Fig. 8–35, *B*). In several instances these features led to the erroneous diagnoses of osteoblastoma or chondroblastoma. The principal histologic clue in differentiating clear cell chondrosarcoma from chondroblastoma and osteoblastoma is that neither chondroblastoma nor osteoblastoma possess cells with the distinctive clearing of the cytoplasm, as shown in Figure 8–35, *A*. Although the clear-cell chondrosarcoma is malignant, it behaves with low-grade virulence. It is an extremely important tumor to recognize and to distinguish from chondroblastoma and osteoblastoma.

Secondary Central Chondrosarcoma

The vast majority of secondary central chondrosarcomas arise from enchondromatous rests. The vast majority of reported cases are those in association with Ollier's disease. There are very few cases reported of solitary enchondroma leading to chondrosarcoma. Absolute proof rests with the radiological or pathological demonstration of a typical enchondroma 5 or more years prior to the development of a biologically malignant cartilage tumor. If we adhere to these strict criteria very few such cases have been reported.[4] Lichtenstein and Jaffe[14] support the point of view that it is not uncommon for a chondrosarcoma to evolve from a solitary enchondroma, particularly in a long bone. If central chondrosarcomas are examined carefully for signs of a preexistent enchondroma by reviewing the clinical and specimen radiographs (Figs. 8–49, *A* and *B*, 8–37) and searching numerous microscopic fields for evidence of typical benign cartilage tissues (Figs. 8–49, *C* and *E*, 8–50, *A* and *C*), the incidence of such lesions rises to between approximately 15 and 20 per cent (personal observations).

Chondrosarcomatous transformation of a preexistent benign chondroblastoma or chondromyxoid fibroma is very rare.

GROUP III. "BORDERLINE" CARTILAGE TUMOR: ENCHONDROMA VERSUS GRADE I CHONDROSARCOMA

This author very much supports the view of Coley, Higinbotham, Jaffe, Lichtenstein and Aegeter[1,3,14] that a solitary enchondroma may transform to a chondrosarcoma and, furthermore, that this change may be much more common than would be expected if only the few reported cases with proof of a benign enchondroma 5 or more years prior to malignant transformation are accepted. The reason for my strong support of this view is that in at least six instances I have seen a lesion showing radiologic and histologic evidence strongly supportive of a diagnosis of enchondroma combined with the atypical clinical

---

Invasive Patterns of Chondrosarcoma

FIG. 8–27. Advancing edge of chondrosarcoma that shows invasion of marrow fat. Note the clear entrapment of host lamellar bone using partial polarized light (x125).

FIG. 8–28. The chondrosarcoma cells insinuate and infiltrate between the fat cells and compress them. This type of fat infiltration is not seen in benign hyaline cartilage tumors (x250).

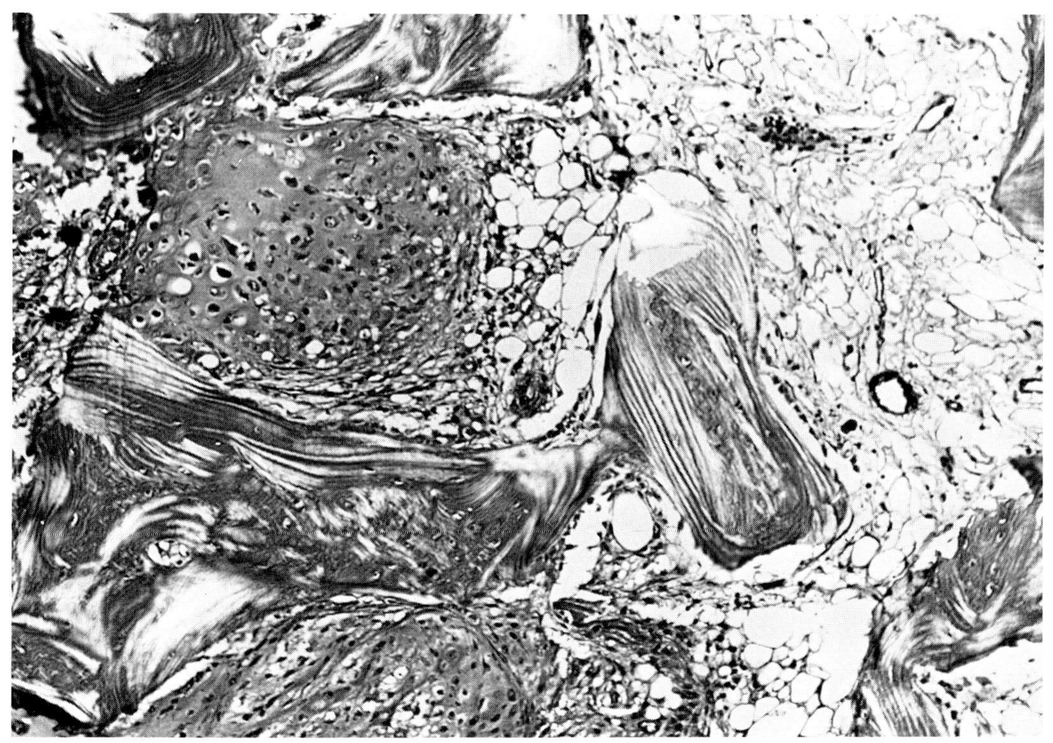

FIG. 8-27

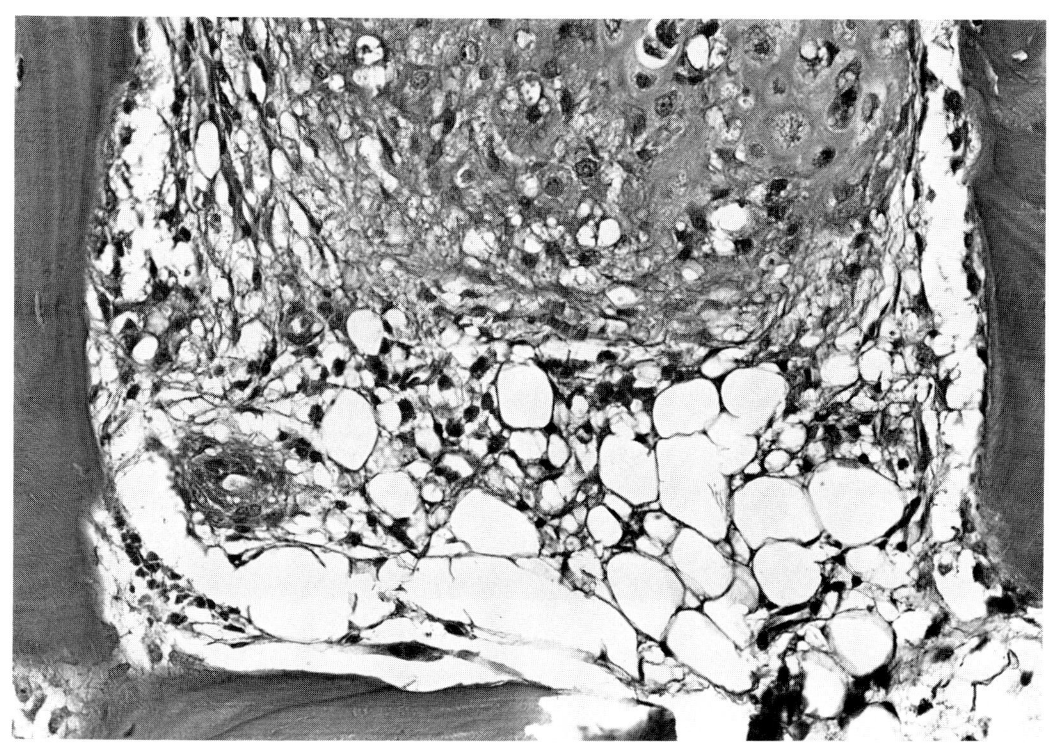

FIG. 8-28

and radiographic features of a chondrosarcoma; these lesions have invariably been associated with biologic evidence of chondrosarcoma within months to a couple of years or have shown evidence of frank chondrosarcomatous, fibrosarcomatous, or osteosarcomatous transformation at the initial biopsy. In only one instance was there a favorable outcome. This patient presented with pain (an ominous sign in relation to cartilage lesions of long bones) and a radiograph of a typical enchondromatous lesion (Fig. 8–36) without any other radiological feature to suggest malignancy. Curettage of the lesion showed chondromatous tissues lacking both anaplasia and invasion of fat. Some lobules were surrounded by plates of lamellar bone. Postoperatively the patient developed a fracture. Two years later the fracture is healing well, with no evidence of sarcomatous transformation (Fig. 8–36). Although the feature of pain was an ominous sign, there were no other features to support a diagnosis of malignancy. Therefore, pain alone is insufficient for a diagnosis of chondrosarcoma, as should be expected.

Clinical Features

The data on "borderline" cartilage tumors of long and flat bones pertain to 27 cases.[4,11,12] (Seven cases are unpublished observations of my own.) All but one of these cases developed frank chondrosarcoma in less than 5 years from initial biopsy. In Coley and Higinbotham's series with long-term follow-up, 10 of 17 patients subsequently died of local or metastatic disease.

Age and Sex. The patients ranged in age from 11 to 71. The mean age was 43. The incidence of females to males was 1.2 : 1.

Site of Involvement. In 13 cases, the femur; in seven, the tibia; in four, the humerus, and one each in the fibula, rib, and ilium. The proximal portion of the long bones was involved more frequently than the shaft or distal end.

Symptoms. The vast majority of patients presented with pain. At first the pain was insidious and intermittent. It gradually intensified and became constant.

Radiologic Features

Basically, these lesions present with one of two features: either as a typical enchondroma with an additional atypical component or with features more in keeping with a chondrosarcoma but lacking a soft-tissue mass or periosteal reaction. Those cases that begin with features of the first may transform to the second in 1 to 2 years, if merely followed by radiographic examinations.

Type I: Borderline Radiographic Lesion-Enchondroma Type With an Additional Ominous Component

The features of this type are as follows:

1. There is the presence of a well demarcated lesion with homogeneous stippled, ringlike, spheroidal to short linear densities (Figs. 3–19, 8–37, *A*, 8–38) identical to that of which we have previously seen in unequivocal enchondromas (Fig. 8–10).
2. There is an additional "ominous" component consisting of focal lysis (Figs. 3–19, 8–37, *A*, 8–38, *arrows*). There may be focal changes in the homogeneous density of the enchondromatous lesion, or "scalloping" of the cortex.
3. There is no soft-tissue mass or periosteal reaction.
4. Significant focal or diffuse cortical thickening.
5. If the lesion is considered benign, follow-up radiographic studies will often show gradual loss of the central enchondromatous lesion and replacement by an expansive, less well-defined lesion with irregular "fluffy," "washed out" to "windblown" patterns of calcification (Fig. 3–19, 8–37, *B*), lysis, or both. In addition, there may be the development of a soft-tissue mass and ominous periosteal densities pathognomonic of chondrosarcomatous transformation (Fig. 8–37, *B, arrow*).

Histologic and specimen radiographic analysis of the lesion described above usually, but not always, shows an enchondroma in association with malignant

(*Text continues on p. 192.*)

Chondrosarcoma

FIG. 8–29. Malignant cartilage lobules are often separated from each other by bands of fibrous tissue. This is a clue to malignancy. The degree of nuclear anaplasia in this case is at least high Grade II (x250).

FIG. 8–30. Whole low-power fields filled with cartilage are common to chondrosarcoma and rare to benign solitary enchondroma. Multiple enchondromatosis (Ollier's disease) may show this degree of cartilage replacement of low-power fields, however. This lesion corresponds to the Grade I plus chondrosarcoma shown in Figure 8–21 (x40).

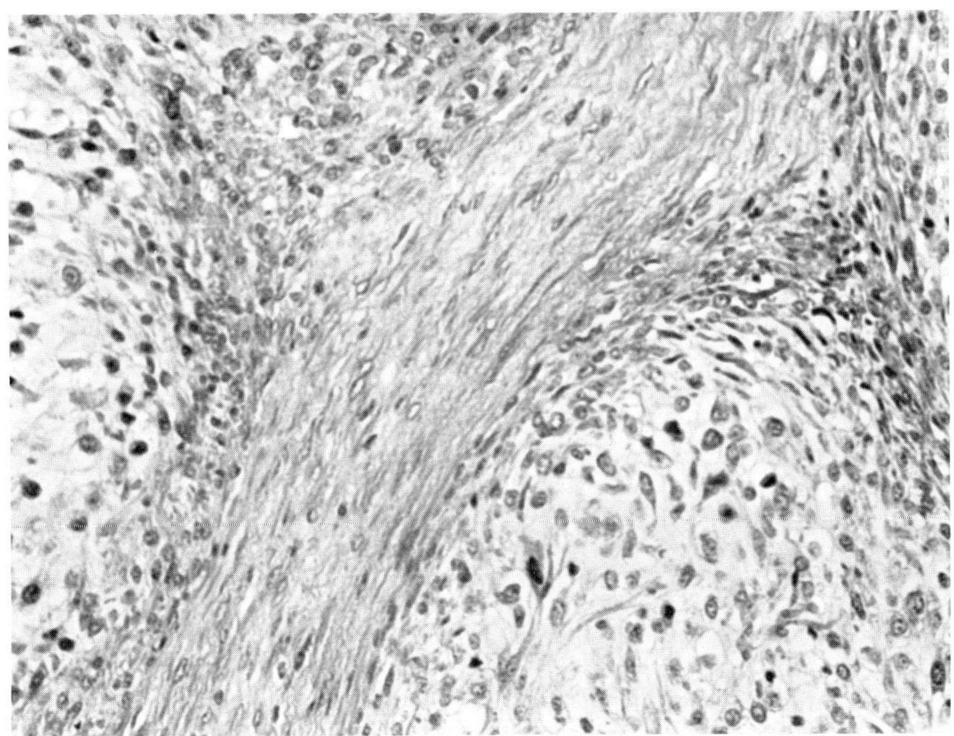

FIG. 8-29

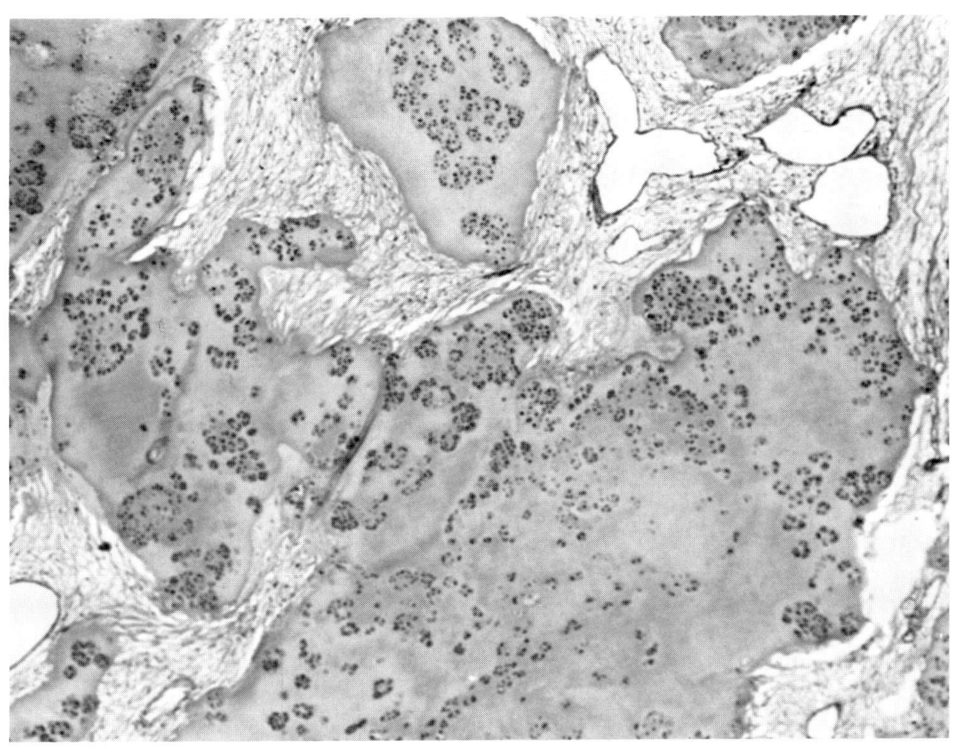

FIG. 8-30

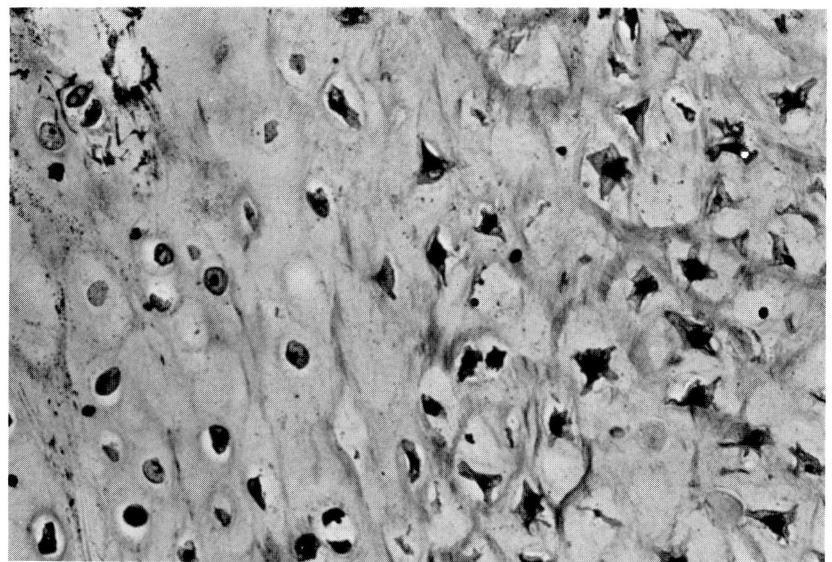

FIG. 8-31

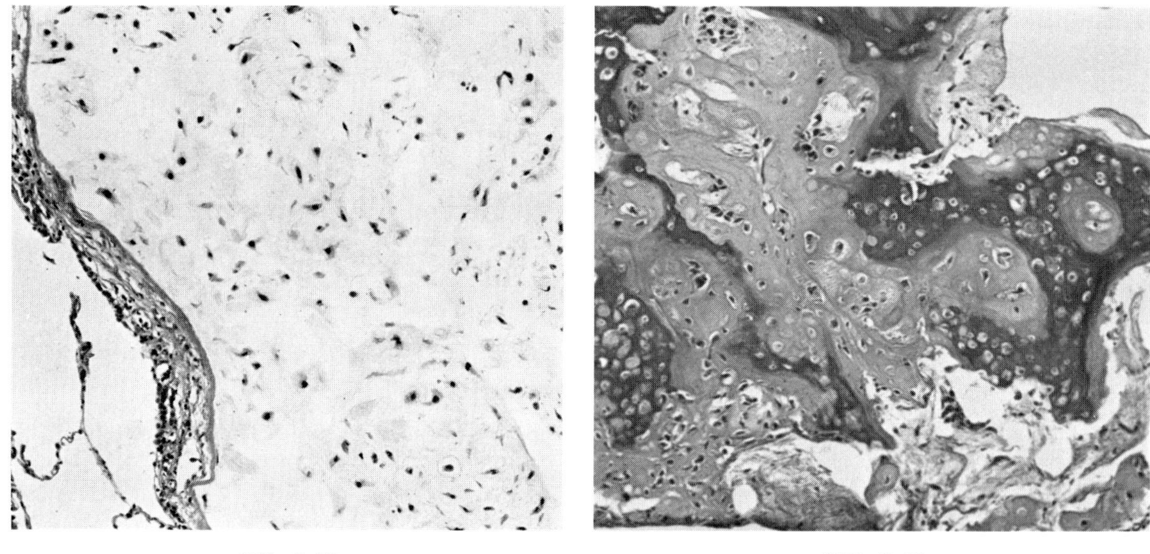

FIG. 8-32 FIG. 8-33

"Borderline" Cartilage Tumor and Chondrosarcoma

FIG. 8-31. Borderline cartilage tumor. Lesions with this degree of cellularity and nuclear atypia are borderline lesions by cytology alone. There is an absence of unequivocal anaplasia. Diagnosing such lesions as enchondromatous or chondrosarcomatous tumors must depend on an assessment of clinical and radiologic features and noncytologic patterns of pathologic involvement (x250).

FIG. 8-32. Grade I chondrosarcoma metastatic to lung. This illustration shows that biologically virulent chondrosarcoma may show surprisingly little in the way of anaplasia. This patient has subsequently succumbed to his lung metastases. The nuclei are small and rounded to ovoid. The most ominous feature is the number of cells per unit area. Compare this feature with that shown in Figure 8-41 *A*, of an unequivocal enchondroma taken at the same power (x125).

FIG. 8-33. Ossification of chondrosarcoma. Quite often the cartilage of chondrosarcoma can be converted to bone. The bone is woven and *not* lamellar. The presence of bony "metaplasia" can cause confusion with osteosarcoma. For the diagnosis of osteosarcoma an area must be found in which the bone must form directly from an undifferentiated malignant stroma without first passing through a cartilaginous phase (x125). Figure 8-51, *C* and *D*, shows the essential differences between a chondrosarcoma and osteosarcoma.

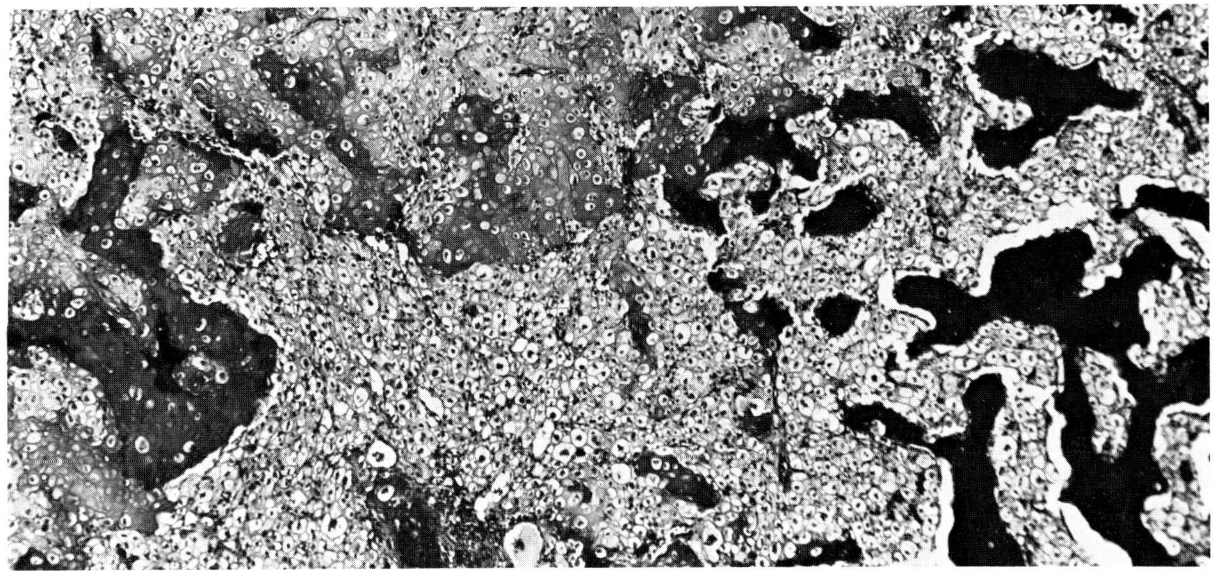

FIG. 8-34

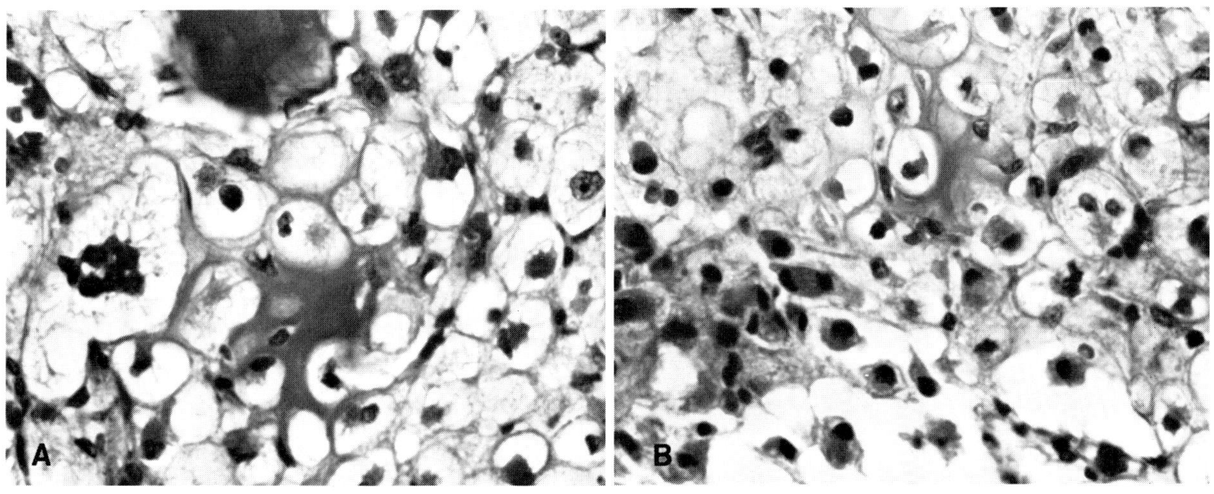

FIG. 8-35

Clear Cell Chondrosarcoma

FIG. 8-34. Clear cell chondrosarcoma. Low-power view of a clear cell chondrosarcoma with extensive bony "metaplasia". Fields such as these may be mistaken for osteoblastoma. Osteoblastomas do not contain cartilage or clear cells, however (H and E, x60) (Figs. 8–34 and 8–35 are from a slide, courtesy of Dr. David Dahlin, Mayo Clinic, Rochester, Minn.).

FIG. 8-35. (*A*) The clear cell chondrocytes that characterize this tumor. The nuclei usually show Grade I plus Grade II anaplasia (x500). (*B*) Foci of small, rounded cells with a granular cytoplasm (most are seen in the bottom of illustration.) Fields such as these may be confused with chondroblastoma. Chondroblastomas do not show masses of clear cell chondrocytes common to the above tumor (x400).

transformation. The enchondroma portion corresponds to feature number 1. Some endosteal scalloping and bone "expansion" is possible in a pure benign enchondroma, but most cases with these features have chondrosarcomatous foci. Although these latter two features (endosteal scalloping and "expansion") are the least reliable radiographic signs of malignancy in a cartilage tumor, if they are present the lesion should be placed in a "borderline" category, because of the probability that it is malignant, at least focally. A large area of lysis in the midst of what otherwise shows typical densifications of an enchondroma usually corresponds to the actual area of malignant transformation. Significant thickening of the cortices is also a highly ominous sign, because microscopic examination of these areas usually reveals insidious invasion of haversian systems by chondrosarcoma. The bone is thickening as a reactive response to infiltrating tumor.

Type II: Borderline Chondrosarcoma-Like Radiographic Lesions

Those "borderline" lesions that show no radiographic signs of absolute malignancy (soft-tissue mass) but that otherwise show the other radiologic features previously discussed under unequivocal chondrosarcoma are, in my experience, incipient chondrosarcomas, provided that biopsy shows it is truly a pure cartilage-producing lesion. On rare occasions there are some benign lesions that can have a "borderline" chondrosarcoma-like radiographic pattern, such as a bone infarct. Therefore, diagnosis of these cases must be backed up with pathologic confirmation.

The radiographic features of Type II "borderline" chondrosarcoma-like lesions are as follows:

1. The lesion usually has expanded the bone (Fig. 8-39, *A* and *B*).
2. It has either a lobulated lytic pattern (Fig. 8-39, *B*) or, more commonly, a fuzzier, less well delineated to "windblown" pattern of calcification (Fig. 8-51), compared to enchondroma (Fig. 8-10).
3. Scalloping of the endosteal side of the cortex may be present.
4. There is an absence of soft-tissue mass or periosteal reaction.
5. The cortices may show focal thickening.

Approximately 10 per cent of chondrosarcomas and enchondromas can be located in the epiphysis. The epiphyseal, lytic, expansive to calcified chondrosarcoma can simulate giant cell tumor or chondroblastoma on radiographs (Fig. 8-39, *A* and *B*). If biopsy shows a tumor entirely composed of cartilage, these latter benign tumors are virtually eliminated from contention. In the case illustrated, (Fig. 8-39) the diagnosis of atypical borderline cartilage tumor was made and en-bloc excision recommended. However, the lesion was treated as an enchondroma and curet-

Enchondroma and Type I Borderline Cartilage Tumors

FIG. 8-36 *Left:* Enchondroma. This patient presented with bone pain, placing her in a borderline cartilage tumor category. However, the radiograph shows a well-circumscribed area of punctate calcifications without zones of lysis, periosteal reaction, or soft-tissue mass. Curettage showed cartilage lobules, many of which were surrounded by plates of lamellar bone. *Right:* Post-curettage, the patient sustained a fracture. Two years later the bone was healing well without evidence of recurrence. With three years of follow-up, bone healing is nearly complete (not illustrated).

FIG. 8-37. Borderline cartilage tumor by radiograph. (*A*) This radiograph shows evidence of a central enchondroma or bone infarct. However, it is surrounded by ominous zones of lysis (*arrows*), an immediate clue to malignant transformation. The clinical diagnosis was benign enchondroma and no biopsy was taken. However, this must be regarded as an ominous type I borderline cartilage tumor. (*B*) Two years later the diagnosis of chondrosarcoma is now obvious. Note the bone expansion, windblown pattern of calcifications, periosteal reaction, and soft-tissue mass (*arrow*). The formerly benign enchondroma pattern is completely gone. Had the patient presented at this time without benefit of prior radiograph, the diagnosis would surely have been primary chondrosarcoma. In all so-called "primary" chondrosarcomas the radiologic and pathologic material should be carefully searched for telltale signs of a preexistent enchondroma. This latter radiograph shows the conversion of a type I borderline tumor to a frank chondrosarcoma radiographic pattern. If the above lesion had not broken out of the bone it should be considered as a very ominous type II borderline cartilage tumor radiographic pattern.

FIG. 8-38. Type I borderline cartilage tumor by radiograph. This radiograph shows an unequivocal extensive enchondroma involving a large portion of the shaft. Note the ominous zone of lysis with focal cortical scalloping (*arrow*). Biopsy from the lytic area showed Grade II chondrosarcoma. Biopsy of the stippled areas of calcification showed typical enchondroma with plates of lamellar bone surrounding bland cartilage lobules. Thus, we have another example of chondrosarcoma arising in a preexistent enchondroma. Please refer to Fig. 3-19 for another classic example of a chondrosarcoma arising from an enchondroma.

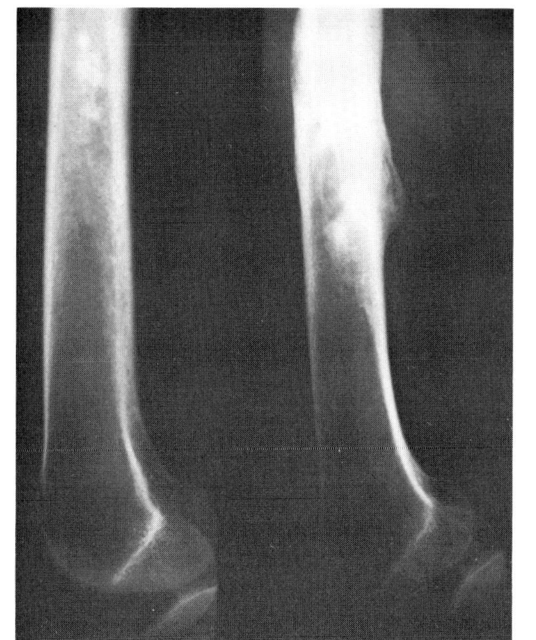

FIG. 8-36

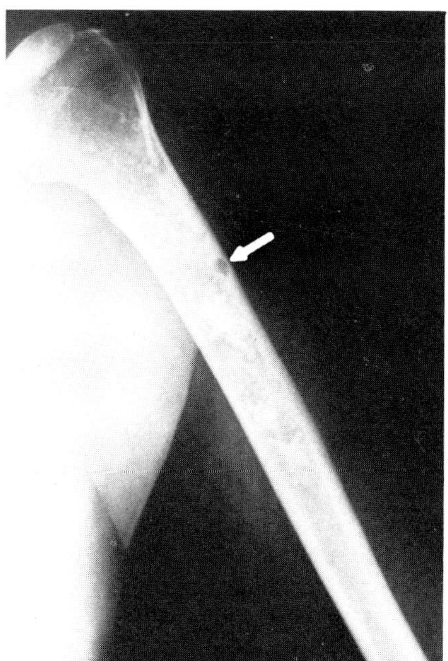

FIG. 8-38

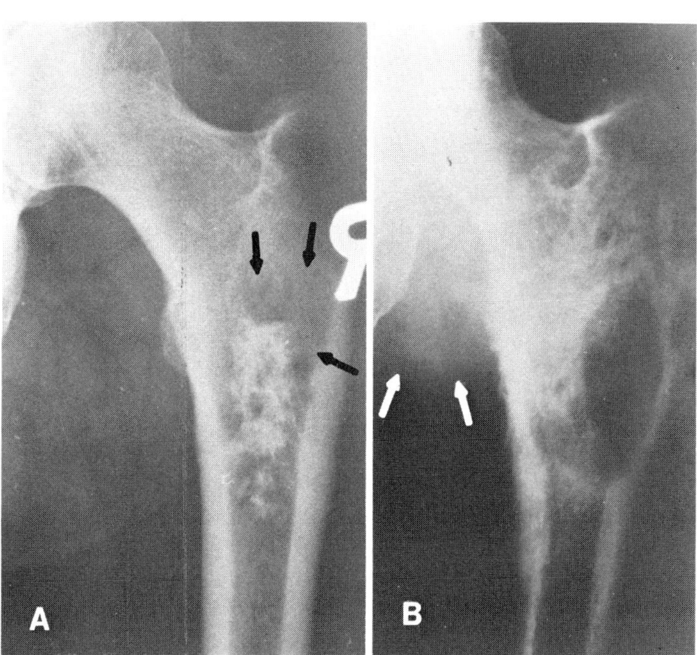

FIG. 8-37

ted and packed with bone chips (Fig. 8-39, *A*). One year later it recurred and even further expanded the bone, thus expressing its biologic malignant potential (Fig. 8-39, *B*). The lesion was removed en-bloc and showed features consistent with a Grade I chondrosarcoma (Figs. 8-39, *C, D, E,* and *F*). Follow-up has been for only one year and there has been no recurrence. In a very similar case of a 22-year-old female, this author reviewed a lytic expansive lesion of the distal femoral epiphysis that produced pure hyaline cartilage without objective anaplasia. It was misdiagnosed as a chondroblastoma. One year later the patient developed pain and swelling in the knee. Biopsy revealed invasion of synovium and capsular tissues by a Grade I chondrosarcoma histologically identical to the primary lesion. Amputation had to be performed. Had the lesion been correctly diagnosed at initial presentation, an en-bloc excision could well have been curative. These cases suggest that lytic, expansive intraosseous lesions of adults composed entirely of cartilage without objective anaplasia and which are initially confined to the bone are best treated with an adequate en-bloc excision or cryosurgery, because they appear to behave with low-grade biologic malignancy. Unless they are diagnosed as consistent with Grade I chondrosarcoma, they are apt to be treated as benign.

Histopathology Seen In Association With Types I and II "Borderline" Central Cartilage Tumors

Correlating histopathology with the radiographic features of Types I and II "borderline" central cartilage tumors is essential to accurate diagnosis. This is a complex group of tumors in which one of the following diagnoses or combinations of diagnoses are possible: enchondroma, and/or chondrosarcoma, and/or chondrosarcoma with fibro- or osteosarcomatous transformation. It is necessary to obtain biopsies from any enchondroma-like, chondrosarcoma-like, and focal lytic areas. It is also necessary to review the radiographs pre- and post-biopsy to be certain that the representative and most ominous areas were biopsied. In order to visualize low-power patterns that are important for diagnosis, the largest fragments of tissue as possible (preferably large wedge biopsies) should be obtained at surgery and submitted whole for section. Only in this way will it be possible to ascertain the relationships of the cartilage lobules to the surrounding host bone and to increase the chances of finding invasion of marrow fat by proliferating chondrosarcoma cells.

In the previous section dealing with unequivocal chondrosarcoma, the histopathology of objective cartilage anaplasia was shown in Figs. 8-21 to 8-24). In dealing with histologically "borderline" cartilage tumors, diagnosis depends heavily upon correlating clinical and pathologic features (see Figs. 8-39–8-47). These illustrations show the subtle, almost insensible gradations between typical bland enchondromas and more cellular enchondromas that overlap with biologically malignant Grade I chondrosarcomas, and also compare and contrast these examples with those cases that show objective anaplasia. This array of illustrations is, therefore, meant to aid in diagnosis and differential diagnosis of a specific cartilage tumor. It should become clear from an analysis of these illustrations that it is virtually impossible, on the basis of cytologic criteria alone, to differentiate an atypically cellular enchondroma from a Grade I chondrosarcoma.

Diagnoses of Types I and II "Borderline" Central Cartilage Tumors

Possible Diagnoses in Relation to Type I (Enchondroma-Like With Additional Ominous Component) Radiographic Lesions

ENCHONDROMA WITH CHONDROSARCOMATOUS TRANSFORMATION. For this diagnosis typical areas of enchondroma (Figs. 8-5, 8-6, 8-11, 8-13) must be

(*Text continues on p. 200.*)

Type II "Borderline" Cartilage Tumor

FIG. 8-39. Type II borderline cartilage tumor by radiograph. (*A*) This 22-year-old female patient presented with pain in the upper arm. Curettage was read as enchondroma and packed with bone chips. (*B*) Some $1\frac{1}{2}$ years later the lesion has expanded the epiphyseal end of the proximal humerus. It has a lytic, bubbly, trabeculated appearance. There is neither an obvious soft-tissue mass nor ominous periosteal reaction. A rebiopsy was performed that showed cartilage with no obvious anaplasia. Nevertheless, its behavior was that of a low-grade chondrosarcoma and en-bloc resection was performed. (*C*) The humeral head is replaced by lobules of hyaline cartilage. It had focally eroded the cortex and was covered in places by only a thin rim of periosteum. (*D*) Specimen radiograph of the tumor showing focal calcifications. (*E*) Low-power view showing huge lobules of cartilage separated by bands of fibrous tissue, a sign most consistent with chondrosarcoma. (*F*) The cartilage was cellular but did not show unequivocal cytologic anaplasia (x500). This case illustrates the slow but incessant growth of an extremely well-differentiated or Grade I chondrosarcoma.

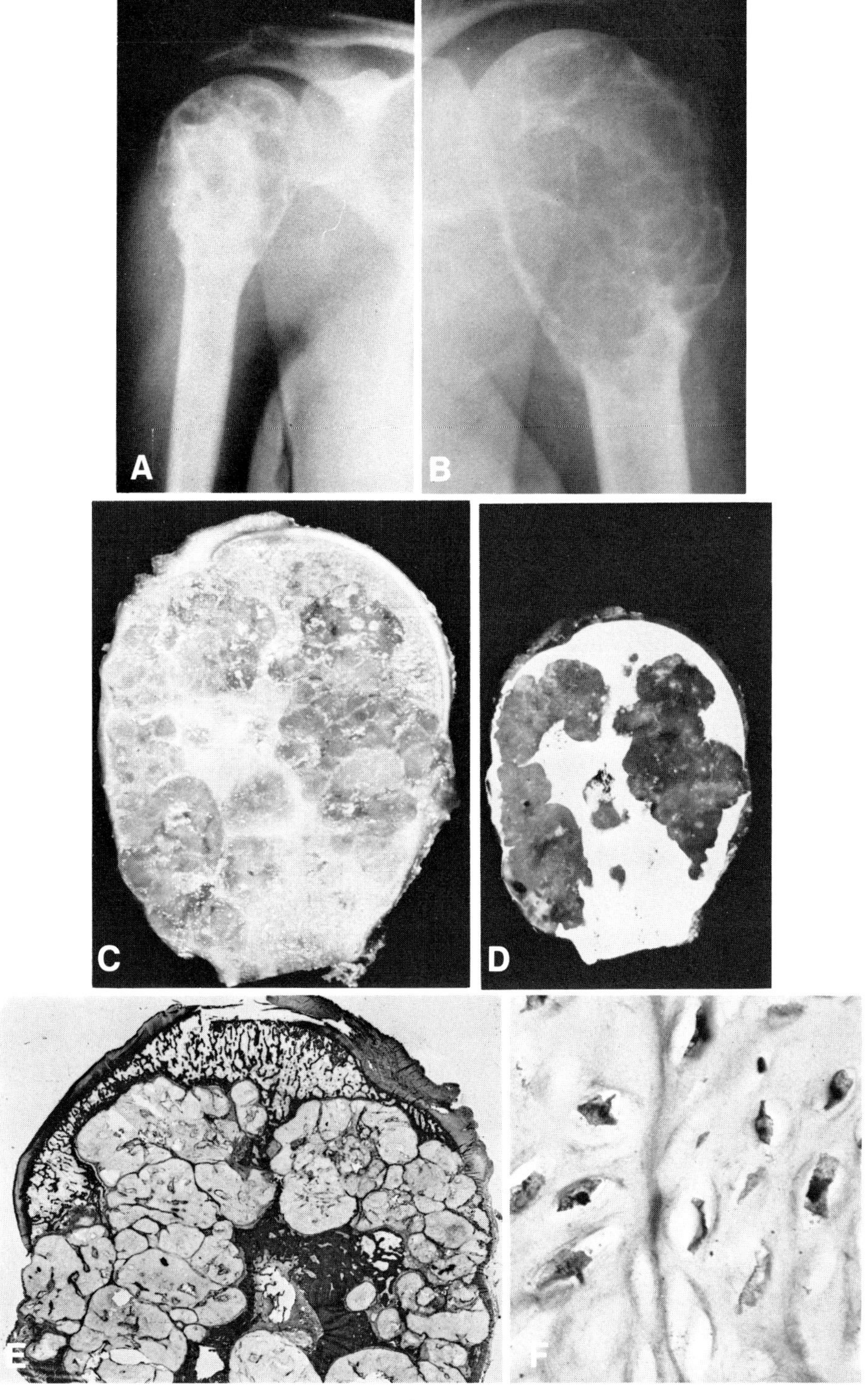

FIG. 8-39

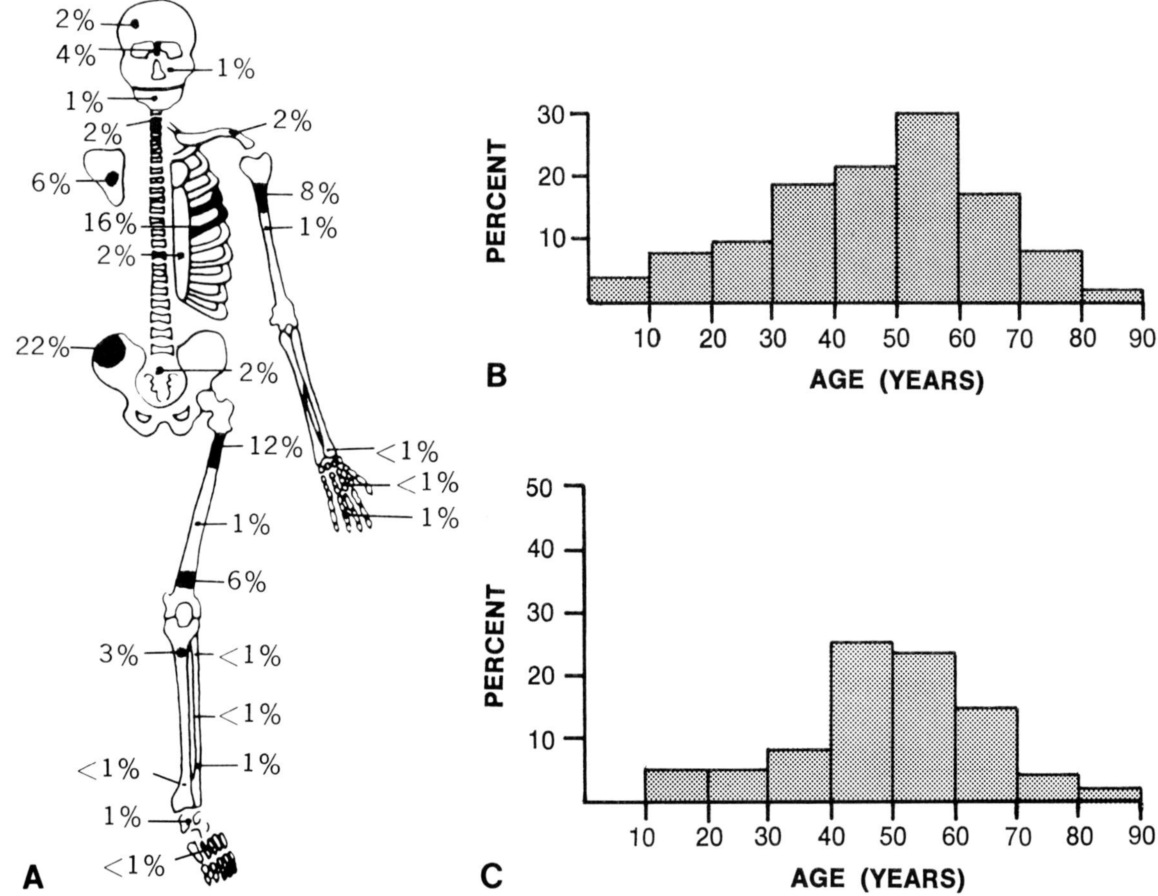

FIG. 8-40. Age distribution of patients with central "primary" chondrosarcoma (325 cases). (*A*) Primary chondrosarcoma. Frequency of areas of involvement in 332 patients. Male: female incidence, 1.6: 1. (*B*) Average age 47 years, male: female incidence, 1:8:1. Data obtained from Dahlin, Barnes and Catto, and O'Neal and Ackerman [6,18,2]. (*C*) Age distribution in patients with chondrosarcoma of the hand and foot (45 cases). Average age 50 years, male: female incidence 1.25: 1. (Data obtained from Dahlin and Salvador, Gottschalk *et al.* and Culver, *et al.* (Mirra, J., Bullough, P., and Freiberger, R.: Orthopedic Diseases, Part II. New York, Famous Teachings in Modern Medicine, MedCom, Inc., © 1972)

Enchondroma Versus "Borderline" Cartilage Tumor

FIG. 8-41. (*A*) Enchondroma with 5-year benign clinical course. Note the plates of lamellar bone (*right*), hypocellularity, and small, round nuclei (x125). (*B*) This field shows increased cellularity and atypically shaped nuclei and cytoplasm. Fields such as these are borderline and not unequivocally malignant (x125). However, search of other fields from this patient showed low grade II chondrosarcoma. The histology and radiographic features were diagnostic of low-grade chondrosarcoma. Nevertheless, within 3 months of en-bloc resection, this seemingly innocuous lesion metastasized to the lungs, eventually leading to the patient's demise (Fig. 8–32).

FIG. 8-42. (*A*) Medium-power fields of an enchondroma with long-term benign course (x250). (*B*) Medium-power field of a histologically borderline cartilage tumor with unequivocal radiographic and clinical evidence to support a diagnosis of Grade I chondrosarcoma (x250). The only essential difference from the former illustration is the increased number of chondrocytes per unit area.

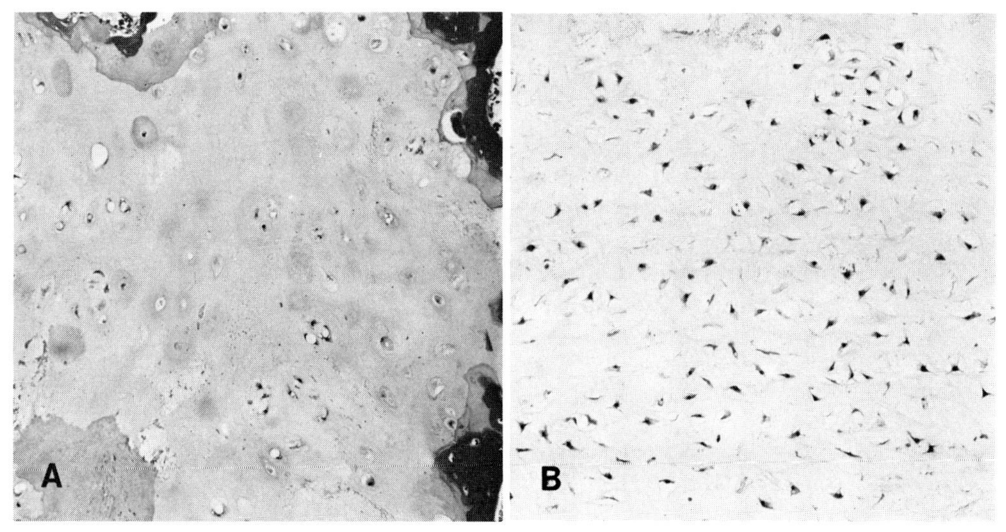

FIG. 8-41

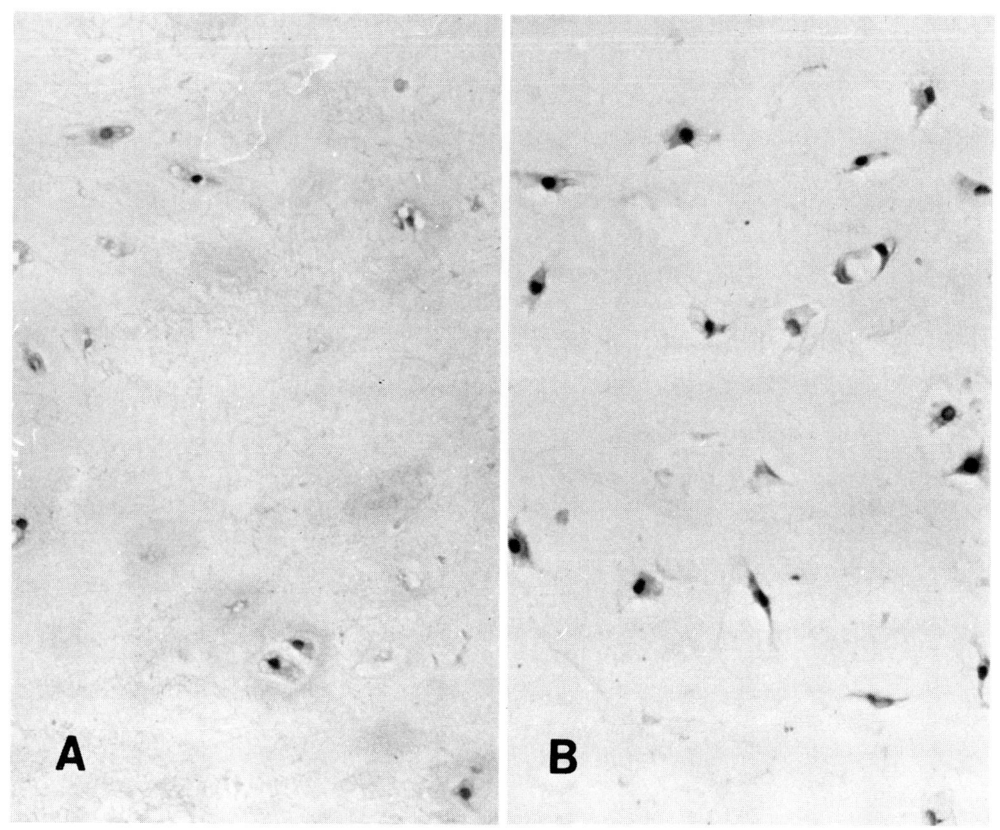

FIG. 8-42

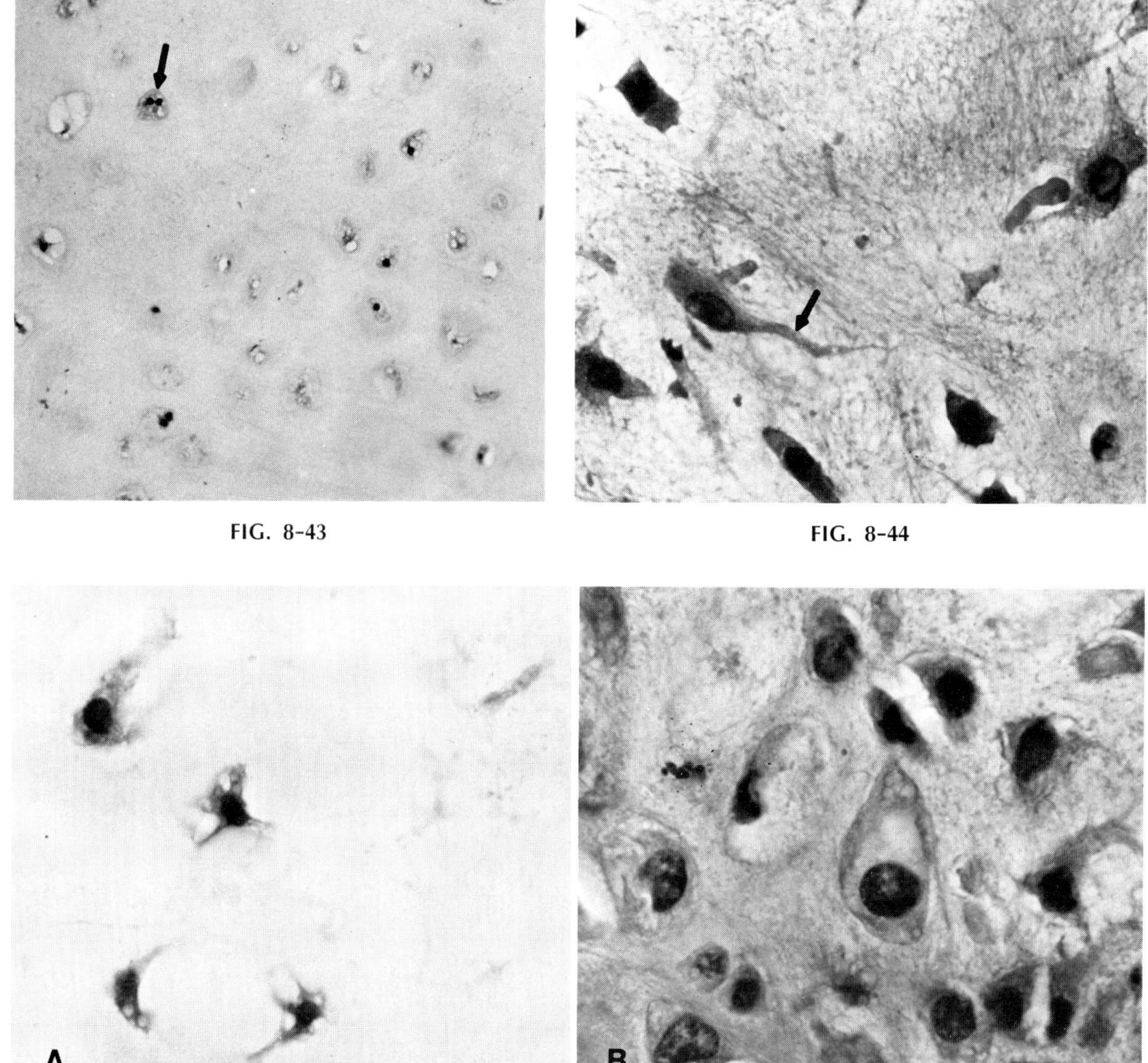

FIG. 8-43

FIG. 8-44

FIG. 8-45

Enchondroma Versus Chondrosarcoma

FIG. 8-43. Enchondroma with a 3-year benign clinical course following curettage. This lesion was relatively hypocellular in regard to the numbers of viable nuclei. An occasional double nucleus was seen (*arrow*) but fewer than one per medium-power field. The finding of an occasional double nucleus is not diagnostic of chondrosarcoma (x250).

FIG. 8-44. Grade II chondrosarcoma. Unequivocal cytologic cartilage anaplasia is characterized by hypercellularity, bizarre cell aggregates, enlarged hyperchromatic nuclei, and occasionally, long, eosinophilic cytoplasmic processes (*arrow*) (x1000).

FIG. 8-45. (*A*) Enchondroma versus Grade I chondrosarcoma nuclei. Although this illustration shows the high-power features of an enchondroma versus a well-differentiated Grade I chondrosarcoma, the patient from which this field was selected had a benign enchondroma (x1000). (*B*) Unequivocal histologic high Grade II chondrosarcoma. The nuclei are at least double the size in length and width and much more voluminous, compared to the nuclei in (*A*). The chromatin is clearly clumped, visible and nuclear size and shape varies considerably from cell to cell. The cytoplasm shows similar variations in size and shape. Compare the marked increase in cellularity of (*B*) with (*A*) (both, x1000).

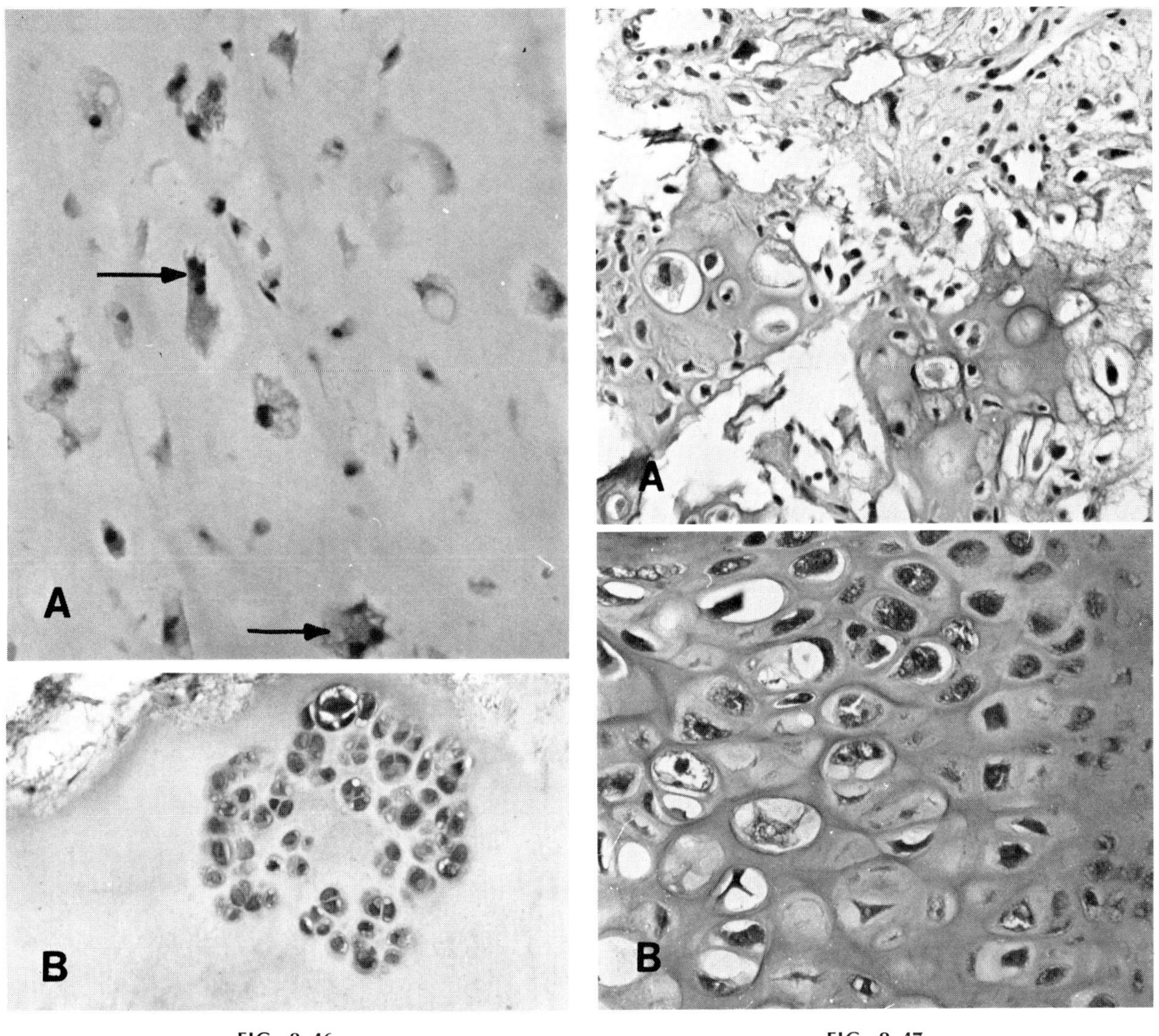

FIG. 8-46 FIG. 8-47

Grade II Chondrosarcomas

FIG. 8-46. (*A*) Low Grade II chondrosarcoma. Although the nuclei are small, the variations in cytoplasm, occasional plump nuclei, triple nuclei (*arrows*), and cellularity are unequivocally anaplastic features (x400). (*B*) Low Grade II chondrosarcoma. Some of the nuclei are too enlarged to be benign in relation to a solitary, long bone cartilage tumor (x250).

FIG. 8-47. (*A*) and (*B*) Unequivocal low and high Grade II chondrosarcomas. The size of the nuclei, cellularity, random distribution of cells, and unusual cytoplasmic characteristics are anaplastic features (A x250, B x400).

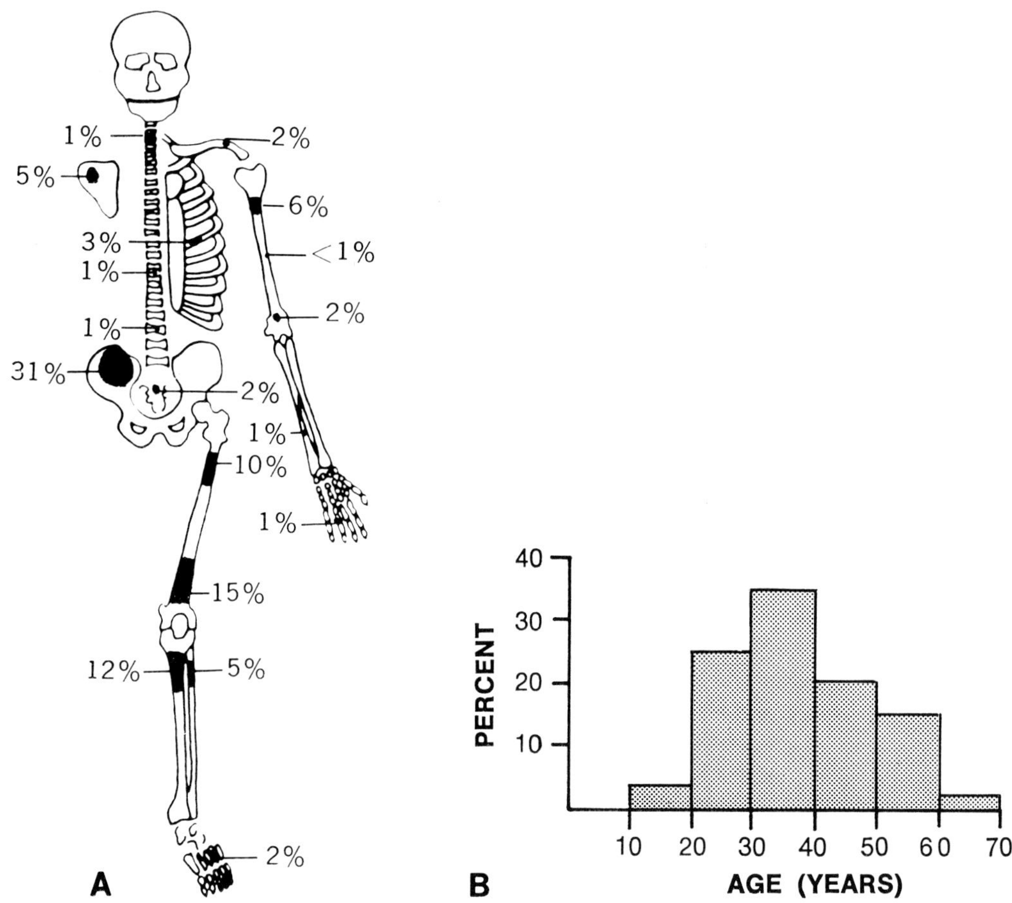

FIG. 8-48. (*A*) Secondary chondrosarcoma. Frequency of areas of involvement in 95 patients. Multiple exostoses (33 cases), solitary exostoses (23 cases), solitary enchondroma (10 cases), multiple enchondroma (29 cases). Male:female incidence, 1.8:1. (*B*) Age distribution of patients with secondary chondrosarcoma [multiple osteochondromatosis (21 cases), osteochondroma (13 cases), Ollier's disease (6 cases)]. Average age; 38 years (Data obtained from Dahlin, Coley, *et al.*, O'Neal, *et al.*, and Barnes, *et al.*[6,4,18,2]. (Mirra, J., Bullough, P., and Freiberger, R.: Orthopedic Diseases, Part IIa New York, Famous Teachings in Modern Medicine, MedCom, Inc., © 1972).

found in association with objective cartilage anaplasia or frank invasion of marrow fat (Figs. 8-27, 8-28).

ENCHONDROMA WITH CHONDROSARCOMA AND FURTHER TRANSFORMATION TO A FIBRO- OR OSTEOSARCOMA. This combination is shown in Figures 8-49, *A-F,* 8-50, *A-C.* Refer to p. 201 for discussion.

ENCHONDROMA ONLY. This is unusual in association with Type I lesions. If there is absolutely no evidence of cytologic or other histologic patterns of malignancy, the diagnosis of chondrosarcoma may not be possible. Such cases are, however, suspect and must be followed up very closely. If curettage or cryosurgery is performed post-biopsy and the lesion recurs, in this author's opinion it should be treated as a biologically malignant lesion and the treatment tailored to the histopathologic findings at recurrence.

Possible Diagnoses in Relation to Type II (Chondrosarcoma-Like) Radiographic Lesions

CHONDROSARCOMA. Cartilage tumors with these radiographic features usually show objective Grade I plus to Grade II anaplasia.

CHONDROSARCOMA WITH ENCHONDROMA. Although the lesion shown in Figure 8-37, *B* was almost totally replaced by a Grade II chondrosarcoma, sections from the center of the lesion showed remnants of the enchondroma seen in Figure 8–37, *A*. Enchondroma remnants are typified by islands of bland cartilage partially to completely encompassed by plates of lamellar to woven-lamellar bone (Figs. 8–6, 8–13). Type I lesions can transform to type II (Fig. 8–37, *A* and *B*).

CHONDROSARCOMA WITH FIBRO- OR OSTEOSARCOMATOUS TRANSFORMATION. These tumors will show a mixture of low-grade chondrosarcoma and spindle-cell fibrosarcoma or osteosarcoma (Figs. 8–51, *A–D*). The osteosarcoma that follows in the wake of a chondrosarcoma can be differentiated from primary osteosarcoma by the fact that these tumors present in a much older age group and that the radiographs and histology show predominant features of a preexistent chondrosarcoma (Fig. 8–51, *A* and *B*).

ENCHONDROMA WITH CHONDROSARCOMA IN ASSOCIATION WITH TRANSFORMATION TO A FIBRO- OR OSTEOSARCOMA. These are similar to the previous examples, with the additional added component of an unequivocal enchondroma (Figs. 8–49, *A–F*, and 8–50, *A–C*).

In summary, from a review of personal cases and those in the literature, most "borderline" intraosseous cartilage tumors of adulthood are in truth chondrosarcomas or chondrosarcoma engrafted upon enchondroma. Approximately 10 per cent may show focal transformation to highly lethal fibro- and osteosarcomas.

Suggested Workup and Treatment

This author would suggest that the following be done in dealing with patients showing radiographic evidence of a borderline central cartilage tumor:

1. The clinician should obtain tomograms to guide biopsy. Biopsy (preferably large wedge biopsy) should include areas that are lytic or areas that do not conform to the typical radiographic appearance of enchondroma. These biopsies should be labeled in relation to the radiographic lesion. Enchondroma-like areas should also be biopsied, appropriately labeled, and then submitted separately.
2. The pathologist should review and correlate the slide material, symptoms, age of patient, and pre- and post-operative radiographs.
3. If the lesion shows Grade II anaplasia and is confined to bone, an en-bloc excision or cryosurgery may be feasible. If the tumor shows a Grade III chondrosarcoma or foci of fibro- to osteosarcomatous transformation, more radical procedures must be employed.
4. If the lesion is a borderline atypical enchondroma versus Grade I chondrosarcoma, the lesion, in this author's opinion, should be locally ablated by either cryosurgery[16] or en-bloc resection. If treated cryosurgically, the margins should be submitted for frozen section to make sure no cartilage is present. If an en-bloc excision is to be performed great care (tomograms) must be taken to ensure that the saw cuts do not pass through tumor.
5. Close follow-up is, of course, essential. Marcove[16] advises that following cryosurgery a "second look" procedure be performed at about 6 months to rule out recurrence (p. 600).

CHARACTERISTICS OF CHONDROSARCOMAS THAT TRANSFORM TO FIBRO- AND OSTEOSARCOMA

Dahlin and Beabout[22] were the first to publish a large series of low-grade chondrosarcomas that had focally transformed to highly malignant fibro- and osteosarcoma. Mirra and Marcove also recognized the importance of this entity and published the second series with this dedifferentiation or transformation process.[25] It is crucial to recognize these transformations, because they behave with extreme virulence and require radical methods of therapy, if there is to be any hope for cure. If the foci of transformation are not recognized, they are usually diagnosed as simple Grade I chondrosarcoma or even as enchondroma, if the spindle cell areas are not biopsied or not recognized as a grave change. Grade I chondrosarcoma can be treated by en-bloc resection or cryosurgery. It would be inviting disaster to perform these lesser procedures on these virulent transformations. Other errors I have noted include mistaking the dedifferentiation process as a primary fibrosarcoma, other sarcoma, metastatic carcinoma, or spindle cell melanoma.

In Dahlin's series fibrosarcomatous transformation outnumbered osteosarcomatous transformation 2 to 1. In my series the ratio is presently 11 to 1.

Clinical Features

The data that follow are based on 50 cases[22,23,24,25] and seven unpublished cases.

(Text continues on p. 204.)

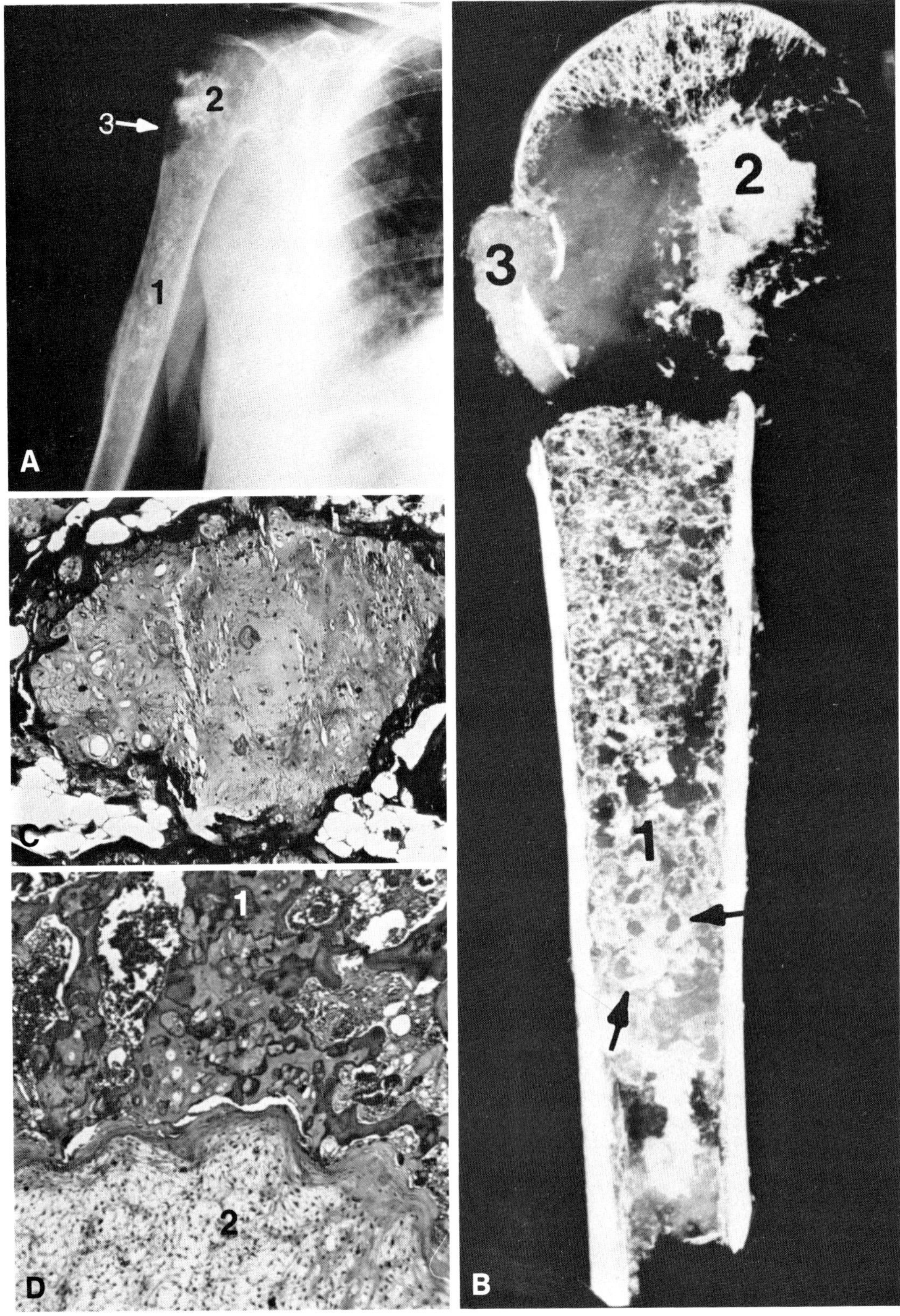

FIG. 8-49

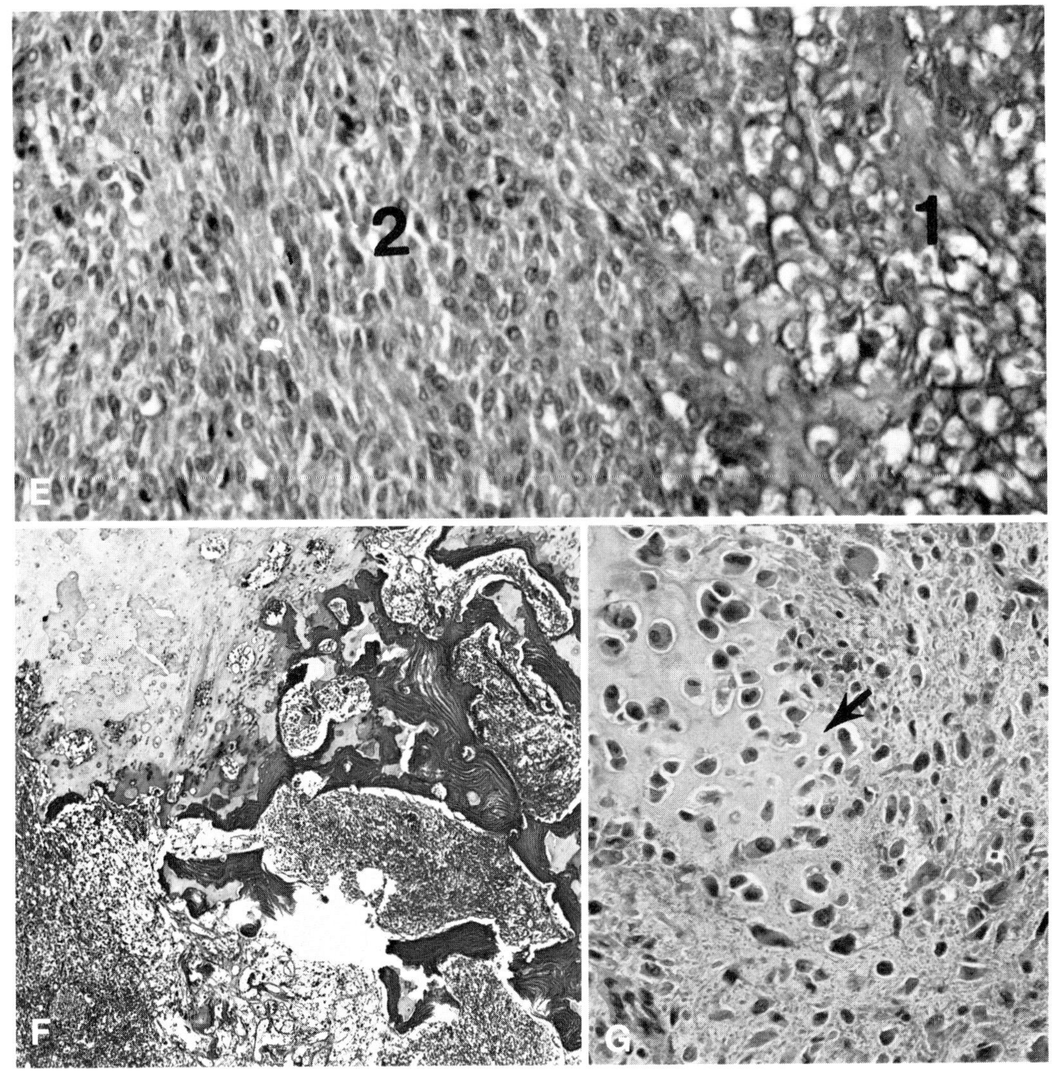

FIG. 8-49

Enchondroma With Chondrosarcomatous Transformation Further Dedifferentiating to a Fibrosarcoma

FIG. 8-49. (*A*) This radiograph shows three distinct areas: (*1*) an area of distinct spheroidal calcifications in the shaft, (*2*) a densely calcified area, and (*3*) a cortical erosion with a soft-tissue mass. (*B*) Specimen radiograph showing the same regions (1,2, and 3). Note that the lesion in the shaft shows circular eggshell-like deposits of density (*arrows*). *These correspond to the ringlike or spheroidal densities seen on radiograph of enchondroma.* Microscopic sections showed that these represented plates of lamellar bone surrounding benign cartilage lobules. (*C*) Field from the enchondroma of the shaft showing circumferential plates of bone surrounding bland hypocellular cartilage lobules (x80). (*D*) Enchondromatous tissues (*1*) in juxtaposition to more cellular chondrosarcomatous tissues (*2*) (x40). The chondrosarcomatous area was found in the metaphyseal portion of the bone and corresponded to the area of the densely calcified metaphyseal mass seen in Figure 8-49, *A* (2). (*E*) Chondrosarcoma (*1*) and high-grade fibrosarcoma (*2*) tissues in juxtaposition (x125). (*F*) Unequivocal enchondromatous tissues (upper field) in juxtaposition to a fibrosarcoma (lower field) (x40). (*G*) A single focus was found in which the chondrosarcomatous portion of the lesion (*arrow*) was apparently loosing its matrix and transforming into a highly malignant spindle cell sarcoma (fibrosarcoma) (Mirra, and Marcove: Fibrosarcomatous dedifferentiation of primary and secondary chondrosarcoma. J. Bone Joint Surg., *56A*:288, 1974)

INCIDENCE. Not rare. In my experience between 10 and 20 per cent of chondrosarcomas may undergo these much very more aggressive transformations. Chondrosarcoma represents approximately 10 per cent of biopsied primary bone tumors. A 20 per cent transformation rate would represent 2 per cent of all primary bone tumors. This, therefore, is an important entity that deserves greater recognition. It is at least twice as common as the chondroblastoma, for example.

AGE. The range is between 10 and 76 years. The mean age is 52.

SYMPTOMS. Pain, swelling, or both.

Radiographic Features

Most cases are indistinguishable from ordinary chondrosarcomas (Fig. 8–51, *A* and *B*) or from chondrosarcomas engrafted upon enchondromas (Fig. 8–49, *A* and *B*). The outstanding clue to their nature is a large soft-tissue mass (Fig. 8–49, *A* and *B*, Plate 6, *C*) devoid of densification in association with a chondrosarcoma and/or calcified enchondroma within the shaft. The soft-tissue mass represents the fibrosarcomatous portion of the tumor. In contrast most chondrosarcomas that invade the soft tissues show densities. Diagnosis depends upon biopsy. Biopsy must include areas of lysis, calcified portions of the shaft tumor, and the soft-tissue mass, if present, since all three of these areas may show strikingly different findings. The instruments used after each biopsy should be discarded in order not to contaminate areas that may be benign.

Gross Pathology

The chondrosarcomas with fibrosarcomatous transformation will show foci of either glistening bluish or gritty cartilage surrounded by soft to firm, grayish to grayish-tan noncalcified fibrosarcoma tissue (Plate 6, *C*). Some fibrosarcoma tissue is intraosseous but most commonly the bulk of it breaks through the cortex into the soft tissue. The distinction between calcified chondrosarcomatous tissue and foci of osteosarcomatous transformation may be impossible to determine from gross examination alone.

In some cases, there may be a longitudinal, tapering, intraosseous mass of smaller cartilage lobules with gross, specimen radiographic, and microscopic evidence of a preexistent benign enchondroma (Plate 6, *C*, Fig. 8–49, *B* and *C*). On radiograph the enchondromatous portion of the lesion shows distinct areas of punctate, ringlike to spheroidal intraosseous ossifications similar to those of other pure long- and flat-bone enchondromatous lesions (Figs. 8–10 and 8–49, *A*).

Histopathology

Fibrosarcomatous Transformation

In fibrosarcomatous transformation of a low-grade chondrosarcoma the fibrosarcomatous tissues are easily distinguished from the chondrosarcomatous areas. Where they abut there is usually a sharp line of demarcation, imparting the appearance of the collision of two tumors (Fig. 8–50, *A* and *B*). The fibrosarcomatous portion is usually high-grade anaplastic (Figs. 8–49, *D, right*). Numerous sections may have to be searched to find the focus where the chondrosarcoma is transforming to the spindle-cell sarcoma (Fig. 8–49, *F*). This is in distinction to mesenchymal chondrosarcoma and osteogenic sarcoma, where areas of spindle-cell sarcoma and chondrosarcoma occur in numerous fields. These latter two malignancies show multiple islands of chondrosarcomatous “metaplasia” from an undifferentiated stroma (Fig. 8–67). In other words, these latter two tumors show multiple focal changes from undifferentiated spindle cells to cartilage or chondroid. In fibrosarcomatous transformation there is a single focus of transformation of chondrosarcoma to the more undifferentiated tumor. The direction of change is from malignant cartilage to malignant spindle cells. The opposite direction occurs in osteosarcoma and mesenchymal chondrosarcoma.

One should also search for regions of enchondromatous tissue. This tissue is composed of small,

(*Text continues on p. 207.*)

Enchondroma With Chondrosarcomatous Transformation Further Dedifferentiating to a Fibrosarcoma

FIG. 8–50. (*A*) This lesion arose in a rib of a 57-year-old male. The low-power view shows a chondrosarcoma (upper half of expanded rib), a fibrosarcoma (lower half of expanded rib), and an enchondroma in the shaft at *D′*. (*B*) This area corresponds to *B′* of (*A*). It shows lobules of Grade I chondrosarcoma and fibrosarcoma with a “collision” appearance. (*C*) Enchondroma with surrounding plates of lamellar bone corresponding to *D′* of (*A*). (McFarland, G.B., McKinley, L.M., and Reed, R.J.: Dedifferentiation of low grade chondrosarcomas. Clin. Orthop., *122*:157, 1977)

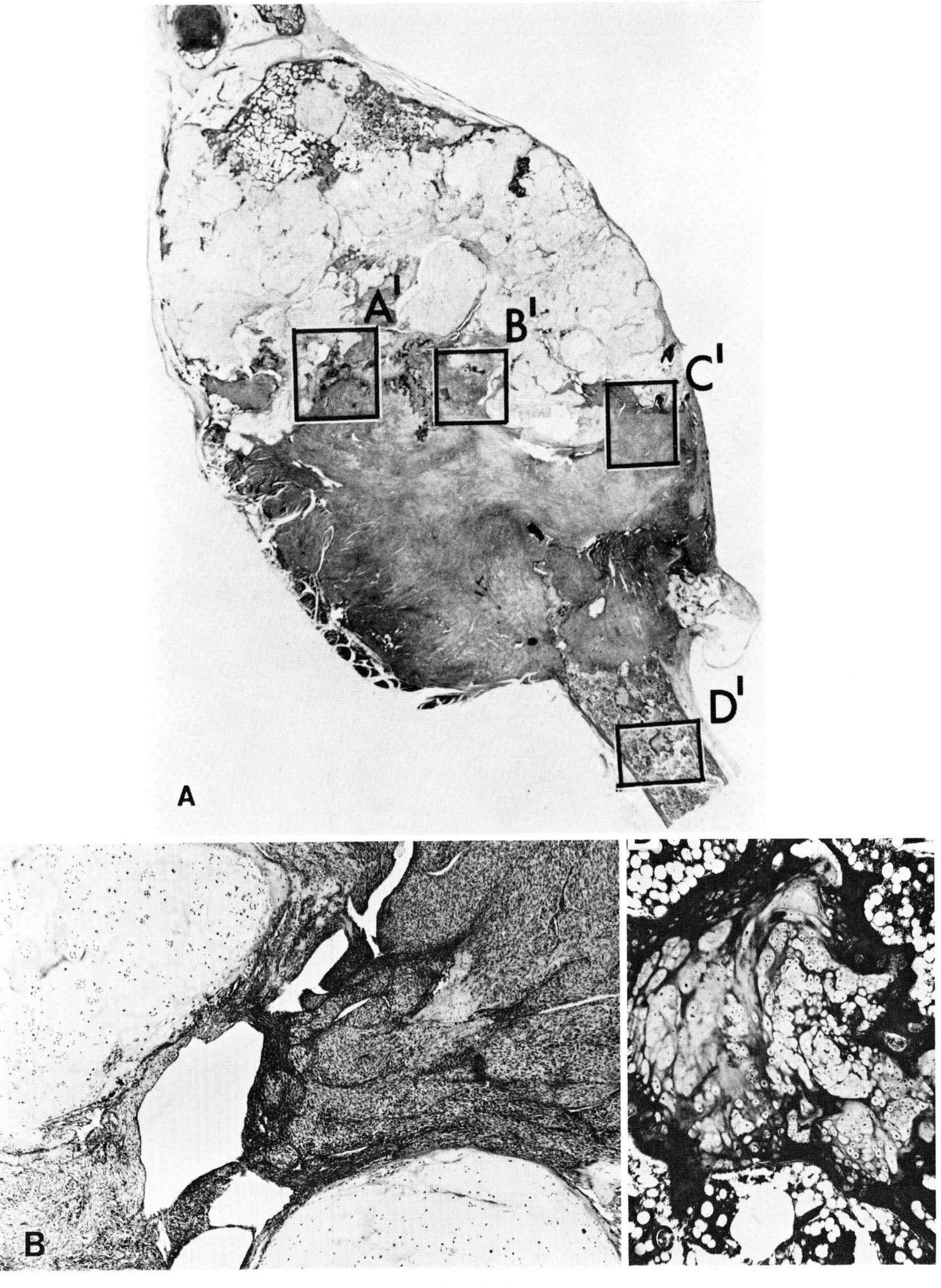

FIG. 8-50

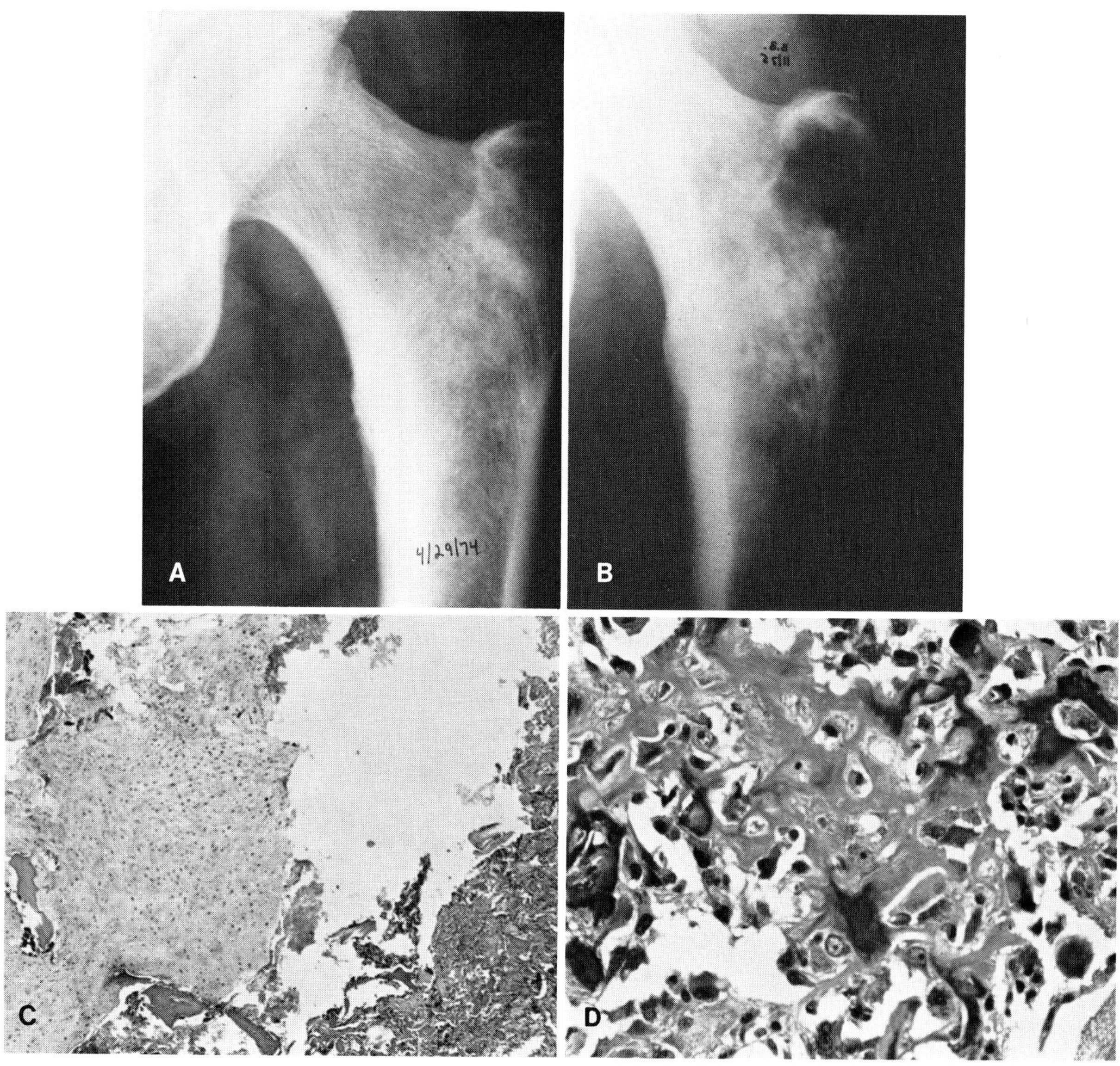

FIG. 8-51

Osteosarcomatous Transformation of Chondrosarcoma

FIG. 8-51. (*A*) "Windblown" pattern of calcifications virtually diagnostic of chondrosarcoma. Biopsy was interpreted as an enchondroma, however. (*B*) An ominous lytic area has developed in the trochanteric region $1\frac{1}{2}$ years later. (*C*) Biopsy showed Grade I chondrosarcoma (*left*). In addition, there was a malignant noncartilagenous component (*right*) (x40). (*D*) Our consultative review of the slides showed areas of malignant osteoid and bone forming without first passing through a cartilaginous phase. This finding is diagnostic of osteosarcoma. The patient's leg was amputated at this time because of the diagnosis of osteosarcomatous transformation of a low grade chondrosarcoma. Nevertheless, he died in 2 years time from osteosarcomatous pulmonary metastases.

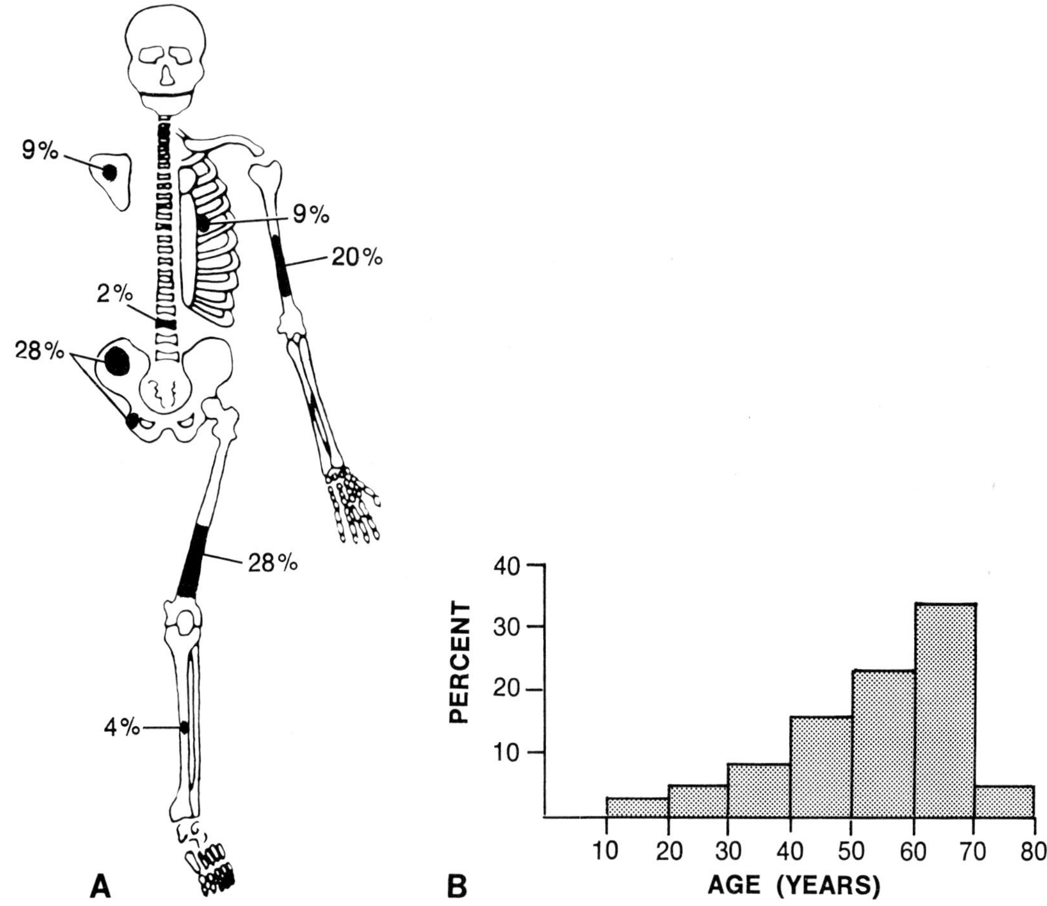

FIG. 8-52. (*A*) Chondrosarcoma with fibrosarcomatous and osteosarcomatous dedifferentiation. Frequency of areas of involvement in 50 patients. Male:female incidence, 1.1/2. Some 37 cases with fibrosarcoma and 13 with osteosarcoma; 3 patients had Ollier's disease, 1, multiple osteochondromatosis and 5 probable antecedent enchondroma. (*B*) Age distribution in patients with fibro- and osteosarcomatous transformation in primary and secondary chondrosarcoma.

round lobules of cartilage surrounded by a sheath of lamellar to lamellar-woven bone (Figs. 8-49, *C;* 8-50, *C*) or larger, bland cartilage islands showing a mosaic or jigsaw pattern of calcification (Fig. 8-49, *C*).

Osteosarcomatous Transformation

The diagnosis of osteosarcomatous transformation of a formerly low-grade chondrosarcoma is a more difficult task. One may justifiably ask, "How would we know whether the tumor was not simply an osteosarcoma in the first place, since this tumor can produce chondrosarcomatous tissues?" This author would restrict the diagnosis of osteosarcoma arising in a preexisting cartilage tumor to those that show the following: remnants of a formerly benign enchondroma, those middle age or older patients who have been followed radiographically for an "enchondroma" for 1 year or more who eventually are shown pathologically to have chondrosarcoma and osteosarcoma (Fig. 8-51), and those elderly patients who show radiographic features typical for a chondrosarcoma but that, nevertheless, show a histologic focus of osteosarcoma clearly separable from a pure chondrosarcomatous area. The great bulk of these lesions may show nothing more than a borderline to low Grade II chondrosarcoma (Fig. 8-51, *C*), which is unusual for ordinary osteosarcoma in which the chondrosarcoma component is usually high Grade II to III. In these low-grade chondrosarcomas with osteosarcomatous transformation, in order to establish the diagnosis, areas must be demonstrated in which an undifferentiated malignant stroma is forming osteoid and/or woven bone (Fig. 8–51, *D*). Using these strict criteria, osteosarcomatous transformation of chondrosarcoma is, in my experience, an extremely rare event (approximately 0.1 to 0.2% of bone tumors).

Course and Treatment

These transformations are highly malignant and metastasize to numerous organ sites, including lungs, skin, adrenals, heart, intestines, and brain. About 80 per cent or more of patients die in less than 2-years time when treated by amputation alone. The metastases show pure fibrosarcomatous elements in those cases of fibrosarcomatous dedifferentiation of chondrosarcoma. Foci of chondrosarcoma are not seen in the metastases. Unless this entity is recognized, the pure spindle cell metastases in association with a primary or secondary bone chondrosarcoma can lead to considerable diagnostic confusion.

Associated Diseases

Of the reported patients, two had Ollier's disease, one, osteochondromatosis, and three, radiographic and microscopic evidence to support solitary enchondromas. I have also seen two other cases arising in solitary enchondromatous tissue and another case in association with Ollier's disease (unpublished observations).

From an analysis of 12 personal cases, at least seven appeared to be associated with antecedent benign enchondroma (five cases) or Ollier's disease (two cases). Those patients with radiographic and histologic evidence to support solitary enchondroma did not present to a physician until after the onset of malignant transformation. In most cases the patients did not present until after fibro- or osteosarcomatous transformation. Those patients with Ollier's disease did present prior to sarcomatous transformation. At some point in their course the enchondromatous lesions transform to a well-differentiated chondrosarcoma. The average length of time for transformation of chondrosarcoma to these even more malignant variants is unknown.

OLLIER'S DISEASE (MULTIPLE ENCHONDROMATOSIS)

Clinical Features

In 1889, Ollier described a disease in which multiple endochondrally formed bones in a predominantly unilateral distribution were involved by large, proliferating masses of cartilage (enchondromatosis). He referred to the condition as dyschondroplasia, implying that it was a developmental defect related to the aberrant growth of cartilage. The disease is not genetically transmitted.

Symptoms usually begin in childhood and vary with the distribution of the lesions and the extent to which they have weakened the bones.

A full spectrum of bony involvement can be seen from as little as two bones to virtually all enchondrally formed bones. The phalanges and the lower limbs are most commonly affected. There is a strong tendency for one side of the body to be more involved than the other. When the long bones are affected, severe deformities and stunting frequently occur.

Ulnar deviation of the hand may be seen in Ollier's disease as well as in multiple osteochondromatosis.

Associated vascular and skin anomalies have been reported, the most common of which are multiple hemangiomas of the soft tissues. This combination is called *Maffucci's syndrome.* Eventually, the hemangiomas acquire phleboliths that appear on radiograph as multiple roundish opacities in the soft tissues (Fig. 8–54). Anomalies of the skin include vitiligo and multiple pigmented nevi.

Radiologic Features

The characteristic radiographic findings consist of rounded, columnar, or bubbly radiolucencies in the metaphyses and shafts of enchondrally formed bones (Figs. 8–53 and 8–54). The lesions are often expansile and show stippled ringlike to spheroidal or more irregular calcifications (Fig. 8–53). The long bones may show pathognomonic longitudinal to "fanlike" linear densities admixed with rounded radiolucent to radiodense cartilaginous islands (Figs. 8–55 and 8–56). These characteristic zones extend from the epiphysis to the shaft. Eccentric or periosteal chondromatous tissues may mimic the periosteal chondroma. The periosteal chondroma, on the other hand, is almost always a solitary lesion and is not associated with multiple, purely intraosseous lesions, as do occur in Ollier's disease. In some patients followed by serial radiography some lesions have been shown to regress after skeletal maturity has been achieved.

Gross Pathology

The bones show numerous islands of glistening cartilage mostly located within the shaft, but the abnormal cartilage may also be seen in any portion of

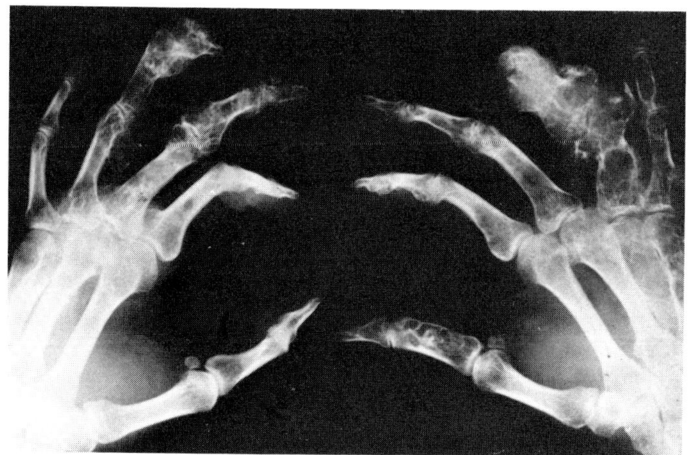

FIG. 8-53

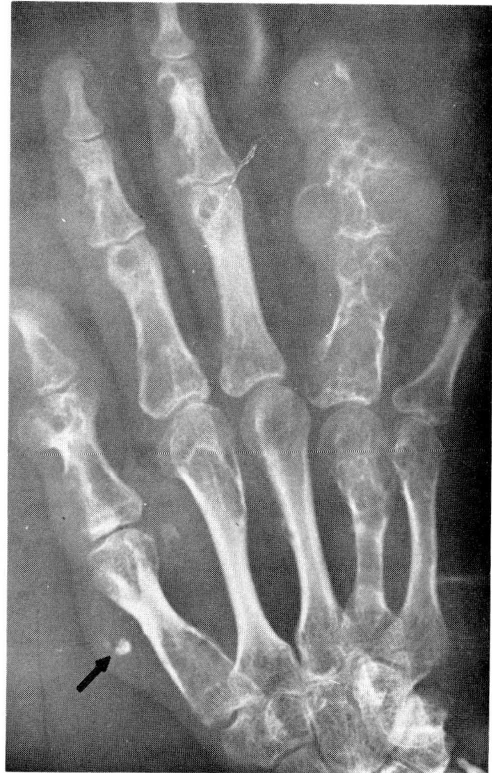

FIG. 8-54

Ollier's Disease

FIG. 8-53. Typical voluminous and expansive trabeculated lesions of the hands of a patient with severe Ollier's disease.

FIG. 8-54. Maffucci's syndrome is multiple enchondromatosis in association with vascular phleboliths (seen here in the soft tissues of the thumb, *arrow*).

an endochondral bone, including the secondary ossification center, articular cartilage, epiphyseal plate, and periosteum (Figs. 8–57 and 8–58; Plate 2–1).

If multiple islands of abnormal cartilage are located within the epiphyseal plate, the following will occur: As the bone lengthens the abnormal regions of the epiphyseal plate leave residua of abnormal cartilage within the metaphysis. This cartilage is typically resistent to normal calcification, cell necrosis, and resorption by osteoclasts. With continued longitudinal growth of the host bone, the abnormal cartilage derived from the epiphyseal plate will, therefore, form long, linear masses within the shaft (Fig. 8–57; Plate 8, *A*). The nondysplastic portions of the epiphyseal plate will develop normally and eventually lead to the formation of the usual metaphyseal bone.

Therefore, if abnormal Ollier's type epiphyseal plate cartilage alternates with normal epiphyseal plate cartilage, the production of long columns of metaphyseal cartilage will occur, alternating with areas of normal bone production. This phenomenon is seen only in Ollier's disease and explains the pathognomonic "fanlike" metaphyseal septations seen on radiograph (Figs. 8–55 and 8–56). The dense lines represent bone formed by normal endochondral ossification and the intervening columns of lucency represent the epiphyseally derived areas of abnormal cartilage.

Histopathology

The histopathology documents the gross pathology. Abnormal foci of variably calcified lobules of cartilage may be found in all portions of the affected bone (Fig. 8–59). Depending on the severity of the disease,

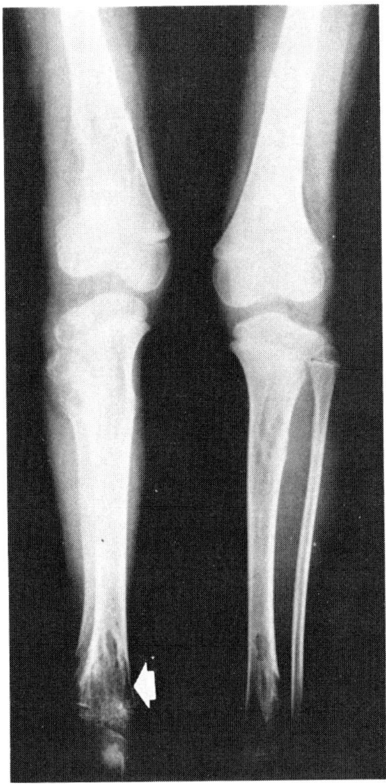

FIG. 8-55

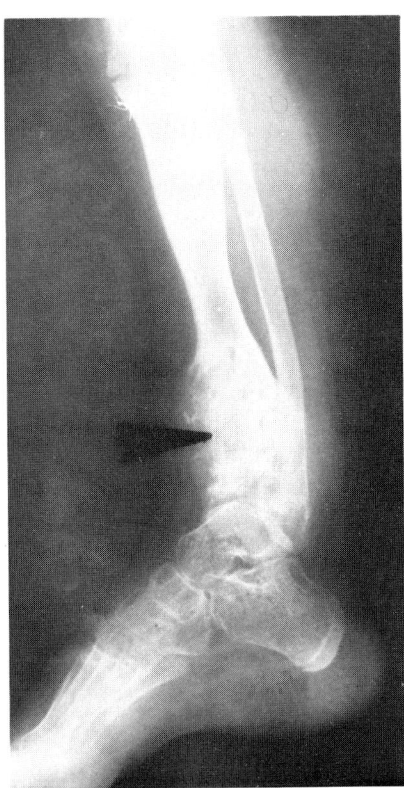

FIG. 8-56

FIG. 8-55. Enchondromatosis of the long limb bones. Note the characteristic fanlike septations of the distal tibia (*arrow*).

FIG. 8-56. Expansive enchondromatosis lesions. The pathognomonic "fanlike" appearance (*arrow*) is consequent to the deposition of long columns of poorly calcified cartilage. Such cartilage arises from abnormally cellular or dysplastic epiphyseal plate cartilage in juxtaposition to thin plates of normal bone that arise from the uninvolved or normal portions of the epiphyseal plate.

the lobules of cartilage may be small and well separated one from another (Fig. 8-59) or they may form massive, confluent lobules separated by bands of fibrous tissue similar to that seen in chondrosarcoma (Fig. 8-60). In contrast to chondrosarcoma, however, the cartilage cells at the periphery of the lobules do not insinuate themselves between marrow fat cells (Fig. 8-28).

Lobules of cartilage may be surrounded by plates of lamellar bone (Fig. 8-61), a feature identical to that seen in solitary enchondroma.

The cellularity and size and shapes of the nuclei may vary from that of ordinary solitary enchondromas (Fig. 8-62) to very highly cellular lesions with ominous nuclei mimicking low-grade chondrosarcoma (Fig. 8-63). The nuclei, however, lack prominent nucleoli, and mitoses, if present, are very rare.

Malignant Transformation

The severely atypical (dysplastic) cytologic features of Ollier's disease may well explain the extremely high incidence (up to 50%) of chondrosarcomatous transformation in patients moderately to severely affected.

Chondrosarcoma is heralded by pain or rapid swelling with or without pathologic fracture. The affected areas shows ominous focal areas of lysis or a chondrosarcomatous "windblown" calcification pattern. The tumor has often broken through the cortex, inciting spiculated or other periosteal reactions (Fig. 8-64). This is the main clue to malignant transformation. Other cases show blatant, malignant radiographic patterns (Fig. 8-65). Any significant change in radiographic pattern in patients over age 20, such

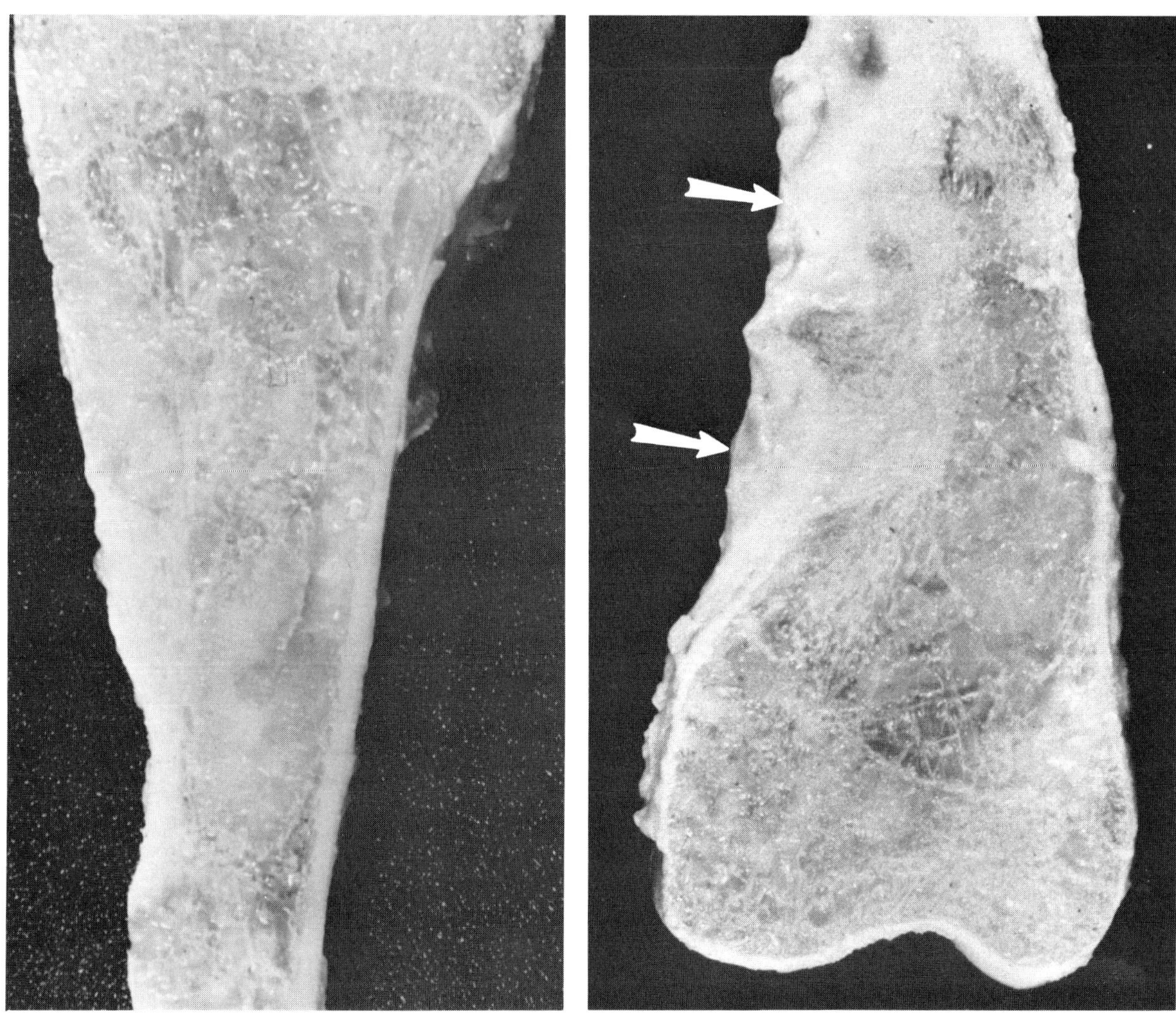

FIG. 8-57 FIG. 8-58

Ollier's Disease

FIG. 8-57. Columns of glistening cartilage can be seen in the metaphysis and diaphysis of this severely affected tibia. The cortex is focally eroded. Although these findings would suggest chondrosarcoma in a solitary cartilage lesion, the actual chondrosarcomatous change in this patient occurred in the proximal femur.

FIG. 8-58. The distal femur of this patient shows the extensive nature of the cartilaginous deposits. It involves the shaft, metaphysis, secondary ossification center, and even the periosteal portions of the bone (*arrows*).

as newly developing foci of lysis or "windblown" calcifications, should lead to a high index of suspicion of malignant transformation. Wedge biopsy from these areas must be carefully analyzed for malignancy. If the clinician waits for the development of a soft-tissue mass on radiograph, it may be too late to save the patient's limb or life.

If the radiograph is not obviously malignant, danger in overdiagnosis can be made, considering the vast range of cellularity and nuclear atypia possible in Ollier's disease. Malignancy by histologic criteria alone should depend upon the demonstration of large, prominent, single and multiple nucleoli, approximately one mitosis per HPF, invasion of marrow fat or soft tissues, or other features of unequivocal anaplasia.

These tumors usually behave with a high degree of virulence. Radical therapy is usually the treatment of choice.

Fibrosarcomatous transformation of the chondrosarcoma of Ollier's disease has been reported by Dahlin and Mirra.[26,27] The incidence of transformation occurs in approximately 10 to 20 per cent of chondrosarcomas (personal observations). Osteosarcomatous transformation of an Ollier's chondrosarcoma has not yet been reported.

TIETZE'S DISEASE

Tietze's disease, also known as costal chondritis, is an uncommon benign disorder characterized by a cartilaginous proliferation at the costochondral junction. The main symptom is a nodular, painful, tumorous swelling. The lesion most often affects women and usually involves the second or third costochondral junction and it may become as large as 4 to 5 cm. On rare occasion, the lesions may be multiple and even bilateral. Personal observations of four cases have shown a bland cartilaginous proliferation arising from the fibrous connective tissue in the region of the ligaments of the costochondral junction. In one case removed by en-bloc excision (mistaken for a possible chondrosarcoma), the costal cartilage showed secondary degenerative changes. In addition, there were marginal osteophytes and chondromatous metaplasia of ligamentous tissues. This lesion may be consequent to repair of a stress injury at the costochondral junction in association with degenerative arthritis. No significant inflammation was seen in any of the four cases.

The importance of recognizing this entity is that the mass can grow rather quickly to an alarming size and be mistaken for a malignant tumor. If the pathologist is swayed by the history of rapid growth, the diagnosis of a well-differentiated chondrosarcoma is possible. I have also seen the lesion called an enchondroma in one instance, and in another, by not recognizing that the bland articular cartilage-like tissue was the cause of the swelling itself, as a benign articular cartilage.

MESENCHYMAL CHONDROSARCOMA

The mesenchymal chondrosarcoma of bone is an unusual neoplasm characterized by undifferentiated mesenchymal cells, islands of malignant cartilage, and areas resembling a vascular tumor such as hemangiopericytoma. This is a rare primary bone tumor, approximately 70 times less common than the intramedullary osteosarcoma and five times less common than fibrosarcomatous dedifferentiation of chondrosarcoma (the two lesions most likely to be confused with the mesenchymal chondrosarcoma).

Clinical Features

The presenting complaints are swelling, pain, neurologic symptoms if the bones of the skull or spine are involved, and rarely, gross pathologic fracture.

Radiologic Features

On radiologic examination the lesions are predominantly lytic, may arise in the medulla of the bone, the periosteum or dura. The intramedullary lesions are sharply or poorly demarcated and may contain foci of stippled calcification. The lesions that arise in the periosteum are frequently rounded in contour and bulge into the soft tissues, where stippled calcifications are usually prominent (Fig. 8–66, *A*). The cortex of the bone is concave and the surrounding intramedullary bone produces reactive new bone. It may be impossible to determine on radiographic examination, as Figure 8–66 illustrates, whether the lesion arises in the soft tissues, secondarily involving the bone; or is from the periosteum. The initial radio-

---

Ollier's Disease

FIG. 8-59. Ollier's disease is a hamartomatous dysplastic cartilaginous process that may affect any portion of the bone or cartilages. In this phalanx, foci of Ollier's type hypercellular cartilage involve the medullary portions of the bone (*1*) the epiphyseal plate (*2*), periosteum (*3*) and even the articular cartilage (*4*) (x10).

FIG. 8-60. Large confluent lobules of cartilage mimicking chondrosarcoma (x2).

FIG. 8-61. Lobules of cartilage (*1*) partially to completely surrounded by metaplastic lamellar bone (*arrows*), a sign of benignancy (x125).

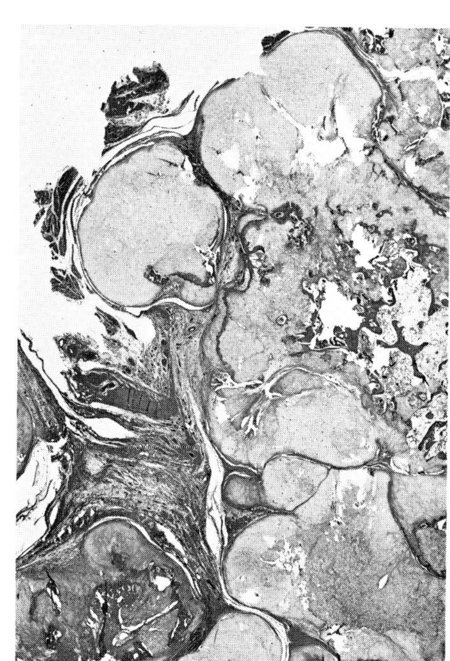

FIG. 8-60

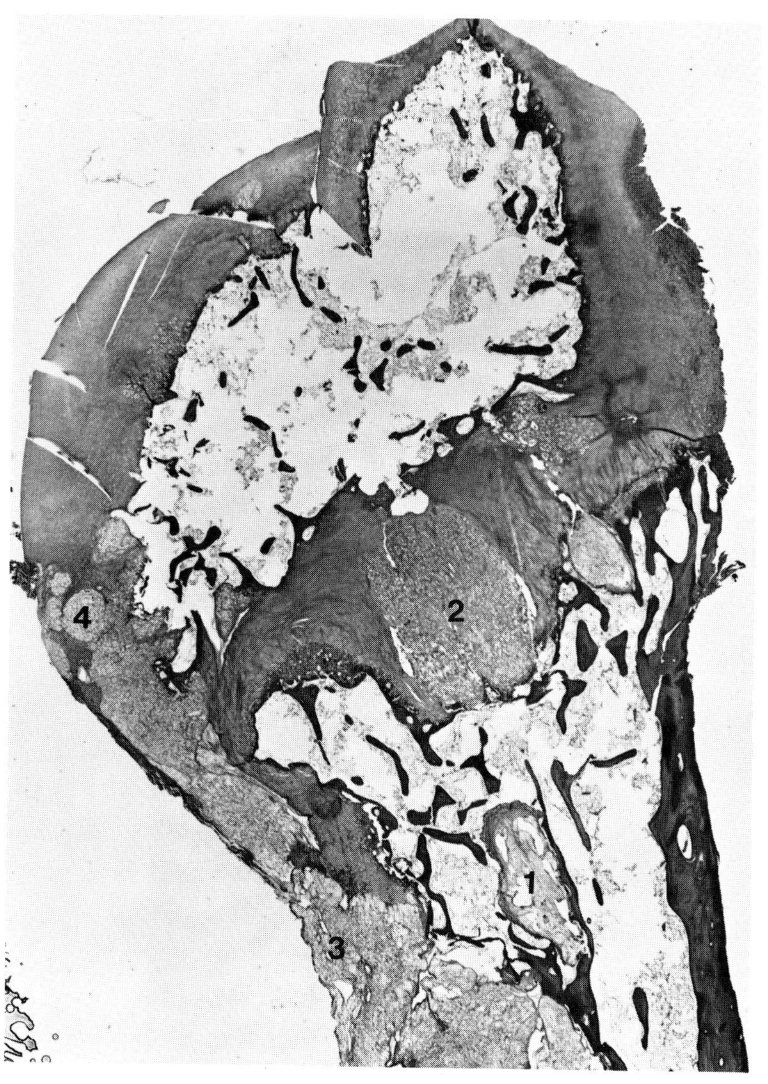

FIG. 8-59

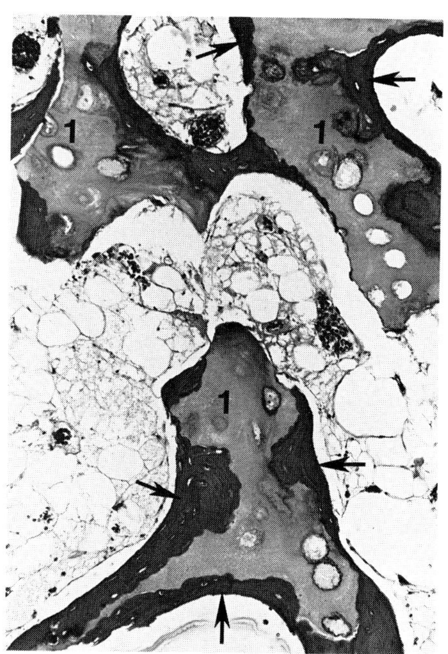

FIG. 8-61

graphic diagnosis of the lesion shown was synovial sarcoma. Only after biopsy, amputation, and gross examination was the diagnosis and site of origin of this particular example possible, particularly since the mesenchymal chondrosarcoma has also been reported as a primary soft-tissue tumor.

Gross Pathology

On gross examination this neoplasm is grayish yellow or pink, firm or soft, and occasionally, lobulated. The gross specimen of the previous case (Fig. 8-66, *B*) showed a firm, yellow-gray tumor that was easily separated from the surrounding soft tissues, was covered with periosteum along its outer margin, and caused a saucer-shaped depression in the shaft along its inner margin. These features established its origin from the periosteum.

Histopathology

The tumor is characterized histologically by prominent sheets of small slightly spindled to overtly spindled undifferentiated mesenchymal cells (Figs. 8-67 and 8-69). For diagnosis islands of "metaplastic" malignant cartilage must be demonstrated to arise from the mesenchymal stromal cells (Fig. 8-67 and 8-69, Plate 6, *D* and *E*). In many cases foci can be found where tumor cells abut on vascular channels (Fig. 8-70, Plate 6, *G*), which are the cells lying outside of the reticulin network. This pattern is hemangiopericytoma-like.

Electron microscopy of the case shown in Figure 8-66, *A*-*C*[32] demonstrated that the cells making up the vascular hemangiopericytoma-like areas did not show features of true pericytes; namely, pinocytotic vesicles and a basement membrane that encircles the tumor cells. Our conclusion was that the vascular pattern in mesenchymal chondrosarcoma is the result of proliferation of undifferentiated cells around vascular spaces rather than being true pericytes. Occasionally, this pattern may also be observed in osteogenic sarcoma and fibrosarcoma of bone. Some of the cases that Hutter, *et. al.*[30] have described under the heading "primitive multipotential sarcoma of bone" are indubitable examples of the mesenchymal chondrosarcoma.

Differential Diagnosis

CHONDROSARCOMA WITH FIBROSARCOMATOUS TRANSFORMATION. This tumor shows chondrosarcoma and a spindle-cell sarcoma in apparent collision (Fig. 8-49, *A*). If numerous sections are taken, a single focus of transformation to the more undifferentiated spindle-cell sarcoma may be found (Fig. 8-49, *F*). On the other hand, mesenchymal chondrosarcoma usually shows numerous islands of chondrosarcoma arising by differentiation of the malignant stroma (Fig. 8-67). The process is the reverse of chondrosarcoma with fibrosarcomatous dedifferentiation. Mesenchymal chondrosarcoma does not, therefore, appear as a collision tumor, but as a lesion with multiple foci of chondrosarcomatous "metaplasia."

OSTEOGENIC SARCOMA. This tumor is usually characterized by marked pleomorphism of nuclei (anaplasia) and woven bone production. Mesenchymal chondrosarcomas do not produce malignant bone and the undifferentiated stromal cells are more monotonously anaplastic than the majority of osteo-

Ollier's Disease and Chondrosarcomatous Transformation

FIG. 8-62. Hypercellular islands of hamartomatous or dysplastic cartilage (*arrows*) interspersed between normal articular cartilage (x125).

FIG. 8-63. Extremely ominous hypercellular areas may be found in Ollier's disease without clinical or other pathologic evidence to support frank chondrosarcomatous transformation, at this site. Dysplastic areas such as these may be presarcomatous, however. Note also the presence of several double nucleated chondrocytes (*arrows*) (x250).

FIG. 8-64. (*A*) This patient with Ollier's disease presented with pain and an ominous lytic area (*arrow*). Because this change was not recognized as malignant, a biopsy was not taken. (*B*) One year later the frank chondrosarcomatous change is readily apparent. The lesion has led to further expansion of the bone; there is cortical erosion and a fluffy soft-tissue mass (*arrows*). Biopsy showed chondrosarcoma with fibrosarcomatous transformation. The patient died after 1 year. Autopsy showed multiple organ involvement by fibrosarcomatous metastases.

FIG. 8-65. An example of a typical high-grade chondrosarcoma that arose in a patient with Ollier's disease.

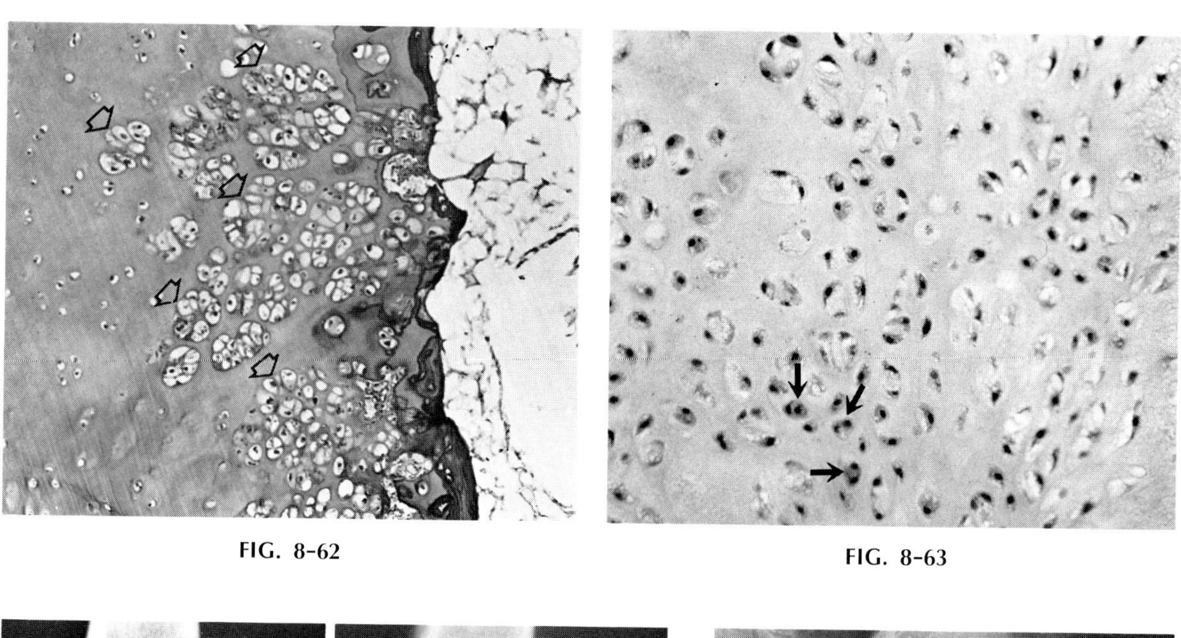

FIG. 8-62

FIG. 8-63

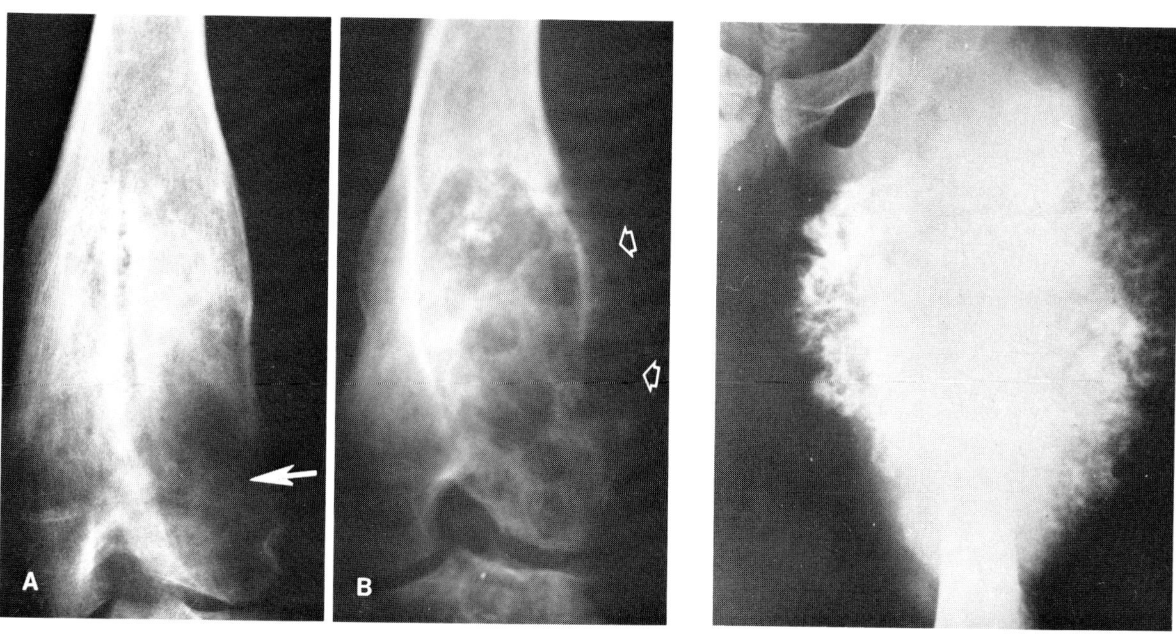

FIG. 8-64

FIG. 8-65

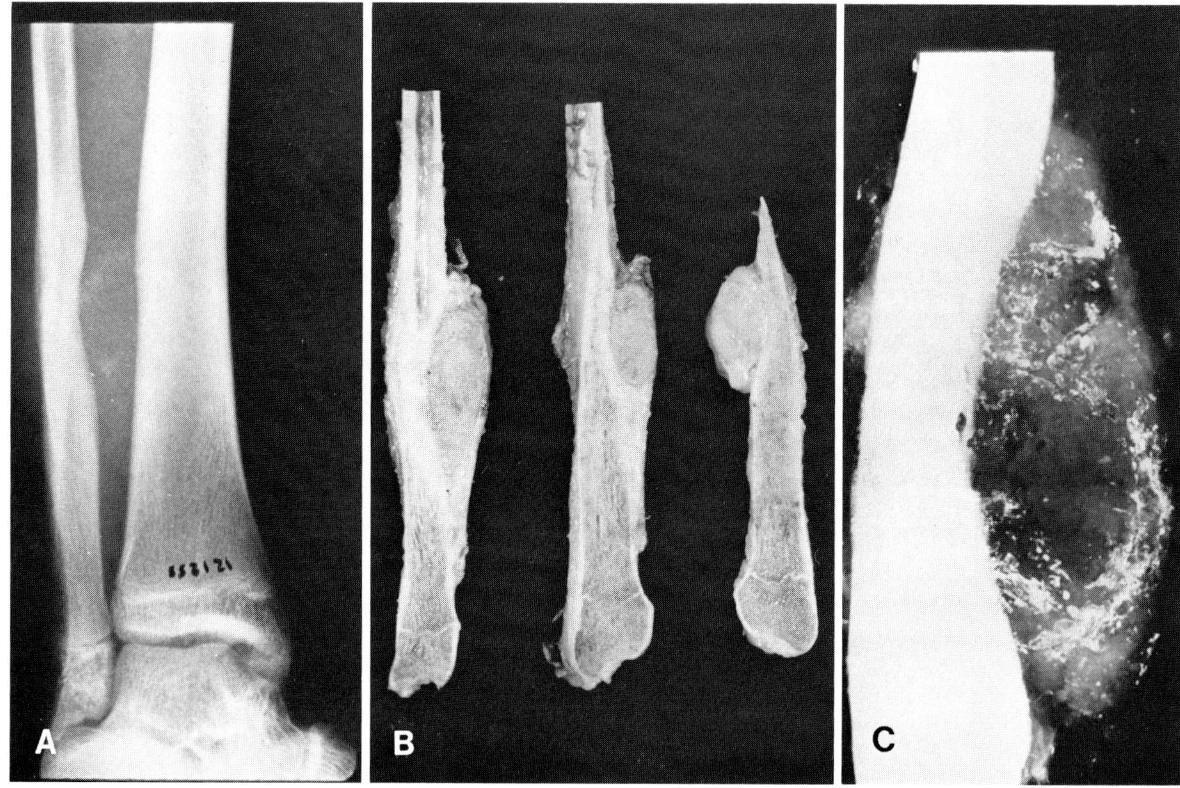

Mesenchymal Chondrosarcoma

FIG. 8-66. Mesenchymal chondrosarcoma. (*A*) Radiograph showed a calcified mass that appeared to arise from the soft tissues, scalloping the fibula. (*B*) In actuality, gross examination showed that the tumor arose from within the periosteum. (*C*) Specimen radiograph of lesions showing irregular calcifications.

sarcomas. The mesenchymal chondrosarcoma often produces an hemangiopericytoma-like component. This is rare in osteosarcoma. Mesenchymal chondrosarcomas may be rich in collagen, which could be confused with osteoid, but conversion to malignant woven bone is not seen. Osteosarcomas usually have a characteristic metaphyseal location with a prominent soft-tissue mass, Codman's triangles, and ominous periosteal "sunburst" and spiculated appearance. Mesenchymal chondrosarcomas have a more variable radiographic appearance and are often found in peculiar locations, such as within the periosteum, spine, ribs, dura, and orbit. It is, however, important to be aware of the features of the much rarer mesenchymal chondrosarcoma, because confusion with the osteosarcoma is common.

Mesenchymal Chondrosarcoma

FIG. 8-67. This tumor consists of small, anaplastic spindle cells with multiple islands of chondrosarcomatous differentiation (x125).

FIG. 8-69. The malignant spindle cells elaborated a cartilaginous stroma, converting them to chondrosarcomatous elements (x400).

FIG. 8-70. Other areas showed hemangiopericytoma-like elements, another characteristic of mesenchymal chondrosarcoma (x125). (Steiner, G., Mirra, J. M., and Bullough P. G.: Mesenchymal chondrosarcoma—a study of the ultrastructure. Cancer, *32*:926, 1973)

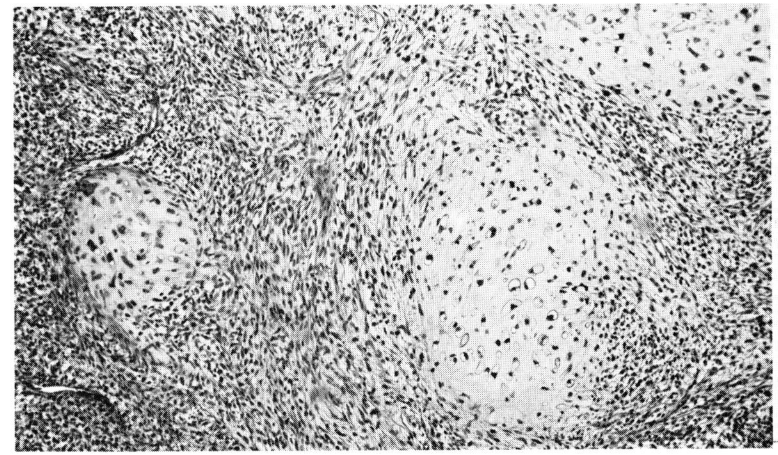

FIG. 8-67

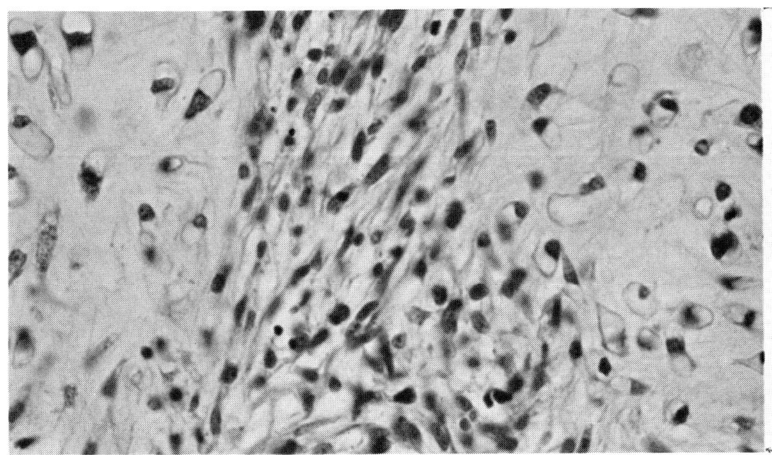

FIG. 8-69

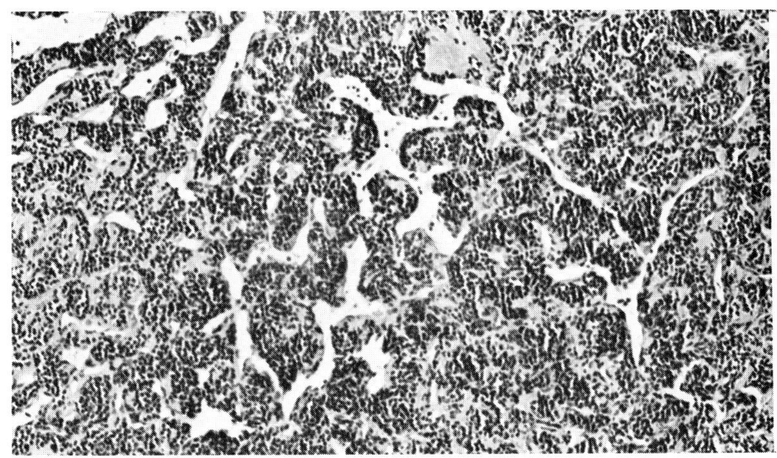

FIG. 8-70

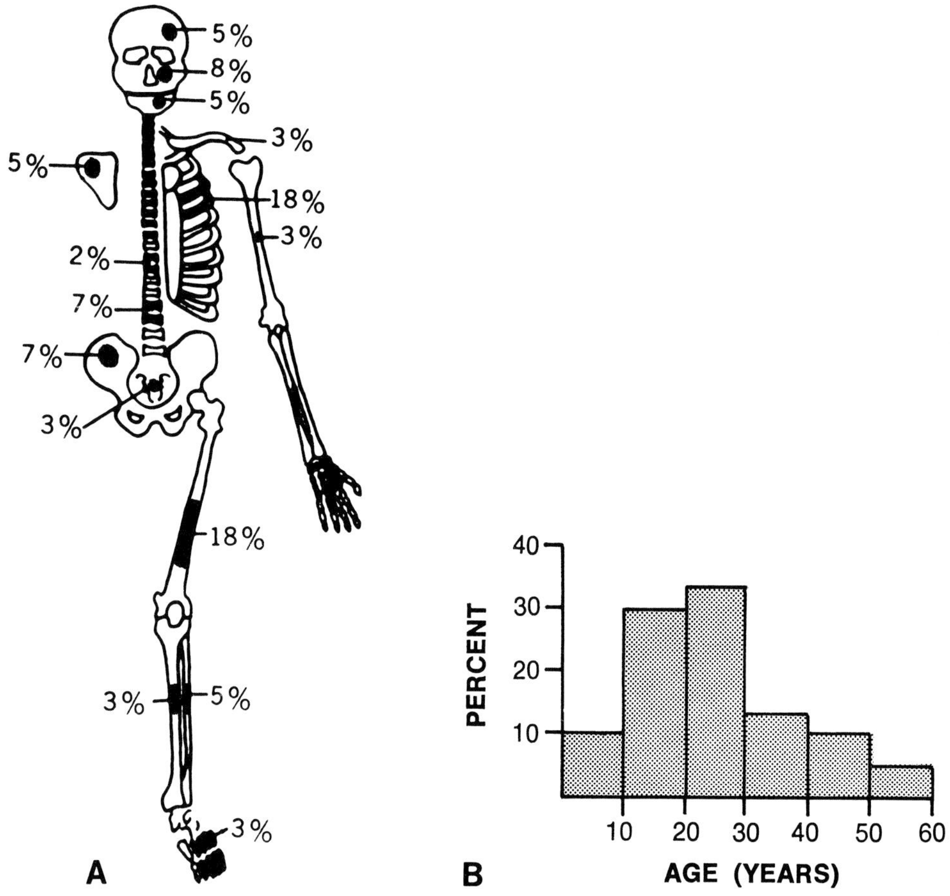

FIG. 8-68. (*A*) Mesenchymal chondrosarcoma. Frequency of areas of involvement in 59 cases. Male:female incidence, 1:1 (*B*) Age distribution of patients with mesenchymal chondrosarcoma (Mirra, J., Bullough, P., and Freiberger, R.: Orthopedic Diseases, Part IV. New York, Famous Teachings in Modern Medicine, MedCom, Inc., © 1977)

FIBROSARCOMA. If the mesenchymal chondrosarcoma produces small amounts of cartilage, a biopsy may miss these areas. But, if any areas of metaplastic chondrosarcoma are seen in association with a spindle-cell sarcoma, the diagnosis of fibrosarcoma must be immediately discarded.

CHONDROMYXOID FIBROMA. See p. 234, Figs. 8-96 to 8-105 and Plate G, 6 *H, I,* and *J.*

Course and Treatment

Mesenchymal chondrosarcoma is a fully malignant lesion with a poor long-term prognosis. Metastases to the lungs and bones (predominantly spine, skull and ribs) may occur up to 10 years or more after amputation. Radical therapy is the recommended treatment.

OSTEOGENIC SARCOMA

Many osteosarcomas produce variable quantities of chondrosarcoma cartilage. The cartilage is most often obviously anaplastic and only rarely Grade I versus enchondroma-like. In fact, in those osteosarcomas with bland, less than objectively anaplastic osteoblasts, analysis of the cartilage may be a deciding factor in the diagnosis of malignancy. Refer to the preceding chapter for those features that distinguish an osteogenic sarcoma from all other cartilage-producing tumors.

CHONDROBLASTOMA

Capsule Summary

Incidence. Approximately 0.5 to 1 per cent of biopsied primary bone tumors. Male to female incidence is 1.8:1. There were over 500 cases reported to 1977. The largest review articles are those of Huvos, *et al.*, and Dahlin, *et al.*[50,39]

Age. Some 65 per cent of patients present in the second decade.

Clinical Features. Pain, limitation of movement, occasionally, joint effusion.

Radiologic Features. Eccentric, usually less than one-half the size of the epiphysis, epiphyseal location, border of sclerosis, and often minute, punctate calcifications.

Gross Pathology. Grayish-pink, soft to variably gritty, has small nodules of chondroid, is occasionally cystic to hemorrhagic and is yellow if it contains histiocytes and/or cholesterol.

Histopathology. This tumor is characterized by polygonal cells (chondroblasts), giant cells, primitive islands of chondroid or hyalin cartilage, "chicken-wire" calcification, and nodules of calcification in the stroma and chondroid. Occasionally it contains cholesterol crystals, xanthoma cells, and aneurysmal bone cyst components. Mitoses may be numerous.

Course. Most cases behave with total innocence. Occasional cases recur and rare cases demonstrate aggressive behavior, including soft-tissue masses and lung metastases.

Treatment. Curettage and packing with bone chips. Refer to p. 226 for a discussion of chondroblastomas with recurrences or metastasis.

Definition. The chondroblastoma was first described in depth by Codman.[37] He called the tumor the epiphyseal chondromatous giant cell tumor. Before his classic description many of the cases were diagnosed as chondrosarcoma. The Codman's tumor is a lesion that almost always originates in the epiphysis and is characterized by a proliferation of chondroblasts and osteoclast-like giant cell in association with the production of chondroid and "chicken-wire" to nodular calcifications.

Histogenesis. Jaffe, *et al.*, Nellmeron, and Welsh, *et. al.*, believe the lesion arises from cartilage "germ cells" or cells of epiphyseal cartilage. This hypothesis is difficult to reconcile with those rare chondroblastomas reported in skull bones or in the middle of a rib, where cartilage "germ cells" or epiphyseal cartilage would not be expected.

Importance. The chondroblastoma is basically a benign lesion that must be distinguished from low- to high-grade malignancies, such as the true giant cell tumor and some variants of chondrosarcoma. An extremely perplexing fact is that some unequivocal chondroblastomas may recur, seed the soft tissues, and even metastasize to the lungs. Whether or not these latter features represent true malignancy with a biologic behavior that will eventually lead to demise of the host is a matter of controversy. A detailed analysis of reported cases of this kind will be covered in the next section. The differential diagnosis of chondroblastoma-like chondrosarcomas will be treated in this section.

Clinical Features

The chondroblastoma is a rare primary lesion. It is about twice as common in males as in females. The vast majority of patients present before age 30. The peak age group is in the second decade.

Symptoms generally consist of pain with local tenderness, followed by swelling and limitation of movement. Joint effusion is seen in about one-third of cases; symptoms are present for between 6 months to several years before treatment. Pathologic fracture is unusual.

Except for slight elevation of the sedimentation rate, laboratory tests are within normal limits.

Radiographic Features

The chondroblastoma is usually located in the epiphysis, but it may extend to the metaphysis. The lesion is eccentric and usually involves less than one-half of the entire epiphysis. There is a border of host bone sclerosis. Small (up to 1 mm.) punctate calcifications are evident in more than half the cases (Fig. 8-72). An open epiphysis is usually present.

These are the characteristic features that are virtually diagnostic of the chondroblastoma, provided that *all* of these features are present. The borders of sclerosis represent a host reaction to the slow growth and benign nature of the lesion. Epiphyseal chondrosarcomas may have calcifications but are not bordered by a rim of prominent host bone sclerosis.

The most common tumor of epiphyses is the neoplastic giant cell tumor (GCT). This tumor lacks calcification, punctate or otherwise, occupies more than half of the epiphysis in most cases, lacks a border of sclerosis, and occurs in older patients in which the epiphysis is closed. Synovial lesions such as pigmented villonodular synovitis and rheumatoid arthritis may penetrate into the epiphyseal end of the bone and form a cystlike lesion with or without borders of reactive sclerosis. They lack calcifications. Tuberculosis may also penetrate into the epiphysis and may even contain spotty calcifications within the granulomas. These lesions, which are of synovial origin, penetrate the bone at the capsular reflection, where the bone cortex joins the articular cartilage. *A*

(*Text continues on p. 222.*)

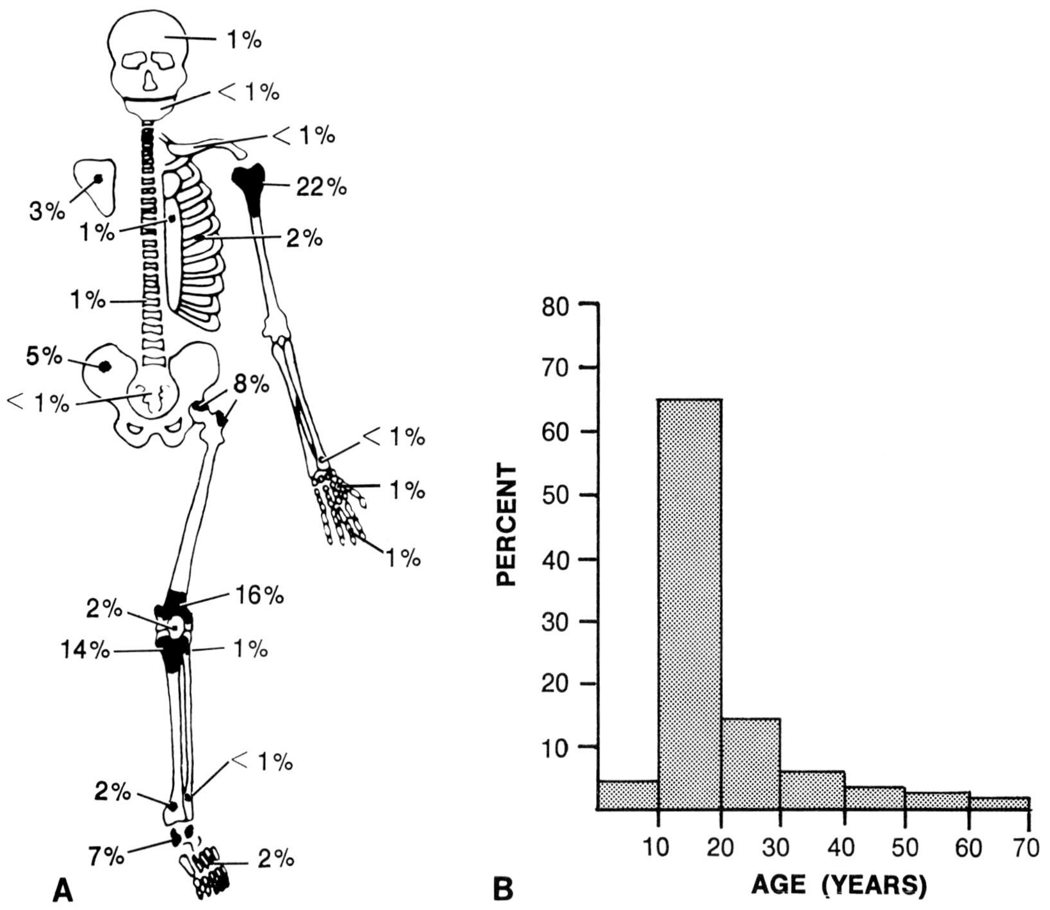

FIG. 8-71. (*A*) Chondroblastoma. Frequency of areas of involvement in 465 patients. Male:female incidence, 1.8:1. (*B*) Age distribution of patients with chondroblastoma (Mirra, J., Bullough, P., and Freiberger, R.: Orthopedic Diseases, Part II. New York, Famous Teachings in Modern Medicine, MedCom, Inc., © 1972).

Chondroblastoma

FIG. 8-72. Classic example of a chondroblastoma. The lesion is eccentric, epiphyseal, trabeculated, contains multiple, small stippled calcifications, and is bordered by benign sclerosis (*arrows*).

FIG. 8-73. Another classical case with all of the above features.

FIG. 8-74. Stippled calcifications and a prominent border of sclerosis are not readily apparent. Note, however, that the lesion is covered by a thin rim of cortical bone (*arrow*).

FIG. 8-75. (*A*) A more atypical example of chondroblastoma. The lesion is larger than usual, more lytic, and benign sclerosis is not clearly seen. (*B*) Tomogram shows lysis, an inferior border of reactive bone (a benign sign), and a pathologic fracture that has resulted in periosteal smooth new bone formation. The inferior border of sclerosis (*arrow*) helps to differentiate the lesion from a giant cell tumor, which does not show reactive bone of any kind, at least not in the vast majority of untreated lesions, at initial presentation.

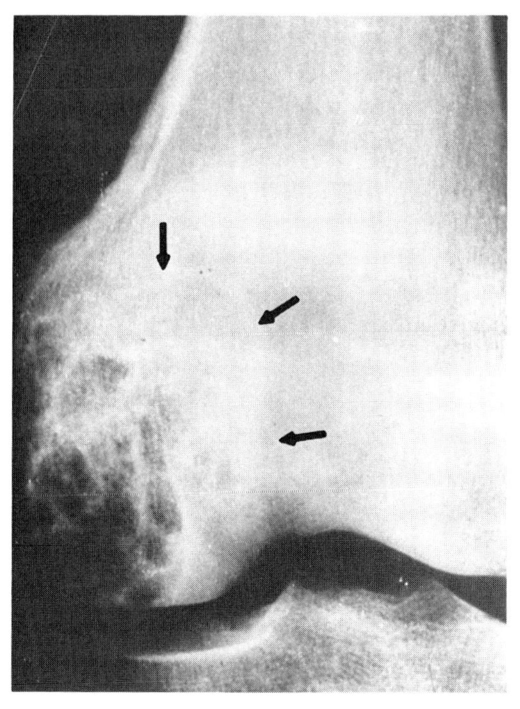

FIG. 8-72

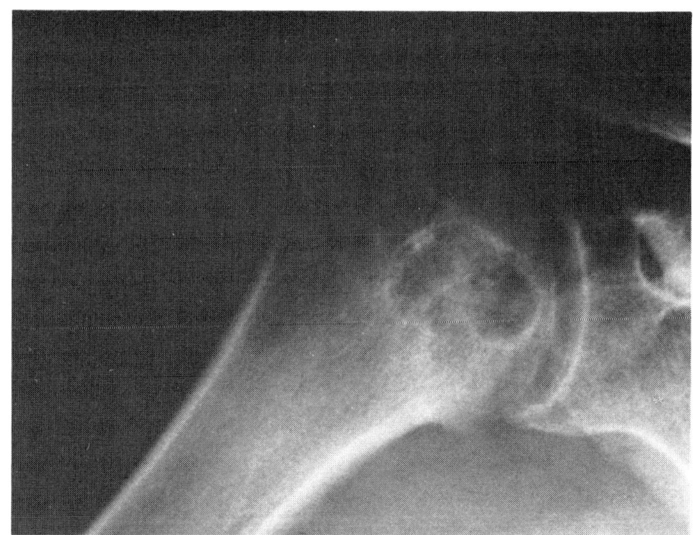

FIG. 8-73

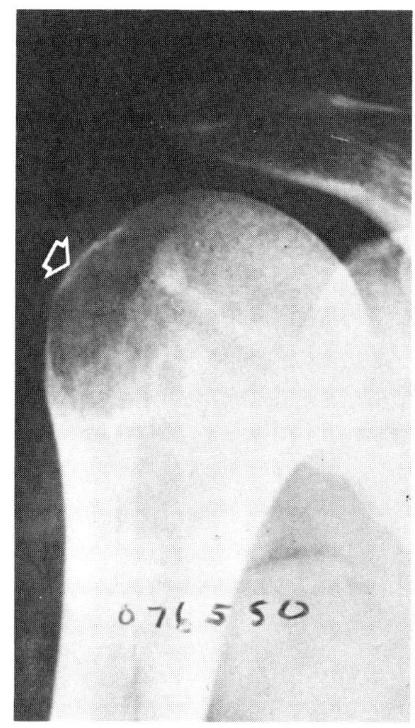

FIG. 8-74

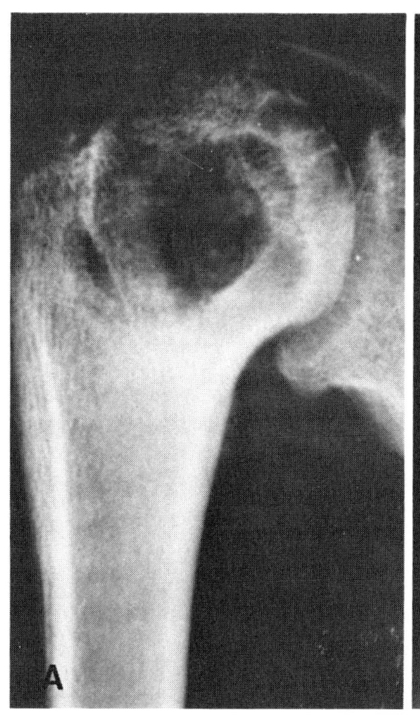

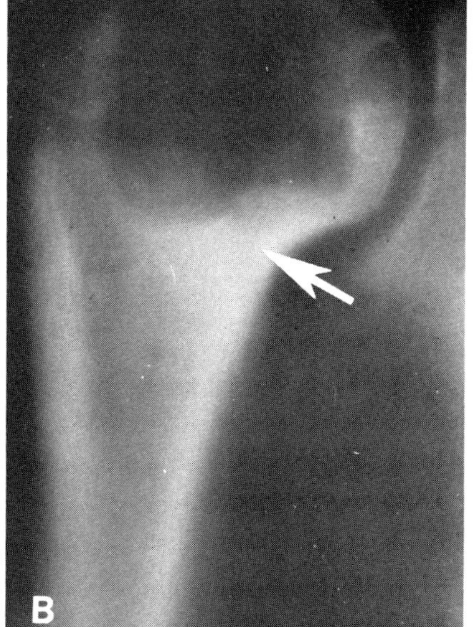

FIG. 8-75

radiologic clue to the true origin of these synovially derived lesions is the presence of focal cortical erosion at the point of penetration (Fig. 8–76, *arrow*).

Chondroblastomas, on the other hand, are almost always surrounded by at least a thin shell of cortical bone. The exception to this rule is in those chondroblastomas in which an aneurysmal bone cyst component has been engrafted (Fig. 8–84). Chondrosarcomas of the epiphysis may mimic chondroblastoma in every radiologic detail, except for the absence of a border of benign host bone sclerosis. Biopsy of each of the primary synovial lesions should readily distinguish them from chondroblastoma. The separation of chondrosarcoma from chondroblastoma depends heavily upon low-power evaluation. Chondrosarcomas are almost always composed of pure cartilage. With chondroblastomas, less than 50 per cent of the total lesional tissue is cartilage or chondroid tissues. They must also contain noncartilaginous areas consisting of chondroblasts, giant cells, and usually "chicken-wire" calcification.

Less common radiographic features of chondroblastoma are that they show pure lysis without punctuate calcifications (Figs. 8–73, 8–74, and 8–75); the absence of a clear-cut border of sclerosis (Fig. 8–74 and 8–75); periosteal new bone consequent to pathologic fracture (Fig. 8–75); large size with involvement of the entire epiphysis and extension to metaphysis (Fig. 8–84); and metaphyseal location without apparent involvement of the epiphysis (rare, less than 5 per cent of cases).

Chondroblastomas with these features are virtually impossible to distinguish from pigmented villonodular synovitis, tuberculosis, rheumatoid arthritis, chondrosarcoma, and giant cell tumor. Biopsy is crucial to distinguish these tumors.

GROSS PATHOLOGY

Curettage specimens are characterized by small pieces of gray-pink to hemorrhagic tissues, occasionally alternating with gritty calcified to yellow cholesterol-laden tissues. Small islands of bluish to white chondroid may be seen. In general, the amount of tissue removed is less than would be expected, considering the size of the lesion on radiograph. This is because the chondroblastoma is often modified by large cystic, degenerative, or regressive areas.

Those rare lesions removed en bloc show a similar admixture of tissues, with foci of cystic softening, small calcifications, and islands of chondroid. Most lesions are soft and resemble the grayish-pink or tan color of giant cell tumors. Areas of regressive changes with cholesterol or xanthoma cell deposits appear bright yellow-orange.

HISTOPATHOLOGY

The microscopic features of chondroblastoma are diagnostic, provided that great care is given to identify all notable features. If all of its features are not identified, the diagnosis must be suspect. In this author's opinion, there are some giant cell tumors and chondrosarcomas that may have chondroblastoma-like features; these lead to serious errors in diagnosis and treatments and hopeless confusion in the literature. Unless the unequivocal chondroblastoma is identified with certainty, the question of whether or not some chondroblastomas have true biologic malignant potential will never be answered. Extreme caution must be taken in the diagnosis of chondroblastoma and great care in obtaining imprints, tissue for electron microscopy, and well-stained sections. Also the radiographic features must be reviewed carefully before arriving at a diagnosis. Even greater care must be given in reviewing all records and material on any case that recurs or metastasizes; the same criteria to the recurrences and metastases of chondroblastoma should be given as for that of primary bone lesion. Only in this way will it be possible to separate those lesions that mimic chondroblastoma, to identify those unequivocal chondroblastomas that have undergone anaplastic transformation from those with aggressive but apparently self-limited growth in local or distant sites.

Microscopic Features of an Unequivocal Chondroblastoma

The following minimum features must be present to diagnose a chondroblastoma with certainty:

1. The lesion must contain two basic cell types: the *chondroblast* and the *osteoclast-like giant cell* (Figs. 8–78 and 8–79). The chondroblast is a polygonally shaped cell with distinct cell borders (Figs. 8–79 and 8–80, *A*). Most of the cells contain a single nucleus. The nucleus is round, oval or slightly indented, or lobulated and fills about one-half of the cell. The chromatin distribution is even and nucleoli are inconspicuous. Mitotic figures are typical and may be quite variable in numbers (in some cases, up to one or two per HPF). The cytoplasm is granular and a deep pink and has rounded sharp borders. The cells

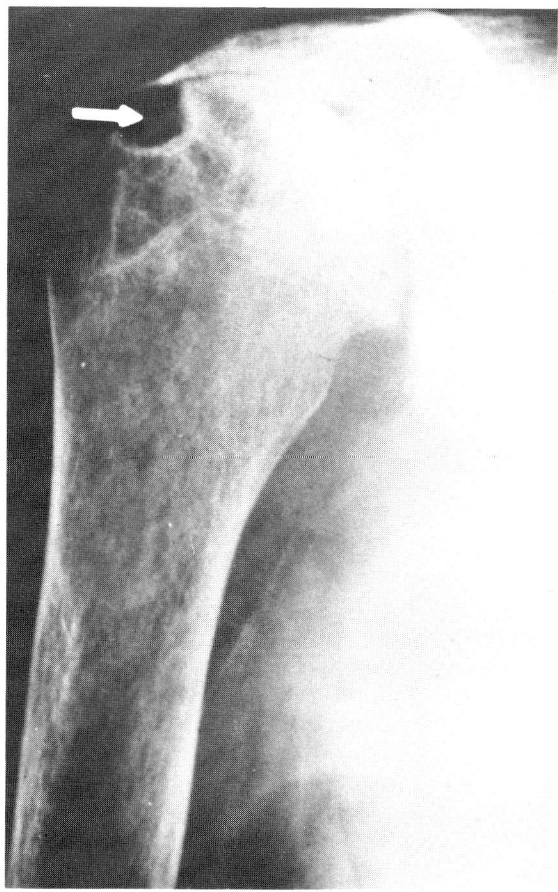

"Invasive" Synovial Lesions Which May Resemble Chondroblastoma

FIG. 8-76. Rheumatoid arthritis: synovium invading bone simulating a chondroblastoma. Note the small defect in the cortex (*arrow*). This represents the area in which the synovium has penetrated the bone at the articular cartilage-cortical interface. Pigmented villonodular synovitis, gout, and tuberculosis may result in similar chondroblastoma-like lesions. A cortical defect similar to that shown in this figure is a clue to radiologic diagnosis of an "invasive" synovial process.

contain variable amounts of glycogen (Fig. 8-79). Although cells with similar shapes may be seen in the stromal cells of the giant cell tumor, the vast majority are spindled in shape (Fig. 8-80, *B*). Spindly cells in chondroblastoma are usually minimal except in areas of reparative scarring. Chondroblastoma-like cells may be seen in the clear-cell chondrosarcoma (Fig. 8-35, *B*). In these tumors there usually is evidence of some degree of unequivocal nuclear anaplasia and, most importantly, cells with a voluminous, distinctly clear cytoplasm (Fig. 8-35, *A*). A chondroblast is, therefore, not a cell which by the light microscope is pathognomonic of a chondroblastoma. The diagnosis of chondroblastoma must depend on its other features as well.

The giant cells seen in chondroblastoma are probably reactive osteoclasts that permeate the lesion and contain from as few as three to 50 or more nuclei per cell section (Fig. 8-78). They usually sprinkle the nonchondroid areas. They may be indistinguishable in number, size, and distribution from true giant cell tumors. Rare cases of chondroblastoma may show so little chondroid that several sections may have to be studied if confusion with a giant cell tumor is to be avoided.

2. The lesion must contain islands of primitive chondroid, fibrochondroid, or hyaline cartilage.

All chondroblastomas produce cartilage or chondroid tissue. The islands of chondroid (Fig. 8-77, Plate 6, *J*) are separated from the adjacent cellular chondroblastic and giant cell areas. *The islands of chondroid rarely occupy more than 50 per cent of the total lesional tissue.* This is crucial in distinguishing epiphyseal enchondromas and chondrosarcomas, which produce pure cartilage with or without osseous metaplasia of the cartilage lobules.

Mesenchymal chondrosarcoma and chondrosarcomas with fibro- or osteosarcomatous transformation may contain islands of cartilage to chondroid that might resemble chondroblastoma patterns on low power. High-power examination will, however, show unequivocal anaplasia in these latter conditions.

The tumor that most closely resembles a chondroblastoma is the clear-cell chondrosarcoma (see p. 186 and Figs. 8-34 and 8-35).

3. The chondroblastoma is also typified by the *deposition of calcium.* It may deposit as calcific nodules within the chondroid islands, but more characteristically, it deposits in the stromal tissue surrounding individual chondroblast cells. The deposition around individual cells imparts an unusual "chicken-wire" type of calcification (Fig. 8-81, Plate 6, *K* and *L*). This type of calcification is almost unique to chondroblastoma but has been described by Unni, *et. al.,*[69] in some cases of clear-cell chondrosarcoma.

The peculiar type of calcium deposition seen in chondroblastoma occurs in the reticulin sheath that surrounds each chondroblast (Fig. 8-82). The reticulin pattern in the chondroblastic cellular areas resembles that of a honeycomb. This reticulin pattern is not, however, found in the chondroid islands (personal observations).

The deposition of heavy calcium salts around each cell probably results in interference with their nutrient supply. As a result the chondroblasts undergo necrosis, which stimulates even more deposition of calcium. The buildup of calcium in these areas leads to the formation of dense calcific nodules (Fig. 8-81), which account for the minute, rounded densities seen on radiographic examination.

Other Microscopic Features

Other features that may be found in chondroblastoma but which are not crucial to diagnosis include:

1. **REACTIONS TO FOCI OF DEGENERATION.** Variable portions of the chondroblastoma may undergo significant degeneration and hemorrhage. As a result, histiocytes may be seen engulfing necrotic debris. Eventually, the smaller histiocytes may convert to large, foamy macrophages. Masses of cholesterol may be deposited in these regions (Fig. 8-83). Similar degenerative features may be seen in nonossifying fibroma and eosinophilic granuloma.
2. **BONY METAPLASIA OF CHONDROID.** In some cases portions of the chondroid lobules undergo bony metaplasia. In most instances the bone is woven. Eventually this bone may be converted to the lamellar type. The degree of osseous metaplasia may be so intense that care should be taken not to diagnose osteoblastoma or osteosarcoma. In order to diagnose these latter conditions, woven bone must form directly from the stroma without first passing through a cartilage phase.
3. **ANEURYSMAL BONE CYST COMPONENT.** In some cases of chondroblastoma an engrafted vascular component occurs (a possible arteriovenous malformation) that resembles an aneurysmal bone cyst. This component consists of cystlike fibrous tissue and its central spaces, which are usually filled with unclotted blood (Fig. 8-85). Focal clotting is possible.

COURSE

The vast majority of chondroblastomas (approximately 95%) do not recur following simple procedures

---

Chondroblastoma

FIG. 8-77. (*A*) A typical area at low power. The tissue consists of stromal cells, osteoclast-like giant cells, foci of stromal calcification, and chondroid islands (*arrows*). The chondroid rarely occupies more than 50 per cent of the entire lesional tissue and may be as little as 5 percent (x40). (*B*) Typical appearance of the chondroid (x125). (*C*) The chondroid consists of small, round cells with hyperchromatic nuclei set in a homogeneously, usually pink stroma. Hyaline cartilage, on the other hand, is usually blue and lighter in staining quality (x250).

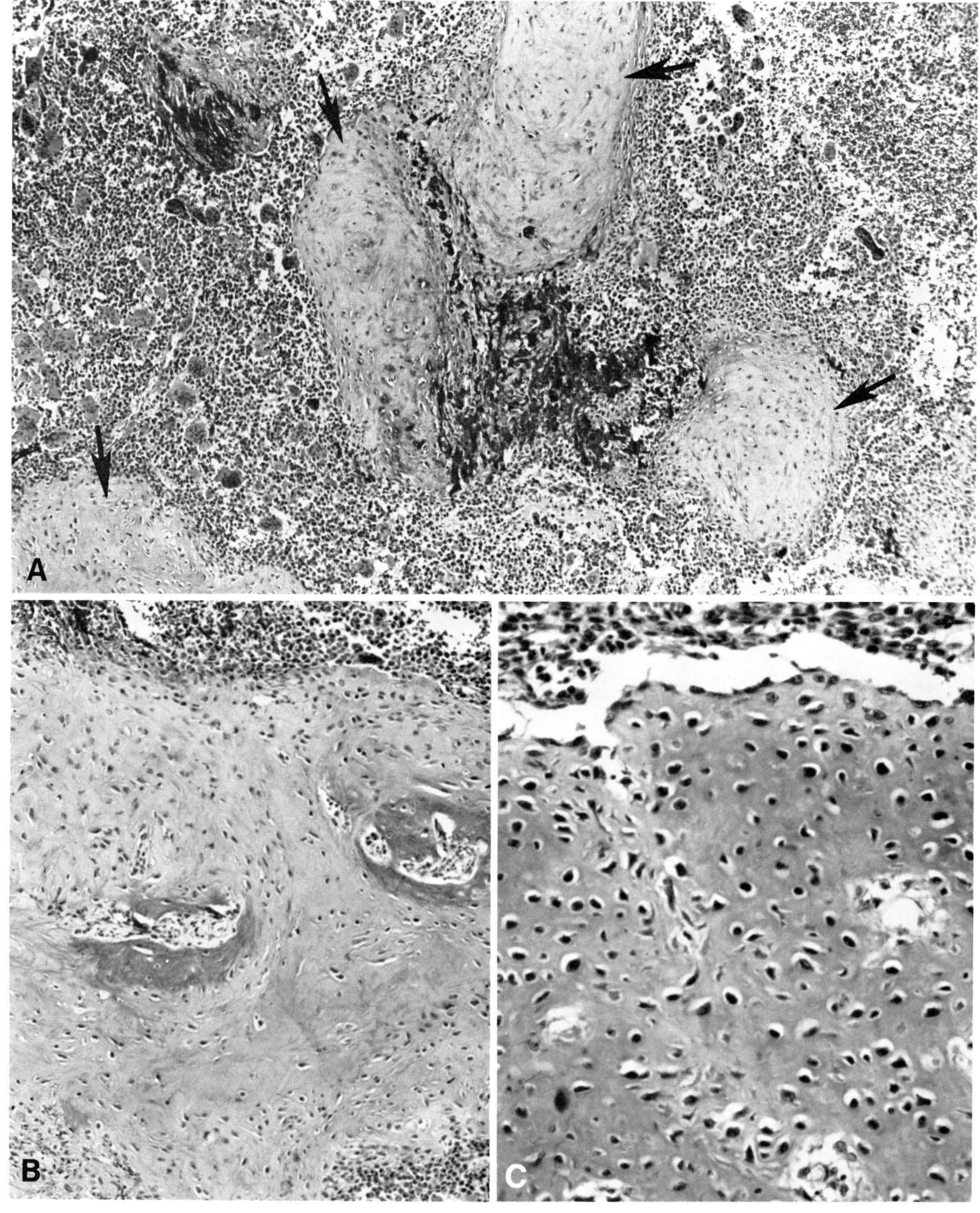

FIG. 8-77

such as curettage and packing with bone chips and/or radiation therapy.[62] Approximately 2 per cent have developed metastasis in addition to one or more local recurrences (see below).

Treatment

The majority of chondroblastomas are unequivocally benign and respond favorably to curettage and packing with bone chips. If the lesion is in the patella or ribs, it is possible to simply resect the lesion.

Irradiation has been used, but there is a distinct danger of sarcomatous transformation years later.

Dahlin and Ivins[39] recommend that chondroblastomas be curettaged and the cavity cauterized with phenol, neutralized with alcohol, and rinsed copiously with saline. This is followed by autogenous iliac bone grafting to fill the defect.

The next section discusses the course of treatment if there is recurrence or metastasis.

MALIGNANT CHONDROBLASTOMA—DOES SUCH AN ENTITY EXIST?

Is there such an entity as a malignant chondroblastoma? In an attempt to answer this question, this author has reviewed all of the reported cases in the literature with the diagnosis of chondroblastoma and metastasis and most of those cases with local recurrence without metastasis. There are slightly over 500 reported cases of chondroblastoma to 1977. From among these cases there are a minimum of 28 with one or more local recurrences, an incidence of 6 per cent of reported cases.[38,43,44,50,53,59,62,64,66] There are nine cases reported with metastasis, an incidence of 2 per cent of reported cases (see Table 8-1).

The series reported by Huvos, *et al.*,[49] showed a recurrence rate of 38 per cent. Some 24 per cent of the recurrences were associated with an aneurysmal bone cyst (ABC) component. None of their patients succumbed to their disease, though one received amputation. These cases of multiple recurrences associated with an ABC component were successfully cured with cryosurgery. All of their patients with long-term follow-up were free of disease. Of the other reported patients with recurrences without evidence of metastasis, all were eventually cured by various modalities of local treatment except for two patients who received amputation.[53,62] Since cure was obtained in these cases by less than radical surgical procedures, their true biologic behavior was, in most instances, benign. Their growth was eventually self-limited. In many of these cases the tumor could not have been totally eradicated by the local surgical procedure (e.g., curettage, partial resection). The fact that cure was eventually achieved in spite of this attests to the fact that these lesions are not malignant, at least not in the usual sense of the term. Therefore, in this author's opinion, these cases do not qualify as examples of malignant chondroblastoma.

Of nine patients with "chondroblastoma" with metastasis, five succumbed to metastatic disease (Table 8-1). Such a clinical course certainly is malignant. But, a critical analysis of these cases reveals the following data. Two patients, both reported by Hatcher,[44,45] developed anaplastic tumors 4 to 5½ years following radiation. In one patient,[42] the malignancy arose in the fibula, while the chondroblastoma had occurred in the tibia.[44] This is clearly a post-irradiation sarcoma of an adjacent bone. It is not possible to state with certainty whether the other case represented *de novo* malignant transformation in a chondroblastoma or radiation sarcoma.[45] It probably was a radiation-induced sarcoma. Sirsat's patient[64] did not receive radiation and 6 years later developed an anaplastic round-cell tumor, which rapidly led to the patient's demise. This case unquestionably qualifies as a chondroblastoma with malignant transformation to an anaplastic small-cell tumor consistent, in my opinion, with a tumor of chondroblastic origin

---

Chondroblastoma Versus Giant Cell Tumor

FIG. 8-78. Areas with numerous osteoclastic giant cells simulating giant cell tumor are common. However, the stromal cells of chondroblastoma are much rounder to polygonal and the cell borders much more distinct (H and E, x400).

FIG. 8-79. (*A*) Imprint characteristics. The nuclei of the chondroblasts are round to lobulated and indented. The chromatin is evenly dispersed. Nucleoli are inconspicuous. Mitoses are usually rare. Note the osteoclast to the left (x600). (*B*) The chondroblast cytoplasm contains dark granules of glycogen (PAS, x1000). However, glycogen may also be seen in the stromal cells of giant cell tumor.

FIG. 8-80. (*A*) Chondroblastoma (x400). (*B*) Giant cell tumor (x400). Note the distinct differences in cytoplasmic characteristics. Giant cell tumor has more spindly cells and indistinct cell borders. (*A*) also shows a fine reticulin sheathe (*arrows*) around many of the cells would not be visible on an H and E section of a giant cell tumor.

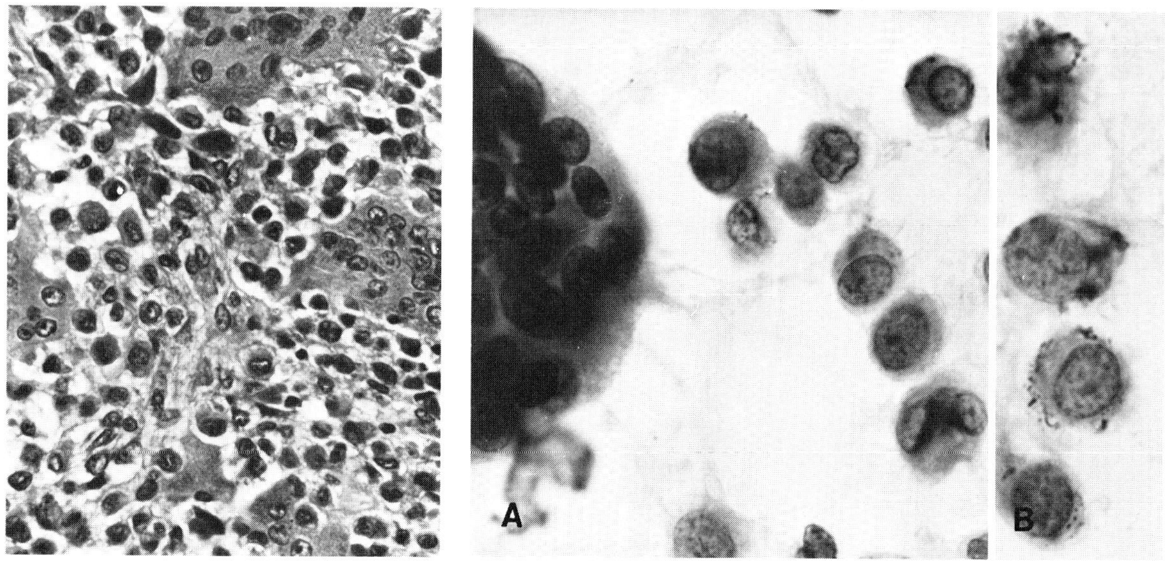

FIG. 8-78

FIG. 8-79

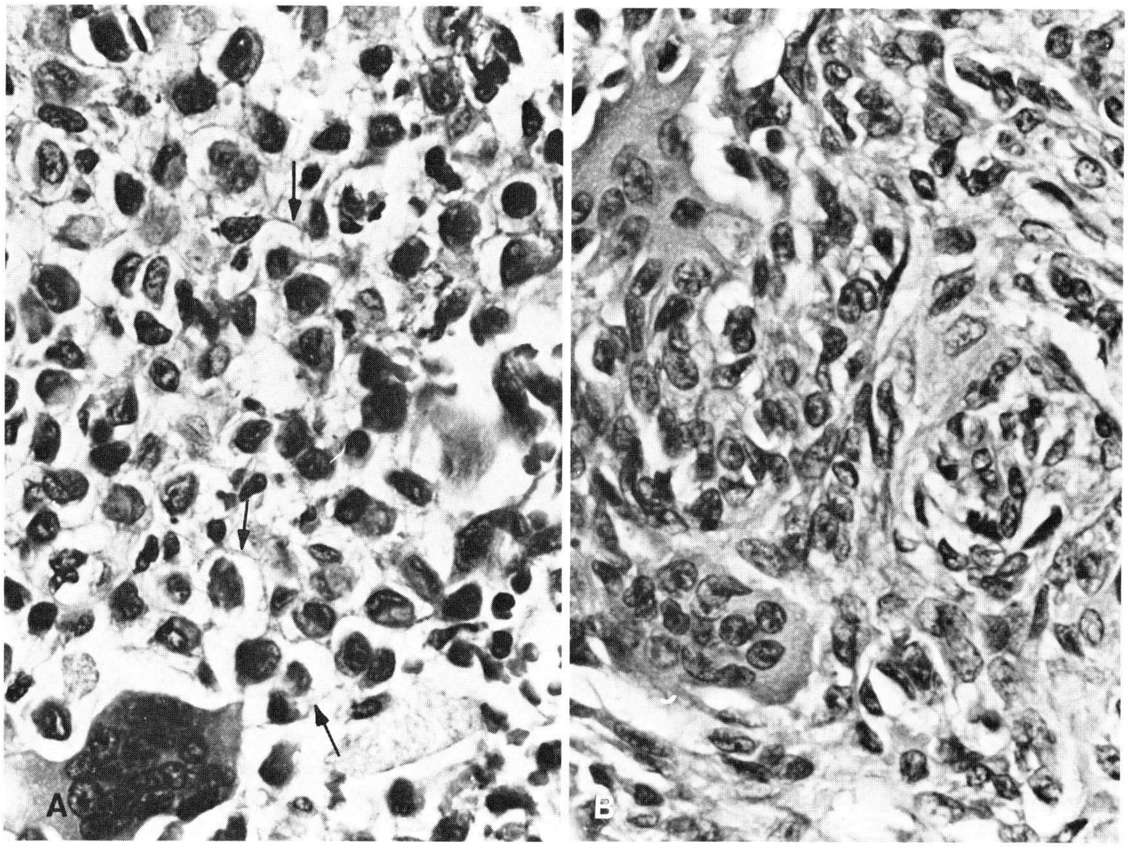

FIG. 8-80

(chondroblastic sarcoma). It is well known that almost any benign condition of bone may undergo malignant transformation in a variable percentage of cases. Sweetnam's case has no illustrations or histological description of the primary tumor or the lung metastasis. Without these data analysis would be purely speculative. Schajowicz's case[62] (Case 6, Table 8–1) shows an unequivocal primary chondroblastoma admixed with atypical spindle cells. Six years after curettage there was "sarcomatous transformation." Amputation showed an anaplastic spindle-cell sarcoma. He died with metastases shortly thereafter and an autopsy was not performed. Unfortunately, there are no histological illustrations of the lesion at amputation. In all likelihood the lesion did represent a sarcomatous transformation in a chondroblastoma, as Dr. Schajowicz has suggested. It is unfortunate that this case has not been more liberally documented.

Of the final four cases, three [43,51,59] are well illustrated and showed unequivocal "benign" chondroblastoma in the primary, recurrent, and metastatic lesions. These are the only three cases with features of ordinary chondroblastoma present at local and distant sites. In all three cases multiple lung "metastases" developed. Most of the lung "metastases" were removed but in two of three cases one or more of the lesions was not removed. All of the remaining lung "metastases" grew to a small size (smaller than 2 cm.) and thereafter ceased growing, even after 2 and 5 years of follow-up. One of the patients received amputation but the other two were treated locally with success. All three patients are alive and well with no progression of the disease. This is a most peculiar phenomenon. The only three cases with unequivocal documentation of ordinary appearing chondroblastoma in all sites had residual self-limited lung nodules in two. In all three there has been neither demise nor progression of the disease. Certainly if these are examples of malignant chondroblastoma, they are most curious. The vast majority of true malignant tumors, when they metastasize lead relentlessly to the demise of the patients. Here we have three out of three cases where the tumors act differently from the vast majority of malignant tumors. Another peculiar fact is that in the chondroblastoma with transformation to an anaplastic tumor without preceding radiation (Table 8–1, Case 5) metastases were to multiple organ systems (liver, lymph nodes, and spleen). All of these facts are explainable by the following hypothesis: in unequivocal chondroblastoma cases, vigorous curettage can result in embolization of tissue into the venous drainage system of the bone and from there, to the lungs. Furthermore, in rare cases this embolization results in benign lung implants with a capacity to grow for a limited time period. In other words the "metastasis" in unequivocal "benign" chondroblastoma may be iatrogenic, benign, and self-limited. This hypothesis would explain the fact that the "metastases" are seen following surgical intervention, are limited to the lungs only, reach a certain maximum size, and fill in with metaplastic bone. It also explains the cure in the primary lesion of Huvos, following cryosurgery, despite soft-tissue implantation.

There would be a vast difference in treatment and prognosis, depending upon which concept is adhered to. On the one hand, the theory that holds that metastatic lesions with unequivocal histological evidence supporting ordinary chondroblastoma are malignant and will lead to the demise of the patient requires that massive en-bloc resection or amputation and surgical removal of each lung metastasis and possibly systemic chemotherapy be implemented. On the other hand, the theory that formulates that this phenomenon seen in association with chondroblastoma is merely benign "metastatic" implants post-curettage would require less radical procedures to control the local and systemic disease. Removal of as many of the lung metastases as possible could be considered an elective surgical procedure, with the expectation that if some are left behind they will be self-limited in growth; this obviates the need for systemic chemotherapy. However, at least one lung lesion must be removed in toto to confirm the presence of ordinary chondroblastoma tissue. The question, of course, is

---

Chondroblastoma

FIG. 8–81. Another characteristic feature rarely seen in any other lesion is pericellular "chicken-wire" type calcifications (left of field). These pericellular reticular calcifications lead to chondroblast necrosis, after which more extensive globular calcification occurs (*arrow*) (x250).

FIG. 8–82. Reticulin stain shows that the calcification in this tumor occurs in reticulin fibers that surround the chondroblasts in a honeycomb fashion (x250).

FIG. 8–83. Foci of necrosis may result in the accumulation of foamy macrophages and cholesterol crystals (x125).

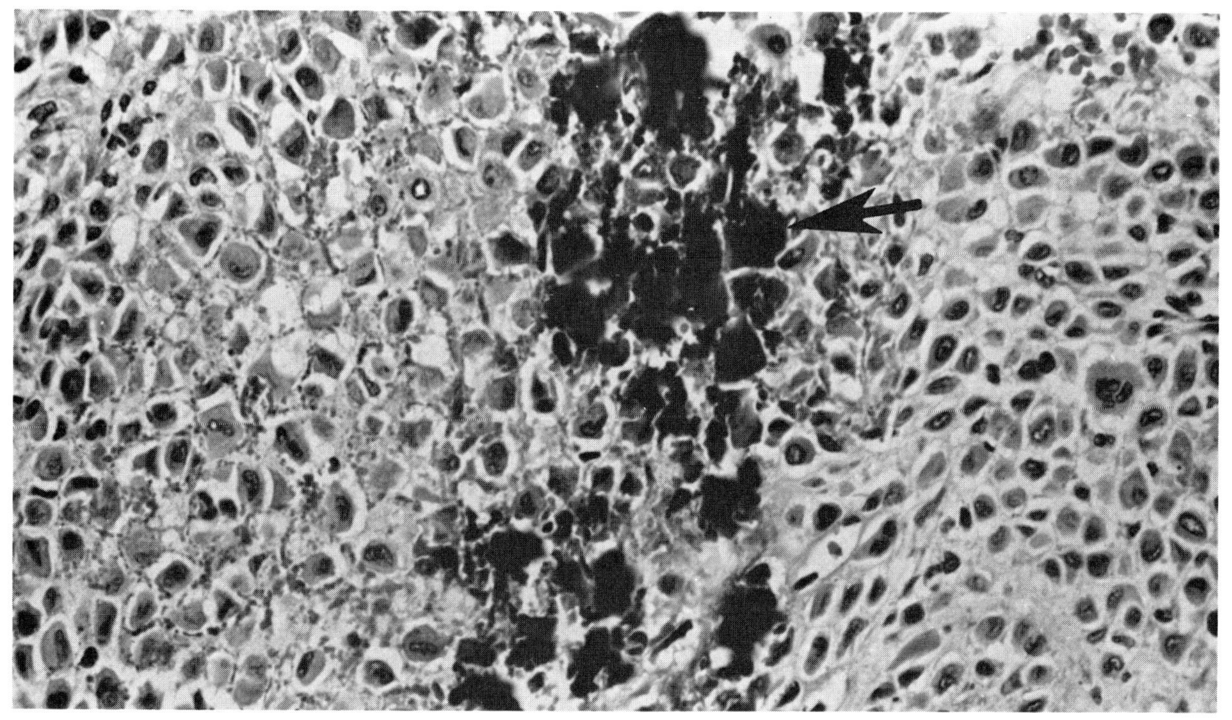

FIG. 8-81

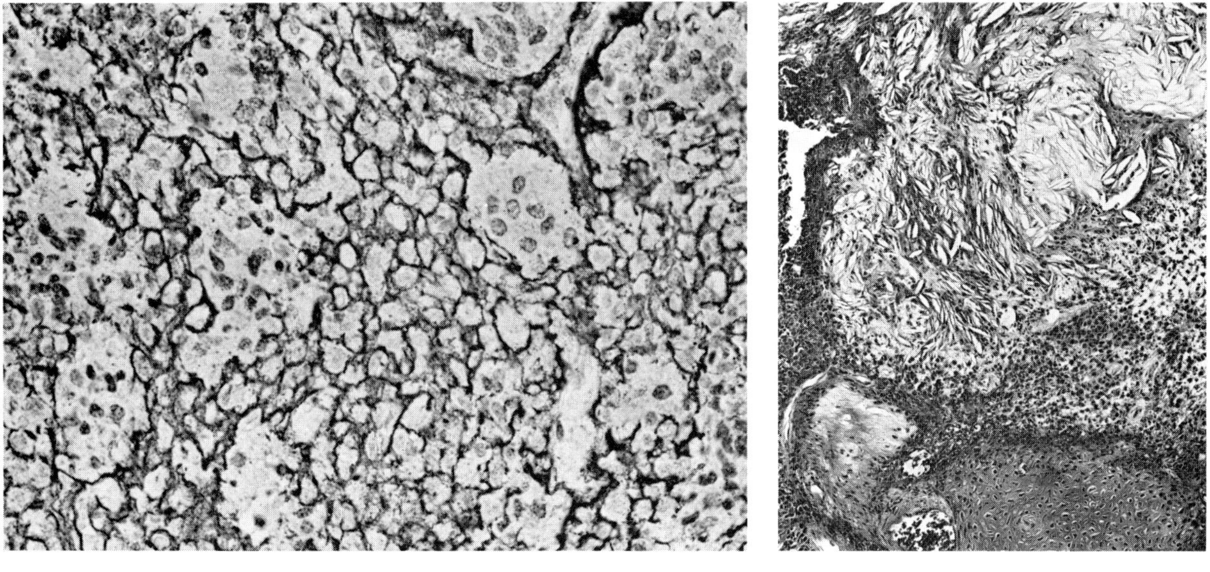

FIG. 8-82

FIG. 8-83

Table 8-1. Reported Cases of

Case	Authors	Age	Sex	Location	Histology	Primary Treatment	Local Recurrence	Histology of Recurrence
1	Hatcher[44]	23	M	Tibia	Probable chondroblastoma (1 illustration*)	Curettage and 9800 rads	4 years post-irradiation developed tumor in fibula	Chondrosarcoma arising in fibula. Lesion composed of round and spindle cells (illustrations poor quality).
2	Hatcher[45]	19	M	Humerus	Probable chondroblastoma (2 illustrations of fair quality)	Biopsy and curettage followed by 3600 rads	+ 4 years	Unequivocal anaplastic (Grade III) chondrosarcoma
3	Sweetnam, et al.[66]	19	M	Fibula	Called chondroblastoma (no illustrations)	Local excision	Not stated	—
4	Kahn, et al.[53]	13	M	Pelvis	Possible chondroblastoma (1 illustration)	Biopsy and curettage	+ multiple to age 29	Highly suggestive of chondroblastoma (1 illustration)
5	Sirsat, et al.[64]	15	M	Tibia	Unequivocal chondroblastoma (well illustrated)	Curettage	+ multiple, 2 to 6 years	Anaplastic round cell tumor (well illustrated)
6	Schajowicz[62]	32	F	Metatarsal	Unequivocal chondroblastoma and spindle cell areas	Curettage	+ 5 months, 1½ years	Not stated
7	Riddel, et al.[59]	14	F	Tibia	Unequivocal chondroblastoma (well illustrated)	Biopsy and curettage	+ 8 months	Unequivocal chondroblastoma (well illustrated)
8	Green, et al.[43]	13	F	Femur	Unequivocal chondroblastoma (well illustrated)	Curettage	+ 7 months	Identical to primary lesion (well illustrated)
9	Huvos, et al.[51]	16	M	Femur	Unequivocal chondroblastoma (well illustrated)	Curettage	+ 7 months, 3½ years. Soft tissue nodules	Identical to primary lesion (well illustrated)

which concept is correct? In this author's opinion, a definitive answer is not yet possible, considering the meager number of cases with excellent documentation. It will obviously be up to future authors to liberally illustrate and fully document such cases so that a unifying concept can be achieved upon which to base therapy with confidence.

Metastasis could be defined as the spread of a malignant tumor from one organ or tissue to another by means of vascular dissemination. Metastasis of a malignant tumor may occur because of the aggressive nature of the lesion or, in some cases, may occur iatrogenically at the time of surgery. In either case the metastases will grow relentlessly and destroy the host in the vast majority of cases. "Benign" metastasis, by strict definition would, therefore, be a misnomer. However, the term *benign* metastasis could be defined as the embolization of a benign tumor by a chance *in vitro* occurrence or as a result of iatrogenic surgical manipulation, such as vigorous curettage. If the lesions progress in size and lead to the demise of the patient, they are obviously not "benign" metastases. But, if the lesions reach a certain maximum size and stop growing and do not lead to the demise of the patient, they could be indicative of a "benign" metastasis or implant. It is well known, for example, that implants of bone and marrow can be found in the lung following rib fracture consequent to vigorous

Chondroblastoma of Bone Associated With Metastasis

Therapy Post-Recurrence	*Metastasis*	*Histology of Metastasis*	*Therapy Post-Metastasis*	*Course*	*Personal Comments*
None	Lungs in $5\frac{1}{2}$ years	None	None	Died $2\frac{1}{2}$ years post-amputation No autopsy	Clearly a post-irradiation sarcoma arising in the fibula, adjacent to the original chondroblastoma of tibia
Wide resection followed by amputation 5 months later	Lung 1 year post-amputation	None	None	Died 1 year post-amputation Total course, 6 years	Probable post-irradiation chondrosarcoma
—	Lungs	Identical to primary (no illustration)	Amputation	Alive and well $5\frac{1}{2}$ years post-amputation	No illustrations to support diagnosis of chondroblastoma
Partial resections	Rib, shoulder, lungs	Very suggestive of chondroblastoma (2 illustrations)	None	Died 15 years after initial diagnosis Pelvic and shoulder masses at autopsy	Chondroblastoma-like chondrosarcoma not clearly ruled out. Radiograph of primary lesion looks like a malignant tumor. Huge size of the lesion mitigates against diagnosis of chondroblastoma
Amputation after 6 years	Liver, lymph nodes	None	None	Died 2 months post-amputation No autopsy	Anaplastic transformation (chondroblastic sarcoma)
Resections	Thigh and neck 6 yrs. after resection	None	None	Died 6 years after initial diagnosis No autopsy	Insufficient documentation for conclusion
Amputation	Lung, 3 months post-amputation	Identical to primary (well illustrated)	3 lungs metastases removed	Well 5 years post-thoractomy Serial radiographs show one remaining and unchanging lung nodule	Chondroblastoma with "benign" metastasis
Curettage and bone grafting	Lungs, multiple	Identical to primary (well illustrated)	Several lung metastases removed, several left	Well 2 years later No progression of remaining pulmonary lesions	Chondroblastoma with "benign" metastasis
Cryosurgery	Lungs, 17 nodules	Identical to primary (well illustrated)	Thoractomy, 17 nodules removed	Well 6 years later No recurrence or remaining disease in lungs.	Chondroblastoma with "benign" metastasis

*Illustration(s) refers to those photomicrographs that appear in the article cited above. Comments about the quality of the illustrations are my own.

cardiac resuscitation and squames and decidua may be found in the lungs as a complication of pregnancy. These cells or implants are entirely self-limited. The rare, benign "metastasizing" leiomyoma to lungs and the rare, benign glandular inclusions in lymph nodes have been formulated to perhaps represent "benign" metastasis by Edlow, *et al.* The concept of "benign" metastasis, therefore, has precedence.

This author has seen one of these three fascinating cases of unequivocal chondroblastoma in bone and lung in 1973 at Memorial Hospital in consultation with Drs. Huvos and Marcove. The concept of iatrogenic implantation of a benign tumor resulted in my belief to resist amputation and to remove the lung "metastases" without follow-up chemotherapy. Drs. Huvos and Marcove concurred. With the kind permission of Drs. Huvos and Marcove I present this very important teaching case.[51]

The patient was a 16-year-old boy who developed a distal femur lesion. It was curetted and showed unequivocal chondroblastoma (Fig. 8-86). It recurred 6 months later and was recuretted and treated cryosurgically. It showed identical tissues. At about the same time a 1-cm. lung nodule was seen on radiograph. Three years later 17 1 to 2 cm.-lung nodules were seen. All 17 were removed at thoracotomy. The lesions showed unequivocal chondroblastoma, most of which were undergoing benign osseous replacement (Figs. 8–87–8–89). Much of the bone surrounding the chondroblastoma was the benign lamellar type. Biopsy of the femur was negative for recurrence. There has been no further progression of the disease with 5 years of follow-up. His extremity functions normally.

This author's working concept in regard to unequivocal "benign" chondroblastoma in the long bones showing unequivocal "benign" chondroblastoma in the lungs from this case and Cases seven and eight from Table 8–1 is the following:

1. Chondroblastoma cells enter the lungs after vigorous curettage.
2. The cells grow in the lung because of unknown favorable conditions.
3. The lesion reaches a maximum size (up to 2 cm.) and stops growing because of an inherent, benign, self-limited growth capacity.
4. The lesion fills in with metaplastic ossification.

The case of Kahn[53] (Table 8–1, Case five) describes a benign chondroblastoma that leads to recurrence and lethal metastases and is a very perplexing case. Anaplasia was not described in the metastases or in the huge local lesion. Mitoses were sparse. There is no doubt that their illustrations strongly resemble an ordinary chondroblastoma. Three of the four basic features are shown: chondroblast-like cells, giant cells, and chondroid. Unfortunately, there is no illustration to show the other crucial feature of "chicken-wire" calcification resulting in cell necrosis and larger masses of calcification.

The first illustration also shows some cells with a clear or vacuolated cytoplasm; this raises the suspicion of clear-cell chondrosarcoma. The illustrations from the metastases do not, however, show this feature. If this case truly represents an unequivocal chondroblastoma in all tissues, then it is the only one of its kind and further emphasizes the need for continued analysis of future cases. The case also raises the possibility that certain host factors that normally contain a benign lesion are not present in certain very rare patients. In other words, what would ordinarily be a benign lesion for most patients may be biologically malignant in very rare cases. This possibility also deserves future consideration.

Let us now return to the original question: "Is there such an entity as malignant chondroblastoma?" From an analysis of the reported data, so-called malignant chondroblastoma appears to fall in the following three categories:

GROUP I. CHONDROBLASTOMA WITH SARCOMATOUS TRANSFORMATION. These cases are characterized by unequivocal chondroblastoma in the primary lesion followed by an anaplastic transformation 4 or more years following radiation or arising *de novo*. This occurs in less than 1 per cent of reported cases.

GROUP II. CHONDROBLASTOMA WITH BENIGN(?) LUNG METASTASIS. Three reported cases are typified by self-limited lung metastases. Whether these cases represent benign iatrogenic lung implantation or true lethal implants is not completely resolved. This occurrence is seen in less than 1 per cent of reported cases.

GROUP III. CHONDROBLASTOMA-LIKE CHONDROSARCOMAS. Unless absolutely strict radiological and histological criteria are met, it is possible that chondrosarcoma variants are confused with chondroblastoma. The malignant radiographic features of Kahn's case would certainly suggest a chondrosarcoma variant.

Some cases of the clear-cell chondrosarcoma variant described by Dahlin and Unni[39,69] (Figs. 8–34 and 8–35) had been mistakingly diagnosed as chondroblastoma prior to their consultation. Varma and Gupta[70], in their 1972 article, describe a case of atypical recurrent chondroblastoma that is histologically similar, if not identical, to a clear-cell chondrosarcoma.

Chondroblastoma With Aneurysmal Bone Cyst Component and a Case With Lung "Metastasis"

FIG. 8-84. Large atypical chondroblastoma with loss of cortical border because of an engrafted aneurysmal bone cyst component.

FIG. 8-85. Aneurysmal bone cyst component in association with chondroblastomatous tissues (x40).

FIG. 8-86. Unequivocal "benign" chondroblastoma of distal femoral metaphysis of a 16-year-old male. Lesion has chondroid, (*arrow*), ordinary chondroblasts, "chicken-wire" calcification, and giant cells (x125).

FIG. 8-87. Multiple lung nodules from the above patient were noted in the lungs 5 years later. The lung nodules were removed and were round in shape and most were surrounded by lamellar bone with central, partially to completely necrotic chondroblastoma tissue (shown *above*). One lung nodule was composed of pure lamellar bone and marrow fat (x10).

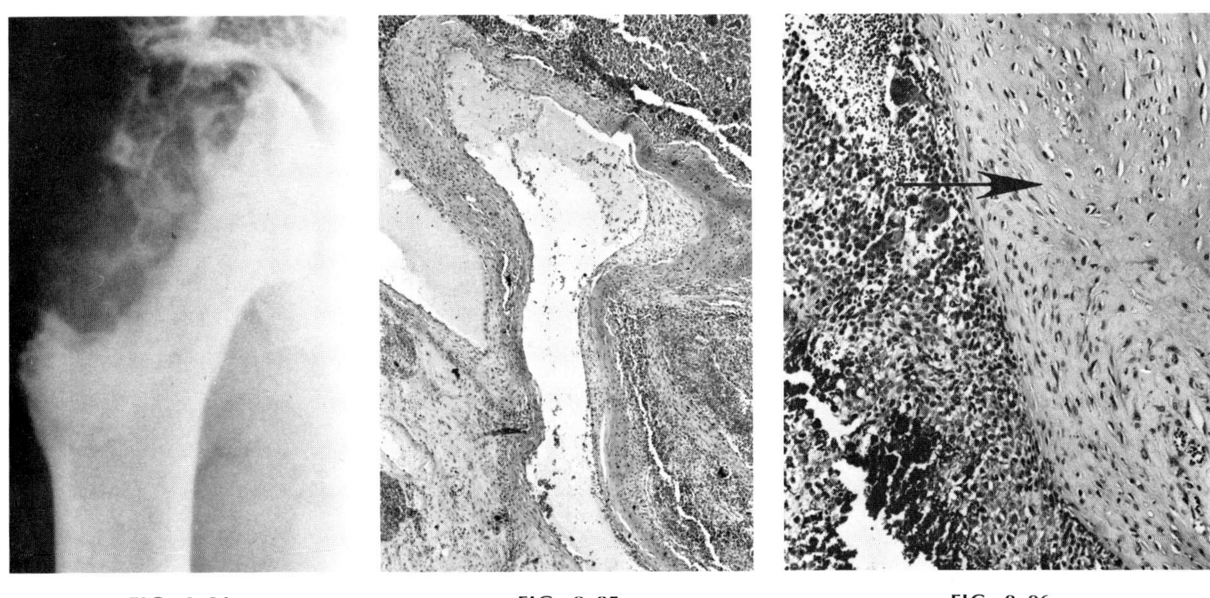

FIG. 8-84

FIG. 8-85

FIG. 8-86

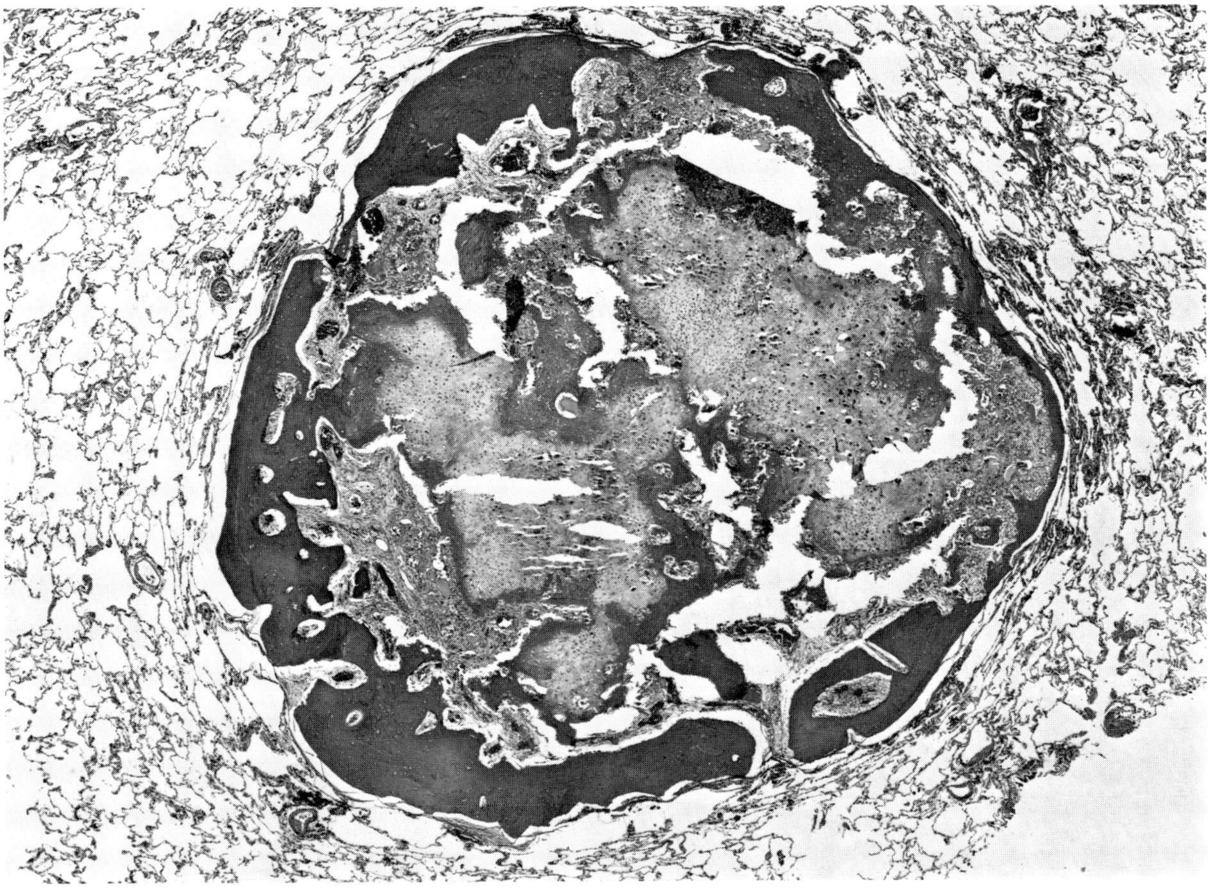

FIG. 8-87

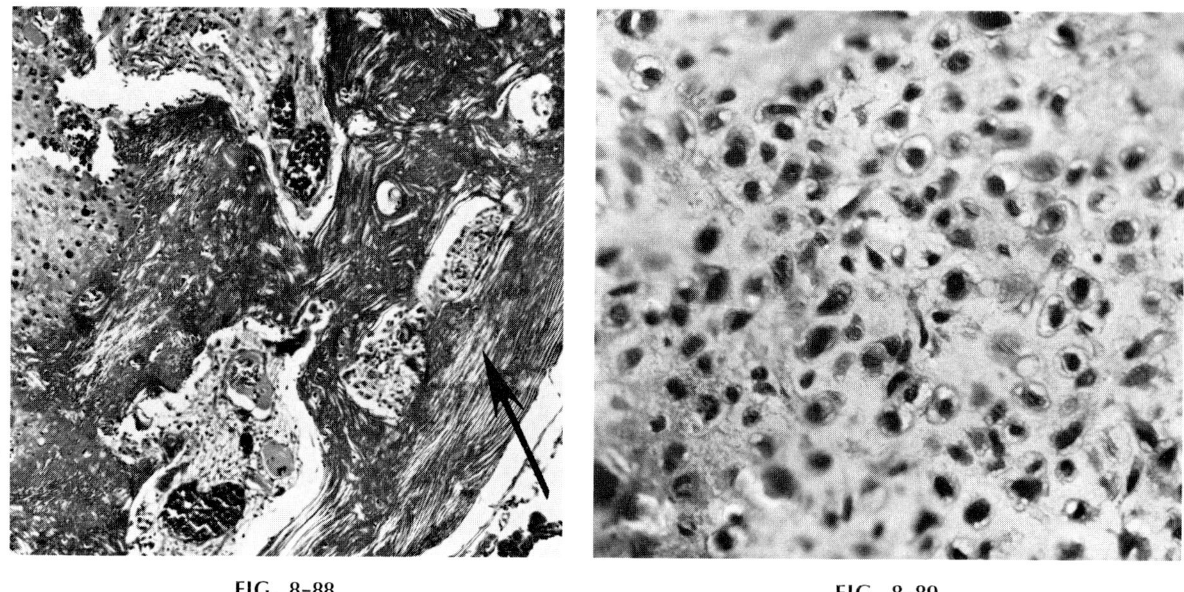

FIG. 8-88

FIG. 8-89

Chondroblastoma With Lung "Metastasis"

FIG. 8-88. The bone surrounding the lung lesion is converting to a benign lamellar form (*arrow*). To the left are degenerating chondroblasts (partial polarized light, x125).

FIG. 8-89. Small focus of viable chondroblasts embedded in chondroid. The nuclei did not show anaplasia (x250). The young man is doing well with no recurrences or further lung metastasis 7 years after thoracotomy. This case probably represents "benign" or "transplant" metastasis with a self-limited growth course. (Huvos, A. G., *et. al.*: Aggressive chondroblastoma. Clin. Orthop., *126:*266, 1977)

FIBROUS DYSPLASIA

On rare occasions, fibrous dysplasia may be associated with variable quantities of cartilage. The typical radiographic and pathologic features of fibrous dysplasia should not, however, lead to confusion (see pp. 128–136).

ANEURYSMAL BONE CYST (ABC)

The ABC can, on rare occasions, be associated with small islands of chondroid metaplasia (Fig. 13–48, *B*). This usually occurs in an aneurysmal bone cyst that is in its healing phase. The degree of fibro-osseous repair tissue may obliterate the usual cystlike spaces of the lesion and lead to problems in diagnosis. The lesion could then be mistaken for fibrous dysplasia or, if seen in association with an "ominous" radiologic pattern and, because of its intense activity and fibroblastic, osteoid, woven-bone, and chondroid matrices, could be mistaken for an osteosarcoma. Usually this stage of the ABC will show a fine peripheral rim of ossification around the portion of the lesion that projects into the soft tissue on the radiographs (Fig. 13–36). This is a particularly useful aid, because osteosarcomas will not show this benign collar.

Histologically, although the healing ABC may be an exuberant lesion, it will not show definite anaplasia. Unfortunately neither do all osteosarcomas; therefore great weight must be given to the radiographic analysis as well as careful observation of the histology and careful search for remnants of an aneurysmal bone cyst in all of the submitted material.

CHONDROMYXOID FIBROMA

Capsule Summary

Incidence. Rare. It represents approximately 0.4 per cent of biopsied primary bone tumors.

Clinical Features. Pain; occasionally, there is swelling and tenderness to palpitation.

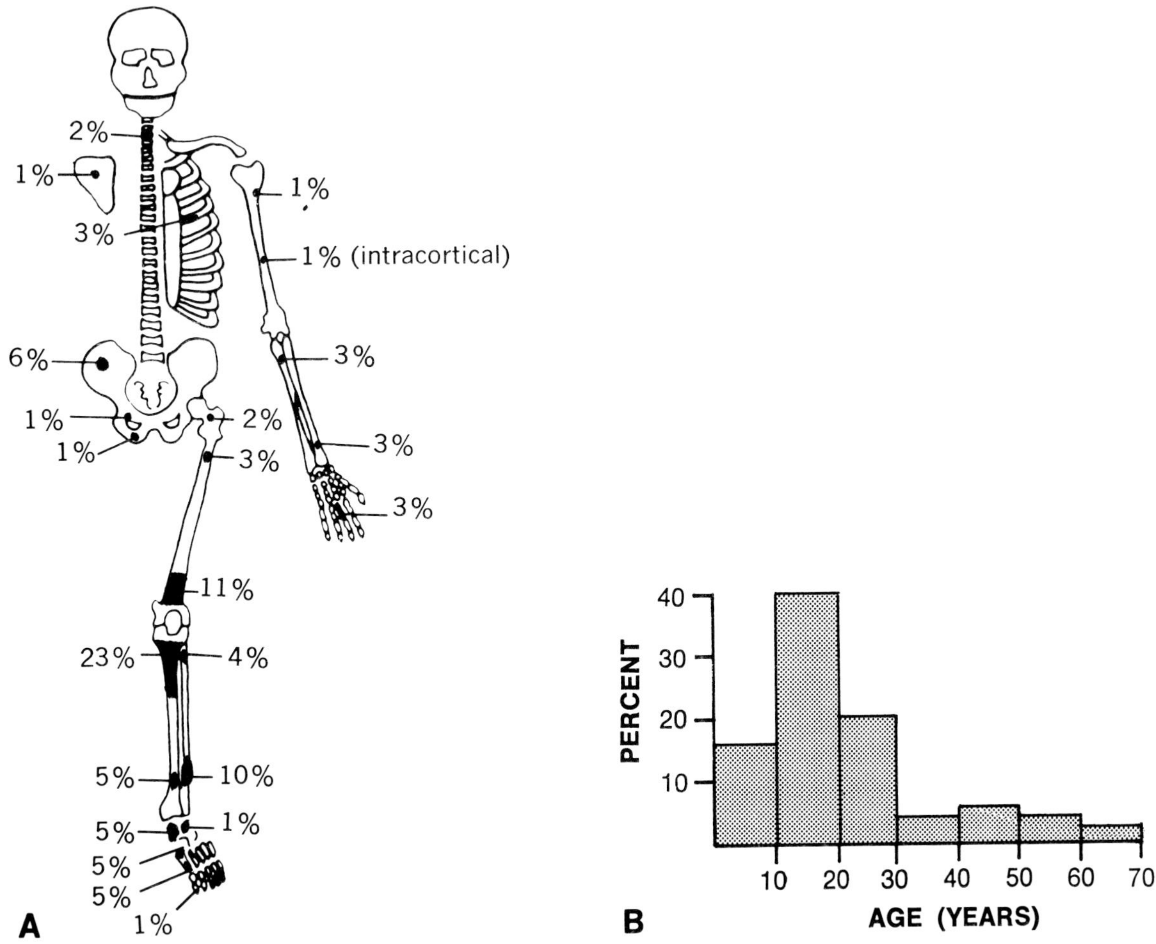

FIG. 8-90. (*A*) Chondromyxoid and myxoid fibroma. Frequency of areas of involvement in 101 patients. Male: female incidence, 1:1. (*B*) Age distribution of patients with chondromyxoid fibroma. (Mirra, J., Bullough, P., and Freiberger, R.: Orthopedic Diseases, Part II. New York, Famous Teachings in Modern Medicine, MedCom, Inc., © 1972)

Radiologic Features. When they occur in large long bones, they are usually lytic, eccentric, and bordered by a rim of sclerosis. In short tubular bones, fibula, and ribs, it usually occupies the entire width of bone, is characterized by fusiform expansion, scalloped borders, and rim of sclerosis. The periosteum may be "blown out" and surrounded by a thin rim of new bone. In large flat bones, it is a bubbly lesion bordered by sclerosis.

Gross Pathology. The color is grayish-white to bluish-gray, is somewhat translucent, resembing cartilage, and is occasionally mucoid and firm. There may be areas of hemorrhage and hemosiderin pigmentation.

Histopathology. It has chondroid, myxoid, and fibrous tissue in any proportions and may be quite cellular. Spindly cells undergo metaplasia to chondroid and myxoid tissue. The nuclei are bland; mitoses, rare; nucleoli, absent to minimal in size. Cellular atypism is rare.

Course. Benign. It may recur in a small percentage of cases. Chondrosarcomatous change is rarely reported.

Treatment. Curettage or block-excision is recommended.

Definition. The chondromyxoid fibroma is a rare, benign, primary bone tumor characterized by the production of fibrous, chondroid, and myxoid tissues in variable proportions. It is important to recognize the lesion in spite of its rarity, since it may be misdiagnosed as a chondrosarcoma or myxoid chondrosarcoma.

Clinical Features

About 75 per cent of cases present in the first three decades of life. Clinical symptoms include mild local

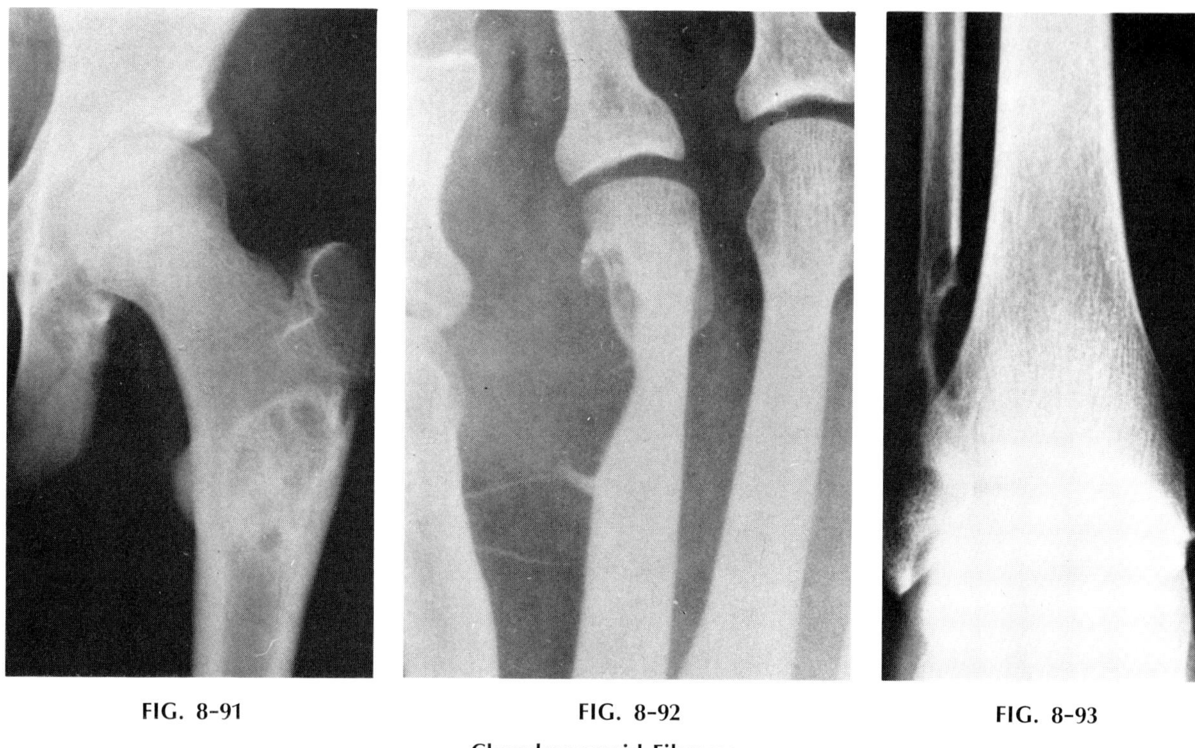

FIG. 8-91 FIG. 8-92 FIG. 8-93

Chondromyxoid Fibroma

FIG. 8-91. Chondromyxoid fibroma. Its usual features include metaphyseal location, eccentricity, rounded trabeculations, and a dense border of reactive benign sclerosis.

FIG. 8-92. Unusual example of an apparently intraperiosteal chondromyxoid fibroma that mimics the "blowout" appearance of an aneurysmal bone cyst.

FIG. 8-93. An example showing a scalloped pattern wrapping around the distal fibular metaphysis.

pain, occasionally with a nontender to tender palpable mass. Many lesions are discovered as incidental findings on radiographic examination.

The chondromyxoid fibroma can have any combination of the following features:

1. ECCENTRICITY. The majority of the lesions are eccentrically placed metaphyseal lesions (Fig. 8–91). This feature is most obvious in the large long bones, such as the tibia and femur. The eccentricity may be so pronounced that it appears in a predominant juxtacortical or periosteal position (Fig. 8–92) and may give a "blow out" appearance. Such lesions will probably be mistaken for the more common aneurysmal bone cyst (A.B.C.), which can have a similar radiological appearance. If the lesion has a distinct fine layer of bone along its periosteal surface and an inner border of intramedullary sclerosis, the diagnosis of chondromyxoid fibroma is more likely than ABC, since this latter lesion usually presents before its slow growth phase and, therefore, before it is contained by a border of reactive host bone sclerosis. Occasionally, the chondromyxoid fibroma may wrap around the peripheral aspects of the bone and have a scalloped lytic appearance. This is most common in thin bones such as phalanges or the fibula (Fig. 8–93).

2. CENTRAL LOCATION. Some lesions will appear centrally placed in the bone. This appearance is most frequent in thin bones such as ribs, phalanges and the fibula.

3. BORDER OF SCLEROSIS (FIGS. 8–91 AND 8–94). These tumors are benign and slow growing and usually elicit a border of reactive host bone sclerosis, a feature rarely seen in malignant tumors. This is a very helpful sign, particularly since the histology of chon-

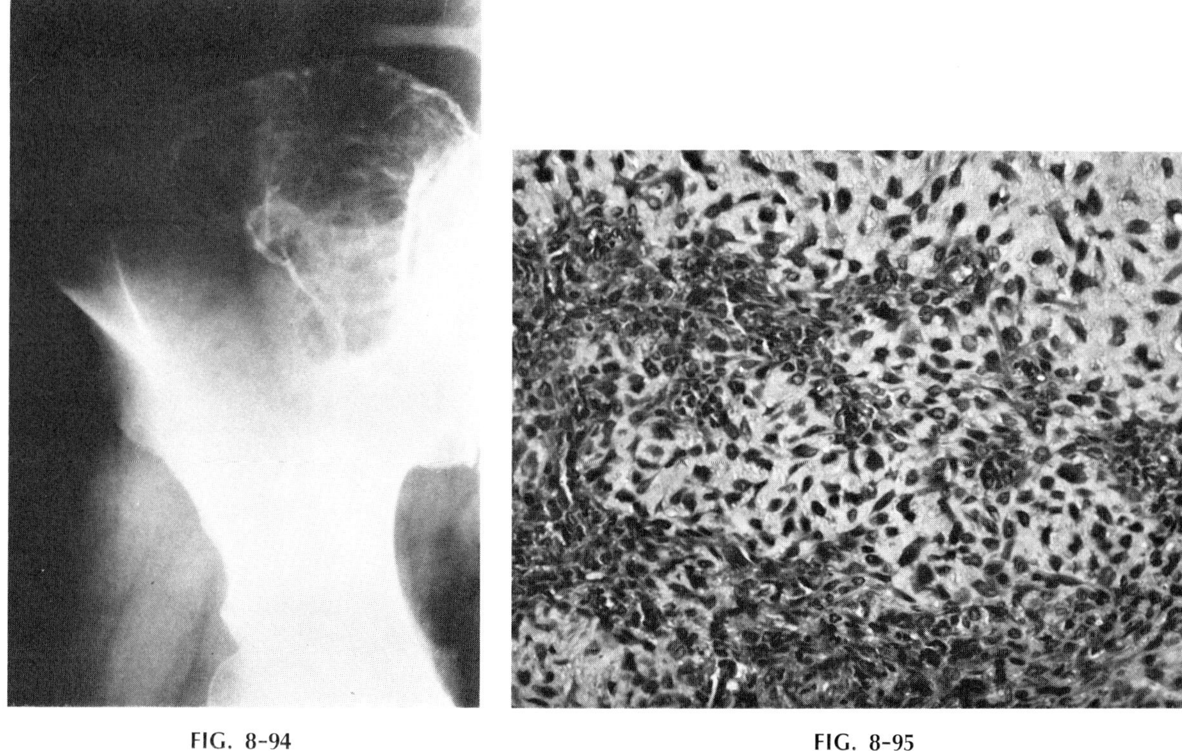

FIG. 8-94   FIG. 8-95

Chondromyxoid Fibroma

FIG. 8-94. Large, bubbly, and trabeculated lesion of the ilium with a border of benign sclerosis on its lower and medial edges.

FIG. 8-95. Intimate mixture of exuberant spindly (fibroid element) and stellate and polygonal cells embedded in a chondroid matrix (x250).

dromyxoid fibroma may be alarming to the uninitiated. The majority will have this sign. This sign is most common in patients over age 20.

4. ABSENCE OF A BORDER OF SCLEROSIS. Some lesions will not show a well-demarcated border of sclerosis. Patients without this helpful sign of benignancy tend to be under age 20 and perhaps reflect the early developmental or growing stage of the tumor. Its growth during this early stage of development might, therefore, explain its absence of a border of sclerosis.

5. TRABECULATED OR "BUBBLY" APPEARANCE. Many lesions will have a trabeculated or "bubbly" appearance (Fig. 8-94).

6. PURE LYSIS. A small percentage of these lesions will show a purely lytic lesional appearance. These also tend to occur in the active growth phase or in the younger patients.

7. PUNCTATE OR OTHER CALCIFICATIONS. Unlike most cartilage-producing tumors, this is a rare phenomenon in chondromyxoid fibroma. The calcifications, if they appear, are 1 to 2 mm. in diameter.

The chondromyxoid fibroma may have various combinations of the above features. It almost always involves the metaphysis, although it may extend to the epiphysis after the physeal plate has closed. Pure epiphyseal lesions are rare and lesions within the midshaft are virtually nonexistent. The chondromyxoid fibroma can, therefore, mimic the features of a nonossifying fibroma, solitary eosinophilic granuloma, parosteal chondroma, enchondroma, aneurysmal and solitary bone cyst, chondrosarcoma, myeloma, or giant cell tumor.

The lesion it most often resembles is a nonossifying fibroma, because both lesions are usually metaphyseal, eccentric, surrounded by a border of sclerosis, and trabeculated. Chondromyxoid fibroma may bulge from the original bone contour. Nonossifying fibroma rarely bulges much into the soft-tissue regions. Histopathology should differentiate the two with ease, however. Similarly, biopsy should permit easy differentiation from all of the various possibilities listed above with the possible exception of a form of chondrosarcoma. The diagnosis of chondromyxoid fibroma should always be considered in any patient under the age of 30 with an eccentric, metaphyseal lesion that is trabeculated and bordered by sclerosis in a long bone.

Gross Pathology

Most chondromyxoid fibromas are less than 5 cm. in size, with the exception of pelvic lesions. The tissue is firm and grayish-white to bluish-gray. It may resemble cartilage or mucoid tissue. Cysts and foci of hemorrhage and hemosiderin pigmentation are not uncommon. The surface of the tumor is distinctly lobulated.

Histopathology

It is virtually impossible to illustrate all of the possible combinations of features a chondromyxoid fibroma may assume. Next to the osteogenic sarcoma it is the most difficult tumor to define histologically. This is because the chondromyxoid fibroma may contain chondroid, fibrous, and myxoid tissues in any and all proportions; furthermore, that the appearance in one field may be significantly different compared to another field of the same lesion.

The histopathologic diagnosis can be simplified if one attempts to understand the complex processes that are occurring in relation to this tumor. From an analysis of several cases, this author has come to the conclusion that the basic process is a proliferation of spindly fibroblastlike cells in its early phases. Eventually, these cells undergo metaplasia and produce a matrix containing mucopolysaccharides, which imparts to the tissues a chondroid to myxoid appearance. Microscopic foci of cystic degeneration may further contribute to the myxoid appearance. Because of these various processes, the tissues can have various combinations of features, such as fibrous, chondroid, and myxoid, fibrous and myxoid, chondroid and myxoid in any or all proportions. Some of these various combinations are illustrated in Figures 8–95 to 8–103, Plates 6, *H*, *I*, and *J*. If the fibroblastic cells predominate, the fibrous tissue component will form a continuum and the chondroid or myxoid tissues will form islands (Fig. 8–97). However, if the metaplastic process to chondroid or myxoid is predominant, the fibrous portions will form the islands and the chondroid or myxoid tissues the continuum (Fig. 8–98).

The chondroid of a chondromyxoid fibroma resembles cartilage in so far as it may have a relatively homogeneous matrix in foci (Figs. 8–95, 8–96, 8–100, and 8–102; Plate 6, *G* and *I*). However, it differs from usual hyaline cartilage in that the entrapped cells tend to maintain the spindly nuclei of its precursor fibroblast-like cell, rather than the round nucleus typical of chondrocytes. In addition, the matrix of chondroid is usually eosinophilic (Plate 6, *I*) rather than basophilic. True hyaline cartilage may be seen in the chondromyxoid fibroma, but in minute amounts. Chondromyxoid fibromas, like chondroblastomas, are never composed of pure cartilage. Rarely does the amount of cartilage or chondroid exceed 75 per cent of the total lesional tissue in chondromyxoid fibroma and 50 per cent in chondroblastoma. On the other hand, rarely does the lesional tissue of an enchondroma or well-differentiated chondrosarcoma contain less than 95 to 100 per cent cartilage.

The cytoplasm of the cells of chondromyxoid fibroma can vary from being indistinct to cells with multipolar eosinophilic tapered processes (Figs. 8–96 and 8–103). Although this latter finding is characteristic of a number of chondromyxoid fibromas, it is not

(*Text continues on p. 242.*)

Chondromyxoid Fibroma

FIG. 8–96. High-power examination of some fields such as this may show the gradual transition of the fibroid to the chondroid elements by the deposition of an abundant intercellular matrix. The cytoplasm of the chondroid cells is polygonal to stellate. Although this is a benign entity, the plump nuclei and cellular "activity" could be mistaken for chondrosarcoma or a mesenchymal chondrosarcoma (x400).

FIG. 8–97. Mixture of fibroid and chondroid elements. In this field, the fibroid portions are interlocking and the chondroid disposed into islands (x40).

FIG. 8–98. In other fields the opposite may be true, that is, the fibroid portions are discontinuous (x125).

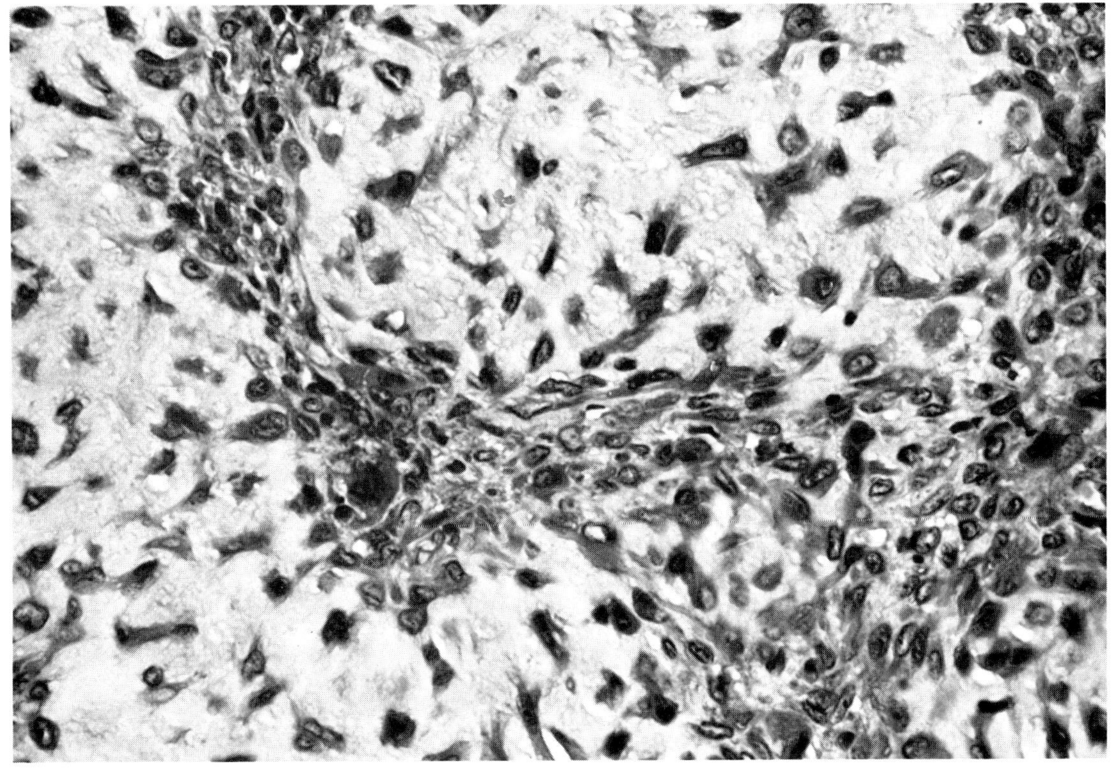

FIG. 8-96

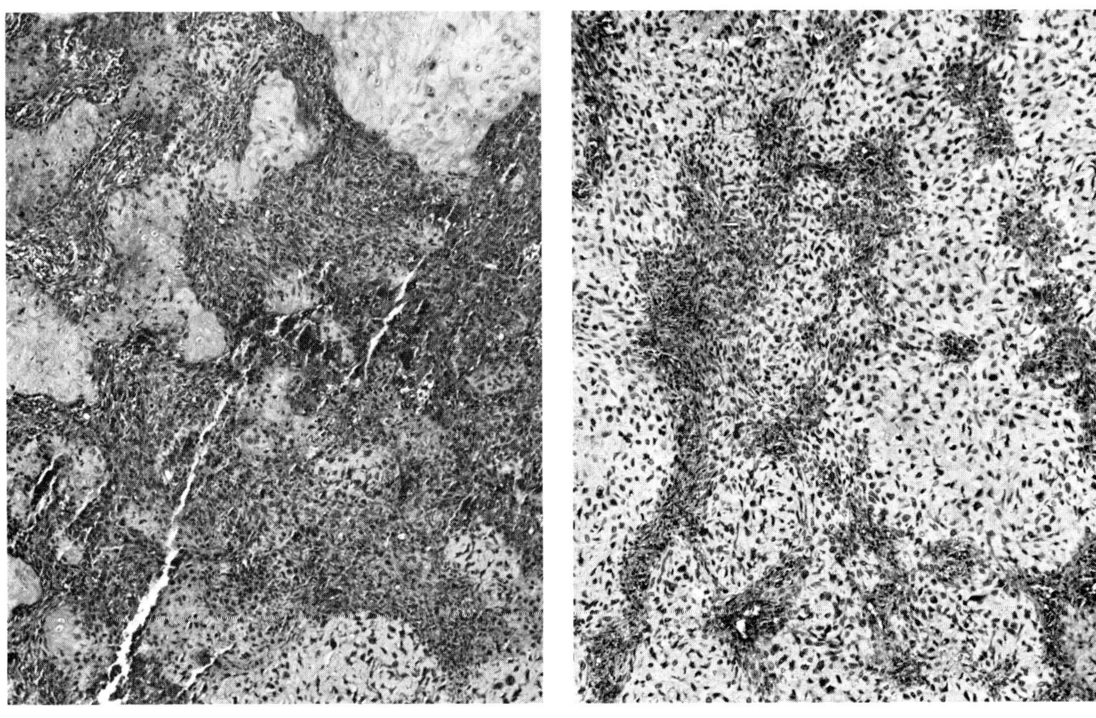

FIG. 8-97

FIG. 8-98

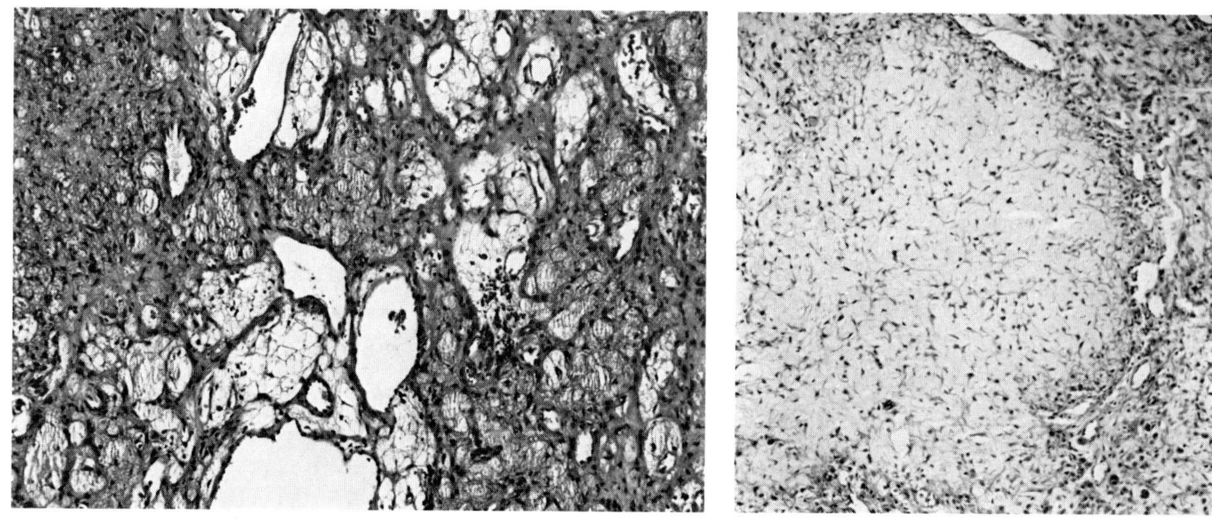

FIG. 8-99

FIG. 8-100

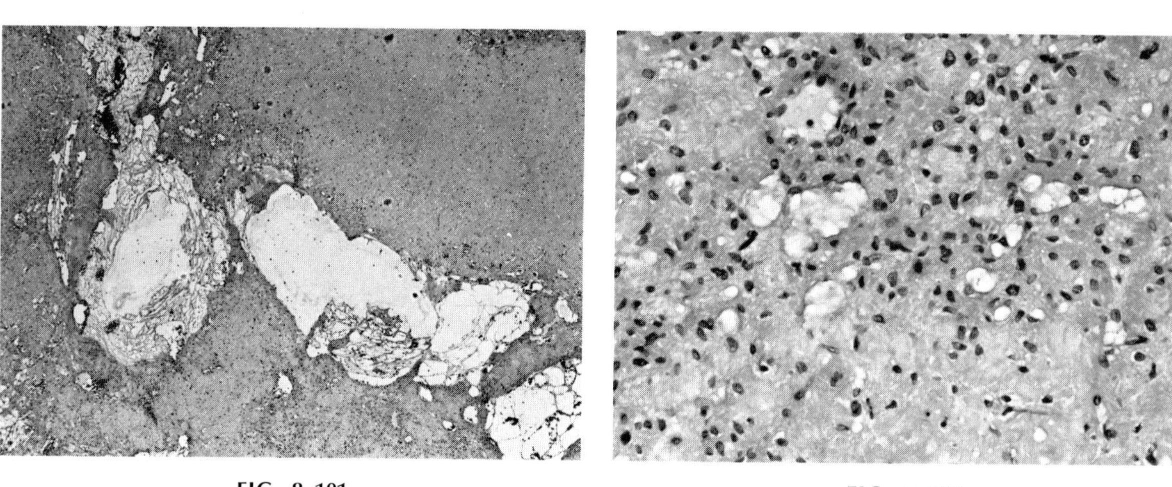

FIG. 8-101

FIG. 8-102

Chondromyxoid Fibroma

FIG. 8-99. An example with a predominantly chondroid-myxoid mixture (x125).

FIG. 8-100. An area with a myxoid-fibroid tissue mixture (x125).

FIG. 8-101. Other lesions may be dominated by bland chondroid and cystic myxoid elements (x40).

FIG. 8-102. High power of most chondromyxoid fibromas show bland, small, oval to polygonal nuclei (x250).

FIG. 8-103. However, some lesions may show areas with exuberant nuclei mimicking a sarcomatous process. The meager to absent mitoses are much fewer than would be expected had this lesion truly been a sarcoma (x400).

FIG. 8-104. Low-power example of a small, circumscribed, chondromyxoid fibroma filling the medullary substance of a rib (x40).

FIG. 8-105. In this field lobulated islands of fibrochondroid are found in the marrow fat. Note that the edges of the lesion are smooth or sharp and not actively infiltrating between fat cells (x125). Active infiltration between fat cells would be indicative of a chondrosarcoma (see Fig. 8-27 and 8-28). Fat cells can be trapped with the lesional tissues of a chondromyxoid fibroma. Even so, this pattern is bland or innocuous looking.

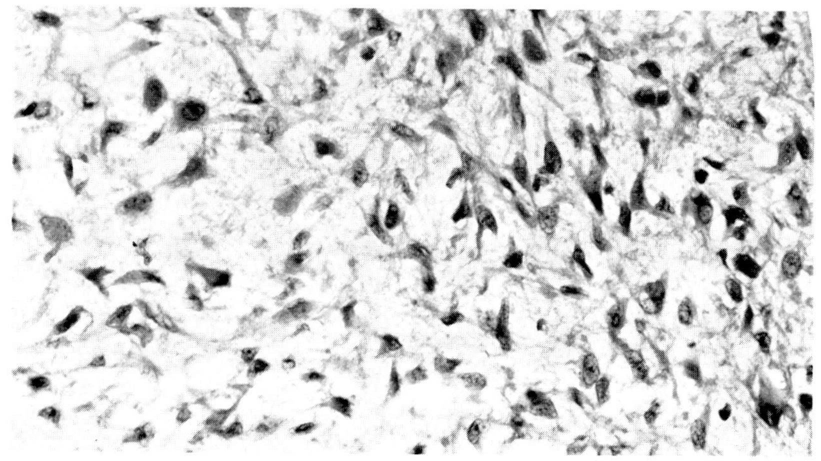

FIG. 8-103

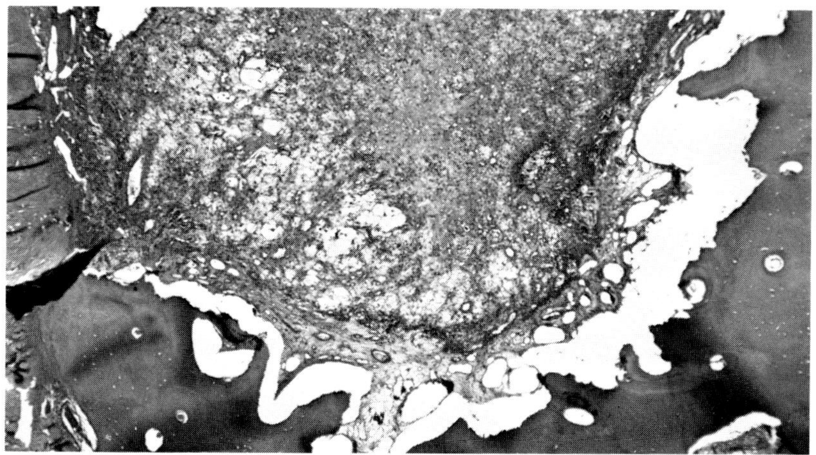

FIG. 8-104

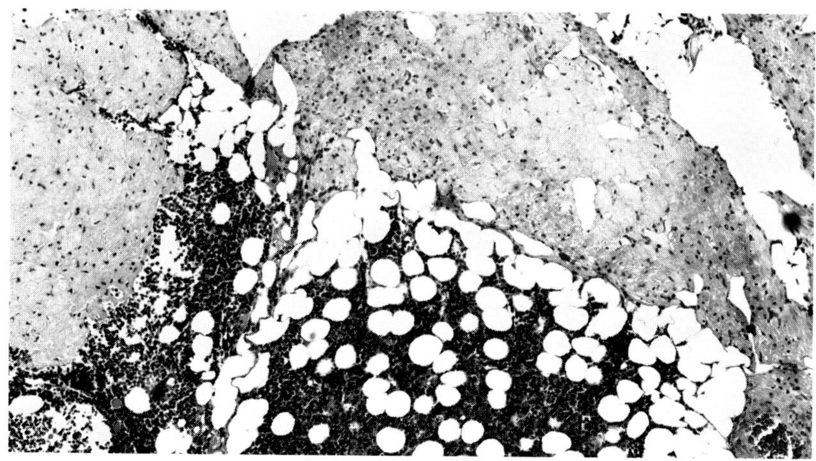

FIG. 8-105

diagnostic and may be simulated to some extent by the mesenchymal chondrosarcoma and Grade II to III chondrosarcomas. (Figs. 8–67 and 8–69)

Other features that may be seen in association with chondromyxoid fibroma are osteoclast-like giant cells, foci of hemorrhage, hemosiderin pigment, cholesterol, macrophages, and lymphocytes. Distinct calcifications are rare.

If the chondromyxoid fibroma is removed intact, its borders are well demarcated to lobulated (Fig. 8–104). It does not invade between host lamellar bone spicules for considerable distances, as observed in osteosarcoma or chondrosarcoma. Small islands of chondroid may be found surrounded by the fatty marrow (Fig. 8–105). However, the edges of the lobules will be quite distinct from the fat. This appearance should be distinguished from the individual cell invasion of the fat with compression of fat cells along the growing edges of a chondrosarcoma (Figs. 8–27 and 8–28).

Dahlin pointed out that an increased concentration of cells at the periphery of the lobules is of "extreme importance" in the diagnosis of chondromyxoid fibroma. Although this feature is present in most chondromyxoid fibromas, it is by no means diagnostic, as this author has seen a similar pattern in lobules of malignant cartilage of some osteosarcomas and chondrosarcomas. The most important histologic features are the following: variable proportions of chondroid, fibroid, and myxoid tissues, bland ovoid to more exuberant stellate to multipolar spindle cells, metaplasia of fibrous to chondroid tissues, blandish nuclei, rare to absent mitoses and the absence of invasion between marrow fat cells.

Differential Diagnosis

Unless one is familiar with the numerous histopathologic patterns of a chondromyxoid fibroma, it is possible to confuse it with chondrosarcomas or possibly even with a chondroblastoma. Radiologically chondrosarcomas will not be bordered by a reactive zone of sclerosis so common to chondromyxoid fibroma. These tumors are usually larger and more destructive.

ENCHONDROMA. These lesions are composed of pure hyaline to fibrocartilage with variable amounts of lamellar to woven-lamellar bone along the periphery of some of the cartilage lobules (p. 174 and Figs. 8–5, 8–6, 8–13, and 8–15). Chondromyxoid fibroma rarely has significant amounts of true cartilage but has cartilage-like tissue (chondroid).

CHONDROSARCOMA. Also composed of pure hyaline to fibrocartilage with variable amounts of anaplasia (Figs. 8–21–8–26, 8–30). Those chondrosarcomas with chondroid rather than true cartilage production are high-grade malignant tumors and show striking anaplasia, in contrast to the blandish nature of the nuclei seen in chondromyxoid fibroma. Myxoid chondrosarcomas show a uniform pattern of cells with variable anaplasia set in a myxoid stroma. The chondromyxoid fibroma is characterized by variable patterns such as chondro-myxoid, fibro-myxoid and chondro-fibro-myxoid, rather than uniformity. In one field, spindly cells may be in juxtaposition to chondroid and in another, to myxoid tissues. The variability in patterns and nuclear blandness are shown in Fig. 8–102 and help differentiate chondromyxoid fibromas from chondrosarcomas.

MESENCHYMAL CHONDROSARCOMA. A mesenchymal chondrosarcoma is composed predominantly of an intimate mixture of spindle cells and chondroid, similar to the chondrofibroid variants of chondromyxoid fibromas. However, mesenchymal chondrosarcomas contain spindle cells in which the nuclei are much more closely packed, about twice as large, as those seen in chondromyxoid fibroma, and contain many more mitotic figures. The chondroid or cartilage produced in mesenchymal chondrosarcoma is usually obviously malignant (Figs. 8–67 and 8–69). Mesenchymal chondrosarcomas often contain hemangiopericytoma-like tissues and lack myxoid or cystic areas.

CHONDROSARCOMA WITH FIBROSARCOMATOUS TRANSFORMATION. These tumors lack the intimate mixture of spindle cells and chondroid seen in chondromyxoid fibroma. In essence these malignant tumors contain Grade I to II chondrosarcoma in apparent "collision" with fibrosarcoma (p. 201 and Fig. 8–50, *A* and *B*). The anaplasia of the spindle-cell component is usually striking and replete with mitoses.

CHONDROBLASTOMA. Chondroblastomas also contain chondroid; however, the presence of distinctive polygonal chondroblasts, numerous giant cells, and "chicken-wire calcification" should distinguish these lesions from chondromyxoid fibroma. Chondroblastomas are almost always epiphyseal lesions and rarely metaphyseal. The opposite is true of the chondromyxoid fibroma.

Course and Treatment

The majority of chondromyxoid fibromas do not recur following simple curettage. Scaglietti, *et al.*,[86a] and

Ralph[85] report eight patients with recurrence. None of their cases metastasized and all were eventually cured. These cases all had one factor in common: youth (ages were 5,5,6,9,10,10,14,14 years, respectively). These cases represent the lower age limit of the chondromyxoid fibroma. In this author's estimation, the facts would support the concept that in the younger age group the lesion is still in an active growth phase and incomplete removal can lead to recurrence. Although this concept may modify the type of therapy in young patients with chondromyxoid fibroma (i.e., more vigorous curettage or local en-bloc excisions where feasible to ensure against recurrence); nevertheless, the benign nature of this process must temper against radical procedures.

Once a diagnosis of chondromyxoid fibroma is made with certainty, all attempts must be made to preserve the limb, even if it associated with rapid and large recurrences. This may entail more vigorous curettage, en-bloc excision, or bone graft struts. Recognition that the chondromyxoid fibroma is a benign lesion and that the youngest patients afflicted with this tumor may manifest the most alarming recurrences should protect against unnecessary amputations.

A couple of cases of chondromyxoid fibroma have been reported to have undergone chondrosarcomatous transformation (Iwata and Coley, Levy, *et al.*[81,86]). An incidence of 1 to 2 per cent malignant transformation would not be terribly surprising, since almost every other benign tumor of bone, with the possible exceptions of the osteoid osteoma, enostosis, and osteoma of skull bones has been reported to have undergone malignant transformation. However, Spjut, *et al.*[87] have questioned the validity of the original diagnosis of chondromyxoid fibroma in regard to these cases.

CHORDOMA

Capsule Summary

Definition. A low-grade malignant neoplasm originating from notochordal remnants. It accounts for approximately 3 per cent of primary bone tumors.

Clinical Features. The symptoms depend on those cranial or spinal nerve structures involved by the local spread of the tumor. Refer to discussion for details.

Radiologic Features. Osseous destruction and soft-tissue mass involving either the structures at the base of the skull or the spine.

Gross Pathology. The tumor is soft, lobular, grayish-tan, glistening, mucinous, or gelatinous. Cranial tumors are usually less than 7 cm. in size; sacrococcygeal chordomas may attain gigantic proportions.

Histopathology. There are variable histologic patterns; matrix appears mucinous, myxoid or chondroid; the cell cytoplasm is characteristically vacuolated or bubbly (so-called physaliphorous cells) or intensely eosinophilic. The cells are arranged haphazardly, in cords or trabeculae.

Course. It is a locally aggressive neoplasm. Metastases occur late in the course. Less than 10 per cent of patients survive 10 years.

Treatment. Cure depends on early and aggressive en-bloc resection.

The chordoma is a slow-growing malignant neoplasm that develops from the remnants of the primitive notochord.

The notochord is found in the highest phylum of the animal kingdom, the chordata. It is formed by a proliferation of cells at the cephalic end of the primitive streak. At about the third week of human embryonal development it is present as a longitudinal, nonsegmented rod of cells extending along the midline from the region of Rathke's pouch cephalad to the most caudad portion of the future spine. The notochord soon becomes invested by a sheath of mesoderm that undergoes chondrification. (Recent experiments have shown that the notochord is an organizer that induces chondrification and segmentation of the mesenchymal elements of the vertebral bodies.) Figure 8–116 shows the notochord of a 7-day-old chick embryo which is invested in embryonal cartilage. As segmentation proceeds, the notochord becomes constricted in the midportion of the vertebral body. The embryonal cartilage is then invaded by vessels and undergoes degeneration and endochondral ossification. As this process proceeds the notochordal tissue within the vertebral body is finally obliterated. Notochordal remnants are, however, sequestered in the central portion of the nucleus pulposus of the avascular intervertebral disc. For the most part these nests are ultimately obliterated. However, remnants of notochordal tissue referred to as "ecchordosis physaliphora" have been found in 2 per cent of autopsies in relationship to the pharyngeal surface of the base of the skull, the spheno-occipital synchondrosis, and, in and about the sacrum and coccyx.

In relation to sacrococcygeal chordomas, males predominate over females in a ratio of between 3 and 4 to 1, but in cranial chordomas, there is no significant statistical sex difference. Sacrococcygeal chordomas are more frequent than those related to the base of the skull.

Symptomatology depends on the location and direction of spread of the slowly growing tumor mass.

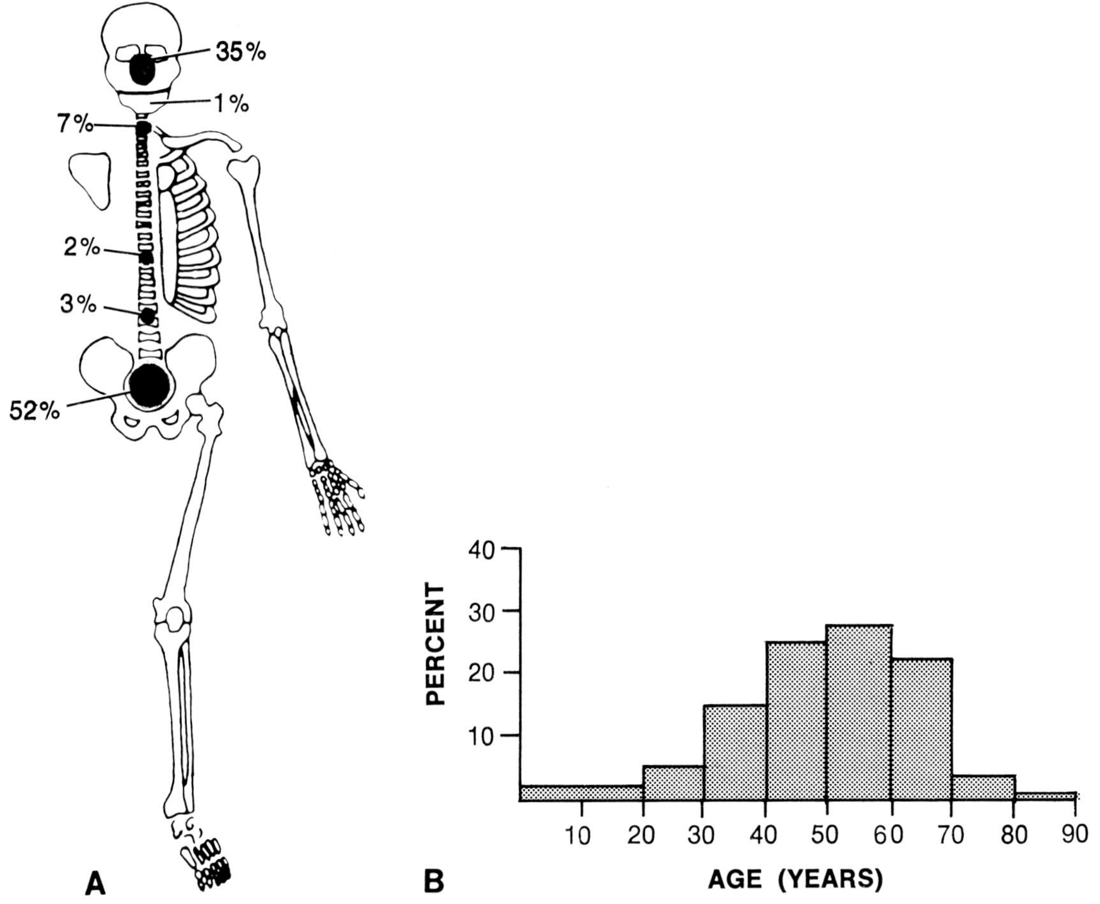

FIG. 8-106. Chordoma. Frequency of areas of involvement in 328 cases. Male: female incidence: cranium 1 : 1; spine, sacrum, and coccyx, 3 : 1.

Chordoma

FIG. 8-107. Most chordomas arise from the sacrum and extend into the pelvis as a variably sized rounded to lobulated mass. Arteriography has been used in this case to better outline the full extent of the lesion.

FIG. 8-108. On low-power examination these tumors are characterized by lobules separated by bands of fibrous tissue (x20).

FIG. 8-109. The lobular nature of the chordoma is reemphasized in this illustration. In this example the cells are arranged in cords. The stroma is bubbly and mucoid (x125).

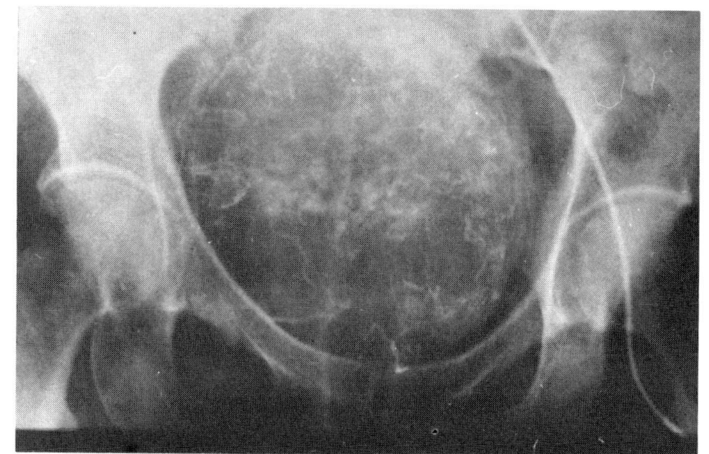

FIG. 8-107

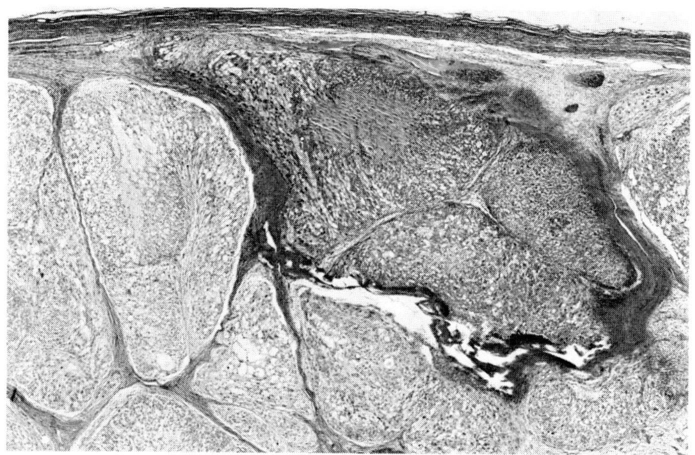

FIG. 8-108

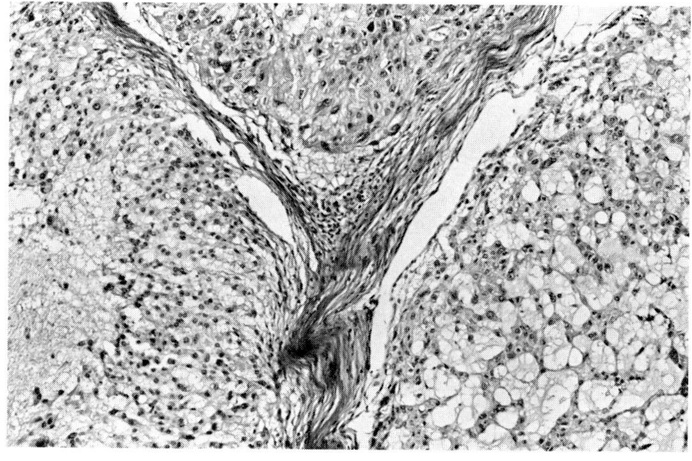

FIG. 8-109

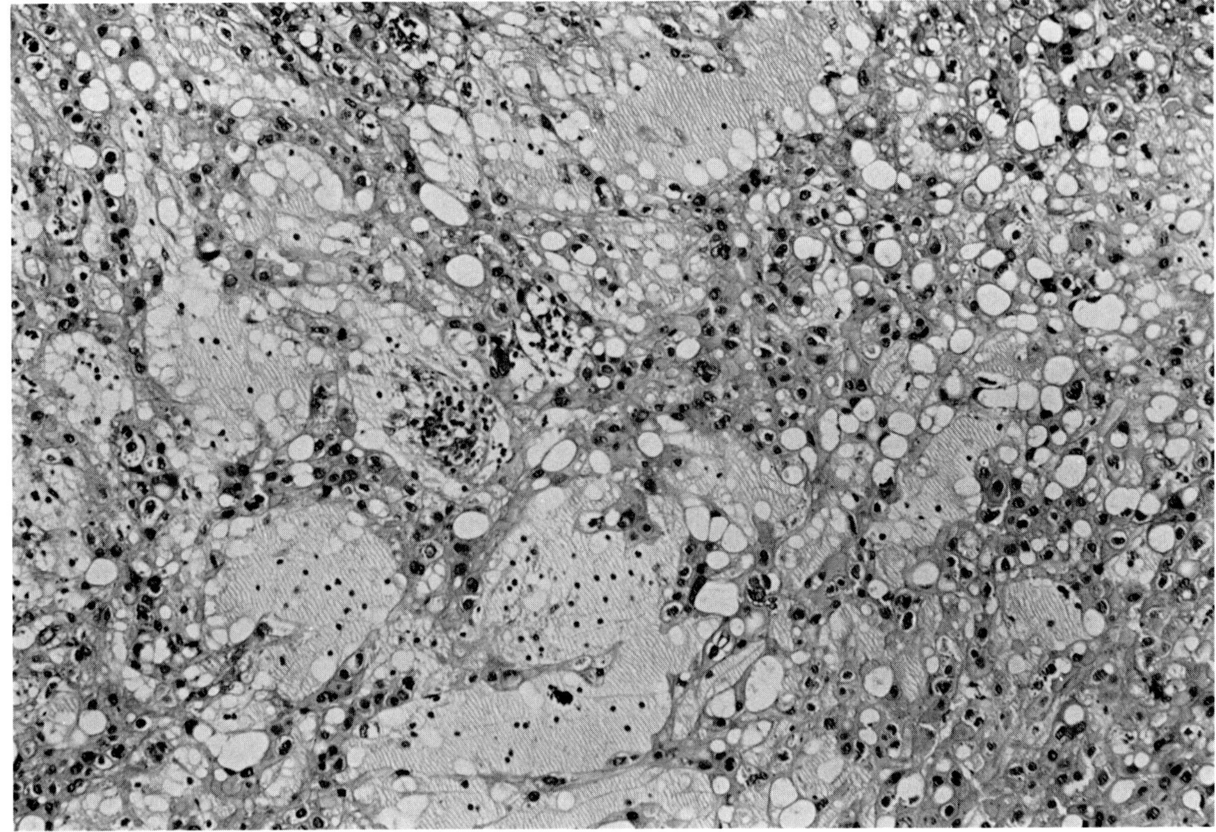

FIG. 8-110

Chordoma

FIG. 8-110. The cells in this example are arranged in trabeculae. The cytoplasm is granular pink to bubbly. Large, mucopolysaccharide-rich mucoid lakes are present (x125).

FIG. 8-111. The cells may be arranged in cords and sheets. Several virtually pathognomonic physaliphorous (basket) cells are present (*arrows*) (x400).

Fig. 8-112. Nests of granular and physaliphorous cells typify this example (x400).

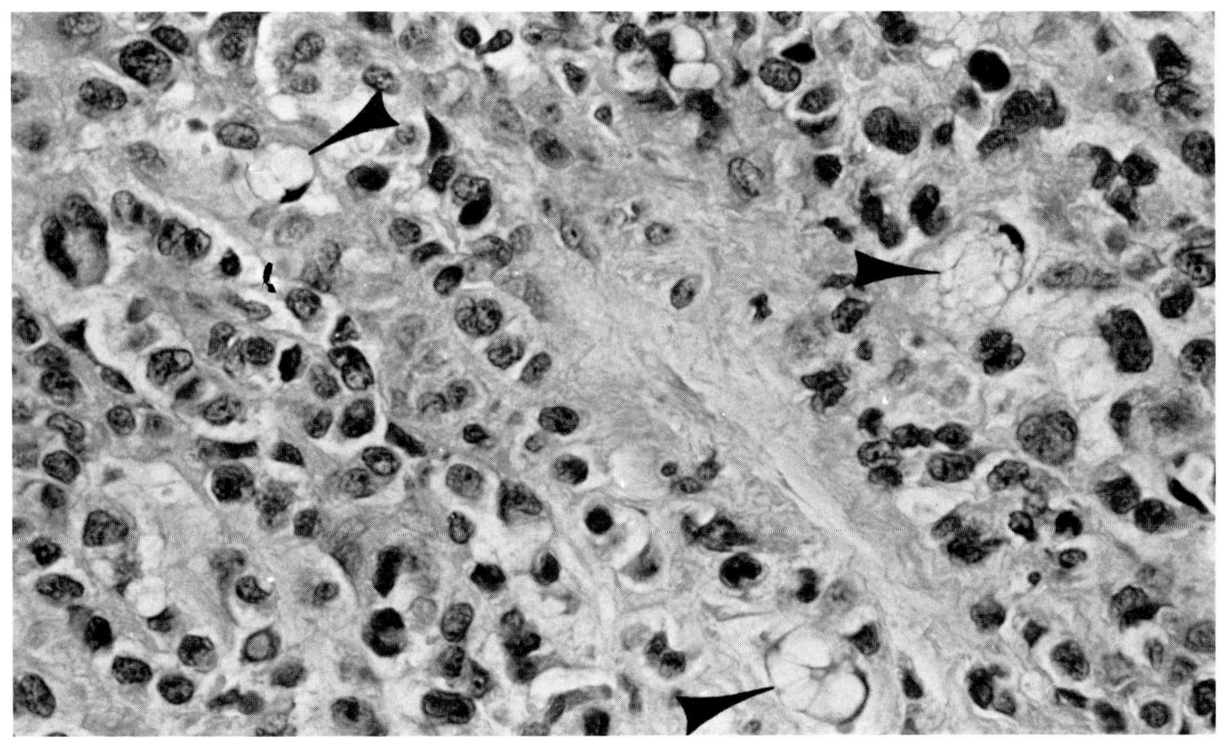

FIG. 8-111

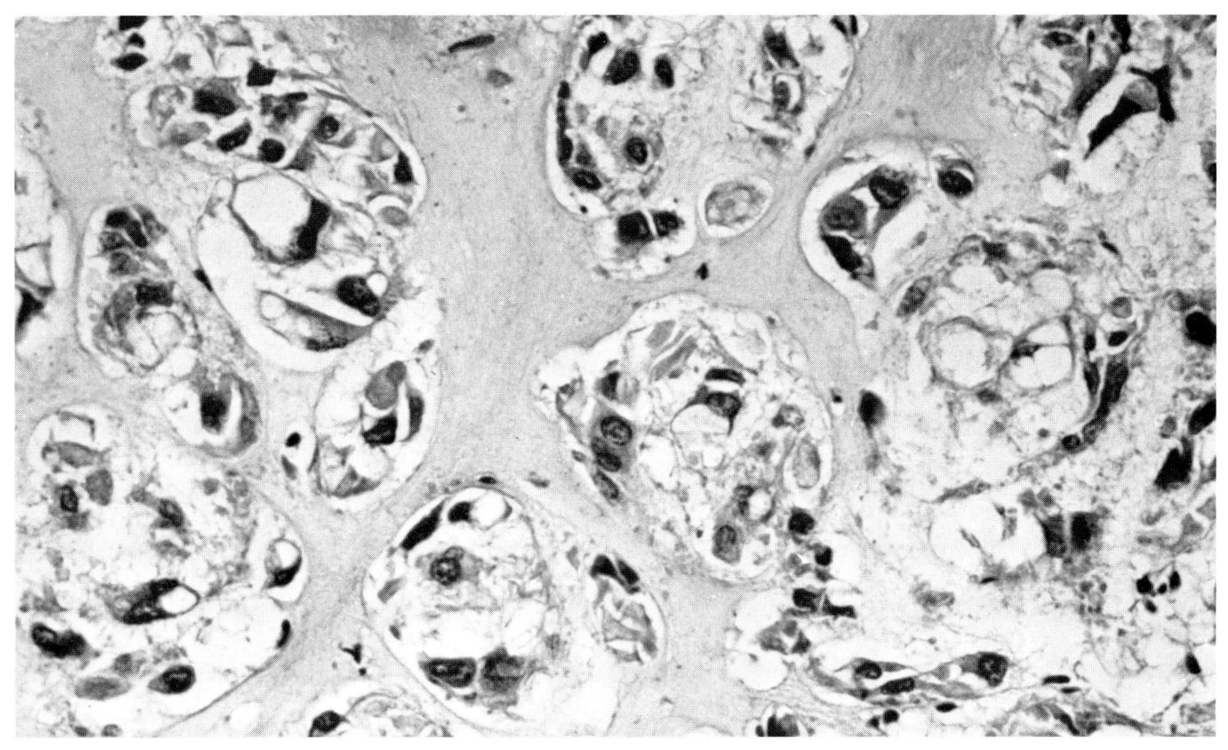

FIG. 8-112

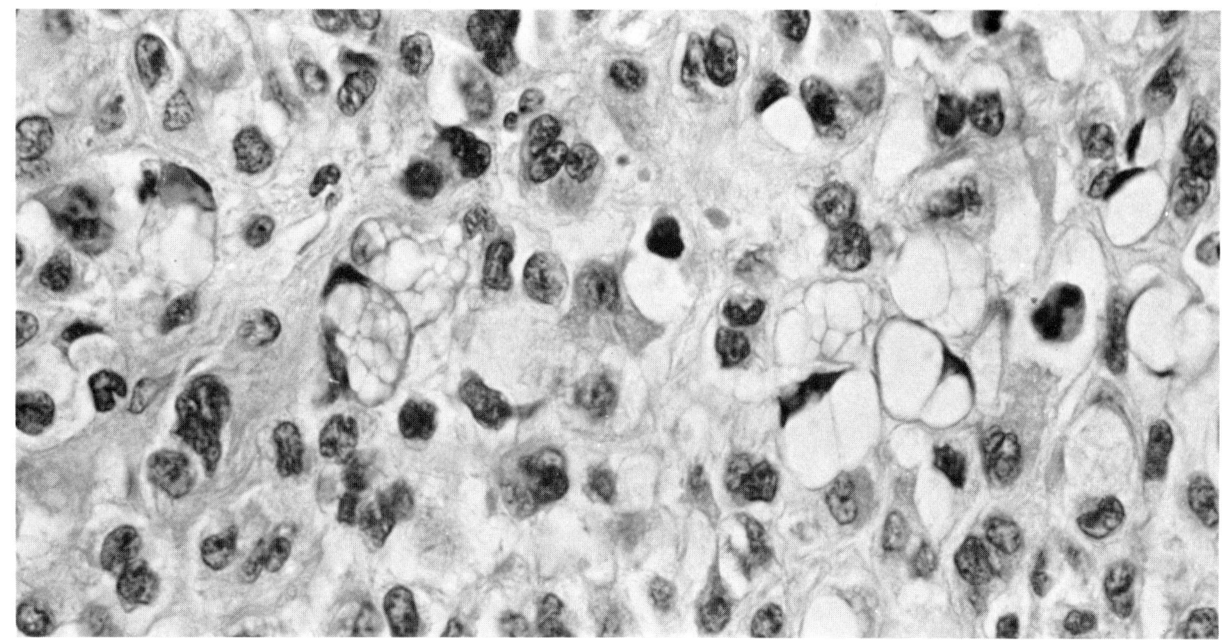

FIG. 8-113

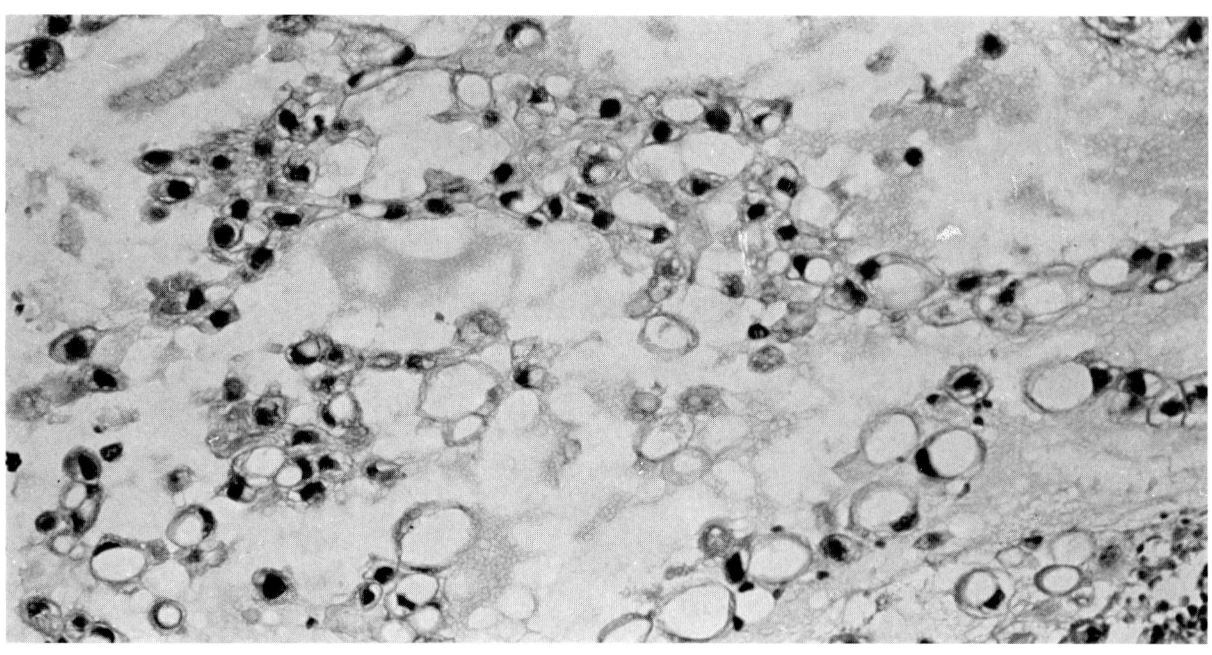

FIG. 8-114

Chordoma

FIG. 8-113. Sheets of pink, granular cells and bubbly physaliphorous cells. The nuclei are plump and oval to multilobulated. Double nucleated forms are present. Chromatin clumping is prominent (x500).

FIG. 8-114. An almost pure collection of strands and nests of bubbly physaliphorous cells. This particular field tends to resemble a liposarcoma or metastatic "signet ring" cell carcinoma (x250).

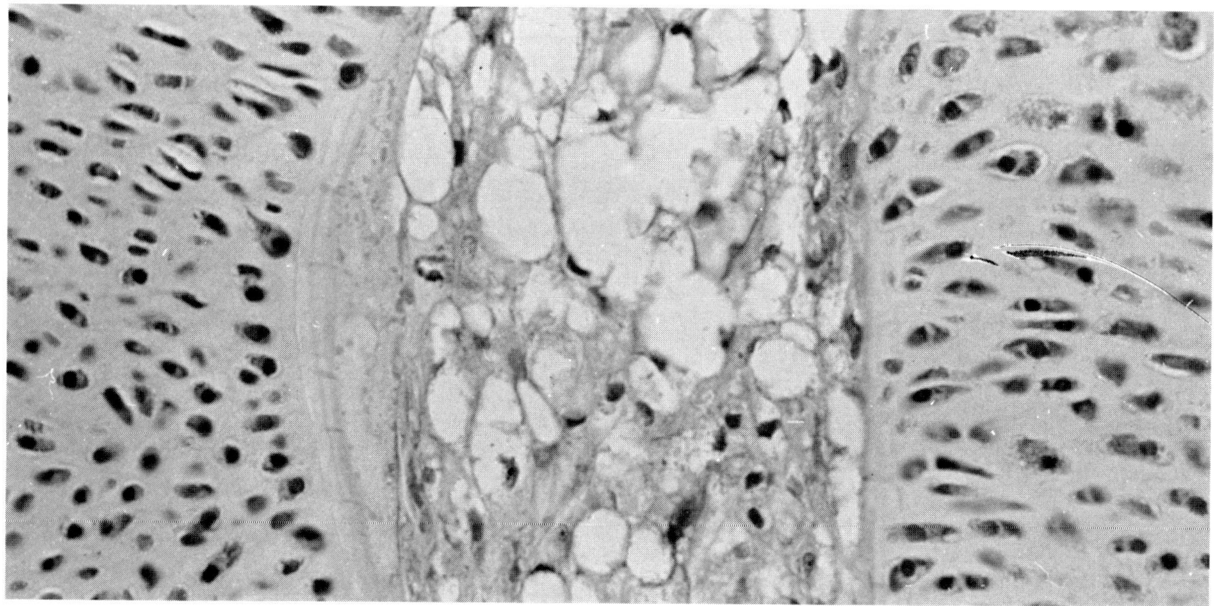

FIG. 8-115

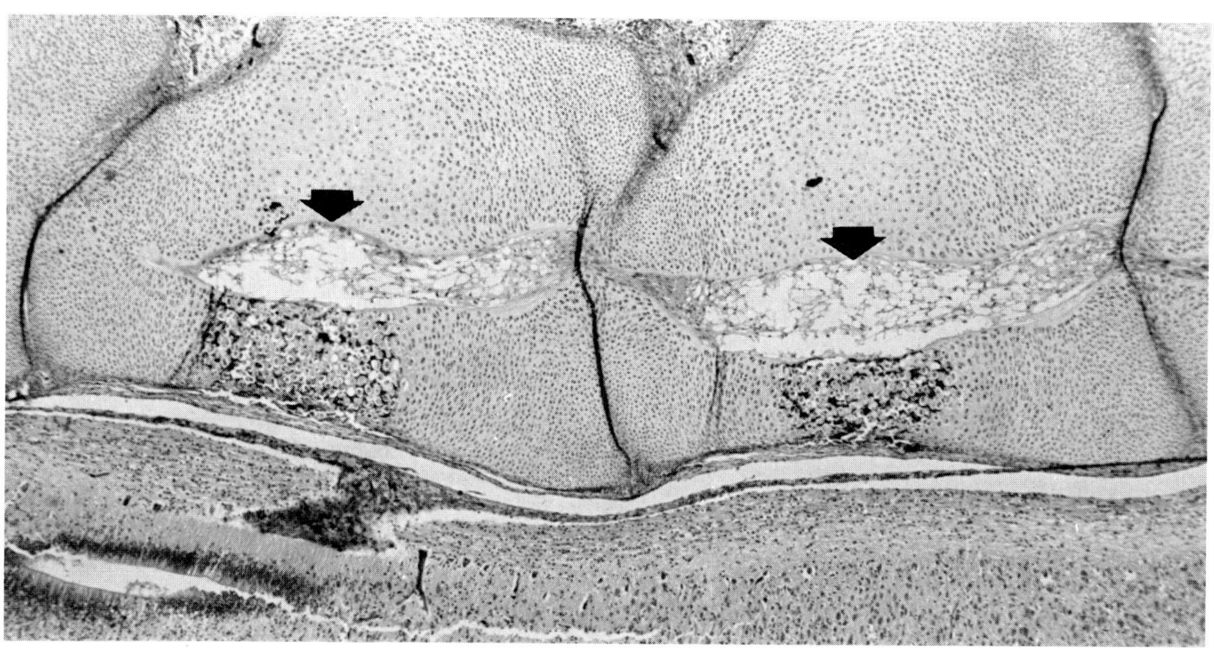

FIG. 8-116

Notochord

FIG. 8-115. The central tube in this illustration containing physaliphorous cells is in actuality the notochord of a chick embryo. The obvious similarities of these cells to the physaliphorous cells of a chordoma are easily apparent (x400).

FIG. 8-116. A tube of notochord (*arrows*) is seen in relation to the developing vertebral bodies of a chick embryo. The notochord is being pinched off at the proximal and distal ends of the vertebral bodies. It will eventually be incorporated as a vestigial remnant in the center of the fully developed disk. Chordomas are believed to arise from notochordal rests. (x125).

The following list gives the location of the tumor and the accompanying symptoms.

Cranial. Headache, vomiting, ocular disturbances, papilledema

Hypophyseal. Disturbances of endocrine function (amenorrhea, sterility, loss of libido, weight gain), abnormal visual fields, blindness

Spheno-occipital. Involvement of Cranial Nerves. Pain, nerve palsies

Nasopharyngeal. Obstructed breathing, nasal discharge, pain, palatiae mass

Vertebral. Dysphagia, difficulty in breathing, pain, numbness, paresthesias, loss of proprioceptive function, loss of muscle power, paraplegia and quadriplegia, palpable mass

Sacrococcygeal. Constipation, difficulty in starting urination, dysuria, frequency, pain, numbness, fecal and urinary incontinence, muscular weakness in the lower limbs, palpable mass

Clinical Features

On physical examination almost every sacrococcygeal chordoma has a presacral extension that can be detected on rectal examination as a firm, roundish, smooth, and occasionally cystic mass. Sacrococcygeal chordomas have a great latitude for expansion before vital structures are involved and thus may attain tremendous size. We have seen one patient where the tumor weighed over 80 pounds. It was located posteriorly on a 30 cm. base or stalk in the region of the sacrum. It was covered by skin and extended as a huge ovoid mass up to the level of the midthorax and as low as the knees. Anteriorly, the tumor filled the pelvis displacing the rectum and bladder and extending into the thighs. This occurrence is not uncommon in long-standing sacrococcygeal chordoma.

Skeletal and age distribution of the chordoma is shown in Fig. 8–106.

Radiologic Features

The radiologic features also depend on the location of the tumor:

CRANIAL. Osteolytic destruction of the dorsum sellae, posterior clinoid processes or clivus, soft-tissue mass in the nasopharynx, dilation of ventricles

VERTEBRAL. Osseous destruction of one to several adjacent vertebral bodies, soft-tissue mass, pathologic fracture of lumbar or lower thoracic spine

SACROCOCCYGEAL (FIG. 8–107). Osseous destruction, anterior bulging of the contours of the sacrum or coccyx, soft-tissue mass predominantly presacral with or without amorphous masses of calcium in the lesional tissue

Gross Pathology

On gross examination a chordoma is a soft, lobulated, glistening grayish-tan gelatinous tumor. The lobules are separated by bands of fibrous tissue. It is likely to be modified by areas of necrosis, hemorrhage, and cyst formation.

Chordomas of the cranium are usually much smaller (less than 7 cm.), compared to those of the spine. This difference is ascribable to the fact that in the head the space available for the tumor growth is naturally restricted.

Cranial chordomas destroy adjacent bony structures, may penetrate the dura to invade the brain substance, may involve cranial nerves, or extend into the nasopharynx, orbits, or nasal sinuses.

In the vertebral column, usually more than one body is involved by either spread along the posterior longitudinal ligament or through direct extension and destruction of the intervertebral disc. The dura is usually not penetrated, although local nerves are

---

Chordoma and Metastatic Adenocarcinoma to Sacrum

FIG. 8–117. Some chordomas may show bizarre nuclei simulating a high-grade sarcoma. These nuclei are probably due to degenerative changes that as are common to endocrine tumors (parathyroid adenomas, pheochromocytomas, adrenal adenomas, and others). This change does not correlate with a higher metastatic potential or a poorer course, compared to chordomas that do not show these nuclear abnormalities (x250).

FIG. 8–118. A female patient presented with a sacral tumor. A biopsy was performed and diagnosed as chordoma. Although chordoma is the most common tumor of the sacrum, review of the slide material showed unequivocal acinar structures, as illustrated. Chordomas do not form true acini. Because of this fact, the diagnosis was changed to metastatic adenocarcinoma. Laparotomy revealed an ovarian primary (x250).

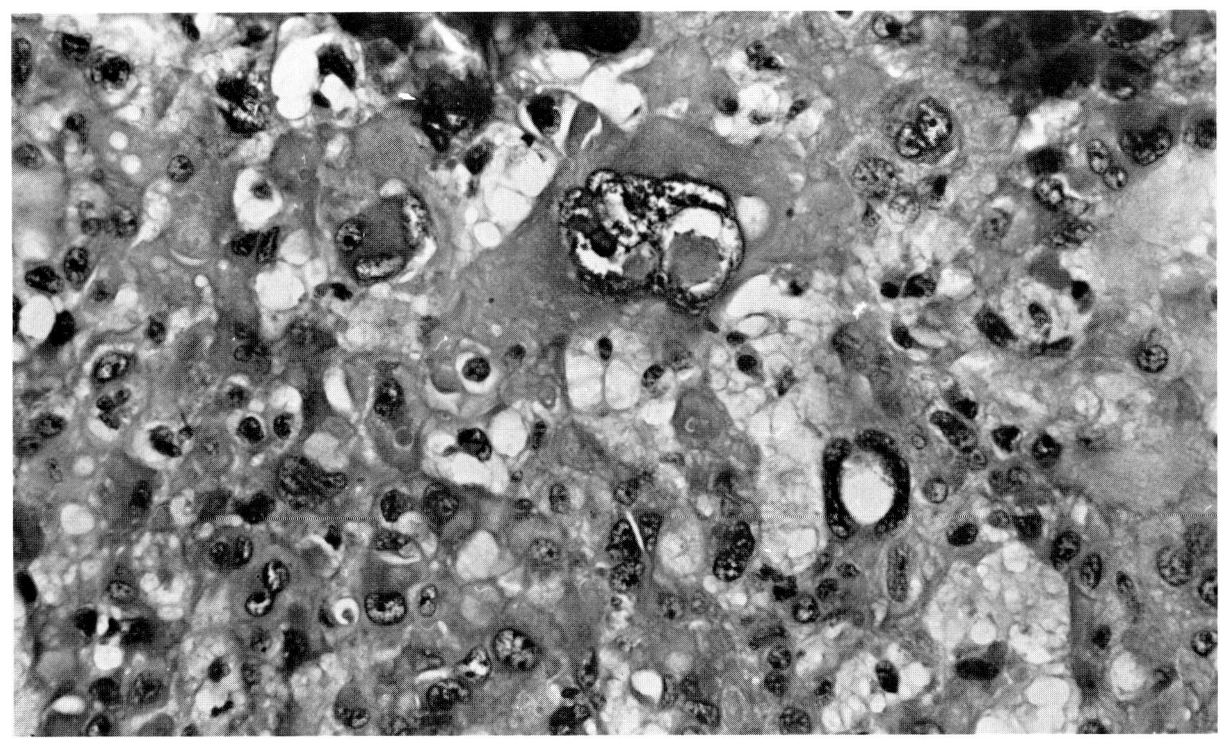

FIG. 8-117

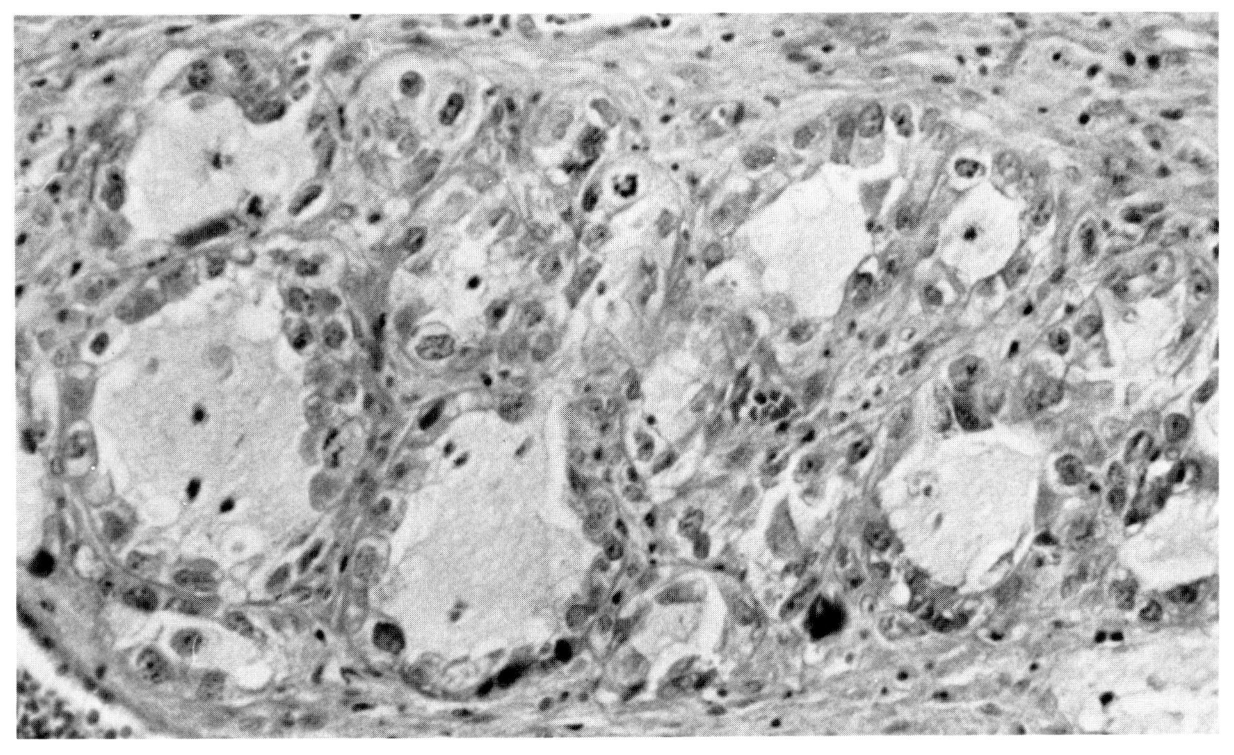

FIG. 8-118

usually embedded in tumor tissue. Anteriorly, the tumor is likely to invade the prevertebral muscle and fascia.

Histopathology

The chordoma is typified by a lobular arrangement, physaliphorous cells, and a mucoid, myxoid or chondroid matrix. The cells may be arranged either haphazardly or in cords or trabeculae.

On low-power examination the chordoma is distinctly lobular (Fig. 8–108). The lobules are separated by thick bands of collagen.

The cells making up the tumor are arranged in either small or long stellate syncytial cords (Figs. 8–109 and 8–110), epithelial-like columns (Fig. 8–111), rounded nests (Fig. 8–112), or as sheets (Fig. 8–113). The pathognomonic feature is the demonstration of the cells that belie their notochordal origin, the so-called *physaliphorous* (meaning basket in Greek) cells (Figs. 8–111–114). These cells contain a voluminous bubbly to clear cytoplasm with slender septae in either a circular or linear arrangement, imparting a feathery or basketlike appearance. These cells resemble lipoblasts to some extent. Cells without these septae will appear as single bubbles with compressed eccentric nuclei mimicking the signet ring cells of gastric carcinoma (Fig. 8–114). In some cases the predominant cell type may be an eosinophilic or pink cell without bubbles or clear spaces in the cytoplasm. Embryologically, the notochord contains two cell types—a pink cell and a bubbly physaliphorous cell. The pink cell is seen in earliest notochordal development and is gradually replaced by the more characteristic physaliphorous cell (personal observations). The importance of recognizing these two cell types is that on rare occasion a chordoma may be encountered that contains the pure pink cell form with no physaliphorous cells identifiable. Usually both cell types are mixed together.

The nuclei are fairly large and round, oval, and multilobulated to multinucleate. It is possible to find in some tumors giant bizarre nuclei with prominent nucleoli (Fig. 8–117). These highly malignant-looking cells are not necessarily associated with a more rapid or lethal course, however.

The matrix may be bubbly, myxoid, or chondroid (Figs. 8–109, 8–112, and 8–114). Large pools of mucinous substances may be deposited (Fig. 8–110). The presence of mucin and cords of cells may mimic a carcinoma; however, true acini are never formed.

Chordomas of the base of the skull are associated with greater degrees of chondroid and cartilage tissues, compared to those in the spine and sacrum.[97]

Chordomas are slow growing and usually show few mitoses. Significant mitoses signify a more rapidly growing tumor that is associated with a worse short-term prognosis.

The diagnosis of chordoma should not be a difficult one if this tumor is always kept in mind when dealing with a lesion that arises in a spinal bone and if a diligent search is made for its pathognomonic cell type.

Differential Diagnosis

LIPOSARCOMA. Liposarcomas of bone are extremely rare entities. The few reported cases occur in long bones, not in the spine. Most so-called liposarcomas of bone usually prove to be metastatic renal cell carcinomas. The odds are vastly in favor of a solitary liposarcoma-like tumor of the spine to be in actuality a chordoma.

CHONDROSARCOMA. Chordomas rarely produce much true cartilage. Chondrosarcomas of the spine are rarer tumors than the chordoma. A chondrosarcoma does not contain physaliphorous cells and its cells do not form columns and cords common in chordoma.

METASTATIC CARCINOMA. On rare occasions a metastatic carcinoma may mimic a chordoma. Metastatic renal cell carcinoma will contain clear and granular cells and possibly, acini or tubules; physaliphorous cells are lacking. The author has also seen a case of a sacral tumor in a middle-aged female diagnosed as chordoma. This tumor mimicked chordoma in terms of its mucinous stroma and cell arrangement. However, careful analysis failed to reveal a single physaliphorous cell and true acini were present (Fig. 8–118), a feature incompatible with chordoma. Exploratory laparotomy revealed a mucinous cyst adenocarcinoma of the ovary.

Course and Treatment

The chordoma grows slowly, often over a period of many years, and metastasizes late in its course to the lungs, bone soft tissues, and liver in 20 to 40 per cent of patients. Some tumors can weigh as much as 100 pounds. Even though it metastasizes late, it is a discouraging tumor to treat because of its close relationship to important and vital structures. More than 90 per cent of patients are dead within 5 to 10 years. To offer any chance of cure, the surgeon must be aggressive in his attempts to remove all traces of the tumor by means of radical block resection. Heffelfinger, *et. al.*,[97] have pointed out that chordomas of the speno-occipital region with significant production of chondroid or cartilage have a much longer course (15.8 years), compared to the noncartilagenous chordomas (4.1 years).

Transformation to a spindle-cell sarcoma (fibrosarcoma?) has been reported to occur on rare occasions.[97]

Alleviation of pain in an inoperable tumor includes radiation, rhizotomy, spinothalamic cordotomy, and narcotics.

REFERENCES

Enchondroma Versus Chondrosarcoma

1. Aegeter, E.: Diagnostic radiology and the pathology of bone disease. Radiol. Clin. North Amer., *8:* 215, 1970.
2. Barnes, R., and Catto, M.: Chondrosarcoma of bone. J. Bone Joint Surg., *48B:* 729, 1966.
3. Coley, B.L., and Higinbotham, N.L.: The significance of cartilage in abnormal locations. Cancer, *2:* 777, 1949.
4. ———: Secondary chondrosarcoma. Ann. Surg., *139:* 547, 1954.
5. Culver, J.E., Street, D.E., and McCue, F.C.: Chondrosarcoma of the hand arising from a preexistent benign enchondroma. Clin. Orthop., *113:* 128, 1975.
6. Dahlin, D.C.: Bone Tumors. pp. 29 and 139. Charles C Thomas, Springfield, 1970.
7. Dahlin, D.C., and Henderson, E.D.: Chondrosarcoma: a surgical and pathological problem. Review of 212 cases. J. Bone Joint Surg., *38A:* 1025, 1956.
8. Dahlin, D.C., and Salvador, A.H.: Chondrosarcomas of bones of the hands and feet—a study of 30 cases. Cancer, *34:* 755, 1974.
9. Gilmer, W.S., Kilgore, W., and Smith, H.: Central cartilage tumors of bone. Clin. Orthop., *26:* 81, 1963.
10. Gottschalk, R., and Smith, R.T.: Chondrosarcoma of the hand. J. Bone Joint Surg., *45A:* 141, 1963.
11. Hamlin, J., and Adler, L: Central enchondroma—a precursor to chondrosarcoma? J. Can. Assoc. Radiol., *22:* 206, 1971.
12. Jaffe, H.L.: Tumors & Tumorous Conditions of the Bone and Joints. Philadelphia, Lea & Febiger, 1958.
13. Laurence, W., and Franklin, E.L.: Calcifying enchondroma of long bones. J. Bone Joint Surg., *35B:* 224, 1953.
14. Lichtenstein, L., and Jaffe, H.L.: Chondrosarcoma of bone. Am. J. Pathol., *19:* 553, 1943.
15. Lindbom, A., Soderberg, G., and Spjut, H.J.: Primary chondrosarcoma of bone. Acta Radiol., *55:* 81, 1961.
16. Marcove, R.C., Stovell, P.B., Huvos, A.G. and Bullough, P.G.: The use of cryosurgery in the treatment of low and medium grade chondrosarcoma. A preliminary report. Clin. Orthop., *122:* 147, 1977.
17. Mirra, J.M. and Marcove, R.: Fibrosarcomatous dedifferentiation of primary and secondary chondrosarcoma. J. Bone Joint Surg., *56A:* 285, 1974.
18. O'Neal, L.W., and Ackerman, L.V.: Chondrosarcoma of bone. Cancer, *5:* 551, 1952.
19. Scherer, E.: Exostosen, Enchondrome, und Irhe Bezienhung Zum Periost. Frankfurt Ztschr. F. Pathol., *36:* 587, 1928.
20. Takigawa, K.: Chondroma of the hand. A review of 110 cases. J. Bone Joint Surg., *53A:* 1591, 1971.
21. Unni, K., Dahlin, D.C., Beabout, J. and Sim, F.: Chondrosarcoma clear-cell variant. J. Bone Joint Surg., *58A:* 676, 1976.

Fibro- and Osteosarcomatous Transformation of Chondrosarcoma

22. Dahlin, D.C. and Beabout, J.W.: Dedifferentiation of low grade chondrosarcomas. Cancer, *28:* 462, 1971.
23. Kahn, L.: Chondrosarcoma with dedifferentiated foci: a comparative and ultrastructural study. Cancer, *27:* 1365, 1976.
24. McFarland, G.B., McKinley, L. and Reed, R.: Dedifferentiation of low grade chondrosarcomas. Clin. Orthop. *122:* 157, 1977.
25. Mirra, J.M., and Marcove, R.C.: Fibrosarcomatous dedifferentiation of primary and secondary chondrosarcoma. J. Bone Joint Surg., *56A:* 285, 1974.

Ollier's Disease (Multiple Enchondromatosis)

26. Dahlin, C.D., and Beabout, J.W.: Dedifferentiation of low-grade chondrosarcomas. Cancer, *28:* 461, 1971.
27. Mirra, J.M., and Marcove, R.C.: Fibrosarcomatous dedifferentiation of primary and secondary chondrosarcoma. J. Bone Joint Surg., *56A:* 285, 1974.

Mesenchymal Chondrosarcoma

28. Dahlin, D.C., and Henderson, E.D.: Mesenchymal chondrosarcoma-further observations on a new entity. Cancer, *15:* 410, 1962.
29. Dowling, E.A.: Mesenchymal chondrosarcoma. J. Bone Joint Surg., *46A:* 747, 1964.
30. Hutter, R.V.P., Foote, F.W., Jr., Francis, K.C., and Sherman, R.S.: Primitive multipotential primary sarcoma of bone. Cancer, *19:* 1, 1966.
31. Salvador, A.H., Beabout, J.W., and Dahlin, D.C.: Mesenchymal chondrosarcoma—Observations on 30 new cases. Cancer, *28:* 605, 1971.

32. Steiner, G.C., Mirra, J.M., and Bullough, P.G.: Mesenchymal chondrosarcoma. A study of the ultrastructure. Cancer, *32:*926, 1973.
33. Stout, A.P., and Murray, M.R.: Hemangiopericytoma—a vascular tumor featuring Zimmermann's pericytes. Ann. Surg., *116:*26, 1942.

Chondroblastoma

34. Aegerter, E., and Kirkpatrick, J.A., Jr.,: Orthopedic Diseases. Physiology. Pathology. Radiology. ed. 4, Philadelphia, W.B. Saunders, 1975.
35. Biesecker, J.L., Marcove, R.C., Huvos, A.G. and Miké, V.: Aneurysmal bone cyst. Cancer, *26:*615, 1970.
36. Castleman, B. (ed.): Case Records of the Massachusetts General Hospital, Case 33. New Engl. J. Med., *271:*94, 1964.
37. Codman, E.A.: Epiphyseal chondromatous giant cell tumors of the upper end of the humerus. Gynecol. Obstet., *52:*543, 1931.
38. Coleman, S.S.: Benign chondroblastoma with recurrent soft tissue and intra-articular lesions. Report of a case. J. Bone Joint Surg., *48A:* 1554, 1966.
39. Dahlin, D.C., and Ivins, J.C.: Benign chondroblastoma. A study of 125 cases. Cancer, *30:*401, 1972.
40. Fechner, R.E., and Wilde, H.D.: Chondroblastoma in the metaphysis of the femoral neck. A case report and review of the literature. J. Bone Joint Surg., *56A:*413, 1974.
41. Gawlik, Z. and Witwicki, T.: Chondroblastoma malignum primarium. Pathol. Pol., *16:*181, 1965.
42. Geschickter, C.F., and Copeland, M.M.: Chondroblastic tumors of bone: benign and malignant. Ann. Surg., *129:*724, 1949.
43. Green, P., and Whittaker, R.P.: Benign chondroblastoma. Case report with pulmonary metastasis. J. Bone Joint Surg., *57A:*418, 1975.
44. Hatcher, C.H.: The development of sarcoma in bone subjected to roentgen or radium irradiation. J. Bone Joint Surg., *27A:*179, 1945.
45. Hatcher, C.H., and Campbell, J.C.: Benign chondroblastoma of bone. Its histologic variations and a report of late sarcoma in the site of one. Bull. Hosp. Joint Dis., *12:*411, 1951.
46. Hellner, H.: Die Klinik der Knochengeschwulste. Helv. Chir. Acta., *26:*621, 1959.
47. Hellner, H.: Semimaligne Geschwulste. Arch. Geschwulstforsch., *18:*107, 1961.
48. Hull, M.T., Crussi, F., De Rosa, G.P., and Graul, R.S.: Aggressive chondroblastoma. Report of a case with multicentric origin, soft tissue invasion, and cytologic features of anaplasia. Clin. Orthop. *126:*261, 1977.
49. Huvos, A.G., and Marcove, R.C.: Chondroblastoma of bone. A critical review. Clin. Orthop., *95:*300, 1973.
50. Huvos, A.G., Marcove, R.C., Erlandson, R.A., and Miké, V.: Chondroblastoma of bone. A clinicopathologic and electron microscopic study. Cancer, *29:*760, 1972.
51. Huvos, A.G., Higinbotham, N.L., Marcove, R.C., and O'Leary, P.: Aggressive Chondroblastoma. Review of the literature on aggressive behavior and metastases with report of one new case. Clin. Orthop., *126:*266, 1977.
52. Jaffe, H.L., and Lichtenstein, L.: Benign chondroblastoma of bone. A reinterpretation of the so-called calcifying or chondromatous giant cell tumor. Am. J. Pathol., *18:*969, 1942.
53. Kahn, L.B., Wood, F.M., and Ackerman, L.V.: Malignant chondroblastoma. Report of two cases and review of the literature. Arch. Pathol. *88:*371, 1969.
54. Lichtenstein, L.: Bone Tumors. ed. 4, p. 76. St. Louis, C.V. Mosby, 1972.
55. McBryde, A. Jr., and Goldner, J.L.: Chondroblastoma of bone. Am. J. Surg., *36:*94, 1970.
56. McLaughlin, R.E., Sweet, D.E., Webster, T., and Merritt, W.M.: Chondroblastoma of the pelvis suggestive of malignancy. Report of an unusual case treated by wide pelvic excision. J. Bone Joint Surg., *57A:*549, 1975.
57. Netherlands Committee on Bone Tumors: Radiological Atlas of Bone Tumors. Vol. 2. Baltimore. Williams & Wilkins, 1973.
58. Onuigbo, W.I.B.: A definition problem in cancer metastasis. Neoplasma, *22:*547, 1975.
59. Riddell, R.J., Louis, C.J., and Bromberger, N.A.: Pulmonary metastases from chondroblastoma of the tibia. Report of a case. J. Bone Joint Surg., *55B:*848, 1973.
60. Ruziczka, O., and Haslhofer, L.: Zur Klinik und Pathologie des Chondroblastoma "benignum," Monatsschrift fur Kinderheilkd., *110:*201, 1962.
61. Salzer, M., Salzer-Kuntschik, M., and Kretschmer, G.: Das Benigne Chondroblastom. Archiv Orthop. Unfall Chir., *64:*229, 1968.
62. Schajowicz, F., and Gallardo, H.: Epiphyseal chondroblastoma of bone. A clinico-pathological study of sixty-nine cases. J. Bone Joint Surg., *52B:*205, 1970.
63. Shoji, H., and Miller, T.R.: Benign chondroblastoma with soft-tissue recurrence. N.Y. State J. Med., *71:*2786, 1971.
64. Sirsat, M.V., and Doctor, V.M.: Benign chondroblastoma of bone. Report of a case of malignant transformation. J. Bone Joint Surg., *52B:*741, 1970.
65. Sundaram, T.K.S.: Benign chondroblastoma. J. Bone Joint Surg., *48B:*92, 1966.
66. Sweetnam, R., and Ross, L.: Surgical treatment of pulmonary metastases from primary tumours of bone. J. Bone Joint Surg., *49B:*74, 1967.
67. Uehlinger, E.: Die pathologische Anatomie der Knochengeschwulste. Helv. Chir. Acta., *26:*597, 1959.
68. Uehlinger, E.: Pathologische Anatomie der Knochengeschwulste. Helv. Chir. Acta., *40:*5, 1973.
69. Unni, K., Dahlin, D.C., Beabout, J., and Sim, F.:

Chondrosarcoma, Clear-cell variant. J. Bone Joint Surg., *58A:*676, 1976.
70. Varma, B.P., and Gupta, I.M.: Atypical chondroblastoma of tibia. Clin. Orthop., *89:*241, 1972.
71. Wellmann, K.F.: Chondroblastoma of the scapula. A case report with ultrastructural observations. Cancer, *24:*408, 1969.
72. Zabski, Z.A., Cutler, S.S., and Yermakov, V.: Unclassified benign tumor of the rib. Cancer, *36:*1009, 1975.

Chondromyxoid Fibroma

73. Aegerter, E., and Kirkpatrick, J.A., Jr.: Orthopedic Diseases. ed. 3. Philadelphia, W.B. Saunders, 1968.
74. Benson, W.R., and Bass, S., Jr.: Chondromyxoid Fibroma; first report of occurrence of this tumor in vertebral column. Am. J. Clin. Pathol. *25:*1290, 1955.
75. Dahlin, D.C.: Bone Tumors. ed. 2. Springfield, Charles C Thomas, 1957.
76. Dahlin, D.C.: Chondromyxoid fibroma of bone with emphasis on its morphological relationship to benign chondroblastoma. Cancer, *9:*195, 1956.
77. Dahlin, D.C., Wells, A.H., and Henderson, E.D.: Chondromyxoid fibroma of bone; report of two cases. J. Bone Joint Surg., *35A:*831, 1953.
78. Feldman, F., Hecht, H.L., and Johnston, A.D.: Chondromyxoid fibroma of bone. Radiology, *94:*249, 1970.
79. Goorwitch, J.: Chondromyxoid fibroma of rib; report of an unusual benign primary tumor. Dis. of Chest, *20:*186, 1951.
80. Hutchison, J., and Park, W.W.: Chondromyxoid fibroma of bone, report of a case. J. Bone Joint Surg., *42B:*542, 1960.
81. Iwata, S., and Coley, B.L.: Report of 6 cases of chondromyxoid fibroma of bone, a distinctive benign tumor likely to be mistaken especially for chondrosarcoma. Surg. Gynecol. Obstet., *107:*571, 1958.
82. Jaffe, H.L., and Lichtenstein, L.: Chondromyxoid fibroma of bone; a distinctive benign tumor likely to be mistaken especially for chondrosarcoma. Arch. Pathol., *45:*541, 1948.
83. Lichtenstein, L.: Bone Tumors. ed. 3. St. Louis, C.V. Mosby, 1965.
84. Lichtenstein, L.: Disease of Bone and Joints. St. Louis, C.V. Mosby, 1970.
85. Ralph, L.L.: Chondromyxoid fibroma of bone. J. Bone Joint Surg., *44B:*7, 1962.
86. Levy, W.M., Aegerter, E., and Kirkpatrick, J.A.: The nature of cartilagenous tumors. Radiol. Clin. North Amer., *2:*327, 1964.
87. Spjut, H.J., Dorfman, H.D., Fechner, R.E., and Ackerman, L.V.: Tumors of Bone & Cartilage. Atlas of Tumor Pathology. second series, p. 59. Washington, D.C., Fasicles Armed Forces Institute of Pathology, 1971.
88. Turcotte, B., Pugh, D.G., and Dahlin, D.C.: The roentgenographic aspects of chondromyxoid fibroma of bone. Am. J. Roentgenol. Radium Ther. Nucl. Med., *87:*1085, 1962.

Chordoma

89. Beaugie, J.M., Mann, C.V., and Butler, E.C.B.: Sacrococcygeal chordoma. Br. J. Surg., *56:*586, 1969.
90. Berdal, P., and Myhre, E.: Cranial chordomas involving the paranasal sinuses. J. Laryngol. Otol., *78:*906, 1964.
91. Cappell, D.F.: Chordoma of the vertebral column with three new cases. J. Pathol., *31:*797, 1928.
92. Dahlin, D.C.: Bone Tumors: General Aspects and Data on 3,987 Cases. ed. 2, p. 285. Springfield, Charles C Thomas, 1967.
93. Dahlin, D.C., and Beabout, J.W.: Dedifferentiation of low-grade chondrosarcomas. Cancer, *28:*461, 1971.
94. Dahlin, D.C., and MacCarty, C.S.: Chordoma: a study of fifty-nine cases. Cancer, *5:*1170, 1952.
95. Falconer, M.A., Bailey, I.C., and Duchen, L.W.: Surgical treatment of chordoma and chondroma of the skull base. J. Neurosurg., *29:*261, 1968.
96. Fletcher, E.M., Woltman, H.W., and Adson, A.W.: Sacrococcygeal chordomas: a clinical and pathologic study. Arch. Neurol. and Psychiatr., *33:*283, 1935.
97. Heffelfinger, M., Dahlin, D.C., MacCarty, C.S. and Beabout, J.W.: Chordomas and Cartilagenous Tumors at the Skull Base. Cancer, *32:*410, 1973.
98. Higinbotham, N.L., Phillips, R.F., Farr, H.W., and Hustu, H.O.: Chordoma: Thirty-five-year study at Memorial Hospital. Cancer, *20:*1841, 1967.
99. Horwitz, T.: Chordal extopia and its possible relationship to chordoma. Arch. Pathol., *31:*354, 1941.
100. Kamrin, R.P., Potanos, J.N., and Pool, J.L.: An evaluation of the diagnosis and treatment of chordoma. J. Neurol. Neurosurg. Psychiatry, *27:*157, 1964.
101. Levowitz, B.S., Khan, M.Y., Rand, E., and Hurwitz, A.: Thoracic vertebral chordoma presenting as a posterior mediastinal tumor. Ann. Thorac. Surg., *2:*75, 1966.
102. MacCarty, C.S., Waugh, J.M., Coventry, M.B., and O'Sullivan, D.C.: Sacrococcygeal chordomas. Surg. Gynecol. Obstet., *113:*551, 1961.
103. MacCarty, C.S., Waugh, J.M., Mayo, C.W., and Coventry, M.B.: The surgical treatment of presacral tumors: a combined problem. Proc. Staff Meet. Mayo Clin. *27:*73, 1952.
104. Minagi, H., and Newton, T.H.: Cartilaginous tumors of the base of skull. Am. J. Roentgenol. Radium Ther. Nucl. Med., *105:*308, 1969.
105. Pearlman, A.W., and Friedman, M.: Radical radiation therapy of chordoma. Am. J. Roentgenol. Radium Ther. Nucl. Med., *108:*333, 1970.
106. Pena, C.E. Horvat, B.L., and Fisher, E.R.: The ultrastructure of chordoma. Am. J. Clin. Pathol., *53:*544, 1970.

107. Plaut, H.F., and Blatt, E.S.: Chordoma of the clivus: a report of four cases. Am. J. Roentgenol. Radium Ther. Nucl. Med., *100:* 639, 1967.

108. Poppen, J.L., and King, A.B.: Chordoma: experience with thirteen cases. J. Neurosurg., *9:* 139, 1952.

109. Rissanen, P.M., and Holsti, L.R.: Sacrococcygeal chordomas and their treatment. Radiol. Clin. Biol., *36:* 153, 1967.

110. Rosenqvist, H., and Saltzman, G.F.: Sacrococcygeal and vertebral chordomas and their treatment. Acta. Radiol. (Stockh.), *52:* 177, 1959.

111. Spjut, H.J., and Luse, S.A.: Chordoma: an electron microscopic study. Cancer, *17:* 643, 1964.

112. Utne, J.R., and Pugh, D.G.: The roentgenologic aspects of chordoma. Am. J. Roentgenol. Radium Ther. Nucl. Med., *74:* 593, 1955.

113. Wright, D.: Nasopharyngeal and certical chordoma—some aspects of their development and treatment. J. Laryngol. Otol., *81:* 1337, 1967.

INTRAOSSEOUS SPINDLE CELL AND COLLAGEN-PRODUCING TUMORS

9

Perhaps every tumor of bone contains some spindle cells, either as a reparative host response or as a slight variation in the shape of the lesional cells. In this chapter only those lesions where the role of spindle cells is an essential component of the tumor or where focal masses of long spindle cells may result in diagnostic confusion, particularly, if they are not considered as a possible, prominent component of the lesion in contention, will be discussed. For example, a simple bone cyst is usually not associated with dominant masses of spindly cells, collagen, and new bone production. But this phenomenon does occur as a reparative response to repair as a result of pathologic fracture through the cyst. Because these tissues may lead to diagnostic error, in that extensive fibroosseous tissue in a simple bone cyst may be mistaken for fibrous dysplasia, this particular phenomenon will be dealt with in this chapter. But if a lesion has dominant characteristics of chondroid, giant cells, "chicken-wire calcifications," and bland polygonal cells, all of which are diagnostic criteria for a chondroblastoma, and a few spindly cells or a focus of reparative scar tissue, diagnostic confusion should not occur; therefore such an entity will not be treated in this chapter. This will eliminate the necessity of discussing every single entity that contains a spindle cell or collagen component.

BENIGN LESIONS

CALLUS

In the early stages of fracture repair, plump, spindly, preosteoblast cells are a predominant feature. These tissues contain plump and crowded nuclei and numerous mitotic figures. Confusing these cells with spindle cells or fibrosarcoma is possible if only a slide reading is used. But because callus differentiates toward bone and cartilage production, the diagnosis of osteosarcoma is possible. In order to rule out this possibility, careful review of history and radiographs is necessary. Refer to pp. 86–97, and Plate 1, *A–I*, for the diagnostic features of fracture callus.

HYPERPARATHYROIDISM AND PAGET'S DISEASE

Both hyperparathyroidism and Paget's disease are characterized by bone resorption and remodeling, where the marrow, in the areas of osteoclastic activity, forms a loose, fibrous tissue (p. 308 and Figs. 10–7, 10–8, 10–10, and 10–11). In the giant cell tumor stage of hyperparathyroidism, the stromal cells are spindled and are usually associated with an abundance of collagen and focal hemorrhages (Figs. 10–7, 10–8, and 10–9). Paget's disease may, after many years, convert to a spindly fibrosarcoma, osteosarcoma, or osteoclastic sarcoma (p. 356 and Figs. 10–62–10–70).

Fibrous Dysplasia

This entity is characterized by bland fibrous tissue in association with variable quantities of curled spicules of woven bone (p. 122 and Figs. 7–53, 7–55, 7–56, 7–57).

Giant Cell Reparative Granuloma

The giant cell reparative granuloma is confined to jawbones and is characterized by bland spindle cells, collagen production, variable quantities of woven bone and osteoclast-like giant cells, and foci of hemorrhage and hemosiderin pigment. (p. 322 and Fig. 10–23). It is very similar in its histologic appearance to the nonossifying fibroma or to the giant cell tumor of hyperparathyroidism. Recent data accumulated by this author suggest that the so-called central giant-cell reparative granuloma may be the jawbone equivalent of the nonossifying fibroma of long bones (p. 260).

Giant Cell Reaction of Bone

This lesion has been described only in the bones of the hands and feet. It is a well-circumscribed lytic lesion characterized by long spindly cells, abundant collagen production, some osteoid or woven bone production, and scattered osteoclast-like giant cells (p. 322 and Figs. 10–24–10–26).

Chondromyxoid Fibroma

The chondromyxoid fibroma contains variable quantities of fibroid or chondroid and/or myxoid tissue (p. 234 and Figs. 8–95–8–105 and Plate 6, (*G–I*).

Eosinophilic Granuloma

In the healing phases of this disease fibrosis or scarring may be a dominant feature, admixed with variable quantities of lipid-filled histiocytes (p. 376 and Figs. 11–14 and 11–15).

Simple Bone Cyst and Aneurysmal Bone Cyst

The cyst wall of a simple bone cyst is thin and fibrous in appearance. A great deal of fibro-osseous repair tissues may fill the former, fluid-filled cyst consequent to fracture (see Fig. 13–17). In most instances, these patients have been followed radiologically for some time and a tissue diagnosis of simple bone cyst has usually been obtained before the phase of fracture and extensive fibroosseous repair. If a biopsy was not obtained originally, examination of the fibroosseous tissue for possible remnants of the simple bone cyst wall and review of the radiographs is helpful. On radiograph the simple bone cyst fills the entire width of the bone in a symmetrical fashion. Nonossifying fibromas are usually distinctly eccentric lesions. In contrast to fibrous dysplasia, the fibroosseous repair tissues of the simple bone cyst usually show prominent osteoblastic rimming, a feature rarely seen or inconspicuous in fibrous dysplasia. Osteoblastoma may also be confused with healing fracture in simple bone cyst. Osteoblastomas, however, do not contain prominent masses of fibroosseous tissue; instead the stroma between the woven bone and osteoid trabeculae are highly vascular.

The aneurysmal bone cyst (ABC) may contain prominent fibrous tissue areas, but the extremely large, blood-filled cavities are virtually diagnostic of the condition (see Figs. 13–48–13–50). The cells within the wall of the cystlike spaces of the ABC show no anaplasia. The telangiectatic osteosarcoma may resemble the aneurysmal bone cyst on low power (Plate 5, *D* and *E*), but shows distinctly bizarre and anaplastic cells in the walls on high power (Plate 5, *F*).

Fibrous Cortical Defect and the Nonossifying Fibroma

Capsule Summary

Incidence. The nonossifying fibroma accounts for 2 per cent of biopsied primary bone tumors. The fibrous cortical defect is well recognized and rarely biopsied.

Age. Some 95 per cent of patients are under 20 years of age.

Clinical Features. The fibrous cortical defect is usually asymptomatic. The nonossifying fibroma may lead to the development of pain and swelling, due to pathologic fracture.

Radiologic Features. Both are sharply delineated, radiolucent, multiloculated, eccentric, and are outlined by a sclerotic border; they are usually found in the metaphysis or, unusually, in the shaft. They are rarely epiphyseal.

Gross Pathology. They have a bosselated surface, are firm, and may be either tan, yellow, or gray.

Histopathology. Both are characterized by fibrocytes arranged in whorled bundles and sprinkled with small, multinucleated giant cells. Foamy histiocytes may predominate.

Course. Both are completely benign.

Treatment. Curettage and packing with bone chips, if indicated.

Terminology and Histogenesis

Sontag and Pyle[13] described common, cystlike metaphyseal lesions of young children. The average age of appearance of these lesions was 46 months and the lesion persisted for an average of 29 months before disappearing, gradually traveling away from the metaphyseal area as the bone grew in length. They speculated that these cystlike areas were composed of cartilage. However, Jaffe and Lichtenstein[9] and Hatcher[7] showed that biopsy of these lesions revealed fibrous tissue, thus coining the terms *fibrous cortical defect* and *nonosteogenic fibroma.*

The term *fibrous cortical defect* refers to those small ephemeral fibrous lesions that occur in young children. Most of these lesions are eventually obliterated by either rapid reparative ossification or gradual extrusion from the cortex by remodeling and tubulation at the metaphyseal growing end of the bone.[7] In a small percentage of cases these small lesions not only persist but undergo proliferative activity, may attain large size, penetrate into the medullary cavity, become symptomatic, and even induce gross pathologic fracture. Jaffe and Lichtenstein[8,9] consider this to be a tumorous evolutionary form of the fibrous cortical defect, for which they use the term *nonossifying* or *nonosteogenic fibroma.* Hatcher[7] prefers to use the term *metaphyseal fibrous defect,* because these lesions may eventually become obliterated by bone, which would seem to obviate the term *nonosteogenic* or *nonossifying*. In the American literature, however, the term *nonossifying fibroma* is firmly entrenched. This author would not support changing the name that Jaffe has suggested because, as Stansfeld has pointed out, the new bone that is formed and which leads to the obliteration of the process appears to arise by encroachment of reparative host bone at the margin of the lesion and not by bone formation by the lesion itself. I have made similar observations; namely, that if a nonossifying fibroma is in the process of obliteration, the new bone is formed at the margins of the lesion by the host bone. I have not witnessed metaplastic new bone within the center of the lesion removed from contact with host bone. A nonossifying fibroma, therefore, need not always be associated with the total absence of ossification. Therefore, this finding in association with typical radiological and histological features of a nonossifying fibroma should not lead to an incorrect diagnosis, such as one of fibrous dysplasia.

Jaffe[8,9] believes that the process of both the fibrous cortical defect and nonossifying fibroma are basically due to periosteal fibroblastic hyperplasia and that in its later phases of evolution, the matrix fibroblast may imbibe lipids and assume a foamy appearance. The process is benign. It may resolve spontaneously, or if it undergoes further growth, it is usually treated adequately by simple curettage. These lesions are, therefore, not true neoplasms as we have defined them. Most authors now believe they represent developmental defects that begin in the region of the epiphyseal plate, migrate away from the plate as the bone grows in length, and tend to be elongated in the longitudinal axis of the bone. Ponsetti and Friedman[12a] illustrated a patient with three successive fibrous cortical defects arising from the same area of the epiphyseal plate, indicating that the factors producing the defects may act intermittently.

Bosch, *et. al.,*[3] support Jaffe's concept that the basic cell in the process is a type of fibroblast and that the foam cells are transformed mesenchymal fibroblasts. They concluded that the initial stem cell has ultramicroscopic features of a fibroblast and does not have the structures of a histiocyte. These cells eventually synthesized lipids that are stored as droplets inside the endoplasmic reticulum. On the basis of their study they would not classify the nonossifying fibroma as a form of histiocytic fibroxanthoma, as proposed by Phelip,[12] Bahl,[1] and Burman and Zinberg.[4]

Clinical Features

Caffey[5] showed that between 30 to 40 per cent of children develop one or more fibrous cortical defects. They are rarely found in children younger than 2 years of age. Males predominate over females about 1.4 to 1. Patients with the rarer nonossifying fibroma are older children or adolescents, which is in accord with Jaffe's concept of the occasional evolutionary transformation of fibrous cortical defect to nonossifying fibroma.[8]

Fibrous cortical defects are asymptomatic lesions that are found incidentally. Large nonossifying fibromas are symptomatic only if they lead to micro- or gross pathologic fractures.

Campanacci has recently described a new syndrome in four patients, characterized by multiple nonossifying fibromas, jaw cysts, café au lait spots, mental retardation (3 of 4 patients), and eye disorders such as congenital blindness (cases presented at the International Skeletal Society Meeting, Boston, Mass., 1978). Definite neurofibromas have not been seen, although the syndrome suggests a possible neurofibromatosis variant.

I have seen one such patient at UCLA. This adolescent female has multiple large nonossifying fibromas, jaw "cysts," café au lait spots, normal mentation, and increased intraocular pressure but no blindness. No neurofibromas were observed. The jaw lesions were called giant cell reparative granuloma by the oral pathologists. On review, however, they were histologically identical to the long bone lesions. This suggests that the so-called giant cell reparative granuloma may be nothing more than a nonossifying fibroma of the jaw. It is of interest that the giant cell granuloma has been described only in jawbones and the NOF, only outside the jawbones. This author has begun studies to see if two names are being used to describe a single entity. Preliminary investigation shows the probable equivalence of the so-called central giant cell reparative granuloma of jawbones and the NOF of long bones (observations being prepared for publication).

Radiologic Features

FIBROUS CORTICAL DEFECT AND NONOSSIFYING FIBROMA (Fig. 9–1). These lesions are almost always found in the metaphyseal regions of the rapidly growing ends of endochondrally formed long bones. The essential difference between the fibrous cortical defect and the nonossifying fibroma is size and extent of the lesion. The latter are significantly larger and involve the intramedullary substance of the bone, and may be left behind in the diaphysis as the bone grows in length. The fibrous cortical defect is smaller and is confined to the cortical bone.

The following radiographic features are virtually pathognomonic of a fibrous cortical defect (FCD) or the larger nonossifying fibroma:

1. The lesions are *metaphyseal.* The younger the patient, the closer the proximal end is to the epiphyseal plate. (Compare Fig. 9–2 with Fig. 9–7.)
2. The FCD is distinctly *eccentric and either intraperiosteal* or *intracortical* (Fig. 9–2). In order to visualize its eccentricity, the radiograph should be at right angles to the lesions. The NOF is also usually an eccentric lesion that extends to involve the intramedullary substance of the bone. If the radiograph is in the same plane as the lesion its eccentric nature may not be appreciated (Figs. 9–4, 9–5, and 9–6).
3. The center of the lesion is either diffusely *lytic, pseudotrabeculated,* or *"bubbly"* (Fig. 9–8).
4. They are surrounded by a *dense border of host bone sclerosis* (Figs. 9–3, 9–4, and 9–8), unless they are very early in development (Fig. 9–2).
5. The fibrous cortical defect is usually less than 1 cm. in diameter, although they may be as long as 5 cm. in length. Most lesions are longer than they are wide, a reflection of their development in a growing remodeling end of a bone. Nonossifying fibromas may be much larger and extend into the intramedullary substance (Figs. 9–7, 9–8, and 9–9). Very large nonossifying fibromas may result in pathologic fracture (Fig. 9–9). Healing is usually excellent post-curettage. Some lesions may, however, recur and result in less than perfect fracture healing (Fig. 9–10). Both the fibrous cortical defect and nonossifying fibroma usually heal spontaneously or involute without surgical intervention. They usually heal by filling in with bone (Figs. 9–5 and 9–6) and eventually become remodeled, leaving little to no trace of their former presence.
6. Either lesion usually does not bulge from the cortex significantly. It usually grows into rather than out of the bone. Lesions that resemble the FCD or NOF but bulge out of the bone are usually either chondromyxoid fibromas, parosteal chondromas, or other benign periosteal lesions. By "resemble the FCD or NOF," it is meant that the lesions are eccentric, involve the metaphysis, and are bordered by a intramedullary rind of benign bone sclerosis.

Gross Pathology

On gross examination of curettings or en-bloc excisions, the nonossifying fibroma consists of brownish-tan (Plate 7, *F*) or yellowish gray (Plate 7, *E*), firm, fibrous tissue. Considerable quantities of hemosiderin pigment impart the brown color; fresh hemorrhage, the reddish hue; fibrous stroma, a grayish white; and lipid-laden macrophages, the yellowish hue, and in discrete foci form yellow-orange nodules. The tumor is bosselated along its surface and is surrounded by ridges of bone or bony septae (Plate 7, *F*). The latter feature accounts for the pseudotrabeculated radiographic appearance. The dense ridges surrounding the lesion represent reactive host bone sclerosis or residual cortical bone. It is this reactive bone that imparts the dense border of sclerosis on radiograph and is so important to the recognition of this disorder and signifies its benignancy. The periosteum is generally nonreactive, except at sites of pathologic fracture.

A rare example of an intact nonossifying fibroma is

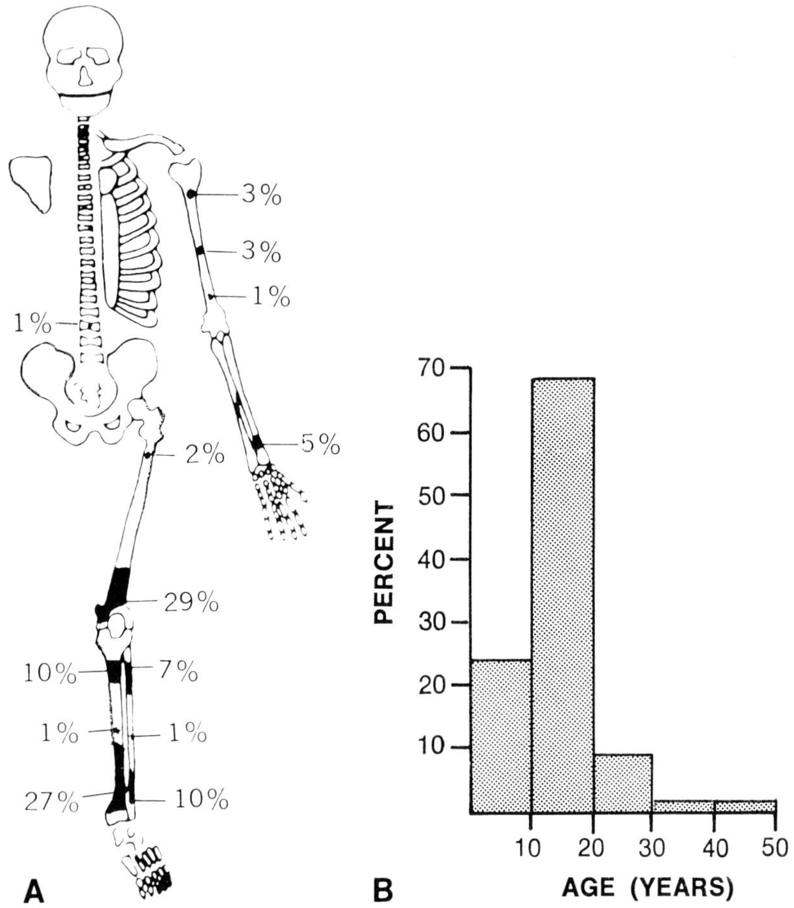

FIG. 9-1. (*A*) Nonossifying fibroma. Frequency of areas of involvement in 88 patients. Male: female incidence, 1.4:1. (*B*) Age distribution in patients with nonossifying fibroma. (Mirra, J., Bullough, P., and Freiberger, R.: Orthopedic Diseases, Part II. New York, Famous Teachings in Modern Medicine, MedCom, Inc., © 1972)

shown in Plate 7, *E*. The radiograph of this particular lesion is shown in Figure 9-7.

Histopathology

The two basic components of either the fibrous cortical defect (rarely biopsied) or nonossifying fibroma (uncommonly biopsied) are the presence of *fibroblastic tissue* admixed with *osteoclast-like giant cells*. The fibroblasts are usually very exuberant and disposed in whorled, storiform, or interlacing patterns (Figs. 9-11 and 9-12). The nuclei are plump and oval and contain small nucleoli (Fig. 9-13). Mitoses are generally infrequent. Marked variations in size and shape, large bubbly nuclei, severe hyperchromatism, abnormal chromatin clumping, and atypical mitoses (signs of anaplasia) are lacking. The giant cells generally contain from three to 10 nuclei and are fairly evenly dispersed throughout the tissue (Fig. 9-12). They usually blend into the tissue so that on low-power examination (Fig. 9-11) they do not stand out as prominently as in the neoplastic giant cell tumor. However, in rare cases large, prominent giant cells with up to 30 or more nuclei may be present (Figs. 9-14 and 9-15).

In about a third of cases small to large collections of *foam cells* with small round nuclei are present (Figs. 9-16, 9-17, and 9-18). The cells appear to form from deposition of lipids within the fibroblastic cells (Fig. 9-18). In rare cases the vast majority of the biopsied tissue consist of foam cells; the remainder of the tissue is fibroblastic. In these older regressive forms of nonossifying fibroma the numbers of giant cells is reduced and the collagen bundles may be quite thick, approaching that of desmoid tumors (compare Fig. 9-29 with Fig. 9-18).

Focal hemorrhages and hemosiderin pigment may be extensive. Vascularity is increased in areas of hemorrhage. Pigment may be found intra- or extracellularly. Both the stromal cells and giant cells may be pigment-laden.

Low-power examination of the margins of relatively intact lesions shows the lobular outer margin of these lesions (Fig. 9-19). The host bone frequently shows osteoclastic resorption along its lesional margin. In those unusual cases when biopsy is taken during a phase of healing, osteoid and woven bone formation may occur at the margin of the lesion with the host bone (Figs. 9-20 and 9-21). Osteoid and woven bone do not form in lesional tissue separated from the surrounding host bone. The bone and osteoid show prominent benign rimming of osteoblasts, identifying it as reactive bone and mitigating against the possible diagnosis of fibrous dysplasia (Fig. 9-21).

Differential Diagnosis

FIBROSARCOMA. The extreme cellularity of the nonossifying fibroma (NOF) is alarming and may suggest a fibrosarcoma to those unfamiliar with its appearance. It does not, however, ever show unequivocal high-grade anaplasia, as is common for most fibrosarcomas (Figs. 9-37 and 9-39). However, distinguishing low-grade fibrosarcoma permeated with giant cells (Figs. 10-73-10-75) may be impossible to distinguish from NOF or even a giant cell tumor from only a slide reading. Fortunately, this form of fibrosarcoma is rare, compared to the more common NOF. The NOF is characterized by a dense border of sclerosis on radiograph and occurs in patients of young age. Low-grade fibrosarcomas may be circumscribed but due to incessant growth, lack a benign border of host bone sclerosis. In addition, fibrosarcoma usually develops in adults, almost always lack benign, foamy histiocytes, and usually do not contain a diffuse sprinkling of osteoclastic giant cells. Nevertheless, fibrosarcoma must always enter into the differential diagnosis and be eliminated by careful consideration of the patient's age and radiographic and histologic features. Bhagwandeen[2] has reported a case of NOF with foam cells which, 18 months after curettage, showed an aggressive fibrosarcoma in a 21-year-old. Whether or not the tumor was from the inception a fibrosarcoma with foam cells or truly a nonossifying

---

Fibrous Cortical Defect and Nonossifying Fibroma

FIG. 9-2. Fibrous cortical defect. This 5-year-old child shows an eccentric, metaphyseal defect of the distal femur, an irregular periosteal reaction, and cortical irregularity. There is no clear border of reactive sclerosis. A biopsy showed a periosteal hyperplastic fibrous reaction admixed with innocuous giant cells. The diagnosis was fibrous cortical defect in early stages of development prior to the sharp margination and border of sclerosis characteristic of most older lesions. The area healed well post-curettage.

FIG. 9-3. This radiograph demonstrates the classical features of a small, fibrous cortical defect of the proximal tibia. It is metaphyseal, slightly lobulated to trabeculated, quite eccentric, and bordered by a dense rim of benign host bone sclerosis. It is 1 cm. from the closing epiphyseal plate of this 17-year-old female.

FIG. 9-4. In this anterior-posterior view, the eccentric nature of the metaphyseal fibrous defect cannot be fully appreciated. It does show a thick, benign border of host bone sclerosis (*arrow*). The lesion is much longer than it is wide, a reflection of its development during the growth-remodeling phase of the host bone.

FIG. 9-5. This 20-year-old male shows a small, dense, eccentric, metaphyseal lesion (*arrow*). Biopsy showed bland scarlike tissue admixed with numerous foamy histiocytes consistent with a late healing phase of a nonossifying fibroma. (Fig. 9-18 is from this patient.) The lesion was also filling in with host bone repair, as its dense appearance on radiograph would suggest.

FIG. 9-6. In this A-P view of the previous case, the circumscribed, lobular nature of the process, surrounded by dense host bone sclerosis, is clearly shown. The lesion is far from the former epiphyseal plate. This is consistent with the relatively advanced age of the patient, considering that most nonossifying fibromas are discovered in childhood or adolescence.

FIG. 9-7. Specimen radiograph showing the typical "soap bubble" appearance of a nonossifying fibroma from the tibia of a 16-year-old girl. Although the lesion is completely benign, the patient had to have an amputation because of a motorcycle accident. The very rare, intact, gross appearance of the nonossifying fibroma, from this unfortunate circumstance, is shown in Plate 7, *E.* (Mubarak, Scott, *et al.:* Am. J. Clin. Pathol., *61:*697, 1974)

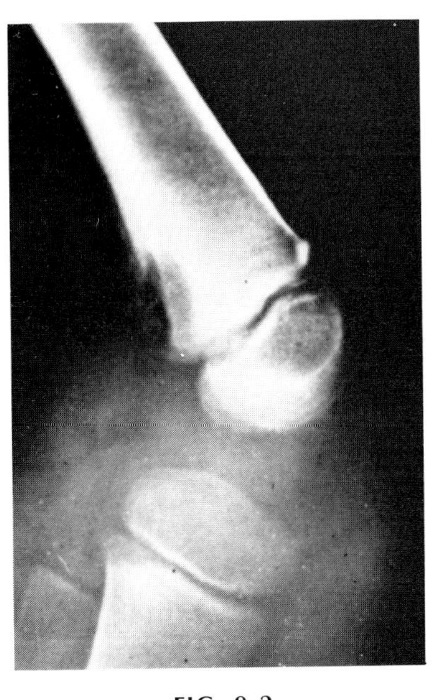
FIG. 9-2

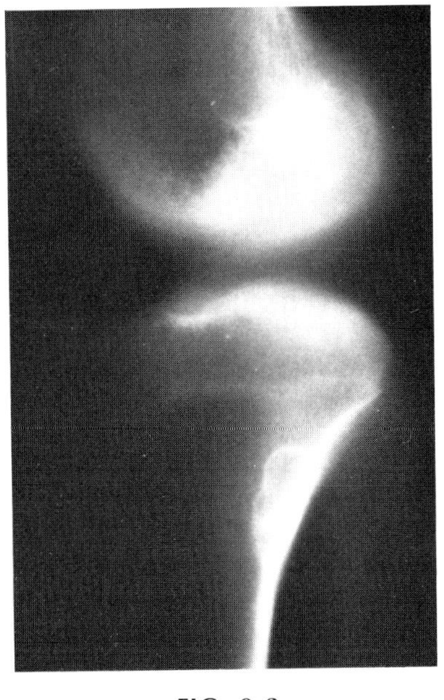
FIG. 9-3

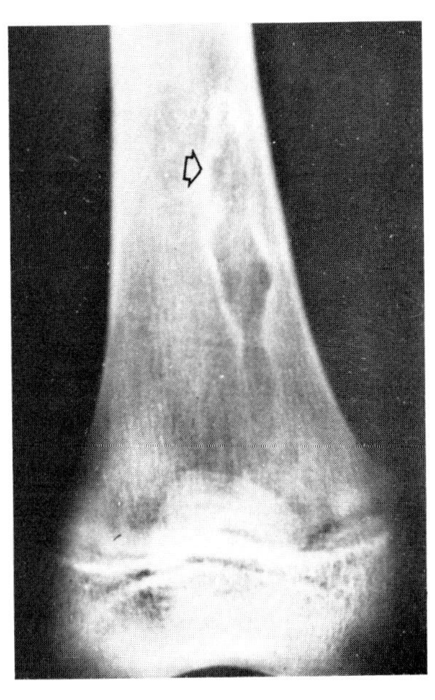
FIG. 9-4

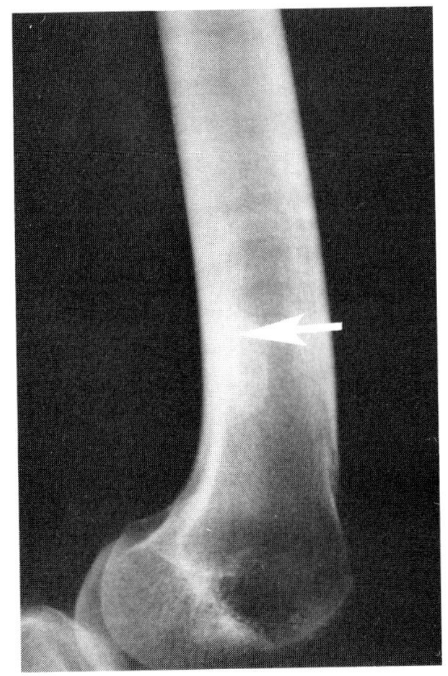
FIG. 9-5

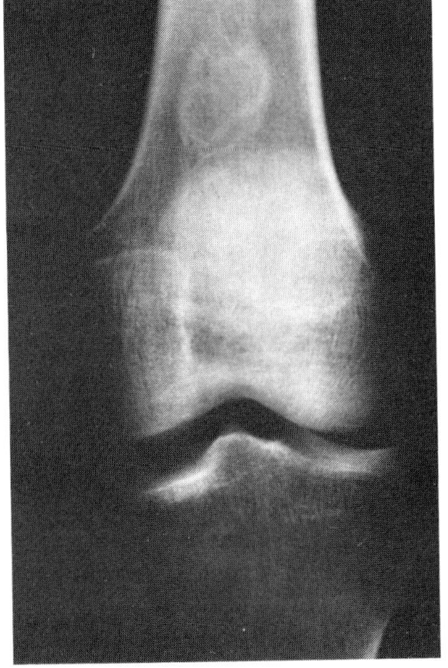
FIG. 9-6

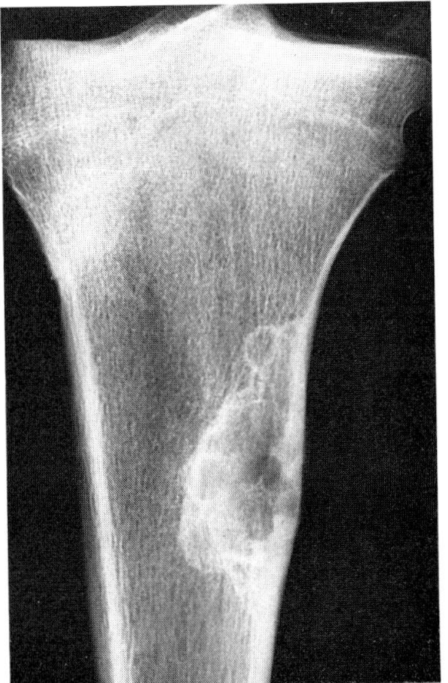
FIG. 9-7

fibroma with fibrosarcomatous transformation is, of course, controversial.

GIANT CELL TUMOR (GCT). Occasionally, nonossifying fibromas contain numerous large giant cells and may simulate a neoplastic giant cell tumor (Figs. 9-14 and 9-15). The vast majority of GCT's are epiphyseal-metaphyseal and almost always extend to the articular cartilage; the nonossifying fibroma is more clearly metaphyseal, rarely extending to articular cartilage. Patients with GCT are usually over 20, while the opposite is true of patients with nonossifying fibroma. GCT rarely has a border of host bone sclerosis. The cells of a nonossifying fibroma are generally much longer, compared to GCT. However, foci of GCT and particularly recurrent GCT may contain long, collagen-producing spindle cells. In nonossifying fibroma the long spindle cells are evenly dispersed throughout the lesions and are not as focally prominent as is the case with GCT. On rare occasions, a nonossifying fibroma could conceivably involve the epiphysis. These should be distinguished from a neoplastic GCT by the usual radiologic and histologic parameters outlined above. All patients younger than 15 years of age with an open epiphyseal plate and a presumptive diagnosis of neoplastic GCT should be reviewed carefully to rule out other lesions, such as a rare epiphyseal location of a nonossifying fibroma.

EOSINOPHILIC GRANULOMA (EG). The late healing phases of EG may be characterized by dense fibrous tissue and an abundance of foam cells similar to those seen in nonossifying fibroma. These late lesions tend to be in older patients and those lesions that are symptomatic are usually multiple, compared to the usual solitary nature of the nonossifying fibroma. The fibrosis seen in the late or healing phase of eosinophilic granuloma is closer to dense, bland, scar tissue than the fibrosarcoma-like cellularity of nonossifying fibroma. Nonossifying fibroma, on radiograph, tends to be metaphyseal and eccentric. EG lesions are diaphyseal or metaphyseal and generally are not placed as eccentrically. The presence of residual eosinophils or the typical granular, basophilic histiocytes common to the early phases of EG are extremely helpful to differentiation.

DESMOID TUMOR (DESMOPLASTIC FIBROMA). In the regressive stages of nonossifying fibroma the degree and thickness of collagen may approach that of desmoid tumors (p. 270 and Figs. 9-27-9-30). However, nonossifying fibroma is distinguishable by the presence of border of sclerosis on radiograph and collections of foam cells and small osteoclast giant cells that are not found in the desmoid tumor.

FIBROUS DYSPLASIA. The fibrous stroma is usually much less exuberant appearing than the NOF. Giant cells are usually focally and not evenly dispersed. The woven bone seen in fibrous dysplasia is not rimmed by osteoblasts.

Nonossifying Fibroma

FIG. 9-8. Although this lesion is quite extensive, the features of eccentricity, multiloculated "soap bubble" appearance, and thin but unequivocal border of benign bone sclerosis are characteristic of the nonossifying fibroma.

FIG. 9-9. On rare occasions, the nonossifying fibroma may attain huge size and even mimic a malignant tumor by radiographic analysis alone. The lesion in the midshaft of this 16-year-old male is lytic and loculated. A pathologic fracture is present in the midshaft (*arrow*). A biopsy showed an exuberant fibroblastic tissue that in some foci contained prominent osteoclastic giant cells. (The histology of the case shown in Figs. 9-14 and 9-15.) Our diagnosis was exuberant, nonossifying fibroma with unusually prominent giant cells. One consultant felt this lesion was a fibrosarcoma with giant cells. Nevertheless, the consensus was that it was benign and the lesion was curetted and packed with bone chips. The patient was then followed closely.

FIG. 9-10. Six months later the radiograph shows good repair of the fracture site; the borders of the curetted lesion show host bone sclerosis rather than continued advance of the tumor, and there is no ominous periosteal new bone or soft-tissue mass. The patient has now been followed for 7 years. The gradual healing of the fracture site supports the diagnosis of a benign but unusually large example of a nonossifying fibroma.

FIG. 9-11. On low-power examination, the nonossifying fibroma or fibrous cortical defect is characterized by interlacing sworls of long, spindly cells. The pattern is highly reminiscent of the "cartwheel" and "storiform" patterns described for tumors of histiocytic origin. The osteoclast-like giant cells are inconspicuous at this power (x125).

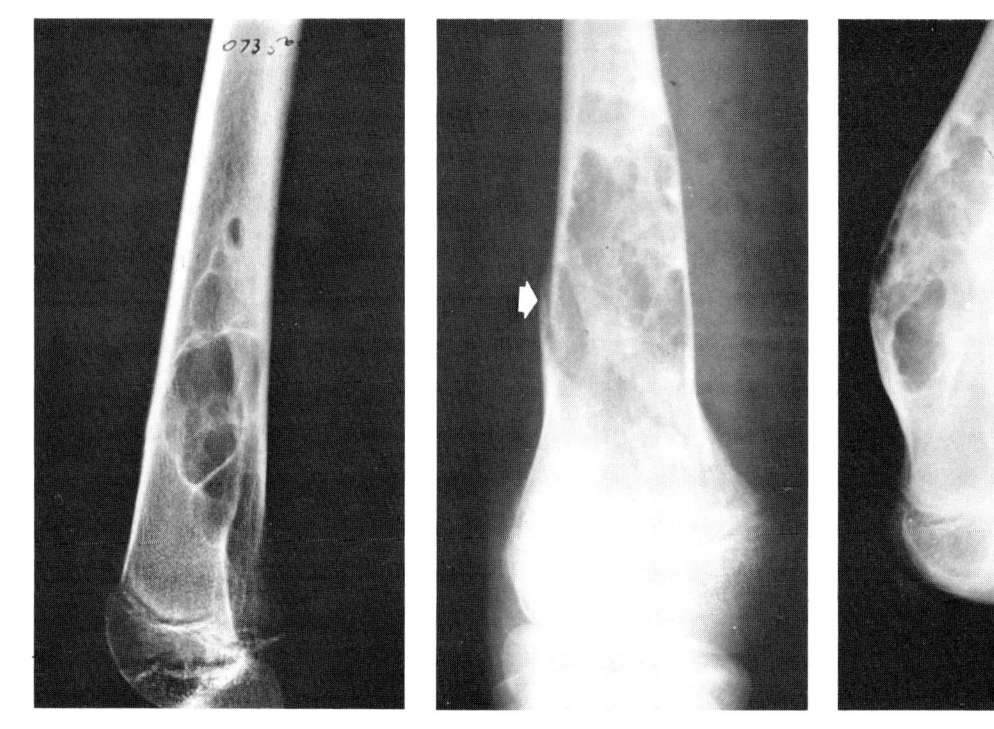

FIG. 9-8

FIG. 9-9

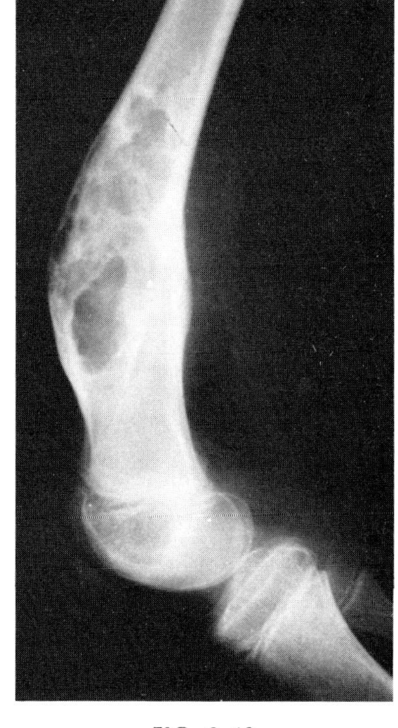

FIG. 9-10

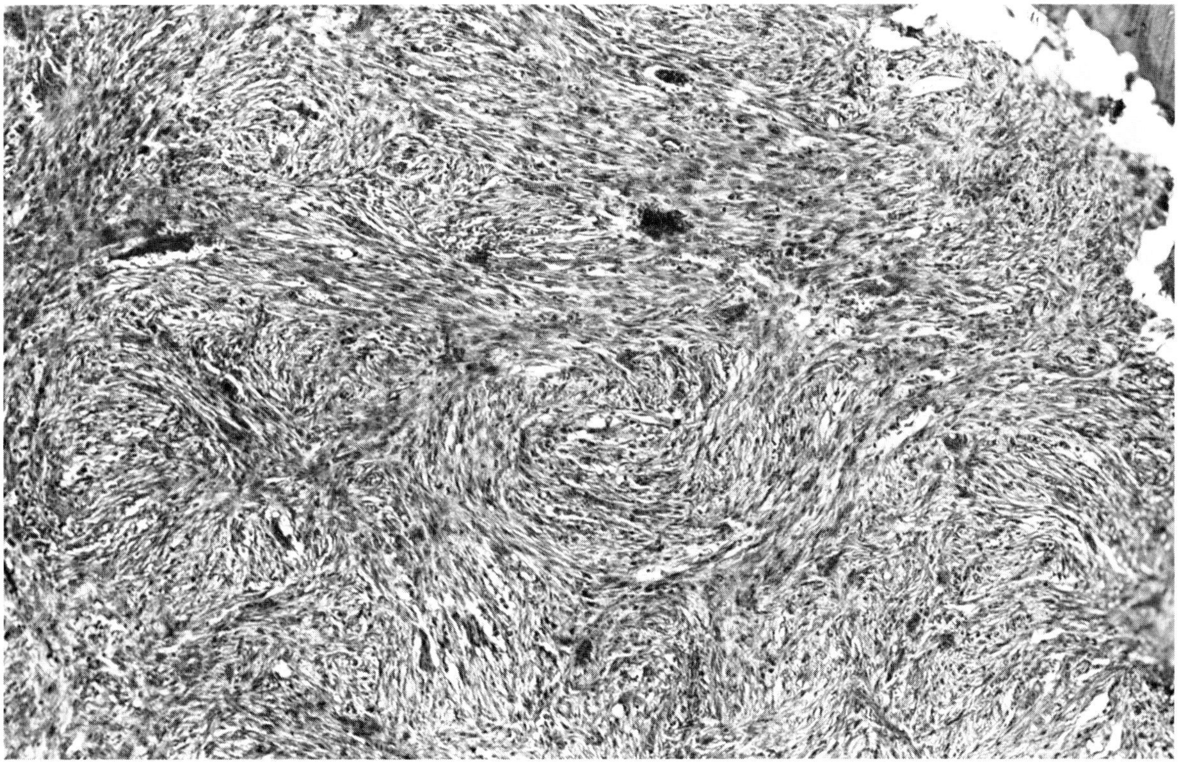

FIG. 9-11

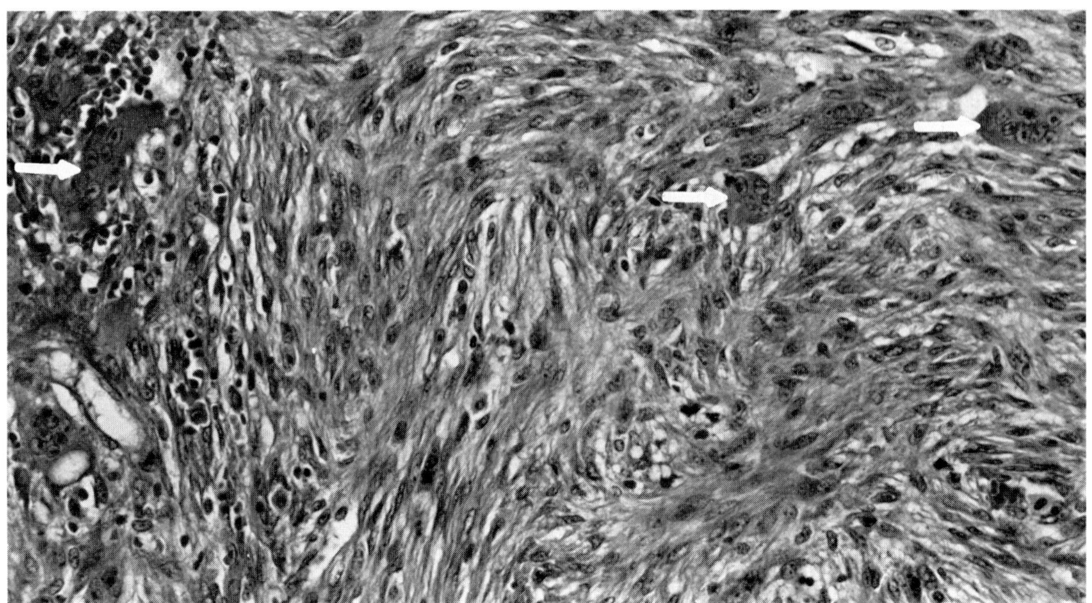

FIG. 9-12

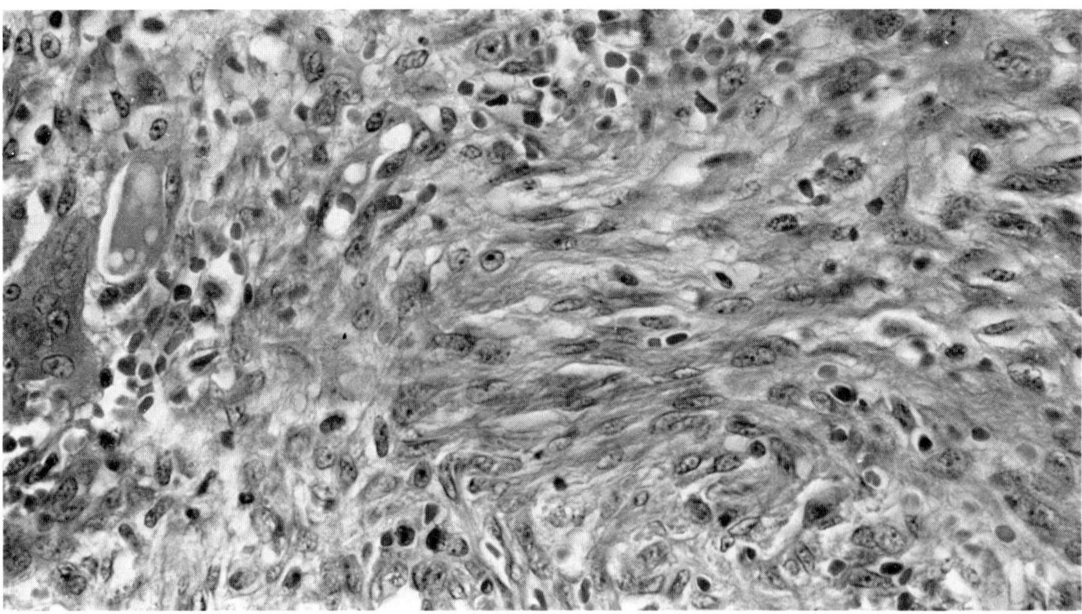

FIG. 9-13

Nonossifying Fibroma

FIG. 9-12. The nuclei of the spindle cells are quite plump and ominous appearing. The osteoclast-like giant cells (*arrows*) are fairly evenly dispersed and blend in with the stromal cells so that they may be difficult to discern at first glance. They generally contain about 3–10 nuclei per cell (x250).

FIG. 9-13. Although the nuclei of the stromal cells are plump, the chromatin is evenly dispersed and the nucleoli are single and small. Bizarre nuclear sizes and shapes and atypical mitoses are absent. Lymphocytes may sprinkle the lesion. Note the small osteoclast-like cells to the left. Figures 9–11 through 9–13 characterize the majority of the spindle and giant cell components of nonossifying fibromas and fibrous cortical defects (x400).

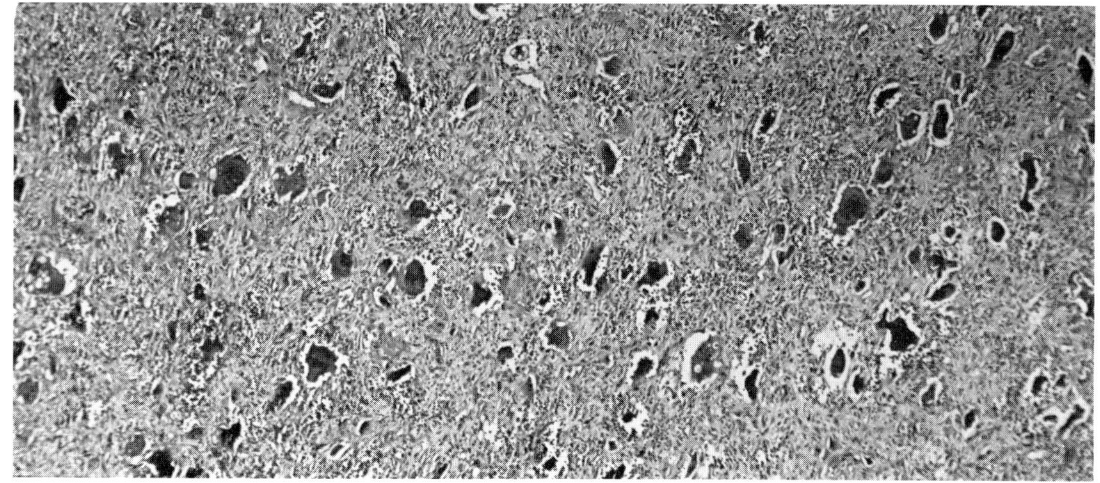

FIG. 9-14

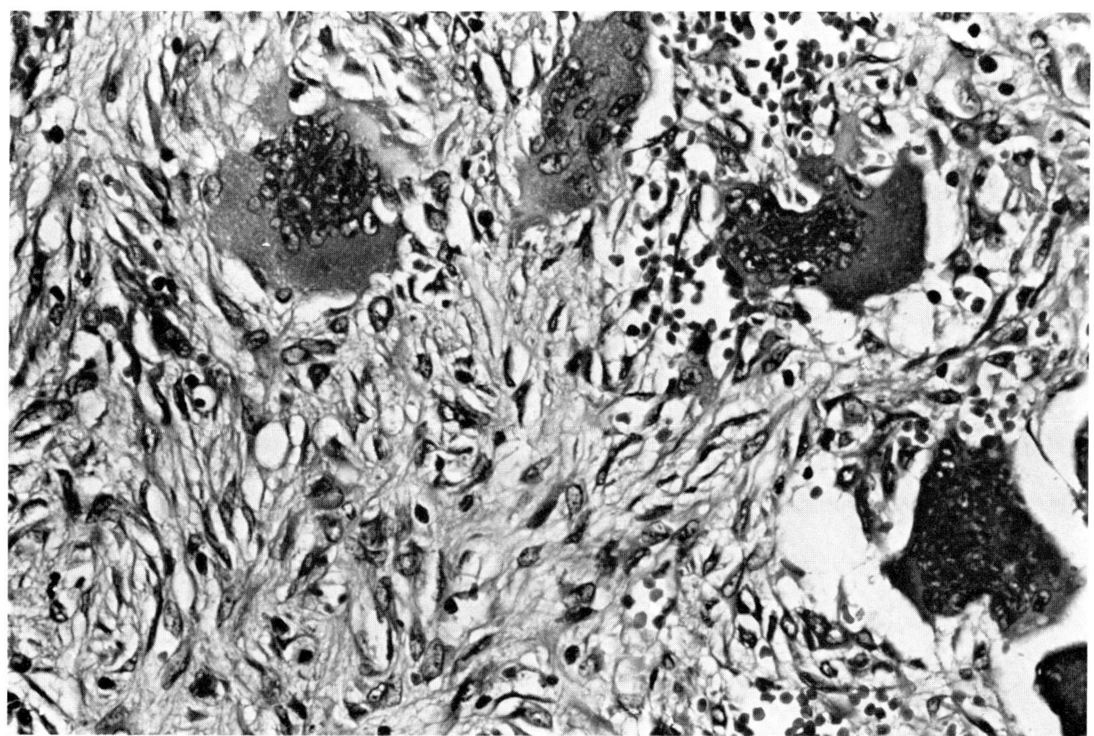

FIG. 9-15

Nonossifying Fibroma

FIG. 9-14. In this unusual example that corresponds to the patient radiographs shown in Figures 9-9 and 9-10, the giant cells stand out much more prominently on low power compared to the usual NOF (x40).

FIG. 9-15. The osteoclasts of the previous case shown contained 20-50 nuclei per cell. These cells stood out much more distinctly from the surrounding stroma than usual. The stroma cells consisted of spindly cells with plump but regular nuclei. The stroma contained abundant collagen. Mitotic figures were typical and rare. Also note the abundant extravasation of erythrocytes, a common finding in NOF. Hemosiderin may be abundant in mononuclear histiocytes and even in the giant cells (x250).

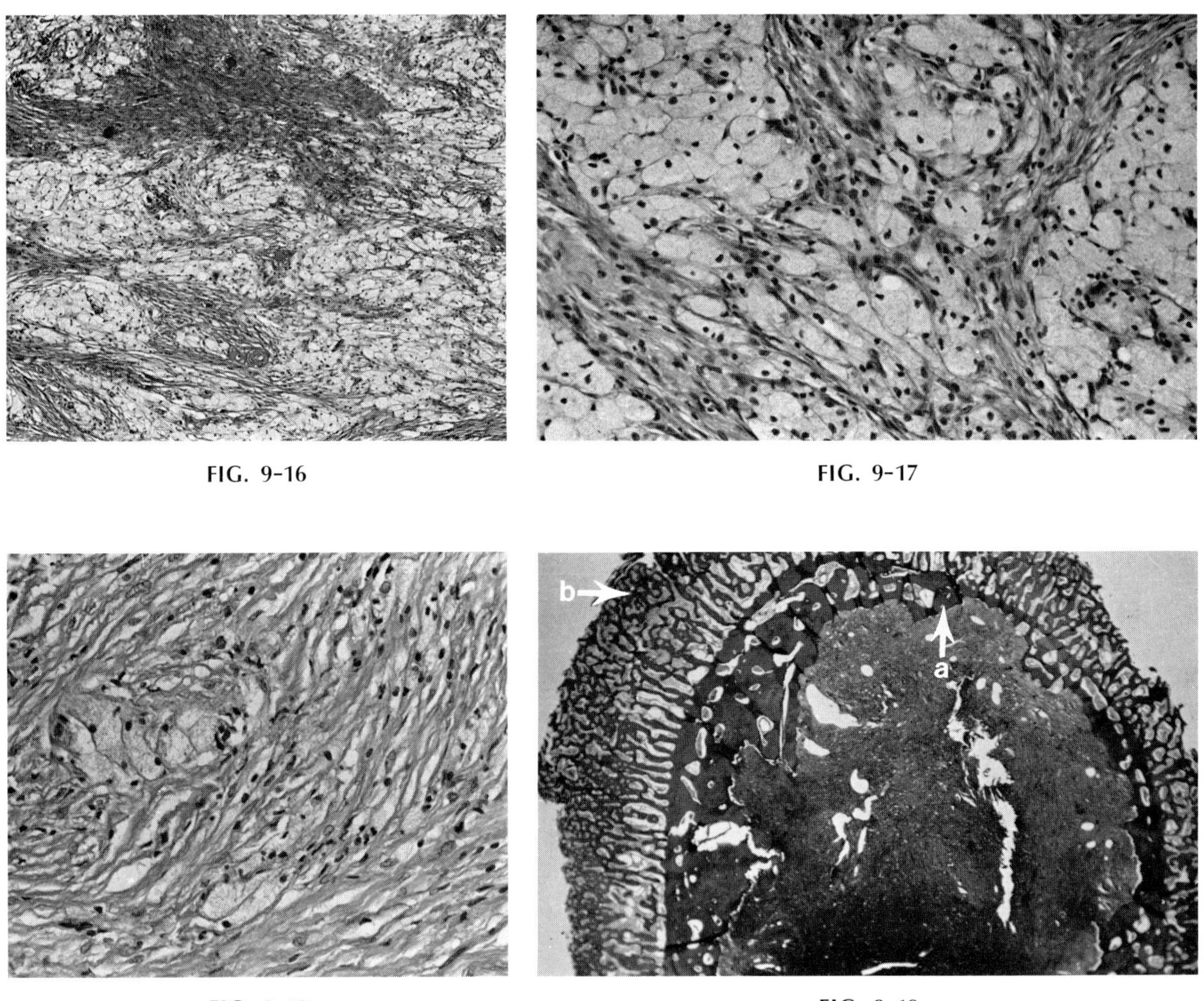

FIG. 9-16

FIG. 9-17

FIG. 9-18

FIG. 9-19

Nonossifying Fibroma

FIG. 9-16. Masses of lipidic macrophage-like cells replace the stroma in the healing phases of the process (x125).

FIG. 9-17. The clusters of foam cells almost seem to arise by lipid deposition within the fibrous stromal cells themselves (x250).

FIG. 9-18. In the very late stages of the disease, the formerly exuberant fibroblastic stroma may be replaced by dense, bland, scarlike tissue admixed with foam cells (x250).

FIG. 9-19. Low-power view of a nonossifying fibroma that has completely filled the metaphyseal region of a fibula. The lesion shows a lobular configuration in relation to the cortical bone (*a*). The peculiar radial bone (*b*) surrounding the cortex represents periosteal new bone, which was induced by pathologic fracture (x10).

FIG. 9-20. In time, these lesions eventually become replaced by host bone, which enters the lesion from its margin (*arrows*) and from there, to reach its center (x40).

FIG. 9-21. Unlike fibrous dysplasia, however, this host bone reparative tissue generally shows prominent osteoblastic rimming, particularly along the outermost margin of the tumor (*arrows*) (x125).

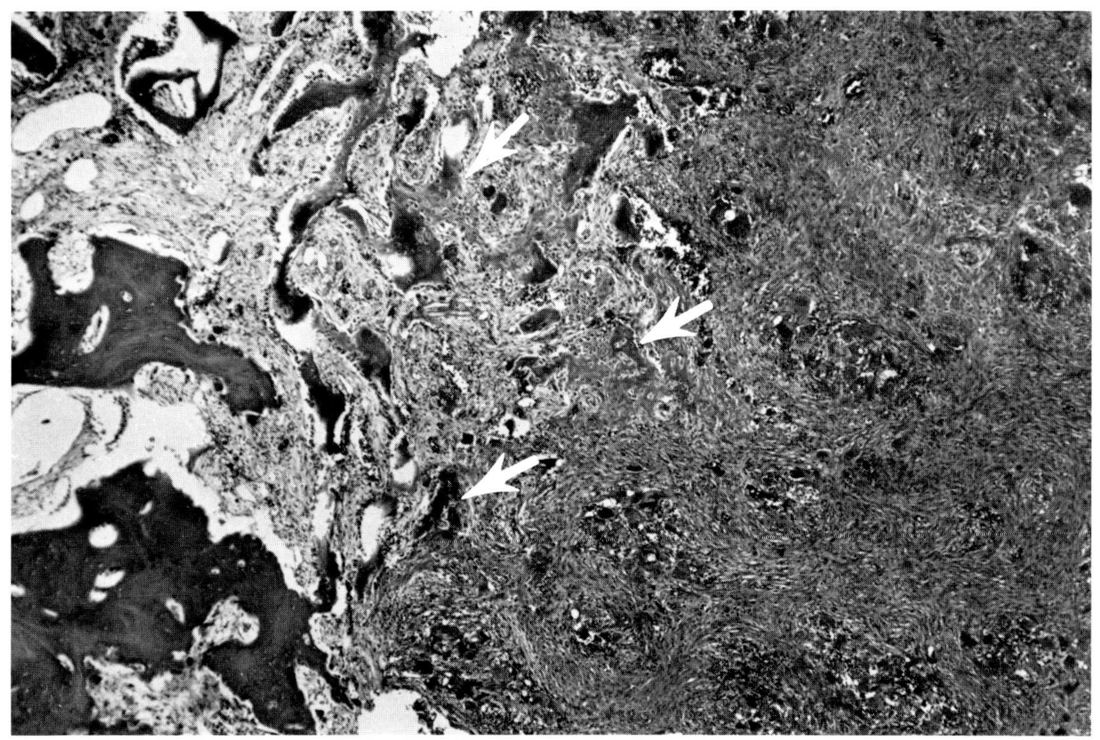

FIG. 9-20

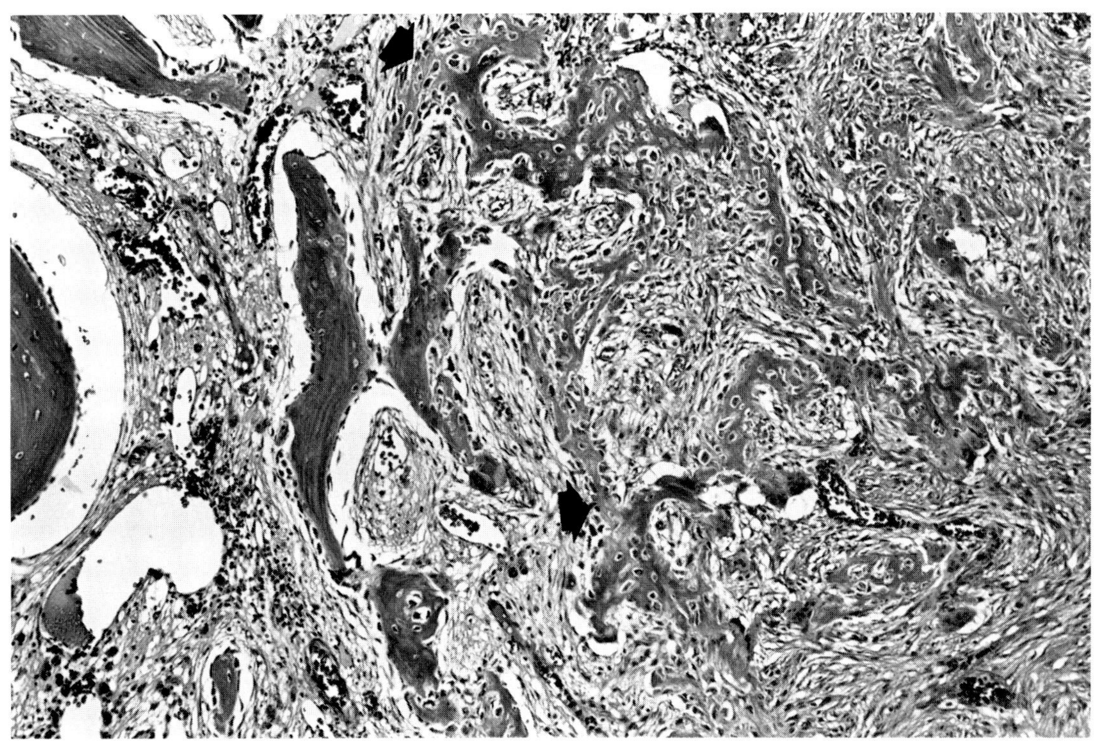

FIG. 9-21

Desmoplastic Fibroma or Desmoid Tumor

Definition

The desmoplastic fibroma is a rare tumor of bone. It may present as an intramedullary or periosteal tumor. Its histological characteristics are essentially identical to the extraosseous desmoid tumor (aggressive fibromatosis).

Clinical Features

AGE. Range is from 8 to 71 years. Approximately 70 per cent below the age of 30.

SYMPTOMS. They include aching pain, painless swelling, and occasionally pathologic fracture.

Radiologic Features

A number of desmoplastic fibromas appear to arise from within the periosteum. From my own collection of four cases, three began as intraperiosteal lesions and only one appeared as a purely intraosseous tumor. The periosteal form is discussed in Chapter 14 (p. 570). These intraosseous desmoids should be distinguished from their soft-tissue counterparts, which may be capable of invading the bone. These latter cases are usually distinguished by the development of a soft-tissue mass first and secondarily by concave cortical erosion and intraosseous invasion. This is particularly prone to occur in areas of soft tissue with tight compartments in close apposition to bone, as, for example, in the regions of the foot, ankle, wrist, forearm (radioulnar compartment), or leg (tibiofibular compartment).

The radiographic features of an intraosseous desmoplastic fibroma are those of a large (over 5 cm.), aggressive-looking, fuzzy to trabeculated lytic lesion with endosteal erosion and cortical expansion (Figs. 9–22 and 9–24). Not infrequently there is associated pathologic fracture. The zone of transition may not be sharp, simulating a fibrosarcoma. Sclerotic reaction around the lesional margins may suggest a form of fibrous dysplasia. On rare occasions the bone may be extremely expanded and resemble a metastasis from a renal cell, thyroid carcinoma, or an aneurysmal bone cyst. Most lesions are metaphyseal and extend into the diaphysis or epiphysis. Some lesions are purely diaphyseal.

Gross Pathology

Upon sectioning those cases removed by en-bloc resection or amputation, the tumor is, because of its rich collagen network, dense, firm, white, and whorled (Fig. 9–26). The margins of the lesion are much rounder and more lobulated (Figs. 9–25 and 9–26) than might be expected on the basis of an analysis of the radiographic features. The mixture of tumor and host bone reactivity at the advancing margins of the lesion probably accounts for its apparent poor delineation or fibrosarcoma-like appearance on radiograph. The more aggressive or recurrent desmoplastic fibromas may totally erode the cortex and present in the soft tissues (Figs. 9–25 and 9–27).

Histopathology

The lesion is characterized by a monotonous arrangement of dense collagen and moderate to low fibroblastic cellularity (Fig. 9–28). The collagen bundles are wavy and may be 10 microns or more in diameter (Figs. 9–28, 9–29, and 9–30, Plate 7, *G*). The nuclei are oval to flattened and contain an even dispersal of fine chromatin. Mitoses are typical and rare (usually no more than one per 20 high-power fields).

Giant cells, bone, and cartilage formation are absent. Cartilage, if present, must be explained either on the basis of fracture callus or another tumor, such as an osteogenic sarcoma.

Differential Diagnosis

FIBROSARCOMA. Refer to Figures 9–30, 9–36, 9–37 and 9–39 for the distinctly different and anaplastic features that characterize the Grade II and III fibrosarcomas. Patients with fibrosarcoma are usually in an older age group than those with desmoplastic fibroma. The Grade I fibrosarcoma is usually discernable from the desmoplastic fibroma by the presence of occasional larger nuclei with ominous chromatin clumping, greater cellularity, evidence of greater mitotic activity, and thin rather than thick collagen bundles (Fig. 9–30). However, from experience with extremely low-grade fibrosarcomas of soft tissues, differentiation from a desmoid tumor may be extremely difficult on occasion. A desmoid tumor may rarely transform into a higher-grade fibrosarcoma or represent, from its inception, a desmoid-like fibrosarcoma with metastatic potential. At the present time it may not always be possible to distinguish a "desmoid" tumor from an innocuous-appearing fi-

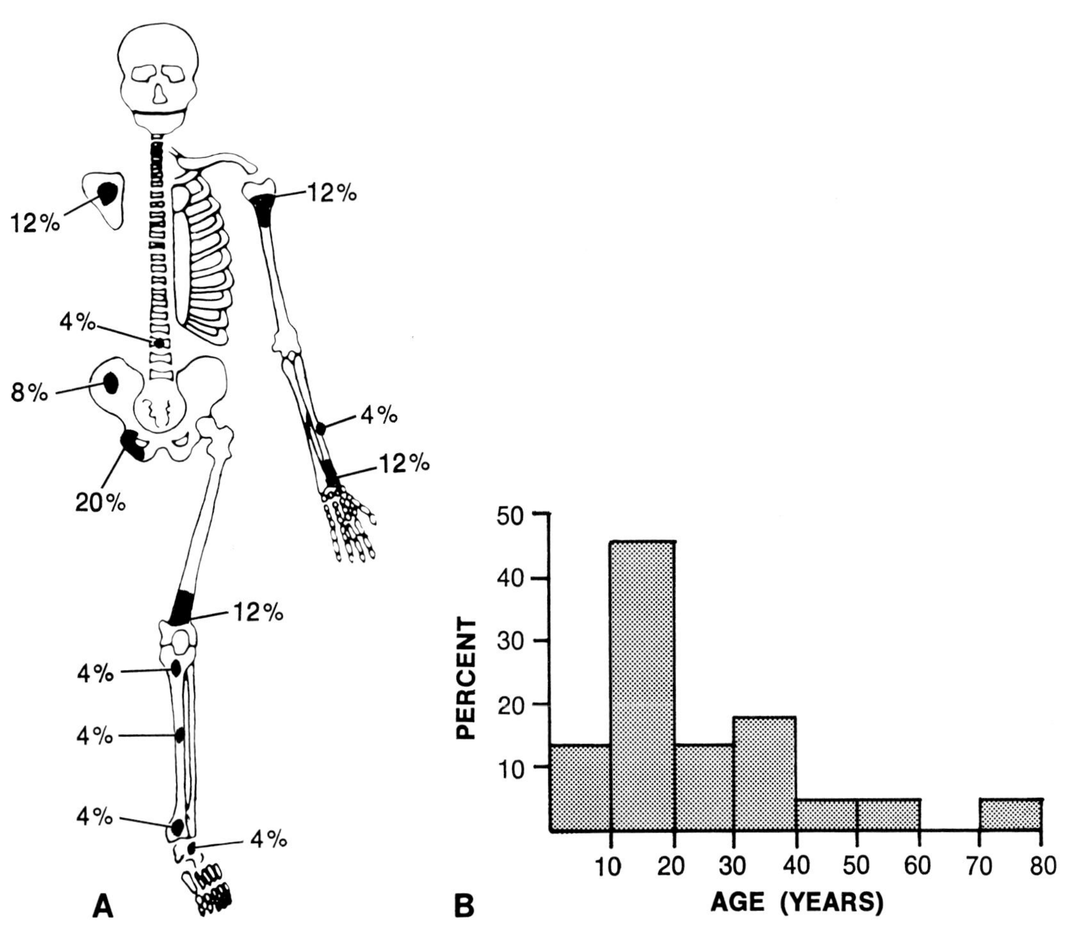

FIG. 9-23. (*A*) Desmoplastic fibroma of bone. Frequency of areas of involvement in 25 patients. Female: male incidence, 1.7:1 (*B*) Age distribution of patients with desmoplastic fibroma of bone.

brosarcoma. Fortunately, this circumstance is very rare.

MALIGNANT FIBROUS HISTIOCYTOMA (MFH). On occasion the bulk of the tissue of a MFH may appear scarlike and resemble a desmoplastic fibroma. Desmoids, however, do not contain prominent storiform patterns or areas of rounded, polygonal cells with prominent cytoplasm and large multiple nuclei. These latter areas may be but a small proportion of the MFH but are almost always present if sufficient tissue is examined. The scarlike MFH areas show a more diffuse homogeniety of the collagen and usually lack the prominent thick bundles common to all desmoplastic fibromas.

THE CORTICAL IRREGULARITY SYNDROME (PERIOSTEAL DESMOID). The so-called periosteal desmoid is not a desmoid tumor at all. It represents a ligamentous or tendinous avulsion leading to the formation of fibrous or fibro-osseous repair tissues. It occurs most commonly on the posterior aspect of the femur of children. The lesion may be bilaterally symmetrical. It can be mistaken for fibrosarcoma, osteosarcoma, chondrosarcoma, or true desmoids. This entity is treated in depth in Chapter 14. (See p. 564 and Figs. 14–74–14–77).

NONOSSIFYING FIBROMA. This benign lesion is easily distinguished by its border of sclerosis on radiograph, dark tan to yellow color, and intense fibroblastic proliferation admixed with small, multinucleate osteoclast-like giant cells. Foam cells may be seen; these are absent in desmoplastic fibroma.

FIBROUS DYSPLASIA. Occasionally fibrous dysplasia may present with a predominance of very bland fibrous tissue. The collagen bundles are not as thick as those of desmoids. Search of enough fields will demonstrate the characteristic foci of fibro-osseous metaplasia (Figs. 7–53 and 7–57).

Course and Treatment

Of the 25 cases of intraosseous desmoplastic fibromas reported, only two patients had one or more recurrences. Jaffe[19] reported one patient with multiple recurrences over a 6-year period. Hardy, *et. al.*,[18] reported one case with recurrence 4 years after initial treatment. The lesion broke out of the bone and involved the ulnar artery. For this reason an amputation was performed. Of the four cases in this author's collection, two were characterized by stubborn recurrences. One was a periosteal tumor of the radius, which was unfortunately treated by amputation (Figs. 14–86–14–88), the other was a tumor of the distal femur that recurred extensively. Pathologic fracture and pseudomonas infection prompted amputation (Figs. 9–22–9–29).

Because of the meager number of cases reported and the variability of their clinical course, it is not possible at this time to accurately classify the desmoplastic fibroma as a benign versus an extremely low-grade malignant neoplasm. In this author's experience and from that of the literature a certain percentage ranging from 10 per cent (literature) to 50 per cent (personal experience) behave similarly to extra-abdominal desmoids; that is, as a low-grade, aggressive nonmetastasizing neoplasm. Unfortunately, it does not appear to be possible at this time to predict which will behave in a totally innocent fashion and which with local aggressiveness.

Perhaps it is justifiable to treat the desmoplastic fibroma by extensive curettage or cryosurgery as the initial procedure. However, if the tumor recurs, either more extensive cryosurgery or en-bloc excision should be the procedure of choice. Amputation is to be avoided, because true desmoids are reported as

(*Text continues on p. 275.*)

Desmoid Tumor (Demoplastic Fibroma)

FIG. 9-22. The intraosseous desmoid tumor is characteristically large and lytic. It may be fuzzy to trabeculated in appearance and may cause endosteal erosion and slow cortical "expansion" because of the deposition of a periosteal collar of new bone. This patient was a middle-aged adult male.

FIG. 9-24. The "expansion" and trabeculated appearance is more obvious from this lateral view.

FIG. 9-25. The lesion was curetted and packed with bone chips after being diagnosed as a benign fibroma. However, it recurred and was associated with a life-threatening severe pseudomomas infection and pathologic fracturing, which prompted amputation. A 3-mm. cut of the femur shows a remnant of the firm white tumor that is eroding the cortex posteriorly (*arrow*).

FIG. 9-26. A fractured portion of the medial condyle shows residual lobulated masses of the tumor, which was firm and whitish-gray.

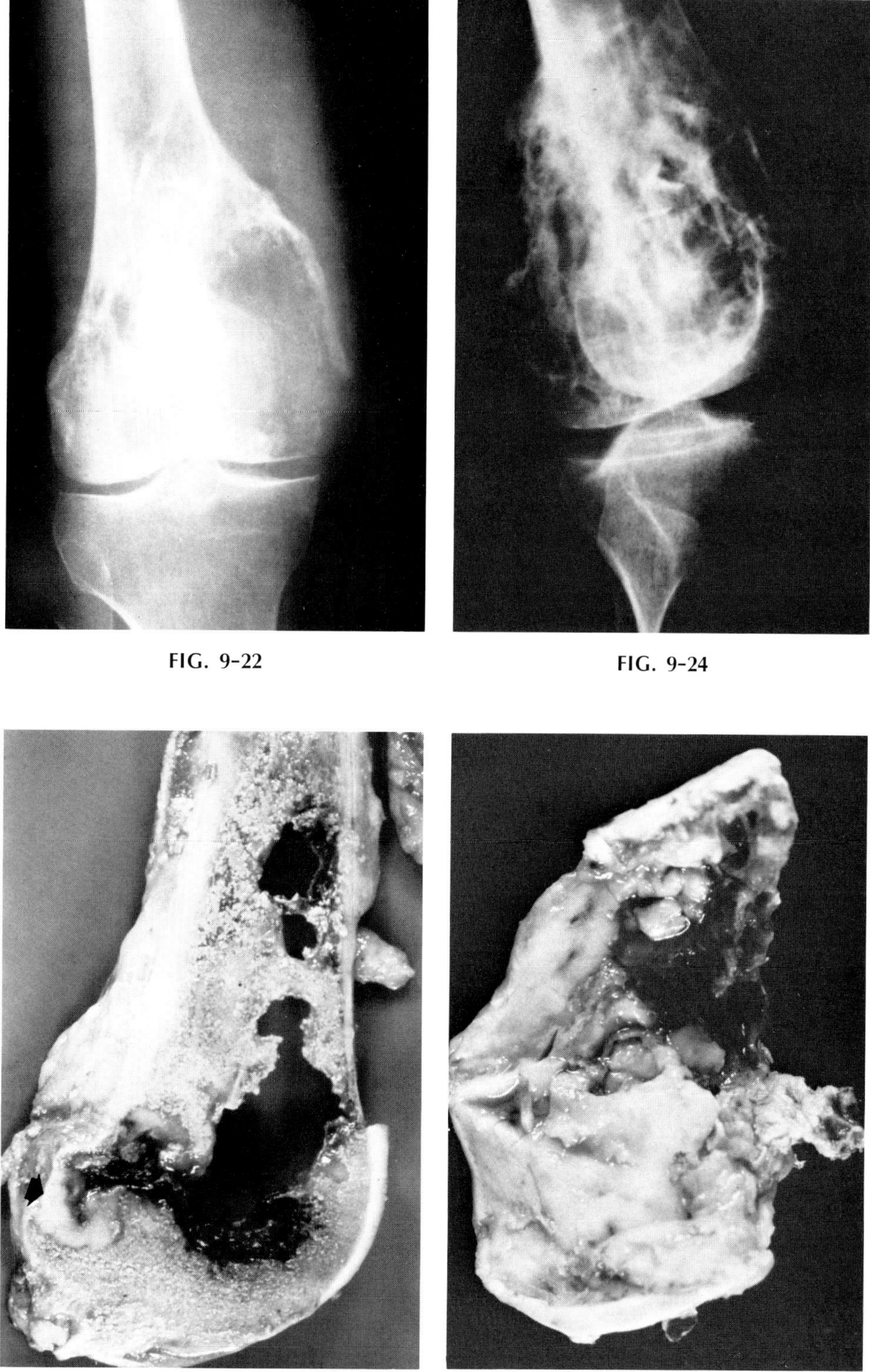

FIG. 9-22

FIG. 9-24

FIG. 9-25

FIG. 9-26

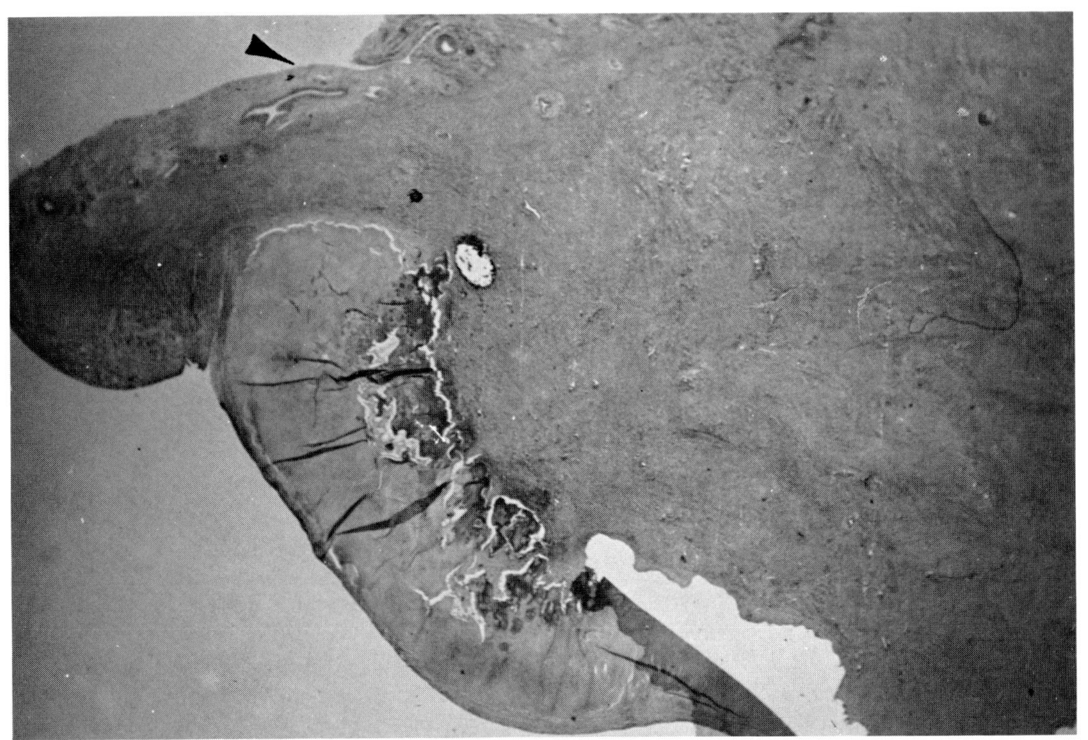

FIG. 9-27

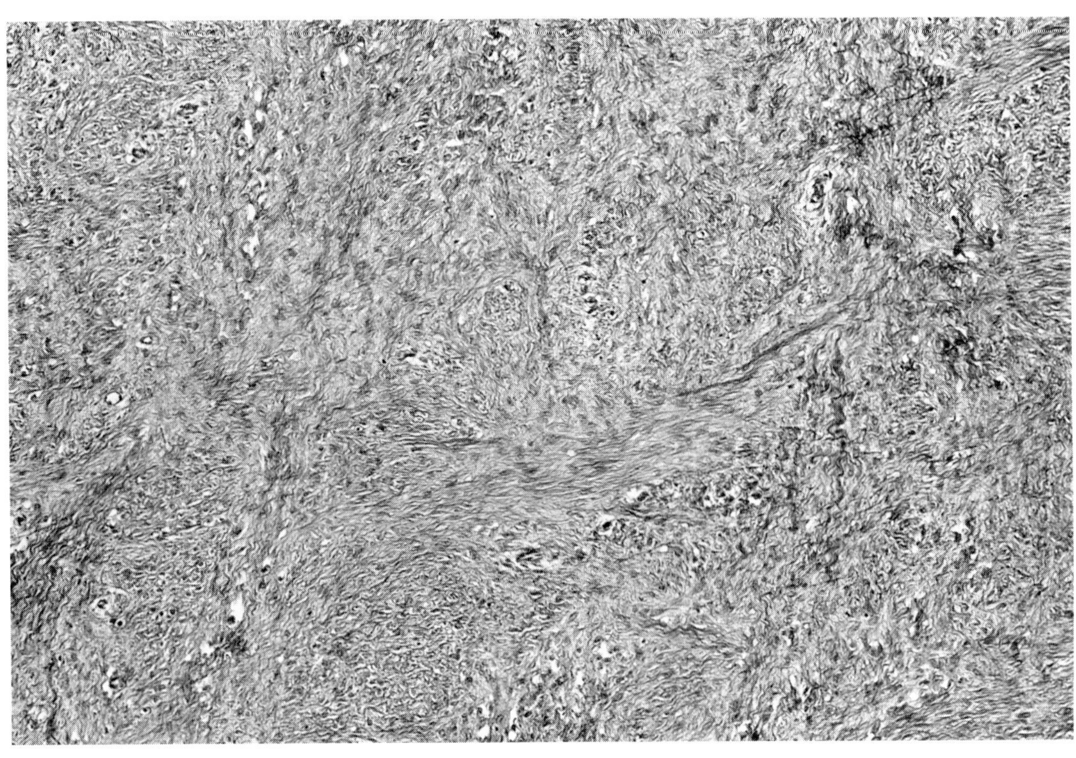

FIG. 9-28

nonmetastasizing. If a "desmoid" tumor recurs, the rate at which it occurs is important. Desmoids are slow-growing tumors. Recurrences do not become clinically obvious for 1 to 2 or more years. However, if a lesion diagnosed as a desmoid recurs as a large mass within 6 months or less, the original diagnosis must be extremely suspect. More likely the tumor is a histologically subtle fibrosarcoma.

LOW-GRADE MALIGNANCIES

Giant Cell Tumor

The giant cell tumor contains spindly cells. In some cases spindling of cells and collagen production is quite prominent, particularly in recurrent lesions. For a more complete description, refer to pages 342–348 and Figures 10–52 to 10–59.

Adamantinoma

The adamantinoma contains dense fibroblastic tissues between which are epithelial-like to carcinoma-like cells. These cells may line slitlike spaces. Adamantinoma is the prime consideration of any cystlike or bubbly tumor that arises in the tibia and/or fibula and radius and/ or ulna that has the above features (p. 440 and Figs. 12–7–12–11). About 91 per cent of adamantinomas arise in the tibia.

HIGHLY MALIGNANT NEOPLASMS

Mesenchymal Chondrosarcoma

The mesenchymal chondrosarcoma contains, in addition to anaplastic spindle cells, foci of chondrosarcomatous metaplasia and often hemangiopericytoma-like areas (p. 212 and Figs. 8–69 and 8–76; Plate 6, *D, E,* and *F*).

Osteogenic Sarcoma

Variable proportions of spindly fibrosarcoma-like areas admixed with foci of malignant bone with or without chondrosarcoma are diagnostic of the osteosarcoma (pp. 138–158 and Plates 4, *A, C, D, F,* and *G;* 5, *A* and *B*).

Fibrosarcomatous Transformation of Low-Grade Chondrosarcoma

This tumor is characterized by low-grade chondrosarcoma in apparent collision with a high-grade fibrosarcoma (p. 201 and Figs. 8–49 and 8–50).

Metastases

Metastatic carcinomas may evoke a severe desmoplastic reaction, particularly in breast carcinoma. Islands, nests, or "boxcar" configurations of malignant epithelial cells found between the dense benign collagen characterize these tumors.

Undifferentiated spindle cell carcinoma may resemble a fibrosarcoma. Most of these cases are associated with a known primary and usually, multiple metastases at initial presentation. Multiple primary fibrosarcoma is an extremely rare entity in comparison to metastatic spindle cell malignancies.

Spindle cell melanoma metastases may be very fibrosarcoma-like. Melanin pigment is usually minimal to absent. A history of a primary lesion is usually present.

Metastatic sarcomas such as leiomyosarcoma of the uterus may be confused with a primary bone fibrosarcoma. The history of a primary nonosseous sarcoma is the key to diagnosis. However, the history is not always clear-cut. For example, this author reviewed a case of a "primary" spindle cell sarcoma of the humerus of an elderly female. It was most intriguing in that the histology and special stains showed an unequivocal leiomyosarcoma. Because of

---

Desmoid Tumor

FIG. 9–27. On low-power examination, the tumor can be seen to be composed of dense fibrous tissue. The lesion obviously eroded through the cortex at the bone-cartilage junction (*arrow*) (x10).

FIG. 9–28. On low-power examination, the desmoid is composed of long, thick, interlacing bundles of collagen. Note the waviness seen in many of the collagen bundles (x125).

the extreme rarity of this tumor as a bone primary, an inquiry was made about whether there was a history of leiomyosarcoma from another primary site. It was ascertained that the patient had a uterus removed for leiomyomas 2 years previously. Review of these slides showed an area of low-grade but unequivocal mitotically active leiomyosarcoma.

HODGKIN'S DISEASE

Hodgkin's disease of bone presenting as a bone primary may be associated with considerable reactive benign fibrosis. An admixture of variable quantities of lymphocytes or plasma cells and/or eosinophils and atypical reticulum cells and Sternberg-Reed cells are the clues to diagnosis (Plate 9, *D, E,* and *F*). If these features are not recognized, then the initial diagnosis will most likely be chronic osteomyelitis or eosinophilic granuloma. The correct diagnosis will become obvious within 2 years, however.

FIBROSARCOMA OF BONE

CAPSULE SUMMARY

Incidence. Approximately 2 to 4 per cent of biopsied primary bone tumors.

Age. Very broad age distribution, from infancy to old age.

Clinical Features. Pain and/or swelling, and/or pathologic fracture. Secondary fibrosarcoma may develop in association with radiation, Paget's disease, fibrous dysplasia, and transformation of chondrosarcoma.

Radiologic Features. Low-grade anaplastic lesions are characterized by circumscription; higher grades show permeative and "moth-eaten" patterns of destruction, soft-tissue mass, and occasionally "ominous" periosteal reactions.

Histopathology. Grade I tumors show minimal anaplasia and may be confused with nonossifying fibroma or desmoid tumors. Grade II and III tumors are characterized by frank anaplasia, lesser degrees of collagen production and nonmirror image mitoses. Sprinkling of benign osteoclast-like giant cells is possible in all grades.

Course. All are potentially metastatic tumors. Survival usually correlates with the degree of anaplasia.

Treatment. Low-grade tumors amenable to en-bloc excision, if feasible. High-grade tumors require radical therapy.

Definition and Introduction

The fibrosarcoma of bone may be defined as a fibroblastic sarcoma that usually begins in the central medullary cavity of the bone and upon which exhaustive examination shows no evidence of malignant bone, cartilage, or origin from histiocytic cells. It

---

Desmoid Tumor and Fibrosarcoma

FIG. 9-29. The desmoid tumor characteristically is composed of thick, occasionally wavy bundles of collagen and regular, oval, fibroblastic nuclei. The numbers of nuclei per unit area are not high, compared to a fibrosarcoma. Nucleoli, if present, are very small and mitoses are rare. Also note the even, innocuous chromatin stippling (x400).

FIG. 9-30. This illustration compares and contrasts a desmoid tumor (*A*) to a low- to moderate-grade fibrosarcoma (*B*). The desmoid contains thick, almost glassy bundles of collagen and oval to flattened nuclei, spaced apart fairly widely. The fibrosarcoma shown here shows less prominent collagen, a great deal more variation in the sizes and shapes of one nucleus compared to another, abnormal chromatin clumping, larger, overall nuclear size, and about 2 to 3 times the numbers of nuclei per unit area. The arrow points to the most obvious malignant nucleus. (*A* and *B*, x250).

FIG. 9-31. Low-grade fibrosarcomas tend to be circumscribed, lytic masses that are not bounded by a rim of host bone sclerosis, as would be expected in benign tumors. The cortex may be eroded and the tumor bulge into the soft tissues, as in this example. This radiograph is by no means specific, because a lytic osteosarcoma would be the more probable choice. On occasion, a giant cell tumor may appear quite similar. The gross appearance of this case is shown in Plate 7, *D*.

FIG. 9-32. Most fibrosarcomas are high-grade tumors and show radiographic features similar to this example. The lesions are large, very poorly defined, and show prominent areas of lysis and moth-eaten or permeative patterns of destruction along their edges.

FIG. 9-33. Although this example of a high-grade fibrosarcoma more closely mimics, in terms of size and location, that shown in Figure 9-31, note that the edges of the lesion within the bone substance (*arrows*) show a permeative pattern of lysis. This is due to the tumor rapidly infiltrating through the cortical haversian systems, resulting in rapid bone lysis. This pattern, when associated with a bone tumor, is usually indicative of high-grade malignancy, although similar patterns can be seen in rapidly destructive osteomyelitis. The most likely diagnoses by a radiographic reading alone for a tumor showing this pattern would be a lytic osteogenic sarcoma followed by fibrosarcoma and reticulum cell sarcoma.

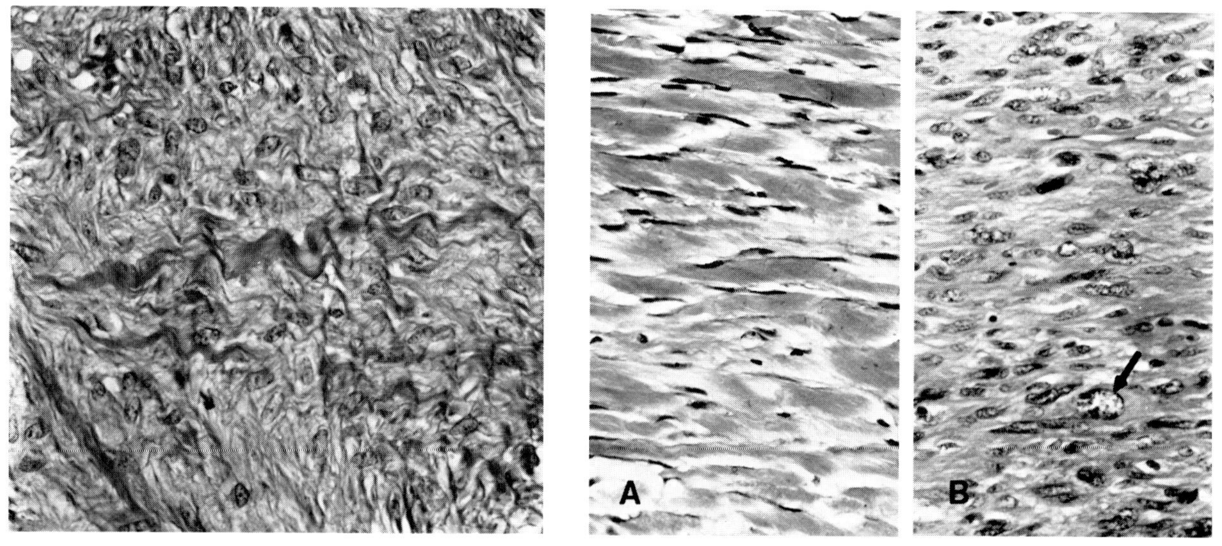

FIG. 9-29

FIG. 9-30

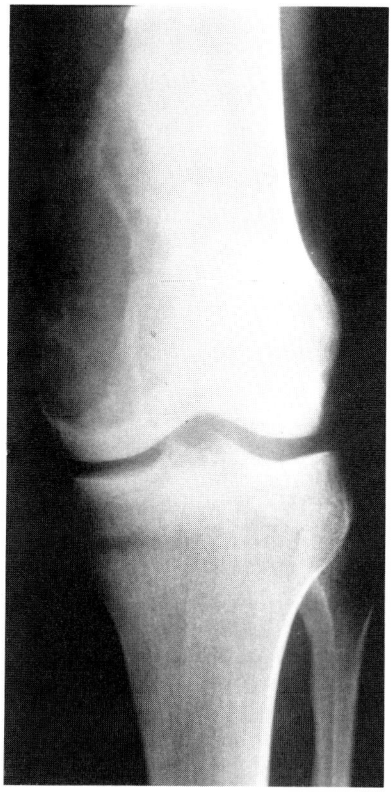

FIG. 9-31

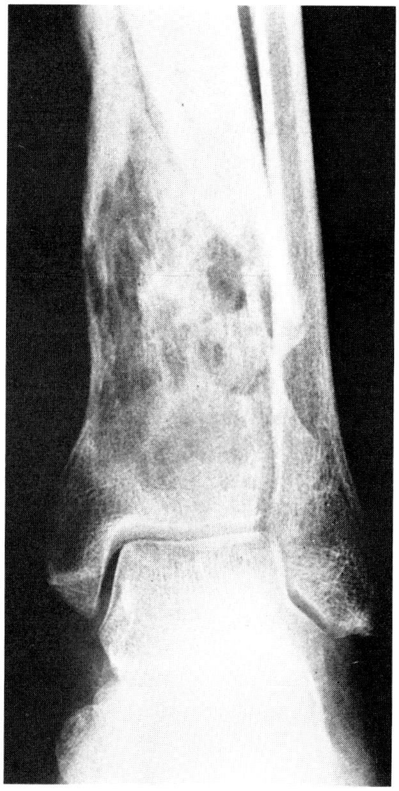

FIG. 9-32

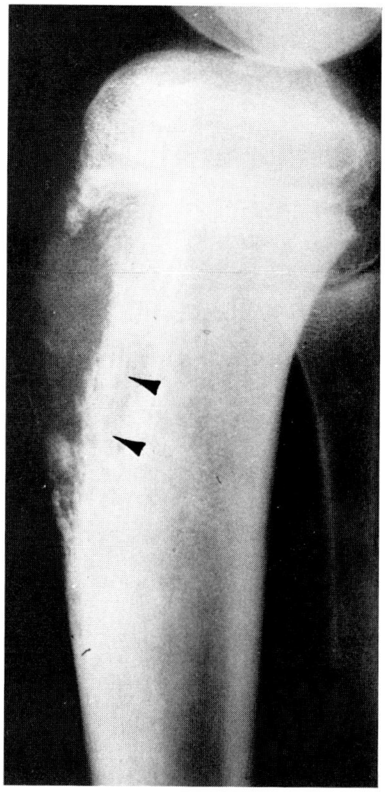

FIG. 9-33

is important to remember that the osteosarcoma not uncommonly shows predominant fibrosarcomatous patterns, yet in some areas will show unequivocal evidence of malignant bone formation. Fibrosarcoma may be either a primary or secondary tumor. Fibrosarcomatous transformation may occur in other benign or malignant tumors, such as fibrous dysplasia, post-radiation, Paget's disease, and fibrosarcomatous transformation of low-grade chondrosarcoma (p. 201 and Figs. 8–49 and 8–50). These transformations are usually associated with a very poor long-term survival.

With the recent description of the malignant fibrous histiocytoma (MFH) of bone, the fibrosarcoma appears to be slipping into oblivion. Spindle-cell sarcomas of bone with a "storiform" pattern of collagen production are being called MFH with increasing frequency. In this author's estimation this pattern alone is not pathognomonic of fibrous histiocytomas, malignant or benign. Usually a "storiform" (cartwheel) pattern of the cells and collagen is present in MFH but on occasion these tumors may present with anaplastic rounded histiocytes to the exclusion of spindling or "storiform" patterns. Unless there is evidence of large, rounded to polygonal granular to foamy, cytoplasm rich, or obviously lipid-laden anaplastic mono- and multinucleate cells, the diagnosis of MFH is extremely tenuous and perhaps not justifiable.

The vast majority of primary fibrosarcomas arise as solitary lesions of the bone. A few cases have been reported which have presented with multiple sites of bone involvement.[31,32] As a general rule, most multiple "fibrosarcomas" or multiple undifferentiated "sarcomas" of bone will usually be found to be spindle cell metastases from either a melanoma or carcinoma, particularly of the lung, kidney, or esophagus.

Clinical Features

Fibrosarcomas have been described in patients of all ages. They occur in an identical distribution and almost identical frequency as the osteogenic sarcoma (compare Fig. 9–38 with Fig. 7–72). No other two tumors of bone have such an identical distribution. For this and other reasons some authors believe the fibrosarcoma may be merely a nonosseous matrix-producing variant of an osteosarcoma arising from the same stem cell line.

As other sarcomas do, these lesions present with pain and/or swelling if the lesion has broken through the cortex and if the bone has been sufficiently weakened with pathologic fracture.

Radiologic Features

LOW-GRADE ANAPLASTIC FIBROSARCOMA. The low-grade anaplastic fibrosarcoma is usually a well-circumscribed lytic mass usually arising in the metaphysis (Fig. 9–31). It does not have a border of reactive host bone sclerosis. The cortex may be completely eroded and it may bulge into the soft tissues. Periosteal reactions are usually minimal.

HIGH-GRADE ANAPLASTIC FIBROSARCOMA. The high-grade fibrosarcomas infiltrate diffusely through the host bone trabeculae and result in "moth-eaten" margins or patterns referred to as permeative (Figs. 9–32 and 9–33). The lesion may be either confined to bone or bulge into the soft tissues (Fig. 9–33). Sunburst, hair-on end Codman's triangle periosteal reactions may be seen, mimicking a lytic osteogenic sarcoma. In general, however, the lytic osteosarcoma will have more rounded margins of growth, compared to the ragged outer margins of a high-grade fibrosarcoma. Borders of benign host bone sclerosis are, of course, absent. The tumor that may mimic the high-grade fibrosarcoma most closely, by radiographic examination, is the reticulum cell sarcoma. Both are predominantly metaphyseal, permeatively destructive lesions. The Ewing's tumor is usually diaphyseal.

Gross Pathology

Because of the presence of collagen, the fibrosarcoma is white to gray (Plate 7, *D*). The more abundant the collagen the whiter and firmer is the gross appearance. Low-grade anaplastic tumors are much firmer and whiter and more circumscribed than is the high-grade tumor. High-grade tumors invade through the marrow spaces much more rapidly than low-grade tumors and produce less collagen, accounting for the difference in the gross pattern of bone involvement and their less white color. Both low- and high-grade tumors may show small to extensive areas of necrosis, cystification, and hemorrhages (Plate 7, *D*). Numerous samples of the tumor and any suspicious areas of bone or other lesional tissue removed from the main tumor mass should be sampled to rule out Paget's disease or any other benign or malignant lesion the fibrosarcoma may have arisen from. Foci of cartilage formation may mean that the tumor arose from a chondrosarcoma with or without an associated enchondroma (p. 201 and Figs. 9–49 and 9–50) or is a mesenchymal chondrosarcoma (p. 212 and Figs. 8–69 and 8–70, Plate 6, *D*, *E*, and *F*) and does not necessarily signify that the tumor in question is a predominantly fibrosarcoma-like cartilage producing osteosarcoma. Numerous samples of the tumor are also necessary to rule out any foci of malignant osteoid or woven bone production, both of which would be diagnostic of an osteosarcoma.

Histopathology

GRADE I FIBROSARCOMA. The well-differentiated fibrosarcoma is characterized by abundant collagen and spindly fibroblasts. The collagen fibers are usually thinner when compared to those of a desmoid tumor (compare Figs. 9–30, *A* and *B*, and 9–34). The nuclei are hyperchromatic and about twice as closely packed per unit area as a desmoid. Mitoses may be infrequent. Most cases will show about one mitosis per 2 or 3 high power fields. This is greater than observed in the desmoid tumor. Numerous sections should be examined to find nuclear atypia of sufficient degree to identify anaplasia. Anaplastic fibrocytic nuclei are closely packed, quite plump, and hyperchromatic and nuclear chromatin is coarse and unevenly distributed (Figs. 9–30, *A*, and 9–35). The nucleoli may be prominent and occasional atypical mitoses can be found. The chromatin of a desmoid is evenly dispersed and prominent nucleoli and atypical mitoses are absent (Fig. 9–29). The nuclear features of a nonossifying fibroma may suggest a low-grade fibrosarcoma (Fig. 9–13). The diagnosis of a Grade I fibrosarcoma is difficult if based upon only a slide reading. The diagnosis of a Grade I fibrosarcoma, as with any Grade I neoplasm, is quite difficult because the range of cytologic atypia may overlap with those of hyperplastic or reparative lesions. All of the radiographic and clinical features must be reviewed in order to protect against error. Only in this way will it be possible to avoid confusion with a nonossifying fibroma, for example.

Unfortunately, the clinical and radiographic features of a desmoplastic fibroma may completely overlap with those of a Grade I fibrosarcoma. Figures 9–29, 9–30, 9–34, and 9–35 show the subtle but essential histologic differences between low-grade fibrosarcoma and the desmoid tumor. The low-grade fibrosarcoma and desmoid tumor are both amenable to en-bloc resection. The metastatic potential of a desmoid is virtually nil, while that of even a low-grade fibrosarcoma is not insignificant (approximately 5–15%). The metastases pursue a lethal course.

On occasion a low-grade fibrosarcoma may show a diffuse distribution of osteoclast-like giant cells closely mimicking a nonossifying fibroma or GCT. The entity of giant cell rich fibrosarcoma has been treated in a separate section (see pp. 351 and 364 and Figs. 10–73, 10–75, 10–79, and 10–80).

GRADE II TO III FIBROSARCOMA. These lesions are characterized by objective anaplasia. Their nuclei are very plump and irregular in shape, the chromatin distribution is quite clumped, and large nucleoli and atypical mitoses are easily found (Figs. 9–36, 9–37, and 9–39). The lesion is two to three times as cellular as a desmoid and the collagen fibers are usually quite thin to inconspicuous. The spindly quality of the cells is maintained, though in severe degrees of anaplasia the cells may become more polygonal. Occasional cells with extremely large hyperchromatic nuclei are present (Fig. 9–37, *arrow*). Multilobulation of nuclei is occasionally seen. Foamy cells, evidence of pigment production, and numerous multinucleate and multilobulated anaplastic giant cells are not seen in fibrosarcoma and would be more indicative of a malignant fibrous histiocytoma (see Figs. 9–50–9–56) or osteoclastic sarcoma (p. 356 and Figs. 10–64–10–70).

Either low-grade or higher-grade fibrosarcomas may show foci where cells veer off in a "cartwheel" or "storiform" pattern resembling the pattern seen in malignant fibrous histiocytoma. However, the fibrosarcoma will show none of the other features diagnostic of the MFH. The storiform pattern may be particularly identifiable in patients with fibrosarcoma complicating Paget's disease (Fig. 9–40).

As with low-grade fibrosarcomas, high-grade anaplastic fibrosarcomas may be infiltrated by small to large numbers of benign osteoclast-like giant cells (see Figs. 10–73, 10–79, and 10–80), the essential difference being the grade of anaplasia of the non-osteoclastic stromal cells. These tumors can be mistaken for so-called "malignant giant cell tumors," when in actuality they are high-grade fibrosarcomas permeated by benign osteoclasts (p. 364 and Figs. 10–73, 10–74, and 10–76–10–80).

The fibrosarcoma is one of the most treacherous tumors to predict behavior of an individual case based upon the degree of anaplasia. On rare occasions an extremely innocent looking Grade I fibrosarcoma that may not even be diagnosed as a malignancy on its initial biopsy can result in multiple systemic metastases in fewer than 2 years. Many sections should be prepared to rule out foci of higher-grade anaplasia. The patient should be treated based upon the highest degree of anaplasia encountered from examination of as much tissue as possible.

Most of the fibrosarcomas of bone are Grade II to III tumors (Fig. 9–38). They outnumber the subtle Grade I tumors by more than 5 to 1 (personal observations).

Secondary Fibrosarcoma

Fibrosarcomas of bone have been reported to occur in other precursor lesions, such as fibrous dysplasia, post-irradiation, Paget's disease, chondrosarcoma, osteomyelitis, and bone infarcts. High-dosage irradiation for giant cell tumor is particularly prone to fibrosarcomatous transformation. Fibrosarcomatous transformation is rarely seen before 7 years from inception of the benign processes from which they stem. Most occur after 10 or more years.

Secondary fibrosarcomas are usually virulent lesions no matter how low-grade anaplastic the bulk of the tumor may appear. In general, however, these tumors show Grade II to III anaplasia.

Differential Diagnosis

NONOSSIFYING FIBROMA. This benign lesion is usually much smaller than fibrosarcoma. Except in the early, rapid growth phases it is surrounded by a border of benign host bone sclerosis. The patients are younger than the majority of these with fibrosarcoma. The lesion is diffusely sprinkled with osteoclast-like giant cells and often some areas have foamy histiocytes. Although exuberant, plump nuclei are the rule, atypical mitoses are not seen. Fibrosarcomas may, on occasion, contain a sprinkling of osteoclast-like giant cells; therefore, distinguishing it from a NOF may not be a simple task based on only a slide reading. The radiological features and experience with the general histologic range of nonossifying fibroma and fibrosarcoma are essential to differentiation.

GIANT CELL TUMOR. The GCT with prominent, spindly, stromal cells and fibrosis may be difficult to distinguish from a low-grade fibrosarcoma admixed with osteoclasts (p. 344 and Figs. 10–71–10–78). The GCT is usually a lesion of the bone ends, the fibrosarcoma, rarely so. The GCT stromal cells may contain exuberant nuclei but lack bizarre nuclei, markedly abnormal chromatin clumping patterns, or atypical mitoses. Examples of the bizarrely enlarged nuclei that may be seen in fibrosarcoma but which do not exist in GCT are shown in Figure 9–37, (*arrow*).

DESMOID TUMOR. The desmoid tumor is a rare primary bone tumor. From the over 1,000 bone tumors I have seen, four were desmoplastic fibromas (0.4 per cent). Fibrosarcomas outnumbered desmoids by approximately 5 to 1. However, Grade I fibrosarcomas were almost as rare as the desmoplastic fibroma. Since the desmoplastic fibroma does not have metastatic potential, the distinction from a Grade I fibrosarcoma is important. The differential features are treated on pages 270–275 and Figures 9–28, 9–29, 9–30, 9–34, and 9–35.

FIBROSARCOMATOUS DEDIFFERENTIATION OF CHONDROSARCOMA. This tumor must be associated with an associated focus of chondrosarcoma (see p. 201 and Figs. 8–49 and 8–50).

OSTEOGENIC SARCOMA. Extensive sampling of every "fibrosarcoma" is necessary to rule out malignant osteoid or bone that defines the osteosarcoma. In problem cases, unfixed tumor tissue may be examined for alkaline phosphatase activity. Alkaline phosphatase activity is reported to be negative for fibrosarcoma and positive for osteosarcoma.[24a]

MALIGNANT FIBROUS HISTIOCYTOMA. (See p. 284 and Figs. 9–50 to 9–56). In essence the malignant fibrous histiocytoma usually contains some foci of rounded or polygonal cells with a granular to foamy, lipid-rich cytoplasm and evidence of phagocytosis (pigments, engulfed cells, *etc.*). The fibrosarcoma lacks these cells and is fat negative. A storiform pattern may be seen in both tumors, but is much more often seen in the MFH.

MESENCHYMAL CHONDROSARCOMA. This contains a mixture of fibrosarcoma-like tissues admixed with

(*Text continues on p. 284.*)

Fibrosarcoma

FIG. 9–34. Portions of low-grade fibrosarcomas may very closely resemble a desmoid tumor. This field shows fairly thick collagen bundles and flattened nuclei. These probably represent artifacts of shrinkage from formalin fixation (x400).

FIG. 9–35. Numerous fields from the above tumor had to be searched to find one where the nuclear features were not sufficiently distorted by artifact to identify the true nature of the lesion. In this area, the nuclei were too large, too crowded together, and the abnormalities in chromatin clumping and sizes and shapes too abnormal to be considered anything other than anaplasia. The evidence of collagen production by the cells, absence of woven bone, osteoid, and cartilage indicated that the lesion was a fibrosarcoma. The arrows point to the most malignant nuclei (x400).

FIG. 9–36. With more adequate fixation, the features of a typical grade II fibrosarcoma are shown here. In particular, note the crowding of nuclei, the distinct and abnormal chromatin patterns, and the marked variations in length of the various nuclei. The arrows point to the most malignant nuclei. (x400).

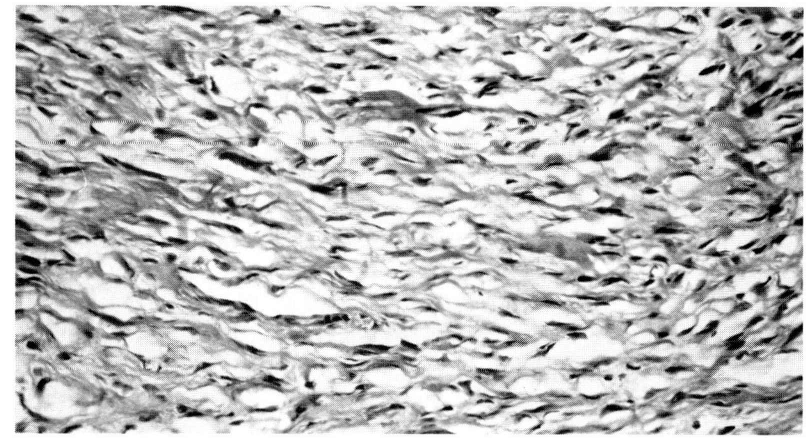

FIG. 9-34

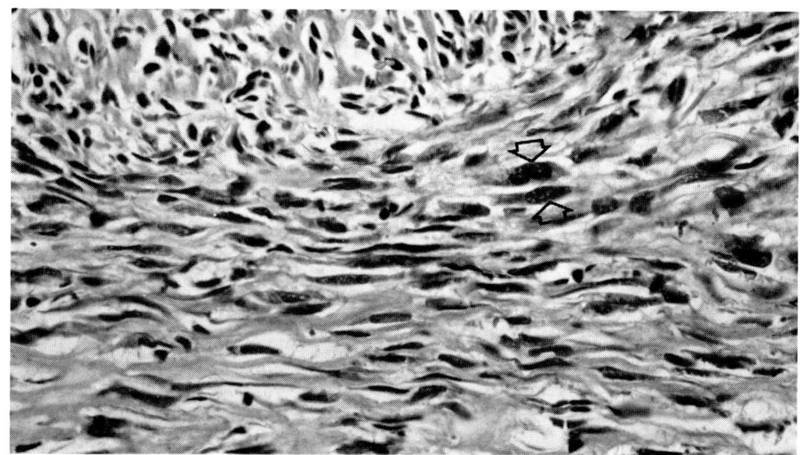

FIG. 9-35

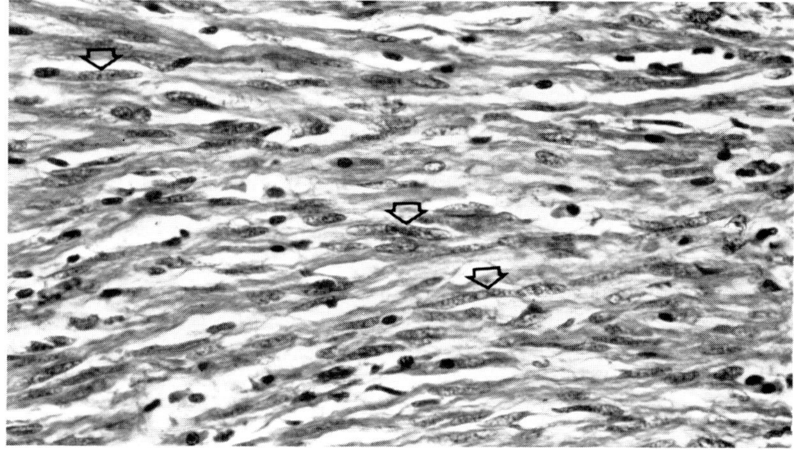

FIG. 9-36

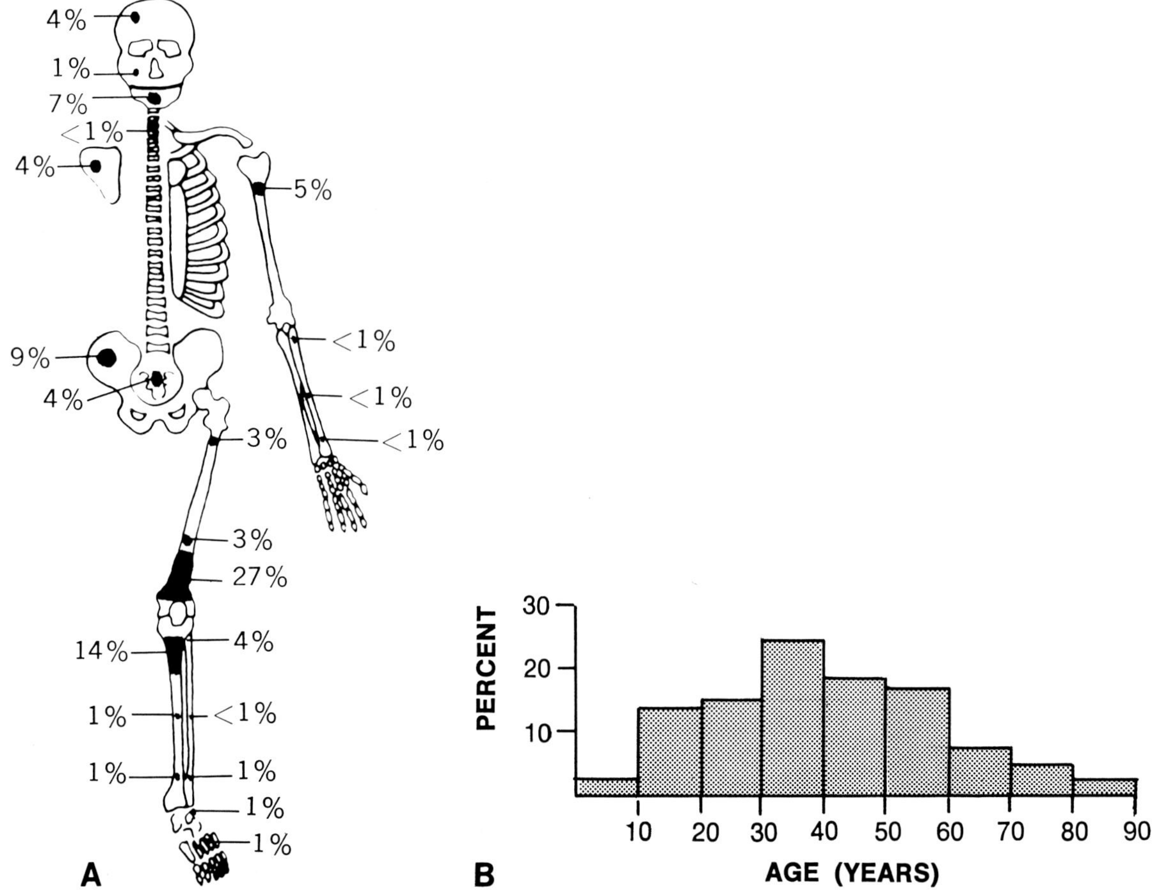

FIG. 9-38. (*A*) Fibrosarcoma of bone. Frequency of areas of involvement in 164 patients. Male : female incidence, 1 : 1. (*B*) Age distribution of patients with fibrosarcoma of bone. (Mirra, J., Bullough, P., and Freiberger, R.: Orthopedic Diseases, Part II. New York, Famous Teachings in Modern Medicine, MedCom, Inc., © 1972)

Fibrosarcoma

FIG. 9-37. High grade II fibrosarcoma. Although the nuclei are not closely packed in this field, note the marked variations in size and shape of nuclei from cell to cell. In the lower field is a huge nucleus with intense hyperchromatism (*arrow*), virtually diagnostic of anaplasia in a spindle cell neoplasm of any type (x400).

FIG. 9-39. Grade III fibrosarcoma. The degree of anaplasia is striking. Note that in the higher grade of fibrosarcomas the degree of collagen production becomes less pronounced (x400).

FIG. 9-40. Fibrosarcoma with a storiform pattern of cells and collagen from a patient with Paget's disease. A storiform pattern may be seen in pure fibrosarcomatous lesions and this finding should not, in and of itself, prompt a diagnosis of malignant fibrous histiocytoma (x125).

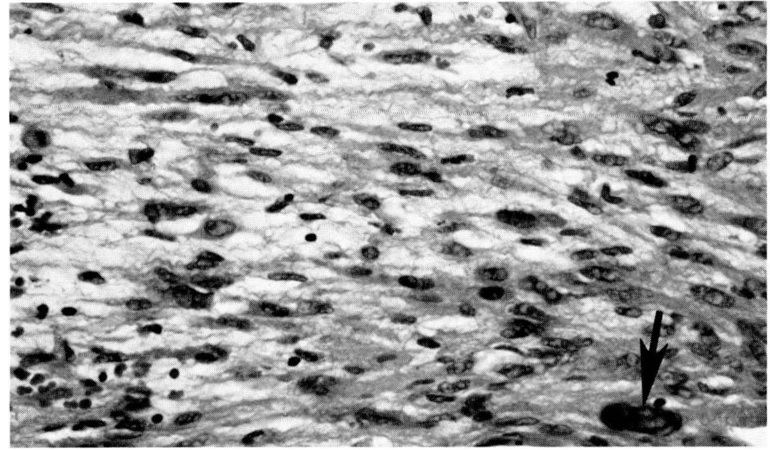

FIG. 9-37

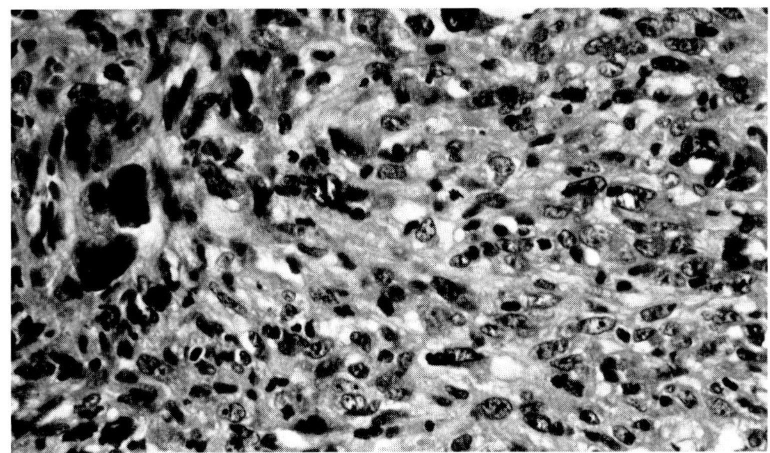

FIG. 9-39

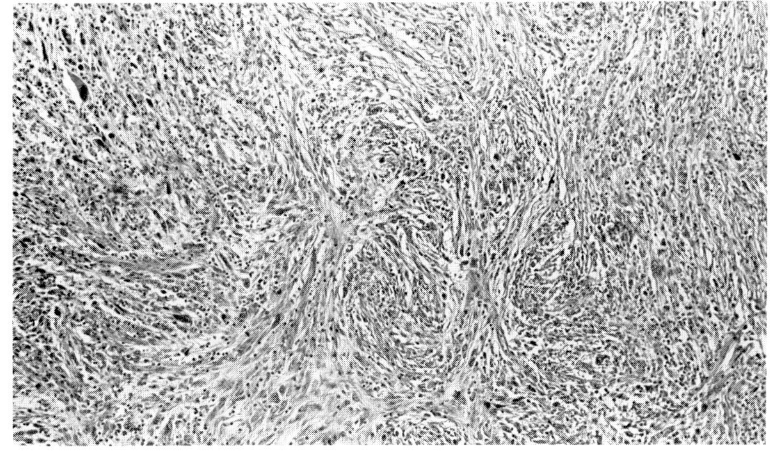

FIG. 9-40

islands of malignant cartilage and hemangiopericytoma-like areas (see p. 212 and Figs. 8–68 to 8–70, Plate 6, *D, E,* and *F*).

METASTASES. On occasion a metastasis from an undifferentiated spindle-cell carcinoma or melanoma may mimic a fibrosarcoma. Careful examination of all "fibrosarcomas" for melanin pigment may distinguish a metastatic melanoma presenting as a primary bone tumor from a tumor where the primary skin lesion had not been identified. For the most part, metastatic tumors have a well-known history of a nonosseous primary. Most patients show multiple bone involvement at initial presentation, even if a primary site of origin is not known or suspected. Do not forget that in adults, metastatic lesions outnumber primary bone tumors approximately 25 to 1 and that multiple primary bone sarcomas, with the possible exception of the osteosarcoma, are an extremely rare event.

Course

Grade II and III and secondary fibrosarcomas behave with as much virulence as the osteogenic sarcoma. Their 5-year survival rate is lower than 25 per cent. Osteosarcoma metastases are often restricted to the lungs. Fibrosarcomatous metastases find any organ system an opportune bed to grow in, including the skin, visceral organs, and lymph nodes.

The well-circumscribed primary Grade I fibrosarcoma in which numerous sections are prepared to rule out foci of high-grade anaplasia have a significantly better prognosis. Lethal metastases from such tumors is in the range of 5 to 15 per cent. Their behavior, therefore, is similar to the low-grade chondrosarcoma. The typical intramedullary osteosarcoma, on the other hand, is a highly lethal tumor, regardless of grade of nuclear anaplasia.

Treatment

Well-documented Grade I fibrosarcomas can be treated with a generous en-bloc resection or possibly cryosurgery, if considered feasible. Nevertheless, the patients must be closely followed to rule out recurrence or metastases. Whether or not systemic chemotherapy should be used as an adjunct to surgery is debatable.

Grade II to III fibrosarcomas necessitate radical treatment, either amputation followed by systemic chemotherapy or possibly chemotherapy and radiation to the primary tumor and en-bloc resection to be followed by a course of systemic chemotherapy.

PRIMARY MALIGNANT FIBROUS HISTIOCYTOMA (HISTIOSARCOMA) OF BONE

Introduction

Feldman, *et al.,*[38] were the first to describe primary intraosseous malignant fibrous histiocytoma of bone (11 cases). Mirra, *et al.,* described the second series of MFH in bone.[45] Since that time at least 92 patients have been reported.[35,37,38,43,45,46] From a review of the literature and personal observations, it is apparent that there are at least two distinct groups: those without evidence of bone infarction and those with. Since the two differ radically with respect to clinical factors, age distribution, sites of involvement and pathogenesis, each will be treated separately.

Soft-tissue malignant fibrous histiocytoma behave with either low or high virulence. Their behavior is said to be extremely difficult to predict by histological features alone. In contrast, the reported cases of MFH reported in bone usually behave with extreme virulence.

Before embarking on a discussion of the MFH of bone, it is necessary to understand how the term evolved and to define the functions and capabilities of the histiocyte. The conceptions and diagnostic difficulties that attend the soft-tissue malignant histiocytic lesions apply to their bone counterparts as well.

A histiocyte or macrophage is a cell with phagocytic ability. It can store vital dyes, has a high content of nonspecific esterase, and is rich in lysosomal acid phosphatases.

The benign or malignant histiocyte may assume many histologic patterns. In their early phase of development, the individual cells appear identical to their blood counterpart, the monocyte. The nucleus is single and lobulated to reniform; the cytoplasm is deep pink and finely granular and its cell borders are distinct. After ingestion of particulate matter (bacteria, tissue debris, foreign material), the cytoplasm begins to swell and becomes less deeply staining. The benign mononuclear histiocytes that are ovoid and have a dense, granular cytoplasm are referred to as *epithelioid cells.* Eventually, as a result of the accumulation of lipids, the cytoplasm becomes vacuolated, foamy or clear, and lipocyte-like. These are referred to as *foamy histiocytes.* By means of syncytial fusion, benign histiocytes become recognizable as giant cells (*Langhans' cells, foreign body giant cells, etc.*). Finally, in the stages of healing the cells lose their lipid, become spindled out, and produce collagen, making them virtually indistinguishable from fibroblasts. These are referred to by Stout as *facultative (histiocytic) fibroblasts.*

A basic problem in diagnosis is that just as cells of any mesenchymal origin, be they muscle, osseous, or synovial, can transform to fibroblasts (so-called facultative fibroblasts), so can similar cells (particularly those that are malignant) acquire tremendous phagocytic ability and become facultative histiocytes while losing many of those specific features that identify them as being from another origin. However, there may be foci in any tumor considered primary histiocytic, where specific structures identifiable as components of other origins may be found. Therefore, it becomes essential to examine many fields and perform special stains and electron microscopy, if necessary, in histiocyte-like tumors, and to make the diagnosis of a primary histiocytic malignancy only after tumors of a different origin have been eliminated.

The term *histiocytoma* (fibrous and nonfibrous) of the soft tissues has caused much confusion and dispute among pathologists. Bednar[34] believes that the lesion called by most contemporary pathologists dermatofibrosarcoma is of neurogenic origin and coined the term "storiform" neurofibroma. Storiform in Greek means "matted." He applied the term to describe a pinwheel or cartwheel pattern of fibroblast-like cells and their collagen production. Hoffman,[42] and Taylor and Helwig[51] were impressed with the fibroblastic appearance and called the same tumor dermatofibrosarcoma protuberans. Stout and Lattes,[50] on the other hand, thought that the tumor was of histiocytic origin. Stout's thesis to explain several benign and malignant lesions with a combination of fibroblastic and histiocytic components was that histiocytes have the potential to transform to spindle cells producing collagen indistinguishable from fibroblasts. A clue to their origin is the production of collagen and cells with a pinwheel or storiform pattern. To support their thesis Ozzello, Stout, and Murray[47] showed in tissue culture that the histiocyte and the spindle-shaped fibroblast cells from fibrous xanthomas and malignant histiocytomas have a similar potential for fibroblastic or collagenous differentiation. In this author's opinion, this concept is an excellent one and can be applied to an understanding of numerous reparative and neoplastic lesions of the soft tissue and bones where histiocytes and fibroblast-like cells are present. Close examination of malignant fibrous histiocytomas, for example, can show fields of anaplastic, rounded histiocytes; in other fields, these cells become progressively spindled until they look purely fibroblastic. They differ from most fibroblastic-derived tumors, however, by the presence of a prominent storiform pattern and by the presence of rounded, foamy to granular malignant histiocytes. However, several words of caution are in order before diagnosing a lesion as being of primary rather than facultative histiocytic origin. Just as Stout[49] has pointed out that cells indistinguishable from fibroblasts may be produced by a variety of other mesenchymal tumors of osteoblastic, fat, muscle or synovial origin, so may cells of identical origin become facultative histiocytes. Even epidermal cells can become phagocytic and by definition represent a form of histiocyte. Histiocytes have been shown to form *in vitro* through transformation of numerous cell types, including osteoblasts, muscle, liver epithelium, and Schwann cells.[47] Therefore, this author would make the following suggestion: *A tumor with masses of histiocytes should not be diagnosed as being of primary histiocytic origin unless all other possible origins have been reasonably exhausted.* The diagnosis should be one of exclusion, analagous to the diagnosis of sarcoidosis, which is made only after known infections and other noxious agents known to produce sarcoid-like reactions are ruled out. In order to do this it is necessary to be familiar with the appearance of tumors of osseous, muscle, neural, synovial, and vascular origin and to employ appropriate special stains and, where necessary, electron microscopy (EM), to determine whether it is another mesenchymal tumor, where some or most of the cells become facultative histiocytes.

Consequent to the excellent studies of Stout[49,50] and Ozello, *et al.*,[47] showing that histiocytes may produce collagen assuming a storiform pattern (Fig. 9–50), this finding has begun to assume an aura of pathogenicity. But nowhere in these papers is it stated that the storiform pattern is pathognomonic of cells of primary histiocytic origin. That this pattern is assuming pathognomonic proportions is most unfortunate, because many pathologists are now applying the term *histiocytoma* to lesions of other origins. This author has seen the storiform pattern in indisputable synovial sarcomas, the fibroblastic portions of some osteosarcomas, leiomyosarcoma, neurogenic sarcoma, hemangiopericytoma, and in benign fibroblastic entities such as the nonossifying fibroma (Fig. 9–11). Although the storiform pattern may be seen most often in tumors with no identifiable origin other than histiocytes, it is certainly not pathognomonic, and its increasingly expansive and indiscriminate usage has persuaded some pathologists that fibrous "histiocytic" tumors are nothing more than variants of fibroblastic or lipocytic lesions.

What then is a histiocytic tumor? *A histiocytic*

(*Text continues on p. 288.*)

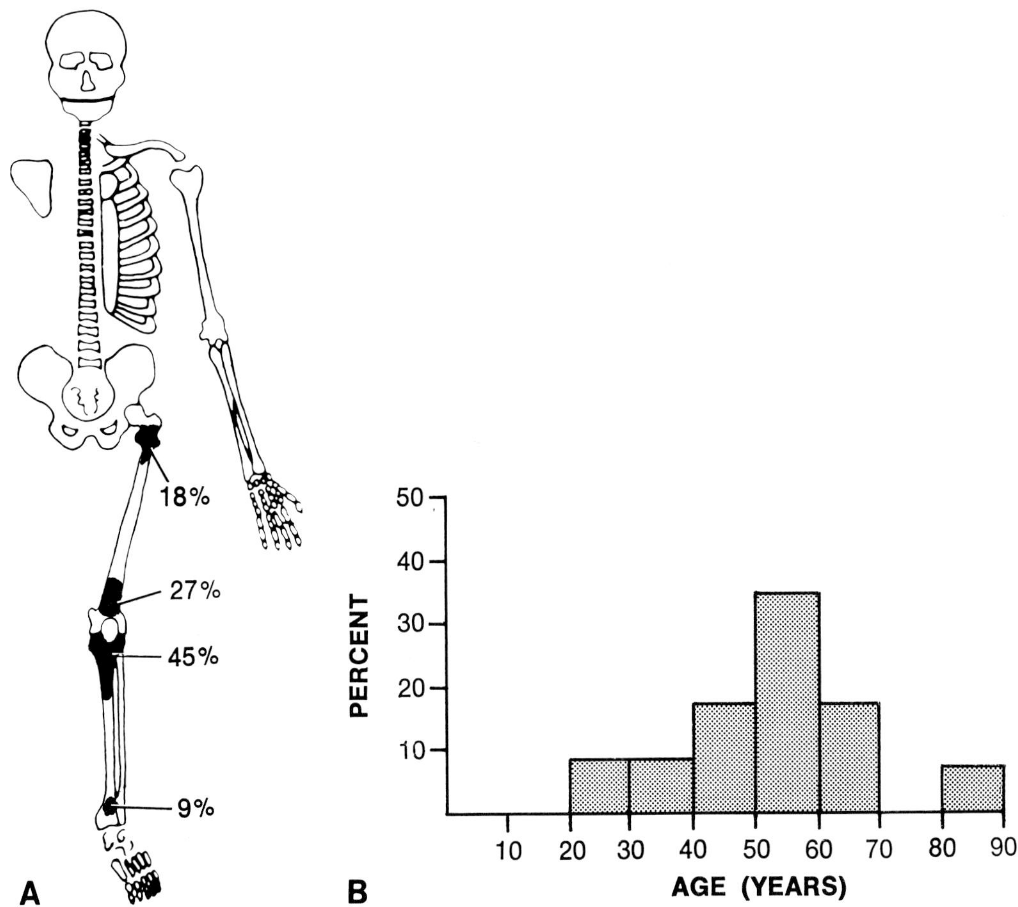

FIG. 9-42. (*A*) Malignant fibrous histiocytoma (histiosarcoma) arising from bone infarcts. Frequency of areas of involvement in 11 patients. All 11 patients were male. Five had malignant fibrous histiocytomas, four, fibrosarcoma, and two, osteosarcoma. Four patients worked under compressed air, one was in a decompression airplane accident at 30,000 feet, one, alcoholic, and one had sickle-cell disease. Male:female incidence, 11:0. (*B*) Age distribution of patients with sarcoma in bone infarcts.

Malignant Fibrous Histiocytoma (MFH) Arising in Bone Infarcts

FIG. 9-41. Malignant fibrous histiocytoma (MFH) arising from bone infarcts. Most patients with MFH arising in bone infarcts show evidence of multiple infarcts. This 86-year-old male quit his employment as a tunnel worker some 20 years prior to the development of pain in his left hip. The right hip showed a triangular-shaped infarct, which is shown in this illustration.

FIG. 9-43. His other hip demonstrated multiple, rounded densities and a pathologic fracture, which was nailed. Biopsy showed evidence of bone infarcts in both hips and a MFH arising from the left hip. (Mirra, J. M., *et. al.*: J. Bone Joint Surg., *56A*:932, 1974)

FIG. 9-44. This 37-year-old male disclosed a solitary infarct in association with a suspicious area of lysis (*arrows*). (Mirra, J. M., *et. al.*: J. Bone Joint Surg., *56A*:32, 1974)

FIG. 9-45. Biopsy and en-bloc resection were performed and the lesion diagnosed as MFH arising in a bone infarct. The specimen radiograph shows a large, circumscribed blastic focus (masses of nonviable Pagetoid bone) and a circumscribed area of lysis and a small cortical infraction (*arrow*). It is from this small cortical infraction, which was not seen on the routine radiographs, that probably incited the presenting symptom of pain in this area.

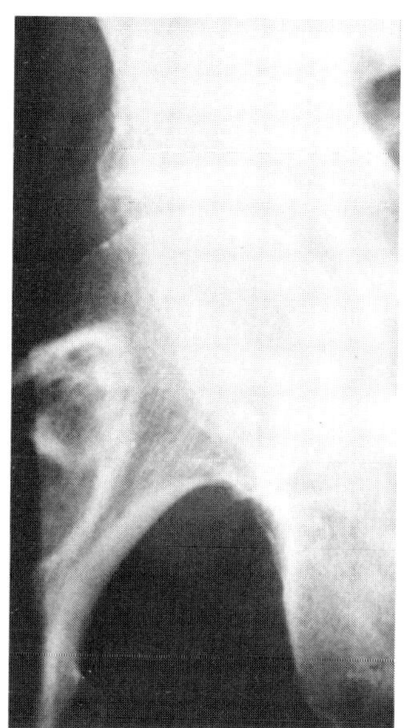

FIG. 9-41

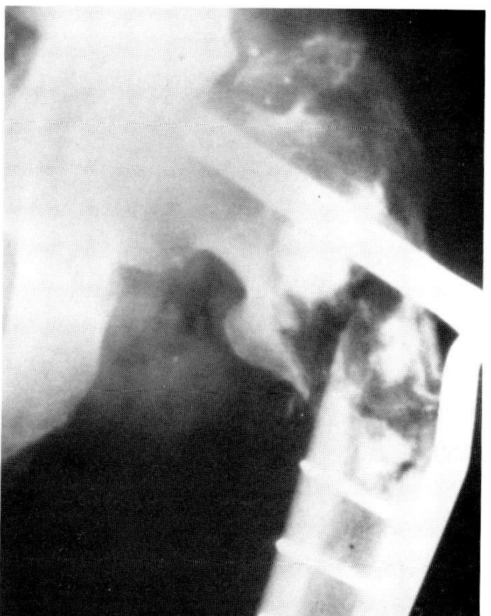

FIG. 9-43

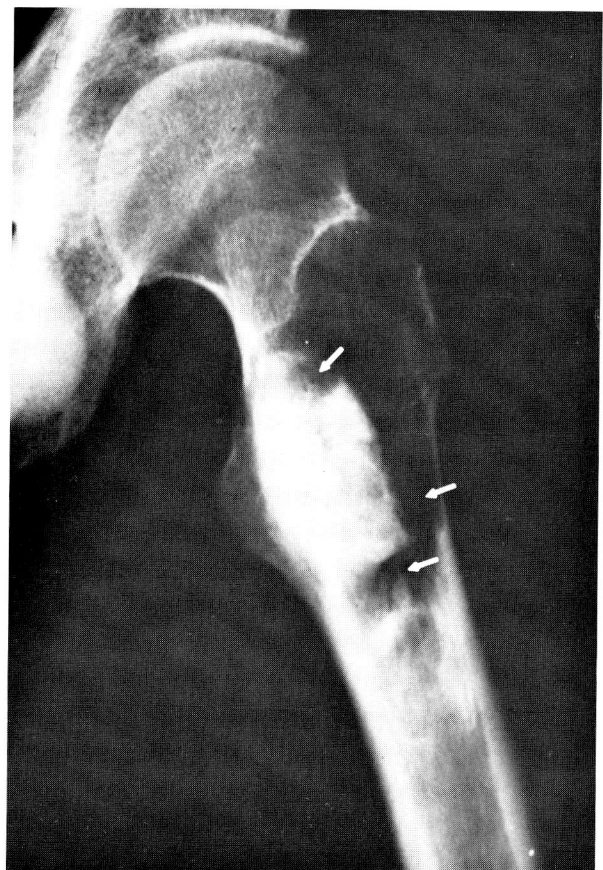

FIG. 9-44

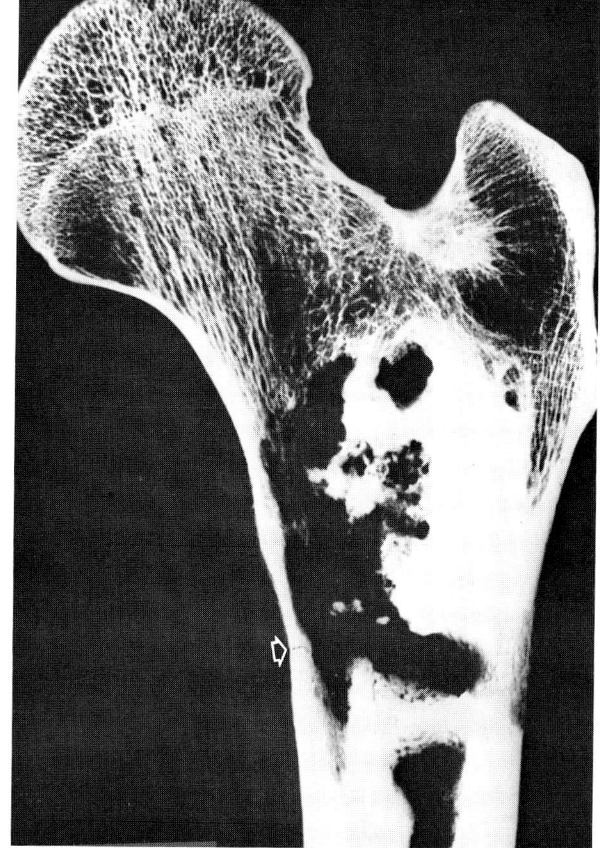

FIG. 9-45

tumor could be defined as one that is composed of mono- to multinucleate cells with pale, vacuolated to foamy cytoplasm that contains fat, are rich in lysosomes by electron microscopy, contain nonspecific esterases, and which have facultative fibroblastic potential, usually with a storiform pattern, and which, after a study of multiple sections, special stains, E.M., and other studies, can be shown not to be derived from other mesenchymal tissue.

In this author's collection of MFH of bone, five of eight were in association with bone infarcts. However, of those reported only five of 92 cases were in association with bone infarcts. The diagnosis of MFH is extremely difficult and the entity has not been proven to the satisfaction of many in the medical community. An example of an osteosarcoma with intensely active phagocytosis and lipid-rich cytoplasm that could easily have been misconstrued as a malignant (fibrous) histiocytoma were it not for the presence of occasional malignant tumor osteoid and even woven bone is shown in Plate 5, *H* and *I*. The reader is, therefore, advised to use this diagnosis with discretion and caution and to obtain numerous sections, fat stains, and even electron microscopy in consideration of other, more likely candidates.

MALIGNANT FIBROUS HISTIOCYTOMA IN ASSOCIATION WITH BONE INFARCT(S) (Fig. 9–42)

Clinical Features

INCIDENCE. Approximately 0.6 per cent of primary bone tumors from among 525 cases at the Hospital for Special Surgery, New York (personal observations), in comparison to an incidence of 0.4 per cent for chondroblastomas at the same hospital over a 15-year span.

SEX. To date, all eleven patients reported have been male (probably because males are most often subjected to occupations where they work under compressed air conditions).

SYMPTOMS. Pain and swelling, occasionally pathologic fracture.

OTHER PERTINENT CLINICAL DATA. Bone infarcts are well known to occur in several disease states, including attacks of the "bends" due to nitrogen embolization from rapid decompression, alcoholism, steroid therapy, sickle-cell disease, systemic lupus erythematosis, and other "collagen-disease" vasculitides. Some cases are idiopathic. In 1974, Mirra, *et. al.*,[45] published four cases of MFH in association with bone infarcts and reviewed the literature. We noted that three patients were former tunnel workers and had quit their "compressed-air" employment 17, 20, and 22 years, respectively, before they developed their sarcoma. This implies that even if these sarcomas were causally related to the infarct, many years usually pass before malignant transformation. In this paper it was speculated that other patients will probably be reported with sarcomas from other causes of bone infarction other than working under compressed air. One of these cases was found in the records at UCLA by simply reviewing all patients with the diagnosis of sickle-cell disease with surgical pathology or autopsy coded data. Seventeen patients were so coded; one had a bone sarcoma (M.F.H) arising in one of multiple infarcts.[46] I believe similar studies should be performed for sickle-cell disease, alcoholism, steroid therapy, Gaucher's disease, systemic lupus erythematosis, and others in order to retrieve those cases diagnosed as spindle cell sarcoma where the infarcts may have been missed by cursory pathologic examination. Our Case 2[45] of a 37-year-old male is interesting in that at the time we wrote the paper we did not know of a subsequent highly important historical finding. The patient recalled an incident in a commercial airplane: while climbing to about 30,000 feet the plane "flamed-out." There was sudden decompression in the plane and he remembers an immediate intense pain in both ears. The plane fell approximately 15,000 feet before "flame-in" and recompression. This incident occurred 8 years before the sarcoma that developed in a solitary bone infarct. (The only patient in the series of 11 patients with a solitary infarct.)

At any rate, of the 11 reported patients, four worked under compressed air, one experienced rapid decompression at high altitude, one had sickle-cell disease, one was a chronic alcoholic, and four were idiopathic. There were six black patients: one was sickle-cell preparation positive, two worked under compressed air, one was sickle-prep negative, one was alcoholic, and in four no sickle-cell preparation was performed.

Radiologic Features

The characteristic radiographic features of the vast majority of the patients are as follows:

1. Signs of blastic to blastic-lytic multiple bone infarcts, particularly in the region of the knee and proximal femur (Figs. 9–41, 9–43, 9–44, and 9–45). Recently, I have had sent to me an MFH arising in a bone infarct of the radius in a 70-year-old Negro male with a history of alcoholism. The distal ulna also showed a bone infarct uninvolved by tumor. A skeletal series for other

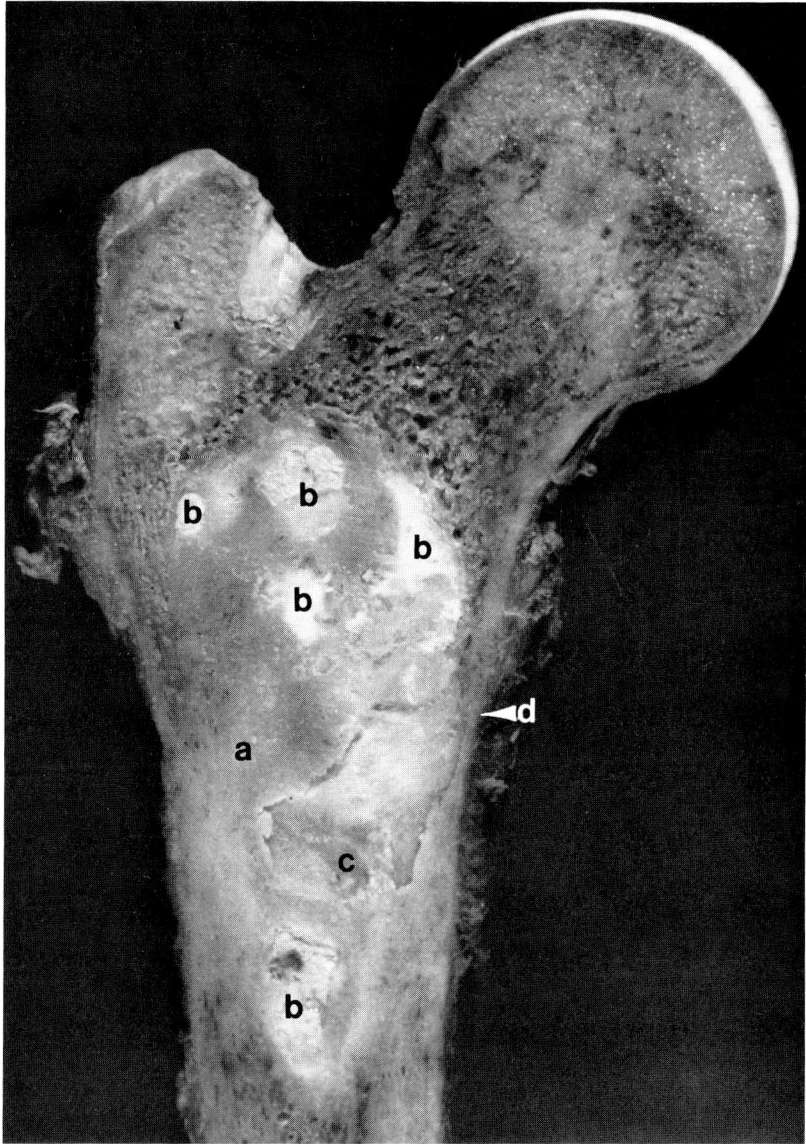

MFH Arising in Bone Infarct

FIG. 9-46. The gross appearance of the resected femur showing the area of dense Pagetoid bone (*a*), bright orange yellow foci of benign foamy histiocytes, and cholesterol clefts (*b*) and the site of origin of the MFH (*c*). The tumor can be seen to erode the cortex (*d*). This tumor is also shown in Plate 7, *I.* (Mirra, J. M., *et al.*, J. Bone Joint Surg., *56A*:932, 1974)

infarcts was not performed, to my knowledge, in this case.

2. An ill-defined focal area of lytic destruction in one of the infarct zones with a permeative moth-eaten or well-defined border along its advancing margins (Figs. 9-43, 9-44, 9-47). Periosteal reactions and a soft-tissue mass are not uncommon (Fig. 9-47). It is the ill-defined or lytic area with or without periosteal reaction that represents the area of sarcomatous transformation.

The patient with sickle-cell disease had ill-defined but definite manifestations of bone infarction in multiple bones.[46] In the humerus there was a fine, linear subcortical radiopacity, localized depression of the end-plates of the vertebrae believed to be due to ischemia, and a lytic infarct with a sclerotic border in the femur (Fig. 9–48). The tibia showed a sarcomatous lytic lesion, periosteal new bone, and a portion consistent with a sequestered fragment of dead bone in an area of bone infarct identified histologically (Figs. 9–47 and 9–49, *A*).

Although most medullary bone infarcts resulting from occlusion of large vessels (such as those related to decompression or steroid therapy) are characterized by a striking increase in radiographic bone density, those infarcts resulting from small vessel occlusion (such as in Gaucher's and sickle-cell disease) usually result in more subtle radiographic changes. Therefore, in patients who develop bone sarcomas with a clinical history where bone infarction is possible, careful scrutiny of the radiographs and multiple sampling of bone adjacent to the tumor is necessary in order not to miss a possible antecedent predisposing bone infarct.

Gross Pathology

Most of the bone infarcts seen in association with this condition showed areas of dense bone or grayish fibrous tissue in which gritty bone or dystrophic calcified debris was deposited (Fig. 9–46, Plate 7, *I*). In all cases the sarcoma is in direct continuity or contained within the area of infarction (Plate 7, *I*). Bright orange to yellow nodules (Plate 7, *I*) represent focal massive collections of benign histiocytes and/or cholesterol crystals. These collections represent chronic histiocytic reparative and degenerative areas of a bone infarct.

The neoplastic portions are usually grayish-white and firm tumefactions, although they may be softer if abundant collagen is not deposited. A softer tumor occurred in the patient with sickle-cell disease. The tumors are usually several centimeters in size and most have broken through the cortex and formed a soft-tissue mass. One case associated with 6-year disease free follow up post-en-bloc resection was small and had led to early symptoms because of a small cortical infarction (Fig. 9–45, *arrow*). The tumor had not yet formed a soft-tissue mass.

Histopathology

Of the 11 cases reported, two showed evidence of malignant osteoid and woven bone diagnostic of osteosarcoma. Four are reported as fibrosarcoma and five as malignant fibrous histiocytoma. Illustrations from those reported as fibrosarcoma, however, showed numerous features highly suggestive of malignant fibrous histiocytoma.

The following characteristics typify the usual malignant fibrous histiocytoma or fibrous histiosarcoma:

1. MONONUCLEAR OVOID TO SPINDLY HISTIOCYTIC CELLS. Of utmost importance to the diagnosis is the demonstration of anaplastic mononuclear histiocytes. These cells will be ovoid to polygonal and have a dense, granular to finely foamy cytoplasm (Figs. 9–51, 9–52, 9–53, 9–54, and 9–55, *D*). The nuclei will be pleomorphic and have oval, reniform, or lobulated shapes (Figs 9–52, 9–53, and 9–55, *D*). Atypical mitoses are usually abundant. In these areas anaplasia will be most conspicuous and collagen least abundant. Such areas may form either a minor or major component of the lesional tissue. At other sites these cells can become tapered and begin to suggest a "storiform" or cartwheel pattern of orientation (Fig. 9–51). The majority of these tumors show areas where the cells have assumed a fibroblastic shape, produce heavy collagen, and become arranged in the classic cartwheel patterns so highly suggestive of cells of histiocytic origin (Fig. 9–50).

MFH Arising in Bone Infarct

FIG. 9–47. MFH arising in one of the multiple bone infarcts in a 27-year-old black patient who had been diagnosed as having sickle-cell disease when he was as young as 1-year-old. The tumor involves the shaft of the tibia, shows considerable permeative destruction, soft-tissue mass, and ominous periosteal new bone (*arrows*) (Mirra, *et. al.:* Cancer, *39:*186, 1977).

FIG. 9–48. Same patient as above. Note the lytic medullary infarct (*arrows*) of the femur surrounded by reactive host bone. (Mirra, *et. al.:* Cancer, *39:*186, 1977)

FIG. 9–49. Bone Infarcts (*A*): The components of the usual bone infarct include nonviable lamellar bone (*a*), fibrosis (*b*), and dystrophic calcification (*c*). This infarct was from the tibia of the above sickle-cell patient (x40). (*B*) This bone infarct corresponds to that shown in Figures 9–44, 9–45, and 9–46 (*a*). This type of infarct is unusual in that it consists of dense masses of nonviable Paget-like bone (*a*) and some fibrosis. The bone on the top (*b*) of field is viable cortical bone (x60). (Mirra, *et. al.:* Cancer, *39:*186, 1977)

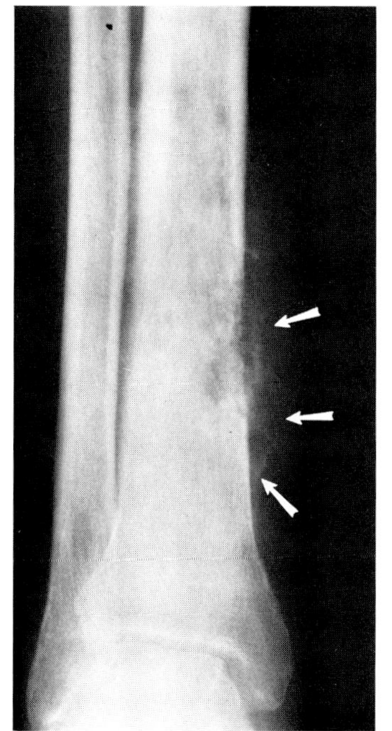

FIG. 9-47

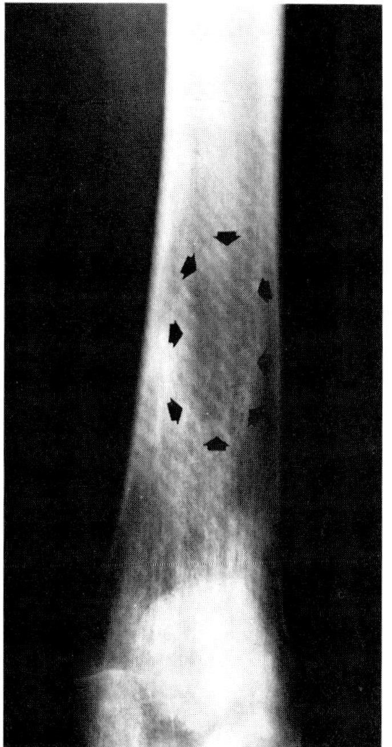

FIG. 9-48

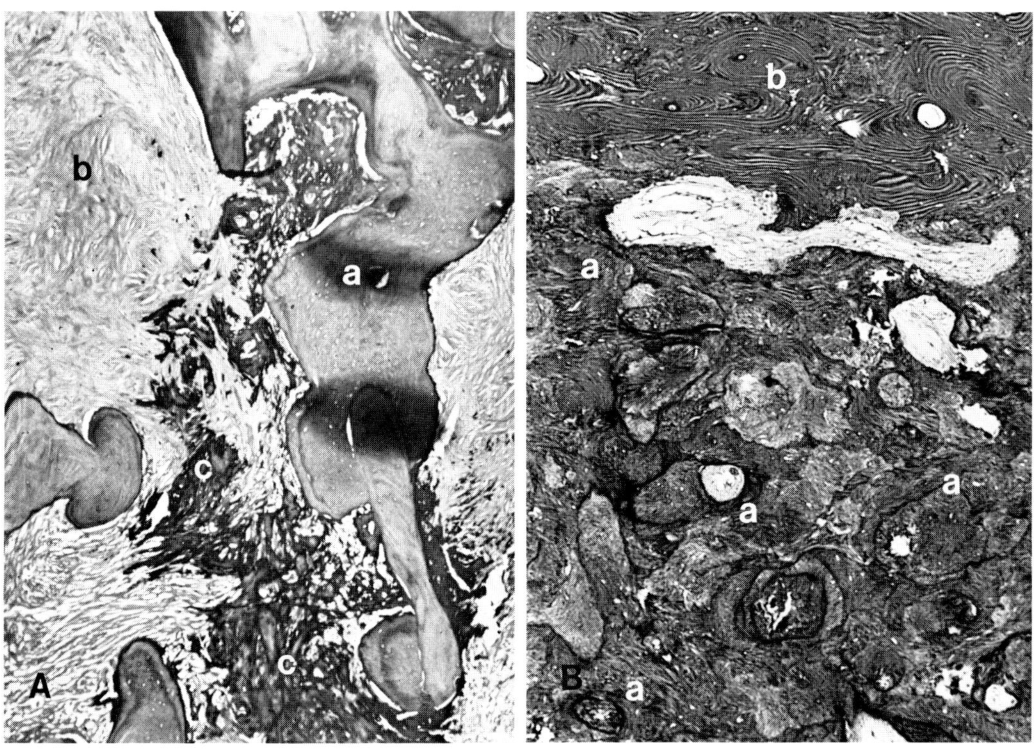

FIG. 9-49

Numerous sections may show changes from areas of benign to dysplastic to obviously malignant histiocytes. The following set of four illustrations from a patient with malignant fibrous histiocytoma arising in a solitary bone infarct is presented. (Refer to Fig. 9-55, *A–D* and Plate 7, *I* for gross correlation.) The heavy orange infiltrates (Plate 7, *I*, demonstrated obviously benign foamy macrophages; also, see Fig. 9-55, *A*). At a site adjacent to the tumor, collections of similar cells were seen. However, some of the nuclei displayed enlargement and atypia (Fig. 9-55, *B*). In an adjacent field numerous atypical cells were seen (Fig. 9-55, *C*), and in the next field transition to frankly anaplastic histiocytes was observed (Fig. 9-55, *D*).

2. ANAPLASTIC MULTINUCLEATE GIANT CELLS. Another crucial pathologic finding is the demonstration of small to large cells with abundant granular to foamy cytoplasm identical to that of the mononuclear stromal histiocytes. The nuclei may be bizarrely multilobulated or even multiple (Figs. 9-52, 9-53, and 9-54). These giant cells are malignant cytologically and do not resemble benign osteoclasts or osteoclast-like giant cells. It may not be possible by histology alone to distinguish MFH from osteoclastic sarcoma, which, in this author's opinion, is a type of histiosarcoma derived from osteoclasts rather than from the usual tissue histiocytes.

3. EVIDENCE OF PHAGOCYTOSIS. The giant cells may demonstrate evidence of phagocytosis of either necrotic debris, dying cells, or erythrocytes or evidence of hemosiderin or hematoidin pigment (Fig. 9-54). Rare cases may show varying sized reddish globules which, by special stains (Sudan black, oil red O, and PAS) are rich in fats and protein (glycolipids). These globules may represent breakdown products of erythrocytes.

4. HEAVY RETICULIN PRODUCTION. The MFH is characterized by an abundance of reticulin fibers that may encase each and every cell.

5. FAT PRODUCTION. Frozen sections show small to large droplets of fat in a variable proportion of the cells. The more vacuolated to foamy cells contain, as we would expect, the greatest fat content. This finding is nonspecific, however, because a variety of malignant bone sarcomas may contain variable quantities of fat, including occasional cases of osteogenic sarcoma.

Bone Infarct Areas

The following characteristics typify areas of bone infarction:

1. *Dense bland fibrosis* of marrow with variable quantities of *dystrophic calcification* (Fig. 9-49, top).
2. Variably sized foci of *nonviable lamellar to woven bone* (Fig. 9-49, *A*). In some cases the amount of dead bone seen is much more than could have been due to the infarction of the original host bone alone. In two cases (personal observations) the amount of nonviable medullary woven to lamellar bone was enormously thickened both on radiograph (Figs. 9-44 and 9-45) and histologically (Fig. 9-49, *B*). This peculiar bone resembled dense Paget bone due to the increased number of cement lines. Obviously, this very thick, nonviable Paget-like bone formed either secondarily upon an infarct area by revascularization and new bone formation or in an area compromised by chronic ischemia. It is generally held that ischemic areas of bone should lead to the development of dense bone, while highly vascularized areas should result in bone lysis. The fact that in these two cases the thick, highly abnormal bone that was identified was itself nonviable implies that some time after its formation, the ischemia must have become complete. The significance of this particular observation is that in dealing with the radiographic features of bone infarcts, the blastic areas seen on radiograph may not be due to only abnormal dystrophic calcification in necrotic fat, but can also be due to dense, Paget-like new bone formation in an area compromised by ischemia, and that later in its development this area may undergo complete avascular necrosis. It is possible that some cases of sarcoma arising in "Paget's disease" are sarcomas arising from focal Paget-like bone infarct areas. I have, for example, noted one autopsy case of bone infarct and sarcoma signed out as arising in Paget's disease. Yet, analysis

---

MFH

FIG. 9-50. This field shows the cartwheel or storiform pattern of cells and collagen that is characteristic, but not pathognomonic, of the MFH (x125).

FIG. 9-51. This field shows numerous pleomorphic spindle and polygonal cells, many with well-delineated cell borders. There is a suggestion of a storiform pattern (x125).

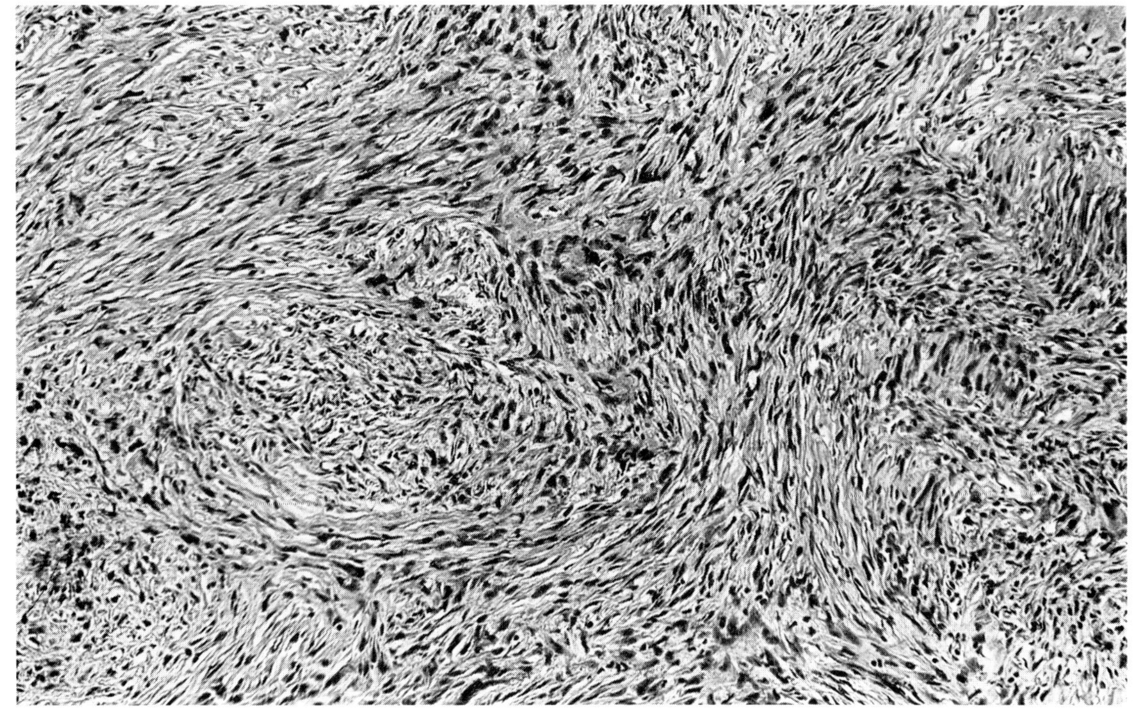

FIG. 9-50

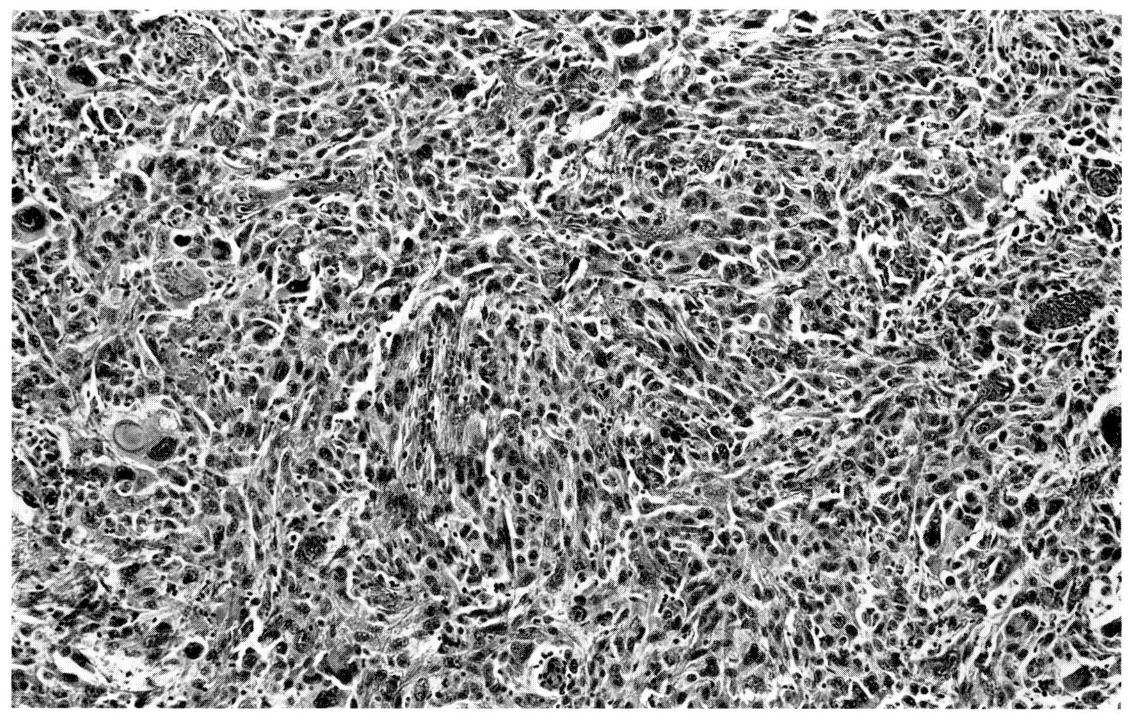

FIG. 9-51

of the radiographs in this patient showed only multiple bone infarcts mistaken clinically for Paget's disease of bone.

3. *Variable quantities of mono- and multinucleate benign histiocytes, cholesterol clefts,* and various blood pigments may be found in association with the infarcted areas. The histiocytes are always seen at the revascularizing margins of the infarct (Fig. 9–56).

Pathogenesis of Malignant Fibrous Histiocytoma in Association With Bone Infarcts

Is it mere coincidence that MFH arises within bone infarcts or are they cause-and-effect related? I proposed[46] that the two are causally related and that these tumors arise as a transformation of a formerly benign chronic reparative process. The data that support this theory are as follows:

1. All of the tumors that have been reported as M.F.H or otherwise have occurred in direct continuity with a bone infarct. None have been reported to have arisen in a site distant from the area of bone infarct.
2. In those patients with known exposure to bone infarct conditions, the tumor developed many years later: 17, 20, 22, and 25 years after the compressed air workers quit their respective employment, 26 years after the development of severe sickle-cell disease, and 8 years after decompression in an airplane. Other chronic reparative and scarring processes are associated with sarcomas after similar periods of time have elapsed. Many cases of sarcomas occurring in chronic burns, chronic osteomyelitis, and scars of tuberculosis have been reported where the cause and effect relationship is now generally accepted.
3. Examination of numerous sections may reveal foci of benign foamy histiocytes blending into dysplastic or atypical histiocytes and finally to frankly malignant areas (Fig. 9–55, *A–D*).

If, as proposed, certain tumors arise within bone infarcts as a complication of the reparative process, these tumors should be related histogenetically to the components of the infarct. The various cell types occurring within bone infarcts were studied in-depth in order to arrive at a definition. Because medullary infarcts of bone are usually asymptomatic they are rarely biopsied. Histologic material from the four medullary infarcts associated with cases of sarcoma previously reported by this author[46] and from a medullary infarct uninvolved by tumor, as well as from 20 infarcted femoral heads resected during total hip replacement, was studied.

The basic pathological process in these 24 cases encompasses necrosis of fat and bone, dystrophic calcification followed by elaboration of granulation tissue beginning at the proximal margin of the infarcts, deposition of new bone with subsequent remodeling, and proliferation of mono- and multinucleate histiocytes and dense fibrous connective tissue. Proliferation of large numbers of mononucleate granular, foamy, and hemosiderin-laden histiocytes was manifest in seventeen cases. Multinucleate histiocytes of foreign-body type were present in ten cases. The histiocytes were usually disposed around small capillaries (Fig. 9–56), or in areas of newly formed fibrous tissue. Spindle-shaped histiocytes were associated with the production of collagen. The histiocytes were concentrated in the proximal revascularizing part of each infarct.

In summary, the basic cells involved in bone infarcts include histiocytes, fibrocytes and histiocytic fibroblasts, and vascular and osseous cells. The neoplasms that could theoretically evolve from these cells

(*Text continues on p. 298.*)

MFH

FIG. 9–52. On higher-power examination of the above, the abundant cytoplasm, large pleomorphic nuclei, and spindle and polygonal shape of the abundant, granular, pink cytoplasm is evident (x250).

FIG. 9–53. On oil-power examination, the granularity and foaminess of the cytoplasm (*a*) and the oval (*b*), multilobulated (*c*) and reniform (*d*) shapes of the nuclei are most consistent with anaplastic cells of histiocytic origin (x1000). Figures 9–51 to 9–53 are from the malignant fibrous histiocytoma associated with sickle-cell disease (Mirra, J. M., *et. al.:* Cancer, *39:*186, 1977).

FIG. 9–54. In some fields of MFH, large, multinucleated or multilobulated anaplastic histiocytes may contain abundant masses of blood-derived pigments. The arrows point to three prominent masses of hematoidin pigment within one such cell. Although the pigment was an intense golden brown, in this illustration they appear a dark black. Note also the characteristic, intense, foamlike quality of the cytoplasm of many of these histiocytes (*b*) (x400).

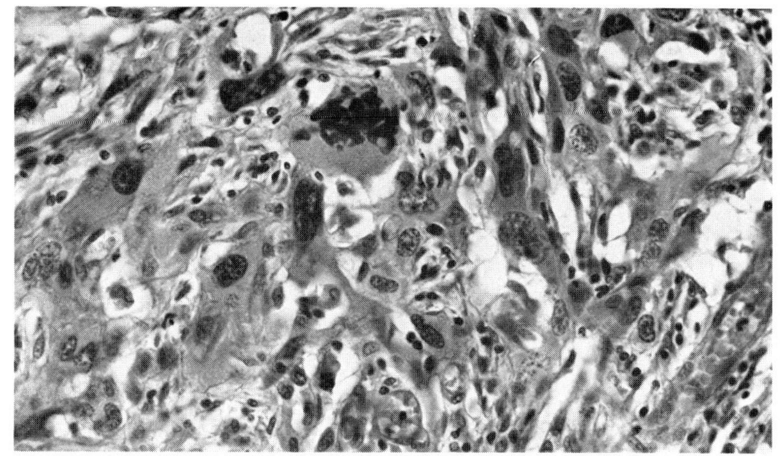

FIG. 9-52

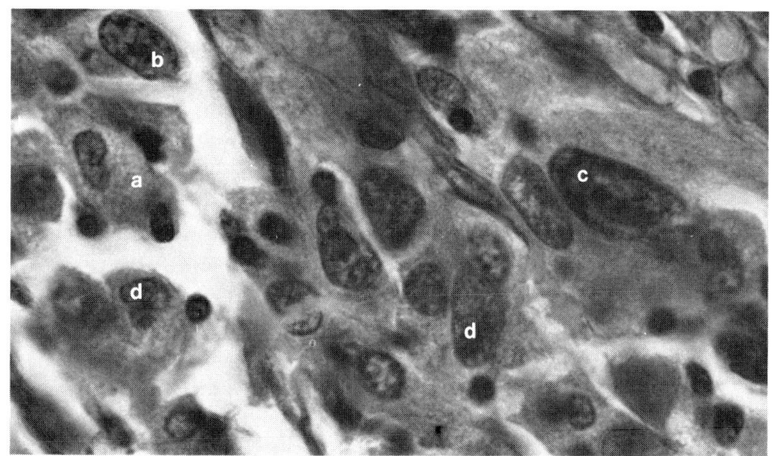

FIG. 9-53

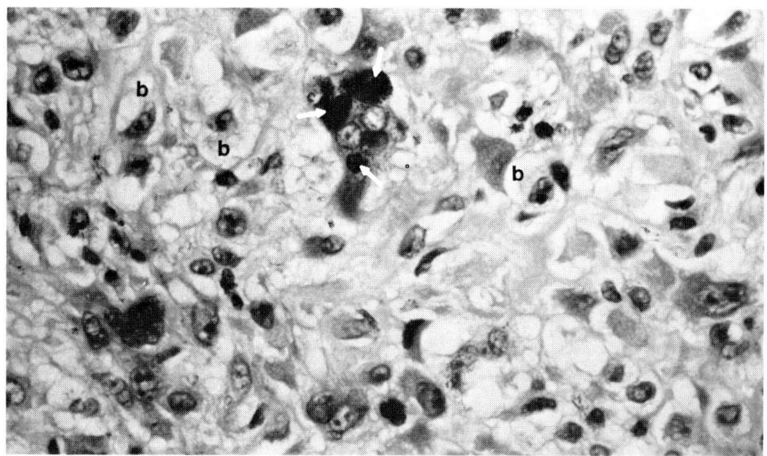

FIG. 9-54

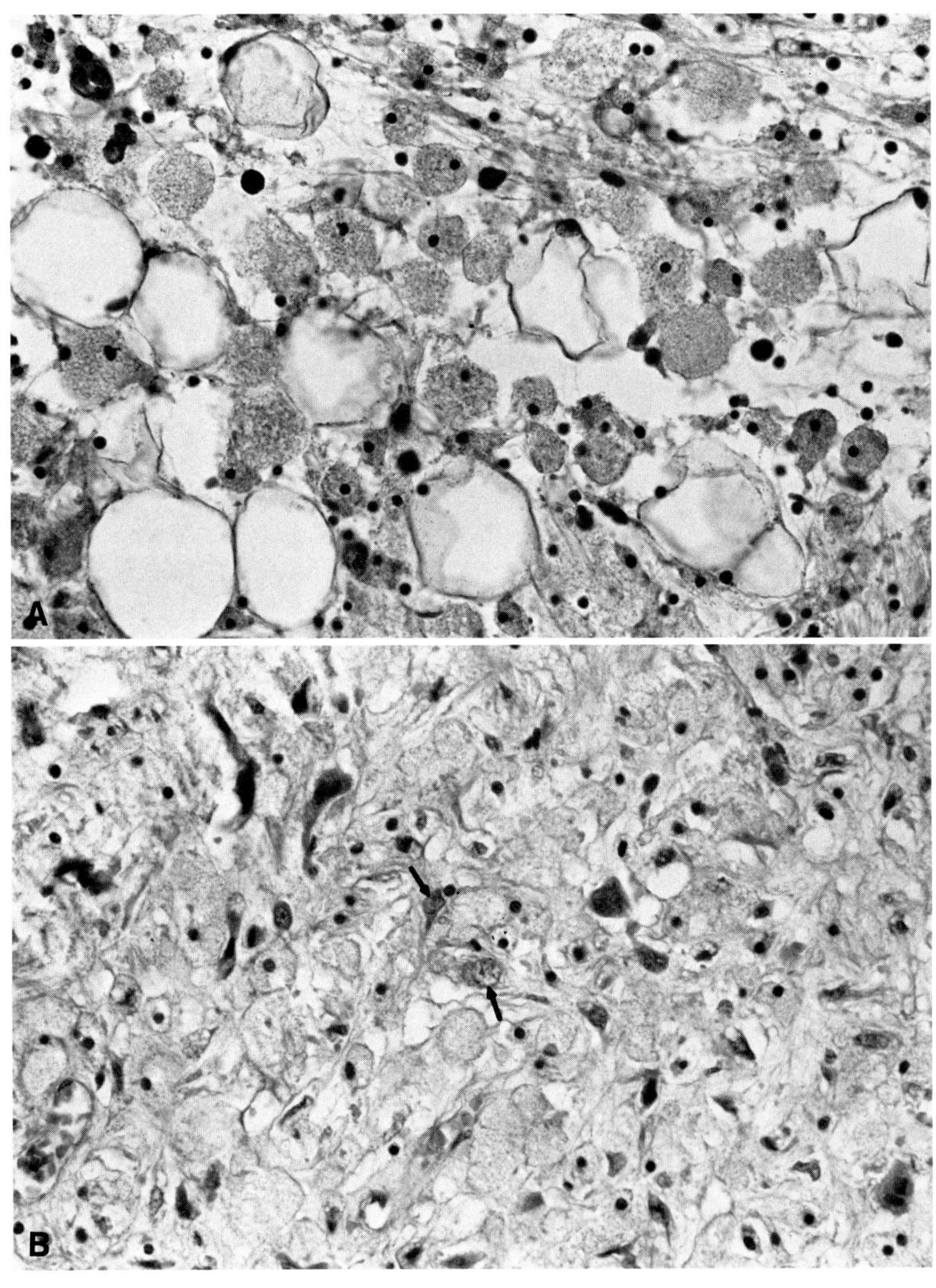

MFH

FIG. 9-55. ***A-D.*** These four illustrations correspond to the tissues of the patient shown in Figures 9–44 to 9–46. They show the insidious conversion of bland, benign histiocytes into a full-fledged histiocytic malignancy. (*A*) Perfectly bland granular histiocytes that correspond to the golden yellow areas shown in Plate 7, *I* (x400). The following three fields were

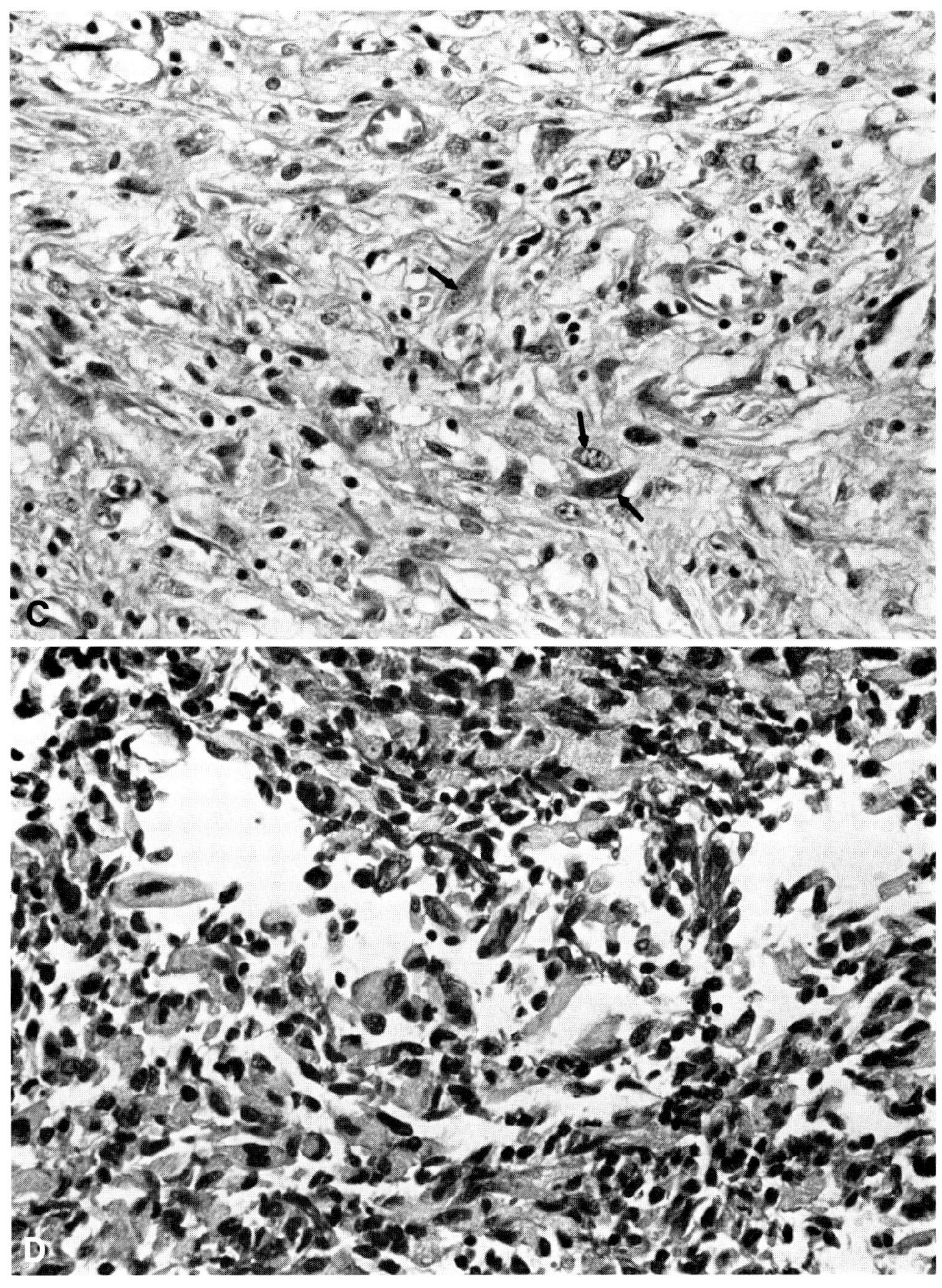

from the region of the development of the MFH. (*B*) Bland histiocytes admixed with histiocytes showing pleomorphic nuclei (*arrows*). (*C*) This field shows a mixture of benign histiocytes and large polygonal and spindle-shaped pleomorphic histiocytes (*arrows*). (*D*) Adjacent to the preceding area, the lesion fully transformed into masses of granular anaplastic histiocytes.

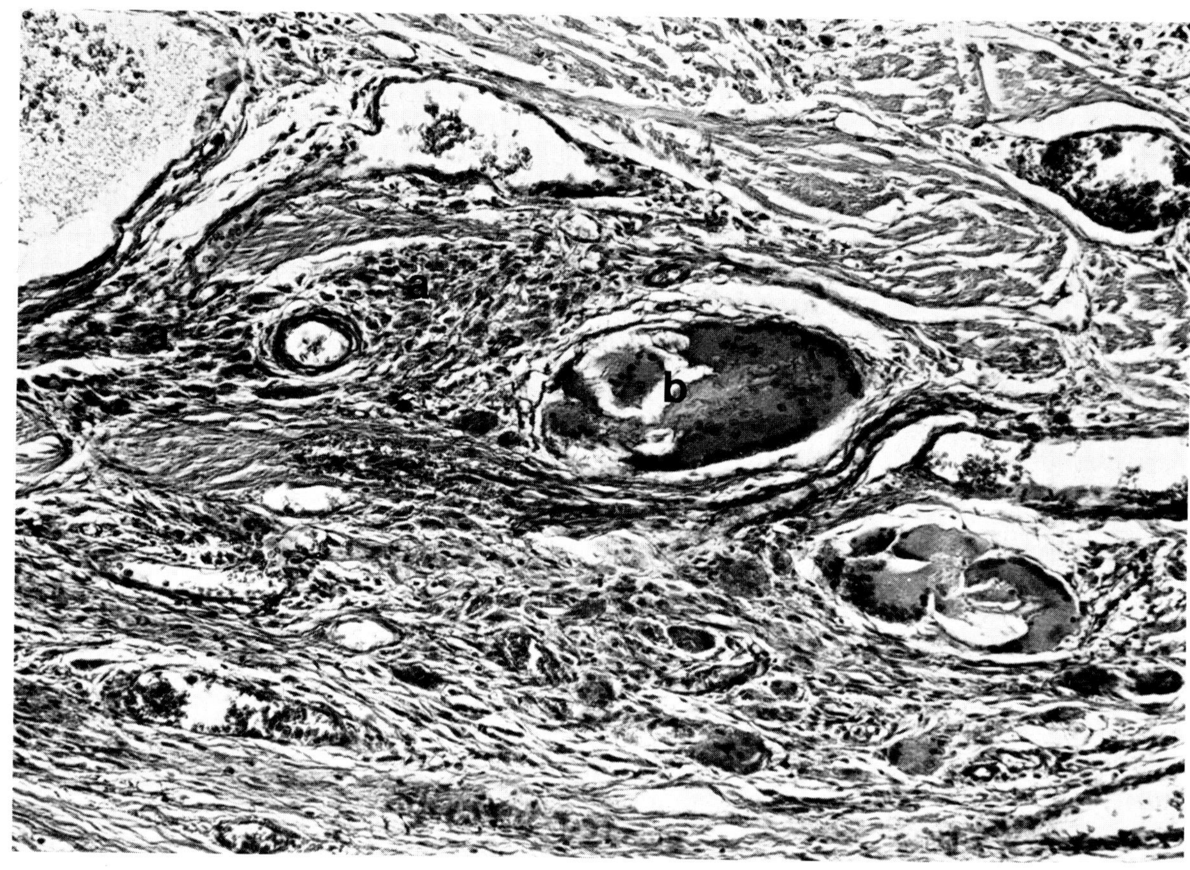

Histiocytes in Repair of Bone Infarct

FIG. 9-56. Analysis of bone infarcts without associated MFH usually show numerous mononuclear (*a*) and even multinuclear (*b*) histiocytes along the revascularizing margin. This patient had avascular necrosis of the femoral head post-steroid therapy for rheumatoid arthritis (x125).

include the MFH, fibrosarcoma, osteosarcoma and angiosarcoma. To date, the first three of these tumors have been reported in association with bone infarcts. As expected, chondrosarcoma, lymphoma, carcinoma, and other tumors deriving from cell types not seen in the organizing of bone infarcts have not been reported.

Thus, we propose that bone infarcts result in a chronic reparative process at their revascularizing margins, an essential component of which is the proliferation of histiocytes. Furthermore, after many years and in rare instances the histiocytic component may undergo sarcomatous transformation. Thus, the MFH associated with bone infarcts probably represents another form of "scar" sarcoma.

Malignant Fibrous Histiocytoma not Associated with Bone Infarcts (Primary MFH)

Clinical Features

The lesions that have been reported as primary MFH of bone have a strikingly different skeletal, age, and sex distribution from those reported in association with bone infarcts (Fig. 9-57). The *age distribution* of primary MFH is about evenly distributed from age 10 to 70. In contrast those patients who get sarcoma in bone infarcts are usually over age 40 as would be expected if there is a cause-and-effect relationship between the benign infarct and malignant

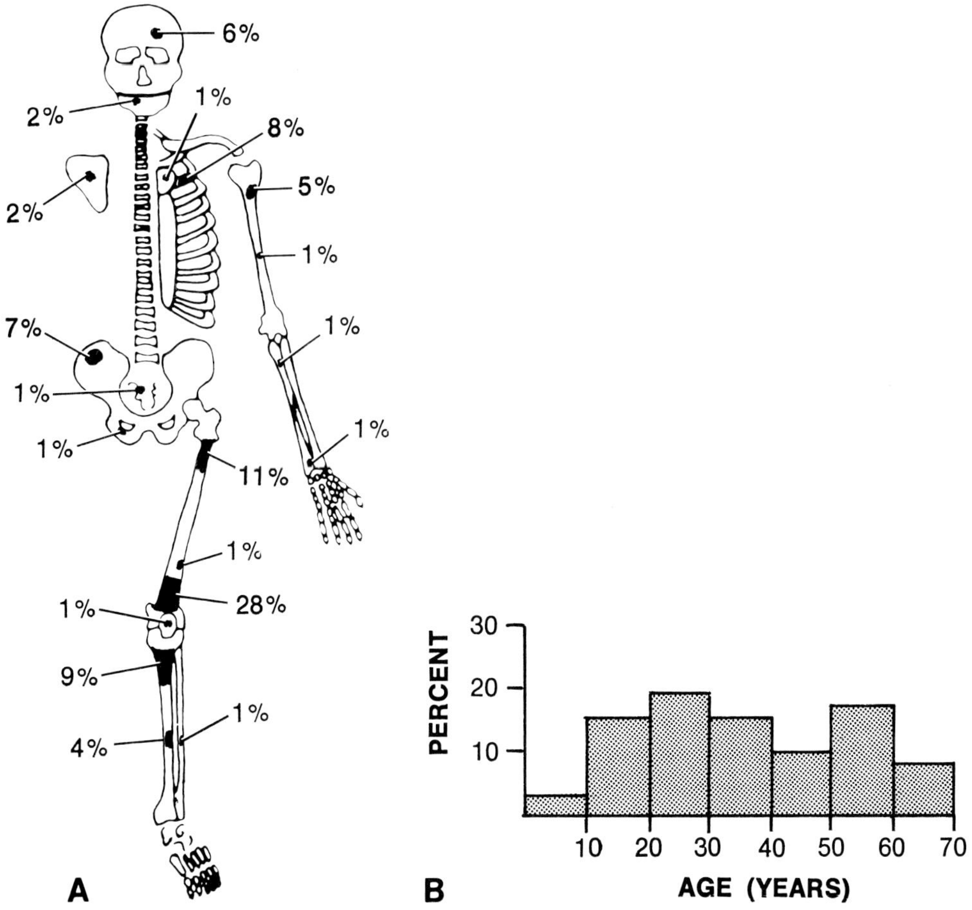

FIG. 9-57. (*A*) Malignant fibrous histiocytoma (MFH) of bone excluding those associated with bone infarcts. Frequency of areas of involvement in 92 patients. Male:female incidence, 1.1:1. (Data obtained from Feldman, *et. al.*, Spanier, *et. al.*, Huvos, Inada, *et. al.*, and Dahlin, *et. al.*) (*B*) Age distribution of patients with primary intraosseous MFH, excluding those arising in infarcts. (Data available on 58 patients.)

transformation. The differences in *sex distribution* are the most striking. All 11 patients with sarcoma (five with MFH) and bone infarct were male. The ratio of males to females with primary MFH is only 1.1 to 1. The *distribution of lesions* is also different. The lesions of bone infarct and sarcoma have a predilection to involve those bones most commonly showing infarcts; namely, the femur and tibia. The primary MFH can apparently affect any bone, including the skull. The syndrome complex of sarcoma and bone infarct appears to be falling within a relatively narrow range of clinical, radiologic, and pathologic features. The primary MFH apparently has a much greater variability in clinical and pathologic presentation.

It is important not to use the term *malignant fibrous histiocytoma* indiscriminately. Numerous sections, special stains, and electron microscopy may be necessary to eliminate certain tumors, such as the intensely phagocytic form of osteogenic sarcoma (Plate 5, *G, H,* and *I*). Also be aware that certain tumors such as the fibrosarcoma may show a prominent storiform pattern but none of the other features characteristic of the MFH. If the MFH becomes a wastebasket term for sarcomas not otherwise specified, phagocytic-rich osteosarcoma, fibrosarcoma, *etc.*, it will be impossible to adequately judge various modalities of treatment or to develop specific diagnostic criteria.

The clinical symptoms associated with the primary

MFH are pain with or without a slowly enlarging mass. Most patients do not present, on initial examination, with radiological evidence of gross pathologic fracture.

Radiologic Features

Almost every bone has been reported to have been involved with the exception of the hands or feet. The distal femur, proximal femur, proximal tibia, ribs, and pelvis account for 63 per cent of reported tumors. Most lesions were centered in the metaphysis, although others were diaphyseal or predominantly epiphyseal lesions. Many of the tumors were eccentric lytic metaphyseal tumors, some of which had eroded through the cortex producing a soft tissue mass most closely resembling (if not in actuality) the lytic osteogenic sarcoma. In the spine the bodies and posterior elements were about equally involved.

The majority of the lesions were lytic, although some showed an admixture of blastic foci. The edges of the lesions are usually ill-defined. The pattern of bone destruction was usually "moth-eaten" or "permeative." Less commonly, the lesions could appear punched out. A border of reactive host bone sclerosis was absent in all but one case.

Gross Pathology

In general, the tumors show extensive permeation between the host bone trabeculae both in the gross and microscopic examinations, as would be expected from the "moth-eaten" or "permeative" pattern of destruction seen radiologically. The tumor has been described as gray-pink to gray-white in color, often mottled with yellow to orange blotches or streaks and with areas of hemorrhage.[38] The soft-tissue mass can be multinodular and associated with a "pseudocapsule." Most often the soft-tissue component infiltrated surrounding skeletal muscles, nerve trunks, and adipose tissue.

Metastases to local lymph nodes are not uncommon.

Histopathology

Except for the absence of infarcted bone the primary malignant fibrous histiocytoma should be no different in appearance from that described in the previous section (see p. 290 and Figs. 9-50–9-55). In summary these features include anaplastic, rounded to polygonal granular to foamy cells compatible with histiocytic origin, bizarre multilobulated and multinucleated giant cells, foci of cells, and collagen arranged in a storiform and cartwheel pattern, occasional foci of phagocytosis of cells, pigment production, intracytoplasmic lipids, and a variable proportion of reticulin fibers which in foci may encompass each and every cell.

In a number of cases benign osteoclast-like cells were described that permeated the tumor not unlike those seen in numerous other benign and malignant primary bone tumors. This permeation of benign osteoclast-like giant cells was not present in five of six MFH's of bone associated with bone infarcts (personal observations).

Differential Diagnosis

LIPID-RICH, INTENSELY PHAGOCYTIC OSTEOSARCOMA. A small percentage of osteogenic sarcomas may assume the aura of a histiocytic sarcoma. The cells may become huge and the cytoplasm extensively filled with reddish lipoprotein rich globules (Plate 5, *H*), which this author has called "sarcoma bodies" (personal observations). These may represent products of erythrophagocytosis. This author has seen these "sarcoma bodies" in eight osteosarcomas: four rhabdomyosarcomas, one fibroxanthosarcoma, and one lymphangiosarcoma of soft tissues. Similar bodies have been described in the Teilum tumor (the endodermal sinus tumor). Fat stains show numerous lipid droplets (Plate 5, *I*).

The first clue to diagnosis is the clinical presentation. Most of these patients show the typical clinical and radiologic features of a lytic osteosarcoma. The patients are generally between age 10 and 25 and show a lytic metaphyseal lesion of the long bones, usually in association with a soft-tissue mass. The crucial histologic feature is the presence of malignant osteoid (Plate 5, *H*), woven bone, or foci of cartilage. The osteosarcoma spindle cell areas may also veer and twist in storiform patterns (Plate 5, *G*). Again, the search for malignant osseous tissue production is crucial to recognition and diagnosis. Between 5 and 10 per cent of osteosarcomas may contain dominant areas of histiocyte-like tissues (personal observations).

FIBROSARCOMA. In this author's estimation the fibrosarcoma is a spindle cell collagen-producing tumor that may on occasion be associated with a storiform pattern of cells and collagen. The storiform pattern is commonly associated with histiocytic tumors but this pattern alone, without other essential identifying features, should not be assumed to be pathognomonic of the malignant fibrous histiocytoma. The other essential features of MFH are granular to foamy lipid-laden polygonal to rounded cells that appear to be of histiocytic origin. In addition, foci of hemosiderin-derived pigments within the tumor cells and evidence of phagocytosis are helpful aids in distinguishing cells of probable histiocytic origin. Cells of this type are essentially absent in the fibrosarcoma.

OSTEOCLASTIC SARCOMA. On the basis of ultrastructural and functional behavior the osteoclast is now believed to be a specialized form of a histiocyte.[41] Therefore, an anaplastic tumor of osteoclastic origin would be a specialized type of malignant histiocytic tumor. In this author's estimation a number of patients with Paget's disease may develop peculiar anaplastic osteoclast-like malignancies most consistent with a diagnosis of osteoclastic sarcoma (p. 356 and Figs. 10–62–10–70). The basic differences between osteoclastic sarcoma and ordinary nonosteoclastic malignant fibrous histiocytomas are the preceding history of Paget's disease and focal or diffuse presence of huge bizarre cells that appear to be histologically most consistent with an osteoclastic origin (see Figs. 10–64–10–66).

Course

The course of the disease is variable depending on whose series is reviewed. There are three major large series in which reasonable follow-up periods of the patients are recorded. In Huvos' series[43] of 18 patients, approximately 40 per cent were dead within less than 1 year. Eight of the patients showed no evidence of disease post-therapy with follow-up periods ranging from 3 months to 2 years. In Dahlin's series,[35] of 35 patients, 28 had follow-ups of 5 years or more. Some 58 per cent of these patients survived 5 years; 43 per cent survived 10 years. In Spanier's series,[49] 82 per cent showed pulmonary metastases in less than 2 years time from initial diagnosis. The 2-year survival rate was less than 50 per cent.

In descending order of frequency, metastases occur to lungs, lymph nodes, other bones, soft tissues, heart, kidneys, adrenals, and skin.

In this author's opinion, the significant differences in sites of distribution, age, incidence, and survival statistics in the different series throw grave doubt on whether the MFH without associated bone infarct, as reported, is a single nosologic entity. These differences are best explained by assuming that the reported cases of so-called primary MFH are a conglomeration of poorly differentiated sarcomas of difficult to impossible to recognize histogenetic types. Therefore, the data abstracted in this section may be useless and not reproducible, because the diagnosis of primary "MFH" is, at present, highly dependent on subjective impressions. Most of the reported cases have not been supported by electron microscopy or fat or esterase stains. Almost all of the tumors reported in these series have been found retrospectively. In some cases, malignant osteoid is reported, which this author would find incompatible with cells of primary histiocytic origin.

Treatment

The malignant fibrous histiocytoma of bone as reported is a highly malignant disorder with a much lower 5-year survival than its soft tissue counterpart.

There is insufficient data upon which to draw conclusions about what constitutes the best mode of therapy in dealing with patients with this tumor.

REFERENCES

Nonossifying Fibroma

1. Bahls, G.: Uber ein solitares xanthoma in knochen. Zbl. Chir., *63:* 1041, 1936.
2. Bhagwandeen, S.B.: Malignant transformation of a non-osteogenic fibroma of bone. J. Pathol. Bacteriol., *92:* 562, 1966.
3. Bosch, A.L., Olaya, A., and Fernandez, A: Non-ossifying fibroma of bone. A histochemical and ultrastructural characterization. Virch. Arch. A Path. Anat. and Histo., *362:* 13, 1974.
4. Burman, A., and Sinberg, S.E.: Solitary xanthoma (lipid granulomatosis) of bone. Arch. Surg., *37:* 1017, 1938.
5. Caffey, J.: On fibrous defects in cortical walls of growing tubular bones. Adv. Pediatr., *7:* 13–51. Edited by S.Z. Levine. Chicago, Year Book Publishers, Inc. 1955.
6. Cunningham, J.B., and Ackerman, L.V.: Metaphyseal fibrous defects. J. Bone and Joint Surg., *38A:* 797, 1956.
7. Hatcher, C.H.: The pathogenesis of localized fibrous lesions in the metaphyses of long bones. Ann. Surg., *122:* 1016, 1945.
8. Jaffe, H.L., and Lichtenstein, L.: Non-osteogenic fibroma of bone. Am. J. Pathol., *18:* 205, 1942.
9. Jaffe, H.L.: Tumors and Tumorous Conditions of the Bones and Joints. Philadelphia, Lea & Febiger, 1958.
10. Mandsley, R., and Stansfeld, A.: Non-osteogenic fibroma of bone. J. Bone Joint Surg., *38B:* 714, 1956.
11. Mubarak, S., Saltzstein, S., and Daniel, D.: Non-ossifying fibroma. Report of an intact lesion. Am. J. Clin. Pathol., *61:* 697, 1974.
12. Phelip, J.A.: Osteite kystigne vasculaire juvenile xanthomatense de l'extremite inferieure de femur. Mem. Chir., *61:* 443, 1935.

12a. Ponsetti, *I.*, and Friedman, B.: Evaluation of metaphyseal fibrous defects. J. Bone Joint Surg., *31A:* 582, 1949.
13. Sontag, L.W., and Pyle, S.I.: The appearance and nature of cyst-like areas in the distal femoral metaphyses of children. Am. J. Roentgenol. Rad. Ther. Nucl. Med., *46:* 185, 1941.

Desmoplastic Fibroma

14. Cohen, P., and Goldenberg, R.: Desmoplastic fibroma of bone. J. Bone Joint Surg., *47A:* 1620, 1965.
15. Dahlin, D.C., and Hoover, N.W.: Desmoplastic fibroma of bone. J.A.M.A., *188:* 685, 1964.
16. Godino, F.S., Chiconelli, J.R., and Lemos, C.: Desmoplastic fibroma of bone. J. Bone Joint Surg., *49B:* 560, 1967.
17. Griffith, J., and Irby, W.: Desmoplastic fibroma. Oral Surg., *20:* 269, 1965.
18. Hardy, R., and Lehrer, H.: Desmoplastic fibroma vs. desmoid tumor of bone. Radiology, *88:* 899, 1967.
19. Jaffe, H.L.: Tumors and Tumorous Conditions of the Bones and Joints. pp. 298–303. Philadelphia, Lea & Febiger, 1958.
20. Nilsonne, U., and Gothlin, G.: Desmoplastic fibroma of bone. Acta Orthop. Scand., *40:* 205, 1969.
21. Randelli, G.: I Fibromi Desmoidi Dell'Osso. Arch. Di. Ortho., *77:* 523, 1964.
22. Scheer, G., and Kuhlman, R.: Vertebral involvement by desmoplastic fibroma. J.A.M.A., *185:* 669, 1963.
23. Unni, K., Dahlin, D.C., McLeoid, R.A., and Pritchard, D.J.: Intraosseous well-differentiated osteosarcoma. Cancer, *40:* 1337, 1977.
24. Whitesides, T.E., and Ackerman, L.V.: Desmoplastic Fibroma. J. Bone Joint Surg., *42A:* 1143, 1960.

Fibrosarcoma of Bone

24a. Brozmanova. E., and Skrovina, B.: Osseous fibrosarcoma-laboratory and clinical evaluation. Acta Chir. Orthop. Traumatol. Cech., *42:* 454, 1975.
25. Cunningham, M.P., and Arlen, M.: Medullary fibrosarcoma. Cancer, *21:* 31, 1963.
26. Dahlin, D.C., and Ivins, J.C.: Fibrosarcoma of bone. Cancer, *23:* 35, 1969.
27. Eyre-Brook, A.L., and Price, C.H.G.: Fibrosarcoma of bone. J. Bone Joint Surg., *51B:* 20, 1969.
28. Gilmer, W.S., Jr., and MacEwen, G.D.: Central (medullary) fibrosarcoma of bone. J. Bone Joint Surg., *40A:* 121, 1958.
29. McKenna, R.J., Schwinn, C.P., Soong, K.Y., and Higinbotham, N.L.: Sarcomata of the osteogenic series. J. Bone Joint Surg., *48A:* 1, 1966.
30. McLeod, J.J., Dahlin, D.C., and Ivins, J.C.: Fibrosarcoma of Bones. Am. J. Surg., *94:* 431, 1957.
31. Nielsen, A.R., and Poulsen, H.: Multiple diffuse fibrosarcomata of the bones. Acta Path. Microbiol. Scand., *55:* 265, 1962.
32. Steiner, P.E.: Multiple diffuse fibrosarcoma of bone. Am. J. Pathol., *20:* 877, 1944.
33. Stout, A.P.: Fibrosarcoma. Cancer, *1:* 30, 1948.

Primary Malignant Fibrous Histiocytoma (Histiosarcoma) of Bone

34. Bednar, B.: Storiform neurofibromas of the skin, pigmented and nonpigmented. Cancer, *10:* 368, 1957.
35. Dahlin, D.C., Unni, K.K., and Matsuno, T.: Malignant (fibrous) histiocytoma of bone—fact and fancy? Cancer, *39:* 1508, 1977.
36. Dorfman, H.D., Norman, A., and Wolff, H.: Fibrosarcoma complicating bone infarction in a caisson worker. J. Bone Joint Surg., *48A:* 528, 1966.
37. Feldman, F., and Lattes, R.: Primary malignant fibrous histiocytoma (fibrous xanthoma) of bone. Skel. Radiol., *1:* 145, 1977.
38. Feldman, F.M., and Norman, D.: Intra- and extraosseous malignant histiocytoma (malignant fibrous xanthoma). Radiology, *104:* 497, 1972.
39. Fu, Y., Gabbiani, G. Kaye, G.I., and Lattes, R.: Malignant soft tissue tumors of probable histiocytic origin (malignant fibrous histiocytomas). General considerations and electron microscopic and tissue culture studies. Cancer, *35:* 176, 1975.
40. Furey, J.C., Ferrer-Torells, M., and Reagan, J.W.: Fibrosarcoma arising at the site of bone infarcts. A report of two cases. J. Bone Joint Surg., *42A:* 802, 1960.
41. Gothlin, G., and Ericsson, J.L.E.: The osteoclast. Review of ultrastructure, origin and structure function relationship. Clin. Orthop., *120:* 201, 1976.
42. Hoffman, E.: Ober das knollen treibende fibrosarkom der haut. Dermatol. Zeitschr., *43:* 1, 1943.
43. Huvos, A.G.: Primary malignant fibrous histiocytoma of bone. Clinicopathologic study of 18 patients. N.Y. State J. Med., *76:* 552, 1976.
44. Michael, R.H., and Dorfman, H.D.: Malignant fibrous histiocytoma associated with bone infarcts. Clin. Orthop., *118:* 180, 1976.
45. Mirra, J.M., *et. al.:* Malignant fibrous histiocytoma and osteosarcoma in association with bone infarcts. Report of four cases, two in caisson workers. J. Bone Joint Surg., *56A:* 932, 1974.
46. Mirra, J.M., Gold, R.H., and Marafiote, R.: Malignant (fibrous) histiocytoma arising in association with a bone infarct in sickle-cell disease: coincidence or cause-and-effect? Cancer, *39:* 186, 1977.
47. Ozello, L., Stout, A.P., and Murray, M.R.: Cultural characteristics of malignant histiocytomas and fibrous xanthomas. Cancer, *16:* 331, 1963.
48. Ponseti, I.V., and Friedman, B.: Evolution of metaphyseal fibrous defects. J. Bone Joint Surg., *31A:* 582, 1949.

49. Spanier, S.S., Enneking, W.F., and Enriquez, P.: Primary malignant fibrous histiocytoma of bone. Cancer, *36:*2084, 1975.
50. Stansfeld, A.G.: Non-osteogenic fibroma of bone. J. Bone Joint Surg., *38B:*714, 1956.
51. Stout, A.P., and Lattes, R.: Tumors of the soft tissues. AFIP Fase. I, Second Series (1967), Washington D.C., p. 44.
52. Stout, A.D.: Fibrous tumors of the soft tissues. Minn. Med., *43:*455, 1960.
53. Taylor, H.B., and Helwig, E.B.: Dermatofibrosarcoma protuberans. A study of 115 cases. Cancer, *15:*717, 1962.
54. Yumoto, T., Mori, Y., Inada, O., and Tanaka, T.: Malignant fibrous histiocytoma of bone. Acta Pathol. Jap., *26:*295, 1976.

INTRAOSSEOUS GIANT-CELL-PRODUCING TUMORS

10

There are numerous giant-cell-producing tumors of the bone. These include benign tumorous conditions, infections, histiocytoses, and "giant cell" neoplasms. Unless a reasonable formulation of giant cells is developed, it will be difficult to determine the histogenesis of each, and the other cells and tissues with which each is associated. It is not difficult with this group of tumors to mistake a benign entity for a malignant one, and vice versa. Quite often therapy differs radically from one entity to another. Accurate diagnosis is of paramount importance.

DEFINITIONS USED IN THIS CHAPTER

HISTIOCYTE. A histiocyte is a cell that functions as a phagocyte. Histiocytes are rich in lysosomes and acid phosphatases. There are at least five kinds of histiocytes: the hematopoietic histiocytes or monocytes; the histiocytes of the connective tissues; the histiocytes of reticuloendothelial organs, which include the Kupffer and littoral cells; the histiocytes involved with bone resorption or the osteoclasts; and the histiocytes of the central nervous system or microglial cells.

The hematopoietic, connective tissues, reticuloendothelial, and microglial histiocytes respond to infection, necrosis of tissues, foreign bodies, and disorders of lipid metabolism. They are involved in numerous benign and malignant processes. The malignant fibrous histiocytoma, for example, is an expression of a connective-tissue histiocyte that has transformed to a malignant neoplasm. Tissue histiocytes may take various guises: mononuclear *epithelioid cells* (sarcoidosis, tuberculosis, fungal infections, eosinophilic granuloma); large *granular, foamy to lipid-rich macrophages* (response to tissue necrosis, Gaucher's disease, eosinophilic granuloma, *etc.*), *multinucleated giant cells* formed by the fusion of mononuclear histiocytes (Langhans' cells of tuberculosis, foreign body giant cells, fungal infections, *etc.*). Tissue histiocytes may also transform from rounded mononuclear to spindle, collagen-producing cells. Stout refers to histiocytes of this type as *facultative fibroblasts.*[2] Because of this tremendous variation in features a histiocytic lesion may be composed in whole, or in part, of granular, monocyte-like mononuclear histiocytes, foamy to lipidic macrophages, foamy to massively lipid-laden giant cells, and fibroblast-like cells. Cells with identical features may be seen in various bone tumors and infections. Lesions of bone in which connective tissue and reticuloendothelial histiocytes play a prominent role include eosinophilic granuloma, tuberculosis, fungal infections, sarcoidosis, Gaucher's diseases, nonossifying fibroma, malignant fibrous histiocytoma, and Hodgkin's disease, and in the reparative or degenerative areas of chondroblastoma, chondromyxoid fibroma, and bone infarcts.

In contrast, the osteoclast is a cell rich in phosphatases and lysosomes and a characteristic brush border whose only well known phagocytic function is the resorption of calcified tissue. Its purpose is the remodeling of bone and calcified cartilage and to aid in calcium homeostasis. The exact origin of this cell is not known but it is presumed *not* to be related to the stem cell that gives rise to the osteoblast or the chondroblast. Cross transfusions in closely bred rats having osteopetrosis with those without this disease have shown that the stem cell is a circulating cell. In osteopetrosis, osteoclasts are present but they are unable to resorb bone. These abnormal osteoclasts lack the necessary brush border and perhaps have one or more enzyme defects, which result in their failure to resorb bone. After cross-circulation with normals the osteopetrotic rats develop bone-resorbing osteoclasts with a normal brush border and the appropriate enzyme systems. The use of millipore filters prevents the reversal of the disease, indicating that a circulating cell is present in the normal donor with the potential to form functioning osteoclasts.

MULTINUCLEATED GIANT CELL. We will define a multinucleated giant cell as a cell that contains two or more separate and distinct nuclei set in abundant cytoplasm. These would include the Reed-Sternberg cells, Langhans and foreign body giant cells, osteoclasts, and osteoclast-like giant cells. The conditions in which these cells may be seen include TB, sarcoid, fungus infections, Hodgkin's disease, eosinophilic granuloma, neoplastic giant cell tumor, benign giant cell tumor of Paget's disease and hyperparathyroidism, osteogenic sarcoma, giant cell or osteoclastic sarcoma, and numerous other conditions to be described in this chapter.

MULTILOBULATED GIANT CELLS. The only giant cell with a multilobulated nucleus common to normal bone is the megakaryocyte. Multilobulated giant cells may be seen in reticulum cell sarcoma, malignant fibrous histiocytoma, Hodgkin's disease, giant cell sarcoma, osteogenic sarcoma, metastatic carcinoma, metastatic melanoma, and megakaryocytic myelosis.

OSTEOCLASTS are cells that contain several oval, separate and distinct nuclei that are found in direct apposition to bone (Figs. 10–8 and 10–10). They are responsible for bone remodeling and maintenance of calcium homeostasis. They are stimulated to activity under the control of parathormone, stress, pressure, and perhaps electrical forces. They are rich in acid phosphatases and can dissolve calcified tissues by secretions of enzymes at the region of their brush-border contact with bone or calcified cartilage. In essence, they are specialized histiocytes whose primary function is bone resorption. They apparently form by syncytial aggregation from mononuclear cells, as mitoses are never observed in the osteoclast. Osteoclasts are usually prominent in osteoid osteoma, osteoblastoma, hyperparathyroidism, active Paget's disease, many osteosarcomas, and at the resorptive margins of almost any bone tumor.

BENIGN OSTEOCLAST-LIKE GIANT CELLS are cells that are histologically identical to osteoclasts, except that they are not found in direct apposition to bone (Fig. 10–53). Although these cells are probably of osteoclastic origin they do not conform to the strict definition of an osteoclast and will henceforth be termed *osteoclast-like giant cell.* They may form large tumor masses in association with excessive parathormone stimulation (giant cell tumor of hyperparathyroidism), Paget's disease, benign giant cell tumor of Paget's, or with the primary low-grade neoplastic giant cell tumor (osteoclastoma). In a number of conditions, benign osteoclast-like giant cells appear to form as "reactive" fortuitous passengers in association with tumors of nonosteoclastic origin, such as the nonossifying fibroma, chondroblastoma, osteosarcoma, fibrosarcoma, eosinophilic granuloma, fibrous dysplasia, solitary and aneurysmal bone cysts, and giant cell reparative granuloma. Rarely do these latter entities produce the diffuse or massive concentrations of benign osteoclast-like cells seen in tumors of probable osteoclastic origin such as the neoplastic giant cell tumor (GCT) or the GCT's of hyperparathyroidism or Paget's disease.

ANAPLASTIC OSTEOCLAST-LIKE GIANT CELLS are cells with individual nuclei that show unequivocal anaplasia and a distribution of nuclei and cytoplasmic characteristics that closely mimic otherwise benign osteoclasts or osteoclast-like giant cells. Cells such as these are seen in the giant cell sarcoma (osteoclastic sarcoma). In some cases myriads of such cells can be seen (Figs. 10–65 and 10–66); in others only a few such cells are apparent to suggest their possible osteoclastic histogenesis.

According to the hypothesis formulated by Ozello, Stout, and Murray,[1] histiocytes can transform to fibroblasts. Since osteoclasts are a specialized form of histiocyte they should also be associated with variable degrees of fibrosarcoma-like malignant fibrous histiocytoma areas with a storiform pattern (Figs. 10–68–10–70). Fibrosarcoma of bone is distinguishable from osteoclastic sarcoma in that it is neither associated with prominent anaplastic, multinucleated, osteoclast-like giant cells nor rounded to polygonal, granular to foamy, malignant, mononuclear stromal cells.

BENIGN HISTIOCYTIC GIANT CELLS. We will define benign histiocytic giant cells as those cells that resemble foreign body and Langhans-type giant cells and tissue histiocytes with abundant foamy, vacuolated or "crumpled paper" cytoplasm (Gaucher's disease). Sometimes it is not possible to distinguish a giant cell as being of either osteoclastic or connective-tissue histiocytic origin by analysis of the histologic features of the giant cells alone. Diagnosis depends on careful inspection of the stromal tissues seen in association with the giant cells.

ANAPLASTIC HISTIOCYTIC GIANT CELLS. These cells may contain multiple separate or multilobulated nuclei. The nuclei must show features of unequivocal anaplasia. Anaplastic giant cells of tissue histiocytic or nonosteoclastic origin are seen in Hodgkin's disease, malignant fibrous histiocytoma, and reticulum cell sarcoma. In Hodgkin's disease the anaplastic cells are characterized by two to eight centrally located, usually separate nuclei with large pink nucleoli and a "spoke-wheel" pattern of chromatin distribution, the so-called Reed-Sternberg cell (Plate 9–*E, F*). Another distinguishing feature peculiar to Hodgkin's disease is that these cells are found in association with variable quantities of benign, chronic inflammatory cells, eosinophils, foamy histiocytes, and fibrous tissue. Malignant fibrous histiocytoma usually contains anaplastic multilobulated histiocytic giant cells (Figs. 9–51 to 9–53) in association with variable quantities of anaplastic granular to foamy macrophages and fibrosarcoma-like tissues. Reticulum cell sarcoma is composed of sheets of anaplastic rounded histiocytes with single to multilobulated nuclei (Plate 9, *G, H*).

ANAPLASTIC GIANT CELLS OF NONHISTIOCYTIC, NONOSTEOCLASTIC ORIGIN. Anaplastic giant cells with either separate or multilobulated nuclei may be found in tumors of nonhistiocytic and nonosteoclastic origin. Bizarre giant cells may be found in high-grade anaplastic metastatic carcinomas, melanomas, and osteogenic sarcomas. In these instances diagnosis depends on the demonstration of such findings as mucin production, glands, squamous "pearls," melanin pigment, malignant osteoid, bone or cartilage, or a history of a proven primary carcinoma or melanoma.

The reader is urged to compare and contrast the illustrations of the various types and range of giant cell features found in each condition that are found in this and subsequent chapters. Numbers of nuclei, separate versus multilobulated nuclei, central versus peripheral placement, size of nucleoli, absence or presence of anaplasia, cytoplasmic characteristics, and the surrounding stromal milieu in which the giant cells are placed are all essential factors in histologic interpretation.

BENIGN LESIONS

Osteoid Osteoma and Osteoblastoma

These two benign lesions are virtually indistinguishable on high-power examination. They often contain numerous osteoclasts in a setting of intense osteoid and bone proliferation (Figs. 7–23 and 7–24 and Plate 2, *G*). They do not form masses of giant cells embedded in a stroma as occurs in the neoplastic giant cell tumor of epiphyses or as in the giant cell tumor of hyperparathyroidism. They must be distinguished from the intramedullary osteosarcoma (pp. 153, 351, and 362, Figs. 7–73–7–77 and Plates 3 and 4, inclusive).

Hyperparathyroidism

FIG. 10–1. Rare epiphyseal presentation of a giant cell tumor of hyperparathyroidism. The lesion is huge, lytic, and has well-demarcated borders. It is surrounded by a thin border of periosteal new bone, a sign of slow growth. High-grade malignant tumors of this size would lack this feature. The striking similarity, both radiologically and pathologically, of the neoplastic and the hyperparathyroid GCT emphasizes the need to obtain serum calcium and phosphorous for all cases of GCT.

FIG. 10–2. Multiple brown tumors of tibia resulting from chronic hyperparathyroidism.

FIG. 10–3. Radiographs of the hands are important to review in suspected cases of hyperparathyroidism. This is because the radiographic changes are often subtle and the obscuring effects to the soft tissues of the hands are relatively minor, compared to those of the leg or arm. This radiograph shows that the bones are osteoporotic and the cortices thinned. The medial portions of the phalanges show resorption (*arrows*), a virtually pathognomonic sign of hyperparathyroidism.

FIG. 10–4. When present, medial resorption of the cortices of the phalanges (*a*) is a pathognomonic sign of hyperparathyroidism. Other characteristic features that are present on this radiograph include blurring of the normally sharp cortical border of the terminal phalangeal tuft (*b*), loss of demarcation between the cortical and intramedullary borders, and cortical resorption canals (*c*) that are thin and smaller than 1 mm. wide by several mm. long. These resorption canals result from osteoclasts tunneling their way through and enlarging the cortical haversian systems.

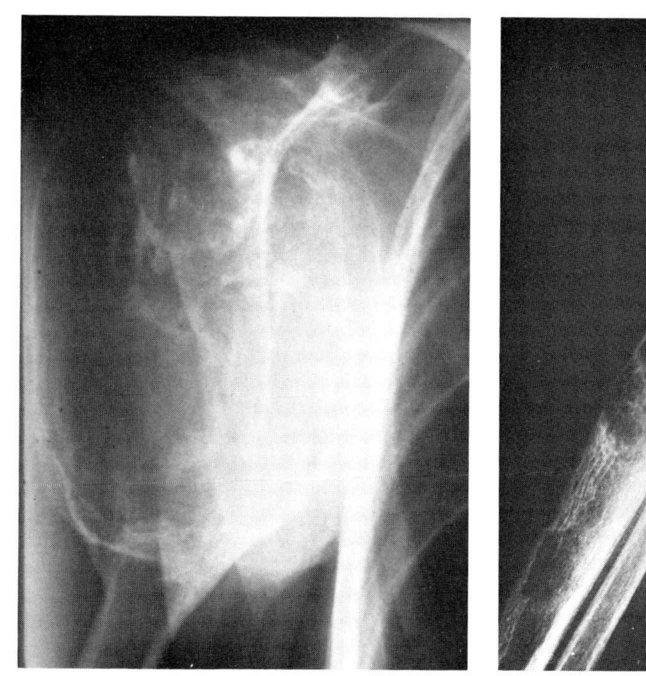

FIG. 10-1

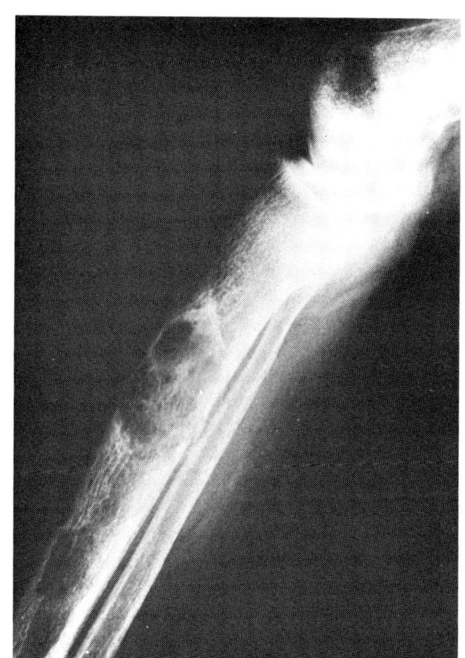

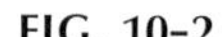

FIG. 10-2

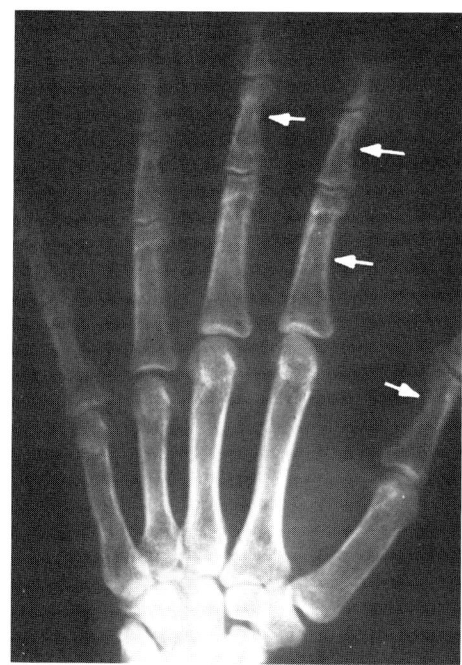

FIG. 10-3

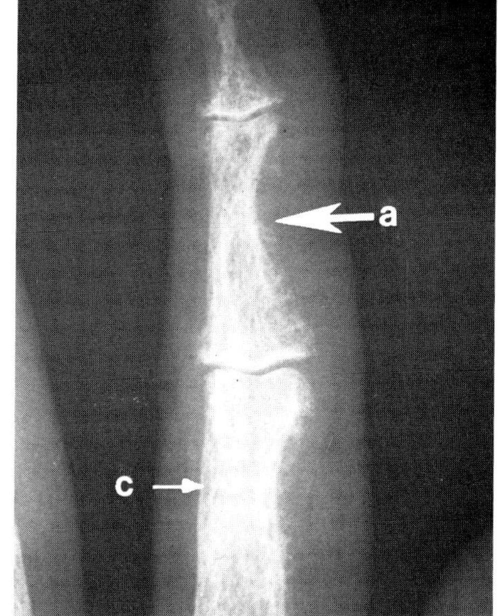

FIG. 10-4

PRIMARY HYPERPARATHYROIDISM

Occasionally patients with hyperparathyroidism may present with a solitary bone tumor that may mimic the low-grade neoplastic giant cell tumor of epiphyses in every aspect, both radiologically and histologically (Figs. 10–1 and 10–9). It is wise policy to have at least three serum calcium's and phosphorous' of every patient with a suspected neoplastic giant cell tumor in order to rule out a hyperparathyroid giant cell tumor. In this author's experience, for every 20 biopsied neoplastic giant cell tumors (GCT) of bone, one is in actuality a GCT of hyperparathyroidism.

The features that should alert the pathologist to the diagnosis of a hyperparathyroid giant cell tumor are the following:

1. Location within the diaphysis or metaphysis of long bones (Fig. 10–2). Most cases of hyperparathyroidism occur in these areas. The neoplastic giant cell tumor almost always involves a bone end and rarely affects the metaphysis or diaphysis alone. It is rare, but nevertheless possible, for the hyperparathyroid GCT to present as an epiphyseal lesion (Fig. 10–1).
2. Multiple "giant cell tumors" of bone. These cases are usually due to either hyperparathyroidism or multifocal eosinophilic granuloma masquerading as a giant cell tumor (Figs. 10–20–10–21). The neoplastic giant cell tumor of bone has been reported as a multifocal entity extremely rarely (<1 per cent of the total).[91a]
3. Focal extensive hemorrhages and broad bands of fibrous tissue (Fig. 10–9). These changes are more usual to hyperparathyroidism than to the neoplastic GCT. However, these features are occasionally seen in neoplastic GCT and represents the weakest aid to diagnosis.
4. If areas of bone are examined away from the main mass of GCT, areas of marrow fibrosis associated with osteoclastic resorption canals are indicative of the osteitis fibrosa reaction of hyperparathyroidism (Figs. 10–7 and 10–8). The neoplastic GCT will not be associated with this reaction at a site distant from the main tumor mass. Hyperparathyroidism is a systemic disease; the neoplastic GCT, a purely localized tumor.

The diagnosis of primary hyperparathyroidism can be confirmed by:

A. Elevated serum calcium and depressed serum phosphorous levels.

B. Elevation of parathormone by assay.

C. Radiological changes indicative of a diffuse metabolic disorder, such as loss of the lamina dura of the teeth, blurring of the distal phalangeal cortical tuft, cortical resorption canals, and medial resorption of the phalanges, a pathognomonic sign (Figs. 10–3 and 10–4) salt-and-pepper skull (Figs. 10–5 and 10–6) and in some patients, increased density of the subchondral bone, compared to the lucency of the centrum of the vertebral bodies similar to the pattern of a rugby jersey (the so-called "Rugger Jersey" spine). Not all of these radiological features may be present in any one case, however.

The basic histologic process in primary hyperparathyroidism is bone resorption. The earliest change histologically is a front of osteoclasts tunneling through either the spongy or cortical bone (Fig. 10–7), which accounts for the characteristic cortical resorption canals seen on radiograph (Fig. 10–4, *C*). The adjacent marrow is converted into a loose fibrous tissue that may cuff a portion or all of a bone spicule (Fig. 10–8). As the process continues, much of the marrow may be converted into fibrous tissue in which are embedded variable numbers of osteoclasts resorbing the bone surface. Bone formation occurs, concomitantly, in an attempt to replace the weakened bone structure. This is evidenced by a flurry of osteoblastic activity and osteoid and woven bone production. However, the new bone that is deposited is resorbed as quickly as it is laid down. During this stage it is impossible to distinguish hyperparathyroidism histologically from the florid, early active phase of Paget's disease (Fig. 10–10).

As the process continues, multiple adjacent but

Hyperparathyroidism

FIG. 10-5. "Salt and pepper" appearance in the skull of a patient with hyperparathyroidism. This is due to innumerable areas of osteoclastic resorption.

FIG. 10-6. Skull with a much more advanced stage of hyperparathyroidism showing a fluffy appearance and large zones of lysis seen in this case particularly in the frontal and occipital areas.

FIG. 10-7. The bone trabeculae show tunnel-like resorption by osteoclasts, particularly at *a* and *b*. The fatty marrow shows conversion to fibrous tissue (x40).

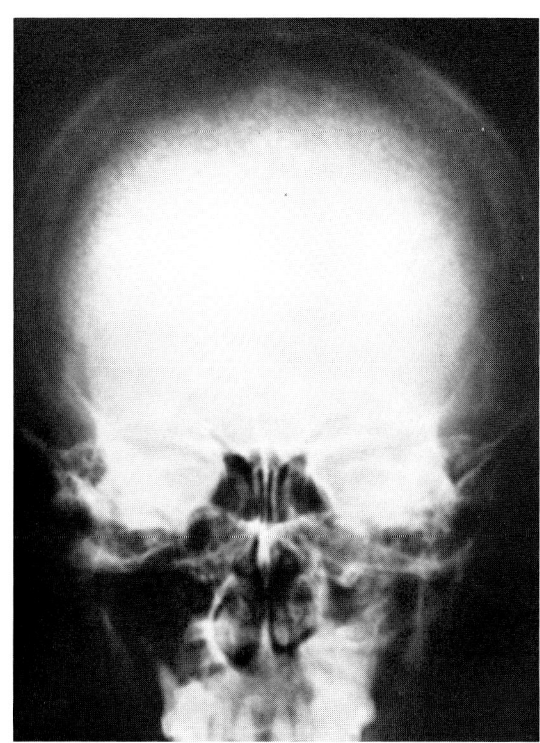

FIG. 10-5

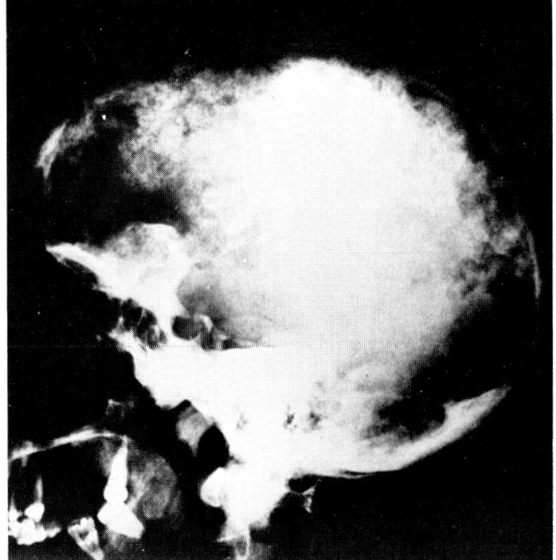

FIG. 10-6

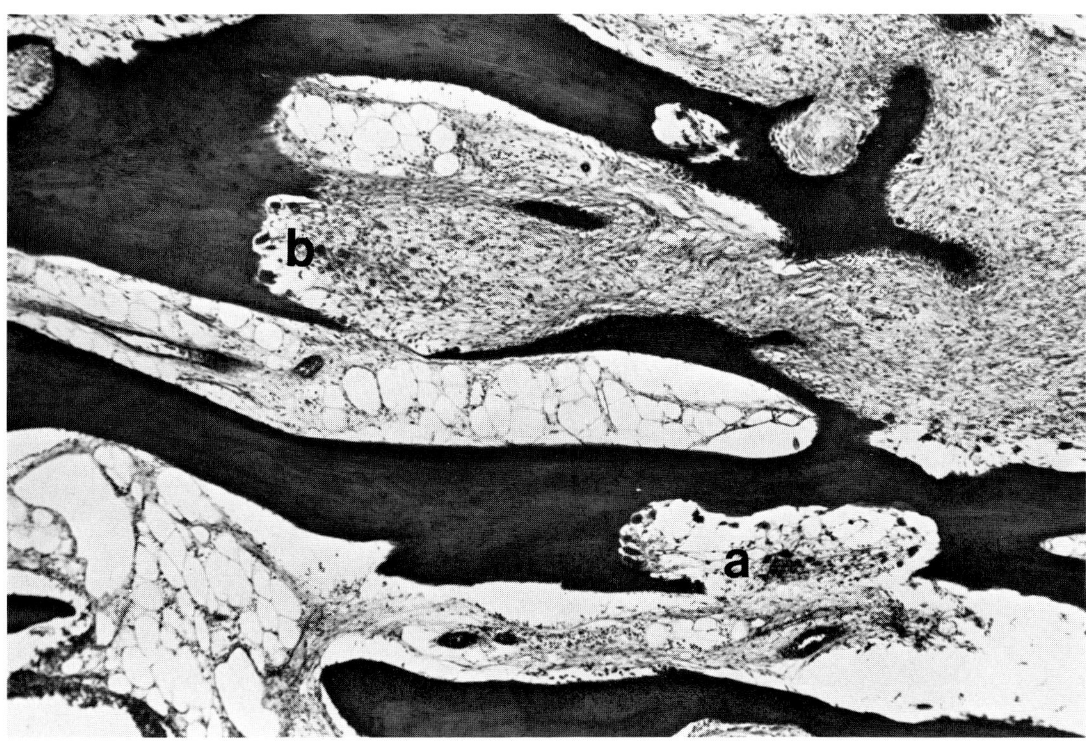

FIG. 10-7

nodular foci of giant cells embedded in a loose fibrovascular stroma develop. These microscopic nodules then coalesce to form macroscopic nodules, the so-called "brown tumors" of hyperparathyroidism; these nodules are readily visible on radiographs as cystic uni- or multilocular lesions (Figs. 10–1 and 10–2). These nodules (Fig. 10–9) may be histologically indistinguishable from the true neoplastic giant cell tumor of bone.

PAGET'S DISEASE

CAPSULE SUMMARY

Incidence. May be an extremely common disease of adults, particularly in its milder forms. In a series of 4,614 autopsies in patients over 40 years of age, Schmorl[14] estimated the incidence of Paget's disease, in persons of European descent to be as high as 3.3 per cent. It occurs frequently in the same family.

Age. Most patients are over 50. Rare before age 20.

Areas of Involvement. Any bone or bones may be affected, but predominantly it affects the long bones, pelvis, and skull. Usually affects the bones bilaterally and symmetrically in polyostotic disease.

Clinical Features. Pain, bone deformities, increasing head size, kyphosis, deafness, prominent temporal vessels, audible bruit over skull.

Laboratory. Alkaline phosphatase usually elevated; this correlates with degree of involvement and activity of the disease process.

Gross Pathology. *Early Stage:* Bone porous and violaceous. *Later stage:* The bone becomes more dense and compact, with a pumice stone appearance. Individual trabeculae and marrow spaces more irregular in size and shape. The cortex becomes irregularly thickened. *Late stage:* There is marked alteration of the normal architecture and loss of demarcation between cortex and spongiosa (Figs. 10–18, 10–19, *B*).

Histopathology. *Early phase:* Marked osteoclastic activity, fibrosis of marrow, thinning of trabeculae, and woven bone production. (This phase is indistinguishable from hyperparathyroidism.) *Later phase:* The bony trabeculae become more compact and cement lines more prominent, imparting a "jigsaw puzzle" or mosaic pattern. *Late phase:* Dense bone with prominent mosaic pattern; diminution of osteoblastic and osteoclastic activity.

Course. Variable. Approximately 10 per cent of patients with severe multifocal disease will develop osteogenic sarcoma, fibrosarcoma, or malignant giant cell (osteoclastic) sarcoma. These tumors result in rapid metastases, with fewer than 10 per cent of patients surviving five years.

Histologic Features

The histologic pattern in the early phase of Paget's may be indistinguishable from hyperparathyroidism (Figs. 10–7, 10–8, and 10–10). The mosaic pattern seen later in the course of Paget's disease is due to woven or lamellar bone deposition and prominent cement lines appearing where one focus of bone deposition meets another (Figs. 10–11 and 10–12). This feature is characteristic of Paget's disease, but not pathognomonic, since it may also be found in chronic repair processes that affect bone, such as fracture callus, chronic osteomyelitis, and chronic or treated resolving hyperparathyroidism. With polarized light the mosaic bone in Paget's disease is usually seen as a mixture of lamellar and woven bone (Fig. 10–13) or pure woven bone. If the bone has been overdecalcified the cement lines may not stain well by routine H and E. Staining for reticulin will usually reveal the cement lines as unstained structures.

Since the histologic features are often subtle and may be mimicked by other entities, a detailed description of the radiological features of Paget's disease are included to help better correlate clinicopathologic findings.

Radiologic Features

Paget's disease can be divided into three radiological phases: an early lytic phase, a mixed lytic and blastic phase, and a late blastic phase.

The lytic phase corresponds histologically to the pattern of marked osteoclastic bone resorption and fibrosis of the marrow (Fig. 10–10). The blastic phase corresponds to a diminution of osteoclastic resorption

Hyperparathyroidism

FIG. 10–8. A front of osteoclasts (left side of illustration) chew away at the bone, forming a tunnel-like dissolution. The results of this tunneling by osteoclasts is seen in high-quality radiographs (Fig. 10–4). Note also the conversion of the marrow to a cellular fibrous tissue. This field corresponds to the area marked *b* on the previous illustration (x250).

FIG. 10–9. Low-power histology of giant cell tumor of hyperparathyroidism. This lesion may be indistinguishable from a neoplastic GCT. As this field shows, however, hyperparathyroidism tends to be characterized by greater degrees of hemorrhage and fibrosis when compared to primary, untreated, neoplastic GCT (x40).

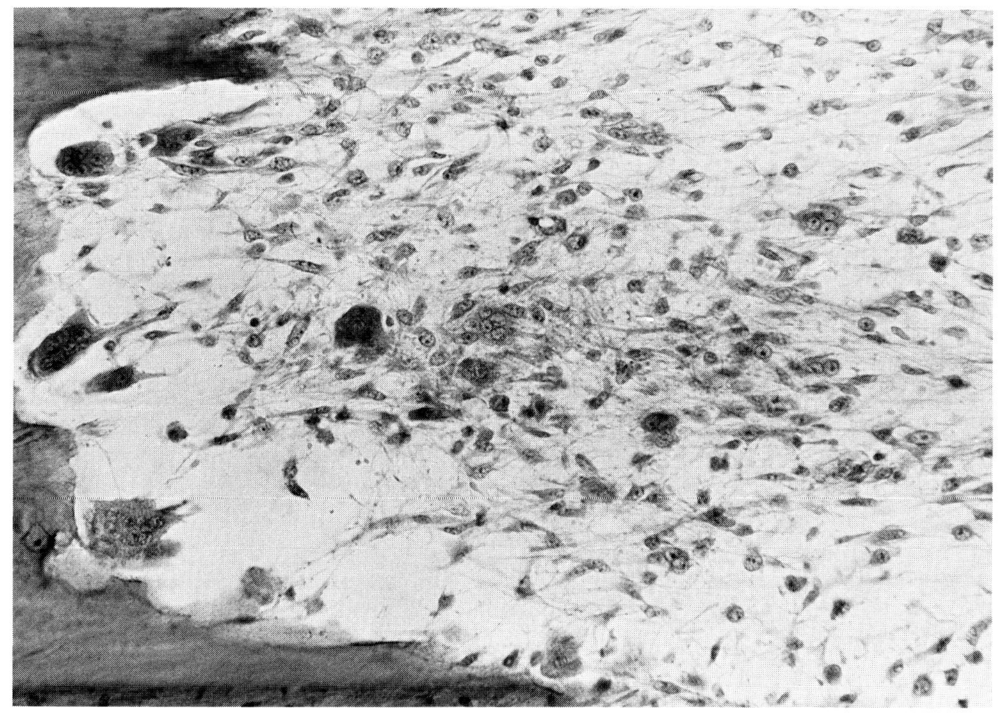

FIG. 10-8

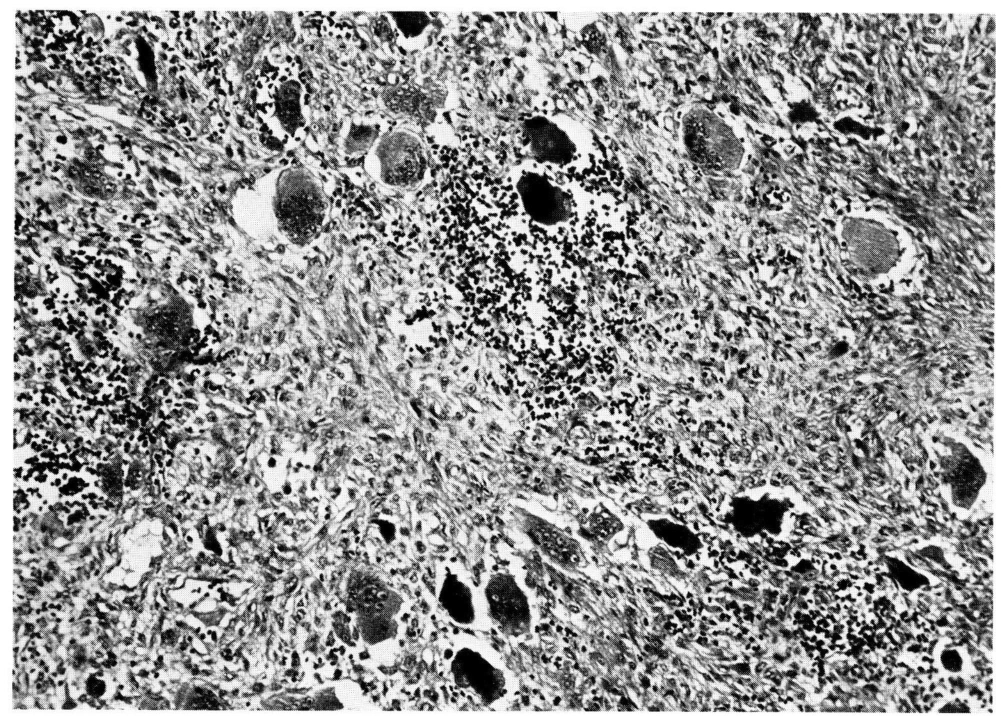

FIG. 10-9

and deposition of dense bone with a mosaic pattern (Fig. 10–12). Radiologically and pathologically, Paget's disease begins as a diffuse advancing osteolysis with sharply defined margins. In long bones the process begins as an advancing wedge with a characteristic "V" or "cutting-cone" shape usually beginning at one end of the bone (Figs. 10–14 and 10–15). In the skull, the early lysis due to Paget's disease results in a lesion referred to as "osteoporosis circumscripta" (Fig 10–16). Later in its course, as new bone is deposited the skull develops the pattern likened to "cotton wool" (Fig. 10–17). The cortical bone and trabeculae become thicker and more irregular in outline. In the late stage the bone trabeculae may become quite thick, particularly those along the lines of stress (Figs. 10–18 and 10–19). The cortical bone thickens and becomes irregular in contour (Fig. 10–19). In very late stages the bone may become so dense that it simulates metastatic prostatic or breast carcinoma, or even osteopetrosis. Affected vertebral bodies may become so sclerotic that they may be designated "ivory vertebrae." The differential diagnosis of "ivory vertebrae" includes Hodgkin's disease and metastatic carcinoma. In the vertebral bodies the subcortical bone may be thickened, imparting a "picture frame" appearance (Figs. 13–53–13–54) or show prominent accentuation of the vertical trabeculae along the lines of stress. Severe Paget's disease may ultimately transform into bone sarcoma of various types, which include the osteosarcoma, fibrosarcoma, and osteoclastic sarcoma (Figs. 10–18, 10–62–10–70). These three tumors are histogenetically related to those cells that proliferate in association with Paget's disease, namely, the osteoblast, fibroblast, and osteoclast.

Giant Cell Tumor of Paget's Disease

Rarely, patients with Paget's disease may form one or more giant cell tumors indistinguishable, on histological grounds, from hyperparathyroidism (Fig. 10–9) or the low-grade neoplastic giant cell tumor (Figs. 10–52 and 10–53). The giant cell tumors associated with Paget's disease have a predilection for the skull and facial bones and not to the epiphyses of long bones, as does the neoplastic GCT.[6] According to Hutter, the course of giant cell tumor of Paget's disease is benign, even with simple procedures such as curettage. However, the number of reported cases is extremely small. A larger series will have to be accumulated before it can be determined whether the giant cell tumor of Paget's disease behaves with complete innocence when only simple procedures such as curettage are performed, or is a locally aggressive tumor similar to the giant cell tumor of epiphyses. Of the few cases reported in the long bones and ilium, some did behave with local aggressiveness.

Speculation About the Etiology and Pathogenesis of Paget's Disease

Sir James Paget considered that the disease that now bears his name was a peculiar form of infection and coined the term *osteitis deformans.* Recent electron microscopic studies[9,11] would suggest that Paget's concept of infection may have been remarkably ahead of his time. These recent studies have shown viral-like inclusion bodies only in the nuclei of the osteoclast of Paget's disease! Other diseases subjected to the same studies have been negative for this finding. These observations would imply that Paget's disease may possibly be a viral infection of osteoclasts. Would this assumption fit the observed clinicopathologic facts? As we have seen, the earliest recognizable phase of the disease is characterized by an advancing radiological zone of rarefaction ("osteoporosis circumscripta") and histologically, by an uncanny resemblance to early hyperparathyroidism, an unequivocal disorder of osteoclasts. Is it possible that a viral infection of osteoclasts causes these cells to be "turned on," so to speak, bypassing the usual parathormone-osteoclast stimulatory cycle? If this were the case, the early features of the disease are certainly understandable. The latter rich, bone-pro-

(*Text continues on p. 320.*)

Paget's Disease of Bone

FIG. 10-10. The early, florid, histologic phase of Paget's disease is characterized by severe osteoclastic activity and bland fibrous conversion of the fatty marrow. This phase is indistinguishable from hyperparathyroidism by microscopy alone and would correspond to an area of osteoporosis circumscripta or advancing wedge of rarefaction, such as is shown in Figs. 10-14 and 10-16 (x125).

FIG. 10-11. Midphase of Paget's disease. The trabeculae are thickened, showing areas of a mosaic or jigsaw puzzlelike pattern (*arrows*). There is considerable osteoclastic and osteoblastic activity and fibroblastic hyperplasia of the former fatty marrow (x125).

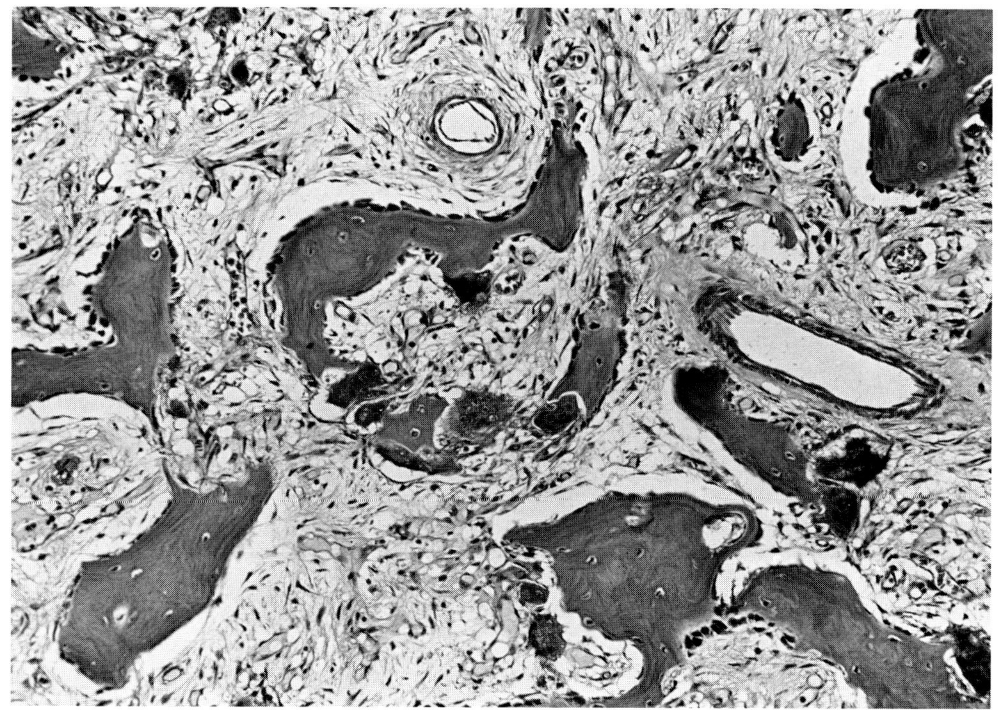

FIG. 10-10

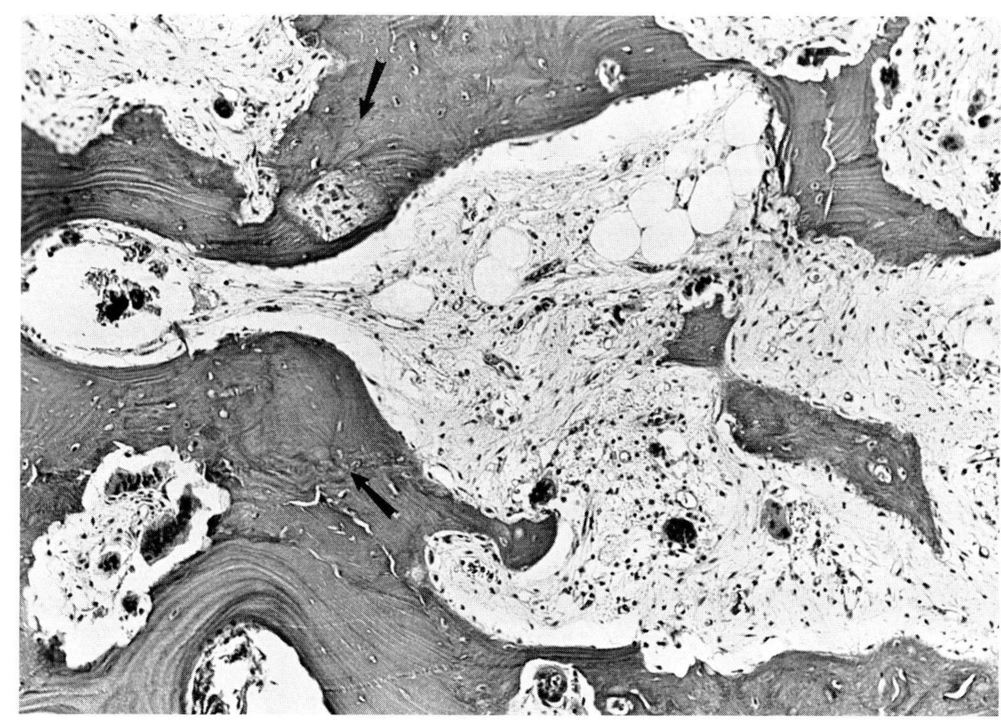

FIG. 10-11

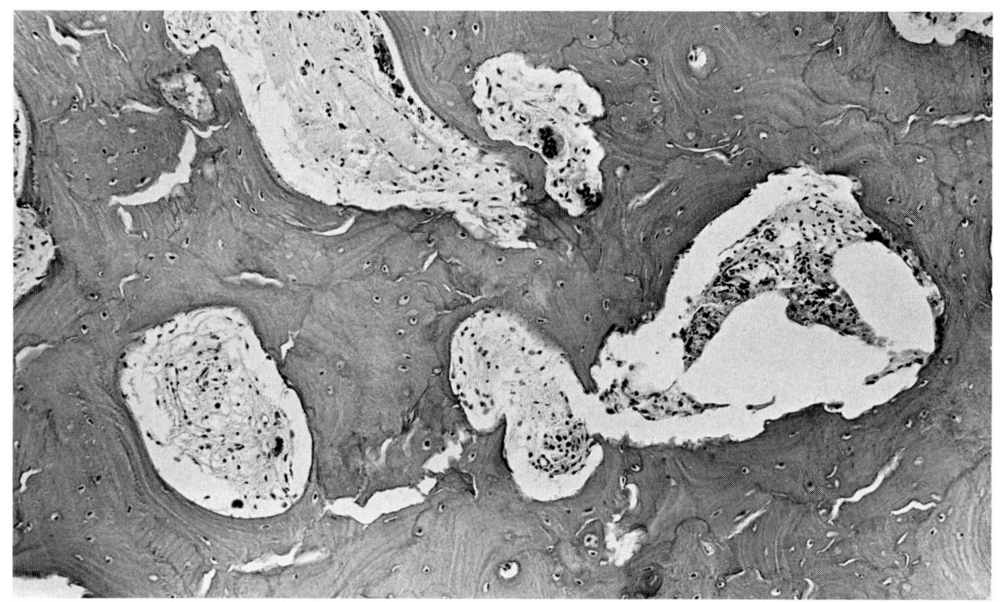

FIG. 10-12

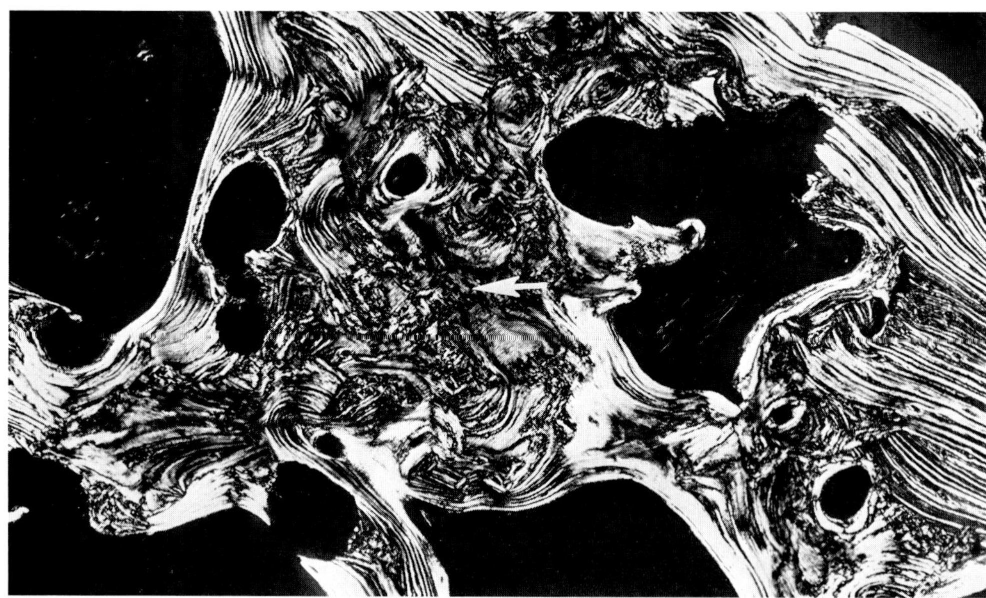

FIG. 10-13

Paget's Disease of Bone

FIG. 10-12. Advanced or late stage of Paget's disease. The trabeculae are very thick and show a prominent mosaic pattern. Osteoblastic and osteoclastic activity abate and the marrow fibrosis is less severe. Blood vessels are still conspicuously dilated, however. This type of bone would appear quite dense or fluffy on radiograph (Fig. 10-17) or as thick bone with a pumice stone quality in the gross (Fig. 10-19, *B*) (x125).

FIG. 10-13. Polarized light of dense Pagetoid bone shows a patchwork quilt of lamellar and weaker woven bone (*arrow*) (x125).

Table 10-1. The Pathogenesis of Paget's Disease of Bone—An Hypothesis

Observations
Viral-like bodies in nucleus of the osteoclasts of patients with Paget's disease only (53 out of 53 Paget's patients. Not seen in non-Paget's control patients).[9,11]
Similar inclusion bodies have been observed in: subacute sclerosing panencephalitis (measle-like virus), Kuru, Jacob-Kreutzfeldt disease, multifocal leukoencephalopathy, systemic lupus erythematosis, and the NZB mouse model system.

Hypotheses	
Let us assume the intranuclear particles observed on the osteoclasts of Paget's disease of bone are viral and they are cause-and-effect related.	Etiological hypothesis based upon recent ultramicroscopic findings[9,11]
Let us also assume that the infection of osteoclasts results in their overactivity.	Hypothesis to explain the tremendously increased osteoclastic activity seen particularly in the incipient and midphases of Paget's disease.

*With the above observation and two hypotheses, the various manifestations of Paget's disease are explainable. In other words, by assuming that the disease is an infectious disorder, as Sir James Paget originally suggested, but more specifically a viral infection of osteoclasts, the clinical, radiologic, and pathologic manifestations can be placed into a coherent system.

	Proposed Pathogenesis	*Comments and Manifestation*
INCIPIENT PHASE	Slow virus infection of osteoclasts that localizes in one or more bones ↓ Pathologic activation of osteoclasts (osteoclastitis) ↓ Severe localized bone resorption that slowly spreads through the affected bone	Osteoporosis circumscripta (earliest radiologic observation) Advancing wedge of resorption Possibility of pathologic fracture Increased numbers of osteoclasts and reactive fibroblasts (Early histologic phase indistinguishable from hyperparathyroidism)
	↓ Increased local stress due to resorption of bone trabeculae ↓	

(Continued)

Table 10-1. The Pathogenesis of Paget's Disease of Bone (Continued)

	Proposed Pathogenesis	*Comments and Manifestation*
MIDPHASE	Activation of osteoblasts (A 2° phenomenon induced by pathologic bone resorption)	Increased osteoblastic activity by microscopy
	↓	
	New bone will be concentrated along lines of increased stress by Wolff's law	Accentuation of stress lines Vertical striations in vertebral bodies, phalanges, *etc.* Woven bone, increased numbers of osteoblasts, osteoclasts, and fibroblasts
	↓	
	Continued assault by osteoclasts	
	↓	
	Massive 2° overactivity by osteoblasts	Increase in bone turnover Increased osteoblastic activity Rise in serum alkaline phosphatase New bone that is laid down is followed by waves of osteoclastic resorption. New woven bone in areas of focal bone resorption, resulting in production of "cement lines." Thick woven bone with numerous cement lines is characteristic of the mosaic pattern of Paget's. The mosaic pattern is merely a reflection of numerous sites of bone resorption and production. Phase of "fluffy" and "cotton-wool" exudates on radiography. All portions of the osseous tissue, cortex, and medulla affected. The bone that is forming rapidly is the weak woven variety. In order to make up for gross weakening, the bone increases in size.
	↓	

Table 10-1. The Pathogenesis of Paget's Disease of Bone (Continued)

	Proposed Pathogenesis	Comments and Manifestation
LATE PHASE	↓ After many years the infection abates or "burns out" in focal sites ↓	Massive bone damage has occurred over the years, leading to the production of a weak admixture of woven and lamellar bone that has a "pumice stone"-like appearance in gross examination. Structural integrity damaged. Increased numbers of pathologic fractures ("banana" and "fissure" fractures). Cortices irregularly thickened and undulating. Abnormal appearance of medullary trabeculae due to thickening and fracturing. Increased bone turnover associated with severe hypervascularity (audible bruits, increased cardiac output, high output failure). The new proliferative bone may interfere with passage of cranial and spinal nerves (in particular, deafness).
	Chronically damaged, high turnover of bony, osteoclastic, and fibroblastic tissue can result in malignant transformation in from 1–10% of patients with extensive disease	Three basic cell types are involved: the osteoblast, osteoclast, and fibroblast. It is from one of the three types that the malignant Paget's sarcomas arise. These would be (1) osteosarcoma, (2) osteoclastic sarcoma, and (3) fibrosarcoma. A benign hyperplastic tumor may develop in rare instances—the so-called benign giant cell tumor of Paget's disease. Usually they arise in skull bones and are indistinguishable on histological examination from hyperparathyroid GCT and GCT of epiphyses.

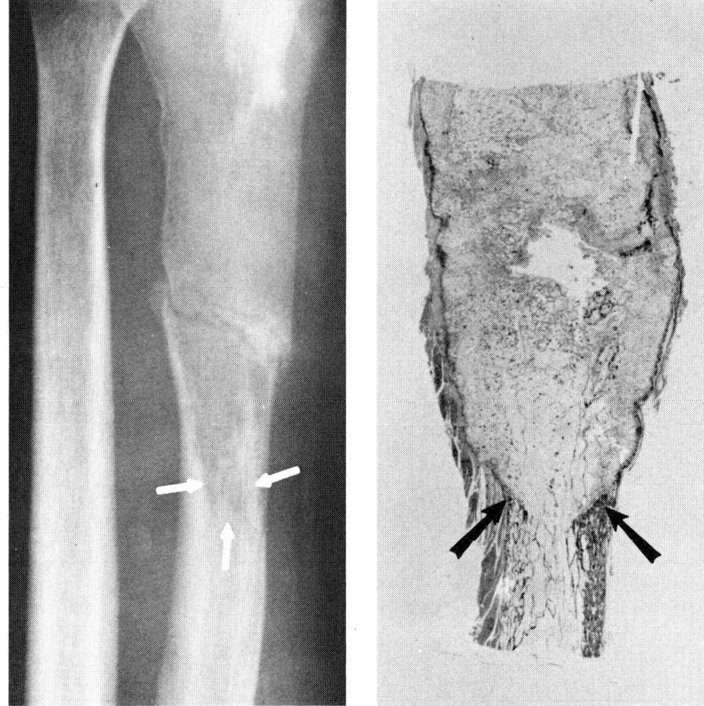

FIG. 10-14 FIG. 10-15

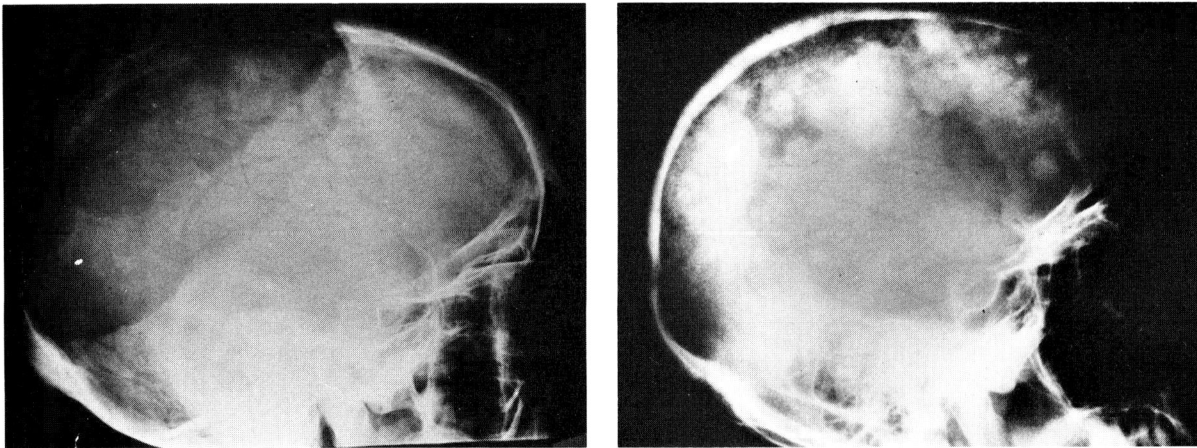

FIG. 10-16 FIG. 10-17

Paget's Disease of Bone

FIG. 10-14. Paget's disease begins as a focal area of lysis. In this patient the disease began in the tibia as an advancing wedge of lysis (*arrows*). Marked bone loss resulted in weakening and pathologic fracture. This appearance is virtually pathognomonic of Paget's disease. The lytic phase of Paget's is referred to as osteoporosis circumscripta.

FIG. 10-15. Low-power view of advancing wedge of osteoporosis (demarcated by *arrows*) and bone "expansion" consequent to early Paget's disease of the tibia (x1).

FIG. 10-16. Osteoporosis circumscripta of the skull, pathognomonic of Paget's disease.

FIG. 10-17. In later phases of the disease, dense Pagetoid bone laid down in areas of former lysis will result in "cotton wool" exudates.

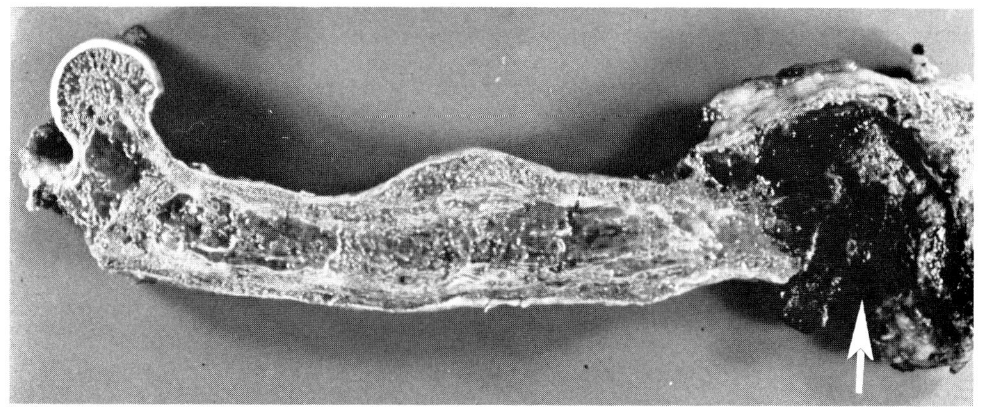

FIG. 10-18

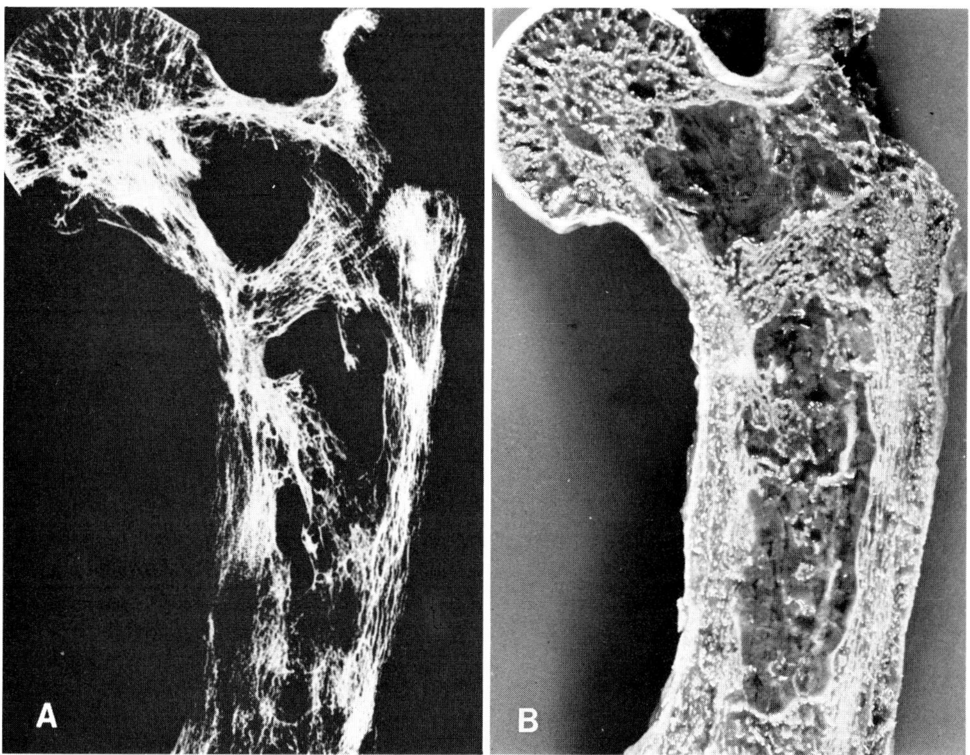

FIG. 10-19

Paget's Disease of Bone

FIG. 10-18. Gross specimen of a femur with an advanced stage of Paget's disease removed because of the development of a highly vascular osteogenic sarcoma of the distal metaphysis (*arrow*).

FIG. 10-19. (*A*) The specimen radiograph shows the characteristic features of advanced Paget's disease; namely, an irregular cortical outline, blurring of the cortical-medullary bone border, thickening of the bone trabeculae, particularly along the lines of stress, and dense, fluffy deposits of bone. (*B*) The corresponding gross specimen area shows the general disorganization, thickening, and the pumice stonelike granularity of the Paget's bone. In some areas there is complete loss of bone trabeculae; in areas of stress the bone trabeculae are two to three times normal thickness. The articular cartilage is unaffected by the disease process.

ductive phase of the disease could then be viewed as a proliferative osteoblastic response to repair by the bone that has been resorbed and weakened by the focal osteoclastic hyperactivity stimulated by the infection. Waves of osteoclastic resorption followed by hasty osteoblastic repair would result in the weakened mixture of woven to lamellar bone seen in this disease. If the disease is essentially one of osteoclasts rather than one of osteoblasts, the bone that is laid down as a secondary response would be expected to conform to Wolff's Law; that is, to be laid down along lines of stress. This is indeed the case in Paget's disease. However, since the bone is laid down in a hasty fashion and is subjected to further waves of osteoclastic resorption, it is less than fully mature and hence weaker than normal bone. It is, therefore, more prone to fracture and is less able to withstand stress. Eventually, however, the process of osteoclastic hyperactivity abates. This is followed by a phase of more intense bone deposition to shore up the weakened osseous structure. The final result is a bone consisting of an irregularly thickened cancellous and cortical structure whose gross appearance suggests pumice stone (Fig. 10–19, *B*). The thick bone merely reflects the weaker quality of the bone in the affected areas; more bone is necessary to withstand the same degree of stress. Normal lamellar bone can withstand ordinary stress with much reduced volume, compared to the abnormal congeries of woven and lamellar bone in areas affected by Paget's disease.

Three basic cell types are involved in the flurry of abnormal activity in association with Paget's disease: osteoclasts, osteoblasts, and fibroblasts. It is from these three cell types that virtually all of the tumors seen in association with this disease derive. These tumors include the benign giant cell tumor (benign osteoclastoma), malignant giant cell or osteoclastic sarcoma (Figs. 10–62–10–70), osteosarcoma (Fig. 10–18), and fibrosarcoma.

Please refer to Table 10–1 for a summary of an hypothesis relating a possible viral etiology to the structural, radiological, and clinical features noted in Paget's disease.

Since inflammation is an uncommon to absent component of Paget's disease, the term *osteitis deformans* is not precise. Unfortunately, we do not have a suffix meaning "infection of cell." However, if from future studies it is determined that Paget's disease is, indeed, caused by a viral infection of osteoclasts, and if, in this instance, it is understood to mean infection of, rather than inflammation of, the name Paget coined for the disease could be changed to a more appropriate etiologic designation standing for infection of osteoclasts leading to deformation (of the bones), namely, "osteoclastitis deformans."

Eosinophilic Granuloma

The solitary and multifocal eosinophilic granuloma (EG) may contain areas with prominent masses of osteoclast-like giant cells (Figs. 10–20 and 10–21). If attention is not given to the other components that characterize EG, such as eosinophils and/or granular, foamy to lipid macrophages, and concentrates on only the large giant cells, an incorrect diagnosis of neoplastic giant cell tumor is possible. The following example demonstrates the gravity of such a mistake.

This author had the opportunity of reviewing a case that began as a solitary lytic lesion in the tibial metaphysis of a 16-year-old female. Because of the giant cells seen (Fig. 10–20), a diagnosis of giant cell tumor was made. Several months later another lytic lesion was noted in the proximal femoral metaphysis. It was interpreted as not only a GCT, but as a metastatic lesion indicative of malignancy, and an amputation was performed. When we ultimately saw the patient 8 years later, she had lytic lesions of the long bones and skull and diabetes insipidus, virtually pathognomonic clinical signs of multifocal EG. The original slides, which showed, in addition to giant cells, eosinophils, plasma cells, and mononuclear macrophages were reviewed (Figs. 10–20 and 10–21). Biopsy of a bone lesion from her recent admission showed, in addition to giant cells, masses of intensely lipid-laden macrophages, fibrosis, and lymphocytes (Fig. 10–22), entirely consistent with the late stages of

---

Eosinophilic Granuloma

FIG. 10–20. On occasion the eosinophilic granuloma (EG) may contain numerous osteoclastlike giant cells and mimic a neoplastic GCT. Analysis of the stroma will usually reveal lymphocytes, plasma cells, eosinophils, and histiocytes rich in granular to foamy cytoplasm. This combination of cellular components is lacking in the neoplastic GCT (x250).

FIG. 10–21. The giant cells of EG can appear to form from or directly abut on vascular spaces (x400).

FIG. 10–22. Large areas of lipid-laden macrophages are very common in older lesions of EG. These cells are rarely found in the neoplastic GCT (x125).

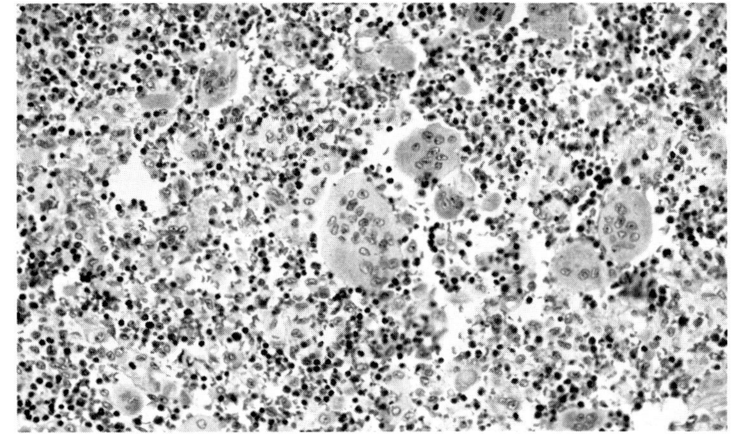

FIG. 10-20

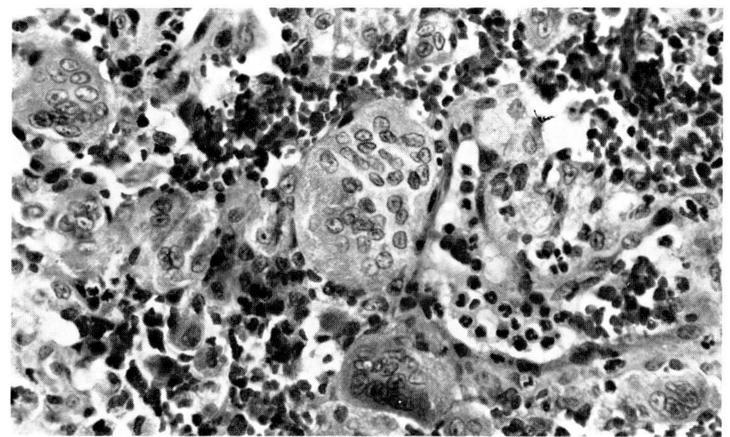

FIG. 10-21

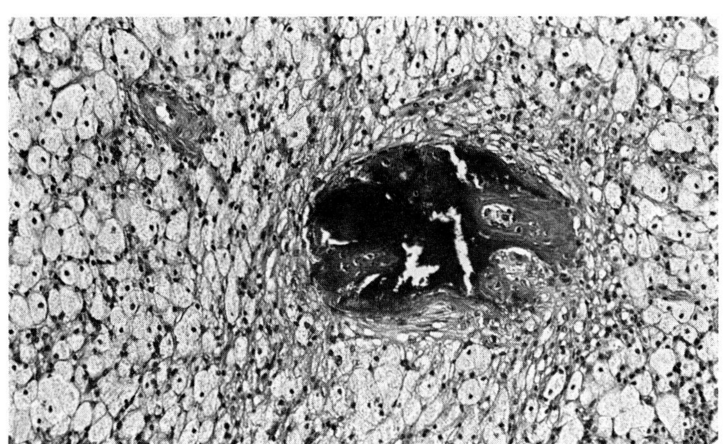

FIG. 10-22

EG. In order to protect against similar disasters in diagnosis and treatment, the diagnosis of an EG with numerous osteoclast-like giant cells should be considered whenever the following parameters are seen:

1. **ANY "GIANT CELL TUMOR" OF METAPHYSIS OR DIAPHYSIS.** EG only rarely involves the epiphyseal end of a bone.

2. **INVOLVEMENT OF OTHER BONES.** Upon skeletal survey, many of these cases show that other bones are involved. Approximately 50 per cent of patients with unifocal eosinophilic granuloma involve the skull. Neoplastic giant cell tumors rarely involve the skull and are almost always solitary lesions of epiphyses.

3. **THE PRESENCE OF EITHER DIABETES INSIPIDUS OR EXOPHTHALMOS.** Approximately 10 per cent of patients with multifocal EG will show the classic Hand-Schüller-Christian triad of bone lesions, diabetes insipidus, and exophthalmos. A higher percentage show bone lesions and only one of the latter two features. These clinical signs in association with lytic bone lesions are pathognomonic of EG.

4. **THE PRESENCE OF VARIABLE NUMBERS OF EOSINOPHILS, LYMPHOCYTES, AND PLASMA CELLS.** In all but the very latest chronic phases of the disease, eosinophils and chronic inflammatory cells can be found to sprinkle the lesion in variable numbers. Eosinophils are not seen in the neoplastic GCT.

5. **THE PRESENCE OF VARIABLE NUMBERS OF GRANULAR, FOAMY TO LIPID-LADEN MACROPHAGES.** In the early phases of EG the granular macrophages may resemble the stromal cells of a neoplastic giant cell tumor. The later phases are characterized by increasing numbers of foamy to lipidic macrophages and increasing fibrosis.

GIANT CELL REPARATIVE GRANULOMA OF JAWBONES

The giant cell reparative granuloma is a benign lesion virtually confined to the jawbones. It is usually a roundish, lytic lesion of the mandible that occasionally may cross the midline. It is composed of dense, spindly fibroblasts, variable numbers of osteoclast-like giant cells that tend to be focal in distribution, numerous vessels, and focal areas of hemorrhage (Fig. 10–23). It is histologically indistinguishable from hyperparathyroidism or the nonossifying fibroma. It should be diagnosed only if abnormal serum calciums and phosphorous, parathormone assay, and other signs of the diffuse skeletal and other visceral organ metabolic disturbances of hyperparathyroidism are eliminated from contention. True neoplastic giant cell tumors of jawbone are exceedingly rare, if they exist at all. Other lesions that may contain giant cells in the jawbone include eosinophilic granuloma, osteosarcoma, aneurysmal bone cyst, fibrous dysplasia, cementoblastoma, ossifying fibroma, osteoid osteoma, and osteoblastoma. These lesions should not, however, be difficult to distinguish from the giant cell reparative granuloma. Whether the so-called giant cell reparative granulomas are nonossifying fibromas of jawbones is open to question (see pp. 258 and 260).

GIANT CELL REACTION OF BONE

The so-called giant cell reaction of bone refers to a rare benign lesion that has been described only in relation to the phalanges of the hands or feet, metacarpals, and metatarsals.[23,24,25]

These lesions are lytic, usually not large, and can be focally expansile. The entire bone is usually not affected. They are covered by a thin shell of bone and occur in the metaphyses and epiphyses (Fig. 10–24). The characteristic findings are those of a proliferation of spindle shaped fibroblasts producing large amounts of refractile collagen (Figs. 10–25 and 10–26). Small, multinucleated osteoclast-like giant cells are interspersed between the fibroblasts and may be sparse to numerous. Some cases produce considerable reactive osteoid and woven bone. Hyperparathyroidism should be ruled out by appropriate measures. Giant cell tumors are reputed to lack the dense masses of refractile collagen described in the giant cell reaction of bone, tend to involve the entire phalanx, and usually lead to considerable expansion. Giant-cell tumors of the bone are soft and brownish-tan (Plate 7, *A*, *B*, and *C*). The tissue in the giant cell reparative lesion is firmer and grey.

Patients with this lesion have ranged in age from 10 to 37. It is curable by curettage alone. Neoplastic GCT, on the other hand, recurs in 50 per cent of cases treated by curettage alone.

"INVASIVE" VILLONODULAR SYNOVITIS AND GIANT CELL TUMOR OF TENDON SHEATH

DEFINITIONS. *Pigmented villonodular synovitis* (PVNS) is a benign lesion that develops in joint linings. The *giant cell tumor of tendon sheath* develops in the fibrous sheath of tendons. Villonodular synovitis may be either localized or diffuse. In *localized villonodular synovitis,* the synovial membrane shows

(*Text continues on p. 326.*)

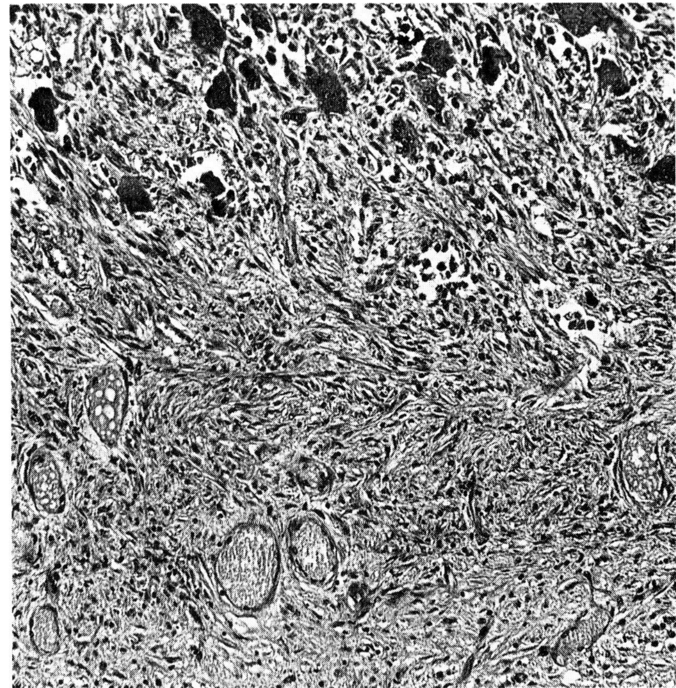

FIG. 10-23

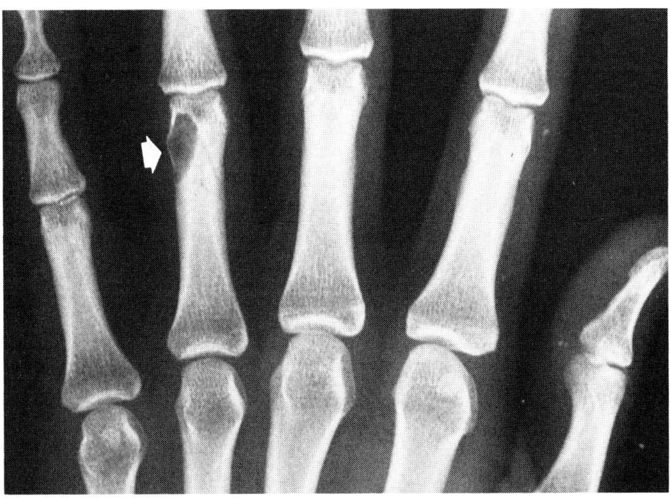

FIG. 10-24

Giant Cell Reparative Granuloma of Jawbones

FIG. 10-23. Giant cell reparative granuloma of jawbones. This lesion is characterized by dense, spindly, fibroblasts, numerous vessels, hemorrhages, and focal clumps of osteoclast-like giant cells. It is histologically indistinguishable from hyperparathyroidism or the nonossifying fibroma (x125).

Giant Cell Reaction of Phalanges

FIG. 10-24. The giant cell reaction of bone has been described only in relation to bones of the hands or feet. The lesion is well circumscribed and lytic (*arrow*) and covered by a thin shell of bone. It may occur in the metaphysis or epiphysis (Courtesy of Dr. Peter Schwinn, Orthopedic Hospital, Los Angeles, and Dr. Harry Pappas, Northridge Hospital, Northridge, Calif.).

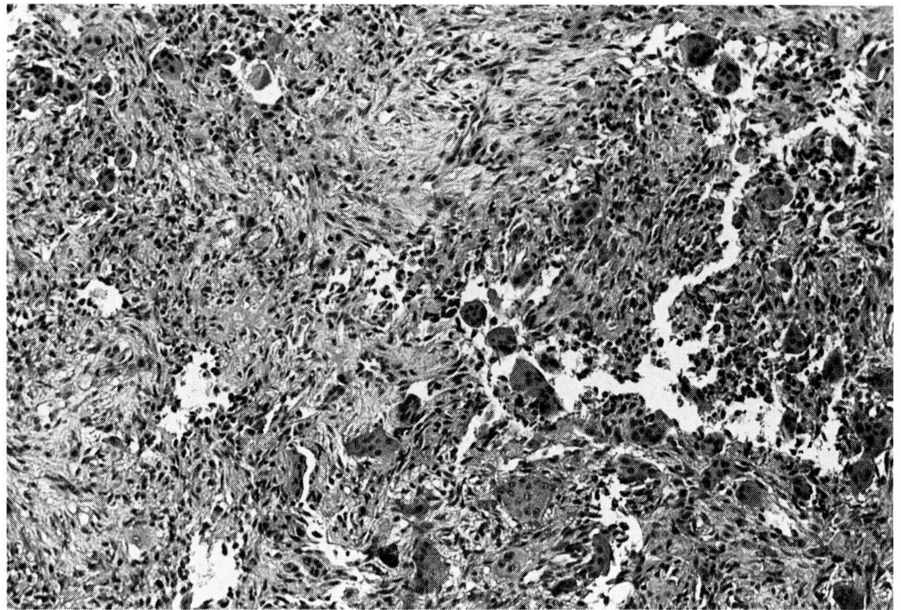

FIG. 10-25

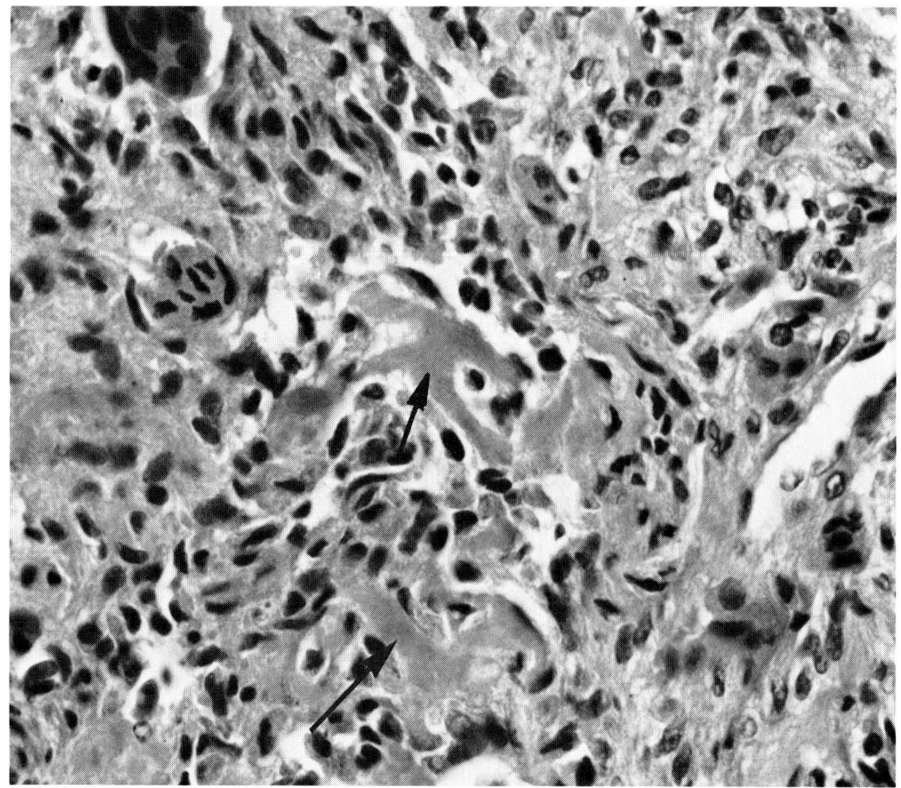

FIG. 10-26

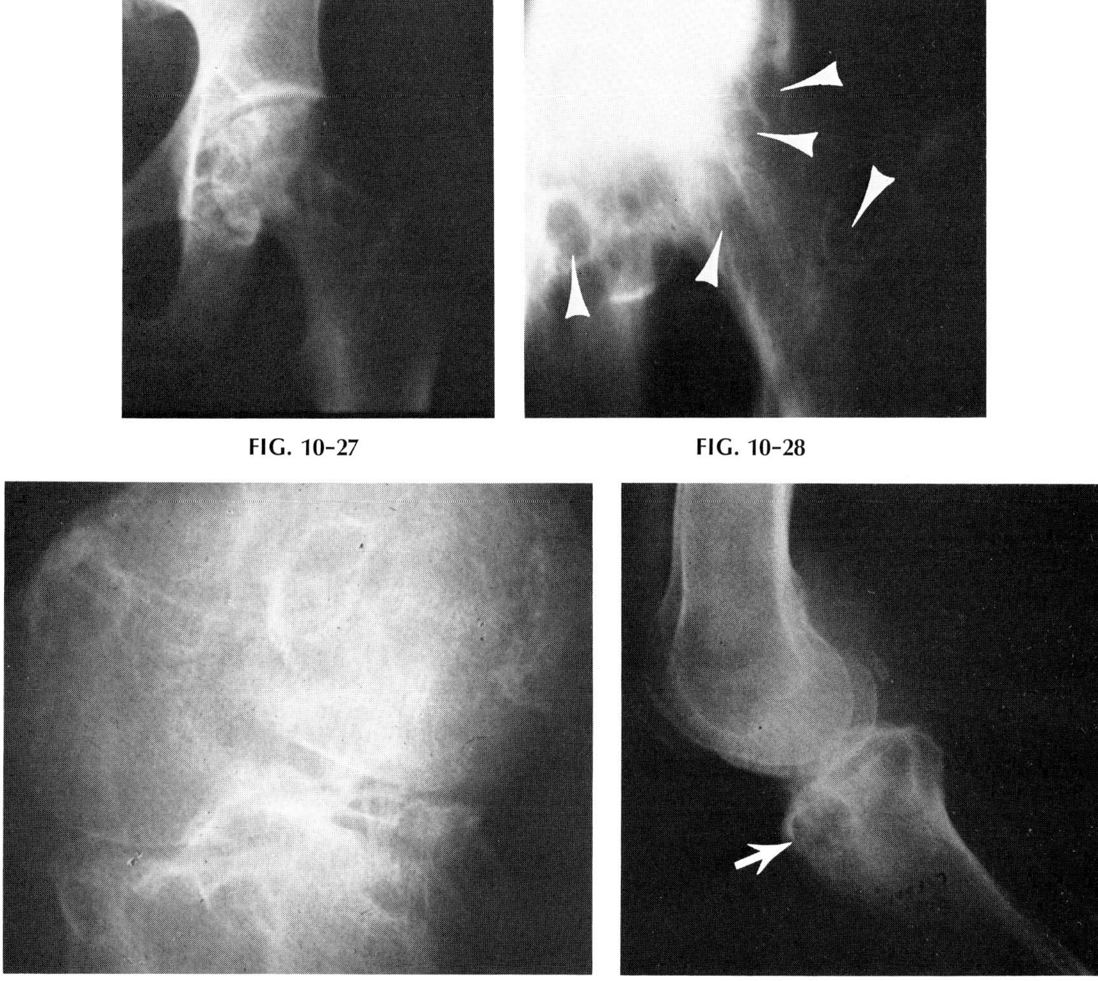

FIG. 10-27

FIG. 10-28

FIG. 10-29

FIG. 10-30

Giant Cell Reaction of Bone

FIG. 10-25. The lesion shows dense, spindly fibroblasts, abundant fibrosis, and focal accumulations of osteoclast-like giant cells (x125). (Courtesy of Dr. Peter Schwinn, Orthopedic Hospital, Los Angeles, and Dr. Harry Pappas, Northridge Hospital, Northridge, Calif.)

FIG. 10-26. High-power examination demonstrates thick, glassy collagen to osteoid-like fibers (*arrows*) (x400). (Courtesy of Dr. Peter Schwinn, Orthopedic Hospital, Los Angeles, and Dr. Harry Pappas, Northridge Hospital, Northridge, Calif.)

Pigmented Villonodular Synovitis Invading Bone

FIG. 10-27. Pigmented villonodular synovitis (PVNS) "invading" bone. Bubbly radiolucencies with sclerotic borders affecting two contiguous bones are the main clue to the diagnosis of a primary synovial lesion. In this case the PVNS involves the proximal femur and acetabulum.

FIG. 10-28. Tomograms to show the clear-cut border of benign host bone reactive sclerosis about the bubbly radiolucencies.

FIG. 10-29. A case of PVNS with massive involvement of the distal femur and proximal tibia.

FIG. 10-30. Cystic lesion of the proximal tibial epiphysis (arrow). Sclerotic borders are difficult to define. There is no clear-cut lesion of either the femur or patella. In such cases the presence of a single bone lytic lesion would rarely lead to the suspicion of "invasive" PVNS. It is usually from lesions such as these that the biopsy may be mistakenly diagnosed as a malignant tumor.

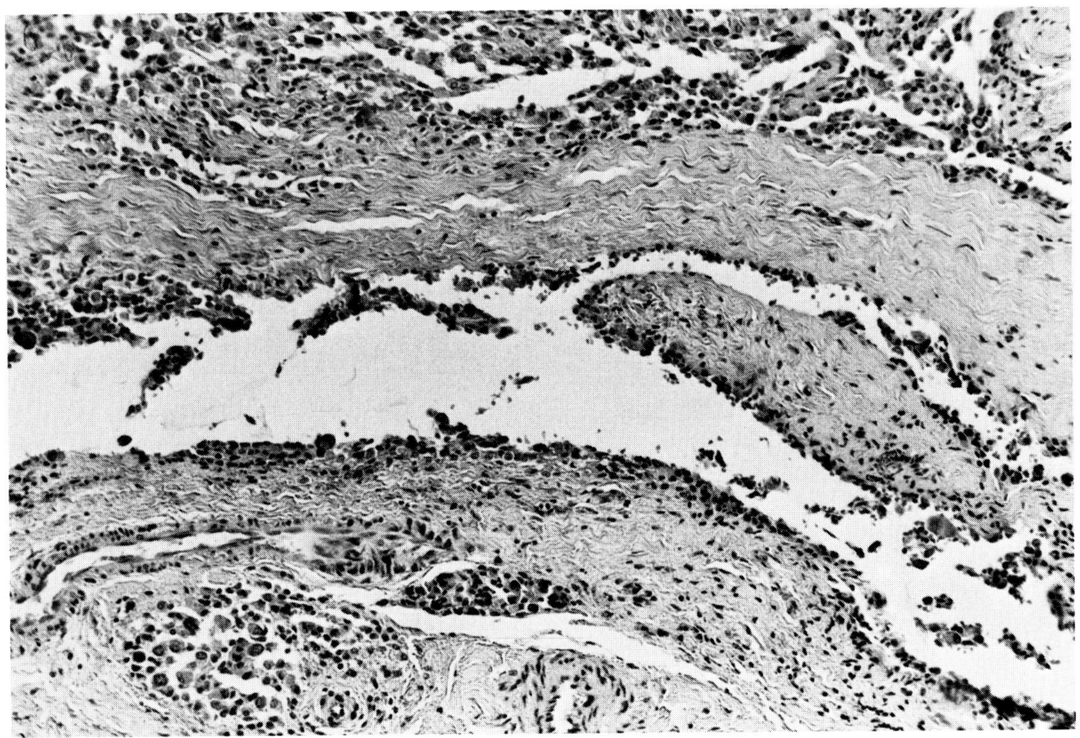

Pigmented Villonodular Synovitis Invading Bone

FIG. 10-31. The presence of slitlike spaces lined by cells is an extremely important clue to the diagnosis of a benign synovial lesion eroding into bone. This histologic sign may not always be present, however. Note also the dense bands of benign fibrous tissue, another common finding in PVNS (x40).

one or more sessile or stalked yellow-brown nodular growths.

Diffuse villonodular synovitis is characterized by numerous fine, brownish, villous and nodular growths basically involving the entire synovial membrane of a single joint.

The giant cell tumor of tendon sheath is similar to the localized form of villonodular synovitis, except for its development in relation to tendon sheaths. These lesions are characterized by similar histological features; namely, granular and foamy macrophages, giant cells, fibrosis, and hemosiderin pigment. On rare occasions, any of these lesions may extend into the bone and simulate a primary or metastatic bone tumor; hence the term *invasive* or erosive. Nevertheless, the lesions are benign and therapy should be conservative.

IMPORTANCE. On rare occasions these lesions may erode into the bone from the joint or tendon sheath area. To the unsuspecting pathologist or clinician

---

Pigmented Villonodular Synovitis Invading Bone

FIG. 10-32. Many fields are characterized by collagenization, spindly fibroblasts, and a sprinkling of osteoclast-like giant cells. Chronic inflammatory cells are common and are rarely seen in the vast majority of primary malignant tumors of bone (x125).

FIG. 10-33. Some fields are usually found that show masses of foamy histiocytes (*a*), prominent vessels (*b*), fibrosis, focal collections of osteoclast-like giant cells (*c*), mononuclear granular histiocytes (*d*) with or without hemosiderin, and a sprinkling of chronic inflammatory cells (x250).

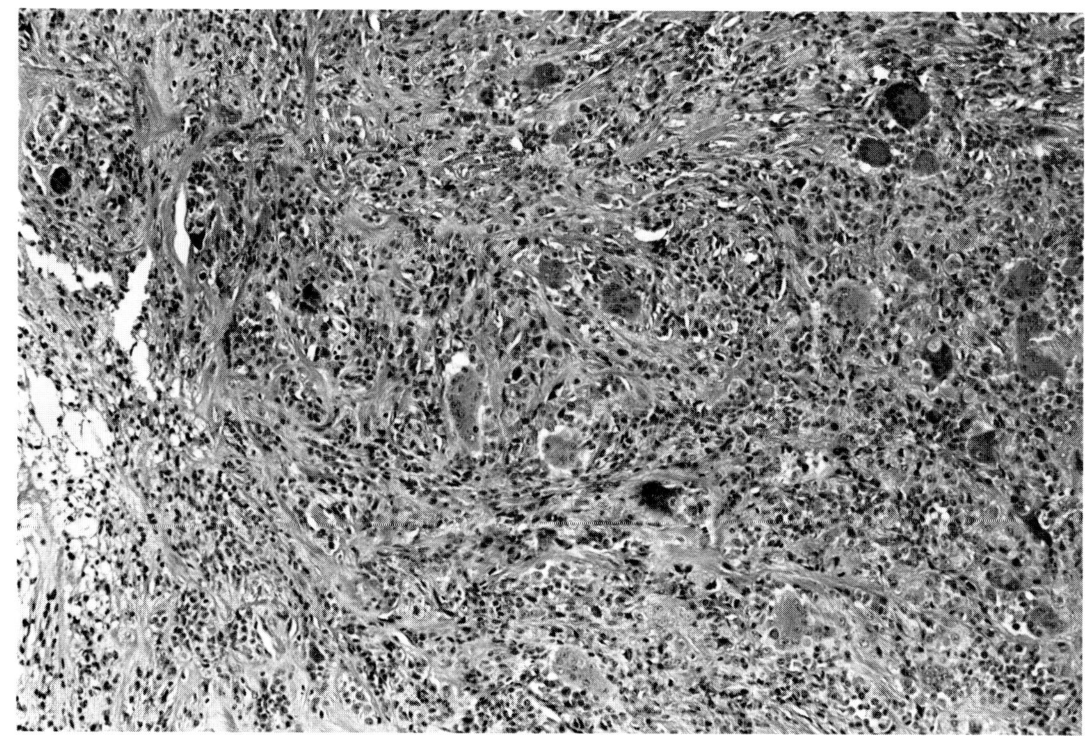

FIG. 10-32

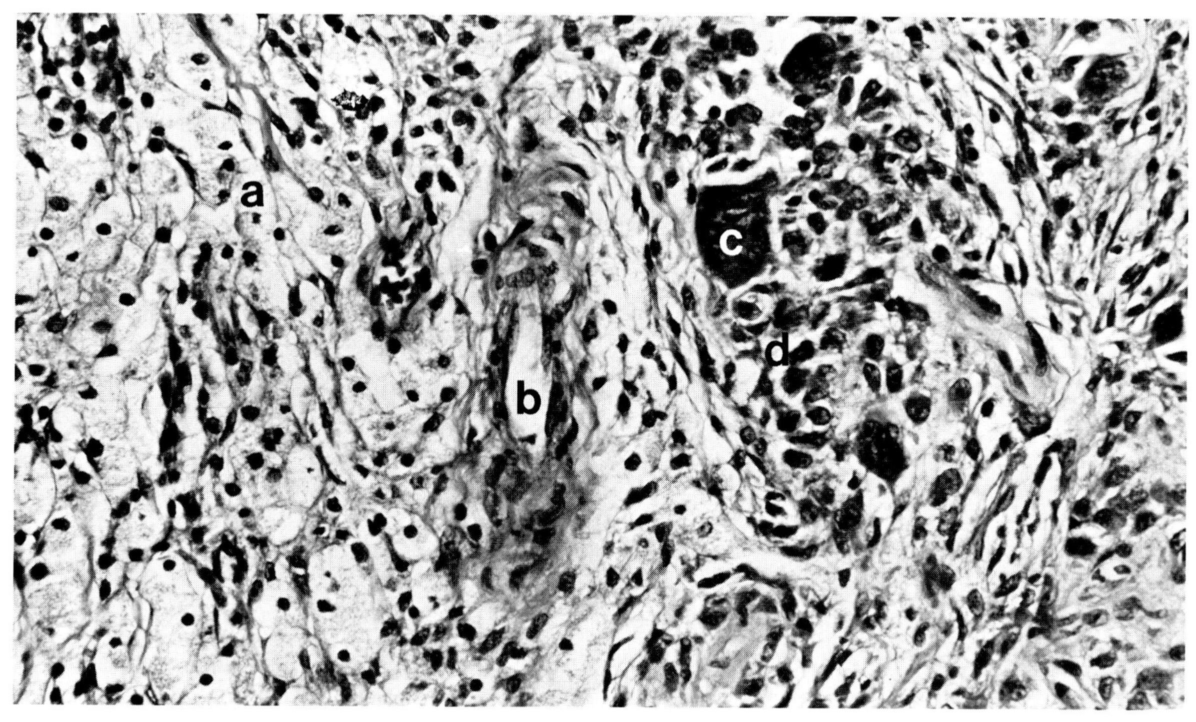

FIG. 10-33

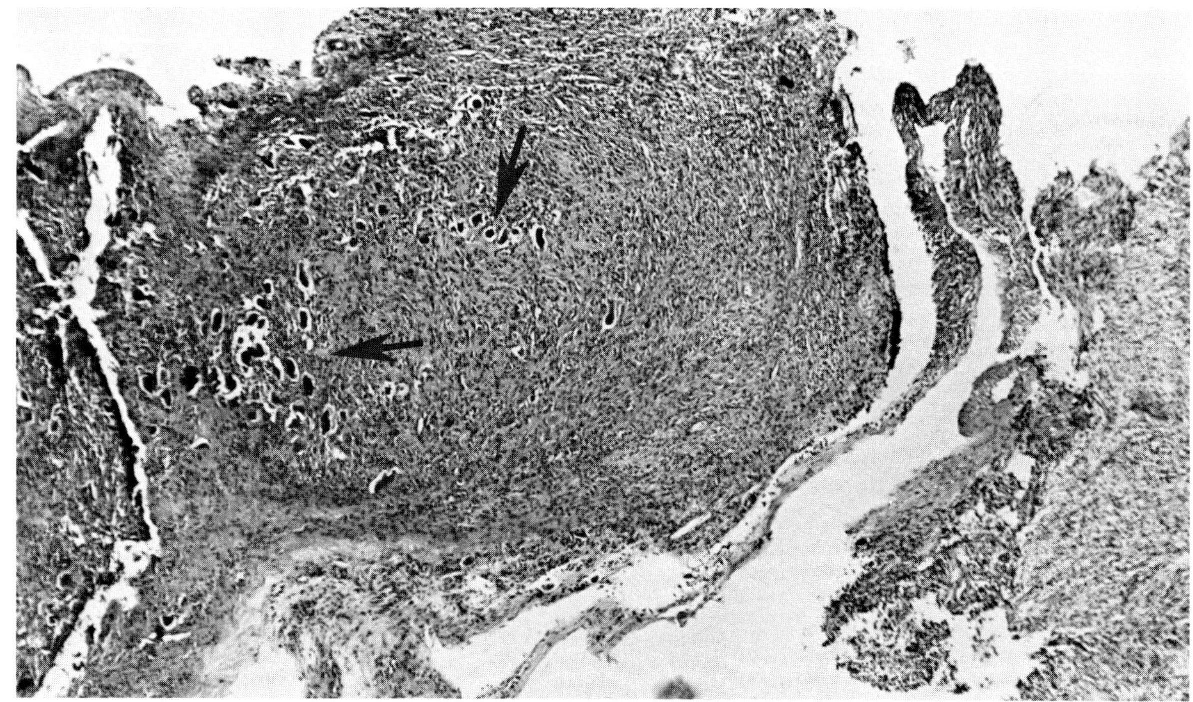

Pigmented Villonodular Synovitis Invading Bone

FIG. 10-34. In distinction to untreated neoplastic GCT, the giant cells of PVNS tend to be focally distributed (*arrows*) (x40).

these lesions may convey an aura of malignancy, both radiologically and histologically. Although these lesions are benign, they are composed of such exuberant masses of fibroblastic and histiocytic tissues that a sarcomatous appearance is simulated. The various diagnoses I have witnessed for these lesions when they present as a primary bone lesion have included fibrosarcoma, neurogenic sarcoma, invasive synovial sarcoma, neoplastic giant cell tumor, liposarcoma, malignant fibrous histiocytoma, fibrous histiocytoma, eosinophilic granuloma, and chondroblastoma. Lack of recognition of its benign nature has lead to disastrous consequences to the patient.

Clinical Features

AGE AND SEX. Most patients are young to middle-aged adults. Males have predilection for this disease.

SITES OF INVOLVEMENT. "Invasive" pigmented villonodular synovitis can affect any bone bounded by a synovial membrane. However, more than 80 per cent of cases involve the knee and hip joint area. Less

Pigmented Villonodular Synovitis Invading Bone

FIG. 10-35. An area of PVNS that mimics the neoplastic GCT. The stromal cells may be either spindly or, as this field shows, quite plump (x250).

FIG. 10-36. This field shows abundant dense bands of collagen formation (*a*), a few osteoclast-like giant cells, and most importantly, masses of dense hemosiderin-laden macrophages (*arrows*). The features of PVNS include, therefore, spindly to plump fibroblasts, foamy to hemosiderin-filled macrophages, bands of collagen formation, synovial slitlike spaces, and focal accumulations of osteoclast-like giant cells (x250).

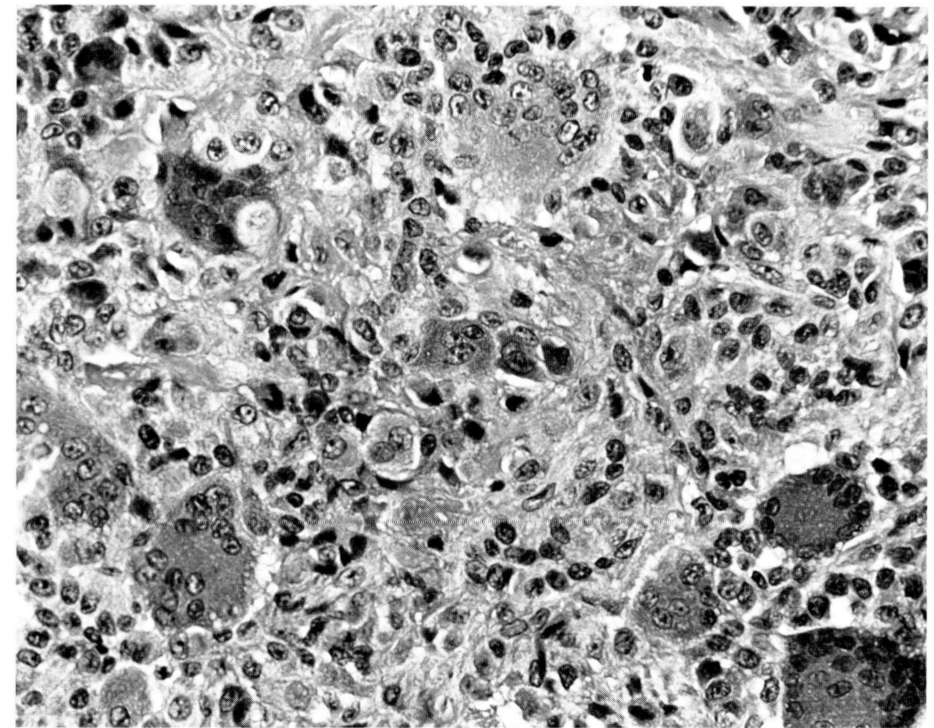

FIG. 10-35

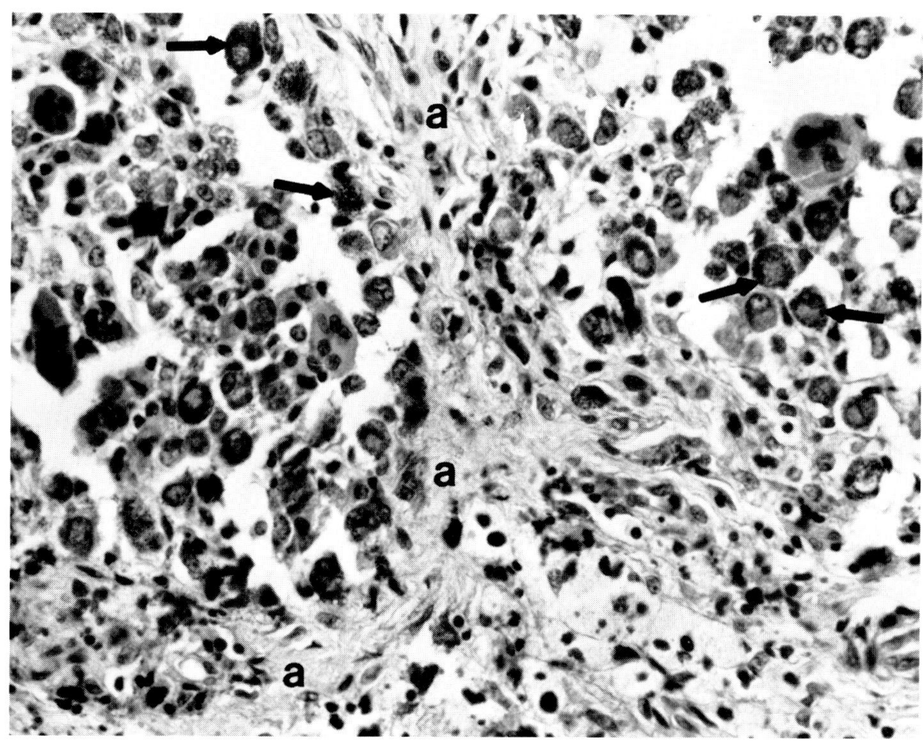

FIG. 10-36

common sites include the wrist and ankle bones. "Invasive" giant cell tumors of tendon sheath have a striking propensity to involve the hand or foot phalanges. Most giant cell tumors of tendon sheath arise in relation to the soft tissues of the hand or foot.

SYMPTOMS. The usual complaints are pain with or without joint swelling. Locking of the joint is not an uncommon symptom. PVNS is characterized by dark brown or serosanguineous fluid upon joint aspiration. If the entity presents as an apparant bone primary, this latter important finding may not be appreciated if the joint is not entered during biopsy. "Invasive" GCT of tendon sheath is usually not associated with effusion.

Radiologic Features

HIGHLY CHARACTERISTIC FEATURES. Characteristic features of invasive PVNS and invasive GCT of tendon sheath are listed below.

"INVASIVE" PVNS. The radiologic features that are highly suggestive, although not pathognomonic, of "invasive" PVNS are the following:

1. Involvement of the epiphyseal and/or metaphyseal ends of two contiguous bones (Figs. 10-27-10-29). It is extremely rare for primary malignant tumors to involve two contiguous bones. This feature usually implies that the lesion has arisen in the synovium and has invaded both bones. A similar radiographic distribution of contiguous bone lesions occurs in rheumatoid arthritis, hemophilia, gout, and infectious diseases, particularly tuberculosis.
2. Bubbly radiolucencies surrounded by a border of benign sclerosis (Figs. 10-27-10-30). This feature in combination with the first is the usual presentation of "invasive" PVNS. The border of sclerosis represents a host response on the part of the bone to contain a slow-growing benign lesion.
3. A cortical defect at the articular cartilage-cortical bone border. This feature is highly suggestive of a synovial lesion that has penetrated into the bone. It is not, however, specific for PVNS (Fig. 8-76).
4. Diffuse swelling of the joint space. This feature may or may not be present and is usually seen only in the diffuse form of PVNS.

"INVASIVE" GCT OF TENDON SHEATH (TS). The characteristic features of this lesion is a single rounded or multinodular cystic zone of rarefaction surrounded by a border of sclerosis in a phalangeal bone. The GCT of TS tends to involve the proximal and middle phalanges more than the distal. Lytic rounded lesions of the distal phalanges are more often consequent to "invasive" glomus tumors or the epidermal inclusion cyst, however.

SUGGESTIVE FEATURES. Suggestive features of invasive PVNS and invasive GCT of tendon sheath are listed below.

"INVASIVE" PVNS. If the lesion presents as a localized area of rarefaction in the metaphysis and/or epiphysis or a single bone without a prominent border of reactive sclerosis or readily appreciable joint effusion, the radiologic diagnosis will be obscured (Fig. 10-30). On radiological grounds these lesions will most probably be called giant cell tumor, chondroblastoma, or possible malignant tumor. Diagnosis depends entirely upon correct histologic interpretation.

"INVASIVE" GCT OF TS. Occasionally these tumors may lead to considerable lytic expansion of the affected phalanx without obvious host sclerosis or a border of periosteal new bone. Such diffusely lytic and expansive lesions simulate osteomyelitis, metastatic, or primary malignant tumors. It is cases such as these that present with a highly ominous radiologic picture that are most commonly diagnosed malignant following biopsy. In rare cases the radiology looks so malignant that ray amputation may be performed prior to tissue diagnosis. However, if the tissue diagnosis remains in error, even more mutilating surgery may be performed for an otherwise totally benign lesion.

Histopathology

These are extremely difficult lesions to describe and illustrate because of the extreme pattern variations from one case to the next. One case may show numerous osteoclast-like giant cells, another but a few. One case may be loaded with hemosiderin, while in another this pigment may be virtually nonexistent. The following features are characteristic of these lesions, but it must be realized that they may vary considerably in extent from case to case or area to area.

"INVASIVE" PVNS

1. Areas of slitlike spaces lined by plump epithelial-like (synovial) cells (Fig. 10-31). This is perhaps the most important histologic clue to diagnosis but it is a feature not present in every case. Synovial sarcomas may show similar slitlike spaces with an epithelial-like lining, but they very rarely invade bone and rarely arise from the joint cavity itself.
2. Extensive areas of collagen-producing spindle cells. The spindle cells may be quite plump and the nuclei closely packed together (Figs. 10-32 and 10-33). These cells are the ones most likely to be confused with a sarcoma. Mitotic figures are usually

scarce and where present, are mirror images. The cells lack large nucleoli and signs of frank anaplasia. The diagnosis of malignancy can be avoided only by attention to all of the radiologic and histologic features. One of the clues to benignancy is the production of dense bands of heavy, collagenized, less cellular tissue (Figs. 10–32 and 10–36).

3. Foci of benign granular, foamy, or lipid-laden macrophages (Fig. 10–33). Malignant tumors are rarely associated with these cells. In malignant histiocytomas the macrophages usually show signs of nuclear anaplasia. In PVNS the nuclei of the macrophages are benign. Almost all cases of "invasive" PVNS show some areas with these cells. It is extremely important, however, to recognize them, because they may be missed by casual inspection. Foamy macrophages are commonly seen in other benign conditions, including nonossifying fibroma, eosinophilic granuloma, and chondroblastoma.

4. Foci of osteoclast-like giant cells (Figs. 10–34 and 10–35). These lesions almost never contain the diffuse masses and numbers of giant cells seen in the neoplastic giant cell tumor. In PVNS they tend to be focal and in association with either plump macrophages or spindly stromal cells or embedded in heavily collagenized tissues. The giant cells rarely contain the myriads of nuclei common to the neoplastic GCT.

5. Foci of hemosiderin pigmentation. In some cases there are huge masses of hemosiderin-laden macrophages, more so than in perhaps any other condition of bone (Fig. 10–36). In other cases the degree of hemosiderin production is minimal.

"INVASIVE" GCT OF TENDON SHEATH (ES). These lesions are histologically identical to PVNS described above. They are composed of variable quantities of spindle cells, giant cells, hemosiderin, macrophages, inflammatory cells, and fibrosis. Slitlike spaces lined by epithelial cells are often lacking, however. Mitoses are rare and frank anaplasia is lacking.

Course and Treatment

These are totally benign lesions. PVNS tends to be a stubbornly recurrent lesion that may lead to considerable morbidity. Radiation has been used to treat stubbornly recurrent lesions. GCT of TS is amenable to cure, in most cases, by curettage alone.

Nonossifying Fibroma

This lesion is composed of spindly fibroblast-like cells admixed with variable numbers of osteoclast-like giant cells. The giant cells are usually inconspicuous and contain from three to eight nuclei. In some cases the giant cells may be large and contain many more nuclei. To help distinguish the nonossifying fibroma from other giant cell and spindle cell lesions, refer to pp. 258–269 and Figures 9–2 to 9–21.

Fibrous Dysplasia and Solitary and Aneurysmal Bone Cyst

These entities may contain small, focal accumulations or sprinklings of osteoclast-like giant cells. The features of these lesions are so distinctive that confusion with lesions that produce masses of osteoclast-like giant cells is negligible. Refer to Figures 7–59, 13–13 to 13–15, and 13–49 to 13–50 for the illustrations of usual maximum extent and appearance of giant cells seen in each of these lesions. If large masses of giant cells and bland stroma cells are seen in association with aneurysmal bone cyst, the diagnosis should be aneurysmal bone cyst arising in association with a neoplastic giant cell tumor.

Chondroblastoma

Chondroblastomas may have considerable areas that mimic the neoplastic Giant-Cell Tumor. The chondroblastoma is distinguished from this latter lesion by the presence of islands of chondroid, no matter how small, polygonal to rounded cells rather than spindly cells and foci of "chicken-wire" calcification (see p. 222 and Figs. 8–77–8–82 and Plate 6, *J*, *K*, and *L*.

Gout

Gout may present with pain and solitary (Fig. 10–37) or multiple bone lytic lesions which, on radiologic grounds, may be mistaken for benign and malignant tumors, osteomyelitis, and eosinophilic granuloma. The pathologic hallmark of the disease is that of urates surrounded by variable degrees of polys, and/or giant cells, and/or mononuclear histiocytes, and fibrosis. The giant cells are of the foreign body type. If the tissue is placed in alcohol, the crystals of urate will not be dissolved. The crystals polarize brilliantly with a "sheaves-of-wheat" pattern (Fig. 10–38). However, if the diagnosis is not suspected, the tissue will, inadvertently, be placed in formalin, a water base in which the diagnostic urate crystals may completely dissolve. If not completely dissolved, the remaining urates will have a brown color and be light polarizable. However, if no polarizable crystals remain, the diagnosis is still possible provided that the characteristic residue consists of small or large masses of pinkish material (Fig. 10–39) in which needlelike spaces arranged in a "sheaves-of-wheat" pattern may be preserved. These spaces represent the former site of urate crystal deposition. In acute gout this material is surrounded by polymorphonuclear leukocytes; in late gout, by variable amounts of multinucleated giant cells of connecting tissue histiocytic origin, fibrosis, and chronic inflammatory cells (Fig. 10–39).

Tuberculosis, Fungal Infections, and Sarcoidosis

Each of these diseases may be associated with giant cells. The giant cells tend to have peripherally located nuclei (Langhans cells). They are always associated with granular epitheloid histiocytes and variable quantities of lymphocytes. These lesions form localized collections of histiocytes known as granulomas. Tuberculosis is most often associated with central caseous necrosis. Fungal infections may or may not be associated with necrosis, and sarcoid is composed of noncaseating granulomas (Figs. 10–41 and 10–42). If any of these lesions present as solitary bone lesions, they may be mistaken clinically for primary bone tumors.

Sarcoid bone disease usually consists of multiple phalangeal lesions (Fig. 10–40) ranging in radiographic appearance from lacey to cystlike. Tuberculosis usually involves the epiphyseal ends of bones, wrists, or the spine. Fungal infections are similar in distribution to tuberculosis.

Appropriate stains are necessary for identification of either acid-fast or fungal organisms. If bone biopsy material is overdecalcified, the distortion of the cellular response may be so great that the granulomas are not readily appreciated. It should be emphasized that eosinophilic granuloma is not exemplified by discrete granulomas; the entire lesion is characterized by eosinophilic and granulomatous inflammation. Discrete granulomas indicate fungal, tubercular, foreign body reactions, or sarcoidosis.

Gaucher's Disease

Gaucher's disease is characterized by the accumulation of large, pale histiocytes with a single or double nucleus. The nuclei are small and round and are usually peripherally located (Figs. 11–33 and 11–34). In most cases the diagnosis is suspected clinically before biopsy. On rare occasions, however, the patient may present with pain and an ominous "onionskin" periosteal reaction mimicking Ewing's sarcoma (Fig. 11–32). Biopsy shows the classic Gaucher histiocytes (Fig. 11–34), in distinction to the much smaller, lymphocyte-like Ewing's sarcoma cells.

LOW-GRADE MALIGNANT NEOPLASMS

The Low-Grade Neoplastic Giant Cell Tumor (Fig. 10–43)

Considerable thought has been given by this author to arrive at the most appropriate designation for this highly controversial tumor. It is the most difficult of all of the lesions of bone to predict, with confidence, the ultimate behavior of any one case. On one end of the spectrum this lesion has been designated benign giant cell tumor or benign osteoclastoma; on the other, because of its unpredictable and rare metastatic behavior, it has been called malignant giant cell

---

Gout

FIG. 10–37. On rare occasions, a gouty lesion of the synovium may erode into the bone and present as a primary lytic bone tumor. In this instance unsuspected gout presented as a lytic tumor of the patella (*arrow*).

FIG. 10–38. Gout is typified by urate crystals arranged in a "sheaves-of-wheat" pattern by polarized light. These crystals will be dissolved by ordinary formalin fixation, however. Alcohol fixation should be used to prevent solubilization (x125).

FIG. 10–39. If the crystals are removed by formalin fixation, the diagnosis can be made by the demonstration of masses of pinkish, proteinaceous debris in which needlelike spaces are seen. These needlelike spaces are arranged in a sheaves-of-wheat pattern and, of course, represent the areas from which the former gout crystals were removed by solubilization. The other feature of gout in this illustration is the presence of mono- and multinuclear histiocytes and foreign body giant cell surrounding the gouty proteinaceous residua (x125).

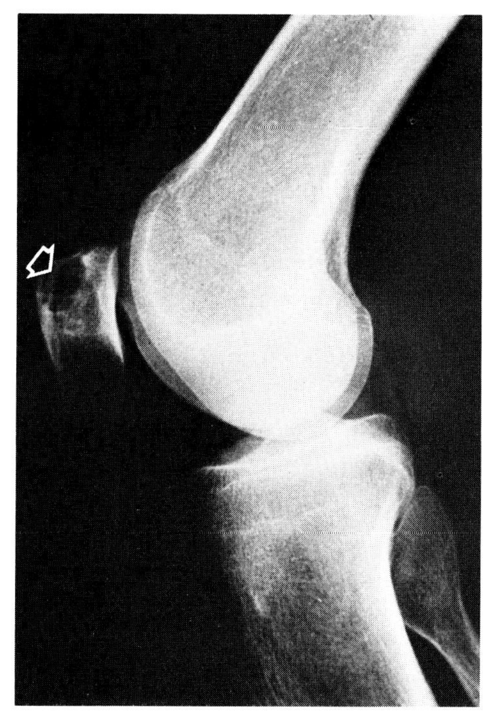

FIG. 10-37

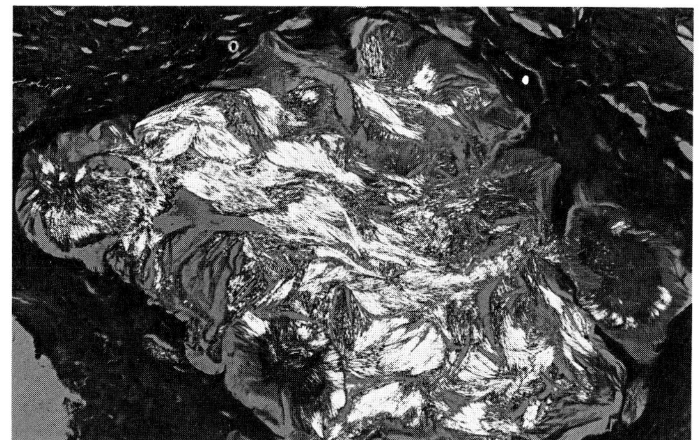

FIG. 10-38

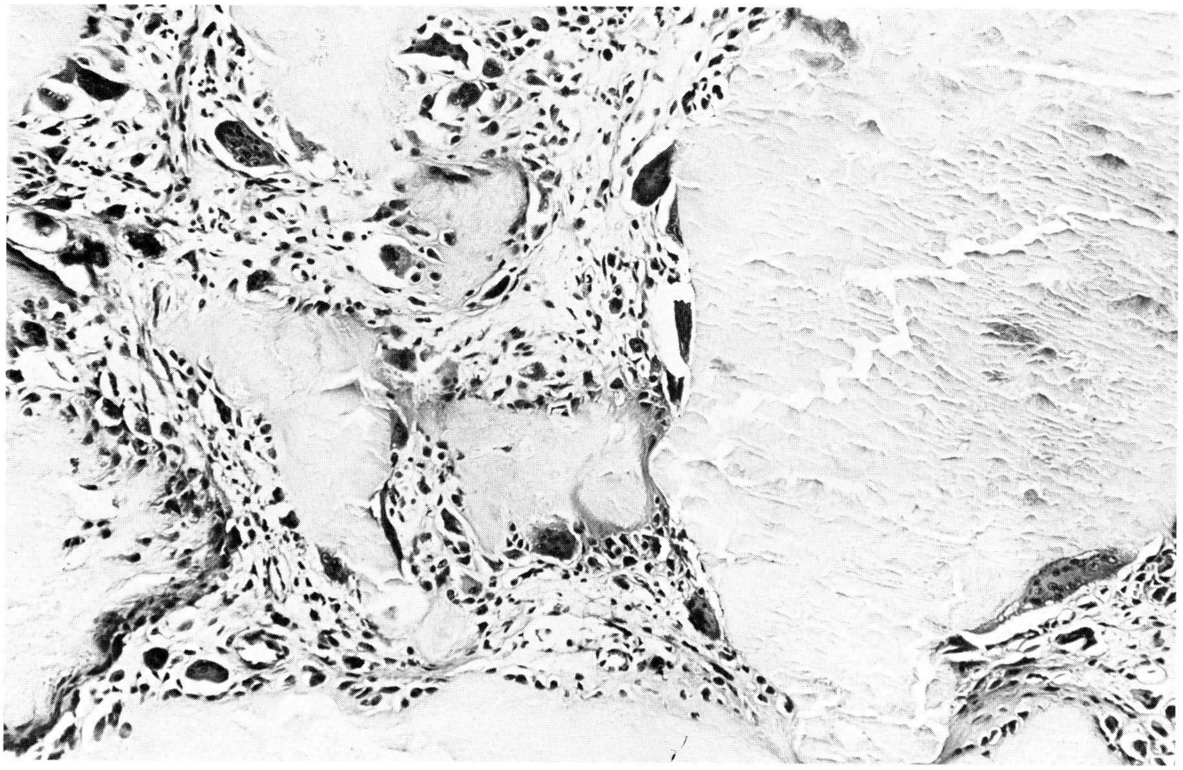

FIG. 10-39

tumor, and even more extremely, giant cell sarcoma. Jaffe[57] preferred to simply use the name giant cell tumor, dropping the designation benign. But he rejected the designation of sarcoma because it does not fit the clinical facts.

The behavior of the giant cell tumor is such that as many as 50 per cent of all cases recur following curettage. Recurrent lesions may require eventual amputation; occasional tumors seed the local soft-tissues; and spinal and sacral tumors may lead to the patient's demise consequent to involvement of vital cord, nerve, vascular or pelvic structures. Some cases even result in metastasis to lungs but only rarely, if at all, to demise if the lung metastasis shows no evidence of anaplastic sarcomatous transformation.

Many of these features fit with our definition of a low-grade malignant neoplasm. In this textbook a neoplasm has been defined as a tumor characterized by an autonomous and continuous growth of cells that will lead to the eventual demise of the patient unless extirpated. A low-grade neoplasm is characterized by slow, relentless growth, a high recurrence rate following less than adequate attempts at local removal, and a low metastatic rate (20% or less). The metastases should also show neoplastic behavior; that is, continued slow growth and ultimate demise of the patient unless extirpated. Because metastases from low-grade neoplasms are slow growing and usually less widely disseminated than those of high grade neoplasms, they are much more amenable to cure by surgical ablation. Other osseous and nonosseous tumors that conform to the behavior designated as "low-grade" neoplasm include the basal cell epithelioma (carcinoma), leiomyoblastoma, mixed tumor of parotid, parosteal osteosarcoma, and chordoma. However, as we shall see in the next section, some cases of well-documented, ordinary nonanaplastic giant cell tumors with metastases to lungs identical to the primary lesion may show regression of some to all of the lung metastases with a benign long-term clinical course after 10 or more years. Other cases have had very long survivals free of disease following removal of all lung metastases, which were generally but a few. These latter findings would tend to cast doubt on whether the ordinary GCT is an unequivocal neoplasm as we have defined the term. However, because of its high recurrence rate, massive local destruction if not adequately treated, local seeding of soft tissues, high morbidity, and occasional demise due to involvement of local vital structures, this author would, at this time, prefer to view the lesion as an unusual variant of a low-grade neoplasm. Because of its locally aggressive behavior in approximately 50 per cent of cases, therapy must be performed as if the tumor were a bona fide, although peculiar, low-grade malignant neoplasm.

A good part of the reason why the literature is in such confusion regarding the lethal potential of the giant cell tumor is that its distinction from other benign and highly malignant tumors rich in osteoclast-like giant cells may be quite subtle. For example, after thorough review of the literature and personal consultation cases, this author is convinced that the so-called malignant giant cell tumor (Grade III giant cell tumor) is a mixture of lesions that includes exuberant, overcalled, but, nevertheless, ordinary low-grade neoplastic GCT's, giant cell sarcomas, osteogenic sarcomas, GCT's with anaplastic transformation, malignant fibrous histiocytomas, and fibrosarcomas rich in giant cells. I have seen occasional osteosarcomas and fibrosarcomas that contain numerous benign osteoclast-like giant cells with minimal or subtle stromal anaplasia that have been incorrectly diagnosed as "benign" or low-grade neoplastic GCT. Nevertheless, they behave with the full biologic virulence common to fibro- and osteosarcomas. One of the purposes of this chapter is to define each of these GCT-like variants in order to reduce the diagnostic error rate to a respectable figure. The error rate in the diagnosis of low-grade neoplastic GCT in some series, upon review by their respective authors, has been as much as 27 per cent in Larsson's series of 75 cases,[66] 13 per cent in Hutter's series of 76 cases,[54] 20 per cent in Schajowicz's series of 55 cases,[85,86] and 18 per cent of Goldenberg's series of 265 cases.[50] The lesions that were originally mistaken for the low-

---

Sarcoidosis

FIG. 10-40. Sarcoidosis of the bones is typified by multiple, cystic, trabeculated lesions of the phalanges (*arrows*).

FIG. 10-41. The bone lesions of sarcoid are similar to those seen in other organ systems; namely, numerous noncaseating granuloma with Langhans' giant cells (*arrows*) (x125).

FIG. 10-42. Asteroid body (*arrow*) found within a large, sarcoid giant cell (x400).

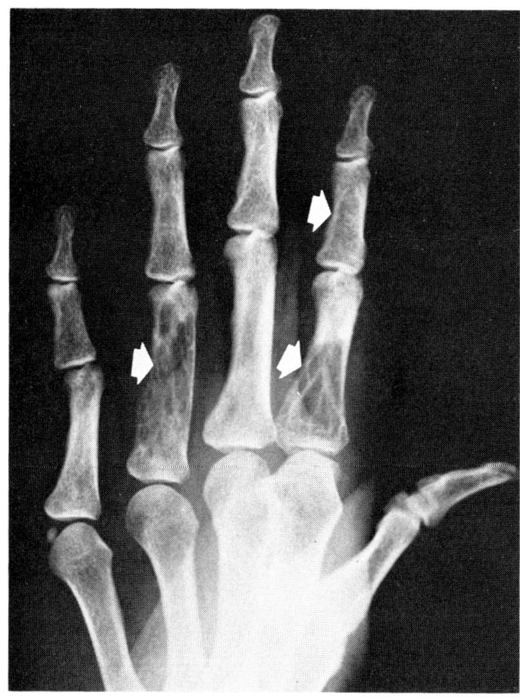

FIG. 10-40

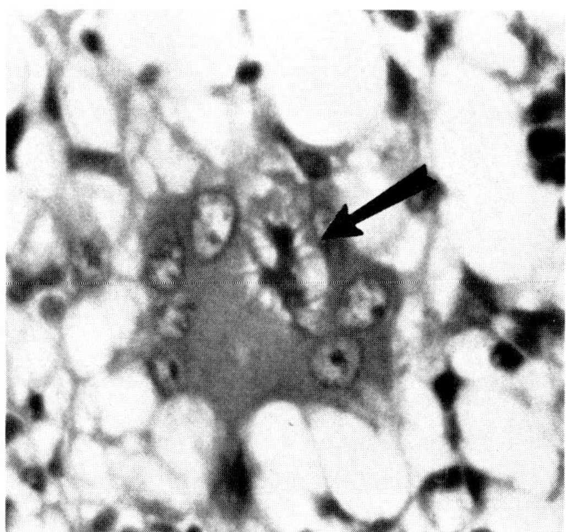

FIG. 10-42

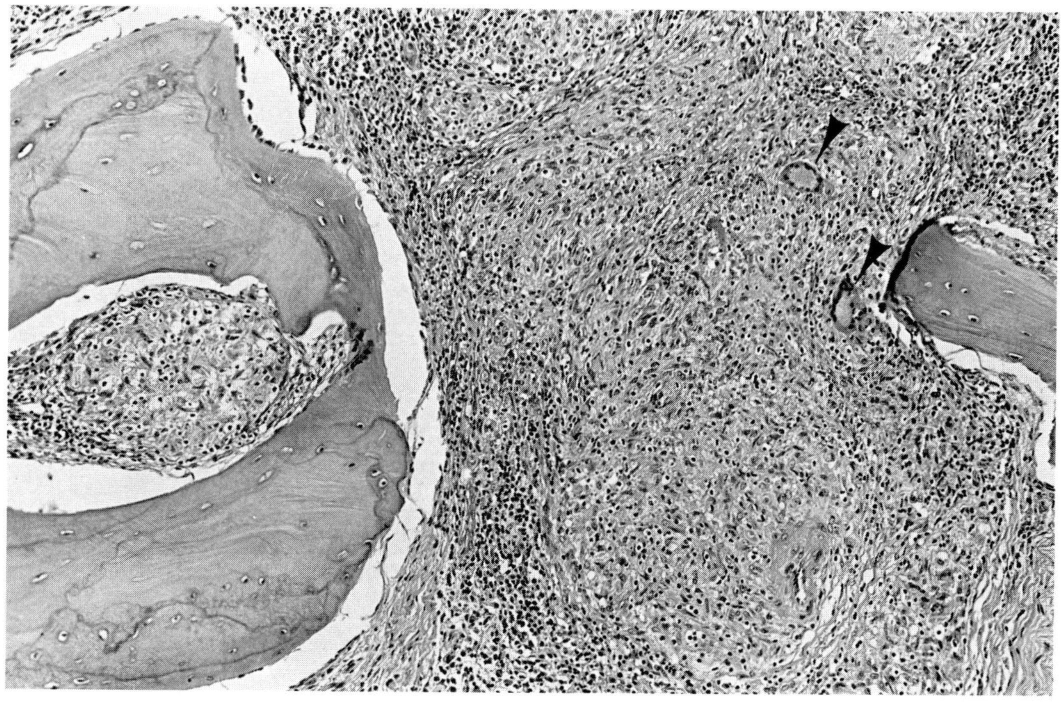

FIG. 10-41

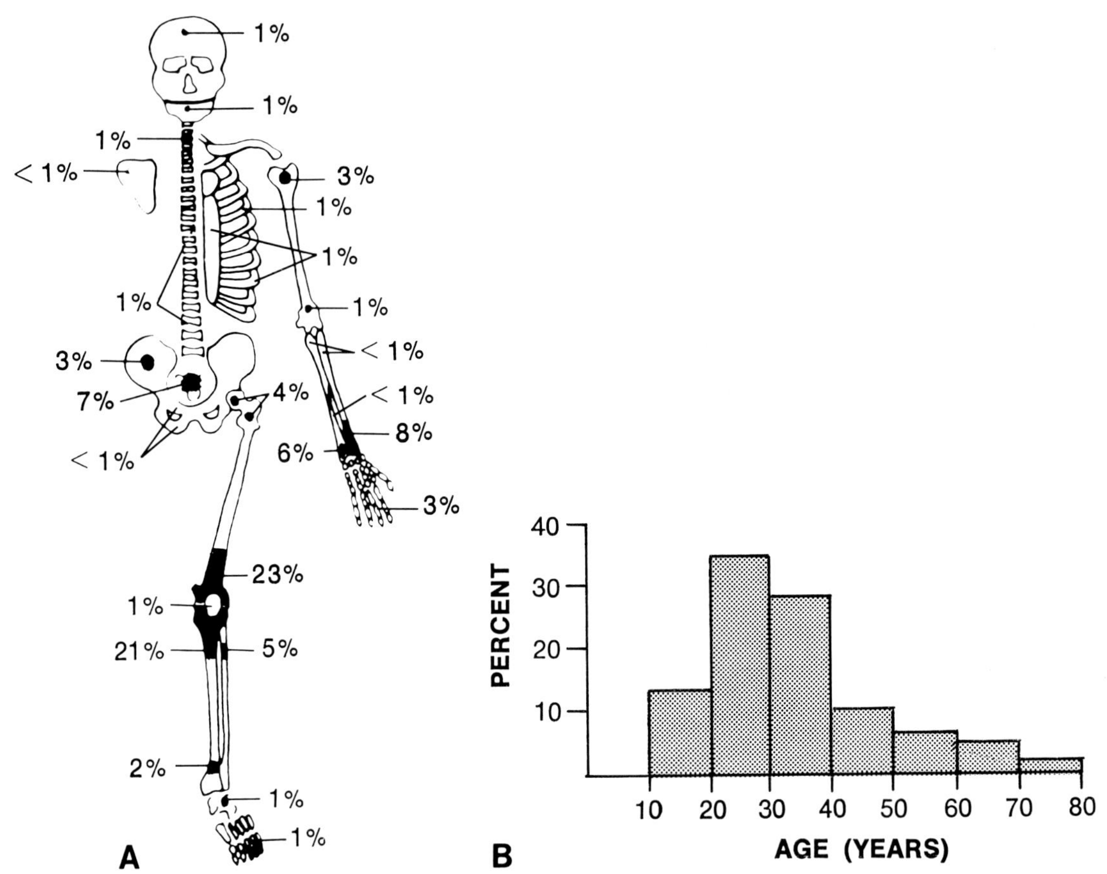

FIG. 10-43. (*A*) Low-grade neoplastic giant cell tumor. Frequency of areas of involvement in 334 patients. Male:female incidence, 1:1.4. (*B*) Age distribution of patients with giant cell tumor. (Mirra, J., Bullough, P., and Freiberger, R.: Orthopedic Diseases, Part II. New York, Famous Teachings in Modern Medicine, MedCom, Inc., © 1972)

grade neoplastic GCT and excluded from their data included chondroblastomas, giant cell reparative granulomas of jawbones, fibroxanthomas, pigmented villonodular synovitis, hyperparathyroidism, bone cysts, and osteosarcomas.

Only with knowledge of the full range of the clinicoradiologic and pathologic variations of true low-grade neoplastic GCT's in comparison to other benign and highly malignant giant-cell-rich lesions can there be any hope of reducing the confusion that reigns and the error rate, which at present is inordinately high.

Capsule Summary

Incidence. Approximately 4.2 per cent of biopsied primary bone tumors. It is the sixth most common of the primary bone tumors.

Age. Wide spectrum of age distribution. Rare under 10 years of age or over 70. Approximately 70 per cent of patients are between 20 and 40 years old.

Clinical Features. Pain, swelling with or without pathologic fracture.

Radiologic Features. Eccentric, expanding, radiolucency usually centered in the epiphysis. Some cases are centered in the metaphysis. However, even these cases usually involve the epiphyseal end of bone and often extend to the articular cartilage in at least one focus. Diaphyseal primaries are almost nonexistent. Lacks a border of benign sclerosis. May appear trabeculated. Lack of calcification and ominous periosteal reactions. Usually a solitary lesion, although there have been rare reports of multiple bone involvement.[91a,95,96]

Gross Pathology. Very soft and tan to tannish red. Variable amounts of hemorrhage, necrosis, fibrosis, and cystic degeneration. Degenerative changes associated with yellow color and fibrosis with a firmer, grey appearance.

Histopathology. Giant cells, plump, spindly to oval stromal cells lacking objective anaplasia. Typical mitoses may be abundant. Variable degrees of collagenization. Variable quantities of osteoid and woven bone may be found in up to 50 per cent of cases.

Course. A 50 per cent recurrence rate by curettage alone. Rare cases associated with lung metastases and/or malignant transformation to a fibrosarcoma. Post-radiation may be associated with radiation induced fibro- or osteosarcoma usually 5 or more years after therapy.

Treatment. Refer to discussion.

Definition. The low-grade neoplastic giant cell tumor (GCT) is a lesion that almost always begins in the epiphyseal-metaphyseal regions of enchondrally formed bones. It is characterized by a monotonous mass of prominent osteoclast-like giant cells and ovoid to spindly stromal cells with variably plump nuclei lacking in objective anaplasia. It must be differentiated from other benign and high-grade malignant entities that may mimic the GCT very closely.

Clinical Features

AGE. It used to be considered that GCT was very rare below age 20. Cases below that age were viewed with skepticism.[57] Review of several large, recent series show that approximately 15 per cent of patients with the GCT are younger than age 20.[50,74] However, even if the patients are teenagers, the majority show skeletal maturity; that is, closure of the epiphyseal plate in the bone affected by the GCT. The opposite is true of the chondroblastoma; that is, it is rarely discovered in patients with closed epiphyses.

In most series the majority (70 per cent) of patients present between the ages of 20 and 40 years of age.

SYMPTOMS. Pain without gross fracture is present in approximately 90 per cent of patients. Approximately 10 per cent present with an obvious pathologic fracture. Local swelling and limitation of movement are common complaints. Patients with involvement of the spine or sacrum may present with neurological symptoms.

LABORATORY EXAMINATION. The neoplastic giant cell tumor is not associated with abnormal chemistries. An abnormally elevated serum calcium and depressed serum phosphorous points to hyperparathyroidism. Since the GCT of hyperparathyroidism may be histologically indistinguishable from the neoplastic GCT, serum calcium and phosphorous tests should be performed. Significant elevation of the serum alkaline phosphatase in association with normal serum calcium and phosphorous should point to the possibility of a benign GCT of Paget's disease. In this author's experience, for every 40 true neoplastic giant cell tumors, there are approximately two GCT's of hyperparathyroidism that may present as an apparant solitary bone tumor and approximately one case of a benign or locally aggressive GCT due to Paget's disease.

Radiologic Features

The neoplastic GCT is a solitary, slow, relentlessly growing neoplasm that results in extensive bone resorption. On very rare occasion, the low-grade neoplastic giant cell tumor may be multiple.[91a,95,96] Therefore, it is characterized by a relatively circumscribed, pure lytic to lytic-trabeculated lesion, with scant periosteal new bone and no border of benign host bone sclerosis. In small bones the lesions usually present with bone "expansion." Although the radiographic features of a GCT are characteristic, they are not pathognomonic. Approximately 10 per cent of

Low-Grade Neoplastic Giant Cell Tumor (GCT)

FIG. 10-44. The neoplastic GCT is characterized by its eccentric epiphyseal location, lysis, circumscription and the lack of host bone sclerosis, periosteal reactions, or punctate calcifications.

FIG. 10-45. Larger lesions may bulge into the soft tissues but are usually covered by a rim of periosteum beneath which may be a very thin layer of periosteal new bone (*arrow*).

FIG. 10-46. This GCT has occupied almost the entire width of the bone.

FIG. 10-47. Very large, lytic GCT of the ilium (*arrow*). In this unusual location the diagnosis of GCT would probably not be entertained on the basis of clinical analysis.

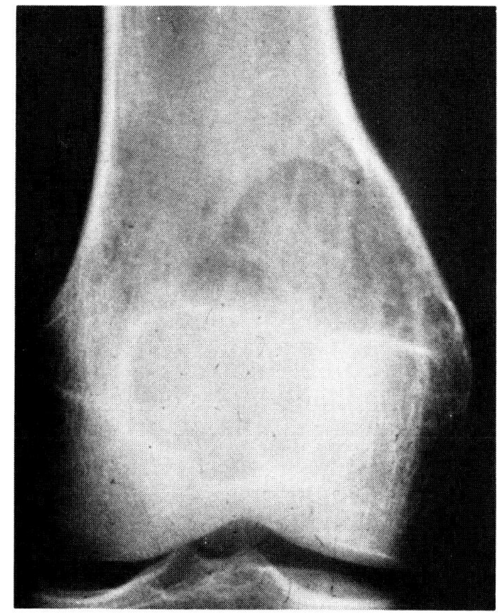

FIG. 10-44

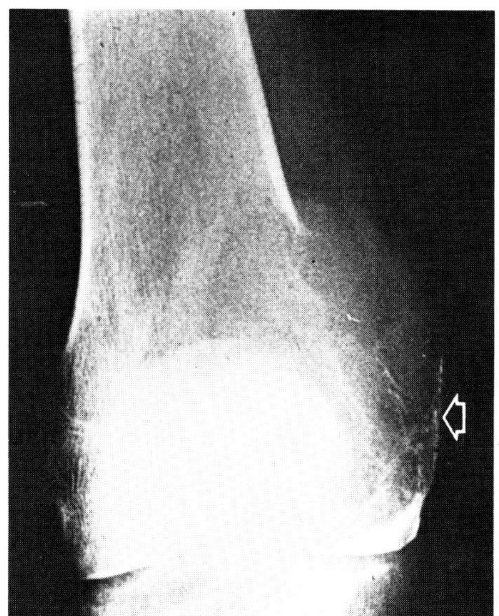

FIG. 10-45

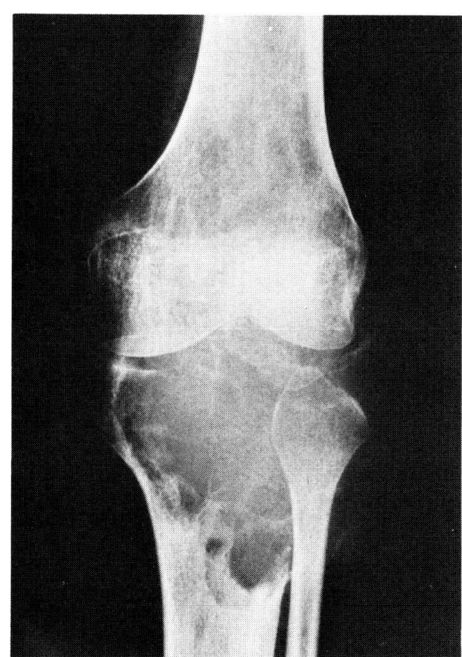

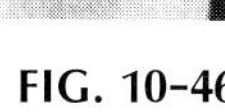

FIG. 10-46

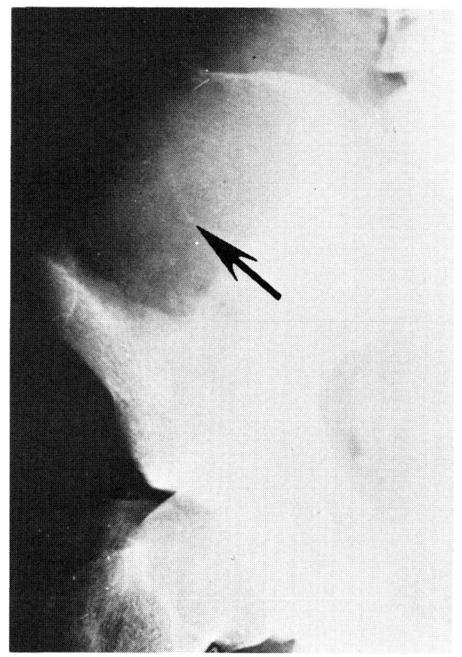

FIG. 10-47

lesions of the epiphysis with radiographic features most consistent with a GCT are in actuality other benign and malignant lesions.

Giant Cell Tumor of the Large Bones

By large bones, it is meant those with a wide diameter such as the ilium, femur, proximal tibia, humerus vertebral body, and sacrum. In descending order of frequency, 50 per cent of GCT's involve the epiphyseal-metaphyseal end of the distal femur; proximal tibia, femur, and humerus.

The characteristic radiographic features of GCT of the large long bones are the following:

1. Epiphyseal location. The overwhelming majority are centered in the epiphyseal-metaphyseal end of the bone (Figs. 10–44 and 10–45). They rarely extend to the diaphysis at the initial presentation. Approximately 1 per cent of all reported cases apparently involve the metaphysis only and do not show involvement of the epiphyseal or diaphyseal portions of the bone; only 0.2 per cent of all cases are centered in the diaphysis.[99]

2. Eccentricity. Most cases present before the lesion had involved the entire bone width (Figs. 10–44 and 10–45). However, large lesions will lose this feature of eccentricity (Fig. 10–46).

3. Confinement to bone. The majority are contained within the original bone contours (Fig. 10–44). Larger lesions may result in eccentric or concentric cortical erosion and bone "expansion." In actuality, although the lesions may at times appear to extend into the soft tissues (Fig. 10–45), at gross examination the lesion is almost always covered by a thin rim of periosteum or periosteal new bone that may or may not be apparent on radiographic examination.

4. Lysis with and without trabeculation. Prominent lysis is common to all GCT's, because they are almost certainly of osteoclastic origin. Many cases show fine lines that impart a trabeculated appearance (Fig. 10–44). The trabeculations usually ramify as a filigree of fine to moderately coarse lines (Figs. 10–50 and 10–51). These patterns are usually not the result of bone deposition within the lesion itself but to irregular cortical erosion or irregular new periosteal bone deposition.

5. Circumscription. The borders of the neoplasm are usually well-rounded or circumscribed. There is usually an absence of a diffuse "motheaten" or permeative pattern of destruction along this border.

6. Extension to the articular cartilage. The vast majority abut a border of articular cartilage (Figs. 10–46, 10–50, and 10–51).

7. Absence of a border of benign sclerosis, punctate calcifications, or ominous periosteal reactions. Primary untreated GCT only rarely shows a containing border of benign reactive host bone sclerosis. Punctate calcifications, "sunburst," "hair-on-end," or other prominent periosteal reactions are rarely, if ever, seen.

Lesions of the large flat bones are similar to those of the large long bones. Because of the width of many of the large flat bones such as the ilium bone, expansion is not observed on initial examination. Lesions of the ilium may be many centimeters in size at presentation (Fig. 10–47). Lesions of the vertebral body or bodies may also be quite extensive (Fig. 10–48). Lesions of the sacrum may be quite large and there may be eccentric expansion (Fig. 10–49).

Giant Cell Tumor of the Thin Bones

The thin bones include the fibula, radius, ulna, distal tibia, and tubular bones of the hands, feet, and ribs. In these bones, most cases of GCT at initial

---

Low-Grade Neoplastic Giant Cell Tumor (GCT)

FIG. 10–48. Large expansive and trabeculated GCT involving at least two vertebral bodies. The lesion is expansive and fairly well circumscribed.

FIG. 10–49. Large, circumscribed, lytic GCT of the sacrum (*arrows*). By radiologic analysis alone a GCT in this location would probably be mistaken for a chordoma or metastatic tumor.

FIG. 10–50. Characteristic appearance of a GCT of a thin bone, in this case, the proximal fibula. It is epiphyseal, lytic, sharply circumscribed, and faintly trabeculated.

FIG. 10–51. Some tumors will show much coarser trabeculation. This uneven trabeculation is peripheral to the tumor and is due to either uneven cortical destruction or the uneven new bone production in periosteum consequent to the slow expansion caused by the tumor's growth. Gross examination of GCT's and specimen radiographs virtually never show coarse, bony trabeculation in the central tumor mass itself. By specimen radiograph the tumor mass is purely lytic.

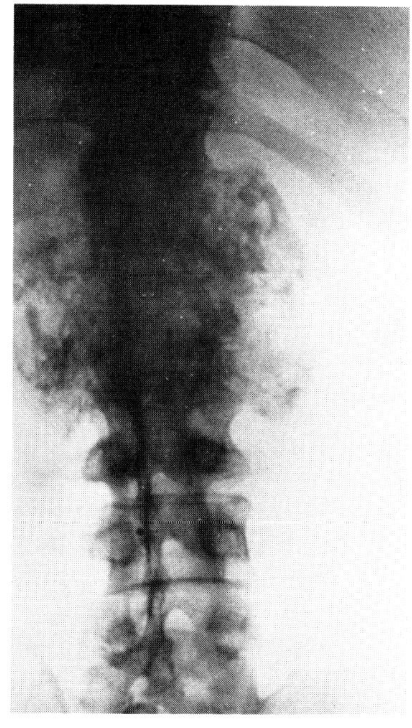

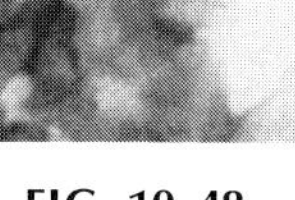

FIG. 10-48

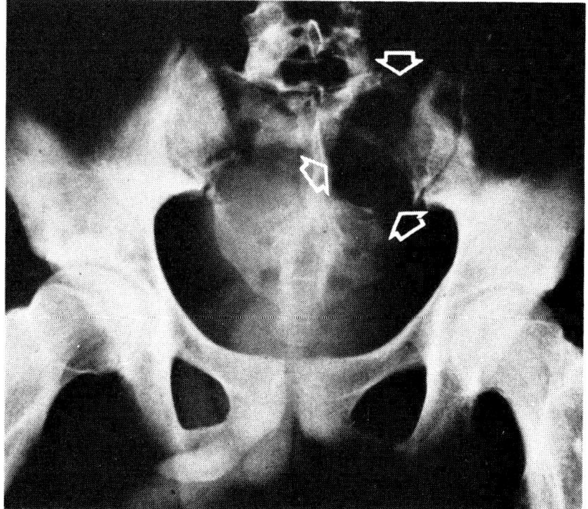

FIG. 10-49

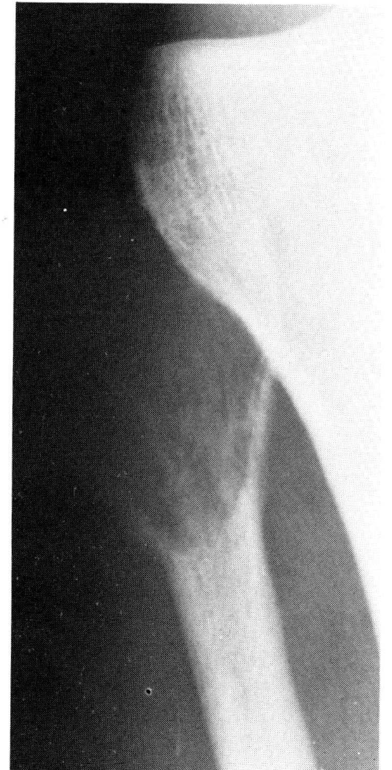

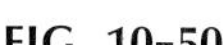

FIG. 10-50

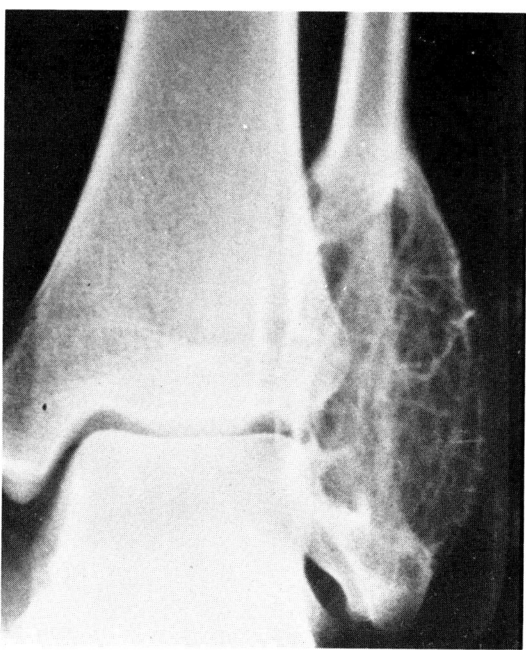

FIG. 10-51

presentation show diffuse symmetric to concentric expansion (Figs. 10–50 and 10–51). Otherwise the features are essentially identical as those of the large bones.

Differential Radiologic Diagnosis

CHONDROBLASTOMA. At the time of initial presentation, the chondroblastoma tends to be about half the size of a GCT in the corresponding site. Chondroblastomas frequently show a border of reactive host bone sclerosis and/or fine 0.5 to 1-mm. stippled calcifications. The GCT is at least about four times as common as the chondroblastoma. The chondroblastoma is the second most common tumor of the epiphysis.

CHONDROSARCOMA. This lesion usually shows more distinct rounded lobulation and rounded trabeculations because of the lobular nature of the growth of cartilage (Figs. 8–18 and 8–19). Approximately 10 per cent of chondrosarcomas (hyaline and clear-cell types) present as epiphyseal lesions. In this author's experience this is the third most common tumor of epiphyses. GCT outnumbers the epiphyseal chondrosarcoma by approximately five to one.

HYPERPARATHYROID GCT. On rare occasions this benign tumor may present as an apparent solitary epiphyseal mass indistinguishable from the neoplastic GCT (Fig. 10–1). Serum calcium and phosphorus tests are always necessary to rule out this exact mimic of the neoplastic GCT. The neoplastic GCT outnumbers the epiphyseal-metaphyseal hyperparathyroid GCT by approximately 50 to one (personal observations). Giant cell tumors of hyperparathyroidism are usually metaphyseal-diaphyseal lesions.

NONOSSIFYING FIBROMA. On rare occasions nonossifying fibromas may present in an epiphyseal location. It is always necessary to consider this lesion in any giant-cell-rich, nonchondroid-producing lesion of epiphysis showing a border of reactive host bone sclerosis in a patient under 20 years of age. The neoplastic GCT outnumbers the epiphyseal nonossifying fibroma by approximately 50 to one.

OTHER TUMORS. For every 50 neoplastic GCT's this author has seen, approximately one each of an epiphyseal-metaphyseal fibrosarcoma, osteosarcoma, reticulum cell sarcoma, Hodgkin's disease, or metastatic tumor present with a GCT-like pattern on radiograph. The histology of each of these lesions is usually sufficiently distinctive to permit easy separation.

Gross Pathology

Most gross specimens consist of curettage specimens. The tissue is very soft to fleshy and distinctly tan in color. Areas of collagenization appear whitish and areas of necrosis appear yellow. Focal hemorrhages and cystification are common.

GCT's removed intact prior to therapy of any kind show, in addition to the above findings, that the contour of the bone is expanded. Nevertheless, it is usually contained by a thin shell of periosteal new bone (Plate 7, *A* and *C*).

Those cases that come to amputation post-surgery or post-radiation where highly malignant transformation has not occurred are quite variable in appearance. There is usually considerably more fibrosis, focal hemorrhage, and areas of cystic degeneration. On occasion the tumor may be seen to have penetrated the bone and to have entered the joint at the articular cartilage bone interface. Some cases may extend to the joint or the contiguous bone by means of interosseous ligaments.

In rare cases, pathologic fracture may lead to total compromise of the vascular supply to the tumor and its total necrosis. Such lesions appear shrunken and yellowish to cystic.

Cases with one or more recurrences may show local seeding of the biopsy tract and even tumefactions in the dermal skin (Plate 7, *B*).

Low-Grade Neoplastic Giant Cell Tumor (GCT)

FIG. 10–52. The low-power histology of a primary untreated GCT is typified by an even distribution of giant cells and few to absent bands of fibrosis. Note the extension to the articular cartilage (extreme right), a characteristic of the neoplastic giant cell tumor of epiphyses (x40).

FIG. 10–53. The illustration represents the usual high-power field from a GCT. The osteoclast-like giant cells are evenly distributed. The nuclei of the giant cells are oval and contain a moderate-sized oval nucleolus. The stromal cells look histiocytic. They are oval to spindled in shape, contain fairly abundant cytoplasm, oval to reniform nuclei, and a smaller nucleolus than those of the giant cells. Typical mitoses (*arrow*) are not uncommon (x400).

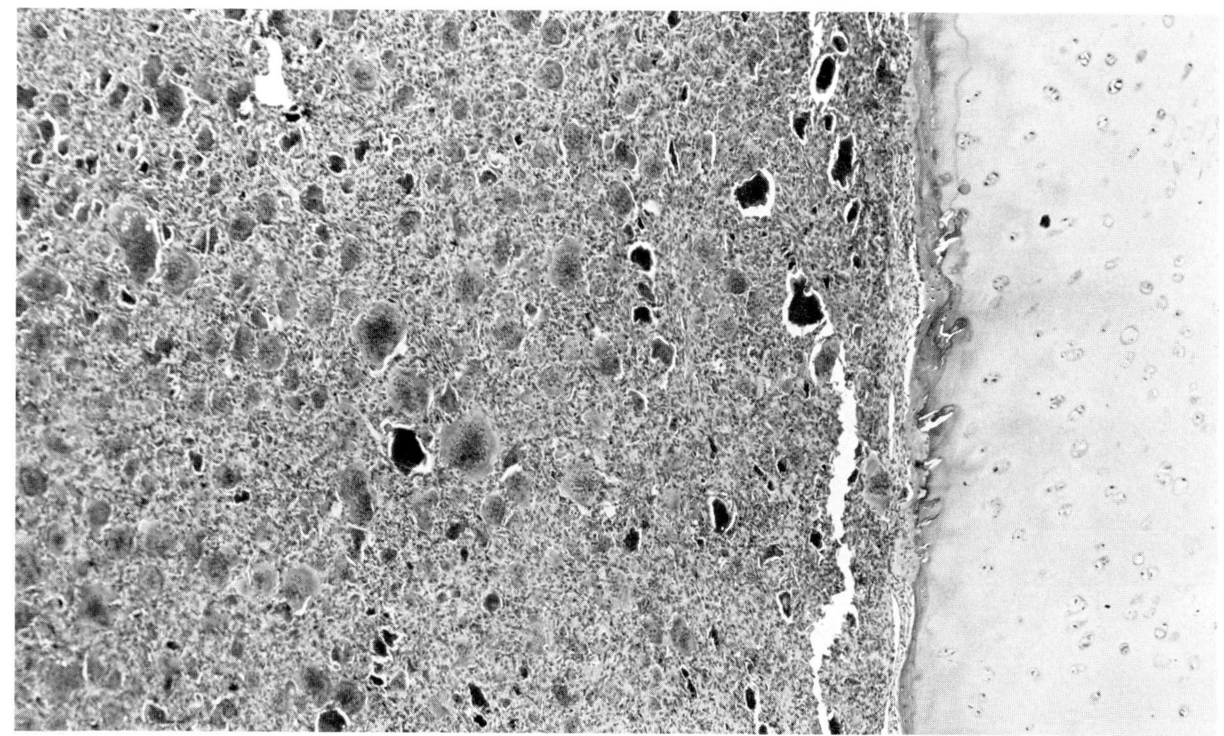

FIG. 10-52

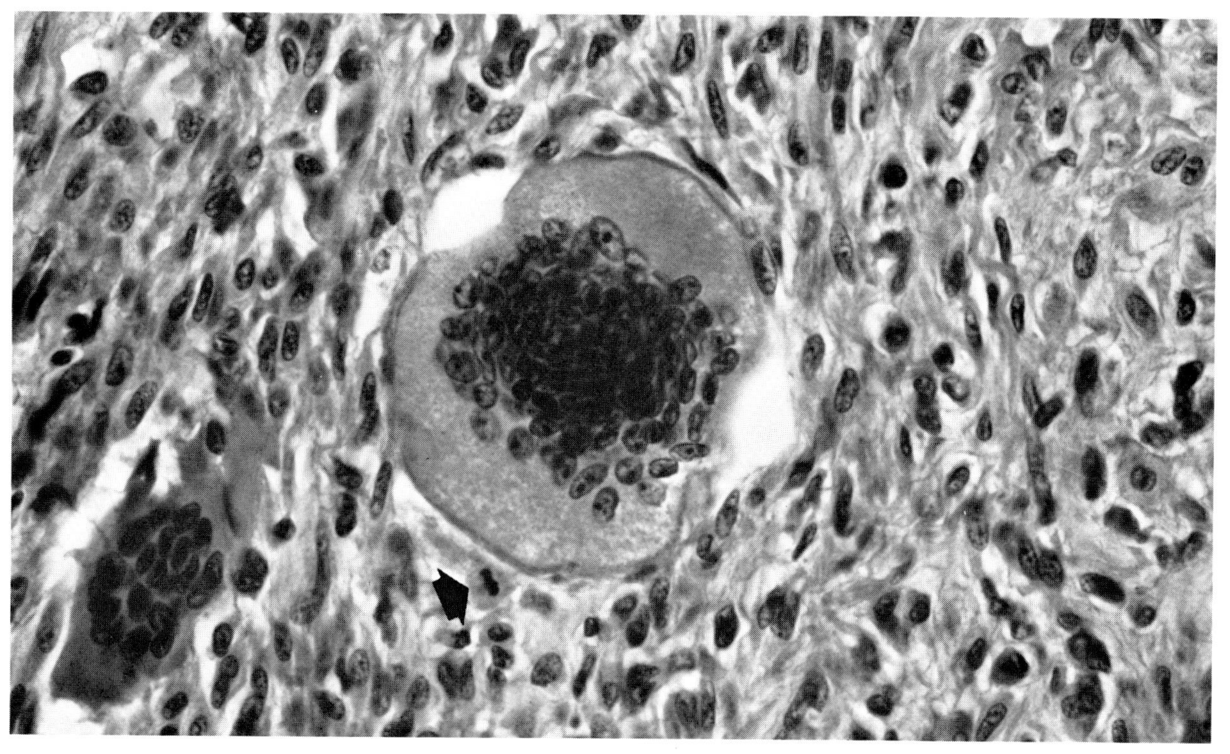

FIG. 10-53

Histopathology

The low-grade neoplastic GCT has characteristic but not pathognomonic histologic features. The benign GCT's of hyperparathyroidism and Paget's may mimic the GCT exactly. In rare cases of osteosarcoma with prominent, benign, osteoclast-like cells, the stromal anaplasia may be so subtle that confusion with GCT is possible without clinical and radiographic correlation. However, the behavior of these low-grade anaplastic osteosarcomas may show the same biologic virulence of their more highly anaplastic counterparts. Therefore, since the histologic diagnosis of the neoplastic GCT is not pathognomonic and other benign and highly malignant lesions may mimic the tumor very closely, we must be aware that the diagnosis may be in error. In order to reduce the error rate to a respectable figure, careful analysis of all clinical, laboratory, radiologic, and pathologic data must be performed. The further an individual case of suspected neoplastic GCT strays from its classical features, the greater must be our effort to eliminate the GCT-like variants. The principal clues to other lesions or malignant transformations are youth, metaphyseal or diaphyseal presentation, reactive border of sclerosis, recurrences 5 or more years post-therapy, prior radiotherapy, systemic or lung metastases, multiple bone involvement, and anaplasia.

The characteristic histopathologic features of a low-grade neoplastic GCT are as follows:

1. MASSES OF PROMINENT OSTEOCLAST-LIKE GIANT CELLS AND OVOID TO SPINDLY STROMAL CELLS. On low-power examination previously untreated tumors are characterized by relatively homogeneous cellularity, except for variable areas of osteoid and woven bone formation and collagenization. Osteoclast-like giant cells sprinkle the lesion in a diffuse and homogeneous fashion (Fig. 10–52). There is little variation in numbers of giant cells per unit area or from field to field except in areas of collagenization. The giant cells are individually placed and do not form local aggregates or isolated clusters.

The numbers of nuclei per cell may vary considerably from cell to cell. Some cells may have as few as three to four nuclei, while others may contain as many as 100 or more (Fig. 10–57). It is rare for any other bone tumor to contain as many nuclei per cell as is present in a considerable proportion of GCT's. The nuclei tend to be aggregated toward the cell's center. The nuclei are oval to slightly reniform and each is separate from the other (not multilobulated). The size and shape of each is uniform. (Bizarre sizes and shapes of individual nuclei are seen in highly malignant giant cell sarcomas and giant cell sarcoma-like entities.) The chromatin is evenly dispersed and the nucleoli are small in size and there are generally not more than two per nucleus. The cytoplasm is abundant, homogeneous to granular, deep pink, and occasionally contains bubbly vacuoles (Fig. 10–58). In many cases, mononuclear stromal cells can be found that appear to enter and fuse with the cytoplasm of some of the giant cells (Figs. 10–57 and 10–58). The nuclei of these fused stromal cells then apparantly migrate to the giant cell's center. It is in this fashion that the numbers of nuclei per giant cell seem to increase. Mitoses are never observed in the giant cells. This latter proposed mechanism appears to fit the observed facts better than the hypothesis of amitotic division.

The stromal cells are oval to moderately spindly in shape (Fig. 10–53), except in areas of collagenization. Each cell contains a single nucleus quite similar in appearance to that within the giant cells. Bizarre variation in nuclear size and shape, atypical mitoses, and large nucleoli are seen in highly malignant GCT-like variants (osteosarcoma, giant cell sarcoma, *etc.*). Mitotic figures may be abundant (up to 2 or 3 per high power field) but are always typical in the low-grade neoplastic GCT.

Low-Grade Neoplastic Giant Cell Tumor (GCT)

FIG. 10–54. High-power view of the ovoid to short spindly stromal cells. The chromatin is finely clumped and nucleoli are small to inconspicuous. Mirror-image mitoses may be abundant but frank anaplasia is absent (x1000).

FIG. 10–55. Recurrences in GCT are characterized by increased spindliness of the stromal cells, more abundant collagen formation, and a more focal rather than diffuse distribution of giant cells (x40).

FIG. 10–56. Higher-power view of a recurrent GCT. There is increased spindliness of the stromal cells and/or masses of collagen production. Note that the number of giant cells per unit area is inversely proportional to the degree of spindliness of the stroma or collagen production. The nuclei, though exuberant, do not show objective anaplasia, such as large, bizarre hyperchromatism or atypical mitotic figures (x250).

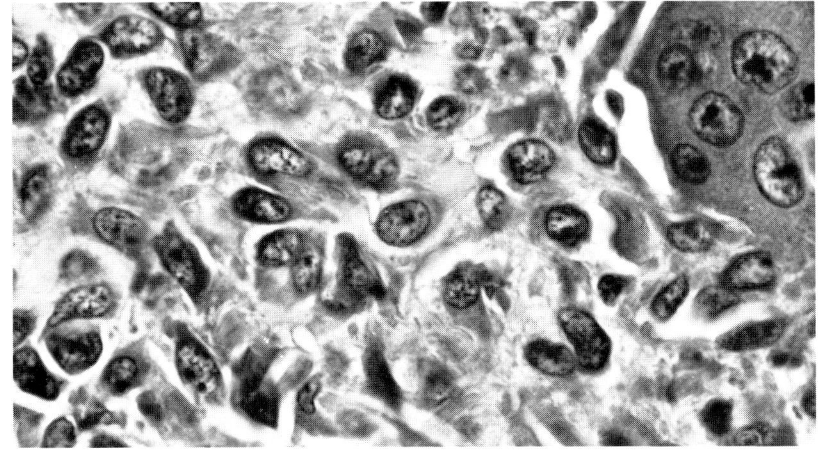

FIG. 10-54

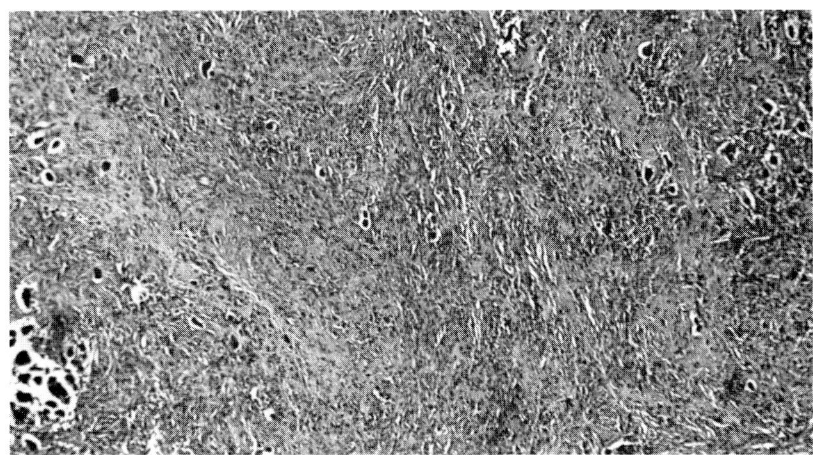

FIG. 10-55

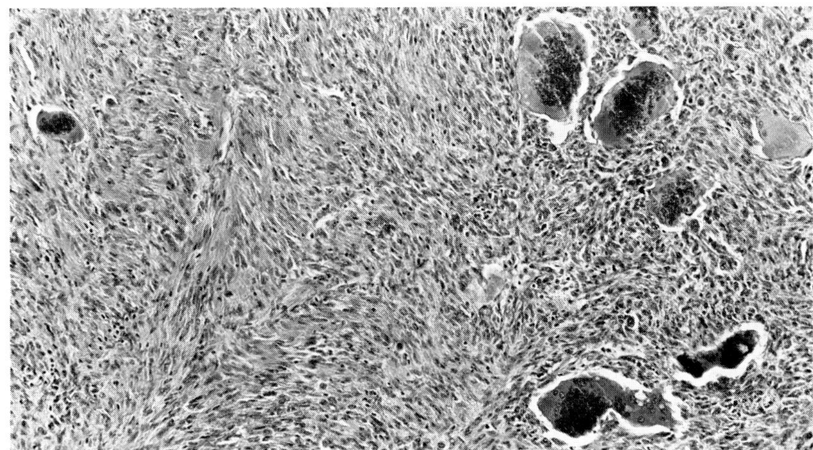

FIG. 10-56

2. FOCI OF COLLAGENIZATION. Most primary untreated tumors show little collagenization. Abundant collagenization or prominently long, spindly stromal cells are suggestive of hyperparathyroidism or nonossifying fibroma. However, each recurrence of GCT is characterized by increasing collagenization (Figs. 10–55 and 10–56). The number and size of giant cells per unit area usually vary in inverse proportion to the degree of collagenization (Fig. 10–56).

3. FOCI OF OSTEOID AND WOVEN BONE. Approximately 40 to 50 per cent of GCT's show variable proportions of osteoid and woven bone. In general, these foci are small and inconspicuous. In rare cases of GCT as much as 50 per cent of the lesional tissue can be osteoid and woven bone (Fig. 10–59). Such cases can be confused with osteoblastoma or osteosarcoma, particularly if they are discovered in atypical locations, such as short bone sites. Osteoblastomas show ordinary osteoclasts—that is, giant cells peppering bone surfaces; they do not show stromal masses of giant cells, as are seen in GCT. Osteosarcomas usually show anaplasia, a more ominous radiographic presentation, and rarely begin in a predominantly epiphyseal location.

The woven bone that is produced in GCT is often rimmed by prominent osteoblasts, a sign pointing to benign reactive bone (Fig. 10–59). The bone is often most prominent at the advancing edges of the GCT. In all probability the bone produced is consequent to trapped reactive host bone or to its production by stimulated periosteum. The GCT is of osteoclastic (histiocytic) origin and should not in and of itself have the ability to produce bone.

4. FOCI OF LIPOPHAGES. Foci of cholesterol-bearing cells and free cholesterol crystals have been described in some reports. These changes generally signify a regressive or healing phenomenon and are common to chondroblastomas, nonossifying fibroma, and eosinophilic granuloma. These tumors respond to treatment well.[57] However, Schajowicz[86] believes that some of these cases may in fact represent rare examples of the nonossifying fibroma (NOF) arising in an epiphyseal location. He diagnoses epiphyseal NOF if the patients are young and the lesion shows the characteristic radiologic and pathologic features of a NOF (Figs. 9–5–9–18), except for its epiphyseal location. The main radiologic clue would be the presence of a border of host bore sclerosis, a sign rarely associated with the GCT. This is a reasonable diagnosis, in this author's opinion, if it satisfies the criteria mentioned by Schajowicz.

5. ABUNDANCE OF THIN-WALLED VESSELS, OCCASIONAL ZONES OF HEMORRHAGE AND HEMOSIDERIN. The GCT is characterized by a prominence of thin-walled vessels. The vascular pattern may explain the occasional presence of abundant hemorrhages, recent and old, and hemosiderin-filled macrophages.[86] The GCT of hyperparathyroidism is almost always characterized by abundant focal hemorrhage.

6. ANEURYSMAL BONE CYST COMPONENT (ABC). Rare cases may show variable portions of the lesion with large, dilated, thick-walled, blood-filled cysts characteristic of an ABC component. If large masses of tumor consistent with GCT are seen in association with an ABC component, the lesion should be treated as a GCT.

7. INTRAVASCULAR OSTEOCLASTS. Occasionally, osteoclasts may be found in vascular lumina.[40,86,92] Although this finding (Fig. 10–60) may be a mechanism to explain rare lung metastasis, Campbell and Bonfiglio stated that some of the cases with this finding survived many years without recurrence of metastasis. This author has observed this phenomenon

(*Text continues on p. 349.*)

Low-Grade Neoplastic Giant Cell Tumor (GCT)

FIG. 10–57. The giant cells may reach enormous proportions and contain myriads of nuclei. With the possible exception of a rare case of chondroblastoma, giant cells with this appearance are usually diagnostic of the low-grade neoplastic GCT. Another fascinating characteristic seen in association with occasional giant cells of the GCT is the incorporation of mononuclear stromal cells within its cytoplasm (*arrows*). In most cases, fixation shrinkage shows a clear-cut space around these mononuclear cells. On occasion, however, the cytoplasm of the mononuclear cell seems to fuse with that of the giant cells. The incorporated nucleus of these cells may then migrate to the center of the giant cell. This feature can account for the huge numbers of nuclei seen in the giant cells in the absence of any histological evidence of either mitosis or amitotic division. A similar phenomenon can be observed in the osteoclastic sarcoma (see Fig. 10–66) (x400).

FIG. 10–58. Giant cells showing prominent vacuolization of the cytoplasm and an occasional mononuclear stromal cell entering their cytoplasm. Vacuolization of cytoplasm is often seen in cells of histiocytic origin and may also be seen in the osteoclastic sarcoma (see Fig. 10–66) (x400).

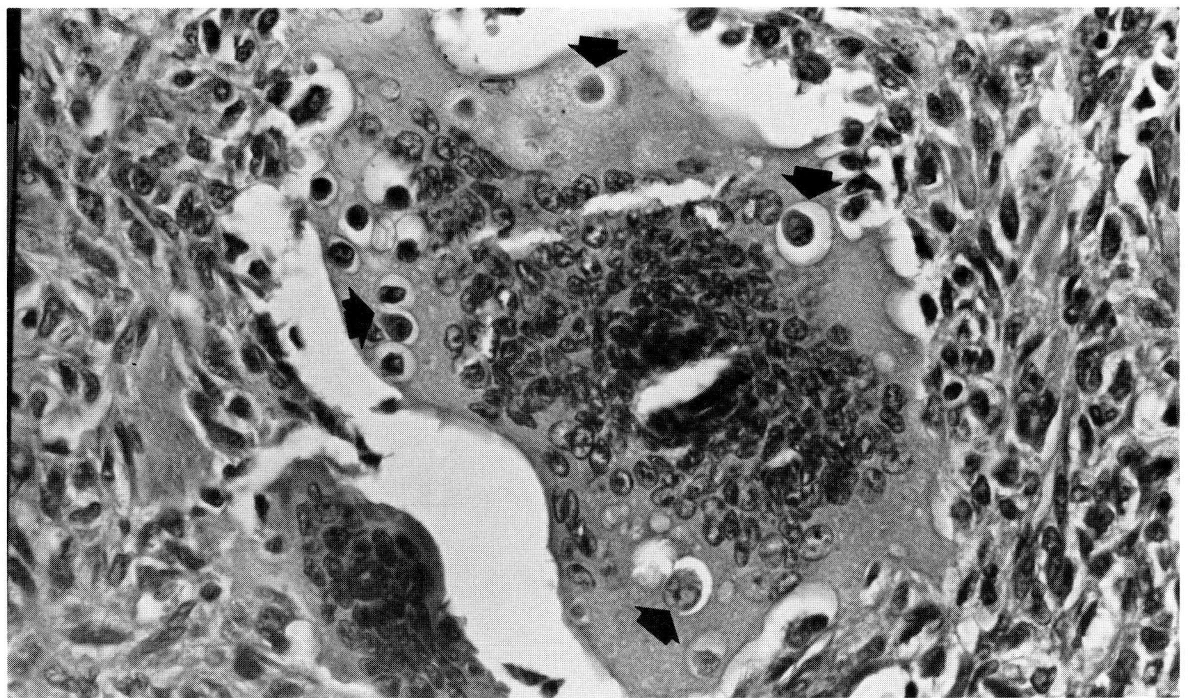

FIG. 10-57

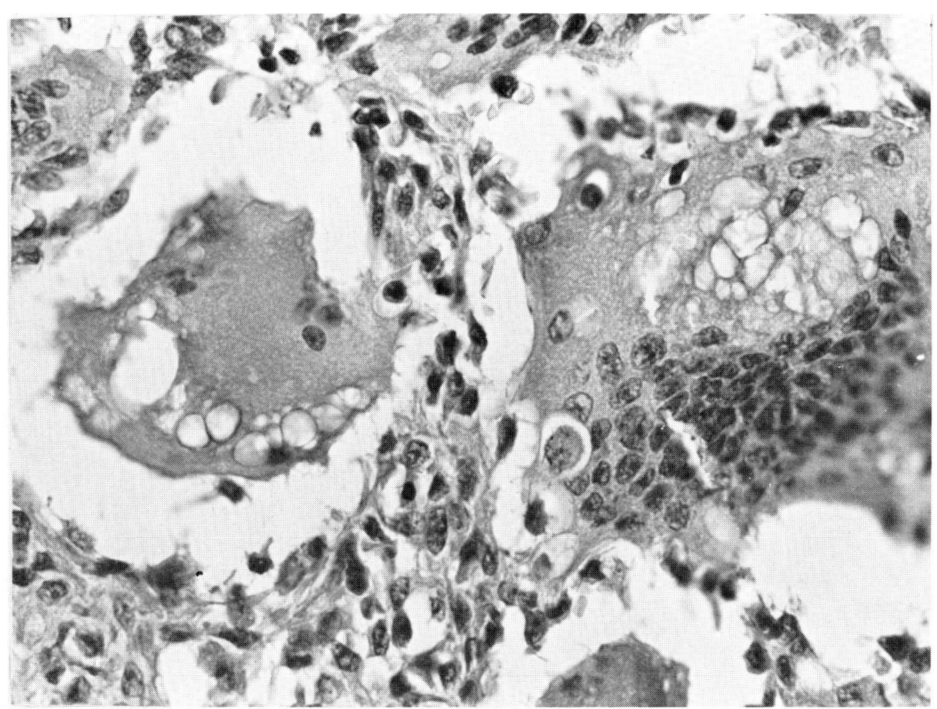

FIG. 10-58

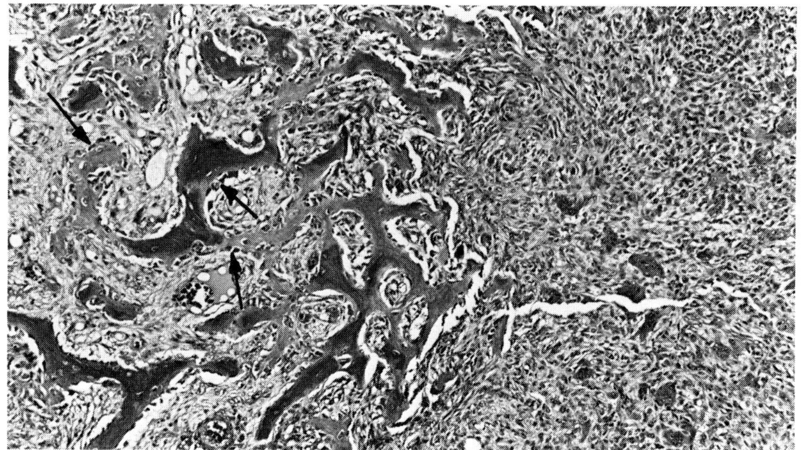

FIG. 10-59

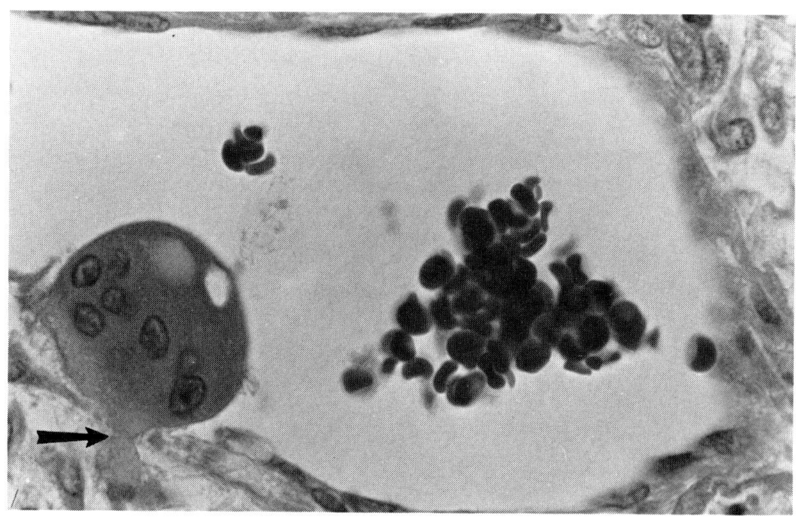

FIG. 10-60

Low-Grade Neoplastic Giant Cell Tumor (GCT)

FIG. 10-59. Approximately 40 per cent of GCT's show a variable degree of osteoid and/or woven bone production, usually concentrated at the margin of the tumor. The bone is benign and often shows focal or extensive prominent osteoblastic rimming (*arrows*). To the right of the field is tissue typical of the GCT (x125).

FIG. 10-60. Careful search will occasionally reveal vessels with osteoclast-like giant cells in their lumen. In this example a giant cell is entering the vessel by diapedesis, a portion of its cytoplasm on the stromal side of the basement membrane (*arrow*). This finding does not correlate with more ominous behavior (x1000).

in approximately 30 per cent of GCT's with no evidence of metastases or more aggressive behavior as compared to those without this finding. Therefore, it appears to have no prognostic significance.

Grading of Giant Cell Tumors

Jaffe[57] proposed grading the GCT by a I, II, III system. Originally he felt that this grading system had prognostic significance. While Jaffe indicates the aggressiveness of GCT by means of histologic criteria, he had discontinued the use of grading because he found that they may recur or metastasize regardless of grade [personal communications to Spjut, *et al.* (1971) and Goldenberg, *et al.* (1970)]. Some pathologists claim that grading was of prognostic significance in their series, while others do not. After perusing the literature thoroughly, I suspect that some series include various entities in their collection. This could explain the differences in grading and survival from one series to another. From my analysis there is little doubt that reported Grade III GCT's include a collection of tumors from exuberant, ordinary, neoplastic GCT's to highly malignant sarcomas. For that reason, this author does not use a grading system, but attempts to distinguish true low-grade neoplastic GCT's from those benign and highly malignant entities that may be confused with it. In this author's experience there has been little prognostic difference between Grade I and II giant cell tumor, provided that they are truly the ordinary neoplastic GCT. Instead of classifying a tumor as Grade III GCT, I prefer to separate these tumors into giant cell sarcomas, osteosarcomas with prominent osteoclast-like cells, malignant fibrous histiocytoma, fibrosarcomas with benign osteoclast-like giant cells, and sarcomatous transformation of a formerly low-grade neoplastic giant cell tumor. These entities will be discussed in detail in pages 352–366 and Figures 10–62 to 10–80.

Differential Diagnosis

In most instances the diagnosis of low-grade neoplastic GCT is not difficult, provided that hyperparathyroidism is ruled out. The typical lesion is epiphyseal-metaphyseal, lytic, lacks of border of host bone sclerosis, and contains monotonous sheets of osteoclast-like giant cells and exuberant oval to spindly stromal cells. Figures 10–52, 10–53, 10–54, and 10–57 characterize the histologic features of the majority of GCT's. Usually at least some of the giant cells contain myriads of nuclei. The histologic features that are atypical and can cause confusion with other entities include extensive blood or hemorrhage (confusion with aneurysmal bone cyst), osteoid and woven bone production (confusion with osteoblastoma and osteogenic sarcoma), extensive collagenization of stroma and long, spindly, stromal cells (confusion with fibrosarcoma and nonossifying fibroma), and osteoclast-like giant cells with no more than 10 to 15 nuclei (confusion with a host of other tumors that contain similar cells).

The differential diagnostic features of those lesions that may mimic GCT to a variable degree are as follows:

GIANT CELL TUMOR OF HYPERPARATHYROIDISM. This lesion may mimic the neoplastic GCT in every detail by histology alone. The differential features are given in Table 10–2.

CHONDROBLASTOMA. On rare occasions a chondroblastoma may produce very little chondroid or cartilage and contain giant cells with myriads of nuclei. Polygonal stromal cells and foci of "chicken-wire" calcification (Figs. 8–80–8–81) should be the stimulus to submit all of the curetted tissue to analysis in order to find the diagnostic chondroid (8–77 to 8–79, Plate 6 *K, L*). Chondroblastomas usually occur in patients with open epiphyses, and are usually surrounded by a border of host bone sclerosis on radiograph. Table 10–1 lists the differential diagnostic features.

ANEURYSMAL BONE CYST (ABC). GCT with extensive hemorrhage may resemble an aneurysmal bone cyst. An aneurysmal bone cyst is typified by large, thick, fibrous-walled structures filled with blood. In the GCT the hemorrhage rests free in the tissue and does not contain cyst walls. If, in an ABC, large fields of giant cells and stromal cells identical to those shown in Figures 10–52, 10–53, 10–54, and 10–56 are seen, the diagnosis should be GCT with an ABC component, provided, of course, that the lesion is centered in the epiphysis or epiphysis-metaphysis. Aneurysmal bone cyst has been reported to occur in association with numerous other entities, including the GCT. A GCT with an ABC component should be treated as a GCT.

OSTEOBLASTOMA. An osteoblastoma is rarely confused with a GCT, but a GCT rich in osteoid and woven bone may be mistaken for an osteoblastoma. An osteoblastoma consists of a rich homogeneous network of osteoid and woven bone peppered with osteoblasts and osteoclasts (Fig. 7–24 and Plate 2, *G*). The stroma contains numerous wide-caliber capillaries and a loose spindly stroma. If the bone, osteoblasts, and osteoclasts along the surface of the bone of

Table 10-2. Differential Diagnosis of Low Grade Neoplastic GCT, GCT of Hyperparathyroidism, and Chondroblastoma

	Low-Grade Neoplastic Giant Cell Tumor	*Giant Cell Tumor of Hyper-parathyroidism*	*Chondroblastoma*
Clinical			
1. Age (% of patients)	20–40 (60%)	20 + (95%)	10–20 (70%)
2. Serum calcium elevated, phosphorous depressed	—	+ (>80% of patients)	—
3. Elevated parathormone level	—	+	—
Radiographic Features			
1. Centered in epiphysis	>97% of patients	rare	>98%
2. Solitary lytic lesion	almost always	usually multiple	always
3. Punctate calcifications	—	—	+ (more than half of cases)
4. Sclerotic border	— (in primary presentation)	—	usually +
5. a. Resorption canals in cortices of multiple bones	—	common (in more advanced stages)	—
b. Loss of well-demarcated cortical borders of terminal phalangeal tufts	—	common (in more advanced stages)	—
c. Medial resorption of cortex of phalanges and long bones	—	not common, but when present is a pathognomonic sign	—
d. Loss of lamina dura of teeth	—	common (in more advanced stages)	—
Histology			
1. Abundant foci of microscopic hemorrhage	+	++	unusual
2. Collagenization	+	++	+
3. Osteoclast-like giant cells	+++	+++	+ to +++
4. Spindle-shaped stromal cells with indistinct cell border	+++	+++	0 to +
5. Polygonally shaped stromal cells with well-demarcated cell borders	unusual and focal, if present	—	+++
6. Islands of chondroid formation	—	—	+ to ++
7. Osteoid and woven bone	0 to ++	+ to ++	0 to +

an osteoblastoma were not considered, the remaining tissue would look nothing like a GCT. This is the principal reason why an osteoblastoma is not confused with a GCT. However, if a GCT contains extensive osteoid and bone production, these tissues are noticeable and if the pathologist is not aware that the GCT may contain significant quantities of these tissues, a diagnosis of osteoblastoma or osteosarcoma is possible. The manner in which a bone-rich GCT can best be identified is by temporarily disregarding the bone production. It is better to concentrate on those areas that show a minimum amount of bone. These areas will show masses of stroma and giant cells never seen in osteoblastoma. In osteoblastoma the giant cells are ordinary osteoclasts; that is, they are applied to the new bone spicules. The giant cells in osteoblastoma do not form masses of giant cells removed from the bone. In fact osteoblastomas never form solid sheets of giant cells where bone and/or osteoid production is not contained in the same high-power field. Both the osteoblastoma and the GCT may show prominent osteoblastic rimming of the osteoid or bone trabeculae, however. Although this feature is not helpful in distinguishing a GCT from an osteoblastoma, it is useful in distinguishing a GCT from a giant cell-rich osteosarcoma.

GIANT CELL-RICH OSTEOSARCOMA. The osteosarcoma may on occasion be diffusely sprinkled with osteoclasts or osteoclast-like giant cells. It, therefore, may resemble a GCT on low-power examination, (Fig. 10–71). However, close inspection of the stroma usually reveals frank anaplasia (Fig. 10–72) never seen in a true GCT. The osteoid and woven bone of an osteosarcoma is not rimmed by a prominent row of osteoblasts. The osteosarcoma may show cartilage production (Fig. 10–71), a tissue not produced in GCT. The GCT always shows some highly cellular fields, even when associated with extensive bone production. The degree of bone production in a GCT may approach 50 per cent of the total lesional tissue, rarely more. Histologic examination of the cellular areas may show exuberant plump nuclei but not frank anaplasia. On the other hand, the cellular nonbone-producing areas of the osteosarcoma almost always show unequivocal anaplasia. It is usually only in dense sclerosing or extensive bone-producing areas that nuclear anaplasia is minimal to absent. An osteosarcoma is in 99 per cent of cases either metaphyseally or diaphyseally located; 98 per cent of GCT's are centered in the epiphysis or epiphyseal-metaphyseal junction. Only 10 per cent of osteosarcomas are purely lytic, while all primary untreated GCT's are pure lytic lesions with or without trabeculations. Most osteosarcomas produce cumulus cloud fluffs of tumor bone. This is never seen in association with untreated or nonirradiated GCT.

NONOSSIFYING FIBROMA (NOF). These lesions contain giant cells with fewer nuclei than most GCT's. The stroma of the NOF is more spindly, associated with greater degrees of collagen production, and they may contain foamy macrophages (Figs. 9–2–9–21). The vast majority are metaphyseal, occur in much younger patients, and are surrounded by a border of host bone sclerosis. However, rare cases of NOF with all of the above features (except location) may be epiphyseally centered.

GIANT-CELL-RICH FIBROSARCOMA. The low-grade fibrosarcoma replete with numerous osteoclast-like giant cells is the most difficult of all to distinguish from a low-grade neoplastic GCT by histology alone. The fibrosarcoma may contain giant cells rarely with more than 15 to 20 nuclei per cell. The giant cells tend to be more unevenly distributed in these tumors than in the GCT. The most important feature is the presence of occasional cells or fields of cells showing large hyperchromatic nuclei and atypical mitotic figures that are beyond the range of cytology of true GCT's (Figs. 10–73–10–76). Fibrosarcomas are usually metaphyseally or diaphyseally centered, are well to poorly circumscribed, are firm, and white to grey. The GCT is epiphyseal-metaphyseal, soft, and dark tan. The fibrosarcoma has a high potential for lethal metastases, even those showing low-grade anaplasia. Any "GCT" with lung metastases with a lethal course must be critically reviewed to rule out a low-grade anaplastic fibrosarcoma rich in giant cells.

Course and Treatment

The giant cell tumor is characterized by a high recurrence rate following curettage or irradiation. The best success has been achieved by either en-bloc resection or cryosurgical techniques.

The recurrence rates with various procedures are as follows:

1. CURETTAGE ALONE. The recurrence rate with curettage alone in most large series is high, averaging 50 per cent (35–70 per cent range).

2. EN-BLOC EXCISION. With en-bloc excision, the recurrence rates are approximately 10 to 15 per cent.[81]

3. RADIATION. With radiation to tumors in inaccessible sites such as the spine the cure rate ascribable to radiation alone in Cambell and Bonfiglio's series[40] of 46 patients was only 17 per cent (dosage range, 1500–5000 R). In 63 per cent of patients radiation therapy was deemed ineffective.

4. CRYOSURGERY. With cryosurgery, the cure rate was 92 per cent in Marcove's first series.[71] Their most serious complication was infection in seven of 25 patients. Two of the infections were ascribed to skin freezing, necrosis, and faulty closure. Those patients required local resection and one resulted in amputation. Five patients required knee fusion because of failure; two because of infection. The patient who required amputation because of infection also developed metastasis but was free of disease $3\frac{1}{2}$ years after pulmonary resection. Fourteen of the cases were recurrent tumors that had been treated previously by curettage. With further refinement of his technique, Marcove has substantially reduced the incidence of complications in 27 additional cases. Except for a single instance of malignant transformation proximal to the treated area which necessitated amputation, the "cure rate" at this time following repeat cryosurgery in this group was otherwise 100 per cent. (Refer to Chap. 15.)

The biologic behavior and ultimate outcome of the ordinary GCT treated by various modalities is summarized in Table 10–2. These observations are based upon review of several large series, Parrish's[81] use of en-bloc excision, and Marcove's use of cryosurgery.[71,73]

Malignant Giant Cell Tumor—Does Such an Entity Exist?

In most large series the incidence of so-called malignant giant cell tumor ranges from 5 to 15 per cent[50,86] to as astoundingly high a figure as 30 per cent.[54] The reasons for this wide discrepancy are manifold. Most of the problem stems from the use of the term *malignant;* another from lumping various types of giant cell rich tumors together. In Hutter's series[54] part of the bias may be due to the fact that the cases sent to Memorial Hospital, the largest cancer hospital in the United States, are probably the worst from the standpoint of size and location, previous treatment (most had already undergone radiation), and those with multiple recurrences and microscopic atypia. Of approximately 60 cases of GCT that this author has dubbed as ordinary low-grade neoplastic type, only 2 have lead to the patient's demise and both were patients who developed radiation-induced sarcomas many years after the initial radiation.

To some authors, malignant giant cell tumor includes those with lung metastases despite the histological appearance; others equate so-called Grade III tumors with this entity; still others use frank anaplasia of stromal and/or giant cells as their criterion; finally, others classify the giant cell tumor as malignant if it leads to demise. It is no surprise, then, that with these vast differences in criteria for the term *malignant GCT* that the statistics concerning this so-called entity are so different and so confusing.

My own particular way out of this mire is to split rather than lump diagnoses. Because of the confusion and differences of opinion concerning the term *malignant GCT,* I would advocate dropping the term altogether or else clearly explaining in a note what is meant by it. From my own experiences and review of the literature this "entity" should be split into at least six groups. The first three of these groups are histogenetically related to GCT; the latter three are tumors of different histogenetic origin that may be confused with low-grade and anaplastic GCT's.

Group 1. Low-Grade neoplastic giant cell tumor with lung metastasis identical to the primary lesion

Group 2. Sarcomatous degeneration of a formerly low-grade neoplastic giant cell tumor. This may occur secondary to irradiation or *de novo.*

Group 3. Giant cell or osteoclastic sarcoma.

Group 4. Giant-cell-rich osteosarcomas

Group 5. Malignant fibrous histiocytoma

Group 6. Giant-cell-rich fibrosarcomas

Each of these entities will be treated individually in the following sections.

Group I. Low-Grade Neoplastic Giant Cell Tumor With Lung Metastasis Identical to the Primary Tumor

From a review of large series, it is apparent that approximately 1 to 3 per cent of otherwise ordinary low-grade neoplastic giant cell tumors can result in metastases (almost always to the lungs) that are virtually identical to the primary lesion.

If the fully documented and illustrated case reports with this occurrence are examined, the highly unusual course of this entity compared to the usual course of malignant tumors as we conceive them becomes apparent (see Table 10–3). Of the 11 patients studied, only one has died of the disease after

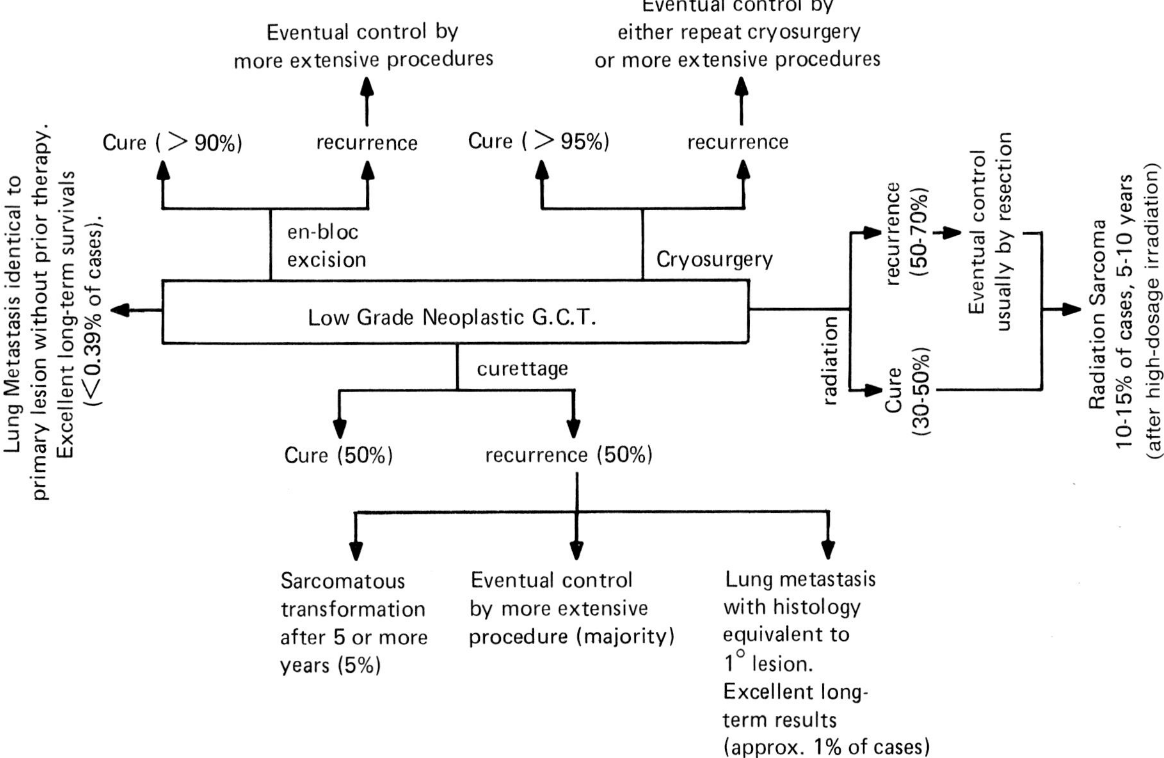

FIG. 10-61. Biologic behavior of the low-grade neoplastic giant cell tumor with different treatment modalities.

follow-up periods of as long as 22 years. Unfortunately, the only case (case 1) with demise had the poorest quality illustrations (in actuality drawings of microscopic fields), upon which no unequivocal diagnosis can be made by critical review. Only the case of Lasser[68] has shown progression of the disease as of the last follow-up examination. In all of the others the metastases were either totally and successfully removed or if there were too many to remove, they did respond to chemotherapy[65] and became stationary or self-limited in growth and/or spontaneously regressed! This bizzare behavior is remarkedly similar to that described for the benign chondroblastoma with lung metastases identical to the primary lesion (p. 226 and Figs. 8-68–8-89). Perhaps as intimated by Pan, *et al.*,[79] the "metastases" of GCT could be considered as "transplants" and possibly as "benign." It is interesting to note that in two of these cases, lung metastases were seen prior to surgical intervention. On the other hand, all of the few chondroblastoma cases with "benign" lung metastases had surgical intervention, implying iatrogenic transplantation. In regard to the low-grade neoplastic GCT the pathogenesis of the lung "transplantation" may be due to the fact that as many as 40 per cent of the lesions show intravascular osteoclasts upon careful search.[92] However, the presence of these intravascular deposits did not adversely affect the prognosis and were not associated with lung metastases in the five cases reported by the above group.[92] Similar findings were reported by Hutter.[54]

In dealing with GCT's showing metastases, this author would suggest removing all lung nodules, providing that respiration would not be compromised severely and by treating any recurrence in the primary bone site by measures short of amputation, if feasible. If the lung metastases are too numerous to remove them all, only the largest can be removed, with the expectation that the course will probably remain self-limited based upon a critical review of published cases (Table 10-3).

It is extremely important to remove at least one lung metastasis to make sure that the lesions do not represent sarcomatous or anaplastic transformation of a

Table 10-3. Reported Patients With Documented, Illustrated Metastasis Associated With Typical Low-

Author	*Age*	*Sex*	*Location*	*Initial Therapy*	*Recurrence(s) (Years)*	*Treatment Post-Recurrence(s)*	*Metastasis To*
Dyke[47]	25	M	Patella	Curettage	3	Amputation. 5 years after initial presentation, 3 years post-curettage.	Lungs, lymph nodes
Pan, *et al.*[79]	61	M	Radius distal	Curettage and 1500 R	1½	1500 R; curettage 1 year later	Lung, solitary
Pan, *et al.*[80]	46	F	10th Thoracic vertebra	Modified excision and 3000 R	None	—	Lung, solitary
Haas, *et al.*[51]	33	M	Femur proximal	Local excision	None	—	Shaft of penis
Lasser, *et al.*[68]	29	M	Femur, distal	Curettage	1½ 7 (recurred in proximal femur and spread to pelvis)	Midthigh amputation (1½) 2000 R to leg (7 years)	Lungs, multiple (6 years) Sternum (7 years)
Goldenberg, *et al.*[50]	27	M	Femur, distal	Curettage	1	Amputation	Lungs, multiple
Stargardter, *et al.*[93]	39	F	Coccyx	Local excision	None	—	Lungs, multiple
Spjut, *et al.*[90a]	44	M	Radius, distal	Amputation	None	—	Lungs, 2 solitary nodules
Kutchemeshgi, *et al.*[65]	23	F	Tibia, proximal	Curettage	2 and 4	3750 R (2 years) Amputation (4 years)	Lungs, multiple
Jewell, *et al.*[59]	22	M	Radius, distal	Curettage	6 months	3000 R	Lung, solitary

Grade Neoplastic 1° Giant Cell Tumor in Which the Metastases Appeared Identical to the 1° Lesion

Metastasis Seen After Initial Therapy	*Treatment of Metastasis*	*Course*	*Quality of Illustrations*	*Comments*
3	None	Demise due to disease 1 year post-amputation	Poor	Quality of illustrations (drawings only) does not permit unequivocal diagnosis.
3	En-bloc excision of lung and diaphragm	Free of disease 6 years after lung resection No recurrence of 1° lesion	Excellent	Unequivocal neoplastic GCT with long-term survival
3	Lobectomy	1 year follow-up. No evidence of further metastasis or recurrence	Good	Typical neoplastic GCT with solitary lung metastasis and short but benign course
2	Excision	1 year follow-up. No further evidence of metastasis or recurrence	Fair	Reviewed by Jaffe[51] and called GCT. Because of metastasis Stout[51] called tumor an osteosarcoma Probable neoplastic GCT with short but benign course.
6 and 7	Lungs, none Sternum, 5000 R.	Progressive regression of many lung mets at 7–10 years. At 10 years new nodules noted in lung and new lesion in pubis. Alive at 10 years with slow progression.	Good	Apparent low-grade neoplastic GCT with relentless, aggressive, but nonlethal, behavior
Present prior to initial therapy Originally were believed to be infectious	Removal of only 2	Alive and well with multiple self-limited lung mets with 18-year follow-up	Excellent Illustrations in Jaffe[57] (pp. 32–33)	Unequivocal low-grade neoplastic GCT with incredible course
Present prior to therapy	Biopsies only	Spontaneous regression of many Self-limited growth in others Last 3 years of follow-up, no change in radiographic appearance Follow-up period of 11 years	Excellent	Unequivocal low-grade neoplastic GCT with incredible course
2 and 4	Lobectomies	Alive and well 22 years after second lobectomy	Excellent	Unequivocal low-grade neoplastic GCT with benign course despite lung mets
2	Cyclophosphamide	Well 5 years after amputation and chemotherapy Lung mets unchanged in size	Good	Low-grade neoplastic GCT with long-term survival despite residual lung mets
3	Segmental resection	5 years after lung resection alive and free of disease	Good	Unequivocal low-grade neoplastic GCT with benign long-term course

formerly ordinary GCT. If lung metastases are noted, it is imperative, of course, to review the original bone neoplasm to rule out an osteo-, fibro-, or other sarcoma with subtle anaplasia misdiagnosed as an ordinary GCT.

Group II. Sarcomatous Degeneration of Formerly Low-Grade Neoplastic Giant Cell Tumors

Post-Irradiation Sarcomatous Transformation

As many as 10 to 15 per cent of ordinary low-grade neoplastic GCT's given radiation may eventually undergo sarcomatous transformation.[54,57] The interval between treatment and sarcoma is generally between 5 and 8 years, with a range of 3 to 23 years. The chances of malignant transformation appear to increase with higher initial dosages of radiation. The above figures for sarcomatous transformation are based upon radiation methods performed several decades ago. With newer radiation techniques these figures may become substantially lower.

Histologically, these anaplastic transformations are either fibrosarcoma with or without benign looking osteoclast-like giant cells, osteogenic sarcomas, or sarcomas with anaplastic spindle-cell stroma and anaplastic giant cells (giant cell or osteoclast sarcoma).

These are all highly malignant tumors that require radical forms of therapy.

DE NOVO ANAPLASTIC TRANSFORMATION OF FORMERLY LOW-GRADE NEOPLASTIC GCT. Transformation of a low-grade GCT to an anaplastic neoplasm without prior irradiation is apparently very rare. Hutter[54] mentions three such cases in his series. Kossey and Cervenansky[64] presented at least three such cases (Cases 6, 7, and 8). One case was associated with a cartilage-producing osteogenic sarcoma, while the other two converted to fibrosarcoma-like lesions. The time intervals for anaplastic transformation were 8, 32, and 10 years, respectively.

There is need for more fully documented examples of this rare occurrence.

Group III. Giant Cell or Osteoclastic Sarcoma

SYNONYMS. Anaplastic giant cell tumor, malignant osteoclastoma, osteoclastic sarcoma, and malignant giant cell tumor.

DEFINITION. This author defines the giant cell or osteoclastic sarcoma of bone as a highly malignant tumor composed of anaplastic stromal and anaplastic osteoclast-like giant cells in which there is no evidence of tumor osteoid, bone, or cartilage. Tumors that conform to this definition are rare and usually follow in the wake of Paget's disease. Other cases apparently arise *de novo* and a few may be associated with malignant transformation of a formerly ordinary low-grade GCT usually many years after initial curettage and/or radiation.

Some authors include this tumor with Grade III giant cell tumors and others like Troup, Dahin and Coventry[97] include them with osteosarcomas. These authors, in comparing and contrasting osteosarcomas to giant cell tumors, stated the following: "Tumors available had been classified either osteogenic sarcoma or as giant cell tumor of bone. Those that included giant cells and had frank sarcomatous stroma throughout we classed with the osteogenic sarcomas. Almost all of these sarcomas bearing benign giant cells produced osteoid in some foci, and in this regard were like osteogenic sarcomas that did not contain benign giant cells. Also included among osteogenic sarcomas were a few highly anaplastic lesions

---

Osteoclastic Sarcoma

FIG. 10-62. Patient with Paget's disease presented with increasing pain of his lower leg. A radiograph showed a faint lytic lesion (*black arrow*) with some degree of soft-tissue extension (*white arrow*), a sign of malignant transformation.

FIG. 10-63. The bone shows the pumicelike quality of Paget's disease and a very soft, tannish grey tumor, causing complete lysis of the involved bone.

FIG. 10-64. This lesion was characterized by huge, osteoclast-like giant cells with individual nuclei tending toward peripheral localization; there are also numerous mononuclear stromal cells (x125).

FIG. 10-65. The giant cells and the stromal cells demonstrate high-grade anaplasia. Note the malignant osteoclast-like cell (*arrow*) (x250).

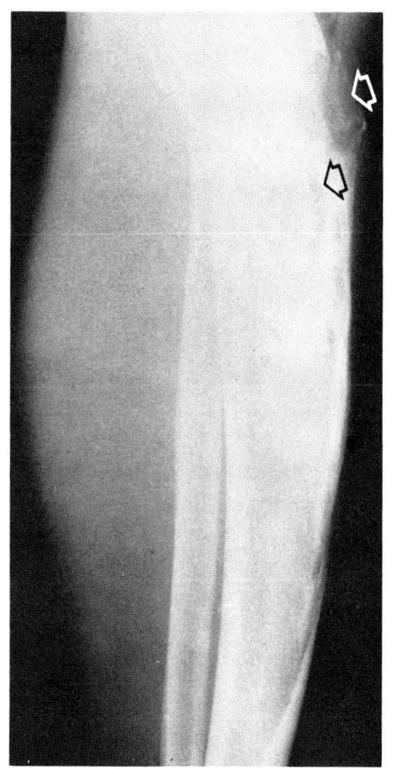

FIG. 10-62

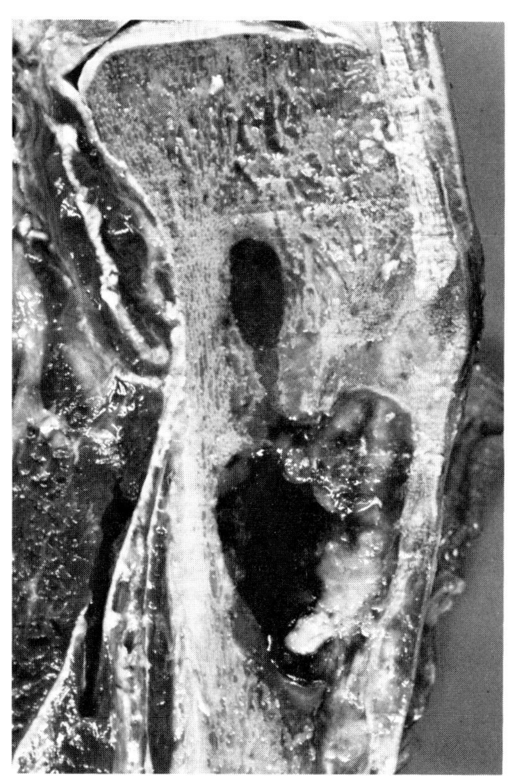

FIG. 10-63

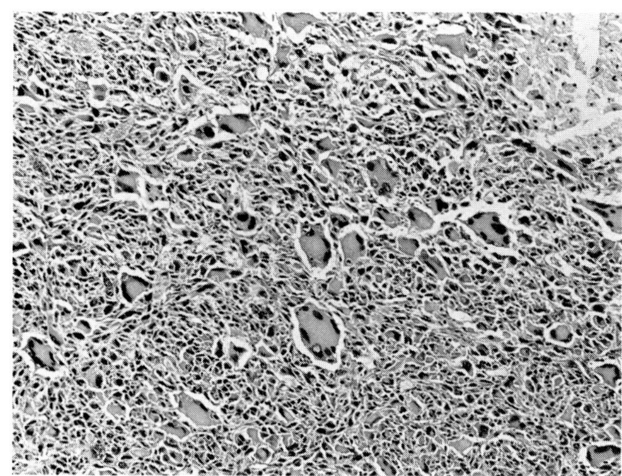

FIG. 10-64

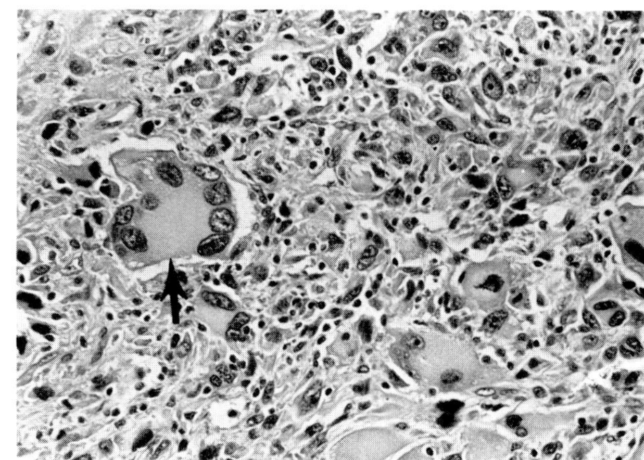

FIG. 10-65

that produced no osteoid but otherwise were similar in histologic appearance to osteoid-producing tumors and would fit in no other category."[97]

My experience is basically similar, in that I have seen occasional highly anaplastic unequivocal bone-producing giant cell-rich osteosarcomas that were similar in many respects to those tumors in which exhaustive review of multiple sections revealed that bone was not produced. Unfortunately, the vast majority of tumor pathologists, including myself, define an osteosarcoma as a highly malignant neoplasm that produces osseous tissues from an undifferentiated stroma. Using this definition it would not be possible to include nonosseous-producing tumors in this category. It is, therefore, contradictory to have a category essentially equivalent to nonosteogenic osteogenic sarcoma. Rather than squeeze these nonosseous-producing osteosarcoma-like tumors into a well-defined category, I believe it would be much more justifiable to place them into separate categories; namely, either giant cell sarcoma, giant cell-rich fibrosarcoma or sarcoma, giant and spindle cell type, not otherwise specified. Russell[84] was the first to recognize that occasional highly anaplastic giant cell tumors that arose in Paget's disease could be completely devoid of osseous tissue production; she called those tumors malignant osteoclastoma. However, this terminology is essentially the same as calling them malignant giant cell tumors since osteoclastoma and giant cell tumor are synonymous terms. If the ordinary neoplastic giant cell is a low grade malignancy, the term malignant osteoclastoma does not distinguish low-grade from highly malignant giant cell tumors. The term *giant cell or osteoclastic sarcoma,* if used as defined above, more aptly differentiates the low-grade neoplastic GCT from the highly malignant variant so that the clinician is not likely to be confused about the kind of therapy to apply in each category or to ask the question of how malignant the tumor is. Ordinary neoplastic giant cell tumors should be treated as locally aggressive tumors by either very thorough curettage, en-bloc excision, or cryosurgery; the giant cell sarcoma must receive radical therapy such as amputation or massive radiation therapy and systemic chemotherapy. The term *sarcoma,* in relation to the category of giant cell sarcoma is, therefore, used in its usual sense of a highly anaplastic neoplasm characterized in most instances by rapid and lethal metastases.

These tumors are rare and most often occur in association with severe Paget's disease. The remainder usually occur as primary tumors or in sarcomatously transformed formerly low-grade neoplastic GCT. An example of the radiologic and gross features of an osteoclastic sarcoma arising in association with Paget's disease is shown in Figures 10–62 and 10–63.

Histopathology

The giant cell or osteoclastic sarcoma is, in essence, a highly malignant histiocytic tumor. It can have any or all of the features common to histiocytic processes; namely, round cells, giant cells, spindly fibrosarcoma-like cells and evidence of collagen production.

On low-power examination the tumor is composed in areas of a striking proliferation of anaplastic osteoclast-like giant cells and ovoid, polygonal to spindly stromal cells. The giant cells tend to have large, separate, anaplastic nuclei (Figs. 10–65–10–68). Histiocytic bubbly vacuolization of the cytoplasm may be observed (Fig. 10–66), similar to that observed in occasional cells of ordinary GCT (Fig. 10–58). Mononuclear cells that seem to enter and fuse with these anaplastic giant cells (Fig. 10–66) are strikingly similar to those described for the ordinary GCT (Figs. 10–57 and 10–58).

The stromal cells may be round (Figs. 10–66 and 10–67), oval (Fig. 10–65) to spindle-shaped (Fig. 10–68). Areas can be observed in which the cells

(*Text continues on p. 362.*)

Osteoclastic Sarcoma

FIG. 10–66. The cytoplasm of the stromal and giant cells are pale and granular to foamy, consistent with their histiocytic origin. (Osteoclasts are in essence specialized bone resorbing histiocytes.) The giant cells may show mononuclear cells entering the cytoplasm from the periphery. In at least one cell the cytoplasm of the mononuclear cell appears to have partially fused with the giant cell (*arrow*). The nuclei of these entering mononuclear cells are viable, arguing against phagocytic digestion by the giant cells. Similar features may be seen in the ordinary low-grade neoplastic GCT (see Fig. 10–57) (x400).

FIG. 10–67. Some fields may show masses of mononuclear histiocytes with polygonal or rounded cell borders (*arrow*) (x250).

FIG. 10–68. In other fields, the polygonal histiocytic cells may taper into longer spindled cells (x250).

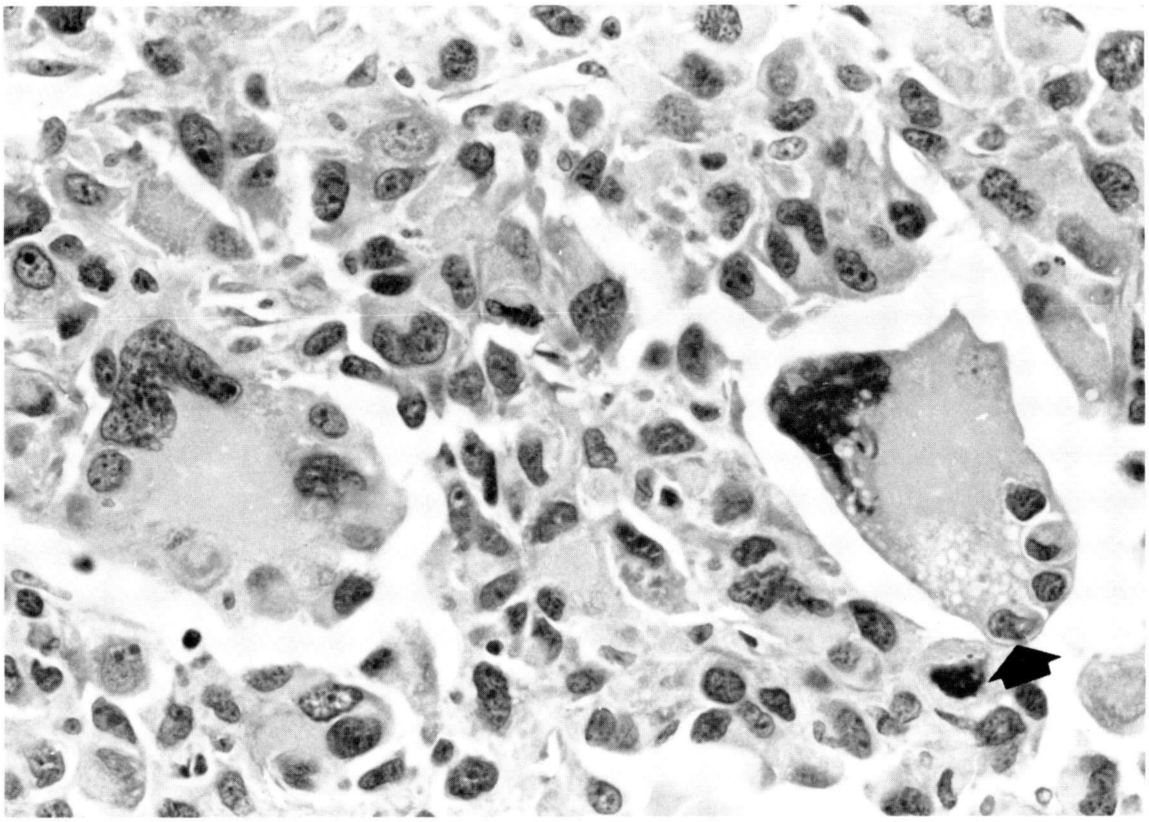

FIG. 10-66

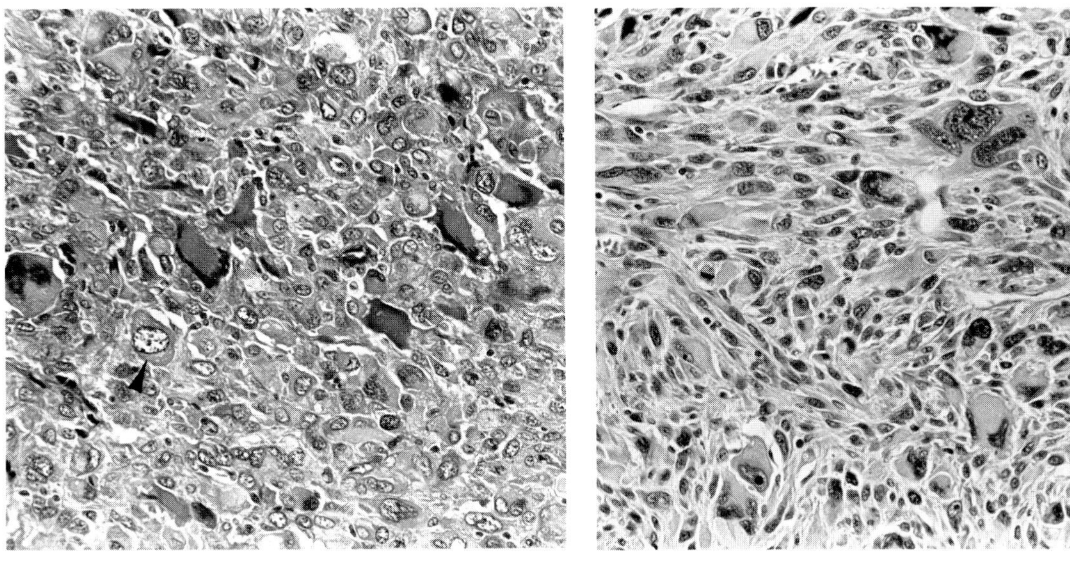

FIG. 10-67

FIG. 10-68

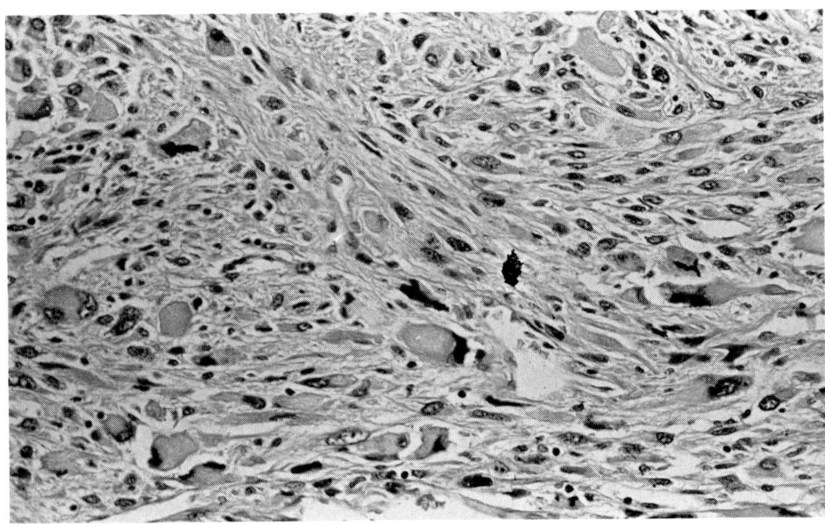

FIG. 10-69

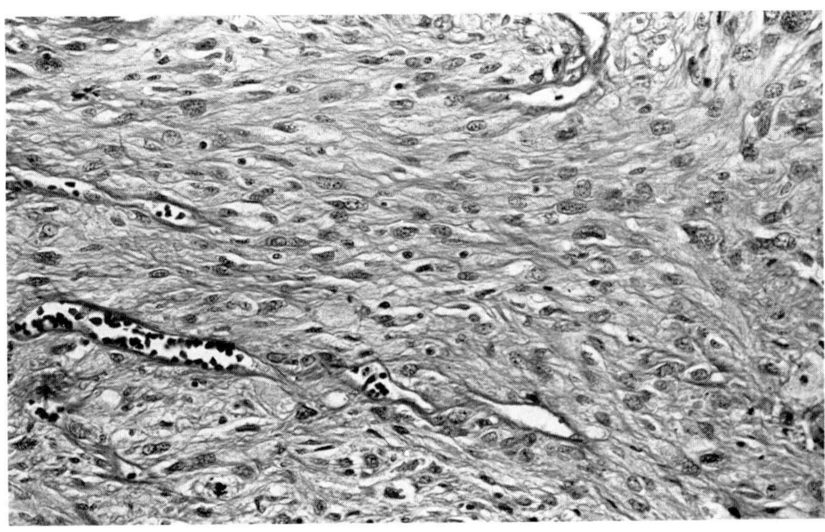

FIG. 10-70

Osteoclastic Sarcoma

FIG. 10-69. The histiocytes may become tremendously elongated and even produce collagen (facultative fibroblasts) (x250).

FIG. 10-70. In other areas, the tumor may resemble a fibrosarcoma (shown above) or a malignant fibrous histiocytoma with a prominant storiform pattern identical to that shown in Fig. 9-50 (x250).

Giant Cell Rich Osteosarcoma

FIG. 10-71. Giant cell rich osteosarcoma. To the right of the field is an area resembling the ordinary GCT. To the left is a focus of tumor cartilage that should immediately make the diagnosis of GCT suspect (x125).

FIG. 10-72 Although some of the giant cells contain benign nuclei and represent ordinary osteoclasts (*a*), individual stromal cells show unequivocal anaplasia (*b*). To the left of the field is a focus of osteoid production (*c*) produced by the anaplastic stromal cells. This finding is diagnostic of an osteosarcoma (x250).

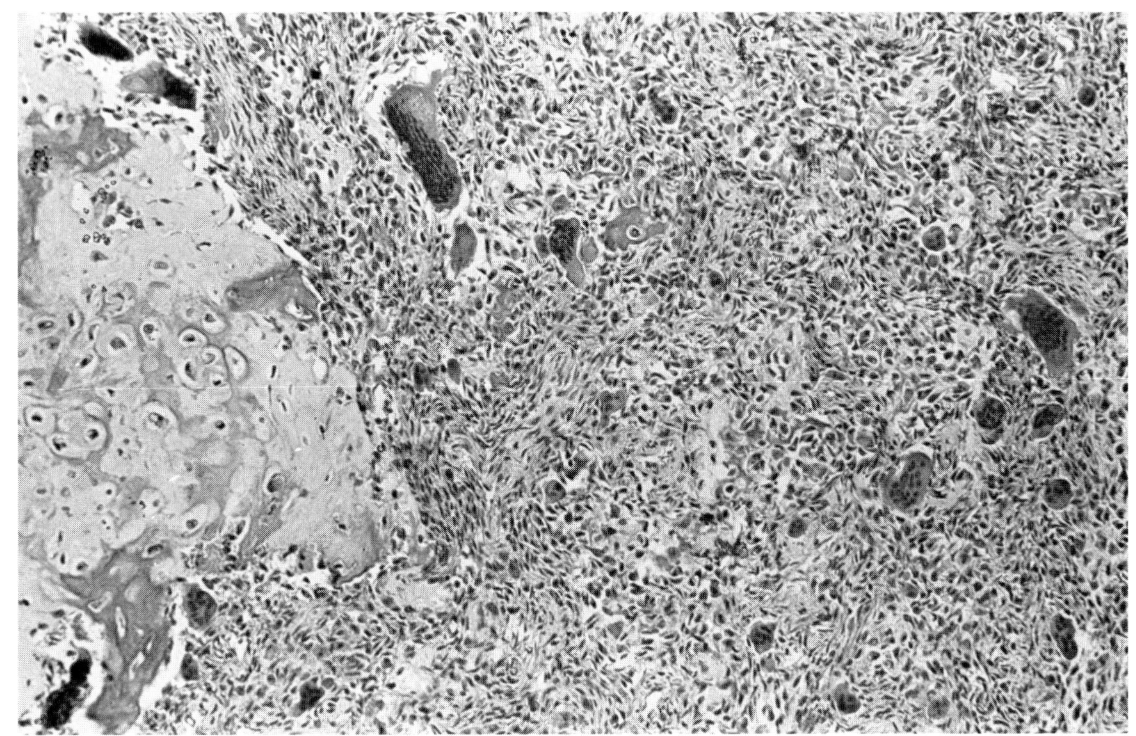

FIG. 10-71

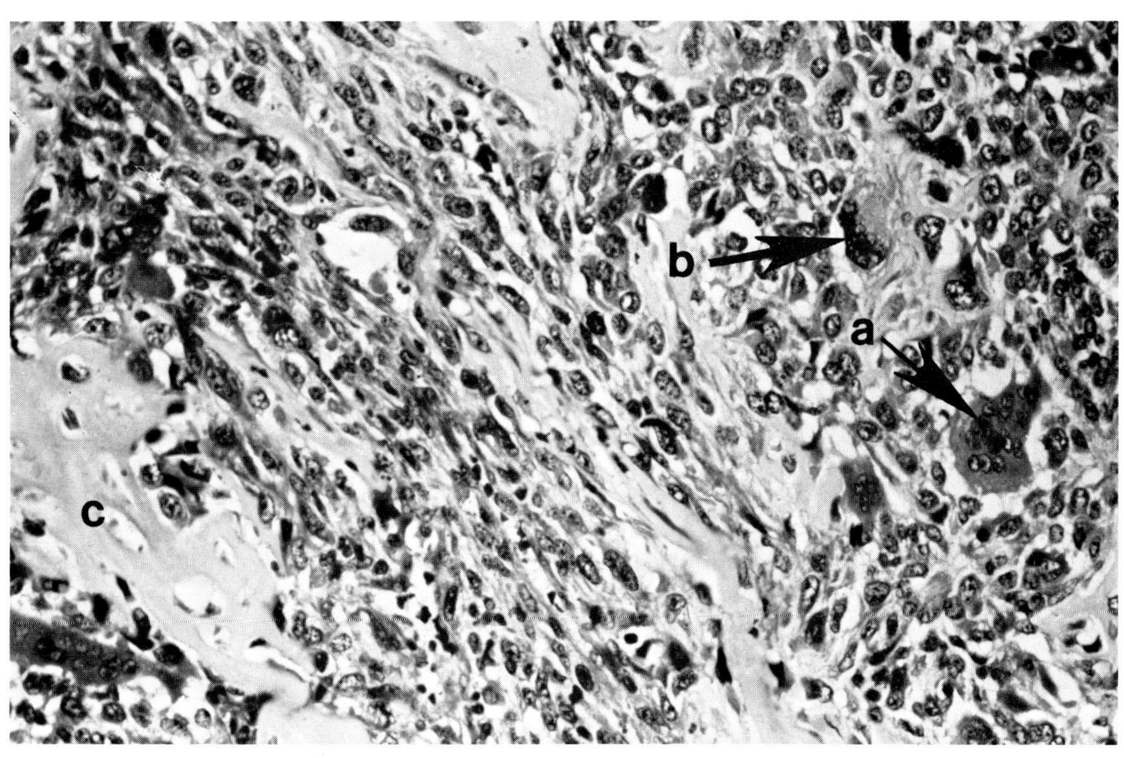

FIG. 10-72

transform from oval to fibrosarcoma-like or malignant fibrous histiocytoma-like tissues with cells and collagen arranged in a storiform pattern (Figs. 10–65, 10–68, 10–69, and 10–70). These cellular transformations are identical to those that may occur in the rare malignant fibrous histiocytoma (MFH) of bone (See p. 285 and Figs. 9–50–9–55). The similarities are explainable based upon the fact that both of these tumors are essentially of histiocytic origin, the giant cell sarcoma of osteoclastic origin and the MFH of connective tissue histiocytic origin. MFH, however, usually does not show the striking osteoclast-like giant cells of the osteoclastic sarcoma and is not associated with Paget's disease. Anaplastic giant cells may be seen in MFH but their features are usually characterized by multilobulation (Figs. 9–51–9–53) and usually by a greater degree of stromal "storiform" patterns (Fig. 9–50).

In giant-cell-rich osteosarcomas, the giant cells are either benign, permeating, reactive osteoclasts or bizarre, multilobulated, anaplastic giant cells of osteoblastic origin.

Course and Treatment

The giant cell or osteoclastic sarcoma is a highly malignant tumor with a very poor 5-year survival. The lesion must be treated by the most radical methods available.

Group IV. Giant Cell-Rich Osteosarcomas

Most of these tumors show unequivocal anaplasia in the stroma, although some to many of the giant cells that permeate the lesion may be benign in appearance (Figs. 10–71 and 10–72). Absolutely essential to diagnosis and separation from the neoplastic GCT's is the finding of the production of osteoid, woven bone, and/or cartilage from an anaplastic stromal component (Figs. 10–71 and 10–72). This essential component, no matter how small, is crucial to proper classification and treatment.

Troup, *et. al.*,[97] found that 13 per cent of osteosarcomas contain large numbers of benign multinucleated giant cells. Eight of 13 cases were originally called ordinary GCT. The chief clinical clue to the error in diagnosis was the fact that the majority of these osteosarcomas that mimicked GCT were located in the metaphysis. Any "GCT" with a pure metaphyseal site of origin, with no involvement of the epiphysis, must immediately be suspect of being another lesion, such as a giant cell-rich osteosarcoma or nonossifying fibroma.

The most treacherous cases are those giant cell-rich osteosarcomas that show minimal stromal anaplasia that could be easily misconstrued as a benign or low-grade neoplastic GCT. Schwinn[87] mentions such a case in a 15-year-old boy. The radiograph showed a metaphyseal lesion. Histology showed numerous benign giant cells and rather innocuous stromal cells. However, because of the unusual location for a true GCT, numerous additional sections were taken and several foci were found where the stromal cells showed large, hyperchromatic nuclei exhibitions variations in size and shape and bizarre mitoses and foci of tumor bone and osteoid formation. The diagnosis was, therefore, appropriately made of osteosarcoma.

Group V. Malignant Fibrous Histiocytoma

The malignant fibrous histiocytoma is a rare primary bone tumor that can be mistaken for an anaplastic GCT (giant cell sarcoma). However, the malignant fibrous histiocytoma does not contain malignant giant cells as clearly of osteoclastic origin as those shown in Figures 10–62 to 10–68. The characteristic features of this tumor are treated in detail in another section (See p. 284).

Giant Cell Rich Fibrosarcoma

FIG. 10–73. Giant cell rich fibrosarcoma versus giant cell tumor. This field is from a patient with a low-grade fibrosarcoma containing a mixture of benign osteoclast-like giant cells (*arrows*) and spindly stromal cells resembling a GCT or nonossifying fibroma (x125).

FIG. 10–74. This field is from a low-grade neoplastic GCT in association with spindly stromal cells showing exuberant but, nevertheless, not frankly anaplastic nuclei (x400).

FIG. 10–75. This field is from an area of Grade I to II fibrosarcoma with exuberant stromal cells and innocuous osteoclast-like giant cells. One nucleus in particular (*arrow*) shows enlargement and hyperchromatism beyond that which is seen in the GCT. This should stimulate a search for fields of greater unequivocal anaplasia.

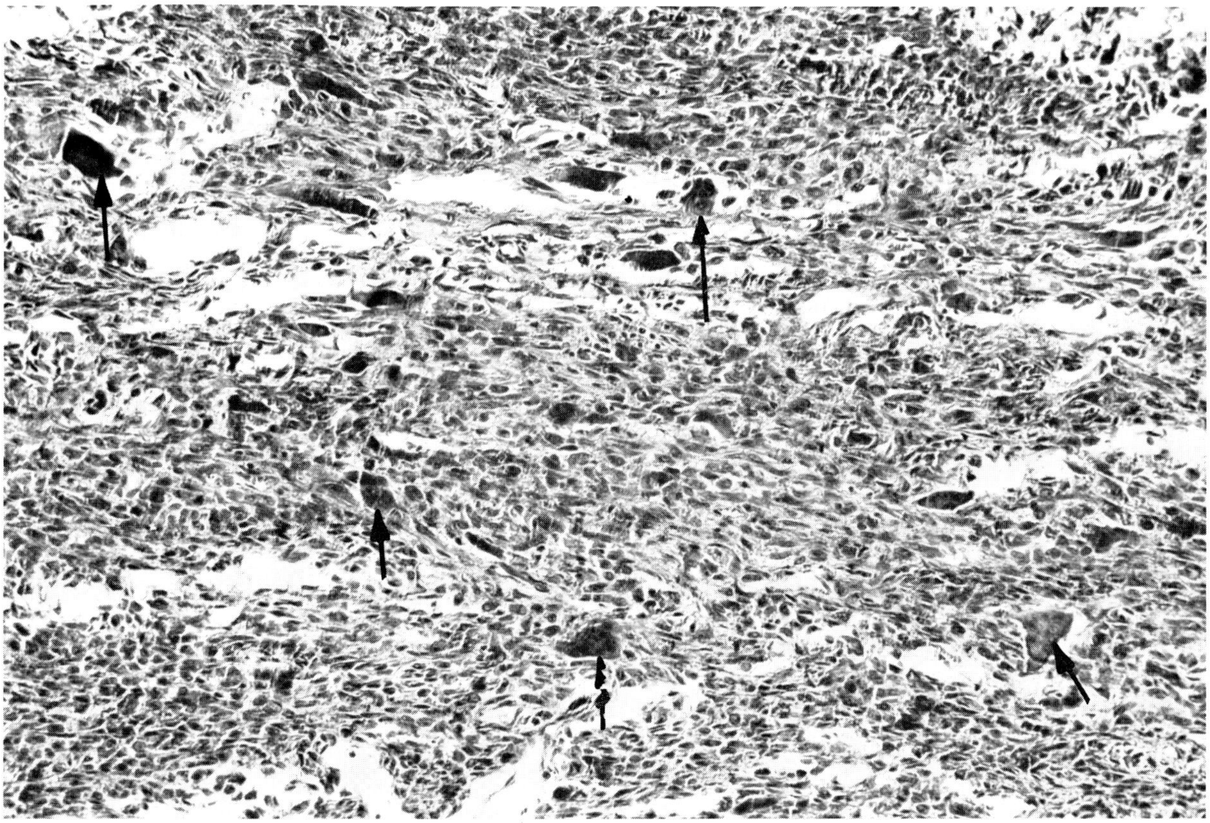

FIG. 10-73

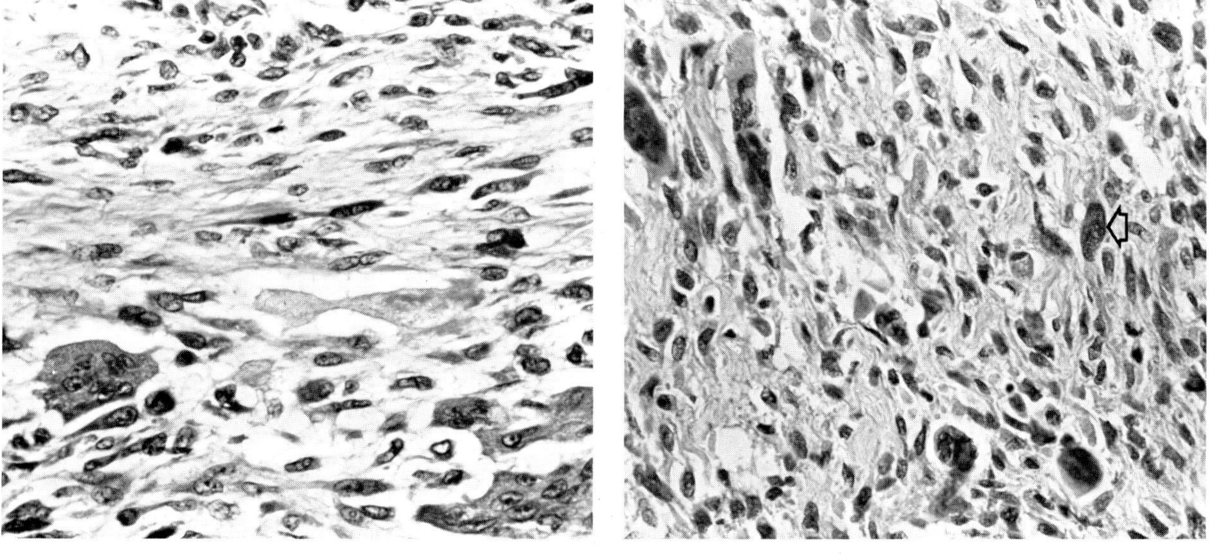

FIG. 10-74

FIG. 10-75

Group VI. Fibrosarcoma in Association With Benign Giant Cells

This tumor is a neoplasm composed of anaplastic collagen-producing spindle cells in which variable numbers of benign osteoclast-like giant cells are found. It is differentiated from giant cell sarcoma by the absence of malignant osteoclast-like cells and from osteogenic sarcoma by the absence of malignant osteoid, woven bone, and cartilage. Benign osseous metaplasia may be found but usually this is at the periphery of the tumor. The treacherous aspect of this tumor is that if the fibrosarcoma is low grade it can be confused with a cellular GCT and graded as II or perhaps III. Those cases with frank anaplasia of the stroma are called malignant GCT or Grade III GCT. This error is not as disastrous as calling it a Grade II giant cell tumor, because fibrosarcomas are all potentially metastatic, lethal lesions that must be treated either by radical en-bloc resection (for low-grade fibrosarcoma) or by more radical procedures.

This author has observed three such GCT-like fibrosarcomas from among 60 true GCT's. Two of these, however, arose in the metaphysis. In other words approximately 5 per cent of histologic "GCT's" are fibrosarcomas with giant cells from the onset. Two of these three cases metastasized with eventual demise of the patient.

The list below outlines the outstanding features of this variant of fibrosarcoma based on an analysis of the literature and my few cases.

Clinical Features

1. They tend to be centered either in the metaphysis or diaphysis.
2. The well-differentiated tumors are circumscribed; the more poorly differentiated ones result in a permeative moth-eaten pattern of bone destruction.
3. The age range is broad, affecting persons between 20 and 70 years of age.

Gross Pathology

On gross examination these tumors are much firmer and grayer or whitish (Plate 7, *D*) than the softer, tan color of true giant cell tumors (Plate 7, *A*, *B*, and *C*). The well differentiated lesions are circumscribed (Plate 7, *D*), and the less well-differentiated, more permeative.

Histopathology

WELL-DIFFERENTIATED GIANT-CELL-RICH FIBROSARCOMA. These lesions are composed of spindly collagen-producing cells that on low-power examination resemble exuberant scar tissue of the fibroblastic portions of ordinary GCT. The collagen that is produced is usually thin and fibrillar, although there may be focal areas with denser collagen production.

Benign osteoclast-like giant cells are usually disposed in a more focal manner compared to untreated

---

Giant Cell Rich Firbosarcoma Contrasted to Low-Grade Neoplastic GCT

FIG. 10-76. This illustration was taken from a better preserved field than shown in the previous figure. Fields such as these demonstrate unequivocal anaplasia and prove the sarcomatous nature of the stromal cell component. The stromal nuclei are considerably plumper compared to the GCT; the chromatin stands out more sharply and is irregularly distributed. The nucleoli vary in number and size from cell to cell. The most malignant nucleus in the field is at *a.* Compare the stroma of this fibrosarcoma, which has permeating osteoclast-like giant cells (*arrows*), with those of the GCT taken at the same magnification (Figs. 10-53, 10-74, and 10-77) (x400).

Low-Grade Neoplastic GCT

FIG. 10-77. Hyperplastic stroma of GCT. The nuclei are elongated and hyperchromatic, but the nucleoli are small, and the chromatin evenly dispersed. Very large, plump, round nuclei are absent and mitoses are mirror image. The nuclei are more widely separated, compared to the packing seen in Figure 10-76 (x400).

Grade II Plus Fibrosarcoma With Benign, Permeating Giant Cells

FIG. 10-78. Grade II fibrosarcoma with benign, permeating, osteoclast-like giant cells (*a*). The sizes and shapes of the stromal cell nuclei are considerably more pleomorphic than is acceptable for a diagnosis of GCT. Arrows point to the most malignant nuclei. Tumors with nuclei as shown here must never be diagnosed as GCT, no matter how many benign osteoclast-like cells are seen. The patient died within 1 year of disseminated metastases, despite correct diagnosis and immediate amputation. It is from cases such as this one and ones shown previously (Figs. 10-73, 10-75, and 10-76) that are partially responsible for the confusion regarding the ordinary neoplastic GCT of epiphyses and its so-called occasional propensity to develop lethal metastases (x400).

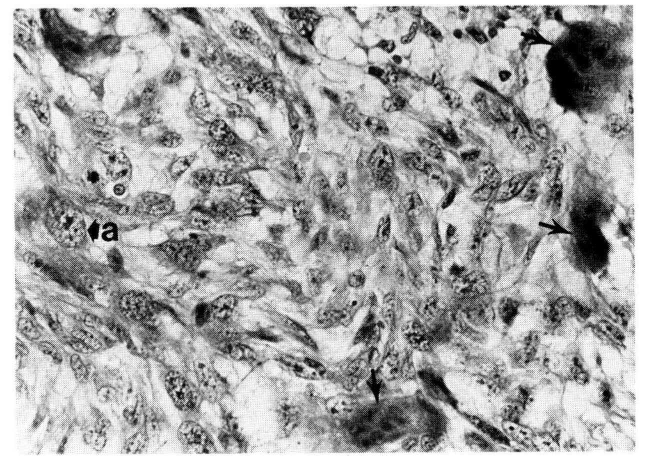

FIG. 10-76

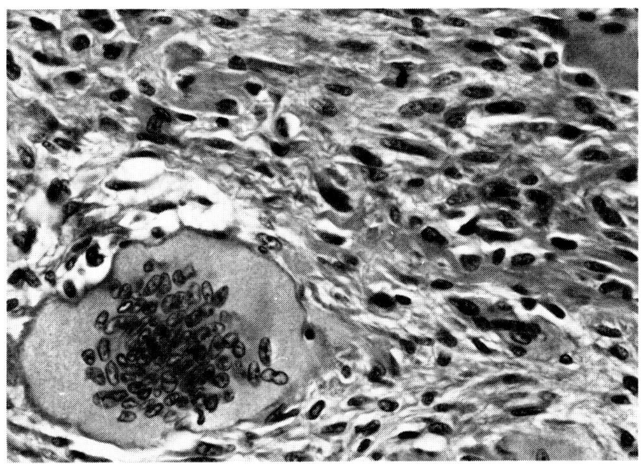

FIG. 10-77

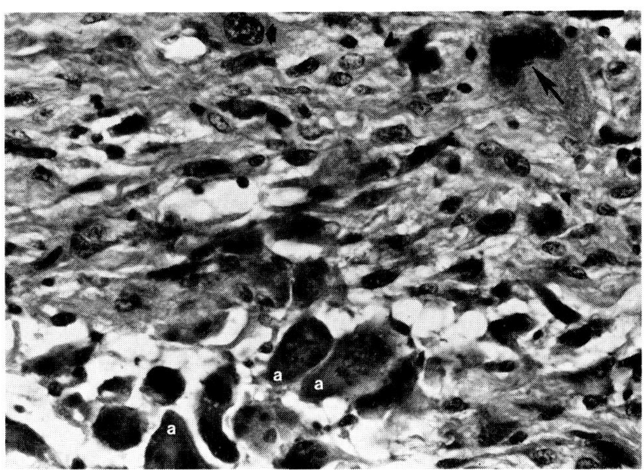

FIG. 10-78

primary GCT's. The giant cells of fibrosarcoma contain fewer nuclei (3 to 15) than most GCT's and do not stand out from the background as prominently as those of true GCT (Compare Figs. 10–52 and 10–55 to Figs. 10–73 and 10–75.) However, these features are by no means diagnostic, since some GCT's may show similar features with respect to the numbers of nuclei per cell and their prominence (Fig. 10–74).

The crucial histologic feature is the demonstration of anaplasia in the fibroblastic stroma. Much of the tumor may show stroma that falls within the range of exuberant GCT's (Fig. 10–75). However, careful search reveals nuclear details and atypical mitoses pathognomonic of an anaplastic or virulent tumor. Figures 10–75, 10–76, and 10–78 show these crucial histologic features. Compare them to the cellular and exuberant fibroblastic but nevertheless nonanaplastic areas of true GCT's (Figs. 10–74, 10–77).

POORLY DIFFERENTIATED GIANT-CELL-RICH FIBROSARCOMAS. Poorly differentiated fibrosarcomas with benign osteoclastic giant cells show frank anaplasia of stromal cells consisting of large nuclei, nuclear crowding, unusual chromatin clumping patterns, large nucleoli, and atypical mitoses (Figs. 10–76 and 10–78). These tumors may be mistakenly diagnosed as Grade III or malignant GCT. However, they lack the anaplastic osteoclastic giant cells of true osteoclastic sarcomas.

The differential diagnostic features of GCT compared to giant-cell-rich fibrosarcoma and Osteoclastic Sarcoma are summarized in Table 10–4.

Possible Origin of the Osteoclast-Like Giant Cells in Fibrosarcoma

What is the origin of the benign osteoclast-like giant cells in relation to a fibrosarcoma, particularly since this tumor is of nonosteoclastic origin? Actually, this question may be asked of any tumor of nonosteoclastic origin associated with prominent benign osteoclast-like giant cells. In this author's estimation the benign osteoclast-like giant cells are in truth osteoclasts that have a peculiar propensity to infiltrate almost any primary tumor or lesion of bone. The osteoclasts apparently represent a benign reactive process rather than a neoplastic component except in the true GCT and giant cell sarcoma. In one of my cases of fibrosarcoma with an extensive permeation of osteoclast-like giant cells (Fig. 10–73), an interesting finding was noted at the margin of the tumor that may shed light upon this phenomenon. At the peripheral destructive edge of the tumor the host bone was being destroyed by unequivocal osteoclasts housed in their distinctive lacunae (Fig. 10–79). High-power examination showed areas in which the osteoclasts appeared to migrate from their site appositional to bone and enter the tumor (Fig. 10–80). The giant cells in the tumor were identical in all histological features to the osteoclasts adjacent to the bone and to those that appeared to migrate from this site (Fig. 10–80).

HIGH-GRADE MALIGNANT NEOPLASMS

The high-grade malignant lesions such as osteogenic sarcoma, fibrosarcoma, and malignant fibrous histiocytoma that could be mistaken for ordinary low-grade giant cell tumor or the so-called malignant giant cell tumor have been discussed in the previous section.

Hodgkin's disease may contain giant cells but they would not ordinarily be confused with a neoplastic giant cell tumor because of the immunocytes they are associated with and the distinctive nuclear features of

---

Giant-Cell-Rich Fibrosarcoma

FIG. 10–79. The next two illustrations show the possible origin of the benign osteoclast-like giant cells that may be found spinkled throughout the stroma of fibrosarcoma or other tumors of bone. The first is a medium-power view showing classical osteoclasts (*arrows*) resorbing bone along the advancing edge of the fibrosarcoma. Note the considerable number of similar giant cells in the stroma of the tumor in the upper half of the field (x125).

FIG. 10–80. This illustration could be interpreted as showing a streaming of unequivocal osteoclasts (*arrows*) into the adjacent stroma of the tumor. Note the exact resemblance of the osteoclasts to those in the stroma of the tumor to the right of the field (*b*). It is from this proposed mingling of benign osteoclasts with almost any primary bone tumor that probably accounts for their ominipresence. In almost every tumor of bone except the giant cell tumor of hyperparathyroidism and Paget's disease, the low-grade neoplastic giant cell tumor, and the osteoclastic sarcoma, the osteoclast-like giant cells seen probably play no role in the histogenesis of the tumor and merely represent fortuitous passengers. It is in the nature of their ubiquity that causes the problems in the diagnosis of the giant-cell-rich tumors of the bones (x250).

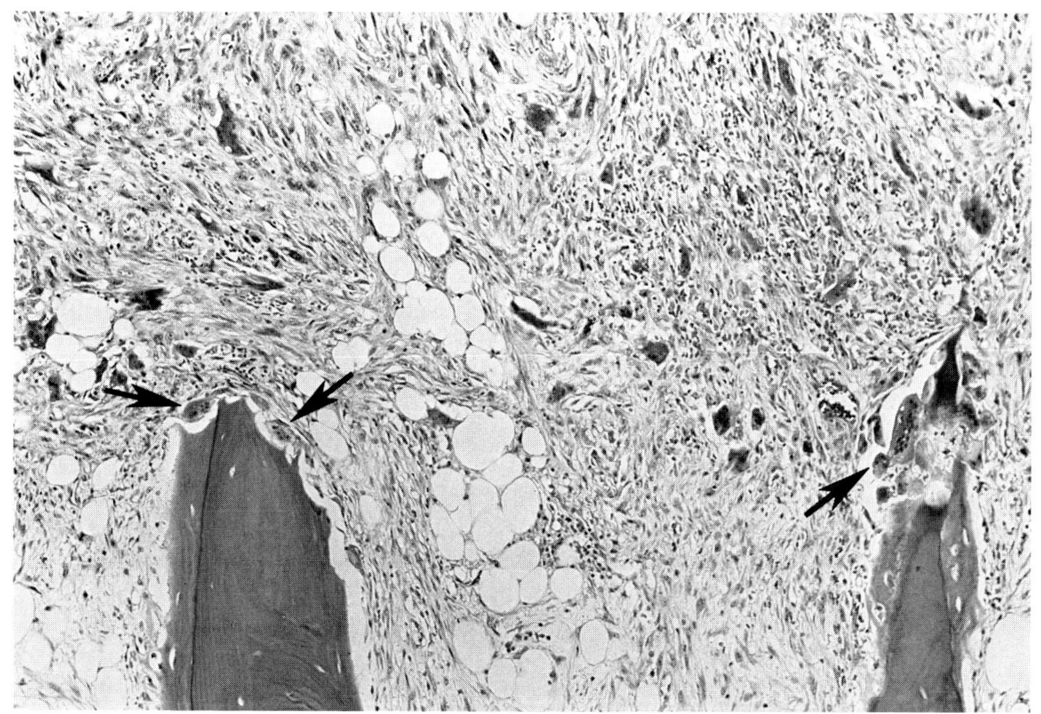

FIG. 10-79

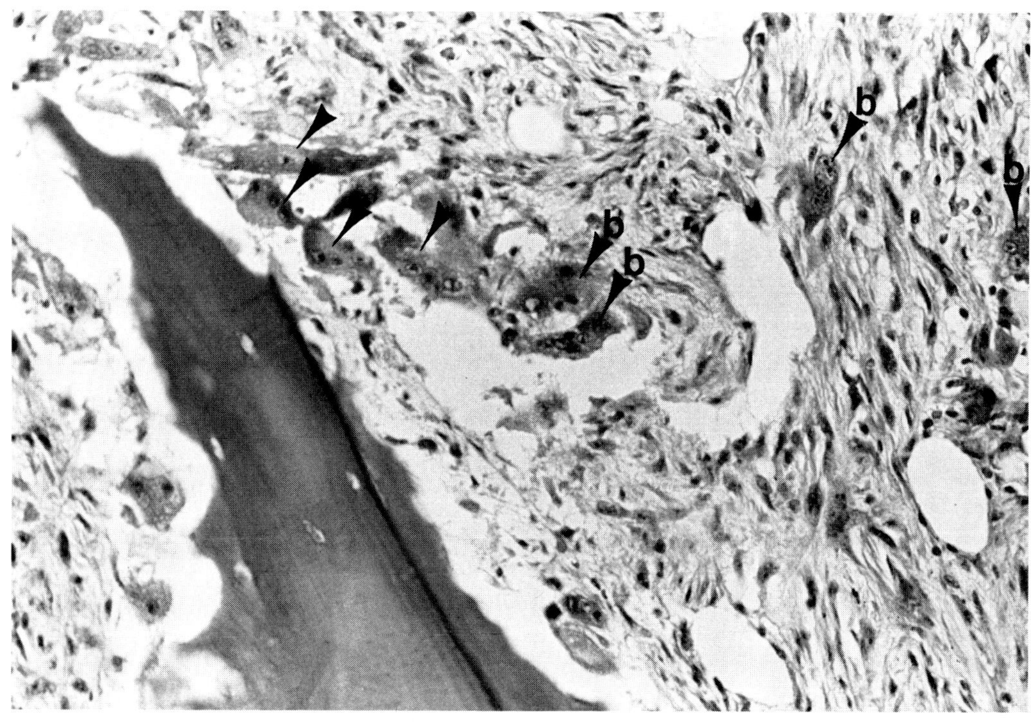

FIG. 10-80

Table 10-4. Differential Features of Ordinary Giant Cell Tumor, Osteoclastic Sarcoma, and Giant-Cell-Rich Fibrosarcoma

	Low-Grade Neoplastic Giant Cell Tumor	*Osteoclastic Sarcoma*	*Giant Cell Rich Fibrosarcoma*
Age	Most between 20 to 40 years	Most over age 40	Any age
Associated Diseases	None	May be associated with Paget's disease or post-irradiation, to low-grade neoplastic GCT	None
Localization	Greater than 95% are epiphyseal-metaphyseal. Rare as pure metaphyseal or diaphyseal tumors.	Most centered in metaphysis or diaphysis	Most centered in metaphysis or diaphysis
Gross Pathology	Very soft, tan	Soft to firm, gray to tan	Firm, gray to very light tan
Giant Cells	Masses of benign looking giant cells. Most cases will contain giant cells with over 40 nuclei cell. Giant cells stand out prominently in most cases.	Anaplastic giant cells with up to ten individually placed nuclei. Tendency to peripheral localization of nuclei.	Focal collections of benign looking osteoclast-like giant cells with up to ten nuclei/cell section. Cells do not stand out from stroma prominently in most cases.
Stroma	May contain exuberant nuclei and numerous mitoses. Moderate variation in size and shape of nuclei. Individual nuclei rarely larger than 20 × 12 microns. Nucleoli small. Osteoid or woven bone will be benign and most often rimmed by a benign layer of osteoblasts.	Bizarre, anaplastic, oval to spindly fibrosarcoma- or MFH-like areas. Numerous atypical mitoses. Large nucleoli.	Even in low-grade fibrosarcomas careful search will often reveal stromal nuclei exceeding 30 × 20 microns with either severe hyperchromatism or marked chromatin clumping. Grade II and III fibrosarcomas show frank anaplasia of the stroma. Atypical mitoses are present. Absence of malignant bone.

the characteristic Reed-Sternberg cells. This entity is discussed later (p. 406).

OTHER LESIONS

In actuality any tumor of bone, either primary or metastatic, is usually associated with some degree of osteoclastic activity. This activity is most pronounced along the expanding margin of the tumor. The "pressure" of the growing tumor is the probable stimulus to osteoclastic induction with consequent resorption of the host bone. Tumor cells themselves, probably, cannot resorb bone, unless, of course, they are of osteoclastic origin.

The same holds for lesions containing osteoclast-like giant cells. Almost any benign or malignant lesion may contain these cells, and, if, in sufficient number, they may lead to diagnostic confusion. These lesions have either been discussed in preceding sections of this chapter or can be found using Table 5 of Chapter 6.

REFERENCES

Definitions Used in This Chapter

1. Ozzello, L., Stout, A.P., and Murray, M.R.: Cultural characteristics of malignant histiocytomas and fibrous xanthomas. Cancer *16:*331, 1963.
2. Stout, A.P.: Fibrous tumors of soft tissues. Minn. Med., *43:*455, 1960.
3. Stout, A.P., and Lattes, R.: Tumors of Soft Tissues. *In* Atlas of Tumor Pathology, series L, Fasc 1, pp. 38–56, Washington, D.C., Armed Forces Institute of Pathology, 1907.

Paget's Disease

4. Brooke, R.I.: Giant-cell tumor in patients with Paget's disease. Oral Surg., *30:*230, 1970.
5. Griffey, L.E., and Tedeschi, L.G.: Giant cell tumor of ethmoid; complication of Paget's disease of bone. Arch. Otolaryngol., *87:*615, 1968.
6. Hutter, R.V.P., Foote, F.W., Frazell, E.L., and Francis, K.C.: Giant-cell tumors complicating Paget's disease of bone. Cancer, *16:*1044, 1963.
7. Jaffe, H.L.: Metabolic, Degenerative and Inflammatory Diseases of Bones and Joints. Philadelphia, Lea & Febiger, 1972.
8. Miller, A.S., Cuttino, C.L., Elzay, R.P., Levy, W.M., and Harwick, R.D.: Giant cell tumor of the jaws associated with Paget's disease of bone; report of two cases and review of the literature. Arch. Otolaryngol., *100:*233, 1974.
9. Mills, B.G., and Singer, F.R.: Nuclear inclusions in Paget's disease of bone. Science, *194:*201, 1976.
10. Paget, J.: On a form of chronic inflammation of bones (osteitis deformans). Med. Chir. Tr., *60:*37, 1877.

10a. ———: Additional cases of osteitis deformans. Med. Chir. Tr., *65:*225, 1882.

11. Rebel, A., Malkani, M., and Bregeon, C.: Osteoclast ultrastructure in Paget's disease. Calcif. Tissue Res., *20:*187, 1976.
12. ———: Nuclear inclusions in osteoclasts in Paget's bone disease. Calcif. Tissue Res. Suppl., *21:*113, 1976.
13. Schajowicz, F., and Slullitel, I.: Giant cell tumor associated with Paget's disease of bone; a case report. J. Bone Joint Surg., *48A:*1340, 1966.
14. Schmorl, G.: The Human Spine in Health and Disease. ed. by E.F. Boseman. New York, Grune and Stratton, 1971.

Giant Cell Reparative Granuloma of Jawbones

15. Ackerman, L.V., and Spjut, A.J.: Bones and Joints. Baltimore, Williams & Wilkins, 1976.
16. Austin, L.T., Dahlin, D.C., and Royer, R.Q.: Giant-cell reparative granuloma and related conditions affecting the jawbones. Oral Surg., *12:*1285, 1959.
17. Bhaskar, S.N., Bernier, J.L., and Godby, F.: Aneurysmal bone cyst and other giant-cell lesions of the jaws; report of 104 cases. J. Oral Surg., *17:*30, 1959.
18. Curtis, M.L., Hatfield, C.G., and Pierce, J.M.: A destructive Giant Cell Lesion of the Mandible. J. Oral Surg., *31:*705, 1973.
19. Dehner, L.P.: Tumors of the mandible and maxilla in Children. I. Clinicopathologic Study of 46 histologically benign lesions. Cancer, *31:*364, 1973.
20. Jaffe, H.L.: Giant cell reparative granuloma, traumatic bone cyst and fibrous (fibro-osseous) dysplasia of the jaw bones. Oral Surg., *6:*159, 1953.
21. Seldin, H.M., Seldin, S.D., Rakower, W., and Selman, A.J.: Giant cell tumor of the jaws. J. Am. Dent. Assoc., *55:*210, 1957.
22. Waldron, C.A., and Shafer, W.G.: The central giant cell reparative granuloma of the jaws; an analysis of 38 cases. Am. J. Clin. Pathol., *45:*437, 1966.

Giant Cell Reaction of Bone

23. Ackerman, L.V., and Spjut, H.J.: Bones and Joints. Baltimore, Williams & Wilkins, 1976.
24. D'Alonzo, R.T., Pitcock, J.A., and Milford, L.W.: Giant-cell reaction of bone; report of two cases. J. Bone Joint Surg., *54A:*1267, 1972.
25. Jernstrom, P., and Stark, H.H.: Giant-cell reaction of a metacarpal. Am. J. Clin. Pathol., *55:*77, 1971.

"Invasive" Villonodular Synovitis and Giant Cell Tumor of Tendon Sheath

26. Breimer, C.W., and Freiberger, R.H.: Bone lesions associated with villonodular synovitis. Am. J. Roentgenol. Radium Ther. Nucl. Med., *79:*618, 1958.
27. Carr, C.R., Berley, F.V., and Davis W.C.: Pigmented villonodular synovitis of the hip joint; a case report. J. Bone Joint Surg., *36A:*1007, 1954.
28. Chung, S.M., and Janes, J.M.: Diffuse pigmented villonodular synovitis of the hip joint; review of the literature and report of four cases. J. Bone Joint Surg., *47A:*293, 1965.
29. Decker, J.P., and Owen, B.J.: An invasive giant cell tumor of tendon sheath in the foot. Bull. Ayer Clin. Lab., *4:*43, 1954.
30. Fletcher, A.G., Jr., and Horn, R.C., Jr.: Giant cell tumors of tendon sheath origin; a consideration of bone involvement and report of two cases with extensive bone destruction. Ann. Surg., *113:*374, 1951.
31. Jones, F.E., Soule, E.H., and Coventry, M.B.: Fibrous xanthoma of synovium (giant-cell tumor of tendon sheath, pigmented nodular synovitis); a study of one hundred and eighteen cases. J. Bone Joint Surg., *51A:*76, 1969.
32. McMaster, P.E.: Pigmented villonodular synovitis with invasion of bone; report of six cases. J. Bone Joint Surg., *42A:*1170, 1960.

33. Phalen, G.S., McCormack, L.J., and Gazale, W.J.: Giant cell tumor of tendon sheath (benign synovioma) in the hand; evaluation of 56 cases. Clin. Orthop., *15:* 140, 1959.
34. Scott, P.M.: Bone lesions in pigmented villonodular synovitis. J. Bone Joint Surg., *50B:* 306, 1968.
35. Schajowicz, F., and Blumenfeld, I.: Pigmented villonodular synovitis of the wrist with penetration into bone. J. Bone Joint Surg., *50B:* 312, 1968.

Low-Grade Neoplastic Giant Cell Tumor of Bone and Osteoclastic Sarcoma

36. Ackerman, L.V., and Spjut, H.J.: Tumors of Bone Cartilage. *In* Atlas of Tumor Pathology, section 2, fascicle 4. Washington, D.C., Armed Forces Institute of Pathology, 1962.
37. Ackerman, L.V., Spjut, H.J., and Abell, M.R.: Bones and Joints. International Academy of Pathology Monograph. Baltimore, Williams & Wilkins, 1976.
38. Adkins, K.F., Martinez, M.G., and Romaniuk, K.: Ultrastructure of giant-cell lesions: mononuclear cells in peripheral giant-cell granulomas. Oral Surg., *33:* 775, 1972.
39. Barnes, R.: Giant-cell tumor of bone; editorials. J. Bone Joint Surg., *54B:* 213, 1972.
40. Cambell, C., and Bonfiglio, M.: Aggressiveness and malignancy in giant-cell tumors of bone. *In* Bone-Certain Aspects of Neoplasia, ed. Price and Ross. London, Colston Research Society, 1973.
41. Cameron, J.A.P., and Marsden, A.T.H.: Malignant osteoclastoma: report of a case. J. Bone Joint Surg., *34B:* 93, 1952.
42. Cares, H.L., and Bakay, L.: Giant cell lesions of the skull. Acta Neurochir. *25:* 1, 1971.
43. Cohen, D., Dahlin, D.C., and MacCarty, C.: Vertebral giant-cell tumor and variants. Cancer, *17:* 461, 1964.
44. Dahlin, D.C.: Bone Tumors. General Aspects and Data on 3,987 Cases. ed. 2. Springfield, Charles C Thomas, 1957.
45. Dahlin, D.C., Cupps, R.E., and Johnson E.W.: Giant cell tumor: a study of 195 cases. Cancer, *25:* 1061, 1970.
46. Dahlin, D.C., Ghormley, R.K., and Pugh, D.G.: Giant cell tumor of bone: differential diagnosis. Mayo Clin. Proc., *31:* 31, 1956.
47. Dyke, S.C.: Metastasis of the "benign" giant-cell tumor of bone (osteoclastoma). J. Pathol., *34:* 259, 1931.
48. Finch, E.F., and Gleave, H.H.: A case of osteoclastoma, myeloid sarcoma, benign giant cell tumor with pulmonary metastasis. J. Pathol., *29:* 399, 1976.
49. Frangakis, E.K.: Soft-tissue spread of giant-cell tumor; a case report. J. Bone Joint Surg., *53A:* 994, 1971.
50. Goldenberg, R.R., Campbell, C.J., and Bonfiglio, M.: Giant cell tumor of bone. An analysis of two hundred and eighteen cases. J. Bone Joint Surg., *52A:* 619, 1970.
51. Haas, A., and Ritter, S.A.: "Benign" giant-cell tumor of femur with embolic metastasis in prepuce of penis. Am. J. Surg., *89:* 573, 1955.
52. Hamlin, W.B., and Lund, P.K.: Giant cell tumors of the mandible and facial bones. Arch. Otolaryngol., *86:* 658, 1967.
53. Hanaoka, H., Friedman, B., and Mack, R.P.: Ultrastructure and histogenesis of giant-cell tumor of bone. Cancer, *25:* 1408, 1970.
54. Hutter, R.V.P., Worcester, J.N., Frances, K.C., Foote, F.W., Jr., and Stewart, F.W.: Benign and malignant giant cell tumors of bone. A clinicopathological analysis of the natural history of the disease. Cancer, *15:* 653, 1962.
55. Jacobs, P.: The diagnosis of osteoclastoma (giant-cell tumour); a radiological and pathological correlation. Br. J. Radiol., *45:* 121, 1972.
56. Jaffe, H.L.: Giant-Cell Tumour (Osteoclastoma) of Bone. Its Pathologic Delimitation and the Inherent Clinical Implications. Ann. R. Coll. Surg. Engl., *13:* 343, 1953.
57. ———: Tumors and Tumorous Conditions of the Bones and Joints. pp. 18–43. Philadelphia, Lea & Febiger, 1958.
58. Jaffe, H.L., Lichtenstein, L., and Portis, R.B.: Giant cell tumor of bone. Its pathologic appearance, grading, supposed variants and treatment. Arch. Pathol., *30:* 993, 1940.
59. Jewell, J.H., and Bush, L.F.: "Benign" giant-cell tumor of bone with a solitary pulmonary metastasis. J. Bone Joint. Surg., *46A:* 848, 1964.
60. Johnson, E.W., Jr.: Adjacent and distant spread of giant cell tumors. Am. J. Surg., *109:* 163, 1965.
61. Johnson, E.W., Jr., and Dahlin, D.: Treatment of giant-cell tumor of bone. J. Bone Joint Surg., *41A:* 895, 1959.
62. Johnson, E.W., Jr., and Riley, L.: Giant cell tumor of bone, an evaluation of twenty-four cases treated at the Johns Hopkins Hospital between 1925 and 1955. Clin. Orthop., *62:* 187, 1969.
63. Kimball, R.M., and Desanto, D.: Malignant giant-cell tumor of the ulna. Report of a case of 18 years duration. J. Bone Joint Surg., *40A:* 1131, 1958.
64. Kossey, P., and Cervenansky, J.: Malignant giant-cell tumors of bone. *In* Bone—Certain Aspects of Neoplasia, ed. Price and Ross. London, Colston Research Society, 1973.
65. Kutchemeshgi, A.D., Wright, J.R., and Hymphrey, R.: Pulmonary metastases from a well-differentiated giant cell tumor of bone; report of a patient with apparent response to cyclophosphamide therapy. Johns Hopkins Med. J., *134:* 237, 1974.
66. Larsson, S.E., Lorentzon, R., and Boquist, L.: Giant-cell of bone; a demographic, clinical and histopathological study of all cases recorded in the Swedish Cancer Registry for the years 1958 through 1968. J. Bone Joint Surg., *57A:* 167, 1975.
67. ———: Giant-cell tumors of the spine and sacrum: a report of 5 cases. Clin. Orthop., *111:* 201, 1975.

68. Lasser, E.C., and Tetewsky, H.: Metastasizing giant-cell tumor; report of an unusual case with indolent bone and pulmonary metastases. Am. J. Roentgenol. Radium Ther. Nucl. Med., *78:* 804, 1957.
69. Lichtenstein, L.: Bone Tumors. ed. 2, p. 133. St. Louis, C.V. Mosby, 1965.
70. ———: Giant cell tumor of bone: current status of problems in diagnosis and treatment. J. Bone Joint Surg., *33A:* 143, 1951.
71. Marcove, R.C., Lyden, J.P., Huvos, A.G., and Bullough, P.G.: Giant-cell tumors treated by cryosurgery: a review of 25 cases. J. Bone Joint Surg., *55A:* 1633, 1973.
72. Marcove, R.C., Miller, T.R., and Cohen, W.C.: The treatment of primary and metastatic bone tumors by repetitive freezing. Bull. N.Y. Acad. Med., *44:* 532, 1968.
73. Marcove, R.C., Weiss, L.D., Vaghaiwalla, M., Pearson, R., and Huvos, A.: Cryosurgery in the treatment of giant cell tumors of bone. A report of 52 consecutive cases. Cancer, *41:* 957, 1978.
74. McGrath, P.J.: Giant-cell tumors of bone; an analysis of fifty-two cases. J. Bone Joint Surg., *54B:* 216, 1972.
75. Mnaymneh, W.A., Dudley, H.R., and Mnaymneh, L.G.: Giant cell tumor of bone; an analysis and follow-up study of the forty-one cases observed at the Massachusetts General Hospital between 1925 and 1960. J. Bone Joint Surg., *46A:* 63, 1964.
76. Mnaymneh, W.A., and Ghandur-Mnaymneh, L.: Giant cell tumor of bone. *In* Progress in Clinical Cancer, vol. 111, pp. 245, Ed: I.M. Ariel, New York, Grune and Stratton, 1967.
77. Murphy, W.R., and Ackerman, L.V.: Benign and malignant giant-cell tumors of bone: a clinical pathological evaluation of thirty-one cases. Cancer, *9:* 317, 1956.
78. Ores, R., Ortiz, J., and Rosen, P.: Localization of acid phosphatase activity in a giant cell tumor of bone. Arch. Pathol., *88:* 54, 1969.
79. Pan, P., Dahlin, D.C., Lipscomb, P.R., and Bernatz, P.E.: "Benign" giant cell tumor of the radius with pulmonary metastasis. Mayo Clin. Proc., *39:* 344, 1964.
80. Pan, P., and Mackinnon, W.B.: "Benign" giant cell tumor of thoracic vertebra with pulmonary metastasis. Can. Med. Assoc. J., *87:* 1026, 1962.
81. Parrish, F.: Treatment of bone tumors by total excision and replacement with massive autologous and homologous grafts. J. Bone Joint Surg., *48A:* 968, 1966.
82. Riley, L.H., Jr.: Soft-tissues recurrence of giant cell tumor of bone after irradiation and excision. J. Bone Joint Surg., *49A:* 365, 1967.
83. Rockwell, M., and Small, C.: Giant cell tumors in South India. J. Bone Joint Surg., *43A:* 1035, 1961.
84. Russell, D.S.: Malignant osteoclastoma and association of malignant osteoclastoma with Paget's osteitis deformans. J. Bone Joint Surg., *31B:* 281, 1949.
85. Schajowicz, F.: Tumors of bone. California Tumor Tissue Registry Semi-Annual Slide Conference, Las Vegas, December 6, 1964.
86. ———: Giant cell tumors of bone (osteoclastoma), a pathological and histochemical study. J. Bone Joint Surg., *43A:* 1, 1961.
87. Schwinn, C.P.: Benign giant cell tumor of bone. Anatomic Pathology No. AP-4, CCE Council and Anatomic Pathology of the American Society of Clinical Pathologists, 1973.
88. Sherman, M.: Giant cell Tumor of Bone. *In* Tumors of Bone and Soft Tissue. A Collection of Papers Presented at the Eighth Annual Clinical Conference on Cancer 1963 at the University of Texas, M.D. Anderson Hospital and Tumor Institute, Houston, Texas. Chicago, Year Book Publishers, 1965.
89. Sherman, M., and Fabricius, R.: Giant cell tumor in the metaphysis in a child. Report of an unusual case. J. Bone Joint Surg., *43A:* 1225, 1961.
90. ———: Bone and Joints. ed. Ackerman, L.V., and Spjut, A.J. International Academy of Pathology Monograph. Baltimore, Williams & Wilkins, 1976.
90a. Spjut, H.J., *et al.:* Tumors of Bone and Cartilage. Atlas of Tumor Pathology, second series, fascicle 5. pp. 299–301. Armed Forces Institute of Pathology, Washington, D.C. 1971.
91. Shifrin, L.Z.: Giant cell tumor of bone. Clin. Orthop., *82:* 59–66, 1972.
91a. Sim, F.H., Dahlin, D.C., and Beabout, J.W.: Multicentric giant cell tumor of bone. J. Bone Joint Surg., *59A:* 1052, 1977.
92. Sladden, R.A.: Intravascular Osteoclasts. J. Bone Joint Surg., *39B:* 346, 1957.
93. Stargardter, F.L., and Cooperman, L.R.: Case reports; giant cell tumour of sacrum with multiple pulmonary metastases and long-term survival. Br. J. Radiol., *44:* 976, 1971.
94. Stewart, M.J., and Richardson, T.R.: Giant-cell tumor of bone. J. Bone Joint Surg., *34A:* 372, 1952.
95. Sybrandy, S., and De La Fuente, A.A.: Multiple giant-cell tumour of bone; report of a case. J. Bone Joint Surg., *55B:* 350, 1973.
96. Tornberg, D.N., Dick, H.M., and Johnston, A.: Multicentric giant-cell tumors in the long bones. J. Bone Joint Surg., *57A:* 429, 1975.
97. Troup, J.B., Dahlin, D.C., and Coventry, M.B.: The significance of giant cells in osteogenic sarcoma: do they indicate a relationship between osteogenic sarcoma and giant cell tumor of bone? Mayo Clin. Proc., *35:* 179, 1960.
98. Verbiest, H.: Giant-cell tumours and aneurysmal bone cysts of the spine with special reference to the problems related to the removal of a vertebral body. J. Bone Joint Surg., *47B:* 699, 1965.
99. Wilkerson, J.A., and Cracchiolo, A. III: Giant-cell tumor of the tibial diaphysis. J. Bone Joint Surg., *51A:* 1205, 1969.

INTRAOSSEOUS ROUND CELL TUMORS

11

INTRODUCTION

This chapter deals with intraosseous round cell tumors. A "round cell" tumor of bone can be defined as a lesion composed of sheets of round to polygonal or oval cells with no signs of osseous matrix differentiation, such as cartilage or bone, or of glandular or of other recognizable epithelial patterns produced by the tumor per se. This definition eliminates such lesions as the chondroblastoma, which may be composed to a large extent of rounded to polygonal cells but which is associated with cartilage or chondroid matrix production by the tumor. Fibrous tissue may be seen as a reactive response to some of the round cell tumors, particularly in Hodgkin's disease. The fundamental cell of origin in Hodgkin's is a large polygonal to oval neoplastic histiocyte (or transformed lymphocyte). In spite of fibrous tissue reaction, Hodgkin's disease will be treated as an example of a round cell tumor, since the basic neoplastic cell is a "round" cell. Tumors with a mixture of round to spindly cells in association with only fibrous tissue and nonosseous-producing tumors are discussed in detail in Chapter 9 or in this chapter. The malignant fibrous histiocytoma (MFH), for example, is usually associated with mononuclear rounded to oval and spindly histiocytes and multinucleated giant cells. However, since the vast majority of these tumors are dominated by a spindle cell element showing a "storiform" pattern of cellular and collagen distribution, this lesion is described in depth in Chapter 9. But in dealing with a specific case of MFH, if the differential diagnostic tables of Chapter 6 are used, this entity will enter in the differential diagnosis of either the round cell tumors, spindle cell tumors, or giant cell-containing tumors, since all three components may be found on histologic analysis.

The principal round cell lesions of bone that are included in this chapter include osteomyelitis, eosinophilic granuloma and Letterer-Siwe disease, Gaucher's disease, myeloma, Waldenström's macroglobulinemia, Hodgkin's disease, Ewing's sarcoma, metastatic neuroblastoma, primary reticulum cell sarcoma of bone, lymphosarcoma and leukemia of bone, and the undifferentiated metastatic carcinoma and melanoma that may simulate primary round cell tumors.

Because of the lack of differentiating matrix components and cellular patterns such as acini, tubules, and cords, the separation of one round cell tumor from another can be extremely difficult. When tissue for histologic examination is scant, necrotic, or poorly fixed, a specific diagnosis is usually impossible. Even under the best conditions, diagnosis is difficult.

Most of the round cell lesions are rare and they generally have no identifying radiologic features or salient features on gross examination. These lesions make it necessary to weigh especially carefully the clinical presentation, the age of the patient, and the radiologic and histologic findings before reaching a final diagnosis.

DEFICIENCY OF H AND E TISSUE SECTIONS ALONE

H and E sections are generally not sufficient to separate the round cell tumors with accuracy. This is principally due to artifacts of fixation that distort nuclear and cytoplasmic characteristics; this may result in a confusing mixture of cells that are difficult to classify. For many years hematologists and hematopathologists have been using bone marrow aspirates stained with Wright's to classify the hematopoietic tumors. Basically, their technique is a cytologic preparation comparable to a Pap smear. Their technique has added a new dimension to classification not possible by ordinary H and E sections of the same tissue after fixation and embedding. One need only compare the H and E preparation of a block of bone removed as a fresh biopsy from a patient with a lymphoma or leukemia to the hematologist's cytological bone marrow preparations to appreciate the vast differences and superior qualities of the imprinted material. For several years this author has been obtaining fresh tissue imprints on all tumors, including those of bone that are processed in surgical pathology. In all instances the imprints are vastly superior with respect to cytology compared to standard H and E sections of the same tissue and in many instances establish a specific diagnosis not possible or dangerously equivocal by analysis of the H and E section alone.

WORKUP OF ROUND CELL TUMORS

The recommended steps in the workup of a round cell tumor of bone are as follows:

1. Obtain fresh tissue. To do this close cooperation between radiologist, surgeon and pathologist is necessary. Any tumor of bone suspected of being a "round cell" tumor should be identified prior to surgery and unfixed fresh tissue sent immediately from the operating room to the surgical pathology suite.
2. A portion of the tissue should be imprinted and immediately fixed in a solution in a ratio of 10 ml. of neutral buffered formalin to 90 ml. of 70 per cent ethyl alcohol. Several slides should be prepared for H and E, Wright's stain, PAS, and other special stains as deemed necessary. A specific method to obtain cytologic imprints of high quality has been treated in Chapter 2, pp. 10–11. Unless attention is given to specific details in the preparation of imprints, poor quality or useless material will be the result.
3. Several small samples of tissue from various sites of the tumor fixed in the standard manner should be set aside for ultramicroscopic analysis, particularly if the imprints and routine sections do not prove conclusive. In most instances, however, diagnosis is possible by review of the tissue sections, imprints, and special stains alone.
4. Half of the remaining tissue should be fixed in 10 per cent neutral buffered formalin and the other half in Zenker's fixative. Zenker's is generally a better fixative for preservation of cytologic details.

If fresh tissue was not obtained for these procedures, a rebiopsy may be necessary if a firm diagnosis cannot be obtained from the fixed tissue. Treatment and prognosis may differ radically from one round cell tumor to another. The usual errors in diagnosis that this author has observed are the following: chronic osteomyelitis confused with Ewing's sarcoma and primary lymphoma of bone mistaken for Ewing's sarcoma; metastatic neuroblastoma mistaken for Ewing's sarcoma; and Hodgkin's disease mistaken for eosinophilic granuloma. A solitary bone metastasis from a neuroblastoma is rarely diagnosed as other than Ewing's sarcoma on initial presentation, and it may be that not until autopsy is the true diagnosis made. This fact has forced one reputable author[104] to conclude from an analysis of a few autopsy cases of so-called Ewing's sarcoma, in which he found evidence consistent with a sympathetic nerve tissue primary, that the Ewing's sarcoma is not a true entity. His belief is that all "Ewing's sarcomas" are in reality metastatic neuroblastomas. Although this conclusion is too radical, the fact remains that a certain percentage of so-called Ewing's sarcomas are other entities that include metastatic neuroblastoma and lymphomas of bone. Great care must be taken to establish an accurate diagnosis by attention to clinical, laboratory, radiologic, and pathologic data; the latter should include special stains and imprint analysis. Where these studies are inconclusive ultrastructural examination may be of benefit.

BENIGN ROUND CELL TUMORS

OSTEOMYELITIS

Osteomyelitis can present with extremely ominous radiographic patterns. The presence of mixed lytic and blastic reactions in the bone and severe periosteal reactions (Figs. 11–1 and 11–2) can mimic bone sarcomas, such as the Ewing's sarcoma, primary reticulum cell sarcoma, or fibrosarcoma. Most patients with osteomyelitis will appear quite ill, manifesting loss of appetite, weight loss, and fever. However, patients with Ewing's sarcoma may have identical signs and symptoms. Some patients with osteomyelitis may appear rather healthy and have little or no fever. This paucity of symptoms is similar in patients with reticulum cell sarcoma and primary lymphoma of bone.

Draining sinuses and the presence of pus at aspiration or open biopsy and positive cultures are the most conclusive clinical signs of infection. The presence of severe synovitis or joint swelling (Fig. 11–2) in addition to bone destruction and periosteal new bone are other signs that are almost always due to osteomyelitis. However, in occasional cases of the rare primary reticulum cell sarcoma of bone, the tumor may break through the cortex to involve the joint. Such cases are generally mistaken for monoarticular arthritis or osteomyelitis until biopsy is performed.

Pathologically, the diagnosis of osteomyelitis is not difficult if significant numbers of neutrophils are present. The only other lesion that could be confused with acute and/or chronic osteomyelitis is eosinophilic granuloma (EG). In general, it is EG that is confused with osteomyelitis rather than the other way around. This error occurs if the eosin stain is weak or not used for a sufficient time, with the result that the eosinophilic granules are poorly stained. The eosinophils that are polymorphonuclear leukocytes can then be confused with neutrophils (also polymorphonuclear leukocytes). This error can be avoided by always considering the diagnosis of EG whenever polymorphonuclear leukocytes are seen by looking for the characteristic histiocytes of eosinophilic granuloma and by ordering phloxine tartrazine or Giemsa stains (see p. 13), which will more clearly stain eosinophilic granules. Imprints of osteomyelitis versus eosinophilic granuloma (Plate 8, *E*) will greatly aid in the differentiation of neutrophils of acute osteomyelitis from the eosinophils and histiocytes of eosinophilic granuloma.

Chronic osteomyelitis may be characterized by sheets of mononuclear cells (Fig. 11–3). If the sections are thick and poorly stained, the lesion can be mistaken for Ewing's sarcoma, reticulum cell sarcoma or lymphocytic lymphoma. These latter sarcomas are generally characterized by a sheet of one cell type only. The principal differentiating histologic feature of chronic osteomyelitis is that various cell types are present. All cases show variable proportions of small lymphocytes and plasma cells (Fig. 11–4) and most cases show, in addition, a few neutrophils. However, as was stated previously, if the sections are poorly fixed, too thick, or not well stained, it will be difficult to decide if one is dealing with a monotony of cells indicative of a lymphoma or sarcoma or a mixture of chronic and/or acute inflammatory cells. This hazard can be avoided by imprint analysis, Zenker's fixation, and by avoiding a final conclusion unless high quality or satisfactory sections are obtained. If these particulars are taken into consideration, the serious error of confusing an osteomyelitis for a Ewing's sarcoma, lymphoma, or an eosinophilic granuloma should not occur.

In long-standing, very low-grade chronic osteomyelitis the tissue generally consists of bland fibrosis, woven bone formation, and often only a very few plasma cells and lymphocytes sprinkled here and there. The relative paucity of inflammatory changes may not be considered sufficient to diagnose or even

---

Osteomyelitis

FIG. 11–1. Osteomyelitis of the adult is most often characterized by "moth-eaten" or permeative destruction and significant periosteal reactions in the diaphysis of a long bone. The differential radiologic diagnosis should include fibrosarcoma, reticulum cell sarcoma in adults, and Ewing's sarcoma and eosinophilic granuloma in younger patients.

FIG. 11–2. In infants and young children osteomyelitis usually destroys the ends of the bones, including the epiphyseal plate. The concommitant association of periosteal reaction and joint involvement are virtually diagnostic of infection.

FIG. 11–3. On low-power examination, chronic osteomyelitis may mimic a round cell malignancy because of massive accumulations of cells. The preservation of marrow fat in this example is a clue to the benign nature of the process. Round cell neoplasms almost always obliterate the marrow fat. However, obliteration of marrow fat may commonly be seen in association with osteomyelitis as well (x40).

FIG. 11–4. On high-power examination, chronic osteomyelitis is typified by a mixture of well differentiated lymphocytes and plasma cells embedded in variable amounts of fibrotic tissue. Occasional poly's are also often present. There is usually evidence of bone repair and nonviable bone sequestra. The only malignant tumor of bone that contains a mixture of plasma cell lymphocytes and fibrosis is Hodgkin's disease. In contrast to osteomyelitis, this condition will contain atypical reticulum and Sternberg-Reed cells (x400).

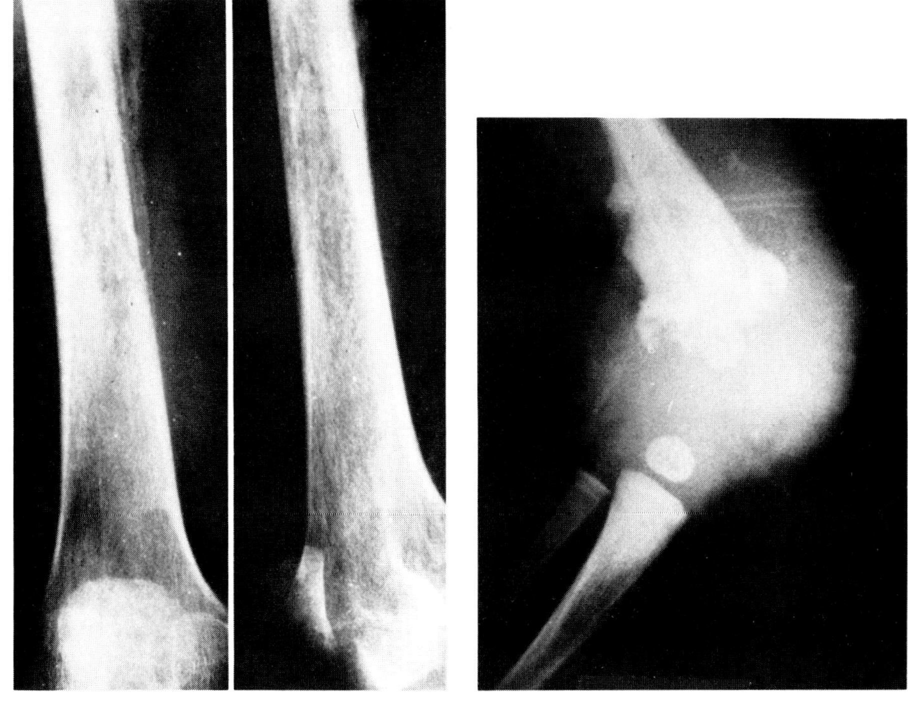

FIG. 11-1

FIG. 11-2

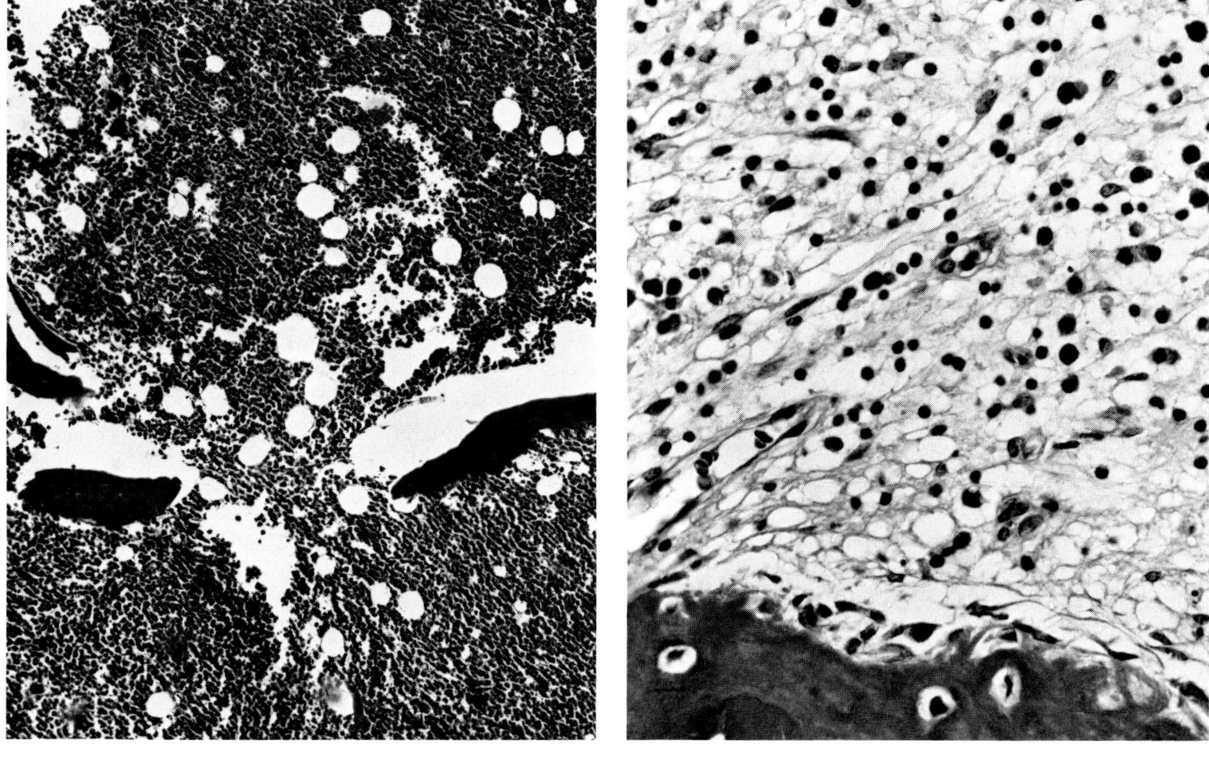

FIG. 11-3

FIG. 11-4

consider osteomyelitis. Nevertheless, a significant proportion of long-standing chronic osteomyelitities may show no more than these meager findings. The presence of marrow fibrosis is an abnormal finding and the presence of even a few chronic inflammatory cells in this tissue is entirely consistent with chronic osteomyelitis. The pathologist should be aware, however, that the histologic changes may be relatively meager. The paucity of inflammatory cells should not interfere with a diagnosis of chronic osteomyelitis, if the history, preoperative clinical diagnosis, and radiographs are supportive.

The Nonlipid Histiocytoses: Eosinophilic Granuloma, So-Called Hand-Schüller-Christian Disease and Letterer-Siwe Disease

Introduction

The *nonlipid histiocytoses* are characterized by a proliferation of histiocytes in which no disorder of lipid metabolism is demonstrable. Historically, the nonlipid histiocytoses include three disorders: eosinophilic granuloma (EG), Hand-Schüller-Christian (HSC) disease, and Letterer-Siwe disease. The histiocytes in these disorders may accumulate lipids in their cytoplasm, but unlike the true lipid metabolic disorders (Gaucher's disease, Niemann-Pick disease, *etc.*), these lipids develop as a consequence to the ingestion of necrotic debris that develops in these lesions, rather than to an inborn error of metabolism.

Jaffe,[22] Lichtenstein and Jaffe,[23,25,26,27] Schajowicz,[35] and others have reached the conclusion that Letterer-Siwe disease, Hand-Schüller-Christian disease, and purely intraosseous eosinophilic granuloma are in actuality three variable expressions of the same disease entity, eosinophilic granuloma. Lichtenstein[25,26] used the term *histiocytosis-X* to relate the three entities. Jaffe believes that while the three conditions differ in their clinical manifestations, they share a common unestablished etiology. On this assumption he considers that solitary EG is the mildest form of the disorder, HSC, the chronic disseminated form, and Letterer-Siwe disease, the acute disseminated and most serious form of EG. The principal reasons that Jaffe believes these three entities are interrelated are the following:

1. Patients with Letterer-Siwe disease, HSC disease, and unifocal EG usually show identical histological features.
2. Approximately 10 per cent of patients with apparent solitary EG will, within 6 months, develop additional bone lesions and extraskeletal involvement or features identical to HSC disease; and rare, nonlethal cases of Letterer-Siwe disease of infancy may develop the clinical and histologic features of HSC disease.

Liebermann,[28] in an extremely thorough review article and from an analysis of his own cases, has arrived at somewhat different conclusions, which are as follows:

1. EG is a benign disorder of bone but in its multifocal form may be responsible for considerable morbidity.
2. The HSC triad is nonspecific.
3. There is no point in using the term *HSC disease* as a synonym for multifocal EG.
4. *Letterer-Siwe disease* is a clinical term that has been used to characterize various malignant histiocytic lymphomas and occasional infectious processes.
5. The term *Histiocytosis-X* is unnecessary and may lead to therapeutic errors.
6. "An analysis of 82 personally followed cases reveals no justification for the current theory that eosinophilic granuloma of bone, Hand-Schüller-Christian disease and Letterer-Siwe disease represent component parts of a single nosologic entity."

Although this author respects many of the concepts formulated by Liebermann in his important article, based upon my own experience and analysis of the literature, my concepts about these three diseases differ to some degree. First of all, the arguments presented by Jaffe and Lichtenstein that at least some of the cases of Letterer-Siwe disease, HSC disease, and EG without extraskeletal involvement are related entities are well formulated and virtually irrefutable. Those cases that evolve from "Letterer-Siwe disease" to "HSC disease", and from "solitary EG" to "HSC disease" are crucial to Jaffe and Lichtenstein's concepts. It would be difficult to consider these so-called entities as not related if such cases occur. Liebermann advocates dropping the term *HSC disease* as having no purpose, but it does have historical precedent and is firmly ingrained in our terminology and in the world's literature. I believe that as long as it is understood that HSC disease is synonomous with multifocal EG with bony and extraskeletal involvement, the term is justified. I concur with Liebermann's view that histiocytosis-X is a mysterious and confusing term and is better dropped from our diagnostic language. This term has been used to cover ignorance and has been applied to lesions with scanty material in which a few histiocytes may be found, while in reality the actual lesion may represent a reticulum cell sarcoma,

Hodgkin's disease, or histiocytic lymphoma. On the other hand, relatively benign EG may be treated too vigorously because the term *histiocytosis-X* has been so bastardized that it now encompasses a disease spectrum that not only includes lethal disorders such as the acute disseminated form of EG (Letterer-Siwe disease) but also histiocytic lymphomas. Another of Liebermann's points is that a certain percentage of so-called "Letterer-Siwe" patients probably include a malignant histiocytic lymphoma group. He considers patients with the clinical symptomatology of so-called Letterer-Siwe disease to actually have a syndrome. We should, therefore, strive to determine whether patients with the Letterer-Siwe syndrome have a malignant histiocytic lymphoma, which would require a form of cancer treatment, or a possible infectious histiocytosis that may respond to steroids and antibiotics. This latter acute disseminated disease may be the form that Jaffe has seen develop into the nonlethal so-called HSC disease. (Multifocal EG with extra-skeletal involvement or chronic disseminated EG [Jaffe].)

Jaffe's formulation is that Letterer-Siwe disease, HSC disease, and unifocal EG are variable expressions of a single etiologic agent; the concept that the manifestations of this agent may be age dependent is most intriguing and may have precedence in another well-known disease entity. For many years the relationship between infants dying with hepatoadrenal necrosis, children with severe gingivostomatitis and adults with "cold sores" was not appreciated. These three diseases were considered to be completely unrelated. Haas, in 1935, discovered in a lethal disease of infancy peculiar intranuclear inclusion bodies in the hepatocytes and adrenal parenchymal cells adjacent to the areas of necrosis. Based upon his review of monkey cells infected by different viral agents only herpes simplex caused identical inclusions. He therefore suggested that the cause of fatal hepatoadrenal necrosis of infancy was due to herpes simplex infection.[20] Many years later his astute observations and conclusions were proven correct. Infantile herpes simplex is the acute disseminated form of the disease, while the childhood and adulthood forms are chronic focal forms of the disease with a variable age dependent morbidity. The younger the patient at the time of initial infection, the more serious the symptoms. The infants die because they cannot produce viral neutralizing antibodies in sufficient time to stem the cytolytic effects of disseminated infection. Similarly, in adults with diseases that interfere with immune competency such as lymphoma or in patients treated with massive steroid therapy, herpes simplex infection may result in death. Adults with "cold sores" reflect the least severe expression of herpes. Clearly there are many similarities between herpes simplex infection and its relationship to the immune competency of the host and eosinophilic granuloma. These similarities would suggest that EG may be due to a viral infection or perhaps to a disseminated "allergen." Jaffe[22] and Schajowicz[35] have suggested that EG is a possible viral infection. Basset, *et al.*,[6,7] have shown cellular inclusions of possible viral type in patients with various forms of EG.

EOSINOPHILIC GRANULOMA (EG), SOLITARY AND MULTIPLE, WITHOUT EXTRASKELETAL INVOLVEMENT

Capsule Summary (Fig. 11-5)

Incidence. Rare tumor. Approximately 1 per cent of biopsied primary tumors of bone.

Age. More than 80 per cent of patients present before age 10.

Clinical Features. Localized, aching pain.

Radiologic Features. Diaphyseal, osteolytic, round-to-oval, ill-defined; new periosteal bone may or may not be present.

Gross Pathology. Scant, tan-red, friable tissue.

Histopathology. *Early phases:* eosinophils and histiocytes in any proportion, sprinkling of plasma cells and lymphocytes; multinucleate giant cells may or may not be present. *Late phases:* may get complete resolution of lesion or large foci of lipid-laden macrophages with scarring.

Course. Benign; 10 per cent of cases develop multifocal disease in less than 6 months.

Treatment. Symptomatic; low-dosage radiation if vertebral body is affected or if fracture is imminent in long bone.

Clinical Features

The mildest and most favorable nonlipid histiocytosis is EG confined to a single bone—or occasionally to several bones—without extraskeletal involvement.

EG generally begins in childhood with localized, aching pain. If the affected bone is near the skin, it also begins with swelling. In multiple bone involvement, it is possible for only one bone to give rise to local complaints. A less common sign is low-grade fever. Laboratory studies may show elevated erythrocyte sedimentation rate, and 6 to 10 per cent of patients show mild, peripheral eosinophilia. Cultures have consistently failed to reveal an infectious agent.

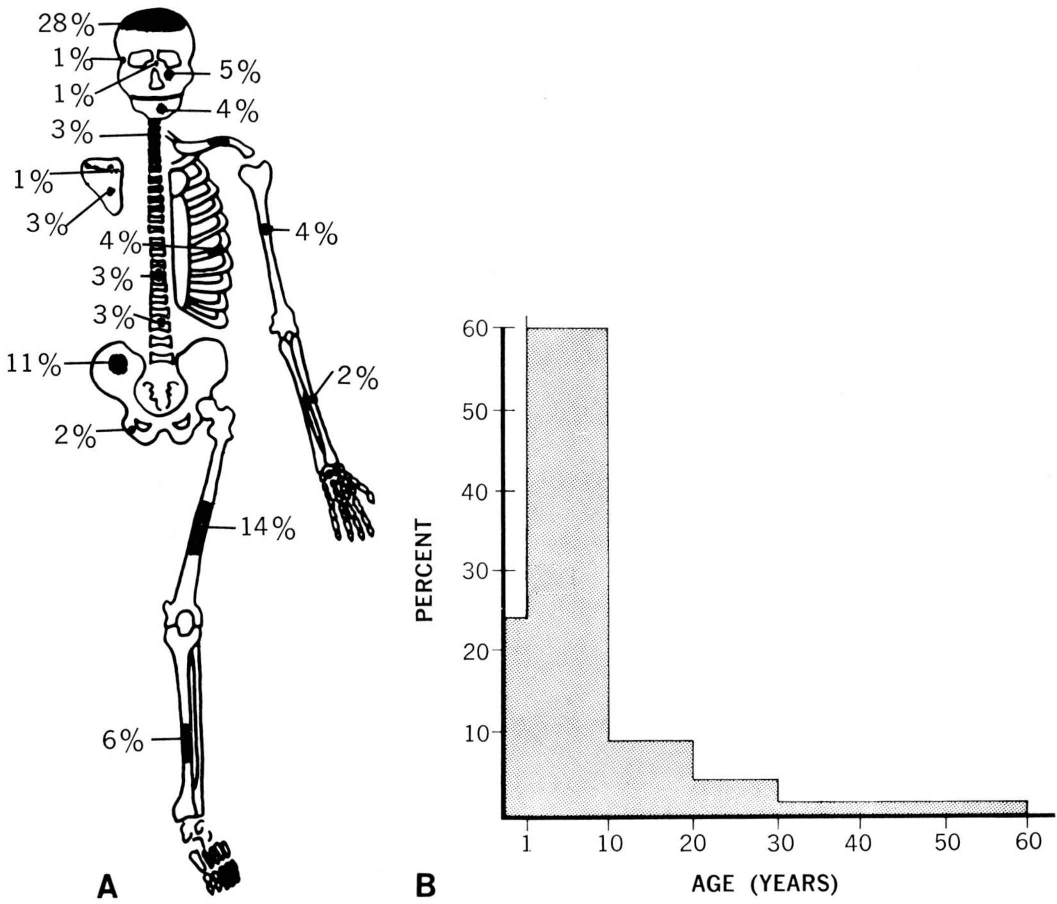

FIG. 11-5. (*A*) Unifocal eosinophilic granuloma. Frequency of areas of involvement in 143 patients. Male:female incidence, 1.5 : 1. (*B*) Age distribution of patients with unifocal eosinophilic granuloma. (Mirra, J., Bullough, P., and Freiberger, R.: Orthopedic Diseases, Part III: Histiocytoses and Round Cell Tumors. New York, Famous Teachings in Modern Medicine, MedCom, Inc., © 1973)

Radiologic Features

The radiologic features of EG are characterized by osteolysis. The lesion is generally 1 to 5 cm. in diameter and nonexpansile. In the early phases of the disease the lesion is poorly delineated or shows a moth-eaten pattern of destruction (Figs. 11–6, *A*, and 11–7). The cortices are often eroded and the periosteum may be stimulated to produce one or more fine lamellations (Fig. 11–6, *A*). It is this phase that most closely mimics osteomyelitis or round cell sarcomas such as Ewing's. In later stages of the disease the process abates and the borders of the lesion become sharp and the contours round or oval (Fig. 11–6, *B*). In this phase sharp delineation of the lesion denotes its benignancy. Eventually the lesion becomes surrounded or walled off by a border of dense or reactive host bone sclerosis. After a few to many years the lesion may disappear completely or leave a small residual defect. In long bones the lesions are usually diaphyseal or diaphyseal-metaphyseal. Lesions centered in the epiphysis are rare (less than 5% of cases). In general, epiphyseal lytic lesions of early childhood are due to osteomyelitis. Pyogenic osteomyelitis also usually leads to focal or complete destruction of the epiphyseal plate and joint swelling. The epiphyseal plate never shows destruction in EG. Cartilage-destroying enzymes are obviously not produced by the eosinophils and histiocytes of EG but are produced by the neutrophils of osteomyelitis.

In a small percentage of cases EG may protrude into the soft tissues as a mass lesion, particularly in the skull. In other bones this is a very rare phenomenon (Fig. 11–8). Usually the presence of a soft-tissue mass is a sign of a malignant tumor. Rib involvement may lead to expansion and pathologic fracture. Fracture is uncommon in long bone lesions, however.

Vertebral body involvement frequently leads to insidious collapse on radiograph (Fig. 11–9, *A*). Eventually the vertebral body may be compressed into a thin wafer (Fig. 11–9, *B*). Extreme flattening of a vertebral body is called *vertebra plana* or *Calvé's syndrome.* Once thought to be due to aseptic necrosis, biopsies from this lesion have shown that most cases are in fact due to EG. Spinal cord and root compression may occur as a result of severe vertebral body destruction and compression.

Most patients without extraskeletal involvement will have only one bone involved (unifocal EG). Occasional patients may have more than one bone involved. One patient is reported to have had as many as eight bones affected[22] without evidence of extraskeletal disease (multifocal EG without extraskeletal involvement).

Approximately 10 per cent of patients who present with unifocal disease will within 6 months develop so-called Hand-Schüller-Christian disease, which is in essence multifocal EG with extraskeletal involvement. Almost any bone can be involved with the exception of those of the hands and feet.

Gross Pathology

Curetted tissue is generally scant and soft reddish to brown. It often shows areas of hemorrhage and cystification. Older lesions will show yellowish areas in streaks or nodules that are due to accumulations of lipid-laden macrophages.

Histopathology

Low-power histologic examination shows the tissue to consist of masses of cells (Fig. 11–10, Plate 8, *A*). The bony trabeculae are often absent from the lesional tissue, accounting for the lytic radiographic appearance.

The term *eosinophilic granuloma*—a granuloma being a collection of histiocytes—aptly describes the histology of this lesion, in which eosinophils and histiocytes occur in any proportion. However, distinct, focal granulomas are not seen in this entity. (Focal granulomas are indicative of tuberculosis, sarcoid or fungal disease.) Eosinophils may predominate as diffuse masses of cells (Plate 8, *C, top*) or as focal masses around vessels (Fig. 11–11), while in an adjacent area histiocytes are the predominant cell type and only a few eosinophils are interspersed (Plate 8, *C, bottom*). In other fields histiocytes and eosinophils may be about equally mixed (Plate 8, *B*, Fig. 11–13).

The eosinophil, a polymorphonuclear leukocyte with prominent eosinophilic granules, requires proper fixation and freshly prepared eosin for accurate granule staining. Tissue overdecalcification and weak eosin often lead to improperly stained eosinophils that may be mistaken for neutrophils. Therefore the disease may easily be misinterpreted as acute osteomyelitis.

In peripheral blood smears the cytologic features of the eosinophil are obvious, but on tissue section it is a small cell (10μ–13μ), usually with a bilobed nucleus and pink or red cytoplasm. The presence of eosinophilic granules on tissue section can be accentuated by using a phloxine-tartrazine or Giemsa stain (see p. 13). Imprints of E.G. stained with H and E, Wright's, Giemsa or phloxine-tartrazine will demonstrate the eosinophils and histiocytes much more clearly than ordinary sections (Plate 9, *E*).

Essential to the diagnosis of EG is the demonstration of monocytoid histiocytes (macrophages). The peripheral blood counterpart of the tissue histiocyte is the monocyte. On H and E section histiocytes have the same characteristics as monocytes: abundant amphophilic cytoplasm, well-demarcated cell borders, and nuclei of various sizes and shapes. Histiocytes may range between 20 and 100 μ, depending on the number of nuclei they contain and the quantity of lipids stored in their cytoplasm.

The nucleus of the histiocyte may be single or multiple and have a round, oval, reniform, or lobulated shape (Figs. 11–12 and 11–13). A bean-shaped or reniform nucleus is often seen and is a characteristic of histiocytes (Plates 8, *C, bottom,* and *D*). The nuclei often show indentations (Plate 8, *C, bottom,* and *E, top*).

The pleomorphism of histiocytes, particularly if they dominate the histologic picture, can lead to the erroneous impression of a reticulum cell sarcoma or Hodgkin's disease. An imprint of curetted EG tissue more clearly shows the ominous cytologic appearance of these histiocytes (Plate 8, *E*). Hodgkin's disease, however, is more likely in middle-aged or elderly patients, and the histiocytes contain even greater nuclear pleomorphism and much larger nucleoli (Plate 9, *E*).

In EG, histiocytes may assume many different histologic forms: they may fuse syncytially to produce multinucleated giant cells (Figs. 10–20 and 10–21, 11–12, and 11–13, Plate 8, *B*), they may phagocytose erythrocytes and convert the hemoglobin to hemosiderin, becoming in the process hemosiderin-filled macrophages; or they may ingest necrotic or damaged tissue and convert it into intracytoplasmic lipids (Fig. 11-14, Plate 8, *E, bottom*).

In months or years, EG lesions can heal both radiologically and histologically, leaving no trace. If healing is incomplete, the proliferative features of the disease—masses of histiocytes and eosinophils—are reduced and the tissue gradually replaced by nests of granular to foamy macrophages in association with some degree of fibrosis. The granular histiocytes are eventually converted into large, confluent masses of pale-staining, foamy, lipid-laden macrophages (Fig. 11-14) or they may disappear completely. Because most lesions of unifocal or multifocal EG are treated by curettage or low-dosage irradiation and heal well, foamy cells are not often seen *in situ.* They are frequently observed in the more extensive, severe, chronically protracted lesions of EG with extraskeletal involvement. In the latest stages of the disease dense fibrous tissue intervenes admixed with variable quantities of oval to spindly lipid-laden macrophages (Fig. 11-15).

Foci of multinucleate giant cells are seen in necrotic and hemorrhagic areas that are being revascularized (Fig. 10-20). In early or late EG they are often attached to capillaries and seem to "bud" from them (Fig. 10-21). The finding of masses of giant cells in association with EG can result in an erroneous diagnosis of giant cell tumor, although the clinical and radiologic features and the total histologic picture should prevent this mistake.

It is clear that EG is one of the great mimics of benign and malignant bone diseases. Examination of even "old" lesions usually shows some residual foci of histiocytes and eosinophils, and correlation of clinical and radiographic findings helps to avoid diagnostic pitfalls. Focal collections of lymphocytes and plasma cells are not uncommonly found in cases of EG. This feature should not result in the diagnosis of osteomyelitis, if careful attention is given to the identification of the characteristic eosinophils and histiocytes of EG.

Differential Diagnosis

OSTEOMYELITIS. Radiographically, the features of EG and osteomyelitis may be identical. Lesions of the skull are common in EG and rare in osteomyelitis. If there is joint swelling, destruction of epiphyseal plate cartilage, or loss of vertebral body disc space the diagnosis is most consistent with osteomyelitis. EG does not result in these changes. Histologically, EG is dominated by eosinophils and histiocytes in varying proportions, although moderate numbers of lymphocytes and plasma cells may be seen. Later stages show foamy to lipid-laden macrophages and fibrosis. Osteomyelitis in acute stages is dominated by neutrophils and in later stages by lymphocytes, plasma cells, and fibrosis. Imprint analysis and well-stained sections may be required to distinguish eosinophilic from neutrophilic polymorphonuclear leukocytes.

EWING'S SARCOMA. Radiographically, both EG and Ewing's sarcoma may be identical. Histologically, there is no resemblance between the two. Ewing's is composed of a monotonous mass of mononuclear cells with numerous mitoses. In EG various cell types are seen (eosinophils, histiocytes, lymphocytes, and plasma cells). Mitoses are rare in EG and abundant in Ewing's.

HODGKIN'S DISEASE. Generally Hodgkin's lesions are larger and more blastic than those of EG. Hodgkin's patients are usually over 20 years of age, while patients with EG are usually younger than 20 years

---

Eosinophilic Granuloma

FIG. 11-6. (*A*) The early radiologic features of EG are one or more foci of ill-defined medullary and/or cortical lysis, usually in association with some degree of periosteal new bone formation (*arrow*). This phase may be indistinguishable from osteomyelitis or Ewing's sarcoma. (*B*) During the healing phase of EG the borders of the lesion become sharp and rounded (*arrow*). Although such lesions can be confused with bone cysts and fibrous dysplasia, biopsy is diagnostic.

FIG. 11-7. Early phase of EG with lytic destruction of a rib (*arrow*) mimicking a malignant neoplasm. Many cases of EG will present with these ominous radiologic features.

FIG. 11-8. On rare occasion EG may erode into the soft tissue (*arrow*) and stimulate considerable periosteal reaction.

FIG. 11-9. EG not infrequently involves the vertebral body, leading to insidious collapse *A*). Eventually the bone may flatten to a wafer thin line (vertebra plana). The syndrome of vertebra plana (*B*) (*arrow*) is now known to be consequent to EG in most instances, although formerly it was believed that this condition was consequent to ischemic necrosis.

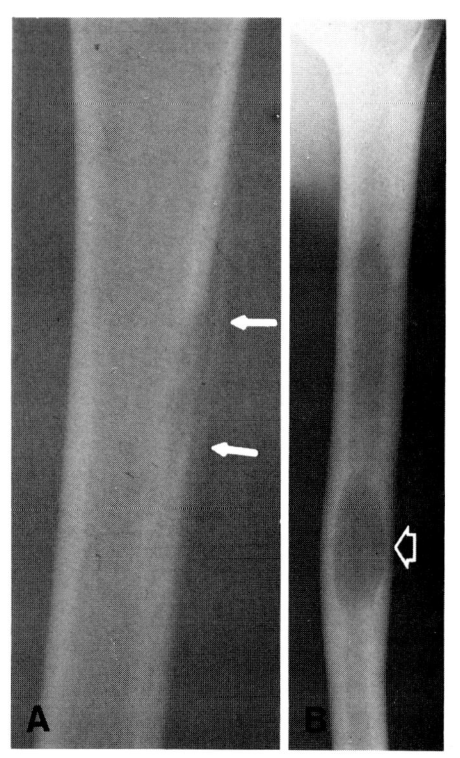

FIG. 11-6

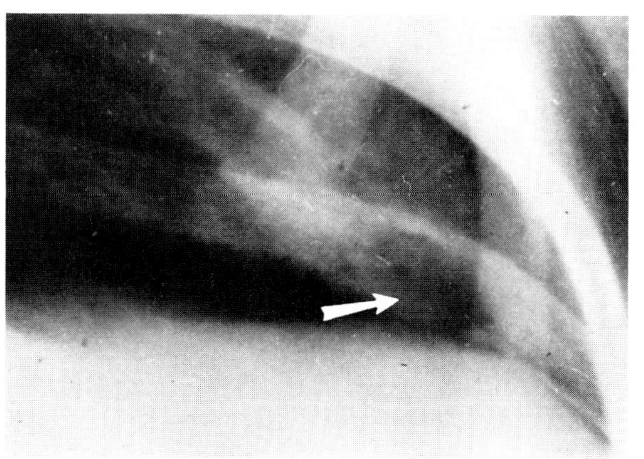

FIG. 11-7

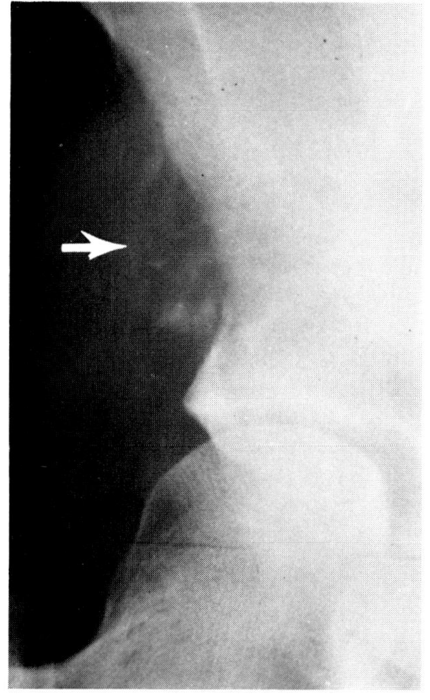

FIG. 11-8

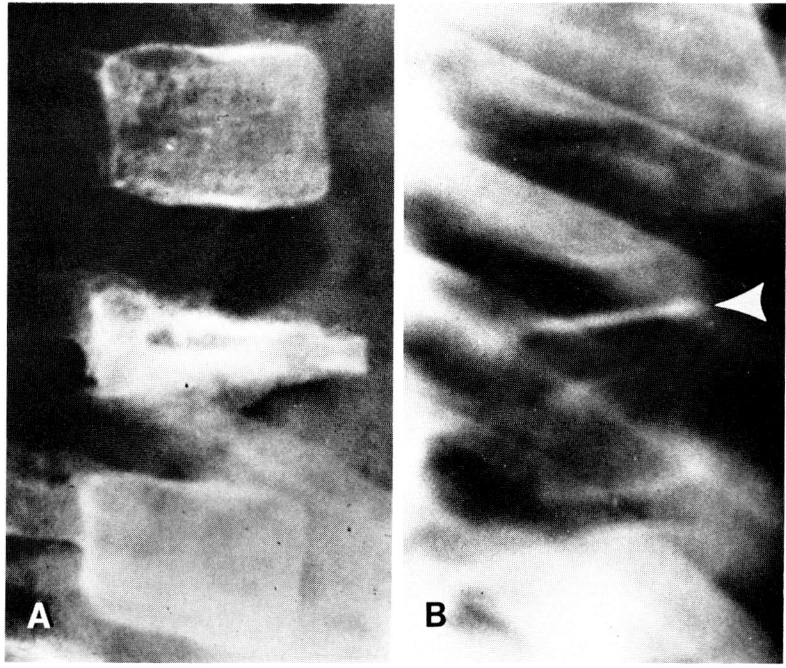

FIG. 11-9

old. Hodgkin's may demonstrate a very similar morphology to EG; namely, histiocytes, eosinophils, lymphocytes, plasma cells, and variable fibrosis. The key feature is the identification of bizarre reticulum cells (Plate 9, *E, top*) and if possible, classic Sternberg-Reed cells (Plate 9, *E, bottom* and *F*). Finding these classic cells may be extremely difficult and even impossible by needle biopsy alone, because many cases of Hodgkin's will show only a few absolutely classical cells per square cm. of tissue. Open-bone biopsy and imprints of marrow are extremely useful to diagnosis. Primary Hodgkin's of bone is rare. Lymphangiography will usually show involvement of the regional lymph nodes.

LOW-GRADE NEOPLASTIC GIANT CELL TUMOR. On rare occasions EG may be dominated by masses of osteoclast-like giant cells (pp. 320–322 and Figs. 10–21 and 10–22). However, careful search will usually reveal lipid-laden macrophages or occasional eosinophils, lymphocytes, and plasma cells. The neoplastic GCT does not show eosinophils and only rarely, foamy macrophages. GCT almost always involves the epiphyseal or epiphyseal-metaphyseal end of a bone; EG rarely involves or extends to epiphyses. GCT tends to affect patients older than age 20 and is only rarely multifocal. EG may be either uni- or multifocal.

GRANULOMATOUS DISEASES. Tuberculosis and other granulomatous diseases are characterized by distinct separable epitheloid granulomas, usually with central necrosis. Eosinophils are usually not seen. In EG small focal granulomas are not present. The histiocytes form indistinct, rather diffuse masses admixed with variable numbers of eosinophils. In eosinophilic "granuloma" the entire lesion is essentially the granuloma. Multiple distinct granulomas are indicative of either tuberculosis, fungal infections, or sarcoidosis.

NONOSSIFYING FIBROMA (NOF). In the late healing phases the NOF closely resembles the late healing phase of EG. The main differentiating feature in these late stages is not histological but radiological. The NOF appears as an eccentric metaphyseal lesion, while EG is usually diaphyseal or if metaphyseal, is not usually distinctly eccentric.

Course and Treatment

The course is benign and the lesion usually heals well after simple curettage. Dangerously large lesions that may lead to pathologic fracture and lesions of vertebral bodies are best treated with low-dosage radiation (600–1500 rads). Healing takes from a few months to a year or more. Steroids or methotrexate have been used to treat multiple lesions. If bone survey after 6 months shows no other lesions in a patient who presented with a single lesion, the disease will probably remain unifocal.

Multifocal Eosinophilic Granuloma With Extraskeletal Involvement: Chronic Disseminated Type (Hand-Schüller-Christian Disease)

Capsule Summary

Incidence. A very rare tumorous process of bone and extraskeletal tissues. Approximately 0.3 per cent of primary bone tumors.

Age. More than 70 per cent of patients present before age 5 (Fig. 11–23)

Clinical Features. Begins in childhood. May develop otitis media, diabetes insipidus and other signs of hypopituitarism; exophthalmos, multiple osteolytic bone lesions usually including the skull; and tooth loosening with man-

---

Eosinophilic Granuloma

FIG. 11–10. On low-power examination, EG is characterized by a massive infiltration of cells in which bone trabeculae are generally absent to markedly attenuated in the center of the lesion (left of field) (x40).

FIG. 11–11. EG is exemplified by variable proportions of eosinophils and histiocytes. In this example, the eosinophils tended to accumulate in a perivascular distribution (x200).

FIG. 11–12. This illustration shows a typical mixture of cells common to EG. The smaller, darker cells are eosinophils, lymphocytes, and plasma cells. The larger cells are granular, mononuclear, and multinuclear histiocytes. The nuclei are folded, occasionally distinctly reniform (*arrow*), and quite variable in shape. Although ominous looking to the novice, they lack the degree of atypia and large nucleoli seen in Hodgkin's disease, or the unequivocally anaplastic size, shape, and dense, very irregular chromatin distribution seen in a well prepared section of reticulum cell sarcoma of bone (Fig. 11–58) (x600).

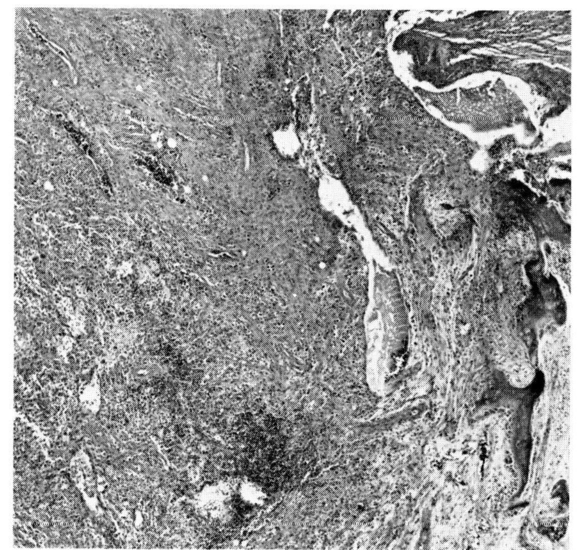

FIG. 11-10

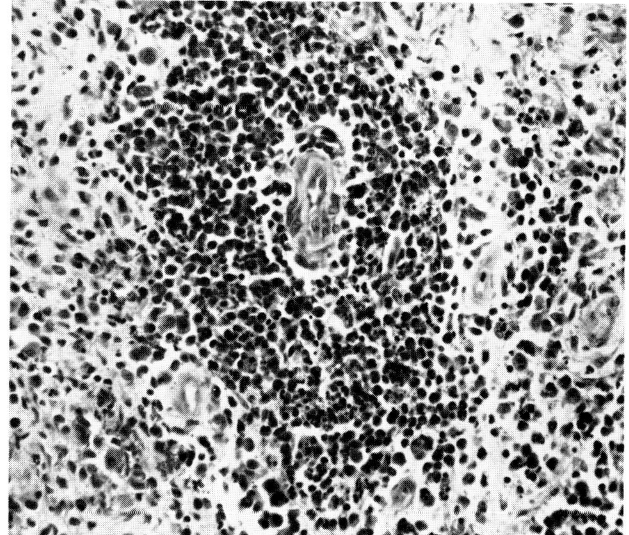

FIG. 11-11

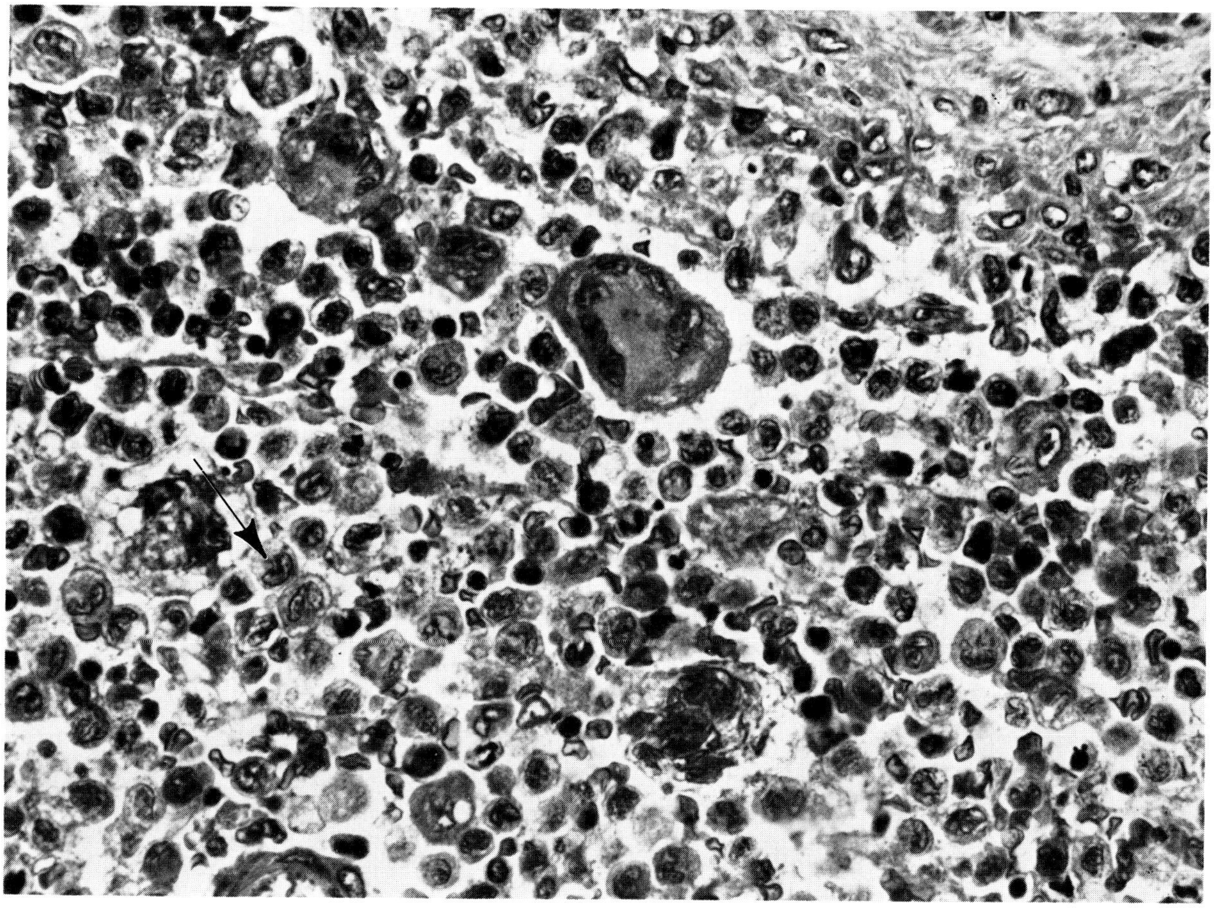

FIG. 11-12

dibular involvement, fever, hepatosplenomegaly, lymphadenopathy, anemia, and abnormal liver chemistries.

Radiologic Features. Multiple destructive lesions of the bones. The lesions may "expand" the bone focally and result in ominous periosteal reactions. Any bone may be involved but the skull is almost always affected. In contrast to solitary EG the bones of the hands and feet may also show involvement. Lesions in the flat bones frequently show beveled edges. Pathologic fractures may occur, particularly of the spine.

Gross Pathology. In early phase, tissue resembles unifocal EG; in the late phase, more extensive lipid accumulates, causing a yellow color.

Histopathology. In early phase, same as unifocal EG; in late phase, more extensive lipid-laden macrophages (lipogranulomas) and scarring.

Course. High morbidity; 10 per cent die of some complication.

Treatment. Chemotherapy, low-dosage irradiation for dangerous or disfiguring lesions, Pitressin, and antipyretics.

Clinical Features

In 1893 Hand described a 3-year-old boy with polyuria, hepatosplenomegaly, cutaneous petechiae, exophthalmos, and destructive skeletal lesions. The boy died after 2 months, and necropsy revealed a yellow substance in the bony lesions. In 1916 Schüller reported a five-year-old girl who had maplike radiolucent defects in the femur, ilium, and skull, in addition to exophthalmos and diabetes insipidus. The lesions of patients whose symptoms and signs correspond to those described by Hand, Schüller, and Christian are histologically the same as those Lichtenstein and Jaffe described for unifocal EG, particularly in the early proliferative phase. Lichtenstein and Jaffe concluded that Hand-Schüller-Christian disease was a disseminated and more severe form of unifocal EG, a view supported by the fact that about 10 per cent of the patients who present with unifocal EG eventually develop multifocal and extraskeletal disease. Although pain and swelling may be present, most patients otherwise appear to be in good health.

Approximately half the patients develop diabetes insipidus early in the course of the disease and respond well to Pitressin. Infrequent associated destruction of the sella turcica suggests that this disorder may be due to involvement of the pituitary stalk or hypothalamus.

Otitis media is a common symptom and the most frequent initial complaint. Radiologic destruction of the mastoid or petrous portions of the temporal bone occurs in half the patients with Hand-Schüller-Christian disease. About one fourth of the patients develop unilateral or bilateral exophthalmos caused by EG of the bony orbit.

The classic *Hand-Schüller-Christian triad*—calvarial defects, diabetes insipidus, and exophthalmos—is present in about 10 per cent of the cases. Fewer than half the patients develop destructive lesions in the mandible, leading to loss of teeth. Ulcerative, bleeding gum lesions are common.

Patients with Hand-Schüller-Christian disease occasionally develop hepatosplenomegaly, lymphadenopathy, and anemia, all of which may simulate malignant lymphoma. Laboratory findings in severely affected patients include abnormal liver chemistries. The alkaline phosphatase is generally not elevated.

Radiologic Features

The most common radiologic manifestation of multifocal EG is involvement of the vault of the skull. This occurs in over 90 per cent of the patients (Fig. 11–17). Due to uneven levels of bone destruction of the tables of the skull the lesions may show characteristic beveled edges. Bone destruction in the occiput can result in platybasia or invagination of the base of the skull caused by pressure from the upper cervical spine. New periosteal bone is not prominent in skull lesions.

Skeletal lesions other than those of the skull and mandible occur in about 40 per cent of patients. The bones show multiple lytic defects, quite often with focal eccentric expansion (Figs. 11–18 and 11–19). At

---

Eosinophilic Granuloma

FIG. 11-13. The histiocytes in this example contain a more voluminous, pinkish-blue cytoplasm, and single to multiple, oval to reniform, "crinkled" or "folded" nuclei. The smaller cells are mostly lymphocytes or bilobed eosinophils (*arrow*) (x1000).

FIG. 11-14. Massive accumulations of pale, foamy macrophages develop in later phases of the disease. (x250).

FIG. 11-15. After several years the tissue may become dominated by fibrosis in which fewer numbers of foam cells are found (x125).

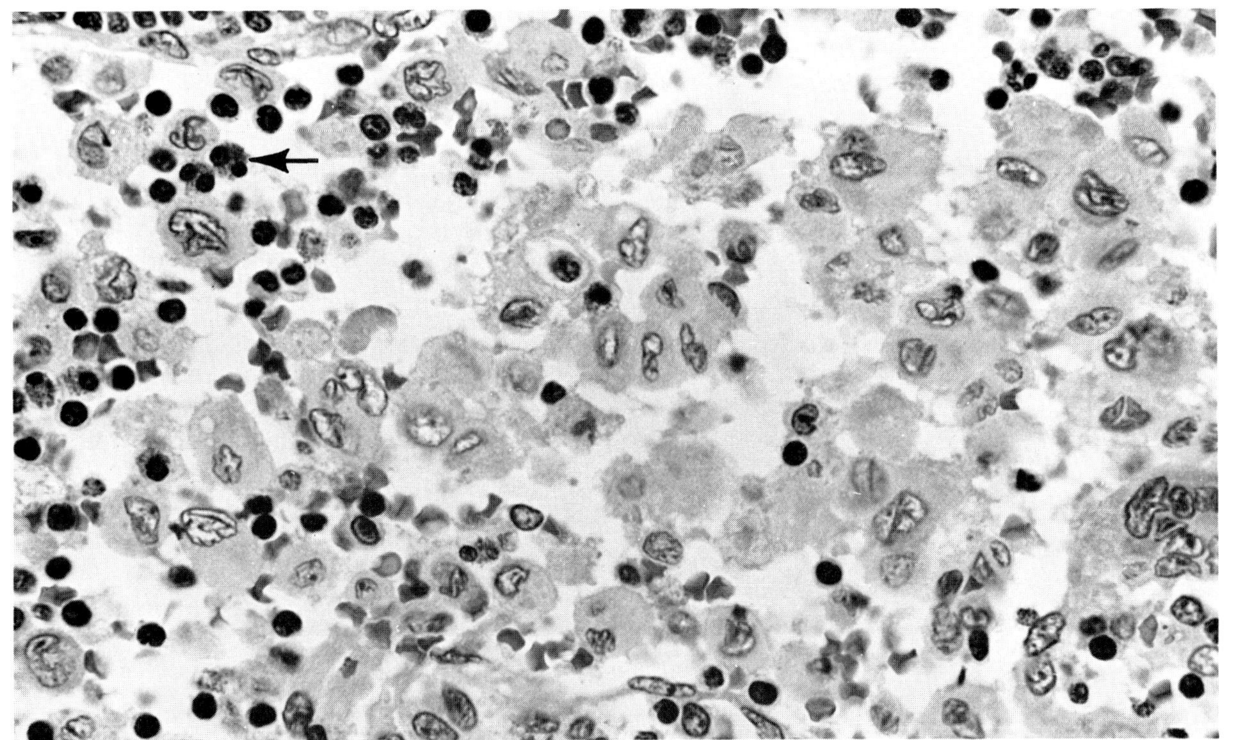

FIG. 11-13

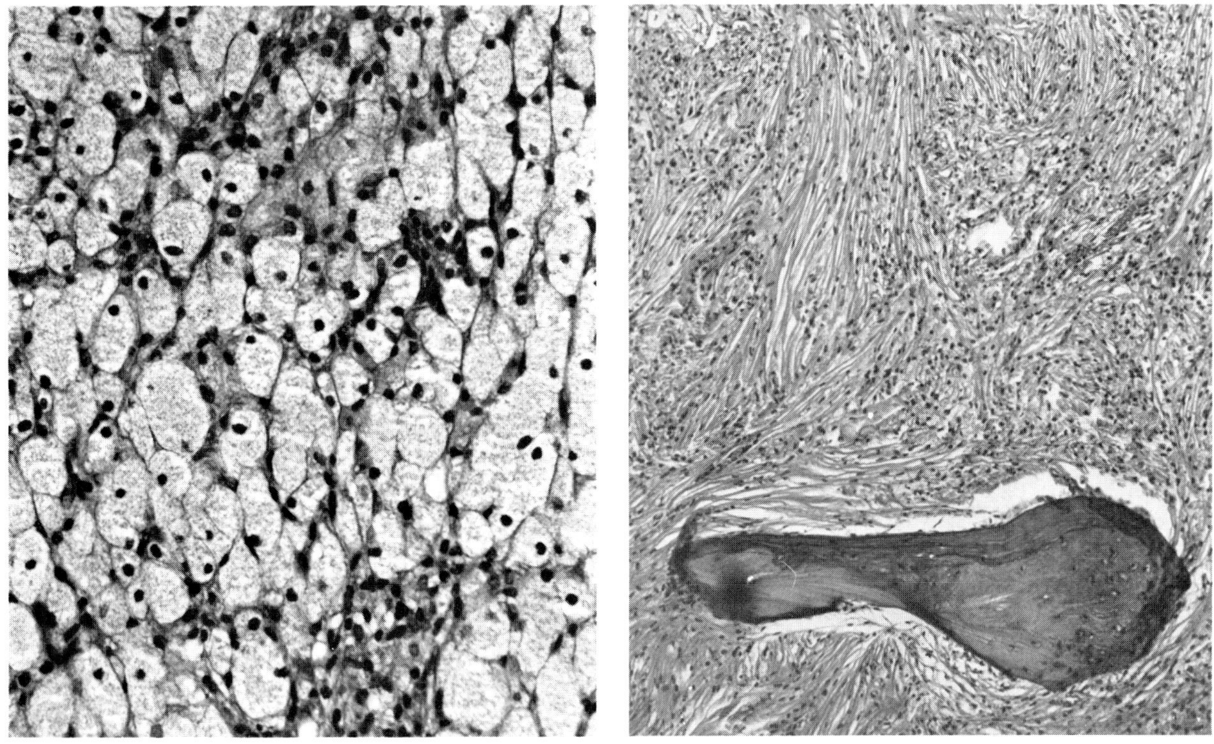

FIG. 11-14

FIG. 11-15

first indistinct, the edge of the defects becomes definite as healing progresses over a period of months to years in the incipient phases of the disease. The periosteum may show considerable reaction and closely simulate pyogenic osteomyelitis. Pathologic fracture in the long bones is uncommon. Involvement of the spine usually leads to compression fracture (vertebra plana).

Most lesions are confined to the diaphyses and metaphyses. Epiphyseal lesions are rare. The epiphyseal plate is not destroyed by the process. In fact, the hyperemia that is associated with the process may lead to long-bone lengthening.

Gross Pathology and Histopathology

The early phase of the disease is identical to that described previously for unifocal EG (Figs. 11-11–11-13; Plate 8, *A, B, C, D*, and *E*). In the later phases of this disease, gross and histologic features are dominated by masses of lipid-laden macrophages (lipogranulomata, see Fig. 11-14), and/or scarring, (Fig.11-15). In some fields foci of histiocytes and eosinophils may be found similar to those seen in the earlier proliferative phases. Foci of multinucleate giant cells may be seen at all stages (Figs. 10-21 and 10-22). The end stage of the disease is characterized by fibrosis or complete healing. The reticuloendothelial organs are commonly affected by the process, resulting in hepatosplenomegaly and lymphadenopathy. These organs will show a diffuse benign enlargement of the sinusoids because of masses of mononuclear and multinuclear histiocytes with occasional eosinophils, lymphocytes, and plasma cells, similar to the histopathology of the bone lesions (Fig. 11-16). Eventually the granular histiocytes convert to large lipid-laden macrophages. Involvement of the lungs can lead to diffuse interstitial fibrosis.

Course

Healing of an individual skeletal lesion usually occurs within a period of a few years. However, new lesions may occur sporadically and the full course of the disease may range from as little as one year to as long as 25 years. The spontaneous resolution of the disease and its known course suggest an inflammatory etiology. Because of the wide range of tissues that may be affected, morbidity is generally high. About 10 per cent of patients die from such related complications as pneumonia, anemia with thrombocytopenia, transverse myelitis, and chronic interstitial fibrosis of the lungs with secondary cor pulmonale.

Multifocal Eosinophilic Granuloma, Acute Disseminated Or Infantile Form (Letterer-Siwe Disease)

Capsule Summary

Incidence. Extremely rare. Fewer than 0.2 per cent of biopsied primary bone tumors.

Age. All patients are younger than 2 years of age.

Clinical Features. Acute onset of symptoms: hepatosplenomegaly, lymphadenopathy, papular rash, bleeding diathesis, anemia, and occasionally exophthalmos and diabetes insipidus.

Radiologic Features. Visible bone lesions usually absent. If present, single or multiple osteolytic lesions with or without laminated periosteal reactions.

Gross Pathology. Gray-yellow, nodular infiltrates in visceral organs and bones.

Histopathology. Two types of proliferating histiocyte masses: benign-appearing and foamy, mixed with eosinophils and anaplastic.

Treatment. High-dosage antibiotics and steroids.

Course. Most cases are fatal. The few survivors develop the chronic disseminated form of the disease (Hand-Schüller-Christian disease).

Clinical Features

Letterer-Siwe disease was named by Abt and Denenholz in 1936 based on a 1924 case report of Letterer and on seven 1933 case reports of Siwe.[1] It nearly always affects infants younger than two years of age and is characterized by acute onset, hepatosplenomegaly, lymphadenopathy, hemorrhagic diatheses, anemia, papular rash, and skeletal lesions associated with a proliferation of histiocytes unre-

Multifocal Eosinophilic Granuloma

FIG. 11-16. Lymph node from a patient with multifocal eosinophilic granuloma with extraskeletal involvement (so-called Hand-Schüller-Christian disease). (*A*) The sinusoids are markedly distended (x40). (*B*) High-power examination showed a mixture of mono- and multinucleated histiocytes and numerous eosinophils identical to the lesions in the bones (x250).

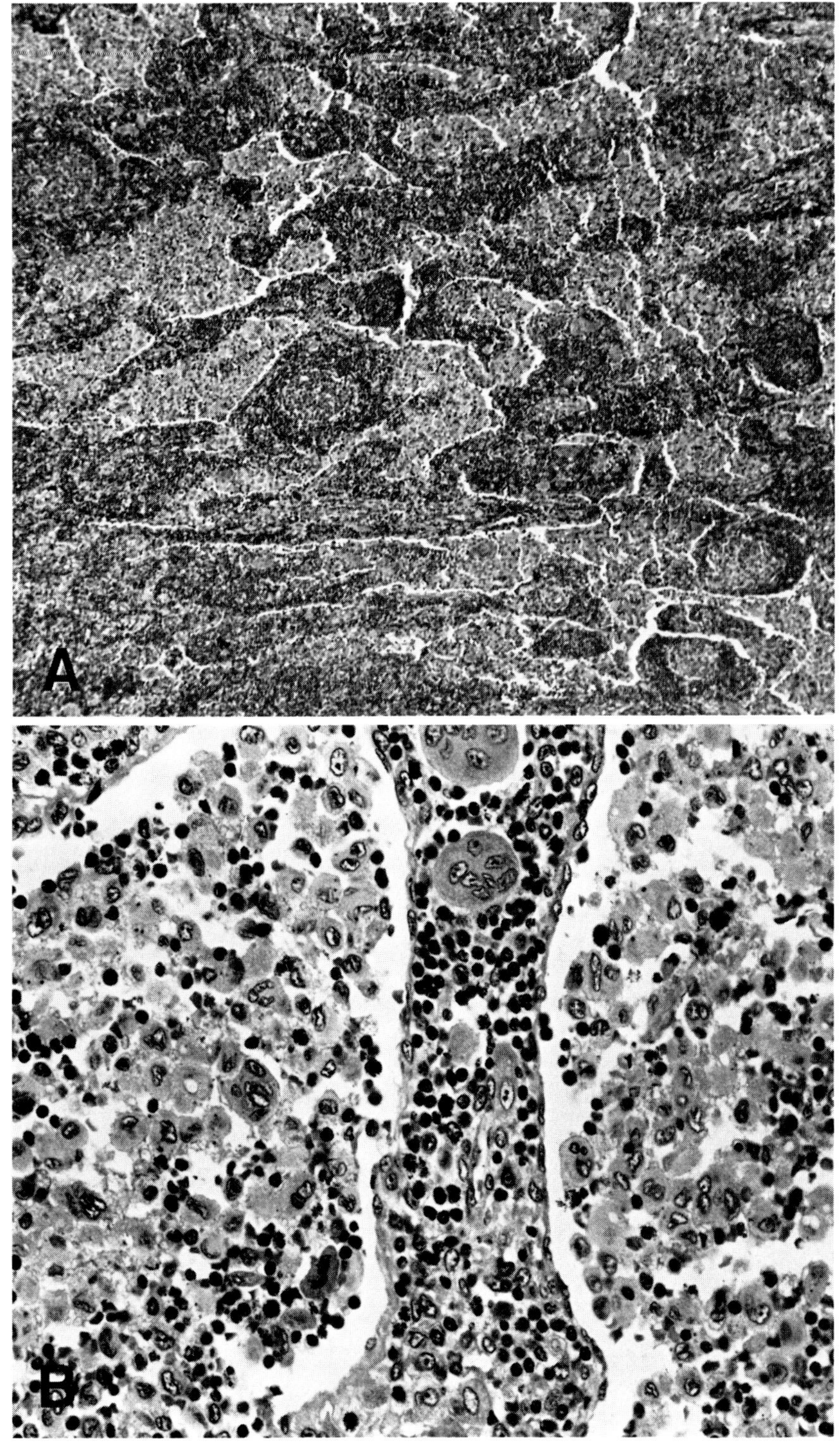

FIG. 11-16

lated to any known infection. In a few cases exophthalmos and diabetes insipidus have developed, bearing at least a clinical resemblance to chronic, disseminated EG. Liebermann's description of two histologic variants suggest that this disease might be more accurately described as a syndrome.[28] The variant containing malignant- or anaplastic-appearing histiocytes seems to be a form of lymphoma and not a severe type of EG, while the benign, cytologic histiocytic type might well be an infantile form of multifocal EG.

Radiologic Features

Only about one third of patients with acute disseminated EG show demonstrable radiographic lesions (Fig. 11-20). In cases that this author has autopsied, although no lesions were clearly visible by standard radiography, specimen radiograph of 2 mm. slices of bone showed numerous small holes (Fig. 11-21) similar to rampant multiple myeloma. With the advent of antibiotic treatment some of the infants are kept alive for longer periods than they used to be. In this group distinct bone lesions may be seen by standard radiography in about half the cases. When lesions are seen they tend to be multiple, poorly defined, and lytic (Fig. 11-20). They tend to involve the diaphyses and metaphyses.

Gross Features

Necropsy shows focal to diffuse infiltrates in the bones, skin, and reticuloendothelial organs (lymph nodes, spleen, and liver). The infiltrates have a bright orange-yellow hue (Plate 8, *F*).

Histopathology

Microscopically, the involved organs show masses of proliferating histiocytes with a quite pale cytoplasm and small, rather innocent nuclei (Figs. 11-22, 11-24). Eosinophils are present in only some cases. Patients who survive consequent to treatment usually develop the classical features of the chronic disseminated form of multifocal EG (so-called Hand-Schüller-Christian disease).

Differential Diagnosis

HISTIOCYTIC LYMPHOMA OF INFANCY. The clinical features may be identical to acute disseminated EG. In this author's opinion the only way to be sure that one is dealing with a malignant or lymphomatous process is to identify nuclear anaplasia in the histiocytes. However, Liebermann[28] classified some of his cases of Letterer-Siwe syndrome that did not show nuclear anaplasia as malignant histiocytic lymphoma. Two of his cases did show distinct anaplasia. Obviously, more research will have to be done on this syndrome complex to develop criteria by which a meaningful classification can be developed upon which treatment must depend.

Course and Treatment

The vast majority of patients succumb to the disease within one year after the onset of symptoms. High-dosage antibiotic regimens and steroids have occasionally resulted in survival. These patients develop the typical bone lesions and extraskeletal involvement of the chronic disseminated form of EG.

(Text continues on p. 392.)

Multifocal Eosinophilic Granuloma

FIG. 11-17. Hand-Schüller-Christian disease. Most patients with this multifocal form of EG show geographic lytic defects in the skull.

FIG. 11-18. Hand-Schüller-Christian disease, an example of the severity of the disease in the long bones. Note the absence of epiphyseal plate destruction, which is never seen in EG.

FIG. 11-19. Another example of a young child with multifocal EG.

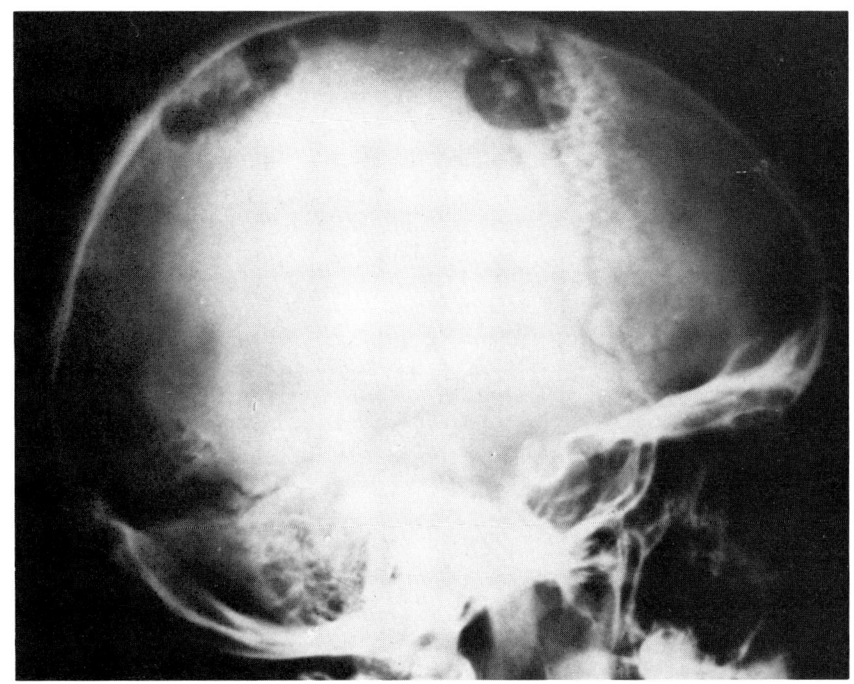

FIG. 11-17

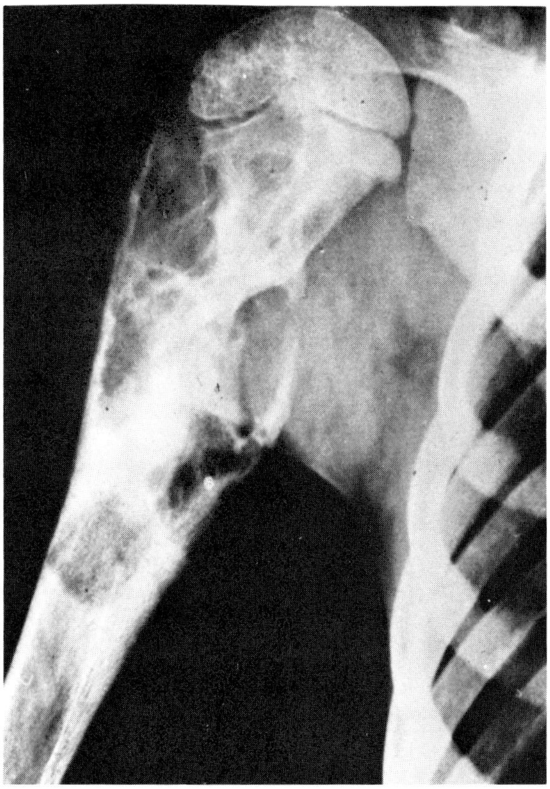

FIG. 11-18

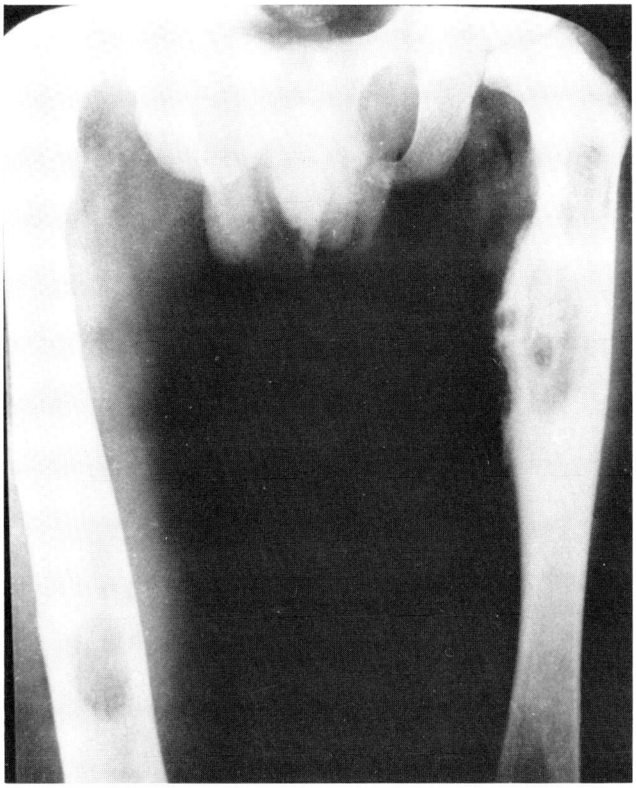

FIG. 11-19

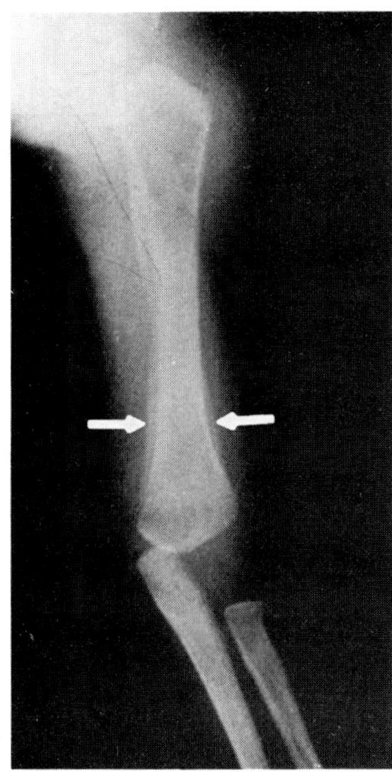

FIG. 11-20

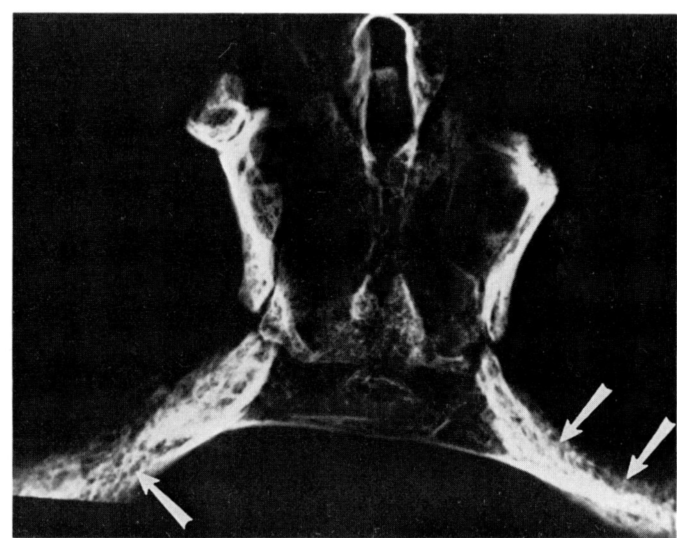

FIG. 11-21

Letterer-Siwe Disease

FIG. 11-20. Most patients with this disease show generalized osteoporosis or, as in this case, ill-defined lytic lesions of the metaphyses and diaphyses. Periosteal new bone may be present (*arrows*).

FIG. 11-21. Specimen radiographs of the bones will usually show multiple, small, punched out defects (*arrows*). This radiograph was obtained from the bones encompassing the sella turcica.

FIG. 11-22. Biopsy of a skin lesion will show an infiltrate of pale histiocytes (x250).

FIG. 11-24. Medium- (*A*) and high power (*B*) illustration of the pale, granular to foamy histiocytes encountered in the bones of patients with acute disseminated EG (x125, x400).

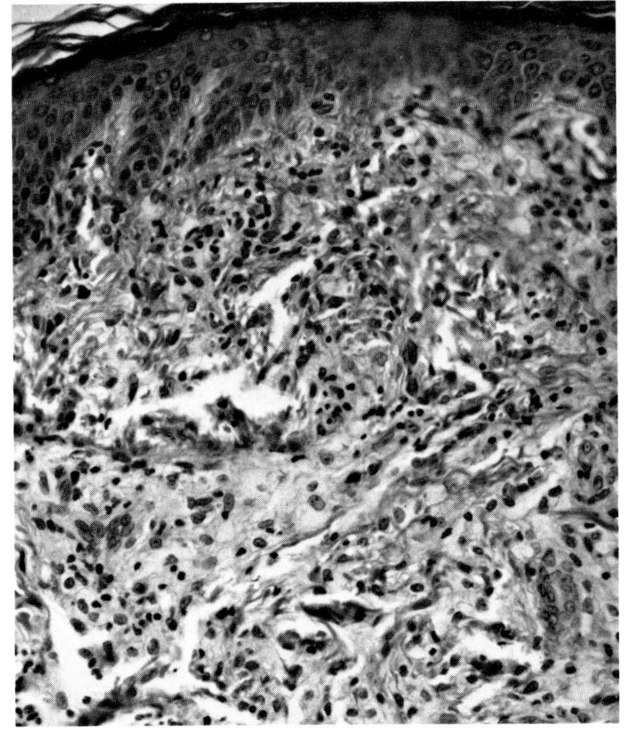

FIG. 11-22

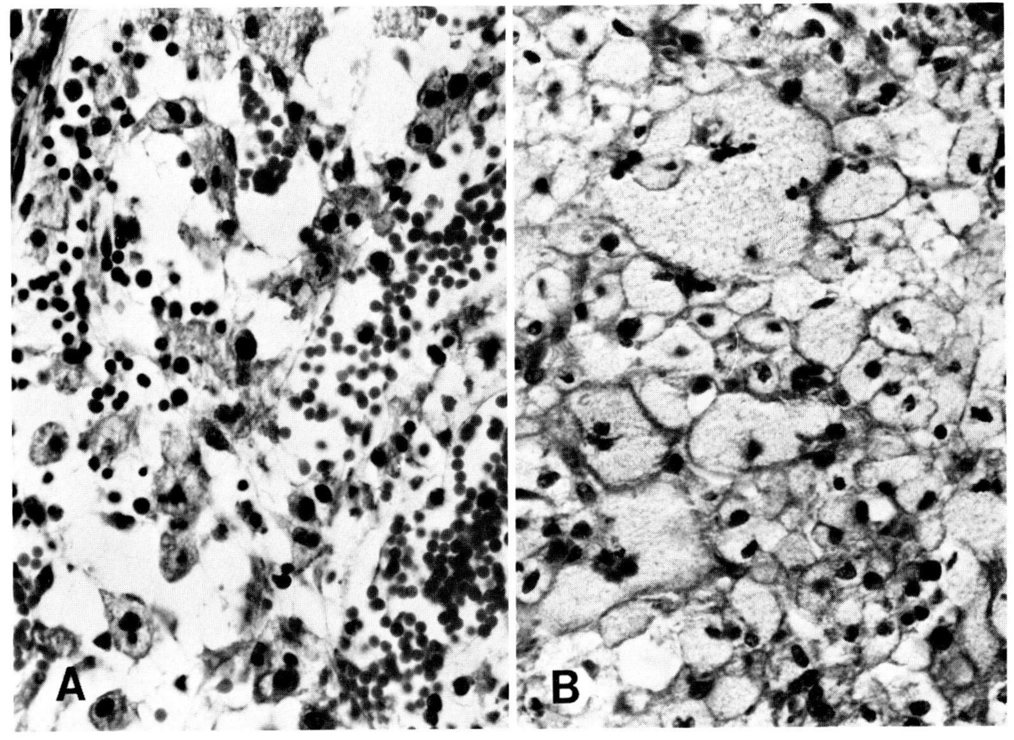

FIG. 11-24

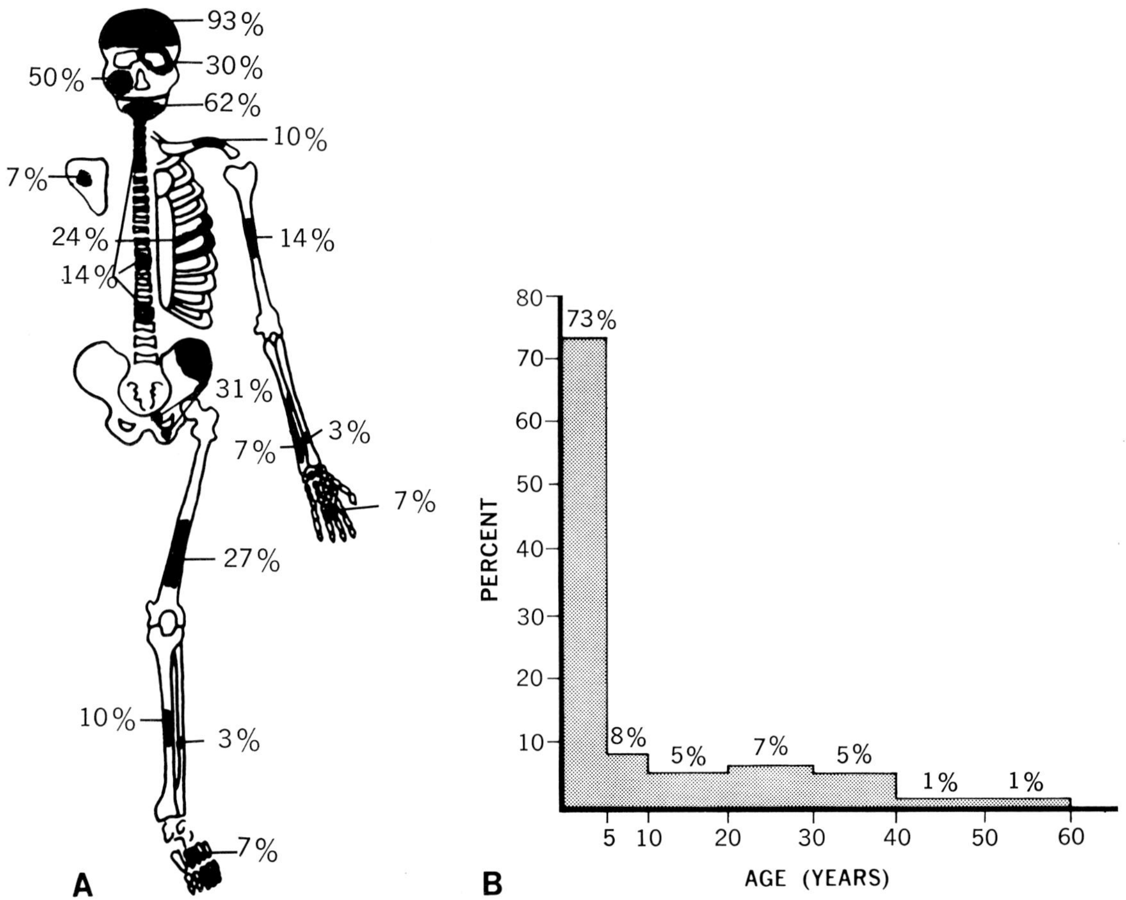

FIG. 11-23. (*A*) Multifocal eosinophilic granuloma (Hand-Schüller-Christian disease) with extraskeletal involvement. Frequency of involvement in 29 patients. Male:female incidence, 1.8:1. (*B*) Age distribution of patients with multifocal eosinophilic granuloma. (Mirra, J., Bullough, P., and Freiberger, R.: Orthopedic Diseases, Part III: Histiocytoses and Round Cell Tumors. New York, Famous Teachings in Modern Medicine, MedCom, Inc., © 1973)

Gaucher's Disease

In *lipid histiocytosis*, an inborn error of metabolism causes complex lipids within histiocytes to accumulate. Gaucher's disease, Niemann-Pick disease, and Tay-Sachs disease are the most common of these, but only Gaucher's disease involves bone as a usual feature.

Capsule Summary

Clinical Features. May affect all age groups. Neurologic involvement (infantile form), hepatosplenomegaly, lymphadenopathy, bone lesions, hypersplenism, possible severe bone pain, fever, and periostitis secondary to microinfarcts. Elevation of serum acid phosphatase.

Radiologic Features. Flask-shaped femurs, cystic or bubbly lesions of the shaft, scalloping of the cortex, avascular necrosis.

Gross Pathology. Yellow-tan deposits in liver, spleen, lymph nodes, and bones. Avascular necrosis, most often of femoral head.

Histopathology. Distinctive, foamy histiocytes, "crumpled-paper" appearance of cytoplasm (Gaucher's cells).

Treatment. Symptomatic

Course. Infantile form: fulminant; adult form: protracted and intermittent.

Clinical Features

Gaucher's disease is a lipid metabolism disorder resulting in excessive accumulation of a complex lipid—mainly glycocerebroside (kerasin)—within histiocytes of the reticuloendothelial system, particularly of the bones and spleen. The enzymatic defect is not fully understood.

Gaucher's disease is not uncommon. As of 1970, over 400 cases had been reported throughout the world, many among Ashkenazic Jews. It is transmitted as an autosomal recessive or autosomal dominant gene with low penetrance.

It may manifest itself at any time of life. The infantile form usually runs a more fulminant course, characterized by neurologic involvement, hepatosplenomegaly, lymphadenopathy, and bone lesions. The adult type has an insidious onset, a long course, and periods of remission.

Symptoms depend on the organ involved and the degree of involvement. Spleen enlargement is nearly always the first sign of disease. The spleen may weigh as much as 8,000 to 10,000 g. Pain, or a dragging feeling in the abdomen, may be serious enough to require splenectomy.

Anemia, leukopenia, and thrombocytopenia may result from hypersplenism or extensive bone marrow replacement by the lipid-filled histiocytes. In cases where pancytopenia is present, it may be difficult to determine which of the above two mechanisms caused it. Gaucher's disease is seldom reported without splenic enlargement.

Careful examination usually reveals changes in the conjunctiva and skin. Deposits of lipochrome pigments in the dermis give exposed skin areas a tan color and tan pingueculae may appear in the sclerae. The yellow-tan deposits in the conjunctiva must be distinguished from the bright yellow, cholesterol-rich deposits seen in primary and secondary xanthomatoses, idiopathic familial xanthomatosis, and biliary cirrhosis.

Accumulated Gaucher's cells in the central nervous system may produce symptoms of progressive decortication: strabismus, difficulty in focusing, spasticity, ankle clonus, seizures, tremors, and increased muscle and tendon reflexes. The symptoms disappear during sleep. Infants who develop the neurologic form of this disease have the gravest prognosis.

Serum acid phosphatase is usually two or three times the normal adult value, probably because the cytoplasm of Gaucher's cells contains lysosomes rich in acid phosphatases.

Radiologic Features

Skeletal changes are usually shown on radiograph after the patient has developed symptoms of an enlarging spleen or depressed marrow function. Because the cells that accumulate abnormal lipid are part of the reticuloendothelial system, lesions may occur in all bones except the basiocciput and facial bones, since the latter do not normally form marrow.

Radiographically, bony lesions generally appear first in the femur and after months or years may develop in other bones such as vertebrae, ribs, sternum, and pelvis. Masses of lipid-laden macrophages in the marrow crowd the intertrabecular spaces and result in resorption of spongy trabeculae. These bone changes are shown on radiograph as diffuse radiolucencies with or without small, punched-out and moth-eaten rarefactions, (Figs. 11–25 and 11–26, *B*). As the disease progresses, cell masses may impinge on the cortex, thinning and scalloping it (Fig. 11–26, *B*).

Because Gaucher's disease commonly affects persons who are growing, it generally interferes with normal tubulation at the metaphysis, flattening and curving the metaphyseal surface convexly instead of concavely. (Compare Fig. 11–26, left, with the right side.) As the fastest-growing part of the skeleton, the distal end of the femur first reflects this change as a "flask-shaped" deformity (Figs. 11–26, *A*, and 11–27). This deformity can also be seen in metaphyseal dysplasia, or Pyle's disease, craniometaphyseal dysplasia, frontometaphyseal dysplasia, dysosteosclerosis, oculodentodigital dysplasia, osteopetrosis, hyperthyroidism, leukemia, osteogenesis imperfecta, and chronic lead poisoning.

In later stages of the disease, the bone shaft and metaphysis may have a soap-bubble or cystic appearance (Fig. 11–27).

Either the expanding masses of Gaucher's cells or lipid emboli resulting from the breakdown of Gaucher cells interfere with the blood supply to the bone and cause infarction. Unilateral or bilateral avascular necrosis of the femoral head is common in Gaucher's disease and may be responsible for the first symptoms (Fig. 11–28, Plate 8, *G*). Avascular necrosis of the bone appears granular and yellow. Degeneration of surface cartilage is caused by collapse of the underlying bone (Fig. 11–29, Plate 8, *G*).

As a result of avascular necrosis in other long bones, coiled, serpiginous radiodense infarcts of the shaft and former epiphyses may become evident (Fig. 11–30).

Gaucher's disease is often characterized by acute episodes of bone pain, fever, leukocytosis, and a high sedimentation rate resembling osteomyelitis. On rare occasions the patient may initially present with pain in association with ominous periosteal reactions (Figs. 11–31 and 11–32). If Gaucher's is not suspected, an erroneous radiologic diagnosis of Ewing's sarcoma or osteomyelitis may be entertained. Biopsy is diagnostic of Gaucher's, however. These periosteal reactions are probably consequent to sterile infarction. Bone aspirations are generally sterile but there is danger that the infarcted bone and marrow may become infected by this diagnostic procedure, since these patients have a very low resistance to even minor numbers of organisms that may be introduced by the diagnostic or surgical procedures. This is probably because of the marked diminution in normal bacterial combative marrow cells that are being replaced by Gaucher cells. Vascular spasm and microinfarction probably cause the periosteal reaction and new bone formation that appear within 2 weeks after the symptoms develop.

Gross Pathology

The spleen is almost always enlarged, firm, and gray-white to yellow-gray. It may contain areas of necrosis and hemorrhage. The liver and lymph nodes are often similarly affected and the liver may be cirrhotic. The marrow spaces of the bones are diffusely infiltrated by intense yellowish or grayish-yellow infiltrates and may in addition show signs of avascular necrosis (Plate 8, *G*). The yellow color is a reflection of the lipid-filled histiocytes; the grayish color reflects fibrosis. The bones may also show areas of hemorrhage and cystification.

Histopathology

Gaucher's cells are of reticular or histiocytic origin and in the early stages of the disease accumulate singly and then form small nests that eventually coalesce into large masses (Figs. 11–33 and 11–34). Portions of the hematopoietic marrow may be relatively uninvolved. Ranging in size from 25 μ to 100 μ, Gaucher's cells usually contain one or two small, round-to-oval, eccentric nuclei. In their cytoplasm they accumulate massive amounts of glycocerebroside that gives a distinctive, "crumpled-paper" appearance (Figs. 11–34, Plate, 8 *H* and *I*). The cells can be extremely pale-staining and unless the observer is aware of the possible diagnosis, cases with only occasional cells may escape attention altogether. The cells can be identified by either open needle biopsy or bone marrow aspirate, because the disorder is metabolic and, therefore, a disseminated one.

Course and Treatment

Except for the infantile form the course of the disease is quite protracted. Patients with Gaucher's disease may live a fairly normal life for many years. Resistance to infection is low. Special care must be taken to avoid osteomyelitis when obtaining bone specimens for diagnostic purposes. The adult patients usually die of either infection, hemorrhagic diatheses, anemia, or cachexia.

Therapy is only palliative. Diet should be low in animal fat. Splenectomy should be avoided unless pain is severe or signs of hypersplenism develop. Operative procedures, such as total hip replacement for avascular necrosis of the femoral head, should be performed under the strictest of aseptic conditions.[40]

Fibro- and osteosarcoma are very rare complications of Gaucher's disease.[52]

Gaucher's Disease

FIG. 11-25. In the early stages of Gaucher's disease, the bones may demonstrate multiple, small, punched-out defects.

FIG. 11-26. (*A*) This femur shows a diffuse lysis and an early "Ehrlenmeyer flask" deformity. (*B*) The shaft of this humerus demonstrates characteristic circular radiolucencies most prominent in the upper shaft and cortical endosteal scalloping (*arrow*).

FIG. 11-27. In the later stages of the disease, the femurs may show gross "Ehrlenmeyer flask" deformity and large, bubbly radiolucencies.

FIG. 11-28. Patients with Gaucher's disease will often develop collapse of the femoral head because of avascular necrosis. The notch in the femur (*arrow*) is due to fracture collapse beneath the acetabular rim. This is the area of the femoral head in which collapse usually begins.

FIG. 11-29. Specimen radiograph of avascular necrosis of the femoral head from Gaucher's disease. Note the white, curved Waldenström's crescent line (*arrow*), which is a pathognomonic radiographic sign of avascular necrosis. This line represents the zone of calcification in the lower portions of the articular cartilage. The dark space beneath this line represents a true space and is consequent to fracture collapse of the underlying bone at the articular cartilage-bone junction. The cartilage often springs back to its original position because of its elasticity; the cartilage's behavior is analagous to the phenomenon one encounters after depressing the surface of a ping-pong ball. The lytic areas in the femoral head represent large aggregations of Gaucher's cells in which the surrounding bone has been resorbed.

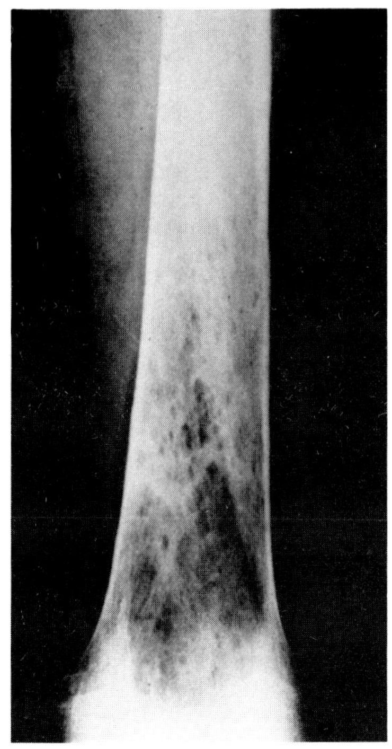

FIG. 11-25

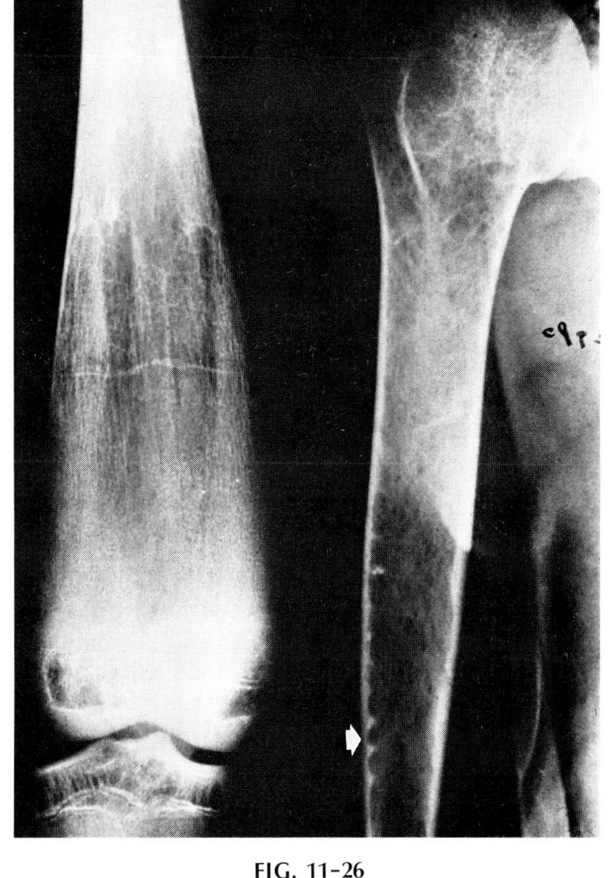

FIG. 11-26

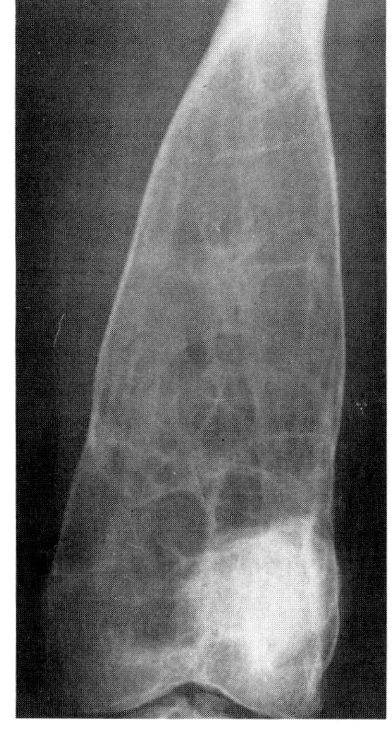

FIG. 11-27

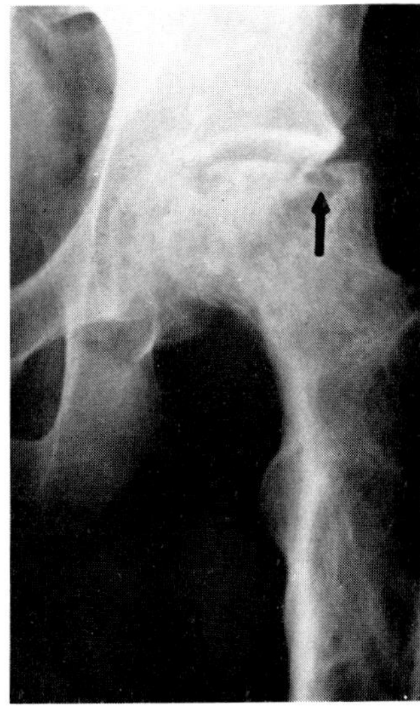

FIG. 11-28

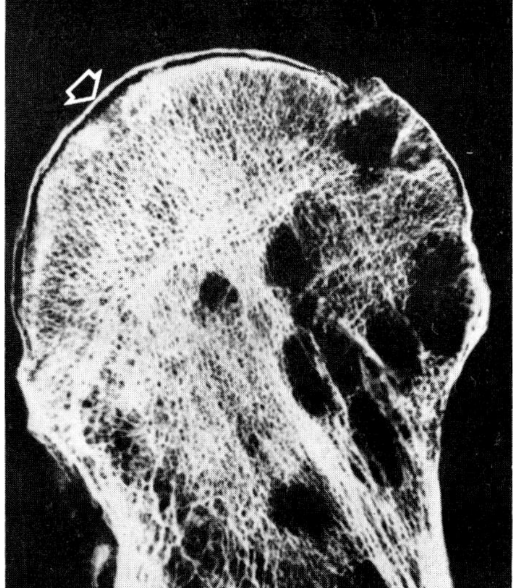

FIG. 11-29

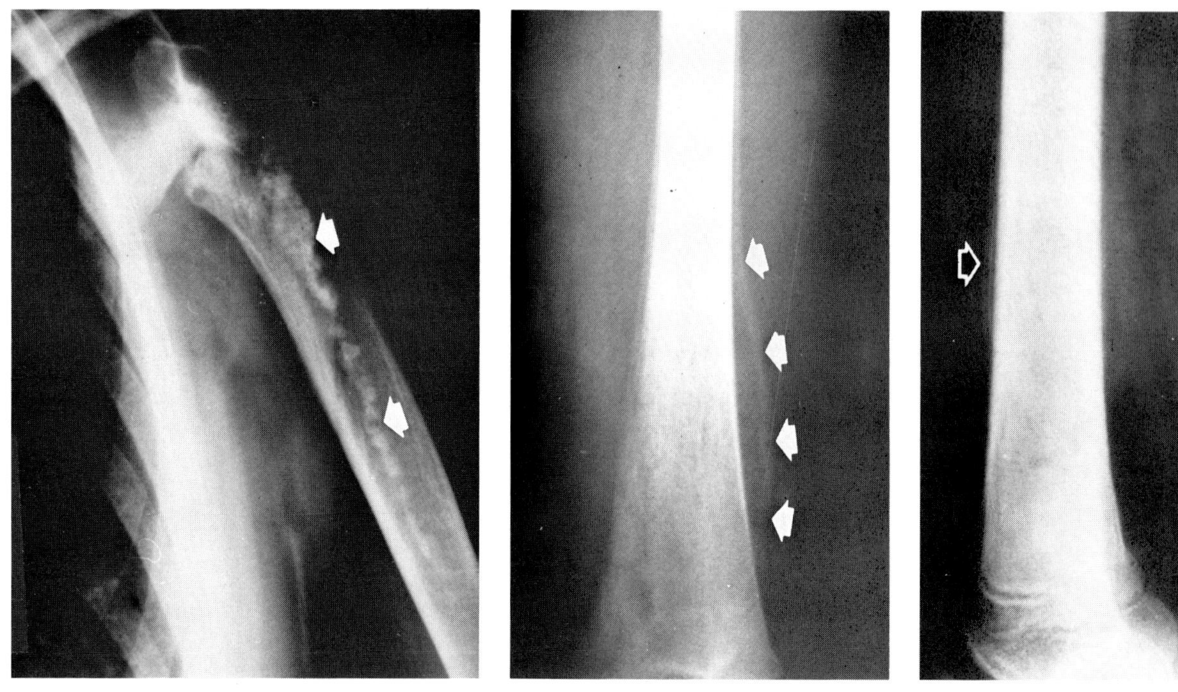

FIG. 11-30

FIG. 11-31

FIG. 11-32

Gaucher's Disease

FIG. 11-30. In this patient with Gaucher's disease, avascular necrosis has led to the almost complete destruction of the humeral head and a characteristic serpiginous or "coil of smoke" sign of bone infarction (*arrows*).

FIG. 11-31. On occasion, Gaucher's patients may develop bone pain and periosteal reactions (*arrows*) because of sterile avascular necrosis. If the disease has not been previously diagnosed and if the bone does not show obvious signs of Gaucher's disease, the lesion may be mistaken, on radiologic grounds, for osteomyelitis or Ewing's sarcoma. Ewing's sarcoma was considered for both this patient and the patient shown in the next illustration. Biopsies were diagnostic of Gaucher's disease, however.

FIG. 11-32. A case of Gaucher's disease presenting with onion-skinning of the periosteum (*arrow*) mimicking Ewing's sarcoma.

FIG. 11-33. Low-power examination will reveal focal (*top*) to diffuse (*bottom*) masses of pale-staining cells (x40).

FIG. 11-34. The cells have one or two small, round, usually eccentric nuclei and a pale histiocytic cytoplasm with a distinctive filigree. These cells are known as Gaucher cells and display the characteristic "crumpled paper" cytoplasm (*arrow, right*), which is indicative of kerasin accumulation (x400, x1000).

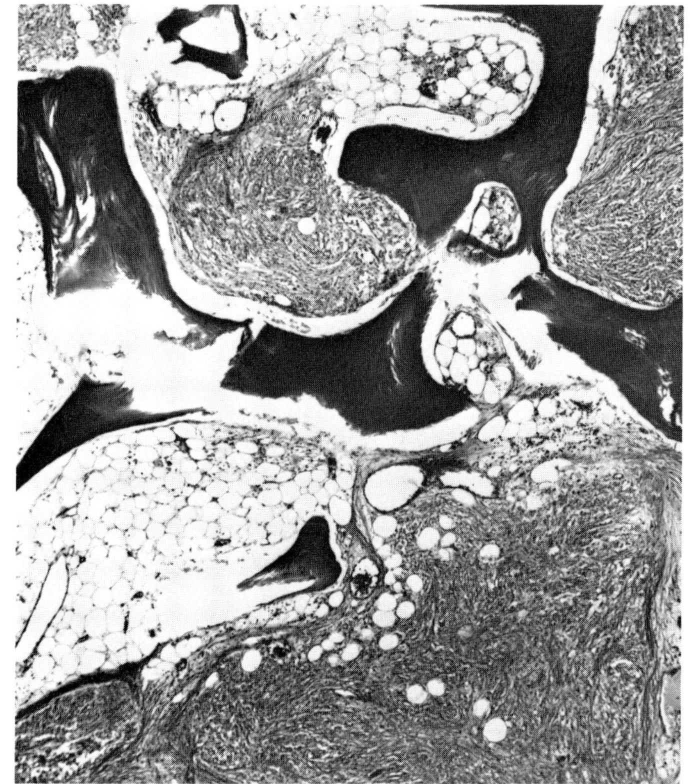

FIG. 11-33

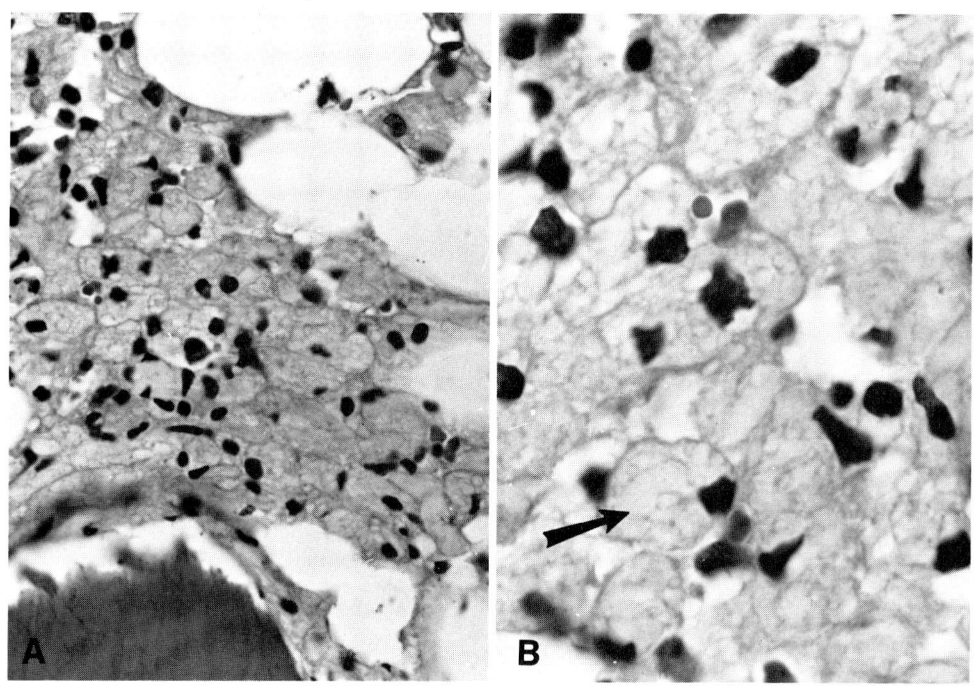

FIG. 11-34

MALIGNANT ROUND CELL TUMORS

Myeloma

Introduction

A neoplastic proliferation of plasma cells, *myeloma,* occurs in several different forms. It is *multifocal* in about half the patients and is generally associated with back pain and anemia. On radiography it shows classic punched-out lytic lesions and is characterized microscopically by nodular aggregates and sheets of plasma cells.

In about 15 per cent of the patients, myeloma is *generalized.* Bone marrow infiltration is diffuse and may be difficult to detect by radiography. It is possible for a patient with back pain and sciatica, without distinct radiologic changes, to be treated for some time for a slipped disk before the malignant nature of the disease is detected.

Solitary myeloma occurs in one fourth to one third of the patients. The affected area is usually the spine and less commonly, the peripheral skeleton. At least two thirds of the patients with solitary myeloma develop multifocal or generalized disease; the rest may remain localized for many years.

Extraskeletal myeloma is rare. When it occurs, it is generally as an extraosseous mass in the nasopharynx.

Capsule Summary (Fig. 11-35)

Incidence. This is the most common primary malignant tumor of the skeleton, accounting for 27 per cent of biopsied bone tumors. Multiple myeloma and osteosarcoma make up almost half (46%) of the primary tumors of bone.

Age. The vast majority (over 90%) of patients are over 40 years of age.

Clinical Features. The initial symptoms are as follows: back pain (approximately 35%); sciatica and paraplegia (approximately 10%); chest pain (approximately 10%); symptoms related to anemia (approximately 10%); bone pain (approximately 10%); pathologic fracture (approximately 5%); abdominal symptoms (approximately 5%).

Laboratory. Elevated sedimentation rate; anemia; hyperglobulinemia with characteristic serum electrophoretic changes; Bence Jones proteins in serum and urine; hypercalcemia and hyperuricemia.

Radiologic Features. Punched-out cystic or trabeculated bone lesions, most commonly in skull, spine, and ribs.

Treatment. Palliative

Course. Five-year survival rates are poor.

Clinical Features

Myeloma is recognized in most patients after age 50. It is rare under age 40, but it has even been reported in children. Pain from a single bone, multiple bones, or the entire skeleton is the most common initial symptom. It is often aching, intermittent at the onset, and aggravated by weight-bearing and lessened by bed rest. The patient frequently describes it as being "like rheumatism." As the disease progresses, the pain becomes more severe, prolonged, and may require narcotics for relief. Pain is most common in the low back, but it is often encountered in the upper spine, pelvis, ribs, and sternum and is frequently associated with bone tenderness. Patients have been treated for sciatica, disk disease, or arthritis before the correct diagnosis has been established. Paraplegia more often occurs with solitary myeloma of the spine than with multiple myeloma, probably because in solitary myeloma the lesions have time to grow much larger. Low back pain in middle-aged or elderly patients in whom radiography shows what looks like osteoporosis of the spine should be investigated for possible myeloma.

Other common complaints are weakness, easy fatigue, weight loss, anorexia, nausea, and vomiting. Less common symptoms are bleeding diathesis—usually due to thrombocytopenia—pathologic fracture, skeletal and extraskeletal masses, low-grade, intermittent fever, and infection.

In the later stages of the disease, renal insufficiency causes death in about 40 per cent of the patients. Renal disease in myeloma is common and can be due to deposits of Bence Jones proteins in the tubules (myeloma nephrosis), hypercalcemia resulting in nephrolithiasis, uric acid deposits; pyelonephritis secondary to decreased immunoresponsiveness, and amyloidosis.

In the differential diagnosis of any patient over age 40 who presents with signs of renal insufficiency, albuminuria, and elevated blood urea nitrogen in the absence of hypertension, myltiple myeloma should be considered.

On initial physical examination, positive findings may be strikingly minimal. Rib cage and spine deformities and pea- or walnut-sized, tender, elastic swelling over the superficial bones are common in the later stages of the disease.

Laboratory Features

Laboratory examination usually reveals many abnormalities. Most patients have anemia. Increased

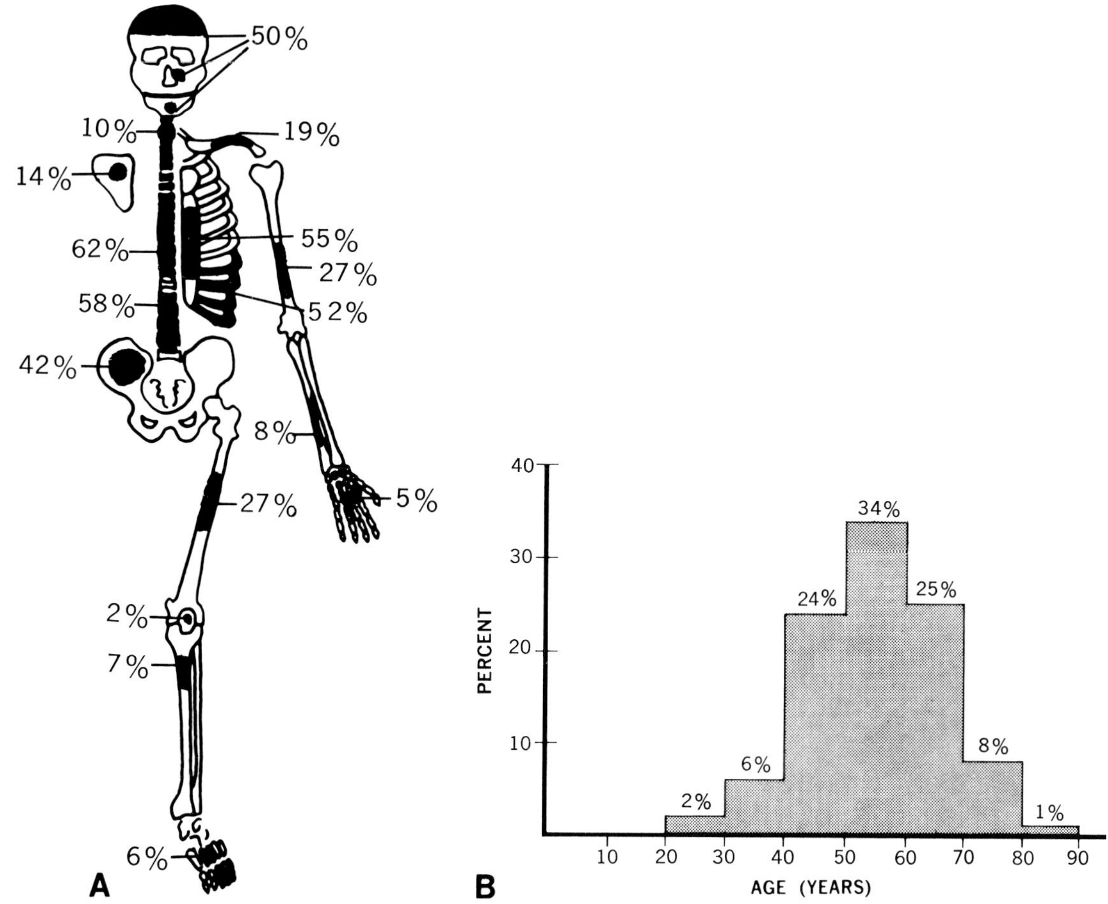

FIG. 11-35. (*A*) Multiple myeloma. Frequency of areas of involvement in the initial presentation of 182 patients. Male:female incidence, 2.5:1. (*B*) Age distribution of patients with multiple myeloma. (Mirra, J., Bullough, P., and Freiberger, R.: Orthopedic Diseases, Part III: Histiocytoses and Round Cell Tumors. New York, Famous Teachings in Modern Medicine, MedCom, Inc., © 1973)

plasma globulins result in rouleaux formation, erythrocyte clumping, and rapid sedimentation rate. Plasma cells are occasionally seen in the peripheral blood but are seldom numerous enough to be considered plasma cell leukemia. Hyperuricemia, which is related to accelerated nucleic acid metabolism, and hypercalcemia, often leading to metastatic calcification, are common. The combination of hypercalcemia and skeletal lesions may suggest primary hyperparathyroidism, but in plasma cell myeloma, serum phosphorus and alkaline phosphatase are normal or slightly elevated.

The most diagnostic laboratory findings are a homogenous spike in the globulin fraction on serum electrophoresis and Bence Jones proteins in the urine and serum.

Serum immunoglobulins are produced almost exclusively by plasma cells. In multiple myeloma, the tumor cells behave as a single proliferating clone producing a homogenous globulin—gamma A or gamma G—and accounting for the spike shown on serum electrophoresis. Because it is not known if the globulin produced in myeloma is the result of a cancerous mutation or is produced in excess in response to an unknown antigenic stimulus, the term *paraprotein* has been suggested instead of abnormal globulin. The globulins produced in myeloma generally have a molecular weight of about 160,000 and a sedimenta-

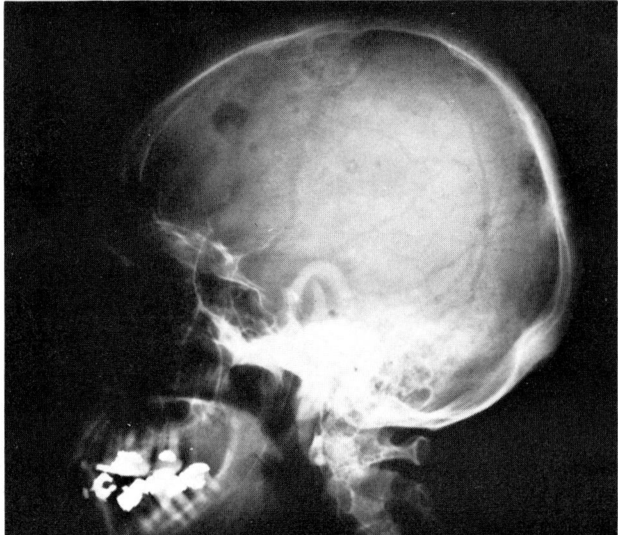

FIG. 11-36

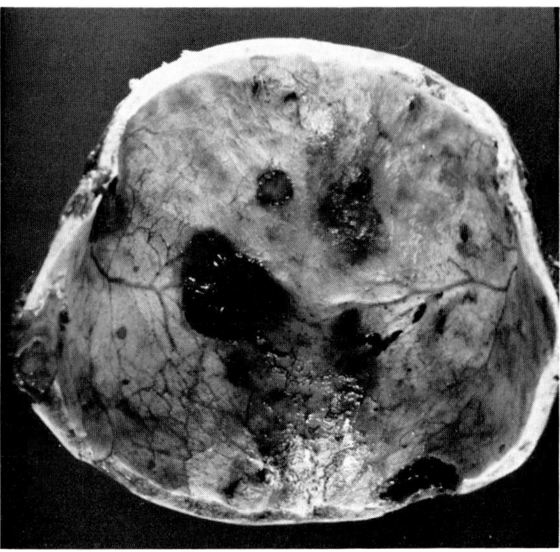

FIG. 11-37

Multiple Myeloma

FIG. 11-36. Most patients with disseminated myeloma will show multiple punched-out rarefactions particularly common to the skull.

FIG. 11-37. Gross appearance of the punched-out lesions in the skull. The lesions are usually dark red to tan in color.

tion coefficient shown by ultracentrifugation to be 7 Svedberg flotation units.

In myeloma, gamma globulins are usually produced, alpha or beta globulins, occasionally, and globulin fragments, rarely. Gamma globulins are proteins composed of two heavy polypeptide chains—H-chains, each with a molecular weight of about 50,000—and two light polypeptide chains—L-chains, each with a molecular weight of about 20,000. Disulfide bonds form bridges between the H-chains and between the L-chains. The H-chains contain the antibody specificity.

Found in the urine of patients with myeloma, Bence Jones proteins have the unique property of forming a cloudy precipitate at temperatures of 50 to 60°C and going back in solution at 90 to 95°C. These proteins consist of only the light chain of the immunoglobulin molecule. Immunoelectrophoresis has shown that they also occur in the serum. Once believed to be pathognomonic of multiple myeloma, Bence Jones proteins are now known to occur in other diseases, such as lymphoma, polycythemia vera, and metastatic carcinoma.

Patients with multiple myeloma occasionally produce only one chain component or the other. In heavy-chain disease (Franklin's disease) serum electrophoresis shows abnormal spikes but not Bence Jones proteins. In the 1 per cent of myeloma patients who produce only light chains, a screening serum electrophoresis fails to reveal a globulin spike. The light chains can be detected as only Bence Jones proteins in the serum or urine.

Multiple Myeloma

FIG. 11-38. Specimen radiograph of the skull to show the numerous punched-out areas of myelomatous infiltration.

FIG. 11-39. On histologic examination, these lytic areas correspond to nodular aggregates of plasma cells. This section was obtained from a skull lesion (x40).

FIG. 11-40. Another common presentation of multiple myeloma is diffuse osteoporosis. The spine is commonly affected and will usually show collapse of one or more vertebral bodies (*arrow*).

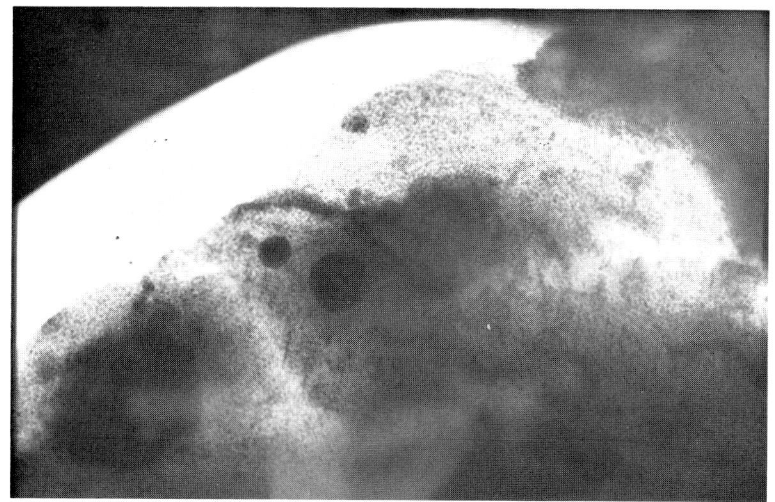

FIG. 11-38

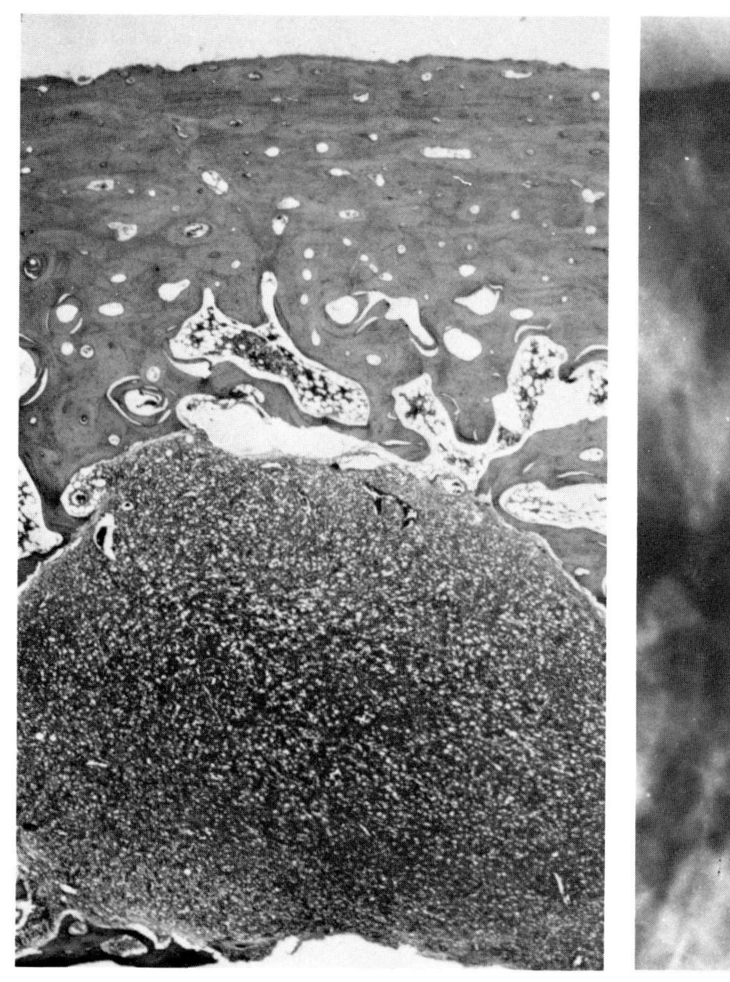

FIG. 11-39

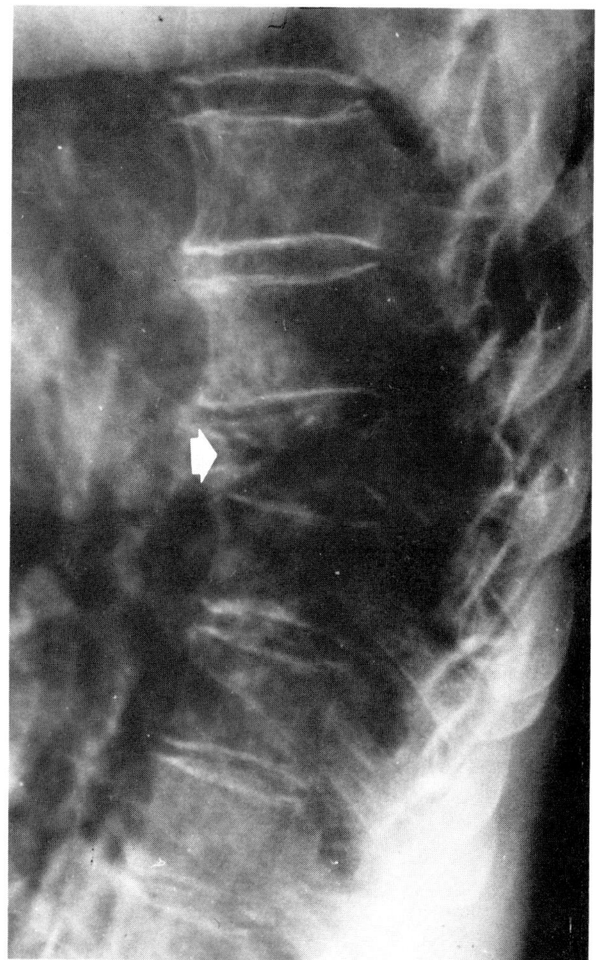

FIG. 11-40

About 5 per cent of myeloma patients produce cold-precipitable globulins called cryoglobulins that cause intravascular occlusion, Raynaud's phenomenon, and hemorrhagic diatheses when the patient is exposed to the cold.

Symptomatology, treatment, and prognosis may be affected by the type and quantity of globulin or globulin fragments produced. Complete globulin molecules with a high molecular weight do not pass the glomerular basement membrane and tend to remain in visceral organs as amyloid-like complexes. These paraproteins may result in red-cell clumping and capillary blood flow sludging, causing intravascular coagulation and bleeding diatheses. Having a molecular weight of only 20,000, light-chain fragments easily cross the glomerular basement membrane. In the dehydrated patient they can deposit very rapidly in the kidney tubules and collecting ducts, causing acute renal insufficiency, or myeloma nephrosis. The patient who produces considerable quantities of light-chain molecules (Bence Jones proteins) must not be allowed to become dehydrated. Intravenous pyelograms should not be preceded by the usual restriction of fluids.

Radiological Features

In contrast to other lymphomas, particularly Hodgkin's disease, myelomatous infiltration nearly always causes cortical and medullary bone lysis without sclerosis. Fewer than 1 per cent of patients show predominant or purely blastic bone lesions.

In multiple myeloma, the bones may be diffusely radiolucent and mistaken for senile osteoporosis (Fig. 11–40). In rare instances, all the bones of the skeleton may be involved, including the hands.

Nodular proliferation of neoplastic tissue causes the classic radiographic appearance of multiple myeloma: diffuse osteoporosis mixed with punched-out radiolucencies several millimeters to several centimeters in size (Figs. 11–36–11–39).

Lesions of the long bones and ribs often appear trabeculated, cystic, or bubbly (Figs. 11–41 and 11–42). The bones may be expanded or balloon out, resembling renal cell carcinoma. If punched-out lesions of the skull and ribs are also present, the diagnosis will likely be myeloma.

Gross Pathology

Gross examination shows that myeloma lesions cause red, diffuse or nodular, gelatinous infiltration of the marrow, or they cause tan tumor nodules (Plate 7, *J*). In over 60 per cent of myeloma patients, particularly those with spinal myeloma, pathologic fracture occurs in the later stages of the disease.

Histopathology

The histologic characteristic of myeloma is nodular or diffuse aggregates of plasma cells. The cells usually contain round nuclei that are clearly eccentric, have an abundance of deep reddish, almost basophilic cytoplasm with distinct cell borders and some show a distinct perinuclear "halo" (Plate 9, *A, B,* and *C*). The "halo" represents the area of the Golgi apparatus. The deep reddish-blue color of the cytoplasm is due to its rich globulin-producing endoplasmic reticulum. In contrast to benign plasma cells, variation of nuclear and cytoplasmic size and shape is often greater, and double and triple nuclei are common.

In distinguishing benign plasmacytoses from myeloma, it is valuable to know that plasma cells of myeloma completely obliterate the normal fatty septae of the marrow.

Normal marrow aspirates contain very few plasma cells (3% or less), while such conditions as chronic infection, rheumatoid arthritis, and cirrhosis have up to 30 per cent plasma cells. It is rare to find more than 30 per cent plasma cells, except in myeloma.

Extreme nuclear and cytoplasmic atypia is occasionally seen (Plate 9, *A, bottom*), and its histologic pattern can be confused with reticulum cell sarcoma or metastatic disease. The diagnosis of myeloma in these cases is made by identifying cells that are clearly of plasma cell derivation, even if they are few in number (Plate 9–1, *bottom, arrows*).

Patients with myeloma may develop systemic amyloidosis. By light microscopy, amyloid stains bright pink with Congo red and a luminescent purple with crystal violet. With polarized light after Congo red staining, amyloid will demonstrate an apple-green to yellow birefringence. On occasion, in areas of myeloma cell infiltration large amounts of a pinkish proteinaceous material appear to form as an extracellular product from the plasma cells. This probably is secondary to a degeneration of plasma cells stuffed with amorphous globulin products. This material is called paramyloid, because it resembles amyloid but neither stains well with crystal violet or Congo red nor polarizes apple-green after Congo red staining. These masses of paramyloid may be surrounded and phagocytosed by histiocytic giant cells, (Plate 7, *K, right*). Polarization studies of these areas after Congo red staining will often show minor amounts of amyloid both in the cytoplasm and stroma immediately adjacent to the giant cells (personal observations, Plate 7, *K, right*). Whether or not these histiocytes are responsible for the conversion of local plasma-cell derived paramyloid deposits into an amyloid by-product, with its systemic disease implications, is under investigation.[58]

Course and Treatment

In patients with multiple or generalized myeloma, prognosis is poor. Over 90 per cent succumb to the disease in fewer than 3 years.

Treatment is palliative. Pain can be relieved and the spinal cord decompressed. Radiotherapy and chemotherapy have been used with limited but increasing success.

Solitary Myeloma With or Without Rapid Dissemination

Capsule Summary (Fig. 11-43)

Incidence. Much less common than multiple myeloma.

Age. Approximately 50 per cent of patients present before age 50.

Clinical Features. Pain at affected site; pathologic fracture, paraplegia. Patients with solitary lesions may not have elevated erythrocyte sedimentation rate, anemia, abnormal or elevated globulins, or Bence Jones proteins.

Radiologic Features. Cystic, bubbly, or trabeculated lytic lesion.

Gross Pathology. Soft, tannish, red tissue.

Histopathology. Masses of well to poorly differentiated plasma cell derivatives.

Treatment. Local irradiation, cryosurgery, or surgical ablation.

Course. Most solitary myeloma patients rapidly develop disseminated disease, sometimes after only a few years. Occasionally the lesion remains solitary.

About 70 per cent of the patients who have what seems to be a solitary focus develop multiple myelomatosis and die within 5 years. In the remainder of the patients the tumor may be localized indefinitely or become generalized after many years.

The host response of patients with solitary myeloma possibly delays or impedes the progress of the disease. Nonneoplastic and chronic inflammatory conditions must be differentiated from myeloma. Inflammatory plasmacytoses are characterized by masses of fully mature plasma cells, proliferation of fibroblasts and capillaries within the lesion (granulation tissue), and a sprinkling of polymorphonuclear leukocytes, histiocytes, and lymphocytes. These changes, which are associated with the inflammatory process, are not seen in myeloma.

Solitary myeloma may be defined as a single focus of neoplastic plasma cells in which a skeletal survey has been performed to exclude other sites of involvement. Also, examination of the sternal or iliac crest marrow has shown no evidence of myeloma and serum electrophoresis may fail to reveal a monoclonal peak.

Radiologically, these tumors are characterized as solitary lytic lesions that may expand the affected bone (Figs. 11-41 and 11-42). They do not have any radiological, gross, or microscopic features that distinguish them from individual lesions of multiple myeloma.

These patients are usually treated with high-dosage irradiation. The tumors may remain localized for many years without dissemination (Figs. 11-41 and 11-42). Perhaps en-bloc excision or cryosurgery should be considered for localized myeloma in order to reduce the risk of dissemination many years later, if radiotherapy is shown by repeat biopsy not to have destroyed all of the tumor cells (see p. 610).

Waldenström's Macroglobulinemia

Waldenström's macroglobulinemia is a rare neoplastic disease of the hematopoietic system. It resembles multiple myeloma and is characterized by a proliferation of lymphoid or lymphoid-plasma cells that produce increased amounts of a homogeneous, high molecular-weight protein called gamma M macroglobulin.

Clinical Features

The disease is twice as common in men as in women and tends to affect individuals over 50 years of age. The principal symptoms are anorexia, weakness, and recurrent infection; visual disturbances; swelling of the uvula; radiculitis, myelitis, encephalitis, and deafness; Raynaud's phenomenon and cold sensitivity; lymphadenopathy and hepatosplenomegaly; and bleeding diatheses and congestive heart failure. Bone pain is not prominent, and amyloidosis and renal insufficiency are unusual.

Laboratory Features

With a molecular weight of 900,000 and a ultracentrifugation sedimentation coefficient of 19 Svedberg flotation units, macroglobulins include the saline Rh antibodies, isohemagglutinins, rheumatoid factor, and heterophil antibodies. Macroglobulins normally make up 5 per cent of the serum globulins but increase to as many as 10 per cent to 20 per cent in such diseases as lupus erythematosus and rheumatoid arthritis.

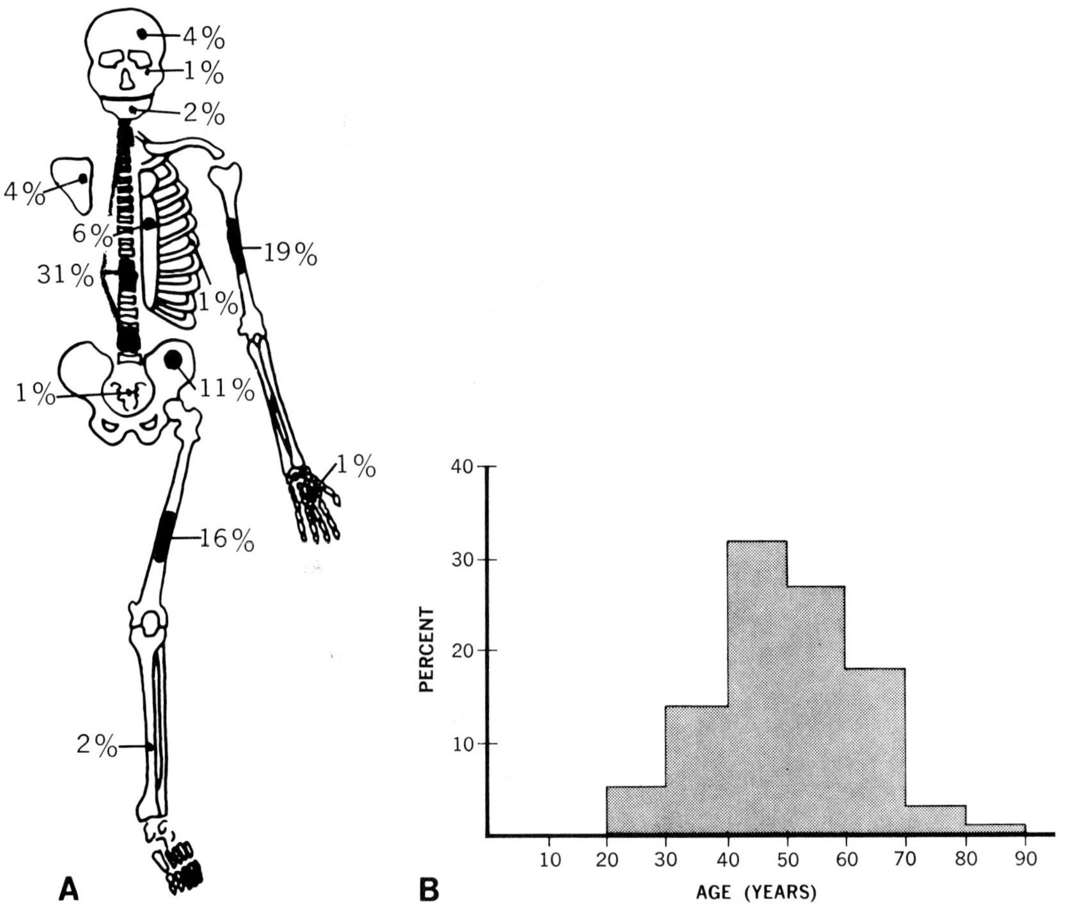

FIG. 11-43. (*A*) Myeloma presenting as a solitary focus. Frequency of areas of involvement in 107 patients. Male:female incidence, 5:1. (*B*) Age distribution of patients with solitary myeloma.

The serum paper electrophoretic pattern of Waldenström's macroglobulinemia shows a spike in the gamma or beta-2 areas indistinguishable from multiple myeloma. Serum viscosity may be increased, and the Sia water test may be positive. Diagnosis is confirmed by immunoelectrophoretic identification of gamma-M globulin or by ultracentrifugation studies.

Laboratory examination reveals rouleaux formation, very rapid erythrocyte sedimentation rate, normochromic/normocytic anemia in over 80 per cent of the patients, thrombocytopenia, hyperproteinemia, macroglobulinemia, positive Sia water test, occasional Bence Jones proteins, and cryoglobulinemia. The macroglobulinemia is believed to cause alterations in blood viscosity. The formation of macroglobulin-protein complexes and the deposition of these complexes in blood vessels and visceral organs are thought to interfere with local circulation and to result in pulmonary hypertension, congestive heart failure, and platelet coating leading to abnormal platelet function.

Radiologic Features

Instead of the punched-out lesion of myeloma, the radiograph of Waldenström's macroglobulinemia usually shows patchy osteoporosis in one or more bones or occasional patchy sclerosis (Fig. 11-44).

Histopathology

Under microscopy the marrow shows a diffuse or nodular proliferation of lymphoid cells or lymphoid-plasma cells. The appearance of the latter is intermediate between lymphocytes and plasma cells. The combination of abundant cytoplasm, which is caused by increased ribosomal ribonucleic acid, and eccentrically located nuclei give the cells the general ap-

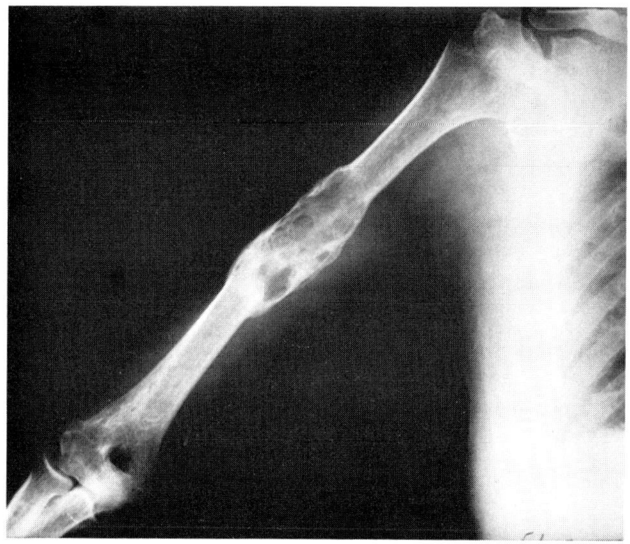

FIG. 11-41

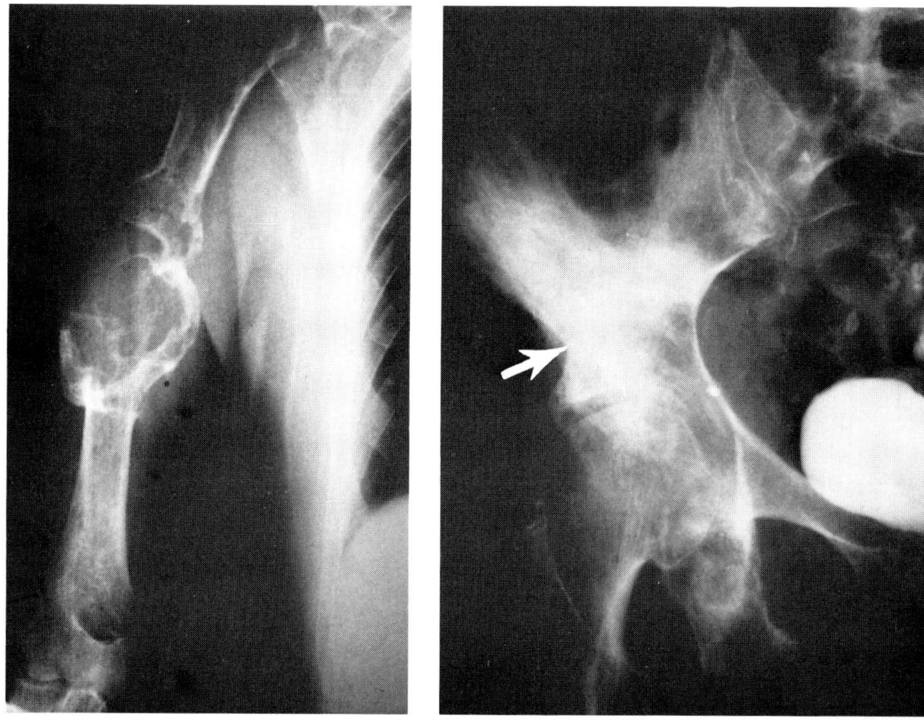

FIG. 11-42

FIG. 11-44

Myeloma and Waldenström's Macroglobulinemia

FIG. 11-41. Myeloma may also present as bubbly lytic lesions. This particular patient had the rare solitary myeloma. Following diagnosis, the patient was treated by irradiation.

FIG. 11-42. Seventeen years later, the lesion showed a greater degree of bubbly destruction. Even though several courses of radiation were given, viable atypical plasma cells were still present. The patient was last seen at the age of 82 with no evidence of dissemination.

FIG. 11-44. Patients with Waldenström's macroglobulinemia tend to show focal areas of patchy sclerosis (*arrow*) or lysis.

pearance of plasma cells. The nuclear characteristics of lymphocytes are retained, however.

Course

Patients with Waldenström's macroglobulinemia have increasing anemia, bleeding diatheses, severe edema, and cachexia. Most patients die between 2 and 10 years.

Hodgkin's Disease

Capsule Summary (Fig. 11-45)

Incidence. A rare primary tumor of bone (less than 0.3%). Most cases of Hodgkin's are secondary; that is, have spread to the bones from involved lymph nodes.

Age. Some 75 per cent of patients present between 20 and 50 years of age.

Clinical Features. Osseous involvement characterized by pain and tenderness with or without palpable mass. May or may not have neurologic involvement from spinal cord or nerve-root compression.

Radiologic Features. Single or multiple lytic, blastic, or mixed lesions. Occasional solitary, dense, ivory vertebrae or compression fractures of spine. Minimal periosteal reaction.

Gross Pathology. Gray-tan focal or diffuse infiltration of bone with or without soft-tissue extension.

Histopathology. Sternberg-Reed cells, atypical reticulum cells, plasma cells, lymphocytes, eosinophils, and variable amounts of fibrosis and bony sclerosis.

The overwhelming majority of patients with Hodgkin's disease of the bone have clinical evidence of lymph node involvement months to years before it is obvious in the bone. Between 12 and 15 per cent of Hodgkin's patients are shown to have bone involvement by either radiography or trephine biopsy.[63,69] However, at autopsy numerous samplings show the disease in the bone in up to 78 per cent of patients.[70]

In a patient with known lymph node disease, demonstration of bone involvement is classified as stage IV disease. O'Carrol, *et. al.,*[69] demonstrated bone involvement in 14 per cent of 107 patients. Two of three patients had lymphocyte depletion, six of 27, mixed cellularity, and five of 64, nodular sclerosis, and two were unclassified. The bone involvement was either focal or diffuse and was characterized by variable mixtures of plasma cells, lymphocytes, histiocytes, eosinophils, mononuclear Sternberg-Reed variants, typical Sternberg-Reed cells, and fibrosis. Some 10 per cent of patients showed nonspecific tuberculoid granulomas. Patients with nodular sclerosis had a markedly increased risk of marrow involvement if their total leukocyte count, absolute lymphocyte count, and hemoglobin and platelet count were depressed. Marrows were considered positive even if classic Reed-Sternberg cells were not found, provided that atypical mononuclear histiocytes with large nucleoli were set in a mixture of chronic inflammatory cells, histiocytes, and fibrosis and provided that the diagnosis of the disease was established on a lymph node or other tissue biopsy.

Hodgkin's disease presenting in the bone is rare.[65] In my own collection I have seen seven such cases. Two presented as vertebral body lesions, two in the humerus and one each in the femur, tibia, and skull. Only two of these patients had true primary lesions. The first patient had a working diagnosis of chronic osteomyelitis of the humerus for several years. The bone marrow was infiltrated by masses of lymphocytes, a few plasma cells, and rare eosinophils. After 5 years the bone was completely infiltrated by bubbly lytic lesions and there was no periosteal reaction, unlike true osteomyelitis (Fig. 11-46). The diagnosis was malignant neoplasm, type unspecified, and the arm was amputated. Gross sections showed replacement by firm, rubbery, pinkish nodules (Fig. 11-47). Sections showed approximately one classic Sternberg-Reed cell in a sea of lymphocytes per slide. The lesion was obviously a rare form of lymphocyte-predominent Hodgkin's disease of bone. The patient is alive and well 15 years post-amputation. The second patient was a 25-year-old black female with a permeative destructive lesion of the right proximal humerus. Biopsy demonstrated unequivocal Hodgkin's disease, mixed cellularity type. She was treated with 8500 rads. Evaluations for generalized disease, including chest radiography, liver-spleen scan, intravenous urography, and metastatic bone survey were negative. She remains free of disseminated disease after 6 years of follow-up.[65a]

The other patients all developed signs of systemic disease within 6 months to two years. Only one of these patients received lymphangiography and Hodgkin's was found in the local lymph nodes. The diagnosis of Hodgkin's was confirmed by biopsy. The difficulty in three of these cases was the delay in diagnosis consequent to small needle biopsies. Before the disease completely manifested itself erroneous diagnoses of eosinophilic granuloma and osteomyelitis were entertained. Hodgkin's disease presenting as a possible primary bone tumor is so rare and the numbers of definitive cells obtained by needle biopsy may be so small that diagnosis is often delayed. The diagnosis should always be suspected in any lesion

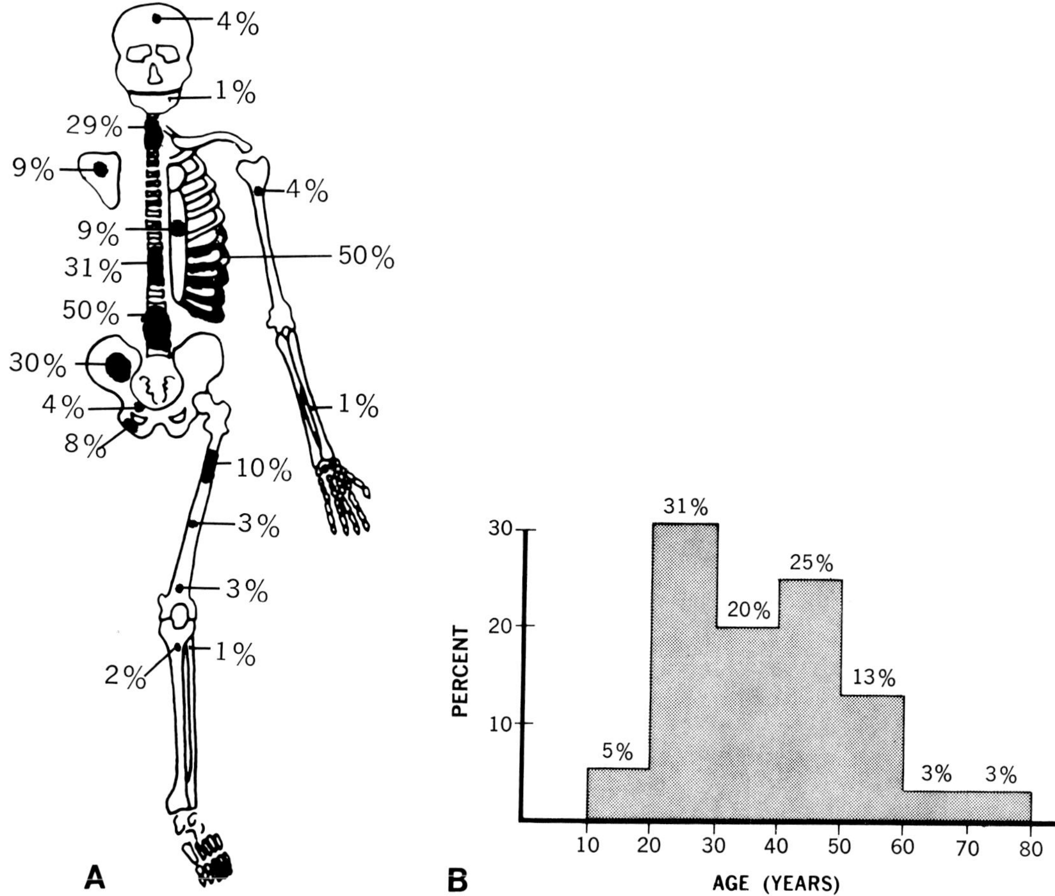

FIG. 11-45. (*A*) Hodgkin's disease. Frequency of areas of osseous involvement by radiologic analysis in 106 of 510 cases with disseminated disease. Male: female incidence, 1.6:1. (*B*) Age distribution of Hodgkin's disease patients who develop osseous involvement.

with a variable mixture of lymphocytes, plasma cells, fibrosis, occasional eosinophils, and most importantly, large atypical mononuclear histiocyte-like cells. If needle biopsy is suggestive, open biopsy should be performed and imprints of fresh tissue made. If Hodgkin's disease is confirmed, lymphangiography, bone scans, and a skeletal survey must be performed to rule out disseminated disease, particularly since the primary bone form of Hodgkin's disease is so extremely rare.

Clinical Features

Pain and tenderness are the early, persistent indications of bone involvement. Because regional lymph-node involvement often prevents tracing the source of pain to bone disease, tenderness to pressure at a bony site is a more reliable sign.

Swelling and a palpable mass are associated with cortical destruction and soft-tissue extension, especially in the ribs and sternum.

Through contiguous involvement with tumor infiltrates in the spinal canal, neurologic deficits often occur with or without vertebral body collapse.

Radiologic Features

Bone lesions in Hodgkin's disease are usually multiple, as observed in 38 patients who had 144 bones involved. The lesions are not distinctive. They may be

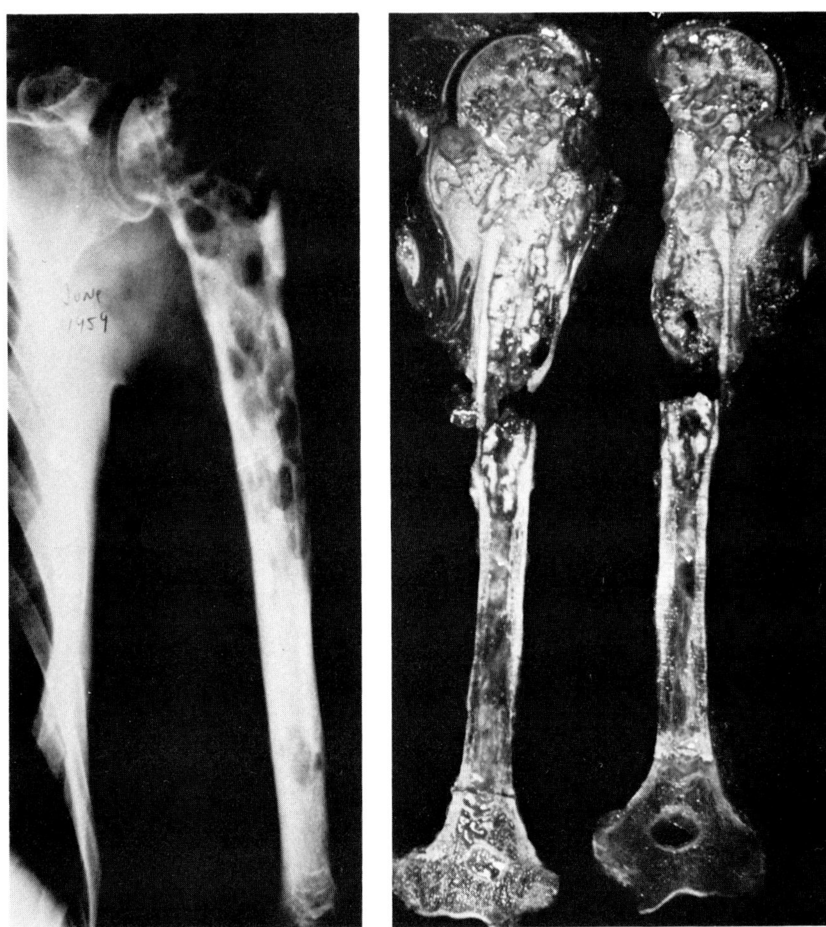

FIG. 11-46 FIG. 11-47

Primary Hodgkin's Disease of Bone

FIG. 11-46. This patient had a rare example of primary Hodgkin's disease, lymphocyte predominant type, confined to bone. It was mistaken for osteomyelitis for several years. The radiograph shows multiple, unusual, rounded lytic defects and no periosteal reaction.

FIG. 11-47. Eventually, the arm was amputated because of multiple fractures and disuse. The tumor was rubbery, pinkish tan, and nodular. The patient is alive and well with no evidence of dissemination many years post-amputation.

FIG. 11-48. (*A*) Bubbly, well-defined lytic lesions may be seen in some cases of Hodgkin's disease. (*B*) More commonly, the lesions show moth-eaten lytic destruction. Both of these patients showed evidence of disseminated Hodgkin's disease.

FIG. 11-49. Occasional cases show a mixed lytic and blastic reaction (*A*) and rarely, a purely blastic reaction (*B*). Both of these patients also had disseminated Hodgkin's disease.

FIG. 11-50. An example of the solitary dense vertebral body (ivory vertebra) that may be seen in Hodgkin's disease. Most of these patients show evidence of disseminated disease.

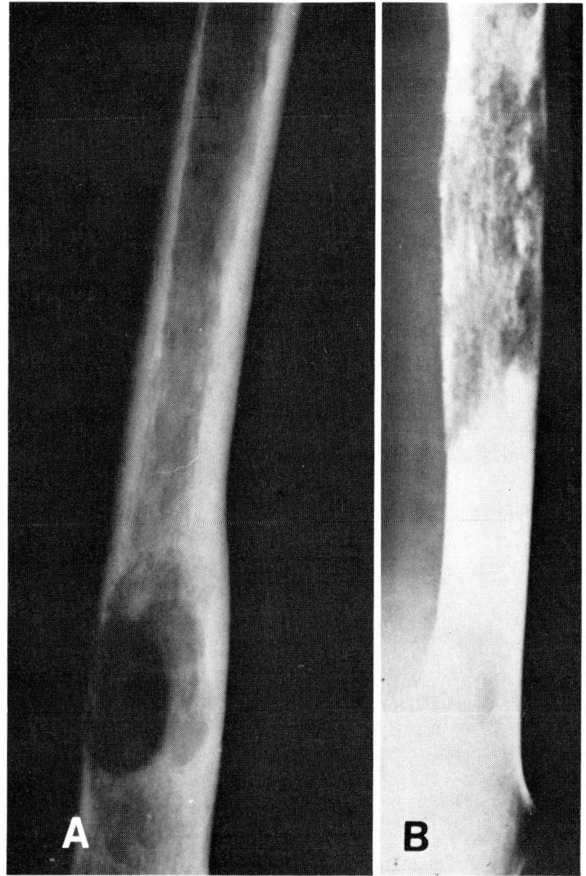

FIG. 11-48

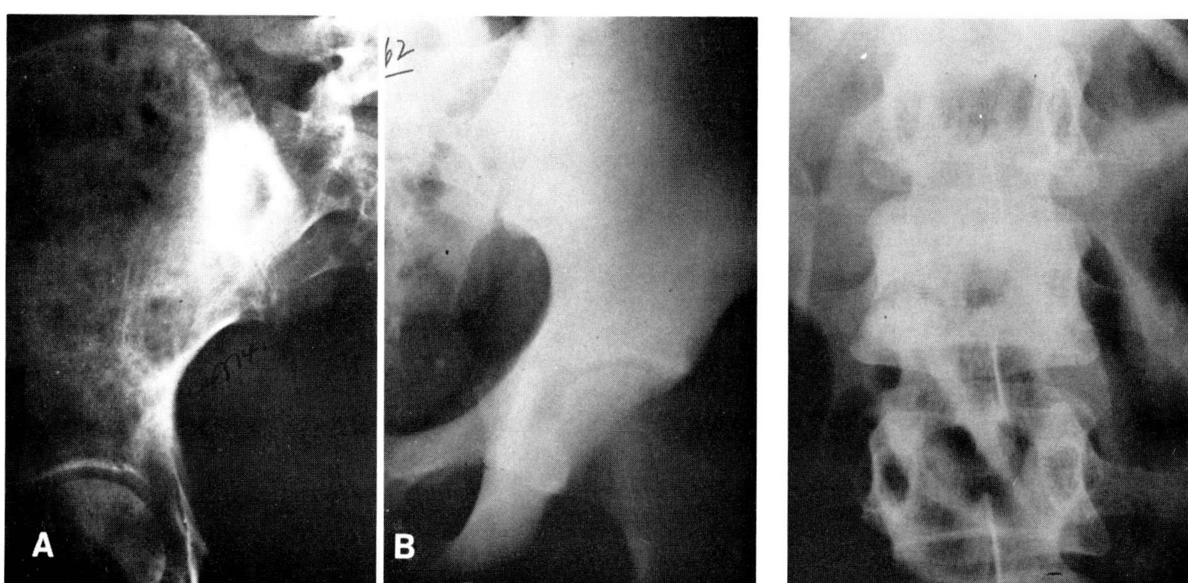

FIG. 11-49

FIG. 11-50

osteolytic (about 25%), osteoblastic (about 15%), or mixed (about 60%) (Figs. 11-46, 11-48, and 11-49). All three may occur in one patient. Diffuse lytic destruction in the spine may lead to compression fracture.

Purely osteolytic lesions usually occur in the flat bones—ribs, sternum, and pelvis—while purely osteoblastic ones generally affect a single vertebral body causing what is known as *ivory vertebra* (Fig. 11-50). About 50 per cent of all solitary, dense, vertebral bodies are caused by Paget's disease; 30 per cent, by Hodgkin's disease; and 20 per cent, by other metastatic diseases.[64] Carcinoma of the breast and prostate usually leads to multiple osteoblastic metastases to the spine. Usually, however, it is carcinomas other than breast or prostate that cause a solitary ivory vertebra. In Paget's disease, solitary, dense vertebrae can usually be identified by dense, peripheral sclerosis creating a picture-frame effect and by vertical trabeculae more defined and thicker than the horizontal trabeculae.

Though it is rare in Hodgkin's disease, periosteal reaction is moderate when it occurs. Fractures are usually of the ribs or vertebrae.

Gross Pathology

Hodgkin's disease ordinarily involves the marrow spaces as separate or confluent firm, gray-tan, rubbery nodules. The tissue may be modified by areas of hemorrhage and necrosis (Fig. 11-47).

Histopathology

On low-power examination the bone may show either focal replacement of the normal marrow (Plate 9, *D, top*) or diffuse involvement. On high-power examination there is usually a diffuse mixture of inflammatory cells, fibrosis, and a variable proportion of large, atypical reticulum cells and classic Sternberg-Reed cells. The benign inflammatory reactive cells include mature lymphocytes, plasma cells, and scattered eosinophils (Plate 9, *E, top*). The degree of fibrosis is variable (Plate 9, *D, bottom*) but occasionally it may be quite extensive and obscure the diagnosis. The principal clue to diagnosis is the presence of focal accumulations of large, atypical reticulum-like cells (Plates 9-4, *bottom,* and 9-5, *top*). These cells generally show one or more small- to moderate-sized reddish nucleoli. The nuclei are large and multilobulated. The chromatin is unevenly distributed, the nuclear membrane is prominent or thick, and areas devoid of chromatin (perinucleolar halo) are seen (Plate 9, *E, bottom,* and *F*). These should be compared with the histiocytes of eosinophilic granuloma (Plate 8, *C, bottom,* and *E*). The nuclei of EG show more even chromatin distribution and darker, smaller nucleoli. Overall, the nuclei of the reticulum-like cells in Hodgkin's are much more atypical than those of EG. The classical Sternberg-Reed cells are similar to the atypical reticulum cells described above, except for the presence of significantly larger nucleoli. Sternberg-Reed cells have been classically described as having a bilobular nucleus but they may be multilobular, with as many as 8 to 10 lobes. In Reed and Sternberg's original paper, their drawings show numerous variants, including the so-called "classical bilobed" Sternberg-Reed cell.

In most cases of Hodgkin's these highly atypical reticulum cells are much more easily found than classic Sternberg-Reed cells. In addition, these cells generally show more numerous mitoses than is present in the histiocytes of EG. The diagnosis of Hodgkin's is confirmed by finding the classic Sternberg-Reed cells (Plate 9, *E, bottom,* and *F*). The problem is that in some cases fewer than one to two such cells may be present per square centimeter of tissue; overdecalcification and artifacts of fixation may obscure their identification. Great care must be taken to avoid these pitfalls and to obtain imprints on fresh tissue whenever possible in order to identify these cells with greater success (Plate 9, *F, bottom*). Because of the meager amount of tissue in needle biopsy, classic Sternberg-Reed cells may be impossible to find. The presence of atypical reticulum cells enmeshed in a mixture of lymphocytes, plasma cells, eosinophils and fibrosis should prompt open biopsy and imprints for definitive diagnosis.

Course and Treatment

The majority of cases of Hodgkin's that present as a bone "primary" will, upon more extensive studies for staging such as lymphangiography, lymph node, spleen, and liver biopsies, usually show evidence of disseminated disease. Long-term survivals are variable but most patients usually succomb to the disease after 5 to 10 years. True primary Hodgkin's of bone may be amenable to cure by local high-dose radiation therapy. With the more advanced radiochemotherapeutic regimens, survival rates in patients with Hodgkin's disease have been substantially increased.

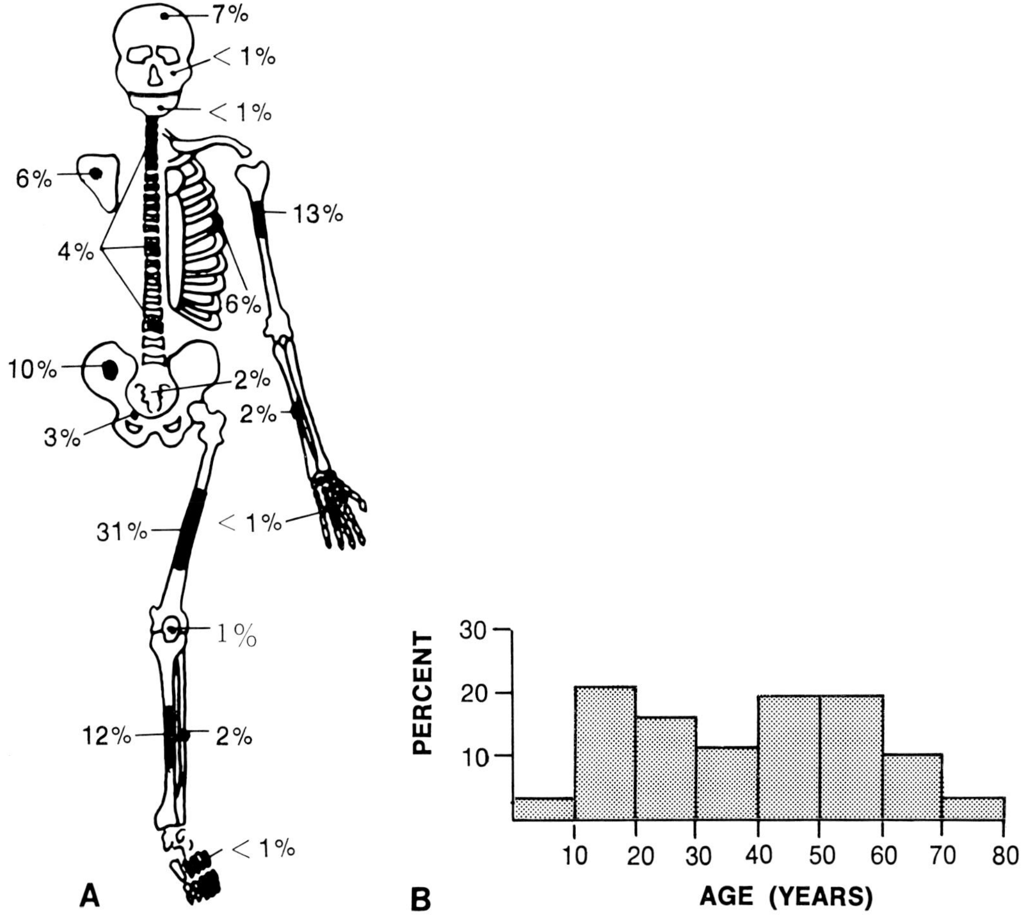

FIG. 11-51. Primary reticulum cell sarcoma of bone (RCS). Frequency of areas of involvement in 162 cases. Male:female incidence, 1.9:1. (*B*) Age distribution of patients with primary reticulum cell sarcoma of bone (Mirra, J., Bullough, P., and Freiberger, R.: Orthopedic Diseases, Part III: Histiocytoses and Round Cell Tumors. New York, Famous Teachings in Modern Medicine, MedCom, Inc., © 1973).

Primary Reticulum Cell Sarcoma of Bone

Capsule Summary (Fig. 11-51)

Incidence. An uncommon primary bone tumor. Approximately, 0.5 to 1 per cent of biopsied primary bone tumors.

Age. Between 10 and 60 years, the disease is about equally distributed among all ages.

Clinical Features. The patients appear remarkably well but have dull bone pain, swelling, tenderness, soft-tissue mass, and pathologic fracture. They have no fever or marked weight loss. Occasional cases with joint involvement mimic monoarticular arthritis.

Radiologic Features. Nonspecific, moth-eaten, lytic destruction; minimal periosteal reaction.

Gross Pathology. Firm, gray-white tissue infiltrating bone and cortex and commonly extending into soft tissue.

Histopathology. Cell sheets with distinct or indistinct borders. Nuclei tend to be reniform. Nucleoli may be prominent. Pleomorphism of size and shape of nuclei usually present. Reticulin stains reveal abundant reticulin separating each cell. PAS is negative for intracellular glycogen.

Treatment. Radiation; rarely, wide local excision or amputation.

Course. Five-year survival of 50 per cent; 10-year survival of 35 per cent. After 20 years, recurrence with widespread metastases have been known.

Not many years ago, most primary malignant, undifferentiated neoplasms in bone were classified as Ewing's tumor. Parker and Jackson[80] recognized they were at least two different tumors: one with an extremely rapid and fatal course (Ewing's tumor) and the other with a much longer course and a much higher cure rate. The more benign tumor produced considerable numbers of argyrophilic reticulin fibers, causing Parker and Jackson to call the tumor reticulum cell sarcoma. This disease, originating in the lymph nodes and metastasizing to bone, must be distinguished from primary reticulum cell sarcoma of bone, which has a much more favorable long-term prognosis. Because they may look the same microscopically, the distinction is a clinical one.

Clinical Features

Males are affected twice as often as females, and most are over age 20. As with Ewing's tumor, the favored sites are the femur, tibia, pelvis, humerus, ribs, scapula, and spine.

Pain, swelling, and local tenderness for several months are common initial complaints. The pain is usually dull or aching and intermittent, frequently worse at night, and seldom relieved by rest. A lesion near a joint may restrict motion. Despite extensive tumor involvement, general well-being is striking.

A definite tumor mass can be palpated in more than 50 per cent of the patients. It is commonly fusiform in the shaft of a long bone, and ovoid or ill-defined in a flat bone. Its consistency is variable. Occasionally the soft-tissue extension is so large and mobile that it resembles a primary tumor of the soft parts. When the tumor affects the distal end of the bone and the soft-tissue mass extends into the joint, resultant swelling and possibly locking, resembling monoarticular arthritis, results. Such patients will usually present first to rheumatologists.

Pathologic fracture occurs in about 10 per cent of the patients; local heat, in 25 per cent.

Physical examination should include a careful survey of regional and distant lymph nodes. Because radiographic findings are rather nonspecific, diagnosis depends on biopsy. If after bone biopsy the diagnosis of reticulum cell sarcoma is established, bone scans and lymphangiography are useful in establishing whether the tumor is primary or metastatic from involved lymph nodes.

Radiologic Features

On radiography the tumor is generally medullary and lytic, occasionally has blastic areas, and shows ill-defined margins with irregular cortical destruction (Figs. 11-52 and 11-53). Soft-tissue extension without calcification is frequently evident (Figs. 11-52, 11-54, and 11-55); and new periosteal bone is usually not a striking radiologic characteristic. Differential diagnosis usually includes osteomyelitis, eosinophilic granuloma, metastatic carcinoma, Ewing's tumor, and fibrosarcoma.

Gross Pathology

The tumor is generally nodular, soft to fleshy, grayish-tan to grayish-yellow, and may be modified by foci of hemorrhage, necrosis, and cystification (Figs. 11-56 and 11-57, Plate 7, *L*).

Reticulum Cell Sarcoma

FIG. 11-52. This illustration shows the typical features of a RCS; namely, moth-eaten destruction, mild periosteal reaction, and soft-tissue extension.

FIG. 11-53. An example of RCS involving a proximal phalanx. The lesion is extremely destructive, with loss of the cortical borders and extension into the soft tissues. The radiograph on the right (*B*) was taken 6 weeks after the one on the left, (*A*).

FIG. 11-54. The RCS may be associated with a huge soft-tissue mass. The bone in this case shows a blastic reaction and the periosteum is forming fine lamellae and Codman's triangles.

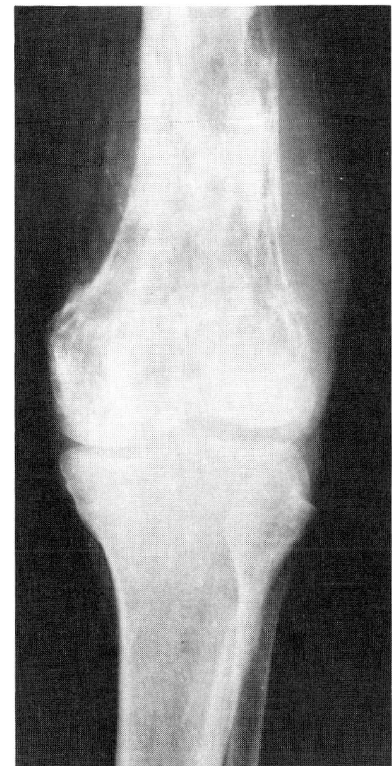

FIG. 11-52

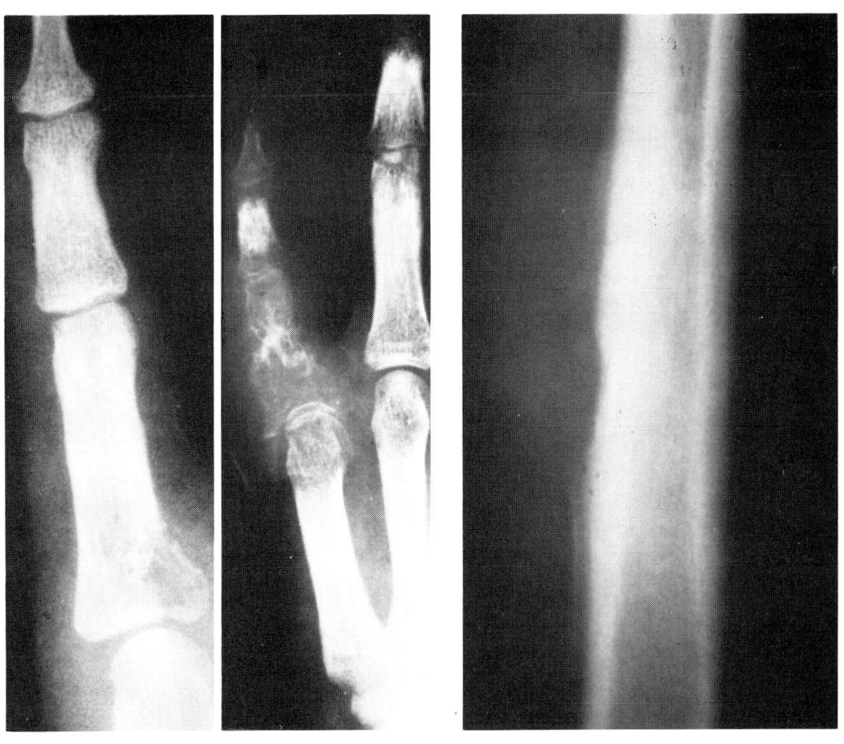

FIG. 11-53

FIG. 11-54

Histopathology

On low-power examination the tumor consists of a sheet of cells. Necrosis is usually of mild degree, compared to Ewing's sarcoma.

The characteristic high-power features are:

1. **MARKED VARIATION IN SIZES AND SHAPES OF NUCLEI.** Some nuclei are strikingly large; others may be as small as those of lymphocytes (Plate 9, *G, H,* and *I*). The nuclei characteristically show distinctive multilobulated and often "mulberry" forms (Fig. 11-58, Plate 9, *H,*) and occasional reniform shapes. Nucleoli may be prominent. Mitotic figures are variable in number. The chromatin pattern is coarse. These features are much more clearly seen on high-quality imprints (Plate 9, *H*). If a reticulum cell sarcoma is poorly fixed and overstained, the cells shrink and are difficult to distinguish from lymphocytic lymphomas, Ewing's tumor, or neuroblastoma (see Figs. 11-59, 11-60, and 11-61).

2. **DISTINCT CELL BORDERS.** On either imprint or well-prepared sections the cells will be separated one from another (Fig. 11-58, Plate 9, *G* and *H*). This feature is a characteristic of lymphoma and often of metastatic neuroblastoma; Ewing's tumor shows indistinct cell borders on H and E section.

3. **RETICULIN FIBERS SEPARATING EACH CELL.** Silver stain for reticulin will usually show a tremendous network of fibers separating each and every cell (Plate 9, *I*). This feature by itself is not pathognomonic, because it may occur in malignant fibrous histiocytoma and occasionally in other tumors. However, tumor cells encased by reticulin in a basketlike network (Plate 9, *I*) is highly characteristic, if not pathognomonic, of the reticulum cell sarcoma of bone (personal observations).

4. **ABSENCE OF INTRACELLULAR GLYCOGEN.** PAS- and diastase-soluble glycogen granules are not seen in the cell cytoplasm of reticulum cell sarcoma.[82] PAS positive and diastase-resistant intercellular material (glycoprotein) is sometimes seen, but it is bound to the reticulin fibers and should not be confused with the intracellular glycogen seen in Ewing's tumor. Electron microscopy can be beneficial in distinguishing Ewing's tumor from reticulum cell sarcoma.[81]

Differential Diagnosis

The entities that may be confused with reticulum cell sarcoma of bone include Ewing's sarcoma, metastatic neuroblastoma, and lymphosarcoma. Refer to Table 11-1 for the principal differential diagnostic features of each.

Metastatic undifferentiated carcinoma or melanoma may mimic the reticulum cell sarcoma histologically. Usually these tumors show involvement of more than one bone and a primary tumor is usually evident. The most important histological feature is the absence of reticulin fibers separating each and every tumor cell in either carcinoma or melanoma.

Course and Treatment

Primary reticulum cell sarcoma of bone is radiosensitive. Radiation has been reported to produce long-term cure in up to 50 per cent of the patients. The others develop metastases to regional and distant lymph nodes, other bone sites, and soft tissue as long as five to ten years after diagnosis and initial treatment. Radiation and chemotherapy is used to treat disseminated disease. Perhaps local excision or cryosurgery should be considered for those cases which, on repeat biopsies, show viable tumor cells post-radiation. The 5-year survival rate is around 50 per cent and the 10-year survival rate, 25 to 40 per cent.

(*Text continues on p. 419.*)

Reticulum Cell Sarcoma

FIG. 11-55. RCS of the talus. The lesion has broken through the bone and resulted in reactive periosteal ossification (*arrow*).

FIG. 11-56. Upon dissection, the tumor was found in the soft tissue surrounding the talus (*arrow*). The gross appearance of the tumor in cross section is shown in Plate 7, *L*.

FIG. 11-57. Note the severe destruction and soft-tissue mass associated with this RCS of a midphalangeal bone. Most reticulum cell sarcomas will show soft-tissue extension.

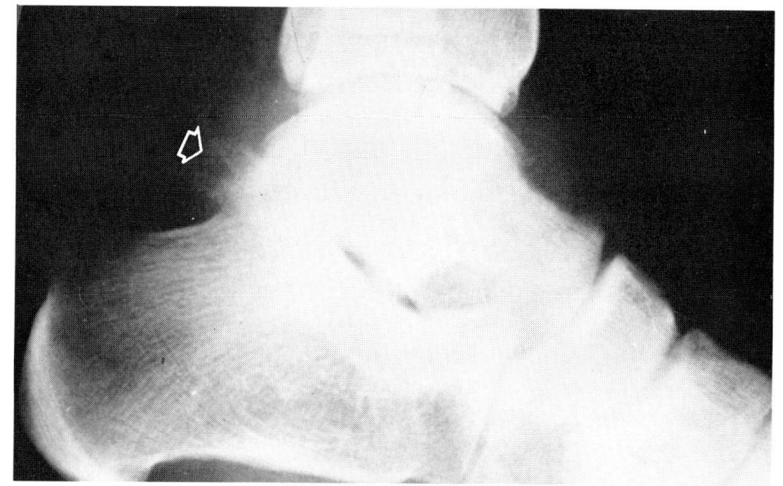

FIG. 11-55

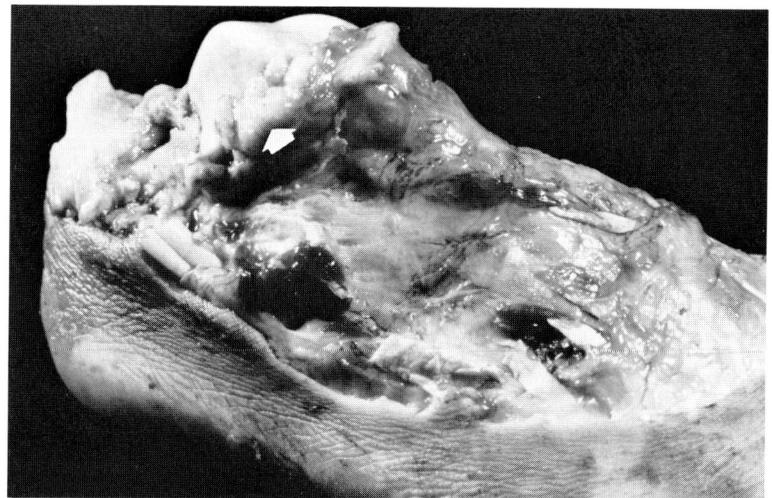

FIG. 11-56

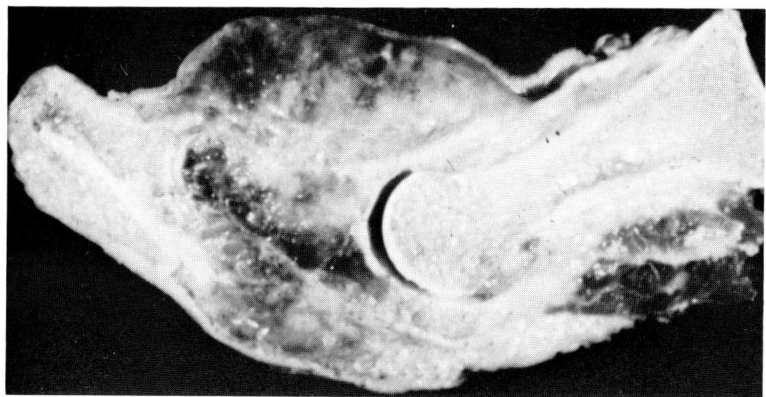

FIG. 11-57

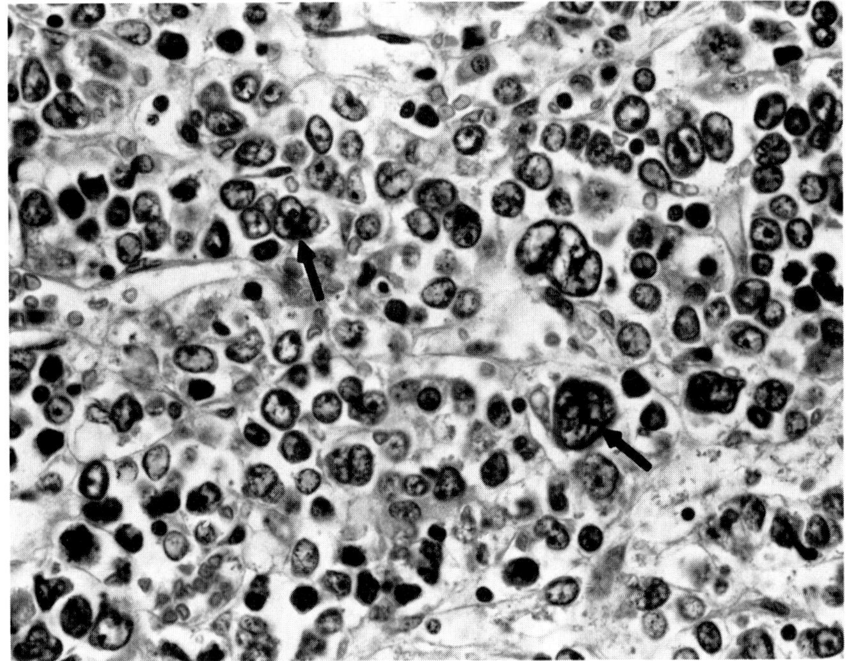

FIG. 11-58

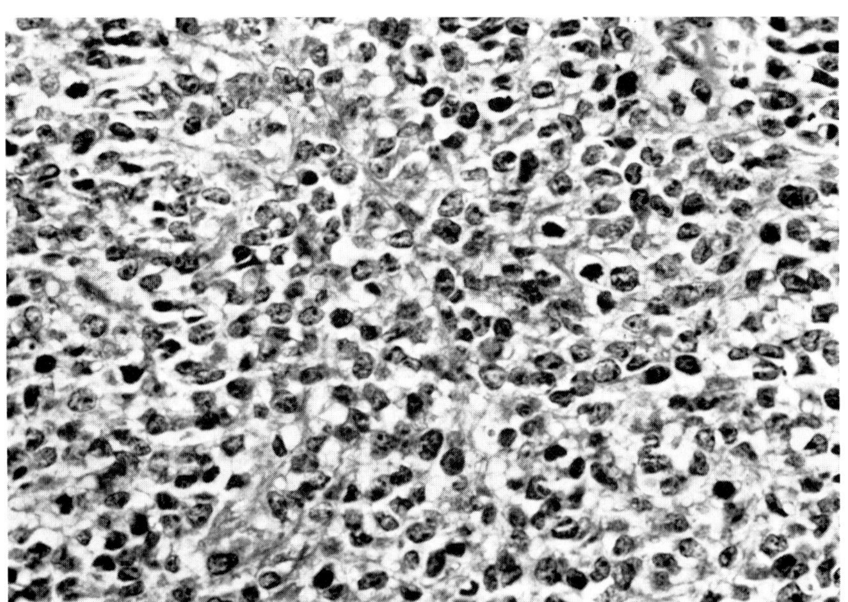

FIG. 11-59

Reticulum Cell Sarcoma Versus Ewing's Sarcoma

FIG. 11-58. Reticulum cell sarcoma (RCS). The nuclei vary considerably in size and shape. Oval, round, lobulated and "mulberry" (*arrow*) forms are prominent. The cytoplasmic borders tend to be distinct. The stroma is not fibrillar (x400).

FIG. 11-59. Ewing's sarcoma. The nuclei are single and monotonously oval to round. The chromatin is smoky or delicate. The cytoplasm is pale, indistinct, and has a fibrillar to lacey quality. The nuclei are larger than those of lymphosarcoma but smaller than those seen in RCS (x400).

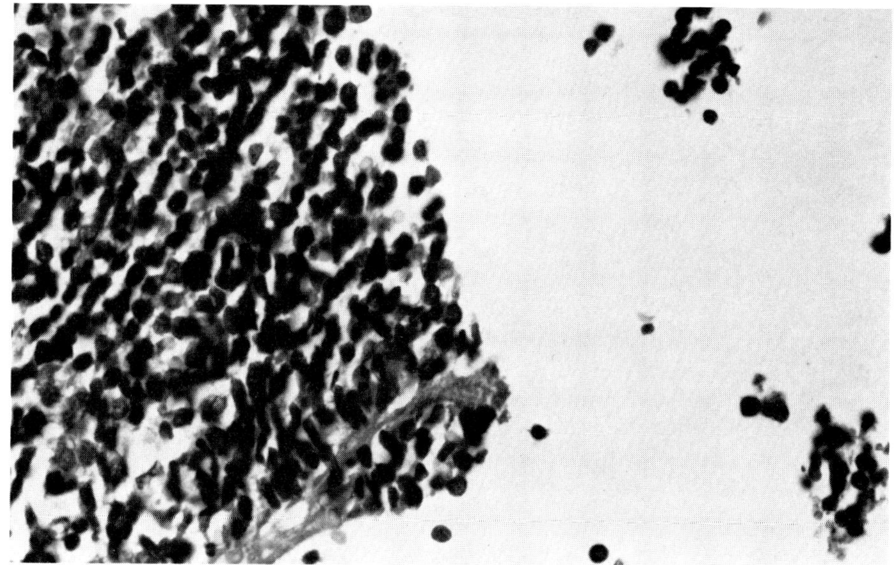

FIG. 11-60

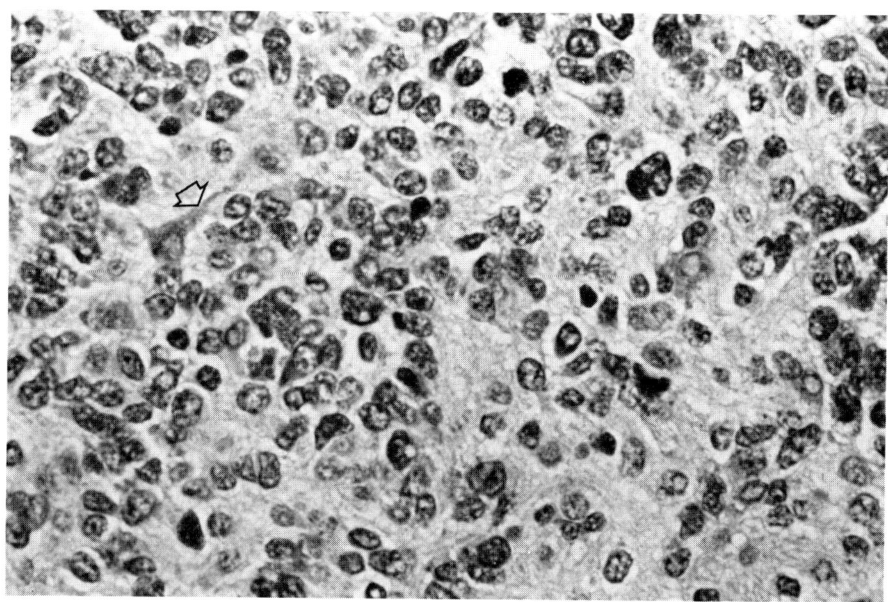

FIG. 11-61

Lymphosarcoma Versus Metastatic Neuroblastoma

FIG. 11-60. Lymphosarcoma. The nuclei are small and very round. The chromatin is dense, hyperchromatic, or clumped. If the observer searches for areas in which the cells are individually displayed (*right*), the cytoplasm will be seen to be scanty and the cell borders quite distinct (x400).

FIG. 11-61. Metastatic neuroblastoma. The nuclei may be lymphocyte-like, Ewing's sarcoma-like or reticulum-cell sarcoma-like. In this example, some nuclei resemble those of Ewing's sarcoma, and the larger multilobulate nuclei resemble those of a reticulum cell sarcoma. Some cells may be multinucleate (very rare in Ewing's and absent in most lymphocytic lymphomas). Rare cells may show prominent cytoplasmic extensions, giving rise to the so-called "pear" or "carrot" shapes (*arrow*). The stroma is often finely fibrillar and resembles brain tissue. The stroma tends to be more clearly fibrillar and more focally abundant, as compared to Ewing's sarcoma (x400).

Table 11-1. Differential Features of the "Lymphocyte-Like" Round Cell Tumors of Bone

Clinical and Laboratory Features	*Primary Lymphocytic Lymphoma*	*Poorly Differentiated Lymphocytic Leukemia*	*Ewing's Tumor*	*Metastatic Neuroblastoma*	*Primary Reticulum Cell Sarcoma*	*Chronic Osteomyelitis*
Age in years	5–20 (50%)	2–5 (50%)	2–25 (75%)	2–10 (80%)	16–60 (90%)	1–10 (70%)
General health	Good	Poor	Poor	Poor	Good	Fair
Anemia	0	+ to ++	0 to ++	0 to ++	0	0 to +
Leukocytosis	0 to +	+ to ++	0 to ++	0 to +	0 to +	+ to ++
Immature cells in peripheral blood	0 to ++	+ to ++	0	0	0	0 to +
Elevated urinary catecholamines	0	0	0	Normal to elevated	0	0
Five-year survival	30%	5%	10%	10%	50%	80%
Radiology						
More than one bone involved at initial presentation	0	Usual	Rare	Usual	0	Rare to +
Metaphyseal bands of radiolucency	0	+	0	0	0	0
Histopathology						
True rosettes	0	0	0	0 to ++	0	0
Rosette-like pattern	0	0	0 to ++	0	0	0
Long uni- or bipolar cytoplasmic extensions ("Pear" and/or "carrot" cells)	0	0	0	+ to ++	0	0
Glycogen in cytoplasm	0 to +	0 to +	0 to +++	0 to ++	0	0 to +
Reticulin surrounding each cell	0	0	0	0	+++	0
Multilobulated nuclei "mulberry" forms	0	0	0	0 to ++	++	0
Multiple nuclei	0	0	0 to +	+ to ++	0 to +	0
Lymphocytes, plasma cells and fibrosis	0	0	0	0 to +	0	+ to ++

Ewing's Sarcoma

Capsule Summary (Fig. 11-62)

Incidence. The fourth most common primary malignant tumor of bone (approximately 5–7% of biopsied primary bone tumors).

Age. Some 75 per cent of the patients present before age 20. Most are usually between 5 and 13 years of age.

Clinical Features. Localized bone pain, swelling, soft-tissue mass, tenderness, heat. Patients may appear quite ill, with mild fever, anemia, leukocytosis, and elevated sedimentation rate.

Radiologic Features. Nonspecific; bone destruction or lysis with or without patchy bone sclerosis; Codman's triangles may be present; large soft-tissue mass is often present. Differential radiologic diagnosis: osteomyelitis, metastatic neuroblastoma, reticulum cell sarcoma, lymphoma, eosinophilic granuloma, and osteogenic sarcoma.

Gross Pathology. The affected bone is widely infiltrated by nodular or diffuse masses of soft, gray-white tumor tissue modified by extensive necrosis and hemorrhage.

Histopathology. Sheets of cells with lacy cytoplasm, indistinct cytoplasmic borders, round-to-oval, usually single nuclei, smoky- or light-staining chromatin appearance. Small nucleoli. Mitotic figures may be abundant. Occasional pseudorosette pattern; frequent PAS-positive intracytoplasmic glycogen.

Treatment. Chemotherapy and radiotherapy.

Course. Extremely poor prognosis; 5-year survival of less than 15 per cent prior to the era of combined chemo- and radiotherapy. 5 year survivals are now projected to be in the range of 50 per cent.

Clinical Features

Ewing's tumor is a highly malignant primary bone sarcoma characterized by sheets of small, round cells of unknown histogenesis. Some 75 per cent of the patients with this disease are under age 20. But the most common diagnosis of a round cell bone tumor in a patient under age 5 will probably be metastatic neuroblastoma; in patients between ages 5 and 30, Ewing's tumor; and in patients over age 35, undifferentiated metastatic carcinoma. Primary reticulum cell sarcoma of bone affects all age groups and must always be considered.

Ordinarily only a single bone is first involved. Multiple sites of bone involvement usually occurs after pulmonary and visceral metastases have become evident.

The most consistent complaint is pain. Localized or generalized, it becomes severe and persistent and is often present for several months before radiographic changes show its seriousness. Less common symptoms are joint effusion with limited mobility or a palpable tumor mass, tenderness at the lesion site, prominent subcutaneous veins, insignificant local heat, mild fever that rises daily to 101°F; mild anemia, leukocytosis, and elevated sedimentation rate. These are often associated with a fulminating course and sudden death.

Radiologic Features

Once considered pathognomonic and characterized by osteolysis with onionskin layering of periosteal bone over the affected site, the radiologic appearance of Ewing's tumor is now recognized as much more variable and relatively nonspecific. Concentric layers of new periosteal bone encircling the shaft—the onionskin effect—is not pathognomonic nor as common as formerly believed.

Clinically, radiologically, and pathologically, Ewing's tumor can be confused with chronic osteomyelitis, malignant lymphoma, and undifferentiated metastatic neoplasms. Any of these lesions may also be mistaken for Ewing's tumor.

In children and adolescents, osteomyelitis tends to begin in the metaphysis, while Ewing's tumor usually starts toward the middle of the bone. In the adult, osteomyelitis is often diaphyseal.

An important radiologic indication of osteomyelitis is the loss of the interface between subcutaneous fat and underlying muscle, as well as obliteration of soft-tissue planes, such as fatty septae between muscle groups resulting from the edema produced by inflammation. Even though a large soft-tissue component is present in Ewing's tumor, the loss of the tissue planes is rare.

Ewing's tumor may present with quite subtle radiologic features such as a minimal degree of permeative destruction (Fig. 11-63) or with one or more thin lines of periosteal new bone that parallel the bone (Figs. 11-65, 11-66, and 11-67). Similar patterns can be seen in occasional cases of osteomyelitis, eosinophilic granuloma, or Gaucher's disease. Within a few days to weeks, however, the degree and extent of permeative bone destruction is intense and the malignant nature of the process becomes more obvious (Figs. 11-64, 11-67). The new layered periosteal bone that may be seen is often delicate, and the bony plates may be thinner than the soft tissue between them. In osteosarcoma and in traumatic periostitis and most cases of osteomyelitis, the bony plates are generally thicker than the intervening lucent areas. Neither layering of periosteal membrane nor a "sunburst" pattern is pathognomonic for a specific tumor.

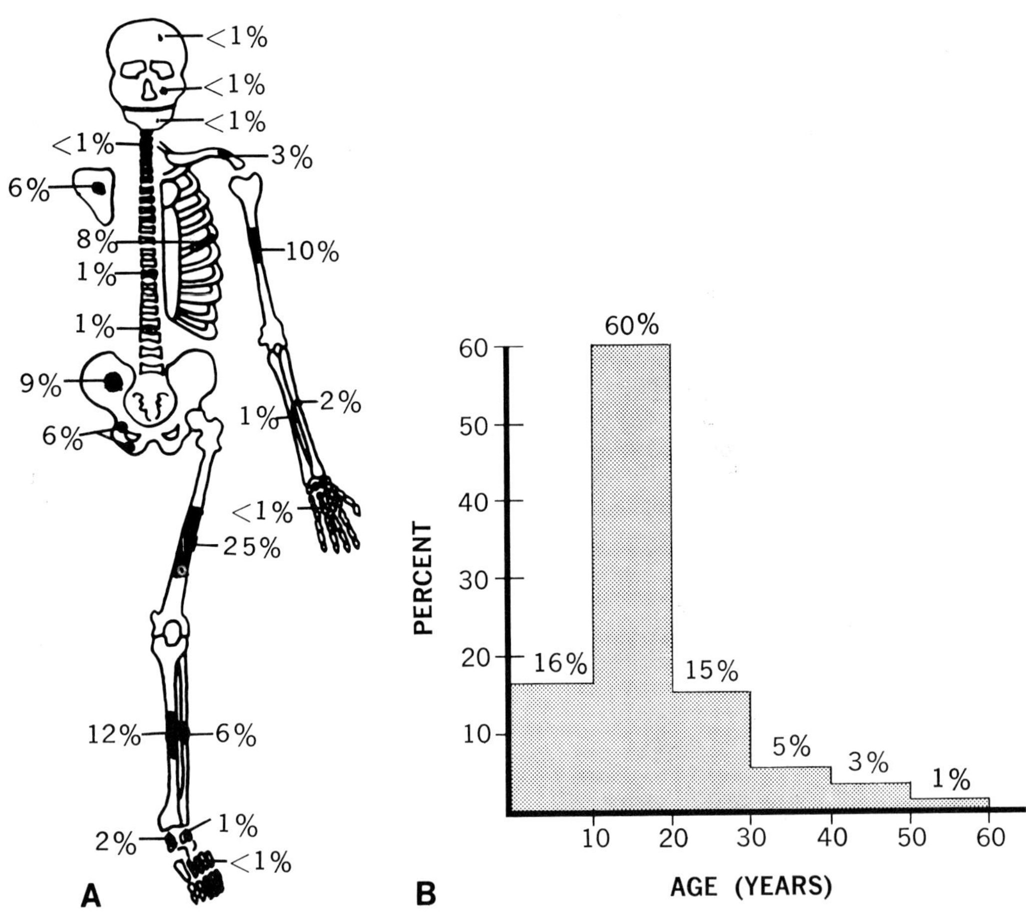

FIG. 11-62. (*A*) Ewing's tumor. Frequency of areas of involvement in 528 patients. Male: female incidence, 2:1. (*B*) Age distribution of patients with Ewing's tumor (Mirra, J., Bullough, P., and Freiberger, R.: Orthopedic Diseases, Part III: Histiocytoses and Round Cell Tumors. New York, Famous Teachings in Modern Medicine, MedCom, Inc., © 1973).

"Onionskinning" probably indicates a pulsating growth pattern; the "sunburst" reaction is indicative of a continuous growth inducing periosteal new bone formation. Both reactions are due to periosteal new bone and are not produced by the tumor cells per se. The former is more commonly seen in patients with Ewing's tumor; the latter, in osteosarcoma.

Most cases of Ewing's tumor begin in the diaphysis or extensively involve this region. Rare cases will present as a metaphyseal primary (Fig. 11-68), which will most often be diagnosed on radiological grounds as a lytic osteogenic sarcoma.

Most cases of Ewing's tumor show lytic destruction. Occasional cases may show blastic reactions from the reactive host bone as a response to the tumor. Prominent blastic reactions in association with an ominous tumorous process in a single bone of a child is more commonly due to osteomyelitis, osteosarcoma, or lymphosarcoma. Histologically, the diagnosis of osteosarcoma versus Ewing's will usually be clear-cut. Unless good sections and imprints are prepared, Ewing's tumor may be difficult to separate from lymphosarcoma or chronic osteomyelitis.

Ewing's usually presents as a solitary bone lesion. Multiple bone involvement is only rarely seen on initial presentation but is common during the patient's subsequent course. On initial presentation, the presence of involvement of more than a single bone in a child is more consistent with metastatic neuroblastoma, eosinophilic granuloma, leukemia, Gaucher's disease, or other entities.

Gross Pathology

Viable tumor tissue is soft, gray-white, occasionally shiny, and diffusely to nodularly infiltrative. It is usually modified by areas of hemorrhage and necrosis. The cortex may be partially or completely destroyed, and the periosteum may be reflected, creating a soft-tissue mass of great proportions. Mottled with areas of necrosis and hemorrhage, the extraosseous mass may contain lamellae of reactive periosteal bone.

Autopsy often shows the tumor widely disseminated throughout most of the skeleton, possibly as the result of metastases from a primary bone site rather than from a multicentric origin. The lungs may be tumor-free or they may be ridden with tumor nodules. The heart and abdominal viscera are often involved, while the lymph nodes tend not to be.

Since radiation and chemotherapy with or without en-bloc resection of the involved bone is now used to treat most cases of Ewing's tumor, amputations are quite rare. They reveal the affected bone to be much more tumor-ridden than radiograph shows, emphasizing the fact that the entire bone must be radiated during therapy.

Histopathology

Essential to the diagnosis of Ewing's tumor is biopsy. Even so, diagnosis is difficult and errors are not uncommon if the available tissue is meager or substantially necrotic. A round cell bone tumor formerly had the same prognosis regardless of whether it is Ewing's tumor, metastatic neuroblastoma, undifferentiated carcinoma, or sarcoma, but a reticulum cell sarcoma has a considerably different prognosis. With proper treatment the 5-year survival rates are as high as 50 per cent for reticulum cell sarcoma, compared to the less than 15 per cent 5-year survival rate for Ewing's tumor in past years. It could be disastrous to mistake osteomyelitis or eosinophilic granuloma for Ewing's tumor, or vice versa.

As an aid to diagnosis, low-power examination often shows the tumor to be modified by large areas of necrosis, hemorrhage, and calcification (Fig. 11-69). Viable tumor areas are usually arranged in monotonous sheets (Plate 10, *A*, Fig. 11-59). High-power examination (Plate 10, *A, bottom;* Figs. 11-59 and 11-70) shows that cytoplasm is lightly stained and lacy, and has indistinct cell borders: nuclei are usually single, of nearly equal size, round or oval, about $1\frac{1}{2}$ times the size of a lymphocyte; chromatin is finely dispersed or powdery; nucleoli are generally small and single; and mitotic figures are usually abundant. Some cases may show considerably larger nuclei, prominent nucleoli, and up to three nuclei per cell. This variant could be called *large cell Ewing's sarcoma.* Radiological and histopathological features are otherwise identical to the more common smaller cell type. A tumor imprint fixed in 70 per cent alcohol more clearly shows the cytologic characteristics of Ewing's tumor (Plate 10, *C*). More distinct than on H and E section, the cytoplasmic borders help to distinguish Ewing's tumor from lymphosarcoma, in which the cells contain at most a thin rim of cytoplasm (Compare Plate 10, *C,* with Plate 10, *F*).

About 10 per cent of cases of Ewing's tumor occasionally show a rosette-like pattern resembling metastatic neuroblastoma (Fig. 11-70). Fragments or ghosts of nuclei seen under high-power examination indicate that the rosette center structure, in some cases as least, is consequent to necrosis as Jaffe had suggested.[108] However, this author has seen occasional cases of Ewing's tumor in which rosette-like structures are present with little to no evidence of central nuclear degeneration or necrosis (Fig. 11–70). These cases are extremely difficult to distinguish from metastatic neuroblastoma. Positive vanyl-mandelic acid studies, radiographic studies to show a sympathetic primary tumor, and the presence of "pear"- and "carrot"-shaped cells and multinucleate cells on H and E sections are the principal features of neuroblastoma. These features are absent in Ewing's tumor.

Red, PAS-positive, diatase digestible glycogen globules are often seen in Ewing's tumor in the cytoplasm of scattered cells or most of the cells (Plate 10, *B*). To bring them out more consistently the tissue should be fixed in 80 per cent alcohol. Glycogen globules have also been seen by electron microscopy. Glycogen granules are not produced in the reticulum cell sarcoma, and they are an important histologic aid in the differential diagnosis. Glycogen may be found in occasional cells of neuroblastoma, however. Price[100] reported an incidence of intracellular glycogen in 0 per cent of reticulum cell sarcomas, 59 per cent of Ewing's tumors, and 18 per cent of neuroblastomas.

PAS- and diastase-resistant intercellular material (glycoprotein) found in reticulum cell sarcoma is believed to be associated with reticulin fibers and should not be confused with the intracellular glycogen seen in Ewing's tumor. Reticulin fibers in Ewing's tumor vary in number and are not prominent or always present. In Ewing's tumor individual cells are not encased in reticulin as they are in reticulum cell sarcoma.

Differential Diagnosis

Chronic osteomyelitis, metastatic neuroblastoma, lymphosarcoma, and reticulum cell sarcoma may be confused with Ewing's sarcoma. The reticulum cell sarcoma, by imprint and high-quality sections, shows distinctly different nuclear and cytoplasmic features and a massive reticulin fiber production. For every 15 "Ewing's tumors" this author has been consulted on there were approximately three that were preleukemic lymphosarcomas presenting as a "primary" bone tumor, one that was a solitary metastatic neuroblastoma on initial presentation, and one that was chronic osteomyelitis. The morphologic features that aid in the differentiation of Ewing's from each of these tumors is treated under each entity. A summary of these features is presented in Table 11–1 and Figs. 11–58 to 11–61.

Course and Treatment

The 5-year survival rate in patients treated by radiation and/or amputation alone is approximately 9 per cent.[87] With the advent of systemic chemotherapy as an adjunct to radiation therapy with or without en-bloc excision or amputation, the course of patients with this disease is being significantly altered. Whether or not there will be significant alteration in the 5-year survival statistics remains to be seen. However, early indications are extremely promising.

Ewing's Sarcoma

FIG. 11-63. The ischial ramus shows a moth-eaten pattern of destruction and no periosteal reaction.

FIG. 11-64. One month later, the area is almost totally destroyed by the tumor and has undoubtedly extended into the soft tissues.

FIG. 11-65. The main clue to the possibility of Ewing's sarcoma in this case is the presence of a fine lamella of periosteal new bone (*arrow*) in the midshaft of the tibia. The degree of cortical destruction is at this time insufficient to delineate clear-cut permeative bone destruction.

FIG. 11-66. This example of Ewing's sarcoma of the humeral shaft shows its classical features; namely, multiple fine lamellae (*arrow*) of periosteal new bone ("onion skinning") and incipient cortical destruction manifested by thin lines of radiolucency.

FIG. 11-67. More advanced phase of Ewing's sarcoma showing obvious cortical and intramedullary permeative destruction in addition to periosteal "onion-skinning." Although highly suggestive of Ewing's, this radiologic pattern can also be seen in osteomyelitis, fibrosarcoma, reticulum cell sarcoma, and rarely, in osteosarcoma and Gaucher's disease.

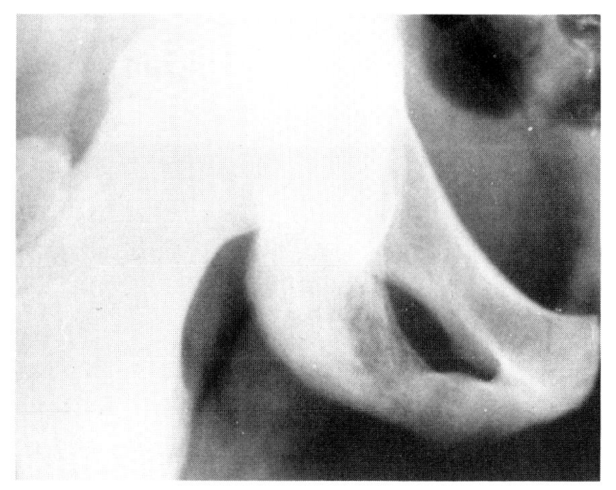

FIG. 11-63

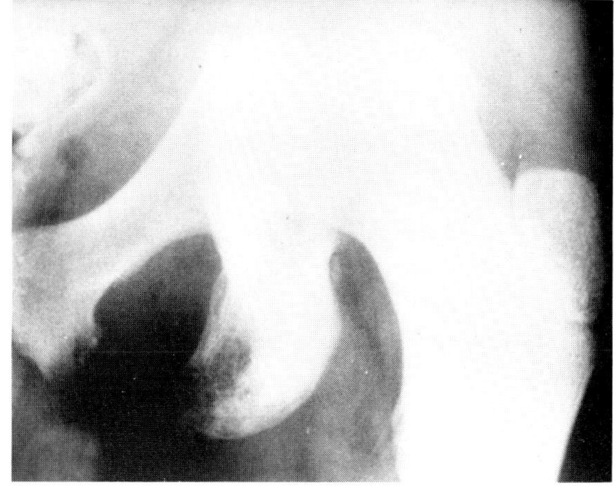

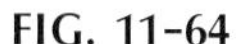

FIG. 11-64

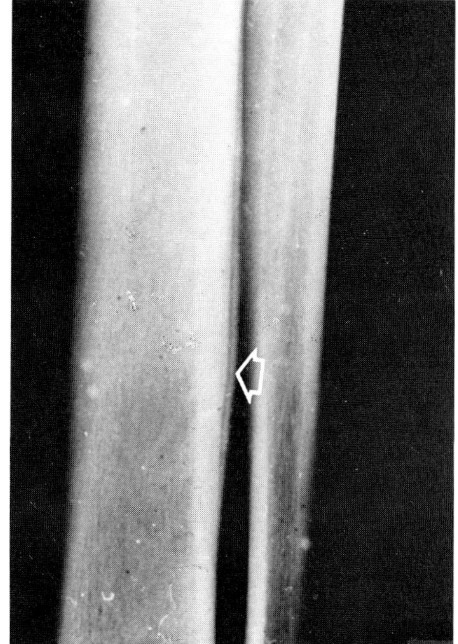

FIG. 11-65

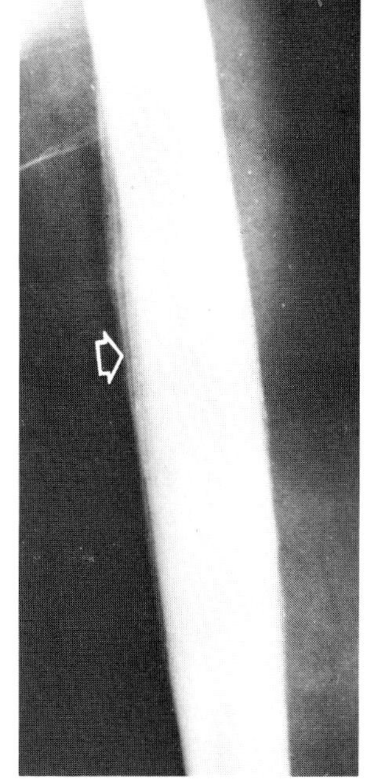

FIG. 11-66

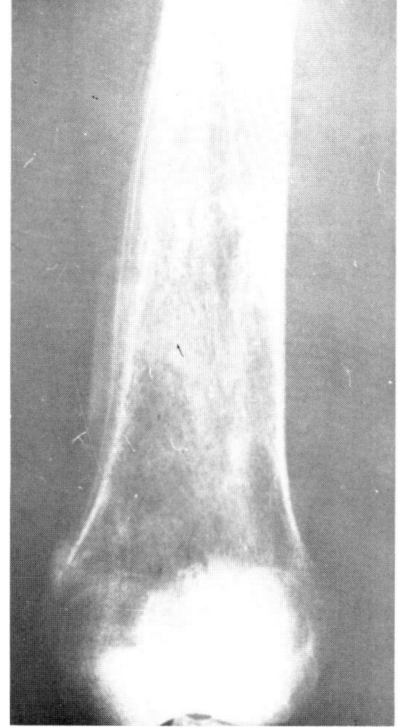

FIG. 11-67

Lymphomas and Leukemia of Bone

The lymphomas of bone principally include the lymphocytic lymphomas, Hodgkin's disease, reticulum cell sarcoma, granulocytic leukemias, myeloma, and Waldenström's macroglobulinemia. The lymphomas, reticulum cell sarcoma, and Hodgkin's disease usually involve the bone by spread from regional lymph nodes. Nevertheless, there remain rare cases that appear to be true primary lymphoma, Hodgkin's disease, and reticulum cell sarcoma of bone. The leukemias (granulocytic, lymphocytic and monocytic) are believed to originate as bone primaries. Myeloma almost always originates as a bone primary, although extramedullary myeloma is seen occasionally.

The discussion that follows discusses the usual initially disseminated lymphosarcomas as well as those lymphosarcomas that usually fall within the domain of the bone pathologist. These will be those cases of preleukemic, leukemic, and primary lymphosarcomas of bone. Generally they present initially as primary bone tumors with little in the way of peripheral blood finding except perhaps for a few "atypical" lymphocytes.

Lymphosarcoma of bone usually presents as a solitary bone lesion and biopsy will often lead to confusion with Ewing's sarcoma. In this author's experience most of these cases develop leukemia within 6 months of initial presentation. The lymphosarcomatous cells in the peripheral blood tend to have indented nuclei; (Plate 10, *F, bottom*). On rare occasions poorly differentiated lymphocytic leukemia may present with clinical symptoms involving a single bone. Biopsy may be confused with Ewing's sarcoma. However, either evidence of peripheral blood leukemia or radiographic signs of metaphyseal bands of radiolucency usually prevent this error. The cells of lymphocytic leukemia tend not to have the nuclear indentation characteristic of primary lymphoma of bone. Only rare cases of lymphocytic lymphosarcoma remain as relatively static mono-osseous neoplasms.

Clinical Features

Males are affected nearly twice as often as females. In about half the patients poorly differentiated lymphocytic leukemia occurs between ages 2 and 5. The primary lymphoma may affect any age group, but the majority of patients are usually younger than 15 years of age.

Over 80 per cent of leukemic patients have pallor, fever, listlessness, hemorrhagic tendencies, and enlarged spleen, liver, and lymph nodes. Bone and joint pain and retinal hemorrhages occur in about half the patients. More than 40 per cent initially have fewer than 12,000 WBC/cu. mm.; almost all show immature white cells on the peripheral smear. These should not be confused with the abnormal white cells regularly seen in the blood of patients who have an infection. Anemia and platelet reduction are generally consistent findings. Diagnosis is confirmed by bone marrow biopsy or aspiration.

Because the first signs of leukemia are fever, joint pains, swelling, and cardiac murmurs, it is often confused with rheumatic fever. Leukemia patients are generally younger and their joint pain and swelling do not usually respond to salicylates. The finding of bone changes on radiography excludes rheumatic fever.

Children with generalized lymphoma may present with signs and symptoms that resemble numerous other diseases, such as juvenile rheumatoid arthritis, infectious mononucleosis, subacute bacterial endocarditis, sickle-cell anemia, purpura, sepsis, tuberculosis, undulant fever, osteomyelitis, osteogenic sarcoma, and Banti's syndrome. Careful assessment of all clinical, radiographic, laboratory, and pathologic data is essential to determine if the disease is leukemia, primary lymphoma, or one of the abovementioned potentially curable disorders.

Rare cases present few symptoms other than bone pain. These patients include those with the true primary lymphocytic lymphoma of bone, as well as minimally disseminated leukemic and preleukemic patients.

Ewing's Sarcoma

FIG. 11-68. An osteolytic, eccentric, metaphyseal destructive mass is perhaps the most uncommon presentation of Ewing's sarcoma. Usually this presentation signifies a lytic osteosarcoma.

FIG. 11-69. On low-power examination, Ewing's sarcoma is often characterized by focal but extensive zones of necrosis (*arrows*) (x40).

FIG. 11-70. Ewing's sarcoma nuclei may be arranged in a circular distribution and resemble the rosettes of neuroblastoma. The reader is referred to the text for the differentiation of Ewing's sarcoma with this pattern from metastatic neuroblastoma.

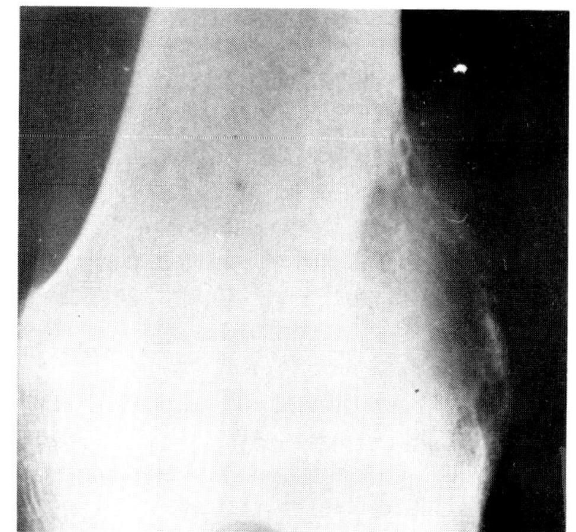

FIG. 11-68

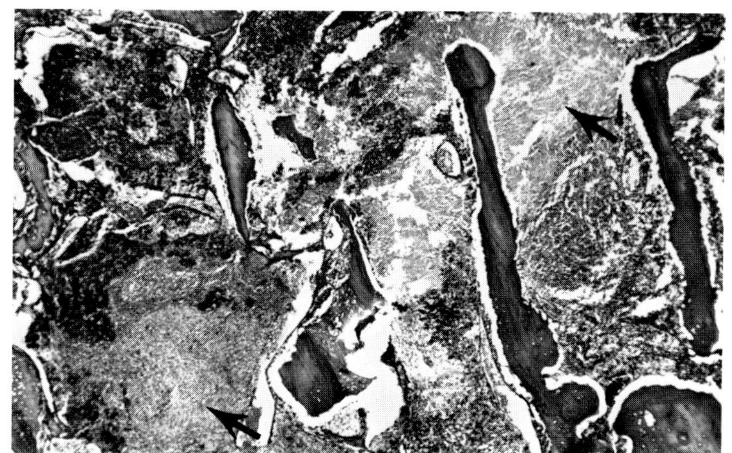

FIG. 11-69

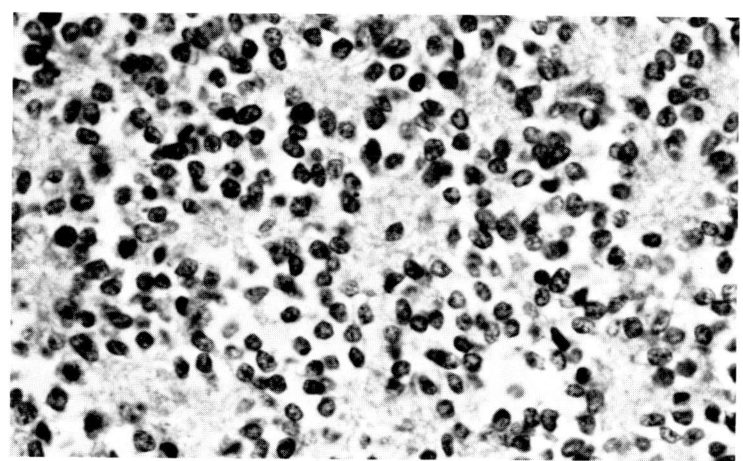

FIG. 11-70

Radiologic Features

OVERT LEUKEMIA. Within 4 to 10 weeks of the first symptoms, 30 to 70 per cent of actively growing individuals with disseminated leukemic infiltrates demonstrate numerous areas of *metaphyseal bands of radiolucency* (Fig. 11-71). These tend to occur most prominently in the regions of the knee and proximal humerus. It is believed that the leukemic infiltrates interfere with normal bone production, which is the most severe in the areas of greatest new bone formation—the metaphyses. On rare occasions patients with an apparent primary lymphocytic lymphoma may present with a so-called solitary destructive, lytic to blastic bone lesion simulating an Ewing's sarcoma. A skeletal survey may show unexpected metaphyseal bands of radiolucency. The sign may be quite minimal and careful radiologic assessment may be necessary to appreciate them.

The bands of radiolucency are nonspecific and before age 2 are usually seen in association with severe malnutrition and other debilitating diseases. After age 2 they are generally associated with leukemia. However, bands of radiolucency in association with a monotonous sheet of cells on biopsy and imprints is indicative of leukemia. Pathologic fracture in the weakened metaphyseal zone often results in a slipped capital femoral epiphysis.

In 30 to 40 per cent of patients the earliest change caused by osteolytic lesions—punctate areas of radiolucency with a moth-eaten appearance—commonly occurs in the metaphyses of the long bones and less frequently in the skull, pelvis, shoulder girdle, and ribs. The moth-eaten appearance may give way to confluent geographic patterns of radiolucency. Entirely osteoblastic lesions are rare, but occasionally they may simulate osteopetrosis.

In about 15 to 20 per cent of patients, periosteal reactions may be the first visible changes and may be easily confused with Ewing's tumor (Fig. 11-72). This new periosteal bone is generally laid down in single or multiple layers parallel to the long axis of the bone. Advanced lesions of childhood leukemic bone infiltration resemble metastatic neuroblastomas. The two lesions may look the same on radiograph if metaphyseal bands of radiolucency are absent. A neuroblastoma generally involves the skull, pelvis and femurs early in the progression of the disease; lymphoma usually involves them later.

Adult leukemia shows little radiographic or clinical evidence of osseous involvement except in the chronic myelogenous and lymphatic forms when it shows generalized porosity, discrete or confluent rarefaction, radiopacity, new periosteal bone, and rib fracture. The bones most commonly affected are the pelvis, long bones, spine, ribs, and skull. Widespread osteosclerosis is usually associated with myelosclerotic anemia.

MONO-OSSEOUS OR APPARENTLY MONO-OSSEOUS LESIONS. Most lesions are osteolytic (about 85%), some are mixed lytic and blastic (about 10%) and occasionally, they are almost purely blastic (Figs. 11-72 and 11-73). Periosteal new bone may be a prominent feature and mimic Ewing's sarcoma or osteosarcoma (Fig. 11-72).

The osteolytic lesions are usually more extensive and invasive than they are in Hodgkin's disease and often advance to nearly complete dissolution. Vertebral body compression and periosteal reaction in long bones are generally severe. Symptoms associated with bony involvement include localized pain and tenderness, swelling or palpable mass, neurologic findings if the spine is involved, pathologic fracture, and elevated alkaline phosphatase.

Histopathology

Whether or not a lymphocytic lymphoma (lymphosarcoma) of bone is primary, metastatic, in leukemic or clinically preleukemic or "aleukemic" phase, it is characterized histologically by the following:

1. SHEETS OF MONOTONOUS CELLS WITH DARK ROUND NUCLEI. (Figs. 11-74, 11-75, Plate 10, *D* and *E*). On low power examination lymphosarcoma shows tightly packed clusters of cells with hyperchromatic nuclei. The nuclear staining and size of nuclei is comparable to metastatic neuroblastoma. Ewing's tumor shows larger nuclei (about $1\frac{1}{2}$ times lymphocyte size) and are usually paler staining and spaced slightly more apart due to their increased cytoplasmic content. Low-power examination is important in that it may give the first indication that a so-called "Ewing's sarcoma" is a lymphosarcoma (Plate 10, *D*). The most crucial histologic features, however, are seen on high-power examination and on imprint analysis.

2. CELLS WITH WELL-DELINEATED CELL BORDERS, A SINGLE HYPERCHROMATIC NUCLEUS, SCANTY CYTOPLASM AND ABSENCE OF CYTOPLASMIC TAPERING. (Plate 10, *D, E,* and *F*). Quite often because of fixation shrinkage problems the cells may appear to be tightly bound to each other and the important characteristic of well-delineated cell borders will be lost (Fig. 11-74, Plate 10, *D, right*). Furthermore, if the cells are overstained and distorted severely, it will be impossible to classify the tumor by H and E sections alone (Fig. 11-74). However, in well-prepared sec-

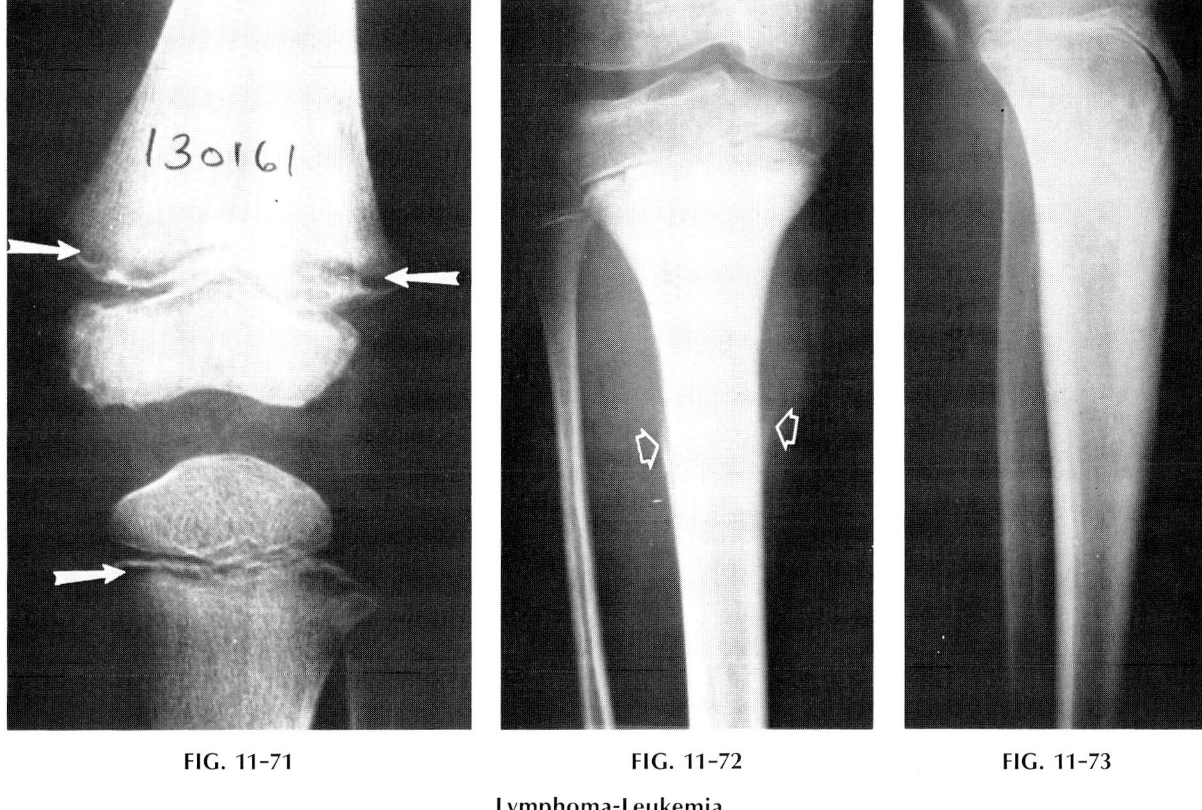

FIG. 11-71 FIG. 11-72 FIG. 11-73

Lymphoma-Leukemia

FIG. 11-71. In children, leukemia is often associated with metaphyseal bands of radiolucency (*arrows*). This sign is not necessarily pathognomonic of leukemia, however, but can be seen in benign, chronic, debilitating diseases of children.

FIG. 11-72. Lymphosarcoma of bone presenting as a blastic focus with two Codman's triangles (*arrows*). This rare presentation will often lead to an incorrect radiologic diagnosis of osteosarcoma or Ewing's sarcoma. Pathologically, the tumor can be mistaken for Ewing's.

FIG. 11-73. Another similar case originally mistaken both clinically and pathologically for Ewing's sarcoma. It shows a diffuse blastic lesion of the proximal tibia.

tions the cells will be recognized much more easily to be of lymphocytic origin (Fig. 11-75, Plate 10, *E*). In less well-prepared sections the best areas for recognizing the tumor is where the cells are lying loosely (Plate 10, *D, right*). Well-prepared imprints stained with H and E or Wright's stain greatly simplify identification of the cells as poorly differentiated lymphocytes (Plate 10, *F, top*). These cells will show an abundance of lacey chromatin, several nucleoli, scanty bluish cytoplasm, and well-demarcated cell borders.

Lymphosarcoma cells usually show a prominent nuclear indentation particularly from imprints or in the leukemic phase of the disease in the peripheral blood (Plate 10, *F, bottom*). Poorly differentiated lymphocytic leukemic cells generally do not show this indentation (Plate 10, *F, top*).

Differential Diagnosis

EWING'S SARCOMA. The radiologic features may be identical. Approximately one in five so-called "Ewing's tumors" of childhood are actually lymphosarcomas (personal observations). These patients usually demonstrate frank leukemia within 6 months of the correct or incorrect diagnosis (Plate 10, *F, bottom*). Well-stained sections and imprints can distinguish a lymphosarcoma of childhood presenting as a bone "primary" from Ewing's sarcoma. Ewing's nuclei are pale-staining, slightly larger, and have pale and lacey cytoplasm on H and E section (Plate 10, *A*). The more abundant cytoplasm results in the nuclei being more widely separated, compared to those of lymphosarcoma. An imprint will show that from 10 to 20 per cent of Ewing's cells show a voluminous cytoplasm that goes beyond that seen in cells of lymphosarcoma (Plate 10, *C*). Lymphosarcoma is characterized by smaller, darker-staining, more tightly packed nuclei, nuclear indentations, and very scant bluish cytoplasm (Plate 10, *D, E,* and *F, bottom*).

METASTATIC NEUROBLASTOMA. The histologic features that serve to distinguish neuroblastoma from lymphosarcoma are the following: the presence of occasional cells with long, tapered cytoplasm ("pear"- or "carrot"-shaped cells) and occasional cells with two or three nuclei and rarely true rosettes (plate 10, *G, H,* and *I,* Figs. 11-61, 11-80).

CHRONIC OSTEOMYELITIS. Well-stained sections show a mixture of plasma cells, lymphocytes, occasional neutrophils, and often fibrosis. The polymorphism of cell types is not, however, seen in lymphosarcoma, and fibrosis is unusual. Poorly stained or thick sections of osteomyelitis may easily be confused with lymphosarcoma or Ewing's sarcoma, and vice versa.

If the marrow fat spaces are not totally obliterated by the round cell infiltrate, the diagnosis of osteomyelitis is suggested, even if staining is poor (Fig. 11-3). However, total obliteration of the fat may be seen in either lymphosarcoma or in most cases of osteomyelitis. This feature is, therefore, only useful in a small percentage of cases.

RETICULUM CELL SARCOMA (RCS). This tumor is distinctly different from lymphosarcoma if careful attention is given to the nuclei and if well-stained sections or imprints are available. The nuclei or RCS are multilobulated, show prominent indentations, may show "mulberry" shapes and vary considerably in size and shape (Plate 9, *H,* and *I;* Fig. 11-58). The only one of these features lymphosarcoma may show is some degree of nuclear indentation. A RCS will show reticulin fibers separating individual cells (Plate 9, *I*). Lymphosarcoma shows sparse reticulin fibers encasing groups of cells.

The features differentiating lymphosarcoma and leukemia from other round cell tumors are summarized in Table 11-1 (also see Figs. 11-58-11-61 and Plate 10, *A-I*).

Course and Treatment

The course of the leukemias, with the exception of chronic well-differentiated lymphocytic and granulocytic leukemia, is dismal. Most of the lymphosarcomas of children who present with a "solitary" bone lesion develop leukemia within 6 months. Adult patients with mono-osseous lymphosarcoma usually have a better prognosis. Treatment by radiation may result in a 5-year survival rate approaching 40 per cent. As I stated for the other primary lymphomas of bone, perhaps en-bloc resection or cryosurgery should be considered for biopsy-proven radioresistant cases, in order to reduce the risk of eventual dissemination.

Metastatic Neuroblastoma

Capsule Summary (Fig. 11-76)

Clinical Features. Over half the patients are age 5 or younger. May have abdominal mass, abdominal or bone pain, fever, anorexia, gastrointestinal disturbances, weight loss, hepatosplenomegaly, lymphadenopathy, exophthalmos, and neurologic symptoms. Urinary catecholamines are frequently elevated.

Radiologic Features. Abdominal or thoracic mass; multiple, symmetrical lytic or blastic bone metastases. The skull is often involved with multiple lytic lesions. Periosteal reaction is common, and intravenous pyelography frequently shows a suprarenal mass.

Gross Pathology. Viscera and bones have multiple soft, white-to-yellow hemorrhagic growths.

Lymphoma

FIG. 11-74. If the sections are inadequately fixed, overstained, or crushed, as this photograph illustrates, it becomes impossible to differentiate a lymphoma from neuroblastoma, reticulum cell sarcoma, metastatic neuroblastoma, Ewing's sarcoma, or osteomyelitis (x400).

FIG. 11-75. A more adequately stained H and E section will show the more obvious lymphocytic features; namely, small, round, hyperchromatic nuclei, scanty cytoplasm, and distinct cell borders (x250). However, occasional metastatic neuroblastomas can mimic cells of lymphoid origin. Differentiation depends heavily on imprint analysis, review of radiographs, vanyl mandelic acid (VMA) studies, and possibly, electron microscopy. Adequate imprints can usually differentiate lymphoma from Ewing's tumor (see Plate 10, *A-I*).

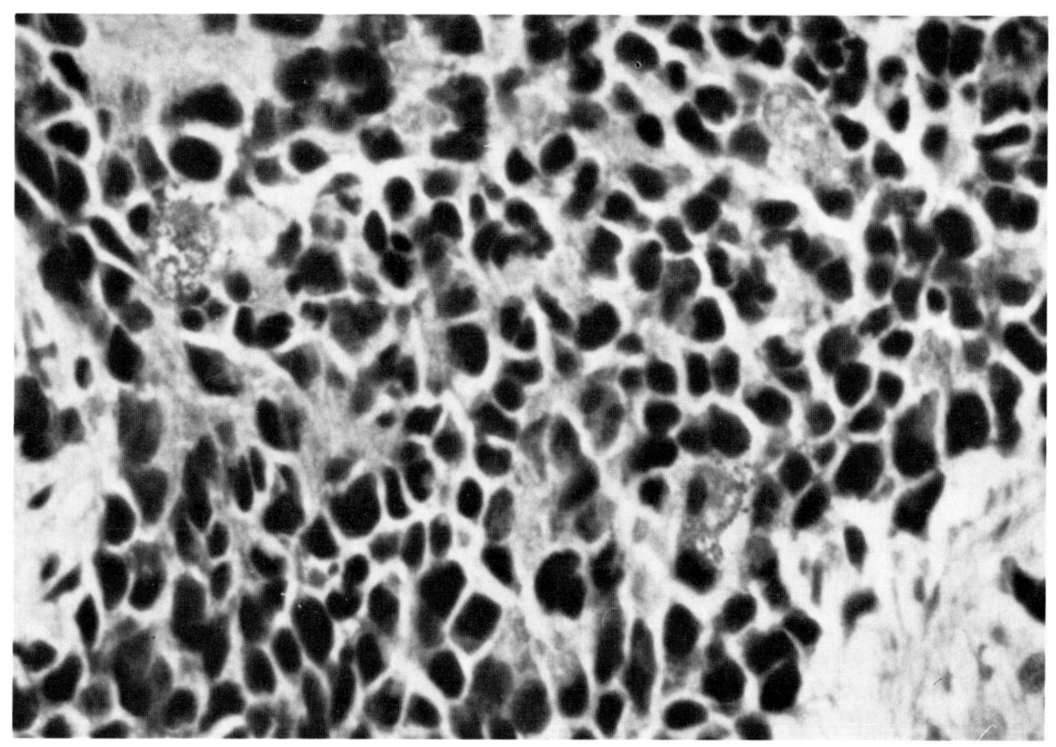

FIG. 11-74

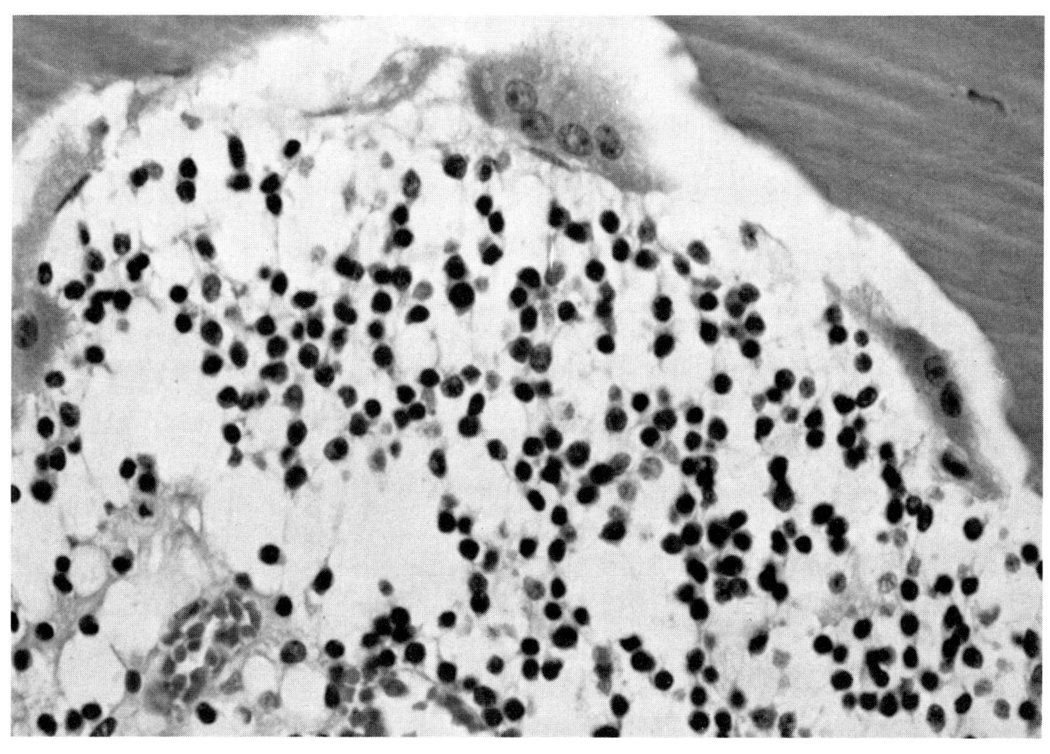

FIG. 11-75

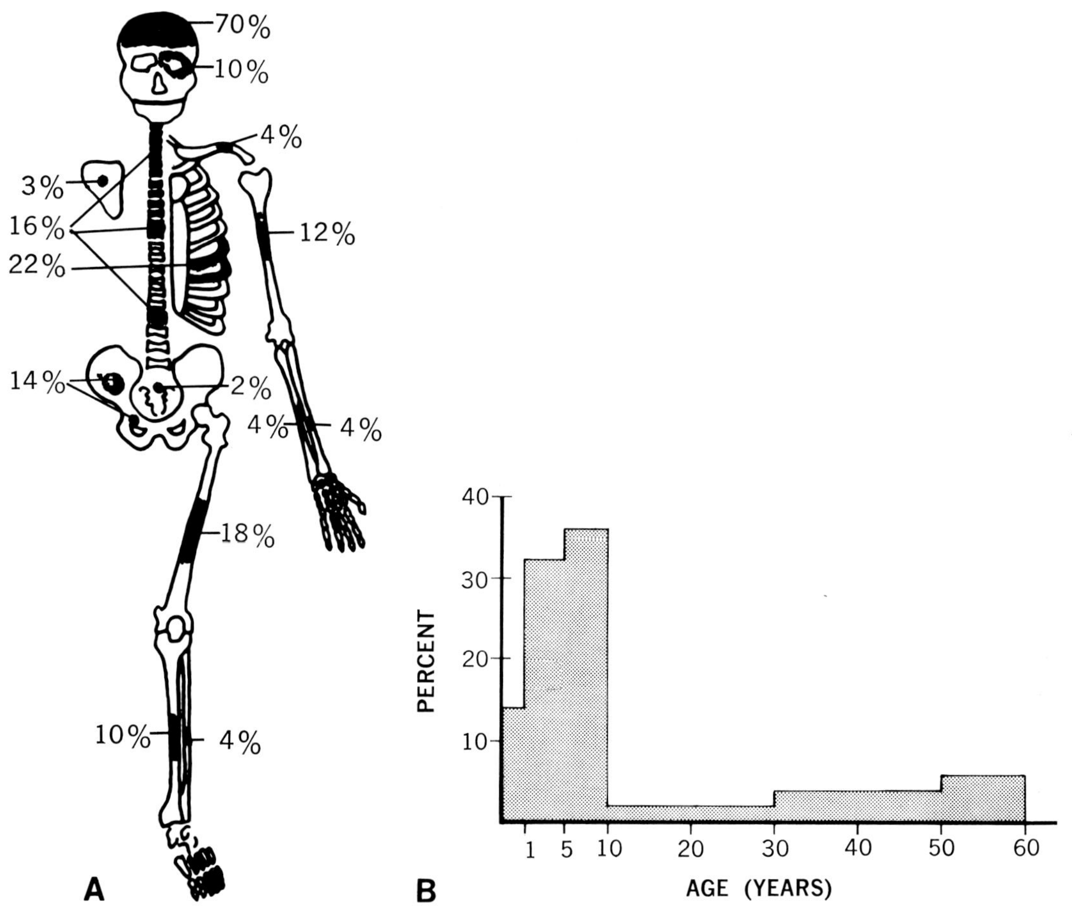

FIG. 11-76. (*A*) Metastatic neuroblastoma. Frequency of areas of involvement in 50 cases. Male:female incidence, 1:1. (*B*) Age distribution of patients with metastatic neuroblastoma. (Mirra, J., Bullough, P., and Freiberger, R.: Orthopedic Diseases, Part III; Histiocytoses and Round Cell Tumors. New York, Famous Teachings in Modern Medicine, MedCom, Inc., © 1973)

Histopathology. Sheets of small cells that simulate small to large lymphocytes. Nuclei are round and hyperchromatic. In 10 to 20 per cent of cases, neurofibrillary rosettes may be seen. Very rarely the neuroblastoma matures into ganglioneuroma, resulting in disease arrest. Cytoplasm tapers out in occasional to rare cells to give rise to "pear"- and "carrot"-shapes.

Treatment. Radiation and chemotherapy.

Course. Five-year survival of about 15 per cent.

Clinical Features

One of the most common malignant tumors of infancy and childhood, the neuroblastoma arises in the sympathetic nervous system, usually in the adrenal medulla but also in sympathetic ganglia, the celiac plexus, and Zuckerkandl's organ adjacent to the origin of the inferior mesenteric artery.

Most patients are under age 5, and their first symptom is usually an abdominal mass. They are likely to suffer from backache or extremity pain secondary to pathologic fracture, abdominal pain, fever, anorexia, hematemasis, diarrhea, constipation, and weight loss.

Primary lesions are generally in the abdominal cavity and posterior mediastinum and occasionally along the sympathetic chain from the cervical region to the pelvis. In 75 per cent of the patients, radiography reveals the primary tumor to be a mass with or without stippled calcific densities displacing the abdominal organs.

In about 40 per cent of the patients, multiple,

symmetrical bone metastases often involve any part of the skeletom but rarely the hands and feet. Orbital metastases are common and cause exophthalmos and hemorrhages. Meningeal metastases cause cranial suture separation secondary to increased intracranial pressure. An important diagnostic feature of neuroblastoma is elevated urinary catecholamines. However, this finding is not present in all patients.

Radiologic Features

Many patients develop lytic skull metastases that are small or large and miliary or confluent (Fig. 11-77). The cranial sutures may become infiltrated with neuroblastoma cells, resulting in apparent suture widening.

In long bones, lesions predominantly involve the shaft, often in a bilaterally symmetrical fashion (Figs. 11-78 and 11-79). Neuroblastomatous metastases are predominantly lytic, moth-eaten, or permeatively destructive. New periosteal bone reaction often parallels the shaft. Solitary lesions showing moth-eaten, predominantly lytic destruction of the shaft and parallel bands of new periosteal bone are easily confused with Ewing's tumor (Fig. 11-79). Sunburst periosteal reactions are not uncommon.

The most important clinical and radiologic distinctions between neuroblastoma and Ewing's tumor or childhood lymphoma are a large single abdominal or posterior mediastinal mass, urinary catecholamines, and lytic lesions in the skull. Ewing's tumor patients are usually over age 5.

Gross Pathology

Gross examination shows visceral and bony neuroblastomas to be soft, white, lobulated, and hemorrhagic and sometimes to have yellow areas secondary to necrosis.

Autopsy has shown metastases to occur as follows: in the liver, 60 per cent; in regional lymph nodes, 55 per cent; in the lungs, 55 per cent; in the skeletal system, 45 per cent; in the gastrointestinal tract, 40 per cent; in the adrenal gland, 30 per cent; in the kidneys, 20 per cent; and in the mediastinum, 10 per cent.

Histopathology

A brief review of the embryogenesis of the sympathetic nervous system will help in the understanding of the classification and histology of neoplasms arising there. The anlage of the adrenal medulla, the sympathetic ganglia, the celiac plexus, and Zuckerkandl's organ are derived from a cell migration from the neural crest tissue of the embryo. The migratory cells, or sympathogonia, are the precursors of the differentiated elements of the sympathetic and parasympathetic nervous systems. Sympathogonia are divided into two cell lines: neuroblasts and lemmoblasts. Neuroblasts are either neuron or ganglion cells, and lemmoblasts are either interstitial or capsular cells of the ganglia. Neoplasms may develop from any of these cell lines. Completely undifferentiated tumors derived from neural crest tissue are called sympathogoniomas; incompletely differentiated tumors are called true neuroblastomas and lemmoblastomas; and fully differentiated tumors are called ganglioneuromas. The more undifferentiated the tumor, the more malignant it is. Tumors that start with an undifferentiated pattern occasionally develop later a more benign or well-differentiated pattern. In rare instances, growth stops.

Fully differentiated tumors of the sympathetic nervous system are easy to recognize histologically and do not metastasize unless they contain less well-differentiated components. In 10 to 20 per cent of the patients, neural differentiation is minimal or absent.

The more completely differentiated metastatic lesions produce diagnostic neural structures called rosettes (Plate 10, *I, top*) that must be distinguished from the rosette-like structures occasionally seen in Ewing's tumor (Fig. 11-70). Nerve stains confirm the well-defined cytoplasmic structures extending centrally as neurofibrils. The nuclei of neuroblastoma tend to resemble those of small lymphocytes or larger lymphoblasts. Particularly in the primary tumor, rosettes may be present in almost pure form, although generally they are most uncommon in the metastases. From a study of eight autopsy cases of metastatic neuroblastoma, only one showed any identifiable rosettes (personal observations). On the other hand, six of eight of the cases showed rosettes in the primary tumor. In this author's estimation too much is made of having to find rosettes in the metastases before one will diagnose or even consider metastatic neuroblastoma. This is unfortunate, because only a minority of cases contain this feature.

In the absence of rosettes, cells suggestive of neural derivation may be seen with tail-like or pointed eosinophilic cytoplasmic extensions creating "*pear*"- or "*carrot-shaped*" *cells* best seen under oil power (Fig. 11-80; Plate 10, *H* and *I*). They were present in seven of eight autopsies of neuroblastoma metastatic to the bone that we have examined. This feature is, therefore, of much more significance to diagnosis than

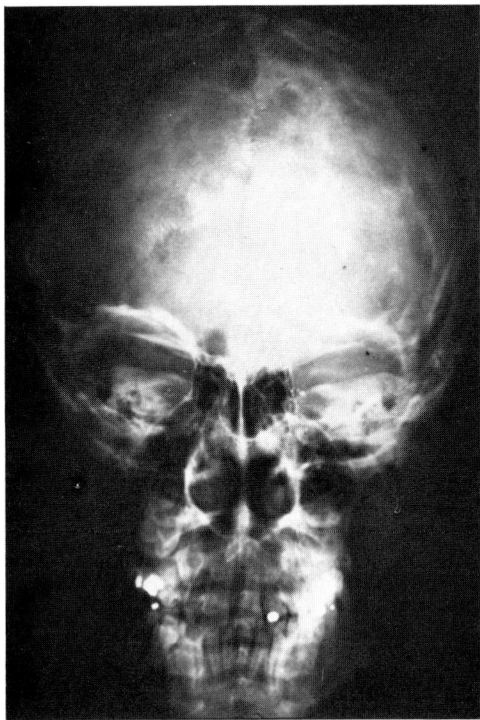

FIG. 11-77

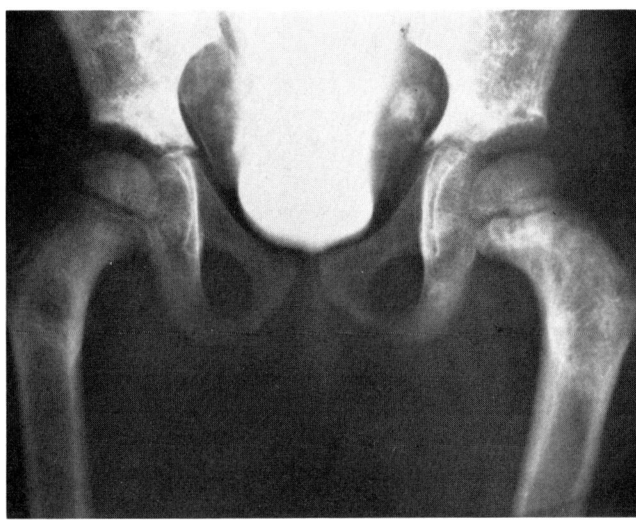

FIG. 11-78

Metastatic Neuroblastoma

FIG. 11-77. The most common malignant tumor in a child under age 10, characterized by multiple, punched-out holes in the skull, is metastatic neuroblastoma. Not all patients with this disease demonstrate this characteristic feature, however.

FIG. 11-78. Even if the skull is not involved, most patients with neuroblastoma will show evidence of multiple bone dissemination.

rosettes because of their greater incidence. In some cases, however, great patience is needed, and well-stained sections. In some slides only three to four such cells can be easily seen; in others, hundreds of such cells can be found. Well-prepared imprints show these cells much more clearly (Plate 10, *I*). Searching for them is similar to looking for tubercle organisms. Oil power should be used and hundreds of cells should be examined. However, it should be stressed that if imprints are not prepared properly, smearing of individual cells may occur. This may cause the originally round cells of Ewing's and lymphosarcoma, for example, to resemble the "pear"- and "carrot"-shaped cells of neuroblastoma. Therefore, their presence is of much more significance in well prepared, noncrushed, tissue sections. Other features of neuroblast cells are the following:

1. Occasional cells with *multiple nuclei* (Plate 10, *I*). Lymphocytic lymphoma does not show this feature of multinuclearity.
2. Exceedingly *long, tapered cytoplasm* and large nuclei with a single large nucleolus resembling ganglion cells (Plate 10, *I*).
3. *Uni- and bipolar cytoplasmic extensions* also a sign of neurally derived cells. The so-called "pear" and "carrot" cells (Plate 10, *H* and *I*).
4. In most cases and in well-prepared sections the cells can be seen to have *distinct cytoplasmic borders.* Lymphomas also have cells with distinctive cell borders. In Ewing's sarcoma, however, the cell borders are indistinct, pale, and lacey.
5. Neural cells often lay down a *fibrillary meshwork between cells,* which probably represents neurofibrillary cytoplasmic extensions (Fig.

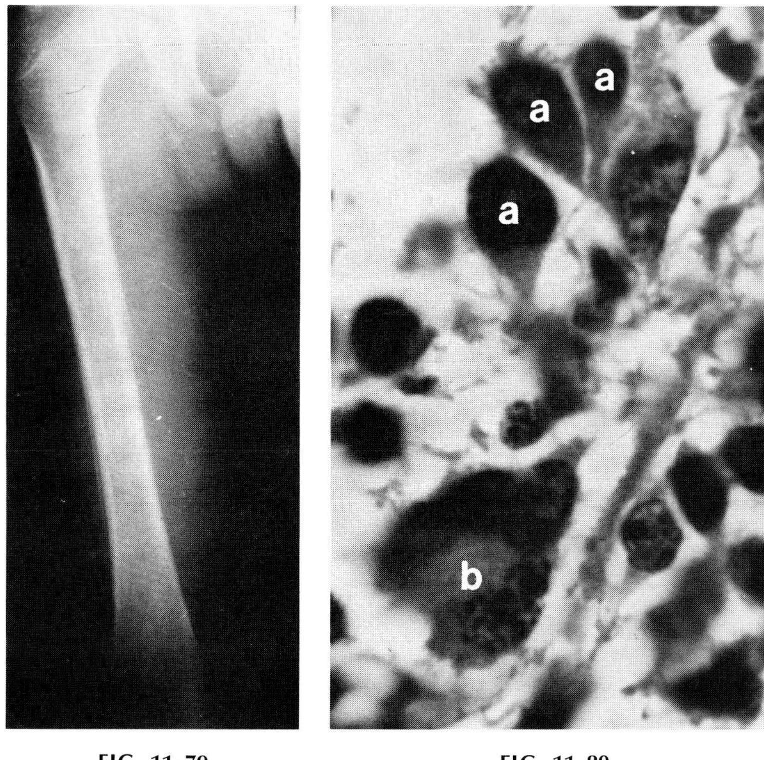

FIG. 11-79 FIG. 11-80

Metastatic Neuroblastoma

FIG. 11-79. On occasion, a patient may show involvement of only a single bone. Usually, these tumors will be mistaken both clinically and pathologically for Ewing's sarcoma. This radiograph shows a diffusely permeative pattern of bone destruction and "onion-skinning" in the midshaft of the femur, certainly compatible with, but not diagnostic of Ewing's sarcoma. Biopsy and subsequent VMA studies proved that this patient in reality had metastatic neuroblastoma.

FIG. 11-80. The virtually pathognomonic features of metastatic neuroblastoma of bone are the young age of the patient and the presence under oil power of the telltale "pear"- or "carrot"-shaped cells (*a*). Prominent multinucleation (*b*) is another characteristic rarely seen in Ewing's sarcoma or lymphocytic lymphomas. Two other malignancies of childhood may show tapered cytoplasm. They are the Wilm's tumor and the embryonal rhabdomyosarcoma. Rarely do these two tumors go undiscovered prior to metastatis. They infrequently metastasize to bone. On the other hand, neuroblastomas frequently metastasize to bone before discovery of the primary tumor.

11–61). Similarly the stromal background can resemble "brain tissue." In some cases neuroblastomas with large lymphoblast-like nuclei and fine fibrillary stroma will closely mimic the large nuclear and lacey pattern common to Ewing's tumor. The differentiation must depend upon careful assessment of all clinical, laboratory, radiographic, and microscopic features.

Differential Diagnosis

Refer to Table 11–1 for a summary of the features that serve to differentiate metastatic neuroblastoma from other round cell tumors of bone and to Figures 11–58 to 11–61 and Plate 10, *A–I*).

Course and Treatment

The 5-year survival rate of neuroblastoma is approximately 15 per cent. Most survivors are those who present before age 1. These infants will usually present with abdominal masses without other symptomatology. The tumor is solitary and encapsulated. Metastases do not develop for reasons that are unknown.

Once metastases have occurred, the course is almost inevitably fatal. In rare instances growth stops after radiation therapy or after further differentiation to well-differentiated ganglioneuroma. Recommended treatment of metastases is radiation and chemotherapy to the involved sites.

METASTATIC CARCINOMA AND MELANOMA

On occasion a poorly differentiated carcinoma may metastasize and present as an apparent pleomorphic "primary round cell tumor" resembling the primary reticulum cell sarcoma of bone. The diagnosis of metastatic carcinoma should be considered in any tumor of bone showing any suggestion of nesting, marked pleomorphism of nuclei, abundant cytoplasm, and large nucleoli. Most patients are adults. A bone survey and scans usually show more than a solitary focus of bone involvement. Mucin stains may be positive. The most common tumors metastatic to bone in which a primary carcinoma is found at a later time are from the lung, kidney, and thyroid. The lung tumors may be completely undifferentiated and show no evidence of acini or nesting. The hypernephroma shows clear and/or granular cells and usually some evidence of acinar formation. Some cancers metastatic to bone may show "innocuous" collections of small clear cells that I have seen numerous pathologists either overlook or mistake for focal collections of histiocytes with no diagnostic significance. There is no such thing as focal collections of "histiocytes" in bone without diagnostic significance. They most often represent Gaucher's disease, old eosinophilic granuloma, or subtly malignant cells, usually from either hypernephorma, prostate cancer, or metastatic paraganglioma. Except for the giant cell carcinoma of thyroid, acini are usually found in thyroid carcinoma metastases. Electron microscopy of these tumors usually shows signs of epithelial derivation.

Metastatic melanoma is characterized by sheets of rounded and/or spindle cells with abundant cytoplasm and prominent nucleoli. Melanin pigment should be searched for in any pleomorphic "round" or spindle cell tumor of bone that is difficult to classify. Special stains for melanin (Fontana stain) and electron microscopy are usually diagnostic for melanin, melanin precursors, and/or melanosomes. In most instances the patient has a history of a melanoma or an enlarging suspicious "nevus." A skeletal series including bone scan most often reveals evidence of multiple bone involvement.

REFERENCES

Benign Round Cell Tumors

1. Abt, A.F., and Denenholz, E.J.: Letterer-Siwe disease. Am. J. Dis. Child., *51:*499, 1936.
2. Aronson, R.P.: Streptomycin in Letterer-Siwe's disease. Lancet, *1:*889, 1951.
3. Avery, M., McAfee, J.G., and Guild, H.G.: The course and prognosis of reticuloendotheliosis (eosinophilic granuloma, Schüller-Christian disease and Letterer-Siwe disease). Am. J. Med., *22:*636, 1957.
4. Avioli, L.V., Lasersohn, J.T., and Loprasti, J.M.: Histiocytosis X (Schüller-Christian disease). Medicine, *42:*119, 1963.
5. Boss, M.H., Sapin, S.O., and Hodes, H.L.: Use of cortisone and corticotropin (A.C.T.H.) in treatment of reticuloendotheliosis in children. Am. J. Dis. Child., *85:*393, 1953.
6. Basset, F., Nézelof, C., Mallet, R., and Turiaf, J.: Nouvelle mise en evidence, par la microscopie electronique, de Particules d'allure virale dans une seconde forme clinique de l'histiocytose X, le granulome eosinophile de L'Os. C. R. Acad. Sci., *261:*5719, 1965.
7. Bassett, F., Nézelof, C., and Turiaf, J.: Présence en microscopie électronique de structure filamenteuses original dan les lesion pulmonaires et osseuses de l'histiocyte X. Bull. Mem. Soc. Med. Hosp. de Paris, *117:*413, 1966.
8. Cancilla, P.A., Lahey, M.E., and Carnes, W.H.: Cutaneous lesions of Letterer-Siwe disease. Cancer, *20:*1986, 1967.
9. Cheyne, C.: Histiocytosis X. J. Bone Joint Surg., *53B:*366, 1971.
10. Christian, H.A.: Defects in membranous bones, exophthalmos and diabetes insipidus: an unusual feature of dyspituitarism. Med. Clin. North Am., *3:*849, 1919–1920.
11. Cline, M., and Golde, D.W.: A review and re-evaluation of the histiocytic disorders. Am. J. Med., *55:*49, 1973.
12. Compere, E.L., Johnson, W.E., and Coventry M.B.: Vertebra plana due to eosinophilic granuloma. J. Bone Joint Surg., *36A:*969, 1954.
13. Dargeon, H.W.: Considerations in the treatment of reticuloendotheliosis. Am. J. Roentgenol. Radium Ther. and Nucl. Med., *93:*521, 1905.
14. Dargeon, H.W.: Reticuloendotheliosis in childhood. Springfield, Charles C Thomas, 1967.
15. Doede, K.G., and Rappaport, H.: Long term survival of patients with acute disseminated histiocytosis (Letterer-Siwe disease). Cancer, *20:*1782, 1967.
16. Enriquez, P., Dahlin, D.C., Hayles, A.B., and Henderson, E.D.: Histiocytosis X. Mayo Clin. Proc., *42:*88, 1967.
17. Farber, S.: The nature of "solitary eosinophilic granuloma" of bone. Am. J. Pathol., *17:*625, 1941.
18. Friedman, B., and Hanaoke, H.: Langerhans cell

granules in eosinophilic granuloma of bone. J. Bone Joint Surg., *51A:* 367, 1969.
19. Green, W.T., and Farber, S.: "Eosinophilic or solitary granuloma" of bone. J. Bone Joint Surg., *24:* 499, 1942.
20. Haas, G.M.: Hepato-adrenal necrosis with intranuclear inclusion bodies. Am. J. Pathol., *11:* 127, 1935.
21. Hand, A.: Defects of membranous bones, exophthalmos and polyuria in childhood: is it Dyspituitarism? Am. J. Med. Sci., *162:* 509, 1921.
22. Jaffe, H.L.: Metabolic, Degenerative and Inflammatory Diseases of Bones and Joints. pp. 875–906. Philadelphia, Lea & Febiger, 1972.
23. Jaffe, H.L., and Lichtenstein, L.: Eosinophilic granuloma of bone. Arch. Pathol., *37:* 99, 1944.
24. Letterer, E.: "Aleukämische retickulose. Frank. Zeit. Pathol., *30:* 377, 1924.
25. Lichtenstein, L.: Histiocytosis X. Arch. Pathol., *56:* 84, 1953.
26. Lichtenstein, L.: Histiocytosis X. J. Bone Joint Surg., *46A:* 76, 1964.
27. Lichtenstein, L., and Jaffe, H.L.: Eosinophilic granuloma of bone. Am. J. Pathol., *16:* 595, 1946.
28. Liebermann, P.H., Jones, C.R., Dargeon, H.W.K., and Begg, C.F.: A reappraisal of eosinophilic granuloma, Hand-Schüller-Christian syndrome and Letterer-Siwe syndrome. Medicine, *48:* 375, 1969.
29. Mermann, A.C., and Dargeon, H.W.: The management of certain nonlipid reticuloendothelioses. Cancer, *8:* 112, 1955.
30. Morales, A.R., Fine G., Horn, R.C., Jr., and Watson, J.H.C.: Langerhans cells in a localized lesion of eosinophilic granuloma type. Lab. Invest., *20:* 412, 1969.
31. Oberman, H.A.: Idiopathic histiocytosis. Pediatrics, *28:* 307, 1961.
32. Otani, S.: A discussion of eosinophilic granuloma of bone, Letterer-Siwe disease and Schüller-Christian disease. J. Mt. Sinai Hosp., *24:* 1079, 1957.
33. Otani, S., and Ehrlich, J.C.: Solitary granuloma simulating primary neoplasm. Am. J. Pathol., *16:* 479, 1940.
34. Schajowicz, F., and Polak, M.: Contribucion al estudio del denominado "granuloma eosinophilico" y sus relaciones con la xanthomosis ossea. Rev. Assoc. Medica Argent., *61:* 218, 1947.
35. Schajowicz, F., and Slullitel, J.: Eosinophilic granuloma and its relationship to Hand-Schüller-Christian and Letterer-Siwe syndromes. J. Bone Joint Surg., *55B:* 545, 1973.
36. Schuller, A.: Über eigenartige schädel defekte Im jugandalter. Fortschr. Geb. Rontgen., *23:* 12, 1915.
37. Siwe, S.: The reticulo-endothelioses in children. Adv. Pediatrics, *4:* 117, 1949.
38. Stern, M.B., Cassidy, R., and Mirra, J.M.: Eosinophilic granuloma of the proximl tibial epiphysis. Clin. Orthop., *118:* 153, 1976.
39. Wallgren, A.: Systemic reticuloendothelial granuloma. Am. J. Dis. Child., *60:* 471, 1940.

Gaucher's Disease

40. Amstutz, H.C., and Carey, E.J.: Skeletal manifestations and treatment of Gaucher's disease. J. Bone Joint Surg., *48A:* 670, 1966.
41. Arkin, A.M., and Schein, A.J.: Aseptic necrosis in Gaucher's disease. J. Bone Joint Surg., *30A:* 631, 1948.
42. Atkinson, F.R.B.: Gaucher's disease in children. Br. J. Dis. Child., *35:* 1, 1938.
43. Fisher, C.R., and Reidbord, H.: Gaucher's disease: pathogenetic considerations based on electron microscopic and histochemical observations. Am. J. Path., *41:* 679, 1962.
44. Geddes, A.K., and Moore, S.: Acute infantile Gaucher's disease. J. Pediatr., *43:* 61, 1953.
45. Greenfield, G.B.: Bone changes in chronic adult Gaucher's disease. Am. J. Roentgenol. Radium Ther. Nucl. Med., *110:* 800, 1970.
46. Groen, J.: The hereditary mechanism of Gaucher's disease. Blood, *3:* 1238, 1948.
47. Jackson, D.C., and Simon, G.: Unusual bone and lung changes in a case of Gaucher's disease. Br. J. Radiol., *38:* 698, 1965.
48. Jaffe, H.L.: Metabolic, Degenerative and Inflammatory Diseases of Bones and Joints. pp. 506–564. Philadelphia, Lea & Febiger, 1972.
49. Kennaway, N.G., and Woolf, L.I.: Splenic lipids in Gaucher's disease. J. Lipid Res., *9:* 755, 1968.
50. Matoth, Y., and Fried, K.: Chronic Gaucher's disease. Isr. J. Med. Sci., *1:* 521, 1965.
51. Morgans, M.E.: Gaucher's disease without splenomegaly. Clin. Orthop., *24:* 213, 1962.
52. Murray, R.O., and Jacobson, H.G.: The Radiology of Skeletal Disorders. pp. 616. London, J. & A. Churchill, 1977.
53. Rourke, J.A., and Heslin, D.J.: Gaucher's disease. Roentgenologic bone changes over 20 year interval. Am. J. Roentgenol. Radium Ther. Nucl. Med., *94:* 621, 1965.
54. Statter, M., and Shapiro, B.: Studies on the etiology of Gaucher's disease. Isr. J. Med. Sci., *1:* 514, 1965.
55. Tuchman, L.R., Suna, H., and Carr, J.J.: Elevation of serum acid phosphatase in Gaucher's disease. J. Mt. Sinai Hosp., *23:* 227, 1958.

Myeloma

56. Carson, C.P., Ackerman, L.V., and Maltby, J.D.: Plasma cell myeloma. A clinical pathologic and roentgenographic review of 90 cases. Am. J. Clin. Pathol., *25:* 849, 1955.
57. Cohen, D.M., Svien, H.J., and Dahlin, D.C.: Long term survival of patients with myeloma of the vertebral column. J.A.M.A., *187:* 914, 1967.
58. Cohen, H.J., Lessin, L.S., Hallal, J., and Burkholder, P.: Resolution of primary amyloidosis during chemotherapy. Studies in a patient with nephrotic syndrome. Ann. Intern. Med., *82:* 466, 1975.

59. Erf, L.A., and Herbut, P.A.: Comparative cytology of Wright's stained smears and histologic sections in multiple myeloma. Am. J. Clin. Pathol., *16:* 1, 1946.
60. Nordenson, N.G.: Myelomatosis. A clinical review of 310 cases. Acta. Med. Scand. [Supp.], *179:* 178, 1966.
60a. Pasmantier, M.W., and Azar, H.A.: Extraskeletal spread in multiple plasma cell myeloma. A review of 57 autopsied cases. Cancer, *23:* 167, 1969.
61. Porter, F.S., Jr.: Multiple myeloma in a child. J. Pediatr., *62:* 602, 1963.
62. Stevens, A.R., Jr.: Evolution of multiple myeloma. Arch. Intern. Med., *115:* 90, 1965.

Hodgkin's Disease

63. Coles, W.C., and Schulz, M.D.: Bone involvement in malignant lymphoma. Radiology, *50:* 458, 1948.
64. Dennis, J.M.: The solitary dense vertebral body. Radiology, *77:* 618, 1962.
65. Falconer, E.H., and Leonard, M.E.: Skeletal lesions in Hodgkin's disease. Ann. Intern. Med., *29:* 1115, 1948.
65a. Gold, R., and Mirra, J.M.: Primary Hodgkin's disease of bone. Skel. Radiol., 1979, *In press.*
66. Horan, F.T.: Bone involvement in Hodgkin's disease. A survey of 201 cases. Br. J. Surg., *56:* 277, 1969.
67. Lukes, R.J., and Butler, J.J.: The pathology and nomenclature of Hodgkin's disease. Cancer Res., *26:* 1063, 1966.
68. Neiman, R.S., Rosen, P.S., and Lukes, R.J.: Lymphocyte depletion in Hodgkin's Disease. New Engl. J. Med., *288:* 751, 1963.
69. O'Carroll, D.I., McKenna, R.W., and Brunning, R.D.: Bone marrow manifestations of Hodgkin's disease. Cancer, *38:* 1717, 1976.
70. Steiner, P.E.: Hodgkin's disease. Arch. Pathol., *36:* 627, 1943.
71. Stuhlbard, J., and Ellis, F.W.: Hodgkin's disease of bone. Am. J. Roentgenol. Radium Ther. Nucl. Med., *93:* 568, 1965.
72. Ultmann, J.E.: Clinical features and diagnosis of Hodgkin's disease. Cancer, *19:* 297, 1966.
73. Vieta, J.O., Friedell, H.L., and Craver, L.F.: A survey of Hodgkin's disease and lymphosarcoma in bone. Radiology, *39:* 1, 1942.

Primary Reticulum Cell Sarcoma of Bone

74. Boston, H.C., Dahlin, D.C., Ivins, J.C., and Cupps, R.E.: Malignant lymphoma (so-called reticulum cell sarcoma) of bone. Cancer, *34:* 1131, 1974.
75. Coley, B.L., Higinbotham, N.L., and Groesbeck, H.P.: Primary reticulum-cell sarcoma of bone—summary of 37 cases. Radiology, *55:* 641, 1950.
76. Dahlin, D.C.: Malignant Lymphoma of Bone (Reticulum Cell Sarcoma) Bone Tumors. ed. 2. pp. 126–137. Springfield, Charles C Thomas, 1967.
77. Francis, K.C., Higinbotham, N.L., and Coley, B.L.: Primary reticulum cell sarcoma of bone. Report of 44 cases. Surg. Gynecol. Obstet., *99:* 142, 1954.
78. Ivins, J.C., and Dahlin, D.C.: Malignant lymphoma (reticulum cell sarcoma) of bone. Mayo Clin. Proc., *38:* 375, 1963.
79. Magnus, H.A., and Wood, H.L.C.: Primary reticulosarcoma of bone. J. Bone Joint Surg., *38B:* 258, 1956.
80. Parker, F., Jr., and Jackson, H., Jr.: Primary reticulum-cell sarcoma of bone. Surg. Gynecol. Obstet., *68:* 45, 1939.
81. Rice, R.W., Cabot, A., and Johnston, A.D.: The application of electron microscopy to the diagnostic differentiation of Ewing's sarcoma and reticulum cell sarcoma of bone. Clin. Orthop., *91:* 174, 1975.
82. Schajowicz, F.: Ewing's sarcoma and reticulum-cell sarcoma of bone—with special reference to the histochemical demonstration of glycogen as an aid to differential diagnosis. J. Bone Joint Surg., *41A:* 349, 1959.
83. Sherman, R.S., and Snyder, R.E.: The roentgen appearance of primary reticulum cell sarcoma of bone. Am. J. Roentgenol. Radium Ther. Nucl. Med., *58:* 291, 1947.
84. Shoji, H., and Miller, J.R.: Primary reticulum cell sarcoma of bone—significance of clinical features upon the prognosis. Cancer, *28:* 1234, 1971.
85. Wong, C.C., and Fleigohli, D.J.: Primary reticulum cell sarcoma of bone—with emphasis on radiation therapy. Cancer, *22:* 994, 1968.
86. Wilson, J.W., and Pugh, D.R.: Primary reticulum-cell sarcoma of bone, with emphasis on roentgen aspects. Radiology, *65:* 343, 1955.

Ewing's Sarcoma

87. Bhansali, S.K., and Desai, P.B.: Ewing's sarcoma. J. Bone Joint Surg., *45A:* 541, 1963.
88. Coley, B.L.: Neoplasms of Bone. Hagerstown, Hoeber Medical Division, 1949.
89. Coley, B.L., Higinbotham, N.L., and Bowden, L.: Endothelioma of bone (Ewing's sarcoma). Ann. Surg., *128:* 533, 1948.
90. Colville, H.C., and Willis, R.A.: Neuroblastoma metastasis in bones, with criticism of Ewing's endothelioma. Am. J. Pathol., *9:* 421, 1933.
91. Dahlin, D.C.: Ewing's Sarcoma and Malignant Lymphoma (Reticulum-Cell) Sarcoma of Bone In Tumors of Bone and Soft Tissue. Chicago, Year Book Publishers, 1965.
92. Dahlin, D.C.: Bone Tumors. ed. 2. Springfield, Charles C Thomas, 1967.
93. Ewing, J.: Diffuse endothelioma of bone. Proc. N.Y. Pathol. Soc., *21:* 17, 1921.
94. Ewing, J.: Neoplastic Diseases. ed. 4. Philadelphia, W.B. Saunders, 1940.
95. Freidman, B., and Gold, H.: Ultrastructure of Ewing's sarcoma of bone. Cancer, *22:* 307, 1968.

96. Kadin, M.E., and Bensch, K.G.: On the origin of Ewing's tumor. Cancer, *27:*257, 1971.
97. Lichtenstein, L., and Jaffe, H.L.: Ewing's sarcoma of bone. Am. J. Pathol., *23:*43, 1947.
98. MacIntosh, D.J., Price, H.G., and Jeffree, G.M.: Ewing's tumor. A study of behavior and treatment in 47 cases. J. Bone Joint Surg., *57B:*331, 1975.
99. Marsden, H.B., and Steward, J.K.: Ewing's tumors and neuroblastomas. J. Clin. Pathol., *17:*411, 1964.
100. Price, C.H.G., and Ross, F.G.M.: Bone—Certain Aspects of Neoplasia. London, Butterworth & Co., 1972.
101. Schajowicz, F.: Ewing's sarcoma and reticulum-cell sarcoma of bone—with special reference to the histochemical demonstration of glycogen as an aid to differential diagnosis. J. Bone Joint Surg., *41A:*349, 1959.
102. Stout, A.P.: A discussion of the pathology and histogenesis of Ewing's tumor of bone marrow. Am. J. Pathol., *50:*334, 1943.
103. Wang, C.C., and Schulz, M.D.: Ewing's sarcoma—study of 50 cases treated at M.G.H., 1930–52 inclusive. New Engl. J. Med., *248:*571, 1953.
104. Willis, R.A.: Metastatic neuroblastoma in bone presenting the Ewing's syndrome, with a discussion of "Ewing's sarcoma." Am. J. Pathol., *16:*317, 1940.
105. Willis, R.A.: Pathology of Tumors. ed. 4. London, Butterworth & Co., 1967.

Lymphomas and Leukemia of Bone

106. Coles, W.C., and Schulz, M.D.: Bone involvement in malignant lymphoma. Radiology, *50:*458, 1948.
107. Craver, L.F., and Copeland, M.M.: Lymphosarcoma in bone. Arch. Surg., *28:*809, 1934.
108. Jaffe, H.C.: Tumor and Tumorous Conditions of the Bones and Joints. Philadelphia, Lea and Febiger, 1958.
109. Lukes, R.J., and Collins, R.D.: New approaches to the classification of lymphomata. Br. J. Cancer Suppl., *31:*1, 1975.
110. Patchechefsky, A.S., *et. al.:* Non-Hodgkin's lymphomas: a clinicopathologic study of 293 cases. Cancer, *34:*1173, 1974.
111. Pear, B.L.: Skeletal manifestations of the lymphomas and leukemias. Semin. Roentgenol., *9:*929, 1974.
112. Rappaport, H.: Tumors of the Hematopoietic System. Atlas of Tumor Pathology. Section III, Fasc. 8, Washington, D.C., A.F.I.P. 1966.
113. Rosenthal, N.: The lymphomas and leukemias. Bull. N.Y. Acad. Med., *30:*583, 1954.
114. Thomas, L.B., *et. al.:* The skeletal lesions in acute leukemia. Cancer, *14:*608, 1961.
115. Vieta, J.O., Friedell, H.L., and Craver, L.E.: A survey of Hodgkin's disease and lymphosarcoma in bone. Radiology, *39:*1, 1942.

Metastatic Neuroblastoma

116. Barden, R.P.: The similarity of clinical and roentgen features in children with Ewing's sarcoma and sympathetic neuroblastoma. Am. J. Roentgenol. Radium Ther. Nucl. Med., *50:*575, 1943.
117. Blacklock, J.W.S.: Neurogenic tumors of sympathetic system in children. J. Pathol., *39:*27, 1934.
118. Bodian, M.: Neuroblastoma. Radiol. Clin. North Am., *6:*449, 1959.
119. Fortner, J., Nicastri, A., and Murphey, M.L.: Neuroblastoma: natural history and results of treating 133 cases. Ann. Surg., *167:*132, 1968.
120. Gitlow, S.E., *et. al.:* Diagnosis of neuroblastoma by qualitative and quantitative determination of catecholamine metabolites in urine. Cancer, *25:*1377, 1970.
121. Goldstein, M.N., and Pinkel, D.: Long-term tissue culture of neuroblastomas. J. Natl. Cancer Inst., *20:*675, 1958.
122. Horn, R.C., Koop, C.E., and Kiescuetter, W.B.: Neuroblastoma in childhood. Lab. Invest., *5:*106, 1956.
123. de Lorimer, A.A., Bragg, K.U., and Linden, G.: Neuroblastoma in childhood. Am. J. Dis. Child., *118:*441, 1969.
124. Murray, M.R., and Stout, A.P.: Distinctive characteristics of the sympathicoblastoma cultivated in vitro: method for prompt diagnosis. Am. J. Pathol., *23:*429, 1947.
125. Murray, M.R., and Stout, A.P.: The classification and diagnosis of human tumors by tissue culture methods. Tex. Rep. Biol. Med., *12:*898, 1954.
126. Price, C.H.G., and Ross, F.G.N.: Bone—Certain Aspects of Neoplasia. London, Butterworth & Co., 1972.
127. Scott, E., Oliver, M.G., and Oliver, M.H.: Sympathetic tumors of the adrenal medulla. Am. J. Cancer, *17:*396, 1933.
128. Stowens, D.: Neuroblastoma and related tumors. Arch. Pathol., *63:*457, 1957.
129. Willis, R.A.: Metastatic neuroblastoma in bone presenting the Ewing's syndrome, with a discussion of "Ewing's sarcoma." Am. J. Pathol., *16:*317, 1940.
130. Willis, R.A.: Pathology of Tumors. ed. 4. London, Butterworth & Co., and New York, Appleton-Century-Crofts, 1967.
131. Wyatt, G.M., and Farber, S.: Neurblastoma sympatheticum. Am. J. Roentgenol. Radium Ther. Nucl. Med., *46:*485, 1941.

INTRAOSSEOUS EPITHELIAL CELL AND EPITHELIAL-LIKE-PRODUCING TUMORS

12

Epithelial or epithelial-like tumors that involve the bone secondarily include the epidermal inclusion cyst, cholesteatomata, epidermidalization of draining sinus tracts of chronic osteomyelitis, and metastatic and directly invasive carcinomas. The low-grade malignant adamantinoma of long limb bones is the only true epithelial-like primary tumor of bone other than the epithelial tumors of the jaw, which fall outside the scope of this text. The adamantinoma of jaw bones is related to the epithelium of developing teeth. Although the name used is the same for both tumors, they should not be confused as having an identical histogenesis. The reader is referred to books of oral pathology when encountering an epithelial tumor of jawbones.

The carcinomas commonly involve bone by either metastasis or by direct invasion. In fact, they are the most common tumor of adult bones, outnumbering primary bone tumors approximately 25 to 1. It should be stated, however, that biopsied material is significantly lower than this ratio, since many metastatic lesions are obvious clinical diagnoses. The epidermal inclusion cyst, adamantinoma of long limb bones, and epidermidalization of chronic draining osteomyelitis tracts extending into bone are in contrast rare bone tumors.

BENIGN TUMORS

Epidermal Inclusion Cyst

The epidermal inclusion cyst may erode into bone by a direct pressure effect. Most commonly these occur in relation to the distal phalanges (Fig. 12–1). Less commonly they may erode the middle phalanges, skull, sternum, or wherever the skin is in very close proximity to bone and where epidermal inclusion cysts are prone to occur. The epidermal inclusion cyst is usually a round tumor and its intraosseous appearance is also usually sharply rounded or circumscribed (Fig. 12–1). The epidermal inclusion cyst and glomus tumor are the two most common tumors that involve the distal tuft. The glomus tumor is clinically distinguishable by the exquisite pain produced upon palpation. Pathologically, the two lesions are easily separable.

Cholesteatoma and Epidermoid Tumor of Calvarium

Cholesteatomas consist of benign squamous epithelium, keratin, cholesterol crystals, macrophages, and chronic inflammatory cells. There is usually a history of chronic mastoiditis. They may erode into the adjacent bony structures.

The epidermoid tumor of calvarium, also called the "pearly" tumor, usually occurs in young adults. The lesion may arise from either table of the skull or from the diploë. Although they contain similar tissues to those described in cholesteatoma, their origin is believed to be congenital rather than secondary to chronic infection. Radiologically, the "pearly" tumor has distinctive features. It is a slowly expanding lytic lesion with a distinctly benign border of reactive host bone sclerosis. Within the lesion the pattern is often mottled. The lesion is usually solitary although satellite lesions may be noted. A soft-tissue mass is uncommon.

Epidermidalization (Pseudoepitheliomatous Hyperplasia) Versus Squamous Carcinoma of Draining Sinus Tracts

Chronic osteomyelitis can result in longstanding draining sinus tracts. The edges of the tracts can become lined by squamous epithelium. After many years the epithelial base may be so undermined by inflammation that extensive infiltration of this granulation tissue base may occur, leading to the pseudoepitheliomatous hyperplasia. In some cases the epithelial process can give rise to extensive acanthosis and a "heaped-up" appearance on gross observation. The clinical appearance of a granular heaped-up epithelial tumefaction, pseudoepitheliomatous hyperplasia within the sinus tract of the dermis and bone can lead to considerable clinical and pathologic diagnostic difficulties.

The problem is in separating pseudoepitheliomatous hyperplasia with mild to moderate inflammatory-induced cytologic atypia from a low-grade or well-differentiated squamous cell carcinoma, especially since squamous carcinoma is one of the well-known malignant complications of long-standing chronic osteomyelitis with draining sinuses.

In a review by Sedlin and Fleming,[5] their conclusions were that carcinoma can occur in at least 0.5 per cent of patients with chronic draining osteomyelitis. The average latent interval was 30 years but could be much shorter.

Johnson and Kempson extensively review the problem of distinguishing pseudoepitheliomatous hyperplasia from carcinomatous transformation.[3] They point out that the best method to avoid carcinomatous or sarcomatous transformation of the wound tissues is by prevention. The physicians should utilize adequate drainage, sequestrectomy, removal of foreign bodies, and antibiotic therapy. If the draining sinuses are healed, there is, of course, no chance for carcinoma to develop.

Whether or not the patients had developed cancer or marked pseudoepitheliomatous hyperplasia, they all experienced a change in signs and symptoms. The various changes included increasing pain, change in the character of the pain to sharp and biting, increase of a foul exudate, development of a mass, and bleeding or loss of function of the limb. Johnson and Kempson recommend a thorough physical examination for regional lymph node metastases and liver enlargement or radiographs to check for increased bone destruction, soft-tissue mass, or pathologic fracture. Extensive bone destruction may be seen with pseudoepitheliomatous hyperplasia; on the other hand, carcinoma may show minimal bone destruction. Therefore, the biopsy is the most important diagnostic procedure. They divided the biopsy findings into three groups: (*1*) benign, (*2*) atypical pseudoepitheliomatous hyperplasia, and (*3*) epidermoid carcinoma. The first and third groups are self-explanatory. The second group was designated atypical pseudoepitheliomatous hyperplasia on the basis of sheets of squamous cells invading tissue widely that could include the bone. The individual cells usually show little to no atypical features, absence of non-mirror image mitoses, and no evidence of lymphatic permeation or vessel invasion. This is the group for which they felt it was impossible, on clinical or histologic grounds, to determine whether the changes were benign or malignant, unless metastases were present. Therefore, errors in diagnosis were confined to this group.

Their recommendations were that patients with atypical pseudoepitheliomatous hyperplasia (Group II) should be treated by amputation because in some instances an epidermoid carcinoma may be missed because the tumor is so well differentiated that a definite histologic diagnosis of carcinoma cannot be made and because almost all patients with this form of hyperplasia have a nonfunctioning limb.

This author is in basic agreement with their recommendations, provided that it were not considered feasible to obtain a functional limb short of amputation by an extensive en-bloc resection of the infected bone, soft tissues, and overlying dermis and skin, to be followed by the use of prosthetic devices and bone and skin grafting.

LOW-GRADE MALIGNANT NEOPLASMS

ADAMANTINOMA OF LONG-LIMB BONES

CAPSULE SUMMARY (FIG. 12-2)

Incidence. Some 0.3 per cent of primary bone tumors.

Age. About equally distributed between ages of 10 and 50.

Clinical Features. Dull, aching pain, gradual swelling of involved area; occasional fracture.

Radiologic Features. Over 90 per cent arise in the tibial diaphysis. Cystic, multiloculated, or bubbly.

Gross Pathology. Grayish white, firm, areas of cystic or hemorrhagic softening.

Histopathology. Cords or islands of epithelial-like cells, slitlike spaces lined by epithelial-like cells, bland, fibrovascular stromal component.

Course. Approximately 60 per cent 5-year survival and 40 per cent 10-year survival rate.

Treatment. En-bloc excision versus amputation.

Clinical Features

The most *common presenting* complaints are dull aching pain and gradual swelling; occasionally a pathologic fracture is present. More than half of the patients give a history of antecedent trauma to the affected site. Rare cases have been reported of the concurrence of fibrous dysplasia in association with adamantinoma of long bones.[10] However, review of these cases shows absolutely no evidence to support fibrous dysplasia in bones other than the involved tibia and/or fibula, nor signs such as café au lait spots or precocious puberty. Several patients died of metastatic adamantinoma. It is much more likely that adamantinoma of the tibia and/or fibula can sometimes give rise to a "reactive" fibro-osseous sclerosis, which histologically, can be mistaken for or mimic fibrous dysplasia. This latter concept, which best explains the facts, is championed by Weiss and Dorfman,[21a] with whom this author agrees.

Radiologic Features

The *radiologic appearance* varies from a small to an extensive, bubbly, multiloculated radiolucent lesion involving the midshaft and occasionally extending into the metaphysis (Figs. 12-3–12-6). Variable degrees of osteosclerosis are seen in the larger lesions. In some cases, both the tibia and fibula or radius and ulna may be affected concomitantly.

The periosteum may be elevated, resulting in "expansion" of bone. The lesions may be centrally or eccentrically located.

Because of the extreme rarity of this lesion the diagnosis is not often made on initial examination. Most commonly the lesion is thought to represent a focus of fibrous dysplasia, nonossifying fibroma, metastatic disease, or vascular sarcoma.

The diagnosis of adamantinoma should always be considered in any cystic to bubbly lesion of the tibial and/or fibular diaphysis. The tumors tend to begin in the anterior portion of the bone (Fig. 12-3). They can be eccentrically placed along the anterior surface, in close proximity to the skin. This supports the contention that they may arise from congenital epithelial rests. The anterior portion of the tibia is, of course, closest to the skin surface.

Gross Pathology and Specimen Radiographs

The tumors are gray to white or yellowish and usually firm; occasionally they are soft or gritty. The external contours are smooth to lobulated. Cystic degeneration and foci of hemorrhage are not uncommon. The tumor may involve cortex and periosteum and even show penetration through the periosteum to involve the soft tissues and dermis.

If specimen radiographs are taken of the gross slabs, quite often areas of bone resorption by small lobular extensions of tumor are seen several centimeters beyond what is apparent on the *in vivo* or standard patient radiographs (Fig. 12-6). The clinical implications of this important finding are discussed in the treatment section.

Histopathology

The key feature is the presence of epithelial-like cells with minimal nuclear atypia embedded in a fibrous stroma. The fibrous stroma is heavily collagenized and contains thin, entirely innocuous-appearing fibroblastic nuclei. The second feature is the presence of plump, rounded, or slightly oval to spindled cells, which to most authors resemble cells of epithelial origin although some believe they more closely resemble cells of vascular or synovial origin. To this author the cells of an adamantinoma most closely mimic those of the basosquamous cell carcinoma, because on rare occasion foci of cells with prickles (Fig. 12-11) can be found. The basal carcinoma-like cells have a round to oval, small- to moderate-sized nucleus with fairly even chromatin distribution, small to absent nucleoli, and rare to occasional typical mitotic figures. The cytoplasm is light pink and usually no greater in volume than the nucleus. The cytoplasmic borders can be either distinct or indistinct.

These cells arrange themselves in the fibrous stroma in a variety of patterns, including rounded nests or islands that most resemble basal cell carcinoma (Figs. 12–7 and 12–8), short to long cordlike or tubular structures in which the nuclei may assume a "boxcar-like" orientation mimicking infiltrating lobular or ductal carcinomas of breast (Figs. 12–9, right, and 12–10), single to multiple layers of cells arranged around a slit-like space (Fig. 12–9, left) resembling a vascular tumor, synovial sarcoma, and on rare occasion squamous metaplasia located either focally within nests of the smaller cells or more diffusely (Fig. 12–11). Within these squamous foci the cytoplasm is pink and two to three times the diameter of the nucleus. On very rare occasion squamous pearls and unequivocal prickles are seen. In the important case reported by Donner[11] focal nests showed intercellular bridges, keratohyalin granules, and pearl formation.

Some cases show considerably more atypia of the epithelial-like cells and the stroma. Perhaps the tumor should be graded as showing minimal (Grade I), moderate (Grade II) or severe (Grade III) nuclear atypia, and the biologic course correlated with these features. The degree of atypia of the epithelial component may be different from that of the stromal component. To this author's knowledge grading of the components of the adamantinoma has not been performed and correlated with this tumor's clinical course. On occasion, the tumor may be associated with a pronounced fibro-osseous response that may be confused with fibrous dysplasia. Multiple sections will usually demonstrate small islands or nests of adamantinoma cells within this stromal response.

The occurrence of a diaphyseal, lytic cystic lesion with a basal cell or metastatic breast carcinoma-like pattern typifies the vast majority of adamantinomas of the long limb bones. The diagnosis is not difficult, but this tumor is often not thought of because it is one of the rarest tumors of bone. Nevertheless, it is wise to confirm the diagnosis by ruling out by clinical investigation any chance that the tumor might be a metastatic breast or other carcinoma. On rare occasion such an investigation may reveal metastasis from a small, originally undetected breast primary. The vast majority of tibial lesions with the above histologic features prove to be adamantinomas after a systemic work-up for a primary carcinoma elsewhere.

Origin of the Adamantinoma

Several theories have been set forth on the possible origin of the adamantinoma. These include embryonic nests of basal epithelium misplaced by budlike growth during embryonal development;[12] trauma with implantation of basal cells (many of the patients have had a history of specific trauma to the area short of fracture); endothelial or angioblastic origin;[9] and synovial sarcoma.[13,16] Electron microscopic studies[19,20,22] favor an epithelial origin to the tumor, because the tumor cells show prominent desmosomes and tonofibrils and bundles of microfilaments. On a light microscopic level, it is hard to refute Jaffe's statement that the "finding of some degree of squamous differentiation of the tumor cells of the lesion is not compatible with the 'angioblastic theory.'"[15] The case reported by Donner shows unequivocal typical adamantinoma associated with pearl formation, prickles, and keratohyalin granules.[11] Squamous differentiation also casts grave doubt on the synovial sarcoma or endothelial histogenetic theories, because endothelial or synovial cells have never been shown to undergo squamous metaplasia in any other lesion. Jaffe doubts the trauma theory because of the fact that not a single case of adamantinoma has ever followed upon an open fracture despite the thousands of such incidents.[15]

To this author the most attractive theory is that of Fischer,[12] who contends that the tumor arises from a portion of epithelium trapped in bone during embryonal development (embryonic "rest" theory) and which after many years in a certain percentage of cases, undergoes transformation to a malignant tumor. Jaffe had doubts about this theory because it was difficult for him to conceive that the epithelium in "rest" retains its capacity for specialized differentiation for so many years before it becomes activated to undergo neoplastic proliferation.[15] Unfortunately, I do not find this objection valid. It is well known, for example, that the embryonic notochord may not become totally obliterated during adult life and may be found in rests (ecchordosis physaliphora). These rests have been found to occur most often in the region of the clivus and sacrum, identical in distribution to the most frequent sites of origin of the notochordally derived tumor known as the chordoma. The chordoma retains its specialized cellular and matrix features, which enable it to be identified as being of notochordal origin, and the tumor usually undergoes malignant transformation in adulthood many years after its embryonic function has ceased. Other benign

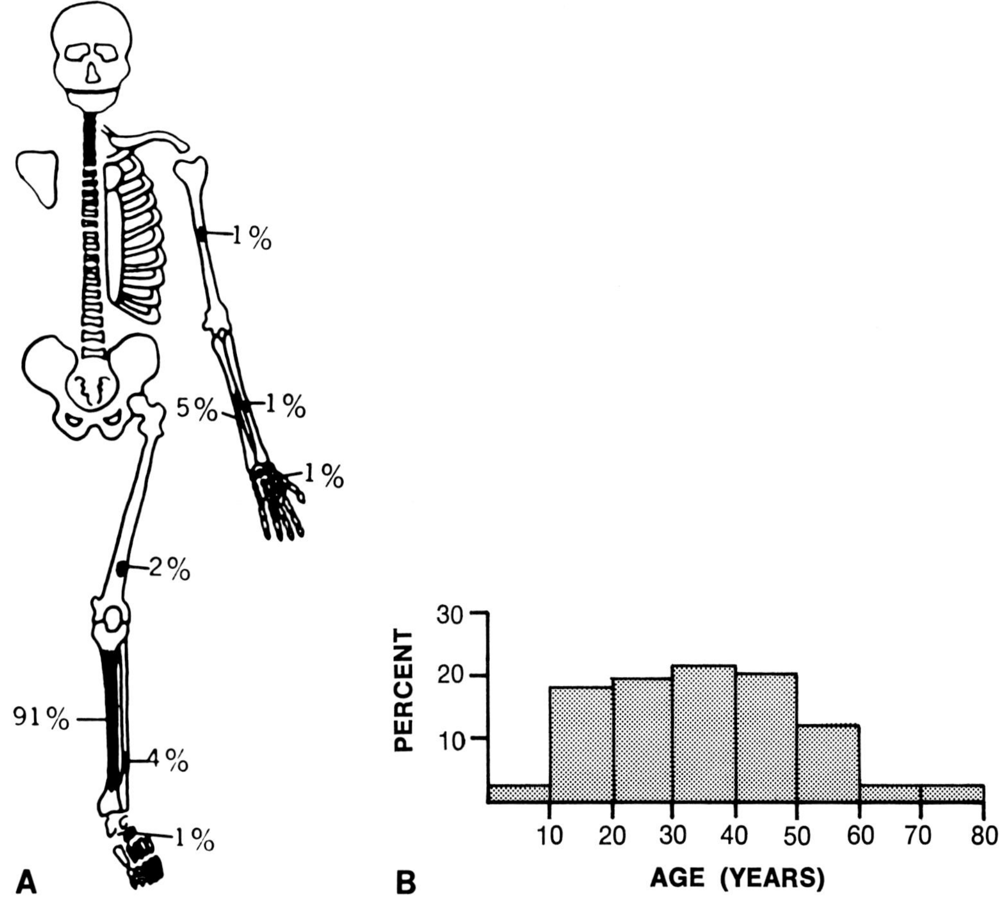

FIG. 12-2. (*A*) Adamantinoma of long limb bones. Frequency of areas of involvement in 101 patients. Male: female incidence, 1.4:1. (*B*) Age distribution of patients with adamantinoma of long limb bones (Mirra, J., Bullough, P., and Freiberger, R.: Orthopedic Diseases, Part IV. New York, Famous Teachings in Modern Medicine, MedCom, Inc., © 1977).

Epidermal Inclusion Cyst

FIG. 12-1. The epidermal inclusion cyst and glomus are the most common tumors of the distal phalanx. These lesions are sharply circumscribed, round, and lytic. Histology of this case showed an epidermal inclusion cyst.

Adamantinoma

FIG. 12-3. The adamantinoma is almost always a cystic, multilocular lesion showing geographic destruction of the midshaft of the tibia. Note the propensity for the lesion to affect the anterior border of the bone most severely. Smaller lesions can be markedly eccentric in the anterior plane. The fibula is also involved in this example, an uncommon but not rare event in relation to the adamantinoma.

FIG. 12-4. Another characteristic example showing extensive cystlike geographic destruction and mild bone "expansion."

FIG. 12-5. An example of an apparent small, single, cystic lesion of the midtibia that fractured. Biopsy showed adamantinoma.

FIG. 12-6. However, a specimen radiograph of a large-bloc resection of the bone showed unequivocal evidence of much greater spread than was apparent on the standard radiograph. Because of the large, radical resection, the patient did not experience recurrence and is completely free of disease after over 5 years of follow-up.

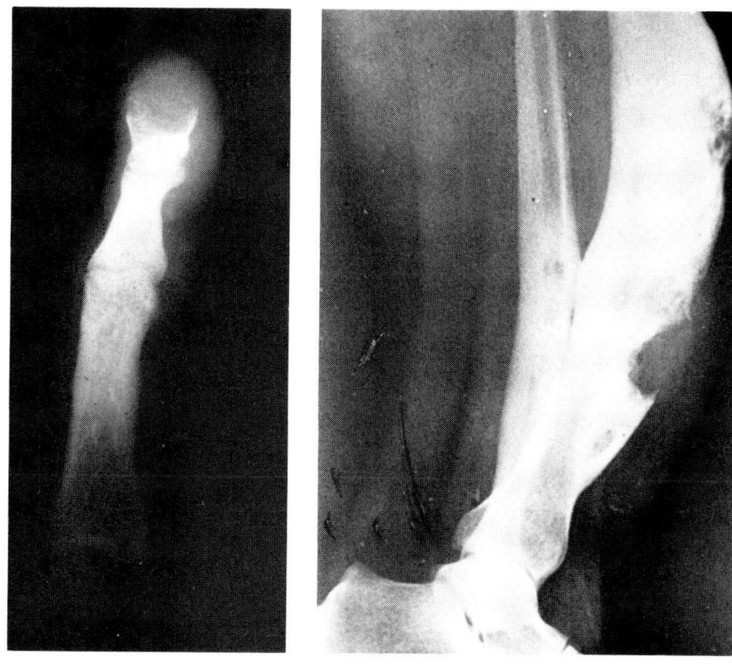

FIG. 12-1

FIG. 12-3

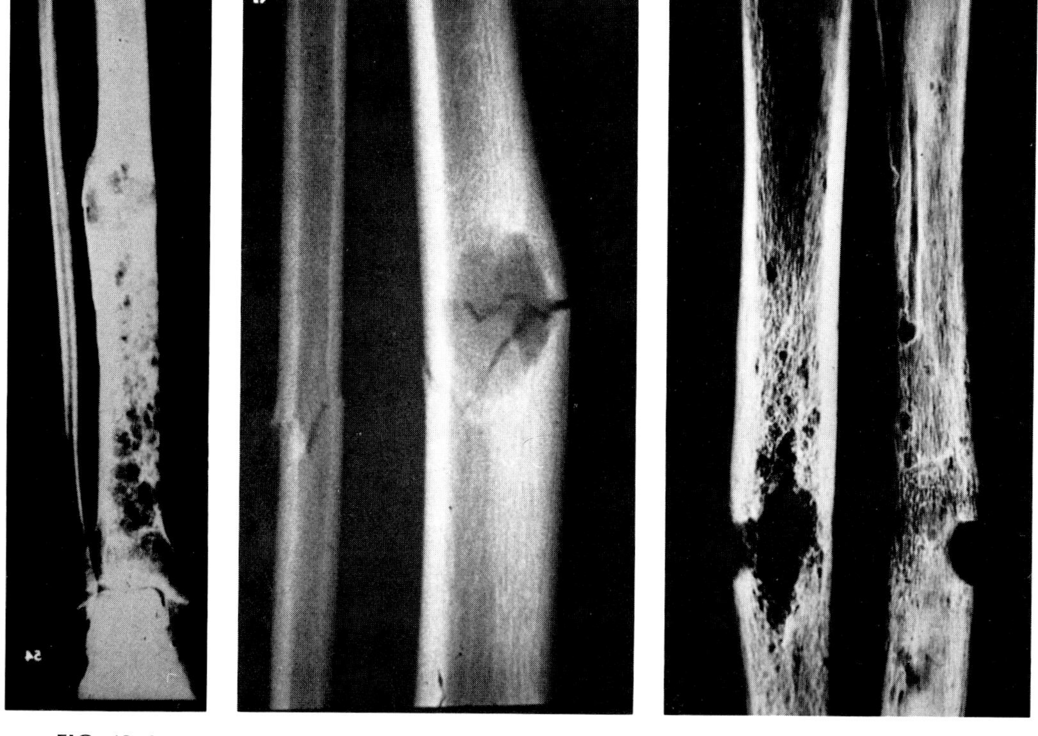

FIG. 12-4

FIG. 12-5

FIG. 12-6

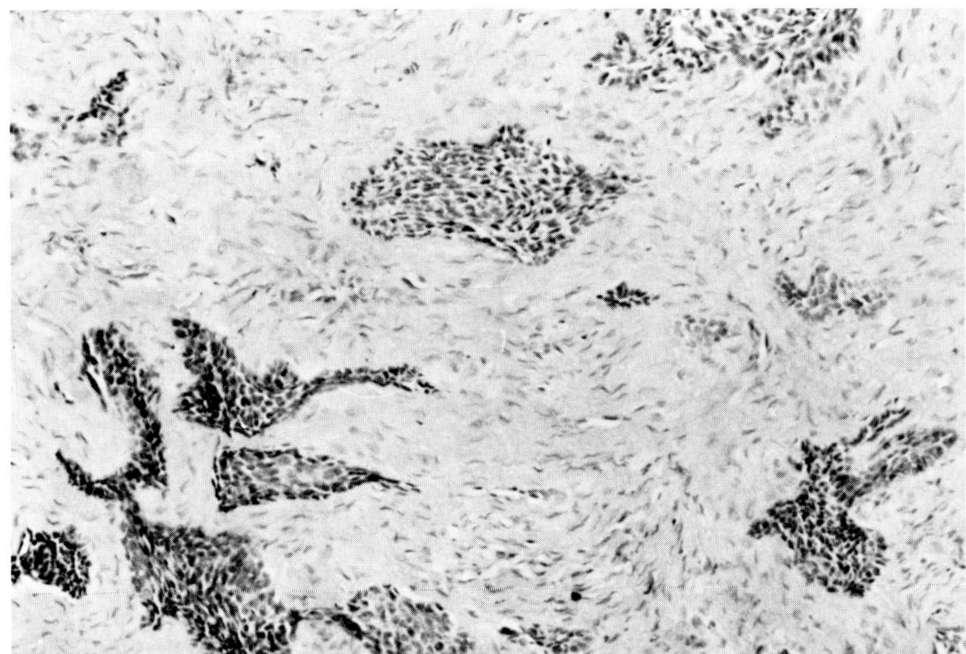

FIG. 12-7

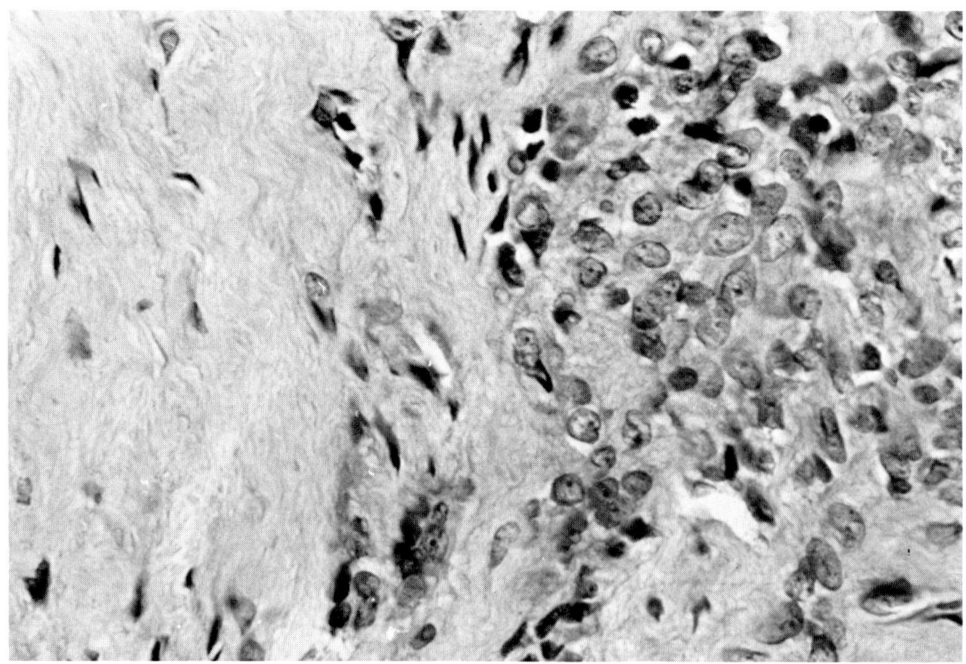

FIG. 12-8

Adamantinoma

FIG. 12-7. Basal cell carcinomalike pattern of cells embedded in a rich collagenous stroma (x40).

FIG. 12-8. High-power examination of the nuclei showing the bland nuclear characteristics common to most adamantinomas (Grade I tumor?) (x400).

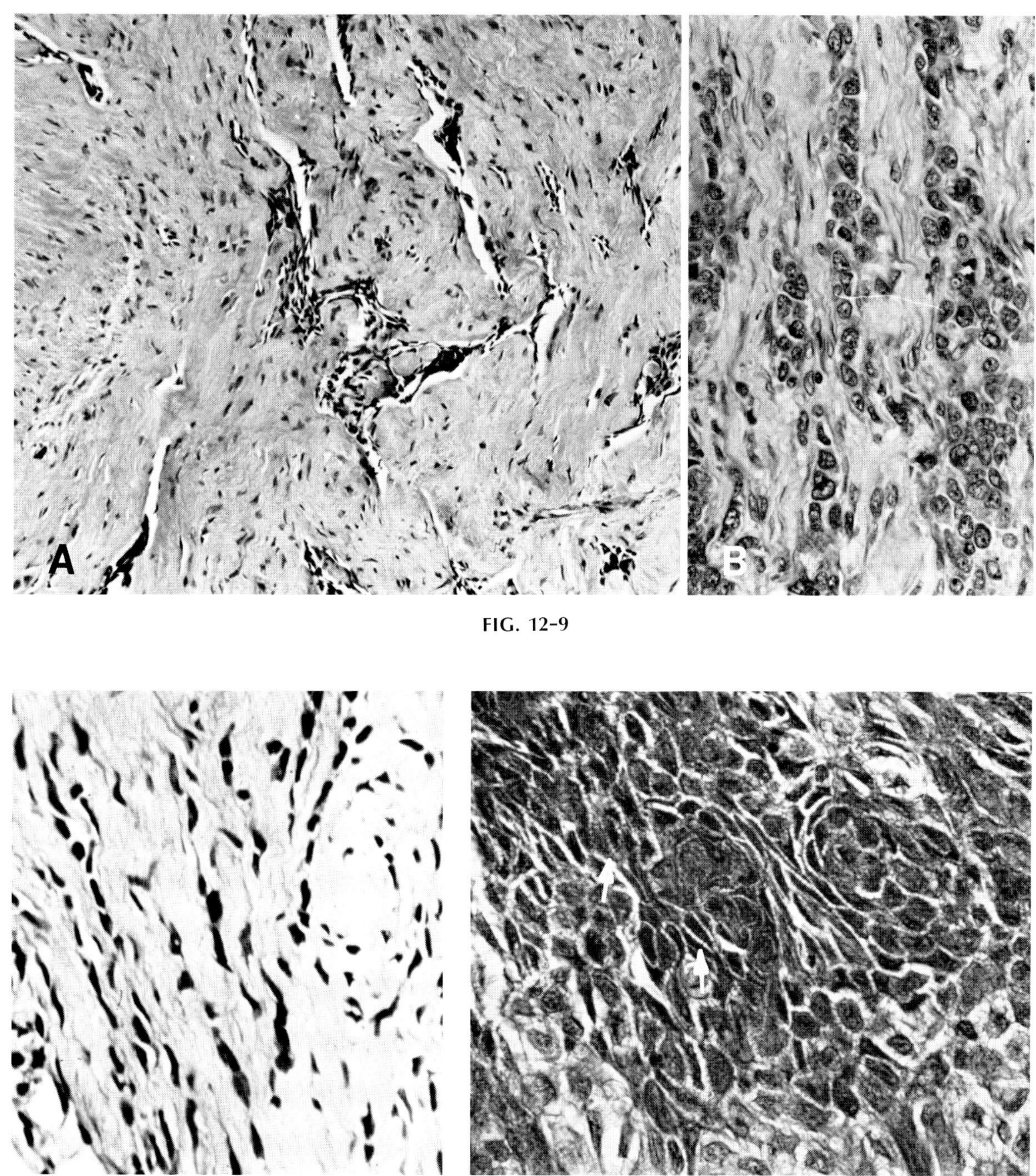

FIG. 12-9

FIG. 12-10

FIG. 12-11

Adamantinoma

FIG. 12-9. (*A*) The slitlike pattern lined by epithelial to endotheliallike cells of an adamantinoma. (*B*) Cords of cells with a "boxcar" pattern.

FIG. 12-10. Typical "boxcar" pattern of an adamantinoma very closely resembling a metastatic breast carcinoma.

FIG. 12-11. A rare example of a focus of prickle-cell production (*arrows*) in an adamantinoma. No primary carcinoma was found. This histologic pattern virtually establishes the adamantinoma as being of epithelial origin.

tumors of bone undergo malignant transformation as well, usually many years after their formation. This is true of enchondroma(s), osteochondroma(s), fibrous dysplasia(s), and others. The other fact strongly in favor of the epidermal "rest" theory is the unique distribution of adamantinoma.The tumor apparently forms in endochondrally formed bone areas closest to the skin; the area closest to the skin is the anterior portion of the midshaft of the tibia. Gross and radiologic examination show that a reasonable proportion of adamantinoma tumors arise precisely in this site (Fig. 12–3).

The other, rarer sites of long, limb bone adamantinoma (radius and ulna) also represent bones separated from the epidermis by only a thin dermal component. However, if this theory is correct, then how is it that embryonic epidermal nests may be incorporated into endochondrally formed bones but never appear to occur in bones of membrane origin even though they may be in close proximity to skin, such as the vault of the skull? Neither a vascular origin explains the very unique distribution of adamantinoma, nor is a tumor that usually arises in the diaphysis compatible with a synovial or synovial "rest" theory. If this latter theory were correct most adamantinomas should arise in the metaphysis and the distribution of lesions would be different. It would be expected that the femur and humerus would have many more than their known share of adamantinomas.

Course

Metastases may be more frequent than was believed from the early literature. Apparently the metastatic rate from this tumor can be as high as 40 per cent in fewer than 5 years' time.[20] The metastases principally spread to the lungs, lymph nodes, abdomen, and other bones.

Although there is not much data in the literature about long-term survival rates, a rough approximation of the 5-year survival rate appears to be in the range of 50 to 60 per cent. The 10-year survival is about 30 to 40 per cent.

Treatment

As innocuous as the tumor may appear microscopically, the behavior of the tumor is more treacherous than formerly believed. Less than adequate en-bloc

---

Metastatic Carcinoma

FIG. 12-12. (*A*) The "loss of the pedicle sign" (*arrow*) is usually due to metastatic carcinoma, in this case from the lung. (*B*) An example of a highly destructive acral metastasis (*arrow*) from a lung carcinoma. Many clinicians rarely recognize this as a metastasis by radiograph and usually consider only osteomyelitis as the inciting cause. Although rare, acral metastases should always be considered in any highly destructive lesion(s) of any bone distal to the elbows or knees. Usually there will also be soft-tissue extension.

FIG. 12-13. Multiple lytic defects in an adult skull are particularly common in myeloma and lung and breast carcinoma. This patient had breast carcinoma.

FIG. 12-14. Large, expansive "blowout" lesions of the bones are not uncommonly consequent to metastatic carcinoma, usually of renal or thyroid origin. The blowout lesions of radius and clavicle shown here were caused by metastatic renal cell carcinoma.

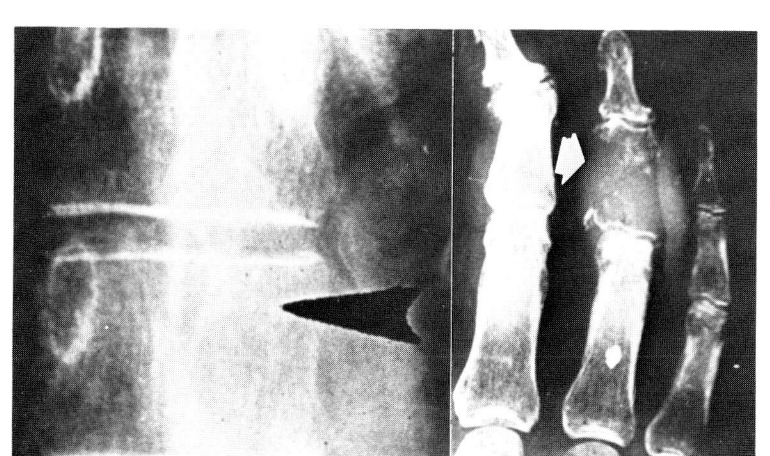

FIG. 12-12

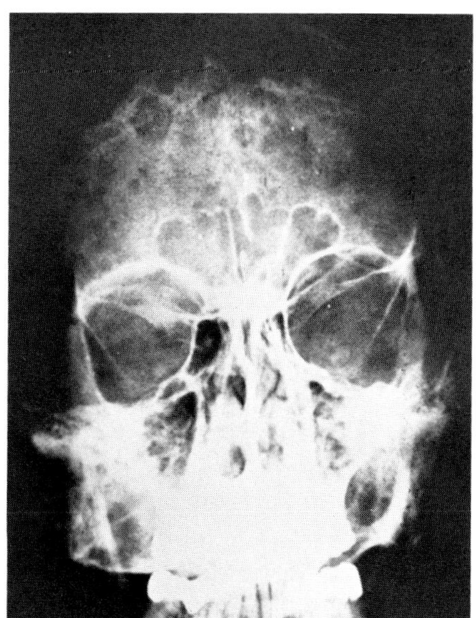

FIG. 12-13

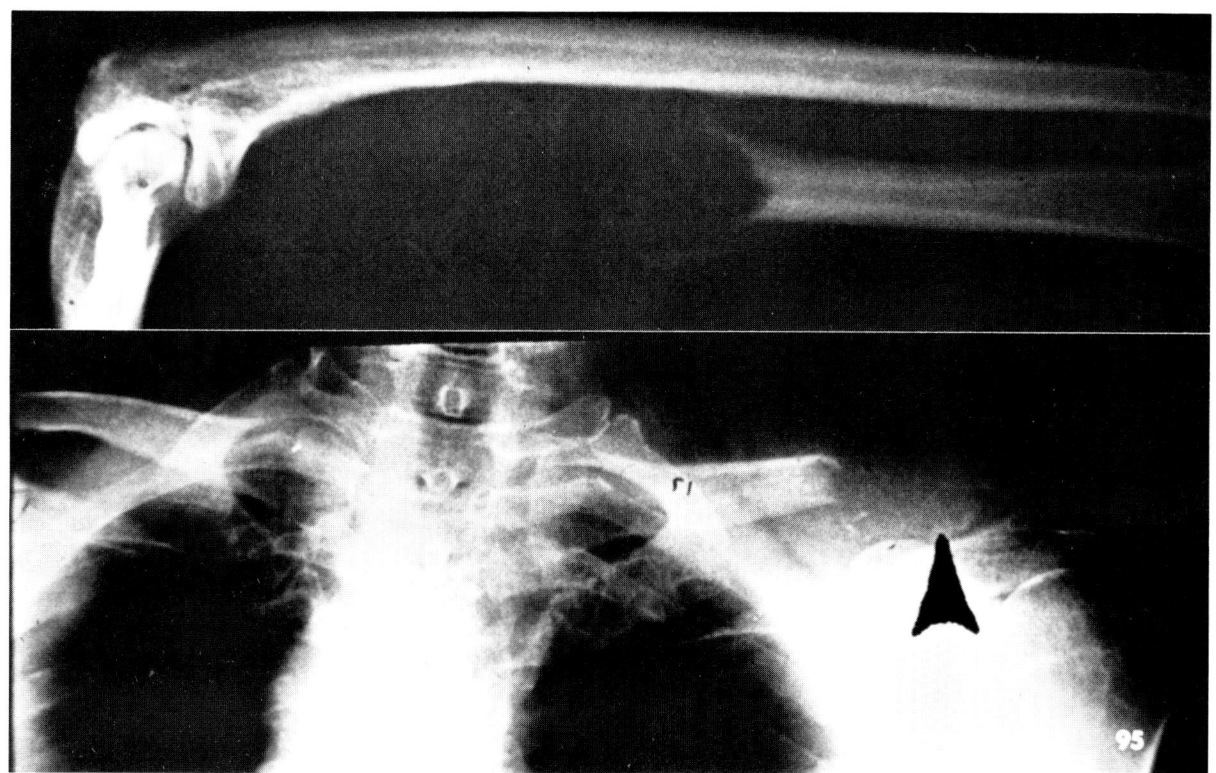

FIG. 12-14

resections and radiation therapy have resulted in numerous recurrences and perhaps have helped to contribute to the relatively poor survival rates. If en-bloc excision is to be performed, all attempts should be made to delineate the true extent of the tumor by our latest techniques, including tomography, CAT scan, or radioisotope scanning. The main problem in treating this tumor is that a seemingly small lesion on standard radiographic films (Fig. 12–5) may, on specimen radiograph (Fig. 12–6) and gross and microscopic examination, permeate many centimeters beyond the main focus or perhaps even involve the bone multicentrically, or in some cases, the adjacent bone. Post-en-bloc resection specimen radiographs of 2- to 3-mm. slab cuts and numerous sampling of margins are crucial to the determination of whether the resection is adequate. Also it may be possible that this lesion can be treated by cryosurgery.

Meningioma

The meningioma may be associated with an epithelial-like tumor. Meningioma is a locally invasive tumor that may affect any portion of the skull. The characteristic whorling and psammoma bodies are common and virtually diagnostic features. This tumor behaves like a low-grade neoplasm.

FULLY MALIGNANT NEOPLASMS

Metastatic Carcinoma

Incidence

Metastases to the skeleton far outnumber primary bone tumors. In large autopsy series the ratio of skeletal metastases to primary bone tumors is approximately 25 to 1. Over 80 per cent of bone metastases are from carcinoma of the breast, prostate, lung, and kidney.

Of patients with metastatic disease, 15 to 20 per cent develop detectable skeletal metastases during their life. If sampling of the bones at autopsy is correct, the incidence of metastases to the skeleton approaches 70 per cent.

Bones with red marrow (trunk bones, ribs, skull, proximal femur, and humerus) are the preferential sites of metastatic deposits for perhaps two reasons:

1. Tumor cells may recirculate in the blood stream for a considerable time and do not necessarily localize in the first organ to which they are transported. Tumor-cell implantation probably depends on many factors, including local blood flow, fibrin deposits, thrombosis, and integrity of the vessel walls. Arteriolar vessels appear to be far more resistant to tumor invasion than veins or capillaries. The vessels of the hematopoietic marrow have unusual anatomic features that may account for the vulnerability of this organ system to tumor metastases. The vessels of the red marrow divide into a rich sinusoidal system. The endothelium of the sinusoids contains larger than usual gaps, apparently to facilitate egress of cells from the hematopoietic marrow into the blood. Moreover, it has been shown that during muscular contraction there is reflux of blood through these gaps, making the marrow particularly vulnerable to circulating cancer cells. Fatty marrow is characterized by intact arterioles and capillaries, the absence of a sinusoidal system of vessels, and a reduced incidence of tumor metastases.

2. A skeletal focus of metastatic cancer is not infrequently the presenting lesion and may be the only demonstrable metastasis. In other cases the skeleton may be riddled with metastases while the lungs and viscera are free of tumor. This apparent dilemma can be largely explained by the discoveries of Batson.[1] His injection studies in the rat, monkey, and human cadaver have demonstrated an extensive communicating plexus of veins surrounding the vertebral column; these veins communicate directly with the lower extremities through the inferior vena cava, and with the upper extremities, head, and neck, through the superior vena cava. This plexus of veins is unique in that there are no venous valves to control the flow of blood. As a result, when pressure in the lungs or

---

Metastatic Carcinoma

FIG. 12–15. Mixed lytic and blastic metastases are usually due to either carcinoma of the breast (pictured here), lung, prostate, bladder, or to a neuroblastoma.

FIG. 12–16. Multiple blastic metastases usually indicate a tumor of prostatic origin.

FIG. 12–17. This example of metastatic prostate carcinoma resulted in such diffuse sclerosis that osteopetrosis is simulated.

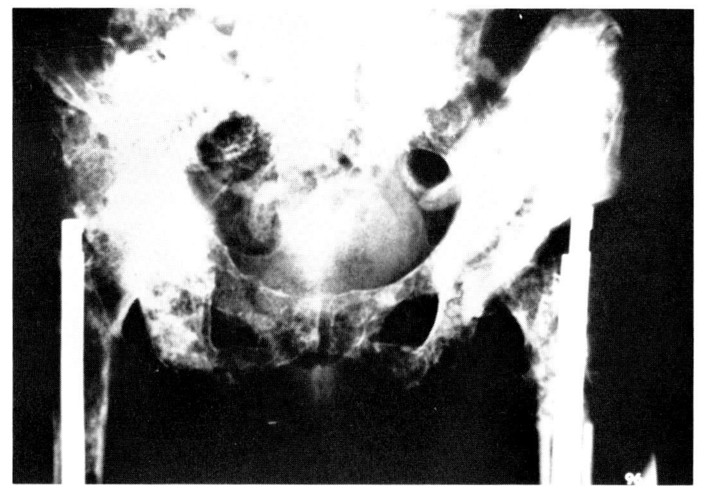

FIG. 12-15

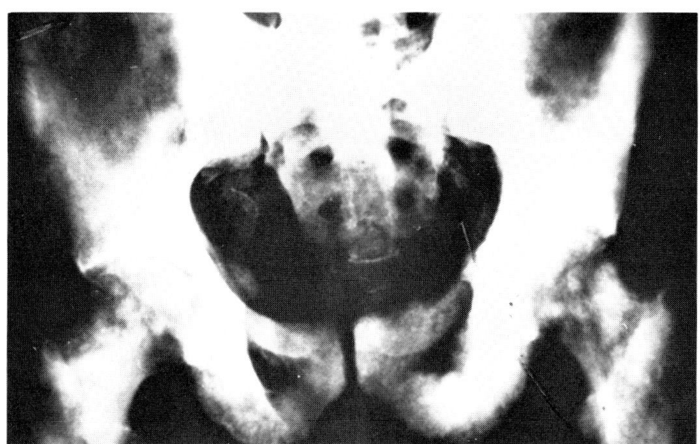

FIG. 12-16

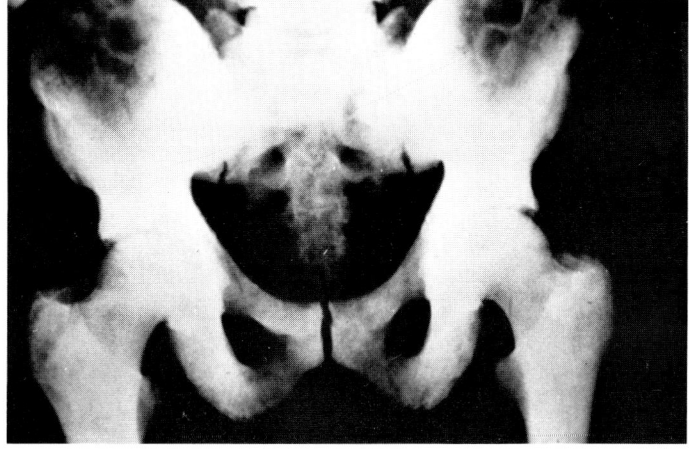

FIG. 12-17

abdomen is increased, as in expiration or during a Valsalva's maneuver, blood may bypass or flow from the caval systems into the vertebral plexus of veins, which in turn communicates with the venous and sinusoidal system of bones of the spine, shoulder girdle, pelvis, skull, or even to the region of the elbows or knees without having to pass through the heart or lungs. It is through this route that the principal skeletal metastases from carcinoma of the breast and prostate are believed to occur, without necessarily involving the lungs, liver, or other parenchymal organs.

Acral Metastases

Acral metastases (i.e., those distal to the knee or elbow joint) are rarely seen. Since Batson's plexus and its communications does not extend beyond the elbows or knees, tumor emboli must reach these sites by means of arterial dissemination. For this reason carcinoma of the lung accounts for over 50 per cent of acral metastases, because a tumor of the lung can disseminate directly into the systemic circulation by means of the pulmonary veins. However, in such cases the clinical or radiologic diagnosis of an acral metastasis is more likely to be mistaken for osteomyelitis (Fig. 12–12, *A*).

Most often metastatic lesions are multiple and present little diagnostic difficulty, since a primary is generally known before metastases become overt.

In patients under the age of 5, metastatic bone lesions are most often due to neuroblastoma. From 5 to 30 years of age multiple cancerous skeletal growths are most often due to lymphoma (leukemia included) and Ewing's sarcoma. Over the age of 40, most malignancies of bone represent metastases from carcinoma.

Kidney and thyroid carcinoma are the two most common tumors presenting with solitary metastases before the primary lesion is discovered. Carcinoma of the lung, breast, and gastrointestinal tract and neuroblastoma also not uncommonly have this presentation.

The *clinical manifestations* of metastatic cancer to the skeleton depend on the bone or bones involved, the extent of involvement, and the rapidity with which the tumor is growing. Metastases to the bone commonly produce pain. Approximately 10 to 15 per cent of patients with demonstrable skeletal metastases on radiographs develop pathologic fractures. Lytic lesions are, of course, much more prone to fracture than are blastic ones.

The decision to perform an aspiration, needle, or excisional biopsy is made after a complete history, physical examination, appropriate radiographs, and laboratory work have provided data for differential diagnosis. Needle core and aspiration biopsy has proved useful in the tissue diagnosis of skeletal metastases. Imprints can be prepared at the time of needle biopsy in order to best appreciate unobscured cytologic details.

Common Metastatic Tumors

It would be impossible to illustrate all the ways in which cancerous metastases affect the bones. However, knowledge of the more common metastatic tumors and their usual radiologic and histologic appearances will aid in establishing reasonable differential diagnosis for tumors in which a primary site has not been clearly established.

On radiologic examination in carcinoma of the *breast,* metastatic lesions may be lytic, mixed, or predominantly blastic; they may be lytic in one or more bones and mixed or predominantly blastic in others. In general, however, the pattern of bone involvement in one bone is similar to that in others. Purely lytic metastases are most often due to carcinoma of the

---

Metastatic Carcinoma

FIG. 12–18. A solitary ivory vertebra can be caused by carcinoma metastasis. Usually solitary lesions are from bladder or colon cancer. The breast or prostate (shown here) are usually associated with multiple metastases, although exceptions, of course, exist. However, the majority of ivory vertebras are caused by Hodgkin's disease, other lymphomas, or Paget's disease.

FIG. 12–19. Massive multiple periostosis (hypertrophic pulmonary osteoarthropathy), in this case resulted from a lung carcinoma. In this example, the metacarpals, distal radius, and ulna are most conspicuously affected.

FIG. 12–20. Pathognomonic features of a metastatic colloid-producing follicular thyroid carcinoma (x250).

FIG. 12–21. Typical tubules and acini of a metastatic clear cell hypernephroma (x250).

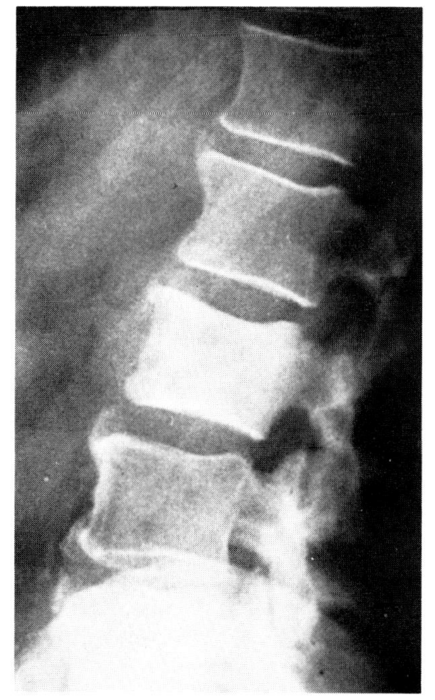

FIG. 12-18

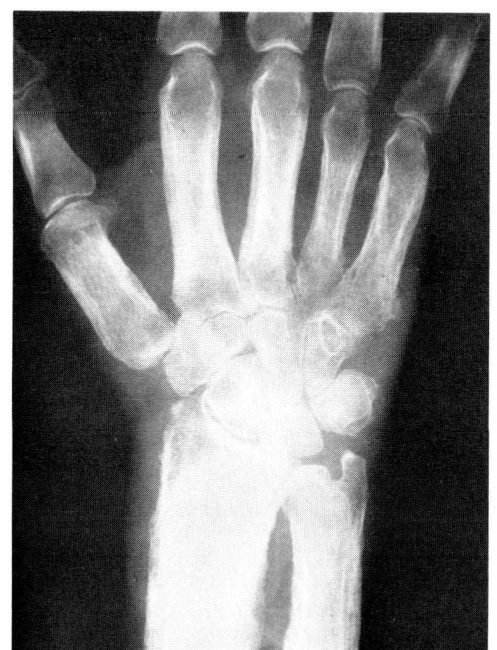

FIG. 12-19

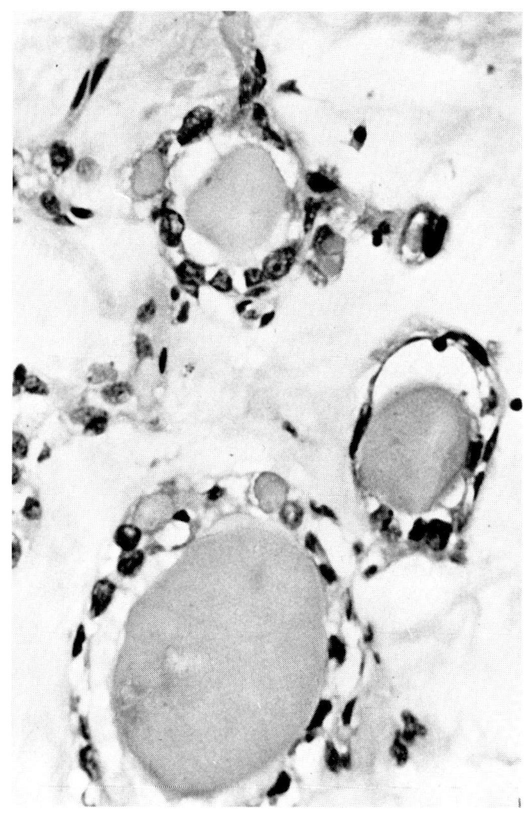

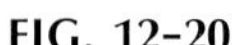

FIG. 12-20

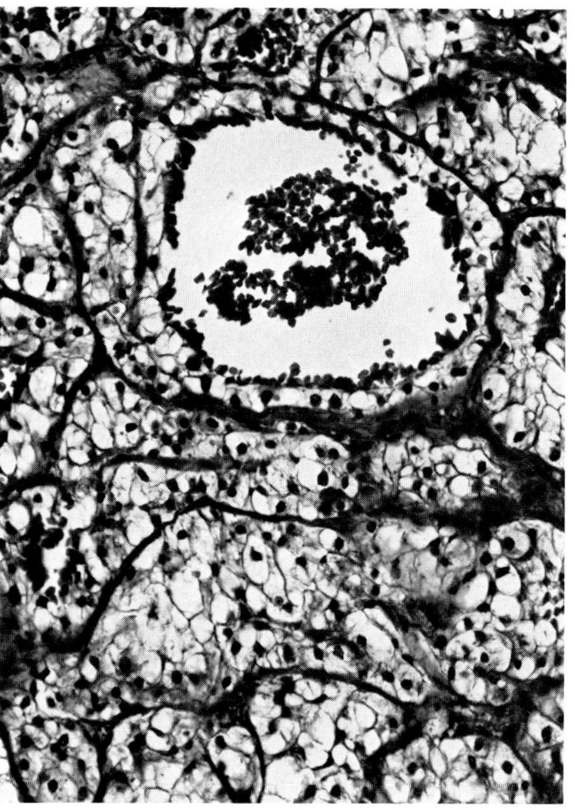

FIG. 12-21

lung, kidney, breast, thyroid, gastrointestinal tract and neuroblastoma, in order of decreasing frequency. Involvement of the pedicles in the spine (Fig. 12–12, *B*) usually differentiates a metastatic process from multiple myeloma, and preservation of the intervertebral spaces excludes infection. Multiple lytic metastases frequently involve the skull, particularly in carcinoma of the lung and breast (Fig. 12–13) and in children with metastatic neuroblastoma.

Carcinoma of the *kidney and thyroid* commonly show "expansion" of the involved bone, imparting a ballooned, blow-out, or even a soap-bubble appearance (Fig. 12–14). This appearance is probably due to a slow, regular rate of growth that has not broken through the periosteum.

Lytic and blastic metastases are most commonly seen in carcinoma of the breast (Fig. 12–15), lung, prostate, and bladder and neuroblastoma. Purely blastic metastases are usually multiple and most often are seen in association with carcinoma of the prostate, breast, bladder, and gastrointestinal tract (often the stomach).

The greatest degree of *skeletal involvement* is usually seen with breast and prostate carcinoma. Metastatic carcinoma of the prostate most often results in multiple blastic nodules, (Fig. 12–16). However, the degree of bone sclerosis induced by the tumor may be so diffuse that it simulates osteopetrosis (Fig. 12–17). The spine is often the first area affected by carcinoma of the prostate or breast, and the lesions are usually multiple. On occasion solitary dense or "ivory" vertebrae may be seen (Fig. 12–18). Most cases of so-called ivory vertebrae are seen in association with Hodgkin's disease, other lymphomatous diseases or Paget's disease.

Pulmonary hypertrophic osteoarthropathy may occur in association with benign or malignant tumors of the lungs and results in clubbing of the fingers and toes, with pain and swelling and periosteal new bone deposition, particularly in the tubular bones of the extremities (Fig. 12–19). The mechanism for these changes is not clear. After removal of the lesion in the lung the osteoarthrophy mends rapidly.

Metastatic carcinoma does not produce a significant *periosteal reaction,* with the exception of rare cases of prostatic, colon, and rectal carcinomas. These tumors on occasion may stimulate a "sunburst" periosteal reaction and appear virtually indistinguishable radiographically from an osteogenic sarcoma.

In patients *without a known primary lesion,* bone biopsy may provide the first evidence of malignancy. An example of a metastatic neoplasm with pathognomonic histologic features is colloid material in thyroid adenocarcinoma (Fig. 12–20) and tubular glands lined by clear cells and granular cells in hypernephroma (Fig. 12–21). Melanin pigments within the cells of a malignant melanoma are also pathognomonic histologic features.

In most instances of metastatic bone disease, *more than one primary site* is suggested by the tumor pattern. Although the presence of keratin pearls establishes the diagnosis of squamous cell carcinoma, the primary site could well be the lung, esophagus, skin, cervix, bladder, or other organs.

Glandular carcinomas (*adenocarcinomas*) make up a large group of metastatic bone cancers but there are some histologic features that may be used to help narrow the range of possibilities of the primary site. For example, glandular carcinomas may or may not produce mucin. Mucin appears pink with mucicarmine stains. Mucin-producing carcinomas are most frequently from the gastrointestinal tract and uterus, infrequently from the lung or breast, and only very rarely from the kidney or prostate.

Metastatic Carcinoma-Epithelioid Osteosarcoma

FIG. 12-22. Metastatic prostate carcinoma usually shows acini and cells with small, regular, innocuous nuclei and a pale cytoplasm (x250).

FIG. 12-23. The typical features of a metastatic "oat cell" carcinoma. Some of the cells do have tapered cytoplasm and resemble the "pear" shaped cells (*arrow*) of a metastatic neuroblastoma. However, the oat cell carcinoma is a disease of adults and will show a parenchymal lung mass (x600).

FIG. 12-24. (*A*) Epithelial-like osteosarcoma. The malignant cells are arranged in a nesting or epithelioid pattern (x40). (*B*) High-power examination shows polygonal cells with abundant pink cytoplasm and well demarcated cell borders. The fact that these are not epithelial cells is demonstrated by careful search to identify focal differentiation to cartilage (extreme right of field) or osteoid to woven bone production. Most patients are adolescents or young adults, much younger than is usual for metastatic carcinoma (x350).

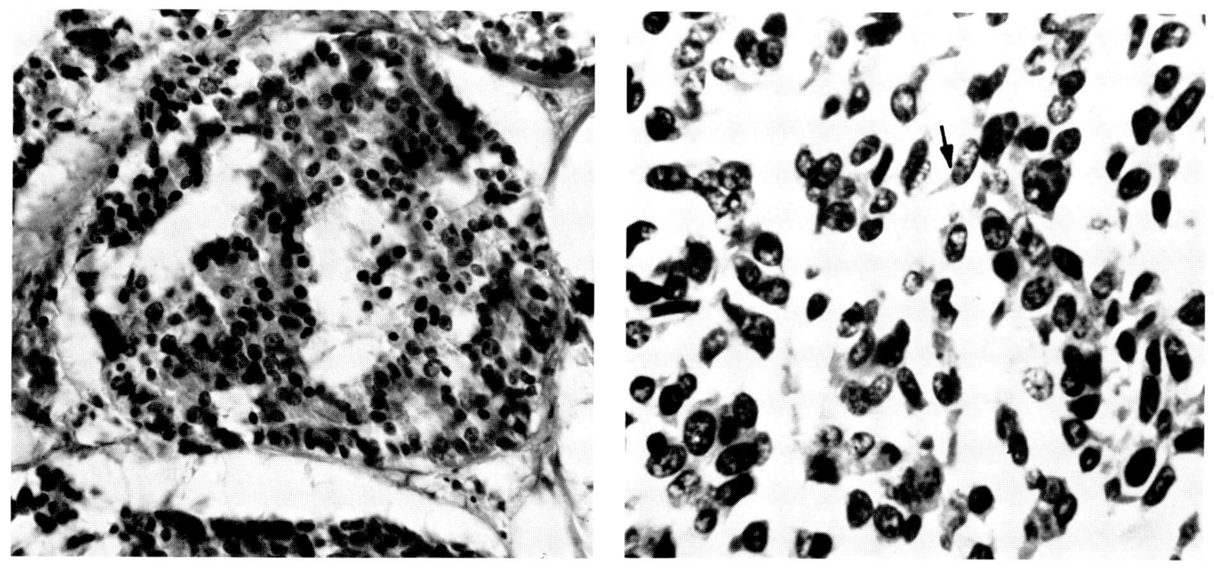

FIG. 12-22

FIG. 12-23

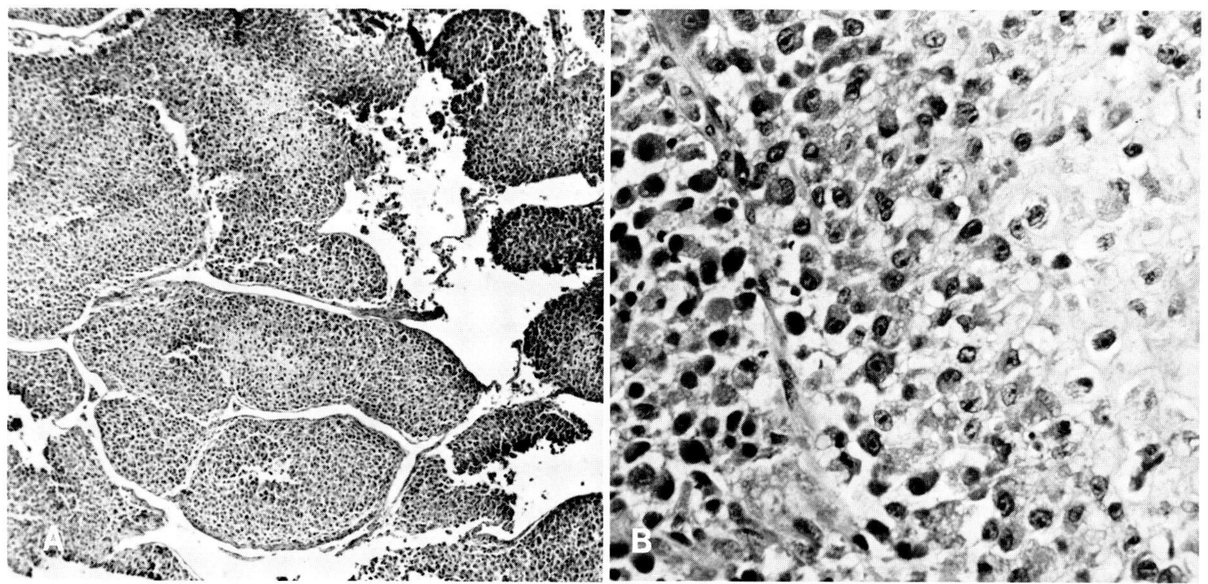

FIG. 12-24

Histologic Appearance

The usual features of carcinoma of the *prostate* are small cells that contain small, round nuclei with an innocuous and deceptively benign appearance. The cells often arrange themselves into cords or small glands or both (Fig. 12–22). If arranged only in solid nests, they may be mistaken for histiocytes.

In *breast carcinoma* the cells usually arrange themselves into an organoid pattern or into elongated tubes in which the nuclei may join end-to-end in a "boxcar" pattern. This pattern is quite characteristic of breast carcinoma. The only primary tumor of bone that can mimic this pattern is the adamantinoma of long limb bones. The breast carcinoma cells can be embedded in extremely dense fibrous or reactive host bone sclerosis. The number of malignant cells may be quite insignificant in relation to the mass of reactive tissue and can obscure diagnosis, particularly on needle biopsy. In any suspected carcinoma the fibrous or bony reactive tissue must be searched quite carefully for the few telltale epithelial cell nests embedded in dense stroma.

In some instances the cellular pattern presented by a metastatic carcinoma is so lacking in differentiation that it offers no clue at all to the site of the primary lesion. Indeed, such tumors may even mislead one into thinking that the bony lesion in question is a primary sarcoma rather than a metastatic tumor. About the only poorly differentiated tumor that has a recognizable cellular pattern is the oat cell carcinoma. The cells, as the name implies, resemble grains of oats; they are small, slightly tapered, and have small oval to tapered nuclei (Fig. 12–23). This tumor may be confused with lymphosarcoma or undifferentiated sarcoma.

Carcinoma Extending to Bone by Direct Extension

It is not uncommon for carcinomas to invade bone by direct extension. This is particularly true of carcinomas of the head and neck or carcinomas forming in chronic, draining osteomyelitis tracts. The diagnosis of head and neck carcinomas invading bone by direct extension is almost never a diagnostic problem, because they will be associated with an obvious large extraosseous primary. The problem of differentiated squamous carcinoma has been treated earlier (see p. 439).

Epithelial-Like Osteosarcoma

On rare occasions an osteosarcoma may produce sheets of cells that mimic an epithelial (epidermoid) carcinoma and that may lead to diagnostic confusion. However, careful attention to the radiologic features and young age of the patient in relation to carcinoma and careful sampling for telltale signs of cartilage (Fig. 12–24) or bone production from the epithelial-like stroma cells should prevent a mistaken diagnosis of metastatic carcinoma.

REFERENCES

Benign Tumors, Carcinoma Arising in Osteomyelitis, and Metastatic Carcinoma

1. Batson, O.V.: The function of the vertebral veins and their role in the spread of metastases. Ann. Surg., *112:* 138, 1942.

1a. Benedict, E.B.: Carcinoma in osteomyelitis. Surg. Gynecol. Obstet.,*103* 1, 1931.

2. Fleming, J.F.R., and Botterell, E.H.: Cranial dermoid and epidermoid tumors. Surg. Gynecol. Obstet., *109:* 403, 1959.
3. Johnson, L.L., and Kempson, R.L.: Epidermoid carcinoma in chronic osteomyelitis: diagnostic problems and management. J. Bone Joint Surg., *47A:* 133, 1965.
4. Murray, R.O., and Jacobson, H.G.: The Radiology of Skeletal Disorders. ed. 2. Edinburgh, London, and New York, J. & A. Churchill, 1977.
5. Sedlin, F.D., and Fleming, J.L.: Epidermoid carcinoma arising in the chronic osteomyelitis foci. J. Bone Joint Surg., *48A:* 827, 1963.
6. Skandalakis, J.E., Goodwin, J.T., and Mahon, R.F.: Epidermoid cyst of the skull; report of 4 cases and review of the literature. Surgery, *43:* 990, 1958.
7. Waldvogel, F.A., Medoff, G., and Swartz, M.N.: Osteomyelitis: a review of clinical features, therapeutic consideration and unusual aspects (three parts). New Eng. J. Med., *4:* 198–206, 260–266, and 316–322, 1970.

Adamantinoma of Long Limb Bones

8. Baker, P.L., Dockerty, M.B., and Coventry, M.B.: Adamantinoma (so-called) of the long bones. Review of the literature and a report of three new cases. J. Bone Joint Surg., *36A:* 704, 1954.
9. Changus, G.W., Speed, J.S., and Stewart, F.W.: Malignant angioblastoma of bone. A reappraisal of adamantinoma of long bone. Cancer, *10:* 540, 1957.
10. Cohen, D.M., Dahlin, D.C., and Pugh, D.G.: Fibrous dysplasia associated with adamantinoma of the long bones. Cancer, *15:* 515, 1962.

11. Donner, R.: Adamantinoma of the tibia. A long-standing case with unusual histologic features. J. Bone Joint Surg., *48B:* 138, 1966.
12. Fischer, B.: Uber ein primaries adamantinom der tibia. Frank. Ztschr. f. Pathol., *12:* 422, 1913.
13. Hicks, J.D.: Synovial sarcoma of the tibia. J. Pathol., *67:* 151, 1954.
14. Huvos, A.G., and Marcove, R.C.: Adamantinoma of long bones. A clinico-pathological study of 14 cases with vascular origin suggested. J. Bone Joint Surg., *57A:* 148, 1975.
15. Jaffe, H.L.: Tumors and Tumorous Conditions of the Bones and Joints. pp. 213–223. Philadelphia, Lea & Febiger, 1958.
16. Lederer, H., and Sinclair, A.J.: Malignant synovioma simulating "adamantinoma of the tibia." J. Pathol., *67:* 163, 1954.
17. Moon, N.F.: Adamantinoma of the appendicular skeleton. A statistical review of reported cases. Clin. Orthop., *43:* 189, 1965.
18. Morgan, A.D., and Mackenzie, D.H.: A metastasizing adamantinoma of the tibia. J. Bone Joint Surg., *38B:* 892, 1956.
19. Rosai, J.: Adamantinoma of the tibia. Electron microscopic evidence of its epithelial origin. Am. J. Clin. Pathol., *51:* 786, 1969.
20. Spjut, H.J., Dorfman, H.D., Fechner, R.E., and Ackerman, L.V.: Atlas of Tumor Pathology. Second Series, Fasc. 5, Tumors of Bone and Cartilage. A.F.I.P., Washington, D.C., 1971.
21. Ummi, K.K., Dahlin, D.C., Beabout, J.W., and Ivins, J.C.: Adamantinoma of long bones. Cancer, *34:* 1796, 1974.
21a. Weiss, S.W., and Dorfman, H.D.: Adamantinoma of long bone. An analysis of 9 new cases with emphasis on metastasizing lesions and fibrous dysplasia-like changes. Hum. Pathol., *8:* 141, 1977.
22. Yoneyama, T., Winter, W.G., and Milsow, L.: Tibial adamantinoma: its histogenesis from ultrastructural studies. Cancer, *40:* 1138, 1977.

INTRAOSSEOUS MYXOID, CYSTIC AND VASCULAR TUMORS

13

MYXOID TUMORS

Myxoma of Jaws and Skull

Introduction

Virchow was the first to use the term *myxoma.* He noted that some tumors seemed to mirror the nature of the Wharton's jelly of the umbilical cord. He believed the umbilical cord contained intercellular mucin and called the tissue of the umbilical cord and its analogues mucinous tissue. Tumors that resembled this tissue he called myxomas. He believed that the myxoma might be a precursor to fat tissue, which would account for myxoid lipoblastic tumors, but that there also remains a variant that does not differentiate further into any other variety of tissue. Dutz and Stout[2] define the myxoma as a "tumor composed of stellate and sometimes spindle-shaped cells set in a myxoid stroma containing mucopolysaccharide through which course very delicate reticulin fibers in various directions. The tumor is poorly vascularized, and the capillaries do not have the plexiform arrangement of embryonal lipoblastic tissue. Like any other tumor it may become fibrosed in some areas. There must be no chondroblasts, lipoblasts, rhabdomyoblasts, or any other recognizable elements."

The myxoma is usually a tumor of soft tissues. According to Enzinger[3] the tumor is benign, although it is rarely associated with recurrence. The myxoma may also be seen in relation to jawbones and the nasal cavity. Those tumors, which are reported as myxomas or fibromyxomas of the long bones, are, in this author's estimation, a variant of chondromyxoid fibroma for reasons that will be dealt with in the differential diagnosis of myxoma.

Myxoid tissue is tissue that resembles the *myxomatous tissue* of true myxomas. However, myxoid tissue is seen in association with identifiable cell types or other matrix not seen in true myxoma. These recognizable cell types may be either of chondrocytic, notochordal, or metastatic carcinoma origin. Myxoid tissue is predominantly mucinous or mucoid, as can be seen in metastatic mucin-rich adenocarcinoma, myxoid degeneration of chondromyxoid fibromas, chondrosarcomas, enchondromas, or in the notochordally derived chordoma. The myxoma of bone is the only one which by definition contains true myxomatous tissue. The other entities that contain recognizable cellular or matrix differentiation may contain a tissue that resembles myxomatous tissue or myxoid tissue. Some lesions not dealt with in this chapter include those with small foci of myxoid degeneration; this may sometimes occur in association with the fibrous stroma of fibrous dysplasia and occasionally in chondroblastoma and a few other tumors. These small foci of myxoid degeneration usually lead to no serious errors in diagnosis.

Clinical Features

The true myxoma of bones has a striking predilection for the jawbones, nasal bones, sinuses, and palate. Patients with myxomas of the jaw tend to be young adults, while those with nasopharyngeal myxomas tend to be children. The tumor of the jaws tends to be associated with uninterrupted or missing teeth and on occasion, with odontogenic epithelium, suggesting that the lesion in this location may arise from the dental tissue.[7] On the other hand, a significant percentage of the children with nasopharyngeal myxomas give a history of significant trauma, such as "bumping" into a door followed by the development of a hematoma and a myxoma within a few weeks. Both groups usually present with painless swelling. The myxoma may grow with amazing rapidity. When this occurs, the clinician is usually sure he is dealing with a highly malignant tumor. Nevertheless, the eventual behavior of the myxoma is benign. Similarly, myositis ossificans and other benign injury lesions may within the first few days to weeks grow with rapidity.

Radiologic Features

The lesions are associated with almost pure lytic destruction of the bone with lobulated to rounded edges. A border of reactive host bone sclerosis is usually absent in the early stages of the disease. The tumors of the jaw and nasopharangeal bones are often associated with a soft-tissue component. The myxoma may fill up entire sinuses.

Gross Features

The myxoma is usually a soft, slimy, mucoid, pallid gelatinous tissue. If the lesion has undergone significant fibrotic change, it becomes firmer and whiter in color.

They usually exhibit well-defined borders but lack a well-developed capsule.

Histopathology

The classic histology consists of stellate to spindly cells set widely apart in a pale mucoid stroma through which course fine collagenous fibers (Figs. 13–1 and 13–2). Capillaries may be very inconspicuous to few in number. They do not contain numerous plexiform capillaries, as would be expected in a myxoid liposarcoma, for example. The cells contain bland, small, oval nuclei that may contain small vacuoles. In some cases cytoplasmic "bubbles" or vacuoles may be seen, resembling to some extent immature lipocytes or possibly physaliphorous cells (Fig. 13–1, *A*). Cytoplasmic "bubbles" were not seen in those chondromyxoid fibromas studied by this author. Mitoses are extremely rare. On low-power examination the distribution of cells is quite homogeneous; that is, the number of cells is quite the same from area to area (Figs. 13–2 and 13–3). There is no condensation of cells around vessels or distinct lobulation, as is common to the chondromyxoid fibroma (Figs. 13–4 and 13–5). Some myxomas contain considerably more fibrous tissue but the numbers of cells per unit area usually remain low (Fig. 13–2, *B*). It is these collagen-rich myxomas that are the most difficult to distinguish from desmoplastic fibromas, very low-grade fibrosarcomas, or chondromyxoid fibromas. Usually, however, the myxoma will show some regions of highly characteristic myxomatous tissue and complete nuclear innocence, always lack cartilage tissue, and show neither lobulation or peripheral nuclear condensations. Their location in jawbones and nasopharyngeal areas is also helpful.

In summary, the characteristic features of a myxoma are as follows:

1. Location (jaw- and nasopharyngeal bones)
2. Slimy to gelatinous gross appearance
3. Myxomatous tissue on histologic examination
4. Homogeneity of nuclei with absence of focal condensation
5. Variable degrees of fibrosis
6. On occasion cytoplasmic "bubbles"
7. No evidence of cartilage production, physaliphorous cells, or clusters, clumps, cords, acini, or nesting of cells
8. Relatively avascular

Course

The myxoma may be associated with recurrence but has never been reported to metastasize.[4,7,13] Myxomas are locally infiltrative neoplasms that can recur if treated by curettage. In two patients with nasopharyngeal myxomas that this author has seen, one (a 17-month female) was treated with an en-bloc excision, and there was no recurrence. The second patient was a 27-year-old female who developed a large myxoma of the nasal bone following significant injury. A large en-bloc excision was recommended following the biopsy diagnosis. The patient refused further therapy. Although the mass, initially, was over 5 cm. in size, during a 9-year follow-up period the mass has gradually decreased in size to the point where only a slight residual nasal deformity is present.

Treatment

Most authors recommend as the procedure of choice a conservative excision of the lesion with tumor-free margins. Kangur, *et al.*,[7] believes that extensive resections should be reserved for either quite large myxomas or for those which have recurred.

Formerly, it was believed that the myxoma of muscle was a low-grade malignancy, perhaps a variant of myxoid liposarcoma. Enzinger,[3] in a study of 34 cases of myxoma of muscle, was unable to corroborate this earlier view. In fact, none of his cases showed recurrence, even though 29 were treated with simple excision. Admittedly the myxoma of skull and jaw bones may not be strictly analogous to the myxoma of muscle, because the former myxomas have been reported to be associated with a locally aggressive course in many instances. However, surgical treatment should remain conservative unless the myxoma of jaws or skull can be shown to be capable of invasion of vital structures such as the brain, metastasis, or persistent unending growth. A large, disfiguring, debilitating en-bloc resection that removes a great deal of functioning tissue must be weighed against the tumor's apparent long-term, essentially benign behavior, and in some instances, at least, spontaneous regression of the tumor after many years.

Differential Diagnosis of Myxoid Lesions

CHONDROMYXOID FIBROMA. The chondromyxoid fibroma often contains prominent masses of myxoid tissue. The majority of chondromyxoid fibromas produce some foci of recognizable chondroid (Figs. 13-4 and 13-5, *B*), which is an important diagnostic aid. However, some cases may show little clearly recognizable chondroid tissues. It is these cases that are the most difficult to distinguish from myxomas of the skull. Indeed, such chondromyxoid fibromas may be classified as fibromyxomas or myxomas by some authors, even though the radiographic, clinical, and certain microscopic features are most consistent with the entity of chondromyxoid fibroma in which little to no chondroid is present. Perhaps the term *chondromyxoid fibroma* is too inclusive in that it leaves little room to accept cases with identical clinical and radiographic characteristics but which do not show focal chondroid differentiation, at least in the sections studied. For this reason some cases appear to have been inaccurately classified as myxoma of long and flat bones.[1,10] Jaffe and Lichtenstein[7a] believe that the chondroid of chondromyxoid fibroma may represent the tissues of a more mature lesion and that on occasion it may be misinterpreted as a "myxoma" of bone.

The confusion resides in the terminology. It would be very confusing, for example, to say nonchondroid-producing chondromyxoid fibroma, because the term implies chondroid, fibrous, and myxoid tissue production. In this author's estimation this error of confusing a myxoma for a chondromyxoid fibroma can be avoided if the terminology is changed to fit the observed facts. The lesion of long and flat bones referred to as *chondromyxoid fibroma* could be changed to fibromyxoma of long and flat bones with or without chondroid differentiation. The term *fibromyxoma* should be recognized as the nonchondroid-producing variant of the so-called chondromyxoid fibroma. The term *myxoma* should be reserved for the different clinical and pathologic entities of the nasopharynx and jaw bones. It should also be recognized that the myxoma may contain variable degrees of fibrous tissue. However, the term *fibromyxoma* for these lesions should be avoided, because this would result in confusion with fibromyxomatous variant of the "chondromyxoid fibroma." There is also a need to prepare numerous sections of the "chondromyxoid fibroma" in order to improve the chances of finding areas of chondroid differentiation.

The most crucial features in distinguishing a myxoma of nasopharynx and jaws from the entity fibromyxoma, with or without chondroid differentiation of the long and flat bones, are the following:

Myxoma of Bone

FIG. 13-1. (*A*) Stellate myxoma cells set in a very loose fibrillar stroma. Note the small intracytoplasmic vacuoles (*arrows*) (x400). (*B*) Myxoma cells set in a much denser fibrillar stroma. Vacuoles are not apparent in this example (x400).

FIG. 13-2. (*A*) Low-power view of a myxoma. Small cells set in a rather loose fibrillar stroma. Note the extreme paucity of capillaries (x100). (*B*) High-power view of same field (x400).

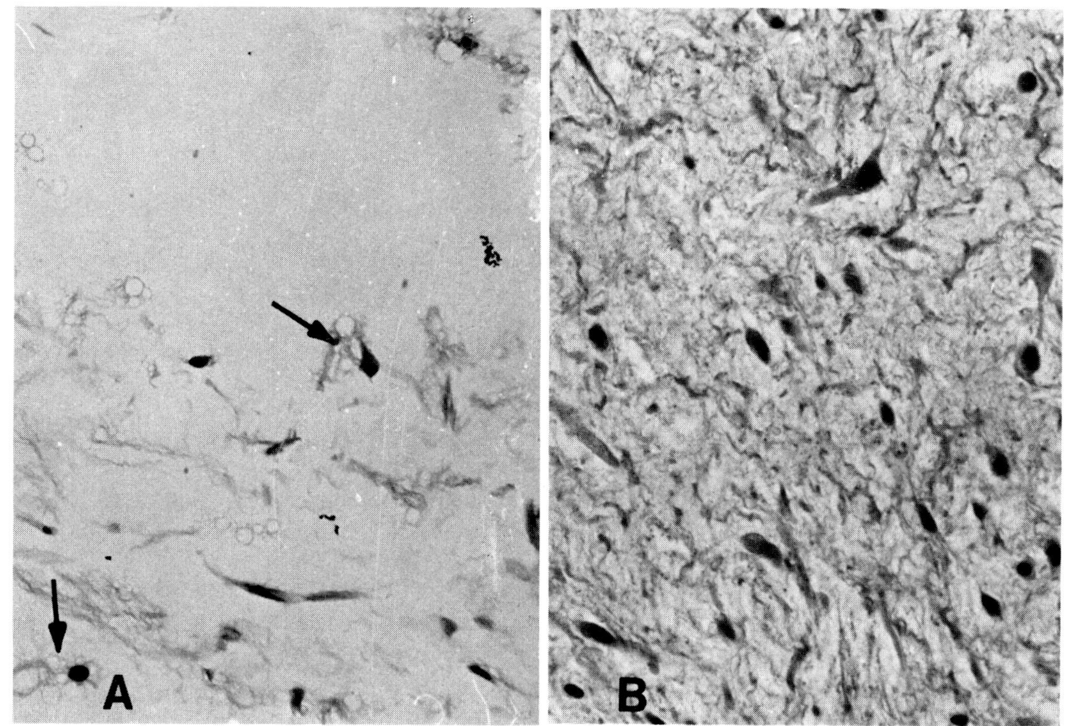

FIG. 13-1

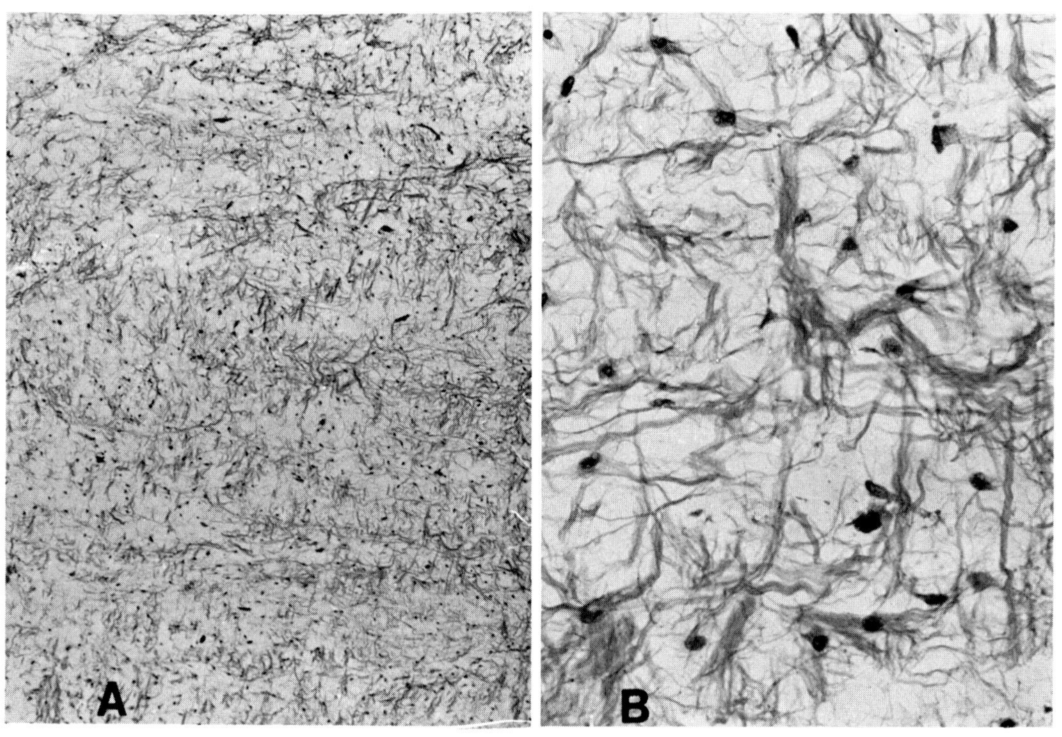

FIG. 13-2

1. Myxomas of bone appear to be confined to the jaw or nasopharyngeal bones. The chondromyxoid fibroma has a propensity to involve the metaphyses of long bones and has not been reported to involve the skull bones. In this author's collection he has seen only one unequivocal chondromyxoid fibroma of the mandible and none in the skull.

2. On low-power examination the myxoma is characterized by a homogeneity of cells, although the degree of collagenous or reticulin tissue may vary from case to case or field to field. On the other hand, with low- or medium-power examination the chondromyxoid fibroma usually always shows, in some fields at least, focal condensations of cells, particularly around capillaries. The focal condensation imparts a lobular pattern to the tissue (Figs. 13–4 and 13–5). This histological difference is as important as the finding of chondroid.

In this author's opinion the majority of the reported so-called myxomas and fibromyxomas[1,10] outside the jaw and skull are variants of the chondromyxoid fibroma, for the following reasons:

1. A significant number of chondromyxoid fibromas may show predominantly fibromyxomatous areas in which chondroid is difficult to find or identify. Apparently the chondroid of a chondromyxoid fibroma represents a later stage of metaplasia from the peculiar fibroblast-like stromal cells. Chondroid is apparently not present in each and every case, or it may be missed on a small sampling.

2. Most of the illustrations of reported myxomas and fibromyxomas of long bones show a distinct to subtle microscopic lobularity due to focal condensations of nuclei. This occurs most often in an identical manner as it does with clear-cut or ordinary chondromyxoid fibromas. This is clearly shown in Figure 4 of Bauer, *et al.*'s article entitled "Myxoma" of Bone.[1] The distinct lobulation due to an unequivocal peripheral nuclear condensation around vessels is identical to that seen in numerous fibromyxoid areas of the chondromyxoid fibroma.

3. The radiographic features and sites of involvement of these reported cases are similar if not identical to those reported for chondromyxoid fibroma.

These observations would support the contention that the chondromyxoid fibroma (fibromyxoma with or without chondroid differentiation) is a separate and distinct entity from the myxoma of skull. In general, the chondromyxoid fibroma is a slow-growing tumor. However, in young patients they may be associated with rapid growth and even recurrence following simple curettage. Scaglietti, *et al.*, report five cases of "myxoma" of childhood, which showed rapid growth of the lesions, recurrence post-curettage, and minimal to absent chondroid tissue.[10] Because of these observations and behavior they believed they were dealing with an entity distinct from chondromyxoid fibroma. Nevertheless, the illustrations are identical to the fibromyxoid portions of chondromyxoid fibroma. The authors themselves admit that other pathologists would probably call these tumors chondromyxoid fibromas. In this author's estimation the absence of chondroid, rapid growth, and recurrence can all be explained by the youth of these particular patients. In young patients the lesion is likely to be in its incipient phase of development and in its rapid phase of growth. If some tissue is left behind recurrence would be expected, because the lesion is rapidly growing. The absence of chondroid can be explained similarly. In early or incipient lesions the development of chondroid apparently depends upon a metaplastic potential of the stroma that may not be present in all cases, particularly in incipient (prechondroid?) lesions. All of the cases reported by Scaglietti and others were eventually cured without evidence of metastasis, which is strong supporting evidence of the benign nature of the process, despite rapid growth and recurrence. Almost any benign lesion, whether they are fibrous dysplasia, enchondromatosis, simple bone cyst, or chondroblastoma, can recur, particularly in younger patients in whom these lesions are obviously in their growth phase,

---

Myxoma Versus Chondromyxoid Fibroma

FIG. 13-3. Myxoma. Note the extreme homogeneity of the cells and stroma. All other fields are similarly homogeneous (x40).

FIG. 13-4. Chondromyxoid fibroma. Note the differences in homogeneity of cells in relation to the stroma. In some areas, the islands or nodules are hypocellular. The intervening more fibrous stromal areas (*arrow*) show increased numbers and condensation of cells in contrast to true myxomas (x125).

FIG. 13-5. (*A*) and (*B*) More extreme examples of the peripheral lobular condensation of nuclei seen in two other cases of chondromyxoid fibroma. This pattern is never seen in true myxomas (x125).

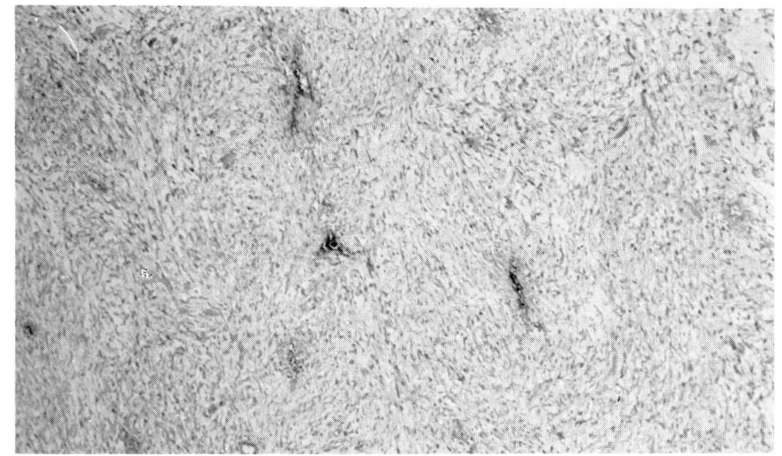

FIG. 13-3

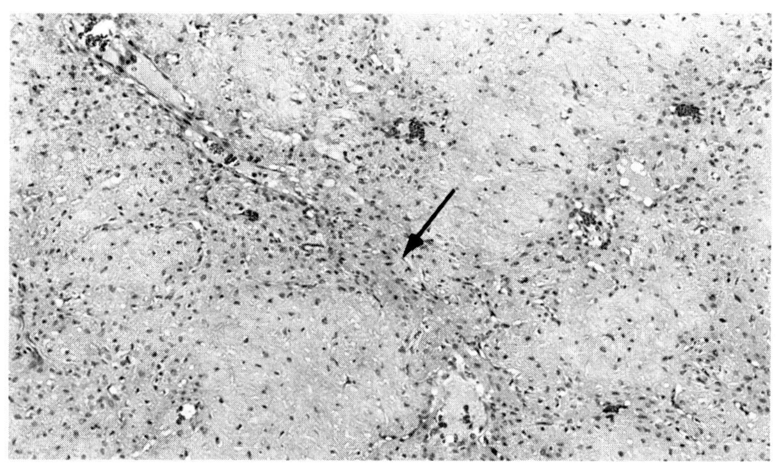

FIG. 13-4

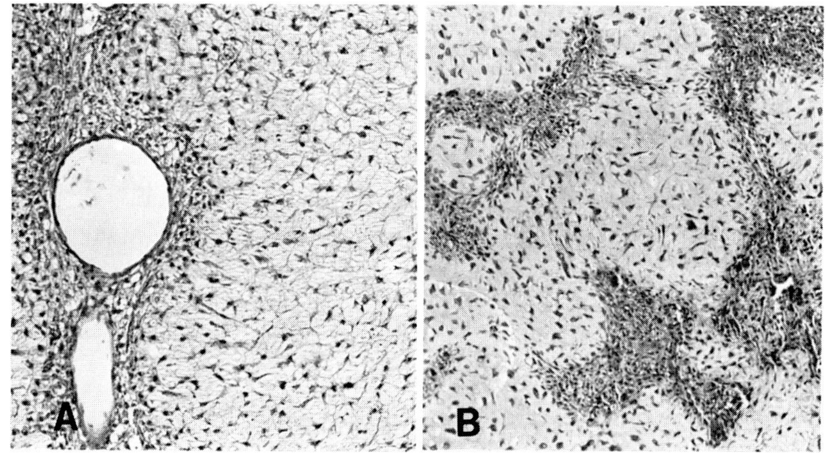

FIG. 13-5

which may not abate significantly until the epiphyses begin to close. Nevertheless, even though these tumors may persist and grow for a number of years, their eventual cessation of growth or cure with non-radical procedures is the essence of a benign lesion. The chondromyxoid fibroma has these same behavioral characteristics and is, therefore, benign. The fact that fibromyxomas (chondromyxoid fibromas) of many youthful patients recur quite often should not necessarily be regarded as a sign of a low-grade malignancy necessitating radical procedures or large en-bloc resections, which may seriously interfere with the function of the patients' limbs.

CHORDOMA. The chordoma is a low-grade malignant neoplasm that takes origin from notochordal rest cells. The stroma may be myxoid but contains nests, strands, cords, and masses of chondrocyte-like or epithelial-like cells with variable degrees of nuclear atypia. The presence of some identifiable bubbly physaliphorous cells is virtually pathognomonic of the chordoma. This tumor always arises in relation to the spinal bones, the sacrum, and the clivus area. This lesion has been described in detail in Chapter 8 (see p. 243 and Figs. 8–107–8–114).

MYXOID CHONDROSARCOMA. Some chondrosarcomas contain variable areas of myxoid degeneration of the stroma. This lesion is characterized by the presence of unequivocal areas of cartilage formation associated with variable degrees of nuclear anaplasia. The myxoid chondrosarcoma may merely represent a myxoid histological variant of a chondrosarcoma. Its behavior and treatment depends upon the degree of nuclear anaplasia and extent of bone and/or soft-tissue involvement. Condensations of cells may be seen along the periphery of the chondrosarcomatous lobules. The presence of some foci of cartilage or chondroid excludes the diagnosis of myxoma, but not a fibromyxoma with chondroid differentiation (chondromyxoid fibroma).

MYXOID DEGENERATION OF BENIGN CARTILAGE TUMORS. On occasion the cartilagenous tissues of an enchondroma or the cap of an osteochondroma may undergo focal myxoid degeneration. The presence of bland nuclear characteristics and at least some easily recognizable hyalin cartilage should not lead to confusion with a myxoma.

MUCIN-RICH METASTATIC ADENOCARCINOMA. Metastatic carcinoma, particularly of the colon, may be characterized by huge lakes of mucicarmine-positive material. The adenocarcinoma cells may be few in number in relation to the abundant mucin present and are often located in small clusters along the periphery of the mucin lakes. In most instances a carcinomatous primary would have been diagnosed prior to the development of metastases.

CYSTIC TUMORS

There are two principal primary tumors of bone that are called cysts; namely, the solitary bone cyst and the aneurysmal bone cyst. The solitary bone cyst is in actuality the only true cyst of bone (i.e., a fluid-filled cyst lined by epithelial-like cells). The aneurysmal bone cyst (ABC) is most likely a vascular malformation that forms secondarily to either benign or low-grade malignant entities or to trauma. The term *cyst* in reference to ABC refers to the multilocular cyst-like appearance in the gross. The "cysts" are actually fibrovascular tissue walls usually filled with free-flowing blood. The interior of the cystlike walls usually lack a lining, although they may undergo endothelialization.

SOLITARY OR UNICAMERAL BONE CYSTS

CAPSULE SUMMARY (FIG. 13–6)

Incidence. Slightly over 3 per cent of biopsied primary bone tumors.

Age. Approximately 70 per cent of patients are between the ages of 4 and 10.

Clinical Features. . Pain in association with gross or microscopic pathologic fracture.

Radiologic Features. Symmetrical radiolucent lesion beginning in the metaphysis and usually extending to but not crossing the epiphyseal plate. In time the epiphyseal plate usually grows away from the lesion. Approximately 70 per cent of lesions occur in the proximal humerus and femur.

Gross Pathology. Unicameral cysts are filled with straw-colored or serosanguineous fluid. After fracture the cyst may become multiloculated or become replaced with blood clot, granulation, or fibro-osseous tissues.

Histopathology. Thin, fibrous wall lined by a thin layer of flattened to plump epithelial-like cells.

Post-Fracture. Blood clot, fibro-osseous, and granulation tissue.

Course. Completely benign. High recurrence rate of cyst after simple curettage.

Treatment. Curettage and packing with bone chips. Recently cryosurgery or local steroid injections into the cyst have been used with reported success.

Clinical Features

The solitary, simple, or unicameral bone cyst is a distinctive benign lesion which is usually discovered

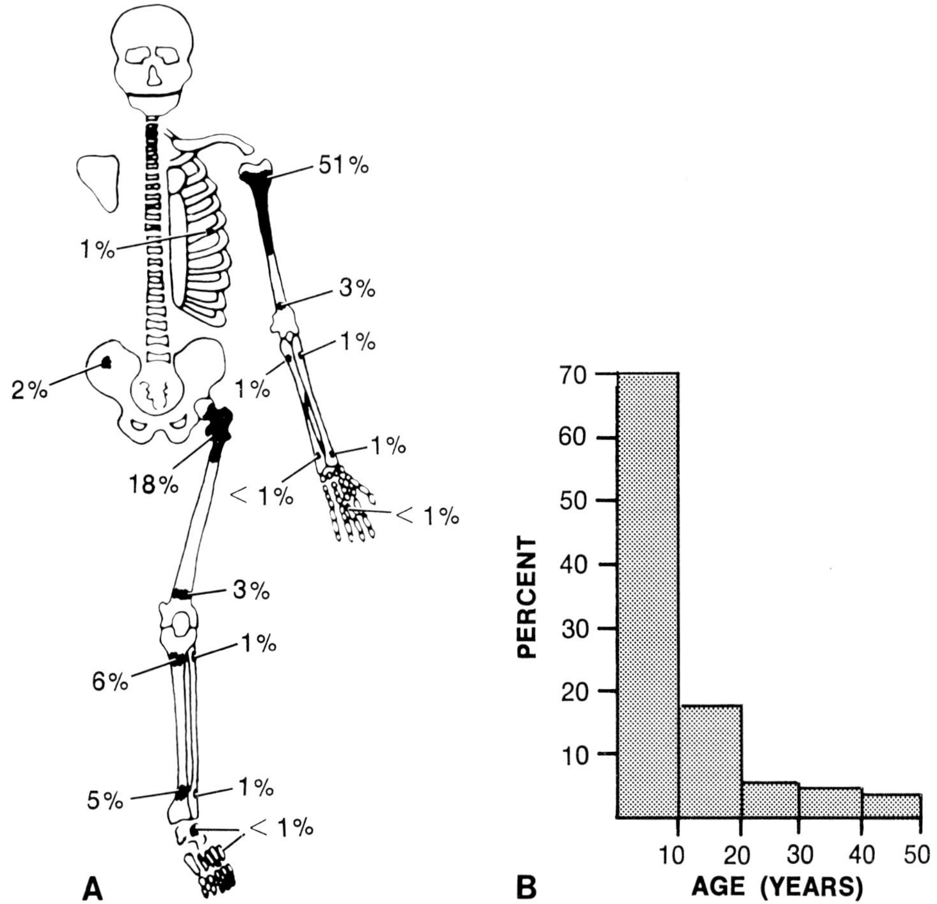

FIG. 13-6. (*A*) Solitary bone cyst. Frequency of areas of involvement in 195 patients. Male:female incidence 2:1. (*B*) Age distribution of patients with the solitary bone cyst. (Mirra, J., Bullough, P., and Freiberger, R.: Orthopedic Diseases, Part IV. New York, Famous Teachings in Modern Medicine, MedCom, Inc., © 1977)

in childhood. The majority of patients present either with pain or less commonly, with swelling. The usual cause of the pain is pathologic fracture with or without displacement and subsequent disability.

Most clinically presenting solitary bone cysts are in the proximal end of the humerus (50%), the proximal end of the femur (18%), or the proximal and distal ends of the tibia. When solitary bone cysts occur in other locations they are apt to remain silent and be discovered only accidentally.

Radiologic Features

The unicameral bone cyst has highly characteristic but not necessarily pathognomonic features, which are as follows:

1. A symmetric lytic lesion of the metaphysis that usually abuts the epiphyseal plate (Figs. 13-7, 13-10, and 13-11). The majority of cases (70%) involve either the proximal humerus or proximal femur.

2. The bone is usually symmetrically "expanded" and surrounded by a fine or thin rim of periosteal new bone (Figs. 13-7 and 13-11). Other cases may show little to no bone "expansion" (Figs. 13-8 and 13-9).

3. In some cases the lesion is seen up to several centimeters from the epiphyseal plate. These lesions are located in a metaphyseal—diaphyseal position (Figs. 13-8 and 13-9). If such cases are followed serially, in the earlier stages of the disease the lesion almost always abuts the epiphyseal plate. Its separation from the growth plate implies that the lesion has entered into a phase of growth slower than the growth of the epiphyseal plate away from it. In essence,

rapid, actively expanding cysts keep up with the growth plate and abut it. When the lesion slows down or abates in expansion the epiphyseal plate "outdistances" the lesion, which then becomes removed from the epiphysis. The lesions that do not abut the growth plate are usually seen in older children, because those represent a later stage of the disease. These cysts are not necessarily fully "latent," because curettage of the lesion even at this later stage can be associated with recurrence.

4. A pathognomonic sign of the simple bone cyst is the so-called *fallen fragment sign* (Fig. 13–8, *arrow*). This represents a portion or portions of fractured cortex that falls to the bottom of the fluid-filled cyst. Since a simple bone cyst is the only unilocular fluid-filled cyst of bone, the sign is pathognomonic. This sign is seen in less than 10 per cent of cases, however.

5. Many cases show evidence of gross pathologic fracture with or without displacement (Figs. 13–8 and 13–10).

With fracture or post-curettage and packing with bone chips the lesions can fill in with fibro-osseous tissues. However, from 35 to 50 per cent of such cases may still go on to develop one or more purely local recurrences (Fig. 13–10). Although the bone cyst is benign, it can be typified by stubborn recurrences. As the children reach young adulthood, the incidence of recurrence abates considerably.

Lesions that can resemble the bone cyst are a lytic expansile osteoblastoma, a poorly ossified fibrous dysplasia, or a small lytic osteosarcoma. One case this author has seen in a publication was that of a small lytic lesion of the distal radius interpreted radiologically as a bone cyst. It was curetted and packed with bone chips from the ilium. The surgical instruments were not changed during the procedure. Unfortunately, the tumor in the radius was an incipient osteosarcoma and seeding of the pelvis occurred because of the failure to change instruments. This author has also seen three identical pelvic transplants in association with three "enchondromas" that were in reality Grade I chondrosarcoma or Grade I chondrosarcomatous transformation of enchondroma. In this author's estimation obtaining bone chips from a distant site for a bone tumor should not be performed without a change of instruments and strict care given to principles of tumor sterility, unless, of course, the surgeon and pathologist are 100 per cent certain the lesion curetted is totally benign. Even then this author would not find it inconceivable to transplant a growing benign lesion to another bony site.

Gross Pathology

Simple bone cysts are rarely removed intact because of their benignity. In the operating room the bone usually shows a bulge in the area of the cyst. The periosteal covering is usually quite thin and fibrous to fibro-osseous. Where the cortical tissue is thinnest, the wall is fluctuant and a bluish tinge from the underlying fluid can be seen, provided that the cyst is relatively intact and the fluid has not been extruded because of extensive fracturing. A rare example of an intact simple bone cyst and its radiograph is shown in Figures 13–11 through 13–13.

Usually the bone cyst shows a solitary cystic compartment if it is intact. In opening the cyst a serous to serosanguineous fluid spurts out under pressure for a brief instant. After the initial pressure is released the fluid simply flows or oozes from the cavity. The wall of the cyst is a thin fibrous membrane generally no more than 1 mm. in thickness. Cysts that have had fractures can fill up with blood. Those cases in which

---

Simple Bone Cyst

FIG. 13–7. This is a typical example of a simple bone cyst. It is lytic with residual cortical bone remnants giving rise to a trabeculated or pseudoloculated appearance. The lesion extends to but does not cross the epiphyseal plate. These are lesions usually seen in association with open epiphyses, because most are discovered in childhood.

FIG. 13–8. The pathognomonic "fallen-fragment" sign. Note the two small slivers of bone (*closed arrow*) that descended in the fluid-filled cyst from a break in the cortex (*open arrow*). This sign is seen in fewer than 10 percent of SBC's.

FIG. 13–9. In this example of a young teenager, the epiphysis has grown away from the cyst, most probably because of a slowing down of the rate of cyst growth or expansion.

FIG. 13–10. These four illustrations show an example of recurrence in a SBC after curettage and packing with bone chips. (*A*) SBC with fracture (*arrow*). (*B*) After curettage and packing with bone chips. (*C*) Recurrence of cyst with dissolution of bone chips. (*D*) Lesion recuretted and packed with bone chips. Although the SBC is benign, in a sizeable percentage of cases there are one or more recurrences. Eventually cure is obtained in virtually every case.

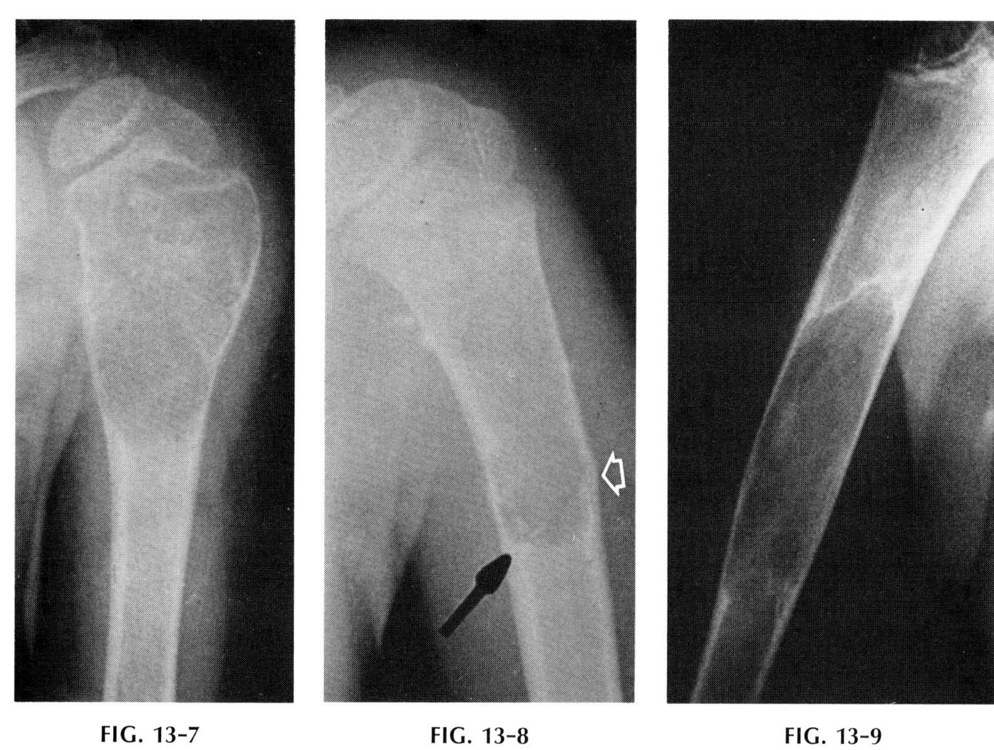

FIG. 13-7

FIG. 13-8

FIG. 13-9

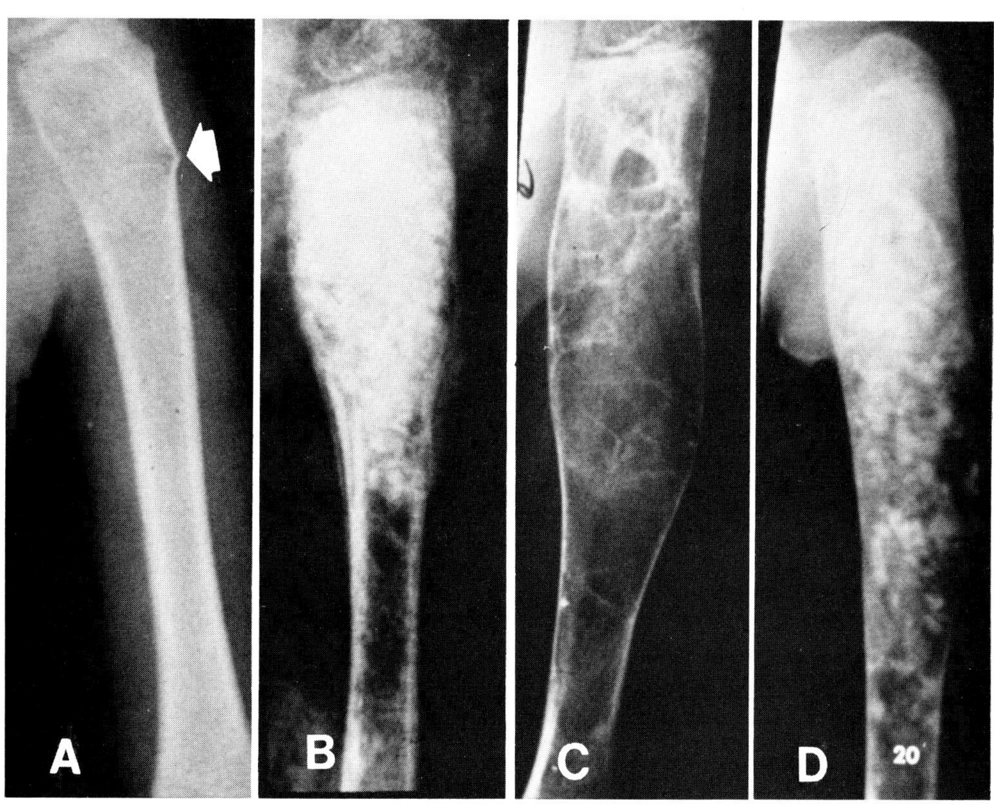

FIG. 13-10

the resolution of the blood is relatively complete may leave thin fibrinous to fibrous membranes that may convert the cyst into a multilocular rather than unicameral structure (Fig. 8–13). In other cases, consequent to fracture the cyst cavity may be completely obliterated and replaced by fibro-osseous repair tissues (a type of callus). Unless serial radiographs or previous biopsy show a precursor simple bone cyst, this "repair" stage of the lesion has been mistaken for other tumors, such as fibrous dysplasia or osteoblastoma both grossly and pathologically. Or even worse, if the repair tissues are particularly exuberant, the bone cyst can be mistaken for the osteosarcoma or fibrosarcoma.

Histopathology

TYPICAL FEATURES. On cut section the simple bone cyst appears thin-walled. It is usually smaller than 1 mm. in thickness (Figs. 13–14 and 13–15). The wall is fibrous and may contain a few slivers of osteoid (Fig. 13–15), woven bone, a mild sprinkling of chronic inflammatory cells, and some osteoclast-like giant cells (Fig. 13–16). Usually the amount of curettage done is meager, because the total bulk of the cyst wall is only a few grams. If bony walls are included in the specimen either from the attenuated cortex or medullary bone surrounding the cyst, the bone should be searched for the fibrous cyst wall (Fig. 13–16). In some sections the entire portion of recognizable cyst wall may be less than 1 or 2 mm. in width and length because of its fragmentation by the curettage.

The side of the cyst wall facing the fluid or interior of the cyst wall show either a single to double or triple layer or flattened to occasionally plump epithelial-like to endothelial-like cells (Figs. 13–20 and 13–29).

FEATURES FOLLOWING FRACTURE. *Consequent to fracture,* secondary features of necrosis and repair may be seen, including small giant cells intermixed with chronic inflammatory cells, hemosiderin pigment, cholesterol clefts, and exuberant fibrous and fibro-osseous repair tissues. The osseous tissue is usually osteoid or woven bone trapped in fairly dense fibrous tissue. Often the appearance of this fracture repair stage of the simple bone cyst can be confused with fibrous dysplasia (Fig. 13–17), osteoblastoma, or nonossifying fibroma. Although the host bone repair tissues may be exuberant, nuclear anaplasia is absent. It is rare to see cartilage in association with simple bone cysts. These extensive fibro-osseous repair lesions can be seen in from 10 to 15 per cent of curetted simple bone cysts. Some cases could be impossible to distinguish from monostotic fibrous dysplasia without previous biopsy showing unequivocal simple bone cyst or serial radiographs showing the relatively classic radiographic features of the simple bone cyst. Consequent to extensive fracture and fibro-osseous repair, great care must, of course, be given not to mistake these tissues for an osteosarcoma and vice versa, and not to confuse a small lytic osteosarcoma for the fibro-osseous repair in a bone cyst.

PRODUCTION OF A CEMENTUM-LIKE SUBSTANCE. Approximately 9 per cent of simple bone cysts (SBC) may be seen to produce a peculiar acellular to hypocellular substance in the wall of the cyst that has been likened to tooth cementum.[31] In fact, in 1969 Friedman and Goldman believed they had found a new entity, which they called "cementoma" of long bones.[23] Refer to Figures 13–20 through 13–23 for the light microscopic features of this peculiar substance. Mirra, Bernard, *et al.*, in one of three cases, subjected this material to ultramicroscopic study, which demonstrated that the calcification of this substance was

---

Simple Bone Cyst

FIG. 13-11. Typical SBC of the proximal fibula in a young teenager. The next three illustrations are from this case.

FIG. 13-12. The lesion was resected in toto and shows the bulging character of the fibula because of the "expanding" cyst contained within its substance. Usually there are areas where the cortex is so thin that a bluish color can be seen because of the fluid contained beneath the stretched periosteum (*arrows*).

FIG. 13-13. On cut section, the cyst is filled with clear to serosanguineous to bloody fluid, depending on whether or not fracture has occurred. When the fluid is removed, a space is left. The edges of the bone are covered by a thin rim of fibrous tissue, the wall of the cyst. If there has been hemorrhage and fibrin exudation, the usual unilocular nature of the cyst may be converted to a multilocular or fibro-osseous tissue consequent to repair. In this case, wisps of fibrous tissue at the bottom of the cyst represent collagenized fibrin, probably consequent to fracture hemorrhage in the past. The thickness of the cyst wall unmodified by significant fibro-osseous repair is generally no more than 2 mm. (*arrow*) and usually it is less than 1 mm. in thickness.

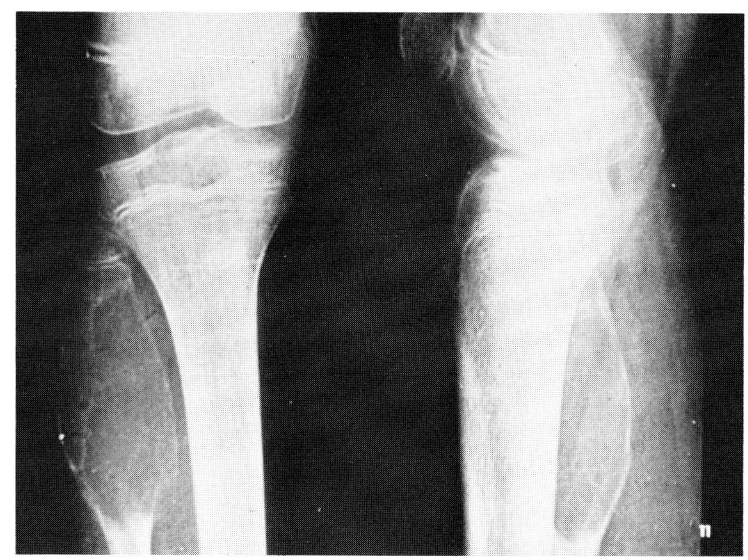

FIG. 13-11

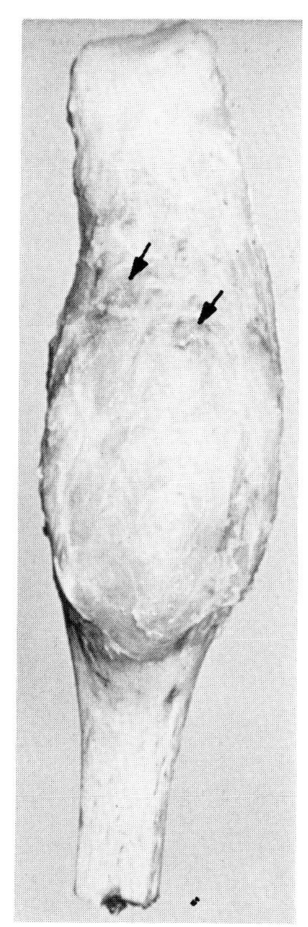

FIG. 13-12

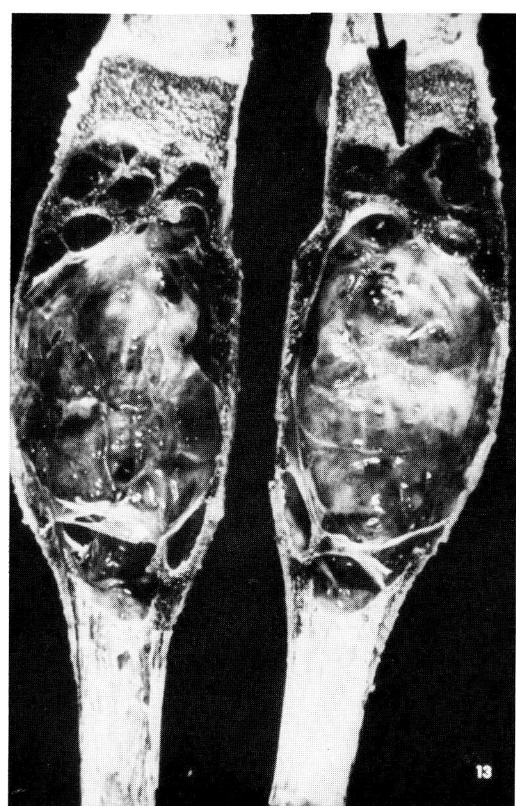

FIG. 13-13

mediated by matrix vesicles (Figs. 13–24 and 13–25), a component produced by either osteoblasts or chondrocytes. True tooth cementum does not contain matrix vesicles and is a product of cementoblasts, not of either osteoblasts or chondrocytes. Therefore, we conclude that this substance is a peculiar form of tissue derived from osteoblasts and is not true cementum but only a substance that has some morphological features that resemble it (cementoid or cementum-like substance).

The pathologist is referred to the paper by Mirra, *et al.*, for the reasons why we believe that the "cementoma" of long bones is a form of simple bone cyst with cementoid production. In short the radiographic, gross, and microscopic features are identical to the SBC, with the single additional component of the cementoid production. Figures 13–18 and 13–19 show the radiological features typical of the simple bone cyst in two patients with concomitant cementoid production in the cyst walls.

We have, however, never noted cementoid production in a lesion other than the SBC, and four of five cases reported to date have occurred in the region of the femoral neck, and one case in the proximal humerus. We do not understand the significance of this substance but to date all five cases have healed well with significantly less recurrence than with the usual SBC. This may be due, of course, to the meager number of cases.

In summary cementoid production is seen in approximately 10 per cent of cases of SBC. It appears to be a unique form of bone and its significance is entirely unknown. It is produced in the walls of the SBC, contains fine reticulin fibers arranged in linear or circular swirls, and by electron microscopy shows that its calcification proceeds upon matrix vesicles that are ultramicroscopic membrane bound cytoplasmic derivatives of osteoblasts.

Theories About the Etiology and Pathogenesis of the Simple Bone Cyst

Any theory relating to the etiology of the simple bone cyst must explain the following facts:

1. Over 70 per cent discovered in childhood
2. Over 95 per cent arise from or involve the metaphysis
3. Some 70 per cent occur in the proximal humerus and femur
4. Its fluid production is rich in protein
5. Cyst wall and lining cells
6. Recurrence
7. Benignancy

The early theories of the simple bone cyst were summarized by Coley and Higinbotham and James, Coley, and Higinbotham.[21,29] These included traumatic hematoma, infection, faulty calcium metabolism, and abnormal hyperplasia of osteoclasts. None of these theories have met with much enthusiasm because they did little to explain all of the observed facts. More recent theories include lymphatic blockage,[18,19] cystic degeneration in a benign tumor such as nonossifying fibroma, with blockage of lymphatics,[17] and degenerating lipoma. Neither of these three theories can explain Numbers 3, 4, or 5 listed above. Other problems exist. Why should nonossifying fibromas undergo cystic degeneration with or without

---

Simple Bone Cyst

FIG. 13-14. Low-power section shows the clear cyst space across which runs a thin wisp of collagenized fibrin (*a*). Note the thinner than 1 mm. cyst wall (*B*) and the attenuation of the cortex (*C*) because of the fact that the cyst is under pressure. (x2)

FIG. 13-15. If curettage is performed, the cyst wall may be completely separated from the underlying bone, as in this example. The wall consists of dense collagen in which may be found small slivers of osteoid (*arrow*), woven bone, and a sprinkling of giant cells and chronic inflammatory cells. On high-power examination, the cyst wall is covered by one to two cell layers of flattened to plump epithelial-like cells that closely resemble synovial cells (see also Fig. 13–29).

FIG. 13-16. In this example, cortical bone had been removed along with the cyst wall. The fibrous tissue to the left is periosteum, the bone is thinned cortex, and to the right is the thin fibrous wall of the cyst liberally sprinkled, in this case, with lymphocytes, occasional osteoclasts, and giant cells (x200).

FIG. 13-17. Consequent to the fracture, hemorrhage into the cyst may become organized into exuberant fibro-osseous tissues, as in this example. Note the extensive osteoid, flattened osteoblasts, and fibrous tissue. If the history or radiographs had not been reviewed, numerous mistakes in diagnosis, such as fibrous dysplasia, osteosarcoma, and osteoblastoma can occur (x125).

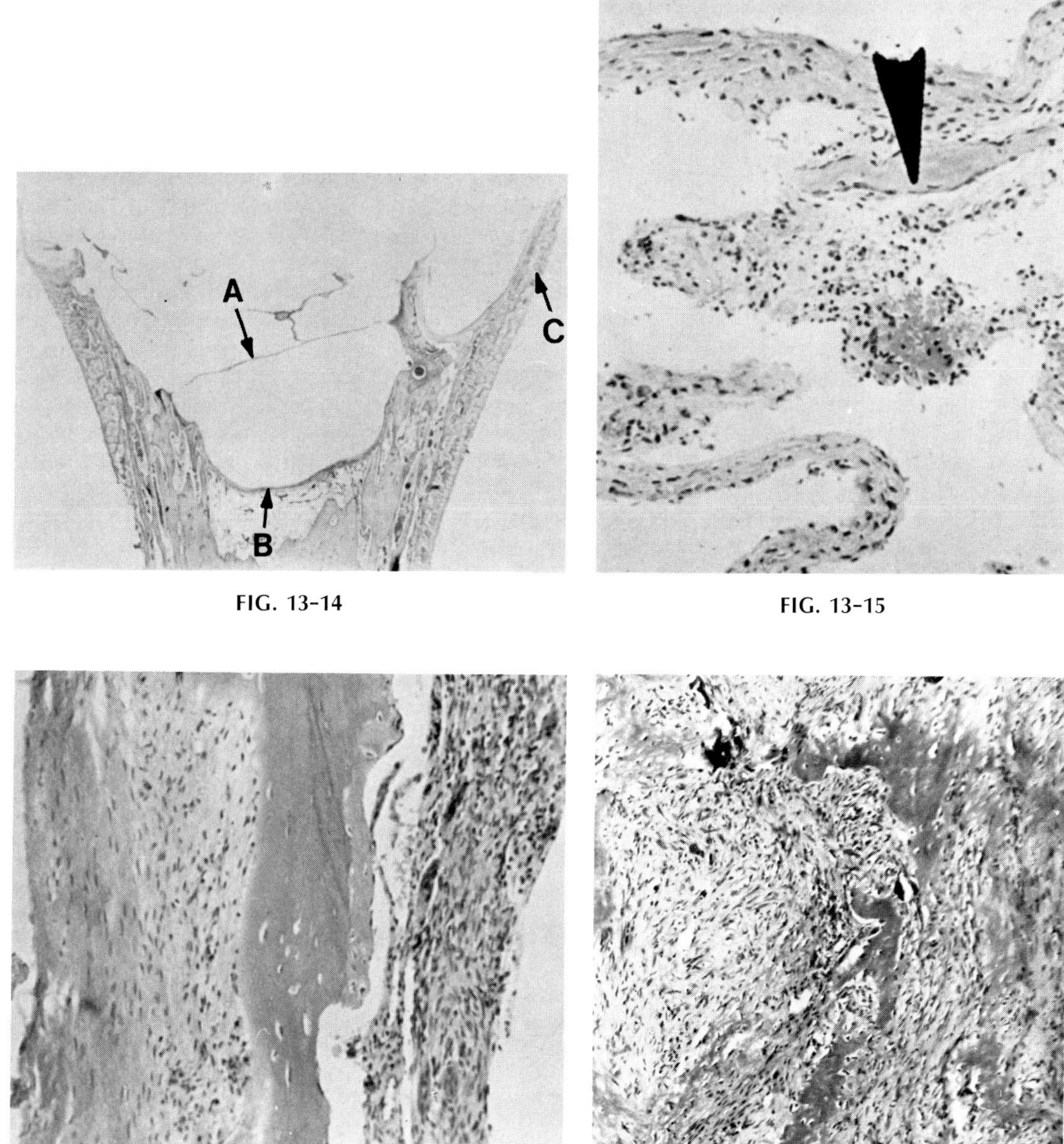

FIG. 13-14

FIG. 13-15

FIG. 13-16

FIG. 13-17

lymphatic blockage in the proximal femur and humerus considering, for example, that only 5 per cent of unequivocal nonossifying fibromas occur in these two sites? True *lipomas* of bone are very rare lesions characterized by "bulls-eye" calcification on radiograph; almost all occur in diaphyses or metaphyses of long bones with no predilection to the proximal humerus or femur and most are seen in adults. Why should degenerating cystic tumors recur as cysts? No one has ever clearly demonstrated lymphatics in bone. Lymphatic fluid is not as rich in protein as is the fluid simple bone cysts. The simple bone cyst is at least 50 times more common than lipoma of bone. Why should lipomas with cystic degeneration be 50 times more common than those without? Why don't we see unicameral cysts in lipomas of the soft tissues?

Electron microscopic observations of one of our simple bone cysts in association with cementum-like production is the first reported case of a simple bone cyst subjected to ultramicroscopic analysis.[31] The cyst lining was three to four cells thick and had the characteristics of mesodermal epithelium. The luminal cells have numerous oriented microvilli as is present in endothelium and synovial cells. The surface cells are elongated and each contain endoplasmic reticulum, mitochondria, free ribosomes, a Golgi apparatus, and vesicles (Figs. 13–26, 13–27, and 13–28). Most of the lining cells have luminal filopodia (Figs. 13–26, 13–27, and 13–28), and some cells contain lysosomes (Fig. 13–27). Beneath all of the cells is an incomplete basal lamina (Figs. 13–26, 13–27, and 13–28). The surface cells relate to each other by minimal intercellular contact (Fig. 13–2, 13–27), gap junctions (Figs. 13–27 and 13–28), and desmosomes (Fig. 13–27).

On a light microscopic level these surface cells closely resemble synovial cells (Compare Fig. 13–29, *A* and *B*). The EM observations show that the luminal cells have features of an epithelium with microvilli, basal laminae, and occasional desmosomes. This lining layer has somewhat the appearance of a venule were it not for the facts that there are numerous areas where there are no cell to cell contacts between the surface cells, a very incomplete basal lamina, and an indistinct lumen containing no blood cells.

The lining has, therefore, more of the appearance of a synovial membrane because of the variations in surface cell to cell contacts and the indistinct basal lamina. These lining cells are surrounded by an amorphous material described in association with synovial cells by other authors. Other authors have reported that cell junctions and basal laminae in the synovial membrane were indicative of pathological changes. Groth, on the other hand, suggests that these might be normal characteristics of synovial lining cells.[26] In our case, the two types of lining cells, "A" and "B" cells reported by Barland, *et al.*,[15] are represented. "A" cells (Fig. 13–26) are probably macrophages and "B" cells (Fig. 13–27) are similar to fibroblasts. The synovium and mesothelium are classified as a mesodermally derived epithelium; this is the same classification as for the pleural, peritoneal and joint cavities. Further support for the concept that the simple bone cyst lining cells are entirely consistent with cells of synovial origin is the fact that Gabbini, *et al.*,[24] have shown by electron microscopy in an unequivocal biphasic synovial sarcoma that the epithelial-like component demonstrated microvilli, specialized intercellular junctions in the form of desmosomes, and distinct basal laminae. These epithelial structures were identical to those found in the lining cells of our case.

The hypothesis we formulate, based partly upon our ultrastructural observations of our Case 3, is that the simple bone cyst is probably an intraosseous synovial cyst. We hypothesize that during fetal or early infant development or perhaps due to trauma at birth, a small nest of synovium becomes trapped in an intraosseous position. If such a "rest" were to occur and if it were to retain some or all of its secretory function, a cyst could develop. As we know from arthritic cysts the host bone will attempt to "wall-off"

Cementum-Like Production in Simple Bone Cyst

FIG. 13–18. Radiograph of a rather classic-appearing SBC of the femoral neck in a 5-year-old boy with cementum-like production in the wall of the cyst.

FIG. 13–19. Pathologic fracture through the neck of an 18-year-old female with a SBC. This patient also had cementum-like production in the exuberant cyst wall.

FIG. 13–20. Wall of cyst with flattened cellular lining (*top*). Globular accretions of accellular cementum-like substance is seen below (x125).

FIG. 13–21. Another example of the pattern and appearance of this peculiar acellular substance (x40).

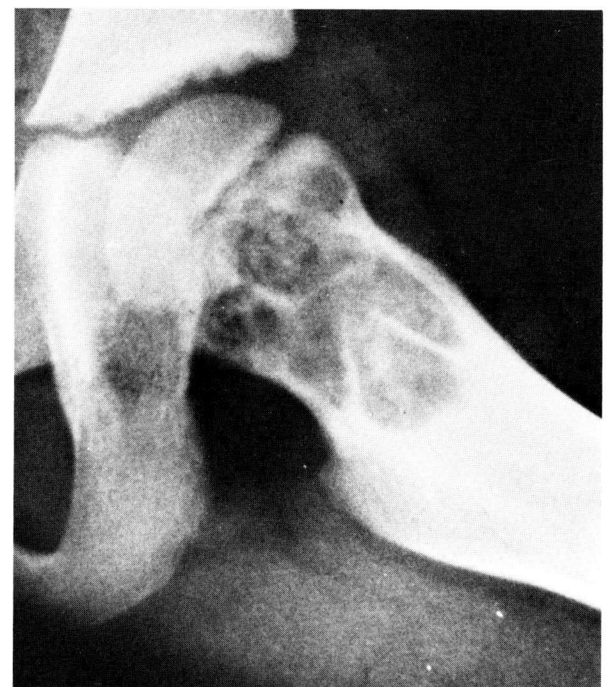

FIG. 13-18

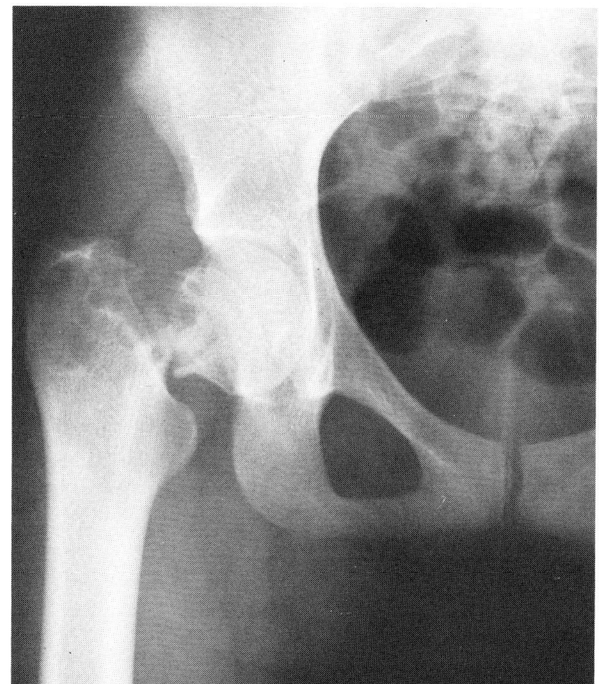

FIG. 13-19

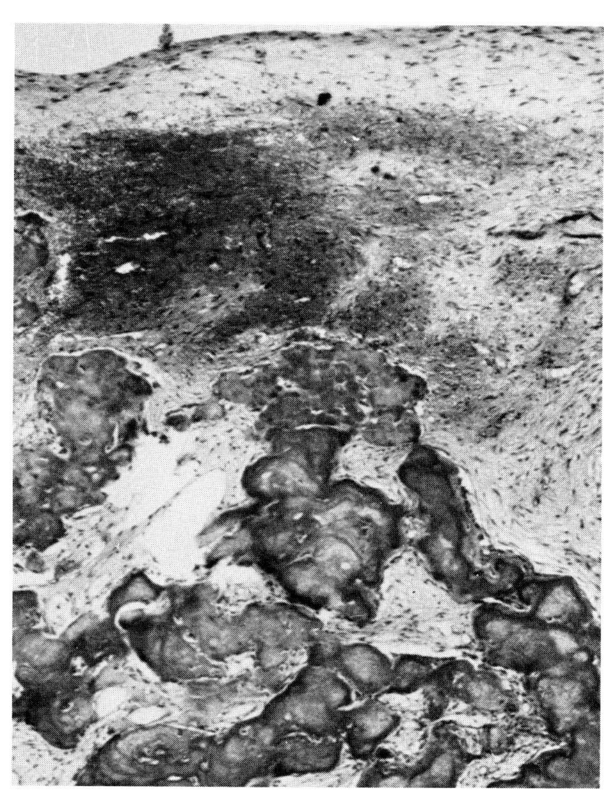

FIG. 13-20

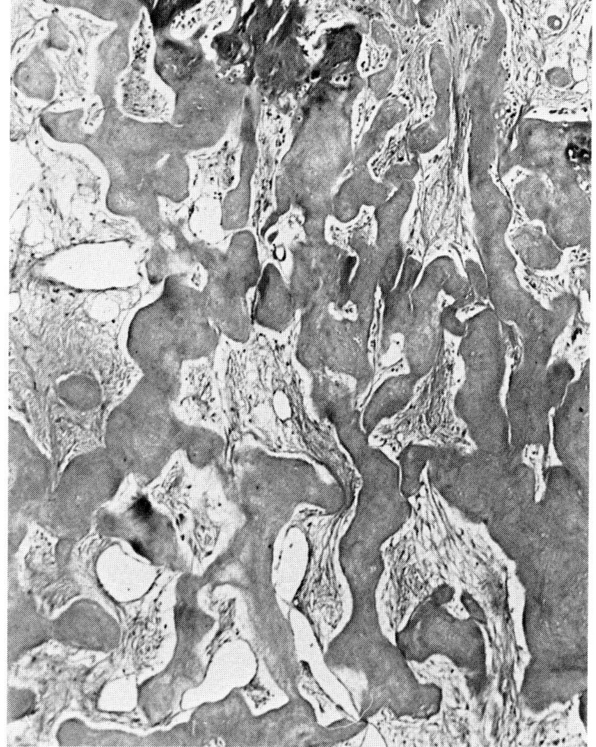

FIG. 13-21

the growing fluid cavity with fibrous or fibro-osseous tissues. All of the morphologic components of a simple bone cyst would, therefore, be explained. The fibrous tissue, giant cells, and slivers of osteoid and bone would be derived from the host bone mesenchyme as a reaction to contain the foreign synovial epithelial cells and the fluid they produce. Simple bone cysts are rich in protein, as is the synovial fluid.[18,19] Lymphatic fluid is much less rich in protein. Therefore, the presence of a rich proteinaceous fluid is much more in keeping with a fluid of synovial origin.

If our hypothetical intraosseous synovial cyst is not contained by the surrounding host bone defenses, it will continue to grow and "expand" the bone and eventually could lead to fracture. The flattened cells lining the cyst could well be due to the increased pressure within the cyst. At surgery the cysts may be seen through the attenuated cortex as a dense, bluish-white structure if they are unmodified by fracture. These cysts will eject fluid when drilled under pressure. Following fracture a bone cyst may fill in with hemorrhage and a reactive fibro-osseous repair tissue that may be confused with fibrous dysplasia.

Let us now consider the age at which most patients with bone cysts present. Most patients are young children, although rare cases may present in infancy or adulthood. The hypothesis of an error in embryonic, fetal, or infantile development fits the observed facts. Simple bone cysts followed by serial radiographic examination are slow growing and would not be expected to produce symptoms until pathologic fracture or marked swelling has occurred. An example of another probable error of early development that is not discovered until childhood or later is the osteochondroma. Virchow hypothesized that the osteochondroma represents a "herniation" of the epiphyseal plate during early development.[36] The osteochondroma, therefore, represents the growth of an aberrant "bone within a bone." His hypothesis explained its discovery in youth, its imperceptible blending with the underlying host bone, its cartilage cap, and the cessation of endochondral ossification of the cartilage cap when the normal epiphysis of the host bone ceased growth. In actuality, this attractive hypothesis was not proven until the experiments of D'Ambrosia and Ferguson. These authors placed a portion of a growing rabbit's epiphyseal plate in the periosteum of the metaphysis in the exact orientation predicted by Virchow. Unequivocal osteochondromas formed (See Figs. 14-2-14-6).[22]

Can a "synovial rest" hypothesis satisfactorily explain the position of the lesion within the bone? The vast majority of solitary bone cysts are metaphyseal in youth and closer to the diaphysis in older patients followed by serial radiographs. Rarely, they are found in the true epiphyseal end of the bone. Our hypothesis formulates that a synovial implant occurs in an intraosseous position. Where would we expect such an implant to occur? Naturally, where bone and synovium are in closest approximation to each other. That would be at the reflection of the capsule with the bone. Generally, the capsule of long bones inserts in the metaphyseal end of the bone, exactly where most simple bone cysts occur. The capsule never inserts in the diaphysis, where no bone cyst ever begins. Another observation we have made is that in human and animal bones the capsule and its synovial recess have the greatest surface area of contact with the thin metaphyseal bone in the two bones with the greatest rotatory motion, namely, the humerus and the femur. These two areas are exactly those sites in which over 70 per cent of the simple bone cysts are found. No other theory fits with this highly unusual anatomic distribution.

Jaffe divided bone cysts into "active" and "latent." He said that a cyst that is in the vicinity of the growth plate possesses potential for growth and hence is an "active" cyst. One which has grown away from the plate is "latent" and no longer has the capacity for growth.[28] We would consider the growth of the cyst to be relatively independent of its relation to the growth

---

Cementum-Like Production in Simple Bone Cyst

FIG. 13-22. (*A*) In some fields, true bone may surround the substance. Note the contrast between the osteocyte, rich woven bone (*1*) and its heavier calcification, compared to the more poorly calcified acellular cementum-like substance (*2*). (*B*) Polarized light shows the differences in the pattern of polarizable fibers in the cementoid, compared to the bone. Note the contrast in fiber thickness between the two (x300).

FIG. 13-23. Under polarized light, the collagen or reticulin fibers in this substance were quite thin compared to the collagen of usual bone. In most fields the fibers were oriented in a linear fashion (*1*) but in some areas the fibers were oriented in a circular distribution (*2*). Note the acellularity and lack of a central nutritive vessel, showing that these structures are not haversian systems (x250).

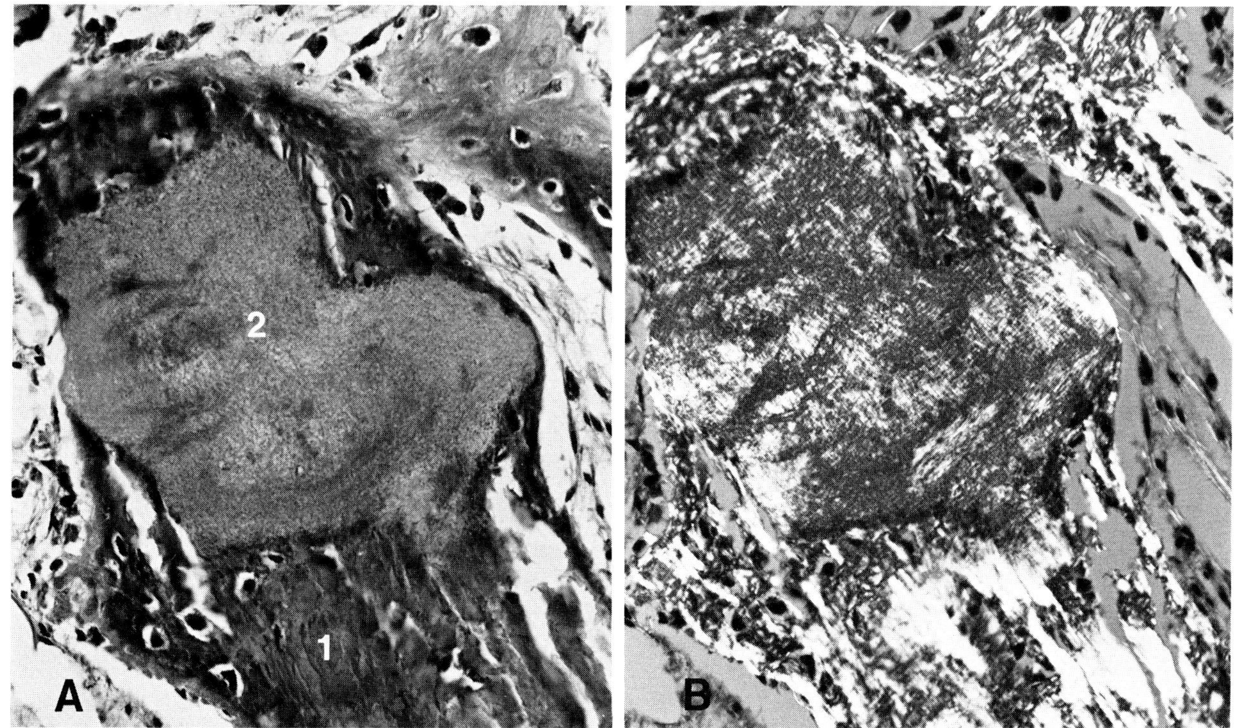

FIG. 13-22

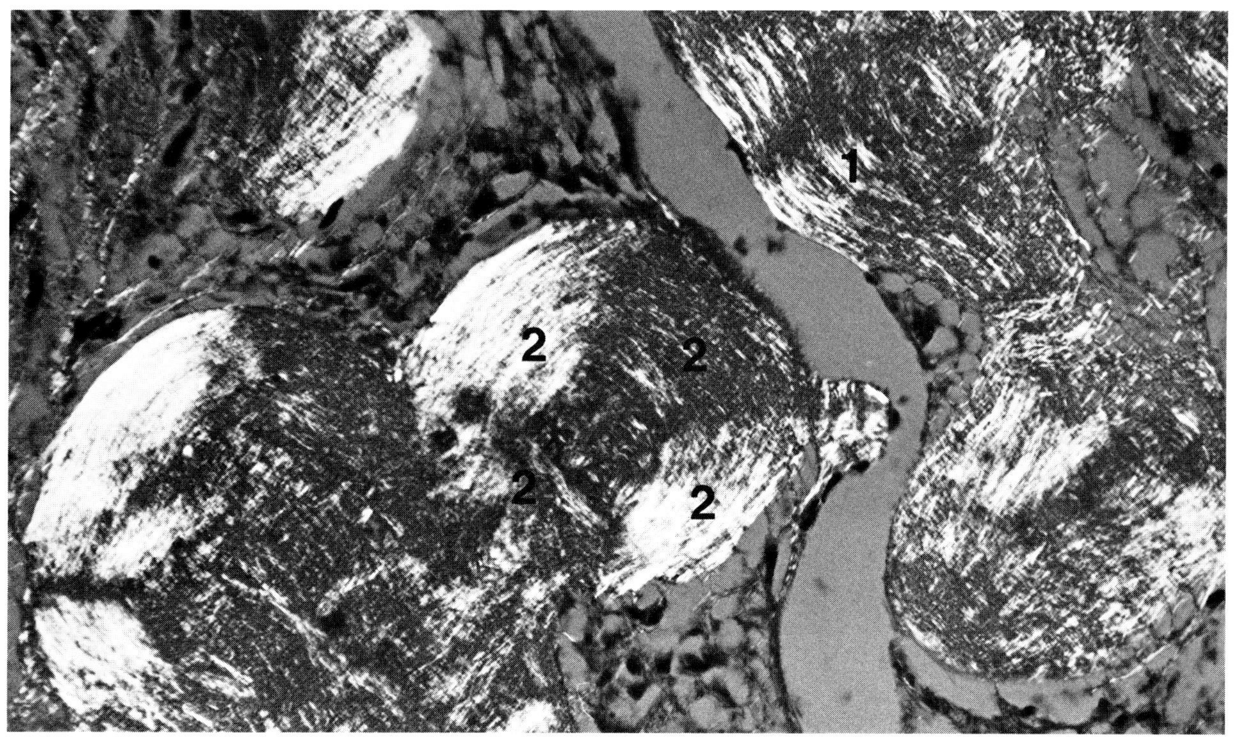

FIG. 13-23

plate. In our hypothesis the only possible relation of cysts to the growth plate is of those that are farther from the plate and are "older" or more slowly expanding, and hence may have entered a phase of less active cellular activity and fluid production. We have seen recurrence and growth in cysts that were far removed from the epiphyseal plate (personal observations). Neer, *et al.*, in a study of 175 cases of simple bone cysts, specifically looked at so-called "latent" versus "active" cysts. They found the following: "Cysts extending to within 0.5 centimeter or less of the epiphyseal plate were compared to those further away in the shaft. When these criteria of activity were used, the results, in terms of recurrence, differed little between the active and latent groups."[33] Our observations coincide with those of Neer and associates in that growth of the cyst and recurrence are not specifically related to its distance from the growth plate. The distance of a bone cyst from the epiphyseal plate may signify a state of less active cellular activity and fluid production as is seen in older patients. According to our hypothesis and the observed facts, these circumstances do not necessarily preclude recurrence, provided that a portion of the cyst lining remains and that some remaining capacity for the lining cells to replicate and to retain their capacity for fluid production. With increasing age, this capacity apparently diminishes to the point where even if a portion of the lining remains, recurrences will not happen.

In summary, using the rule of Occam's razor (the simplest hypothesis which explains the greatest number of observable facts), we believe the most reasonable hypothesis for the simple bone cysts at this time is that it represents a congenital "rest" of synovial tissue displaced into the thin, cortical, metaphyseal region of bones at the synovial-capsular-bone reflection. Its benign nature and slow growth would explain its discovery in early childhood, and the marked preponderance of cysts located at the proximal humerofemoral location can be explained by the fact that these two bones have the largest area of capsular to metaphyseal bone reflection.

Course and Treatment

The simple bone cyst is a completely benign lesion that never metastasizes but is prone to local recurrence. Recurrence following simple curettage is about twice as frequent in children under age 10 as in children over that age. Larger lesions have a greater tendency to recur than smaller ones. The recurrence rate is approximately 30 per cent for lesions of the proximal humerus, 17 per cent in the proximal femur, and 11 per cent in the proximal tibia.

Treatment of the SBC may be complicated by local growth disturbances, an arrest from severe damage of the growth plate resulting from surgery, or occasionally by overstimulation of growth from hyperemia in the region of the epiphysis.

Simple curettage is the usual procedure but cryosurgery has been used by Marcove with success. He protects the epiphyseal plate during freezing with a wad of gelfoam. Campanacci, from the University of Bologna, is using injections of steroids into the cyst and is curing patients, in most cases, without the need for surgical intervention.[17a] The injections are performed under general anesthesia and with radiographic control. Two large needles are inserted into the cyst. The cyst fluid is extracted and one needle removed. A quantity of methylprednisolone acetate equal to the quantity of fluid extracted is introduced through the other needle. This is usually between 2 and 5 ml., that is 80 to 200 mg. The injection is repeated bimonthly two or three times. If there is no pathologic fracture, immobilization is considered unnecessary. There is complete radiologic resolution in about 50 per cent of cases in from 1 to 3 years. In most of the other cases, there is substantial improvement, making surgery unnecessary.

(*Text continues on p. 478.*)

Cementum-Like Production in Simple Bone Cyst

FIG. 13-24. The simple bone cyst and cementumlike substance was subjected to ultramicroscopic study in one of our reported cases. In order to relate this field to the light microscopic level, the reader is referred to Figure 13-20. The area studied by EM in this figure basically corresponds to the lining cells of the cyst, the subcystic loose fibrous tissue, and a portion of the cementum-like substance. (*a*) Cystic lining cells, (*b*) flocculent granular matrix, (*c*) fibroblastic layer, (*d*) dense collagenous zone with a few calcification loci, and (*e*) dense collagenous zone with denser calcifications (x4000).

FIG. 13-25. EM of the cementum-like area showed collagen fibers and matrix vesicles that are becoming calcified (*arrows*). These are the so-called initial calcification loci common to bone and cartilage formation. These structures are not seen in true tooth cementum. Therefore, we believe this substance to be a peculiar acellular to hypocellular type of bone (x35,000).

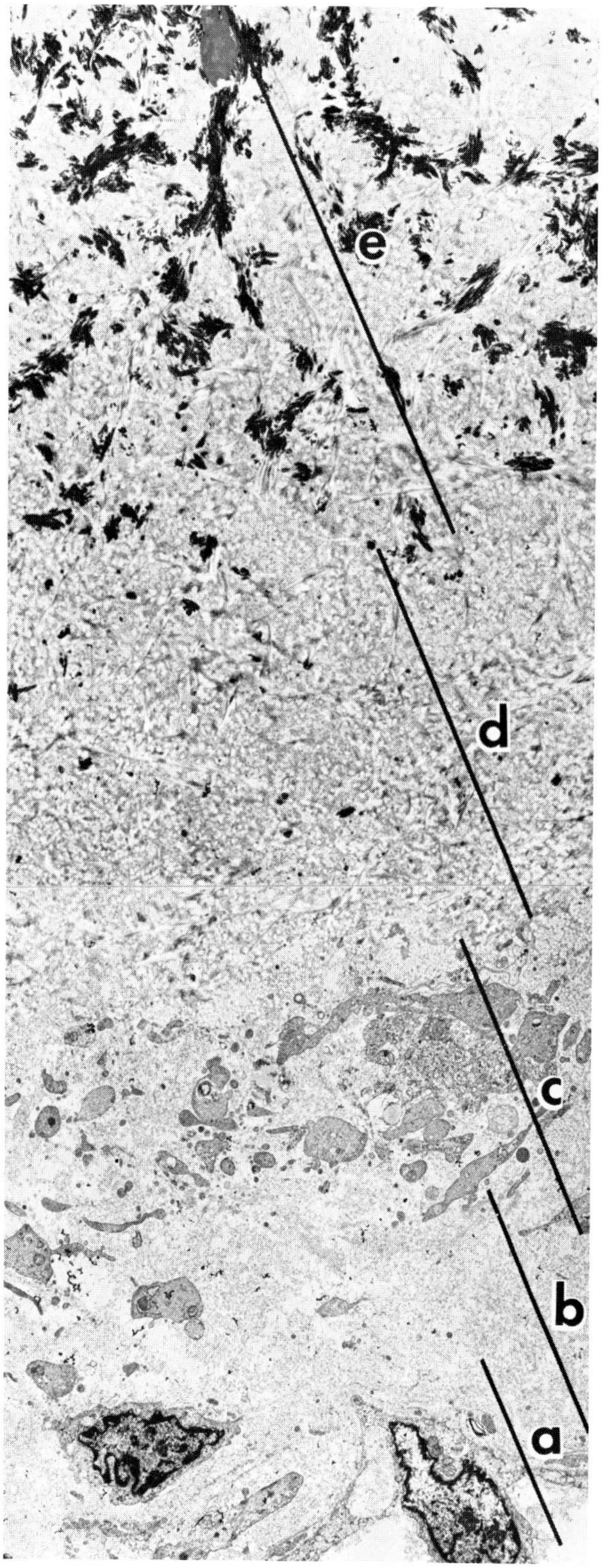

FIG. 13-24

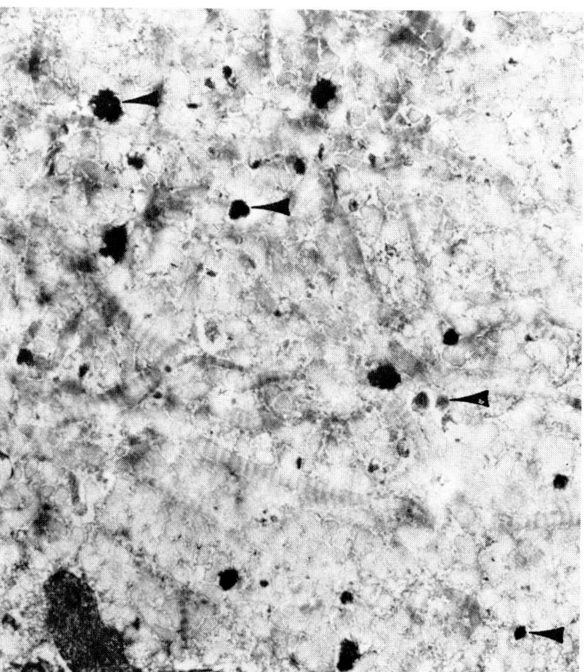

FIG. 13-25

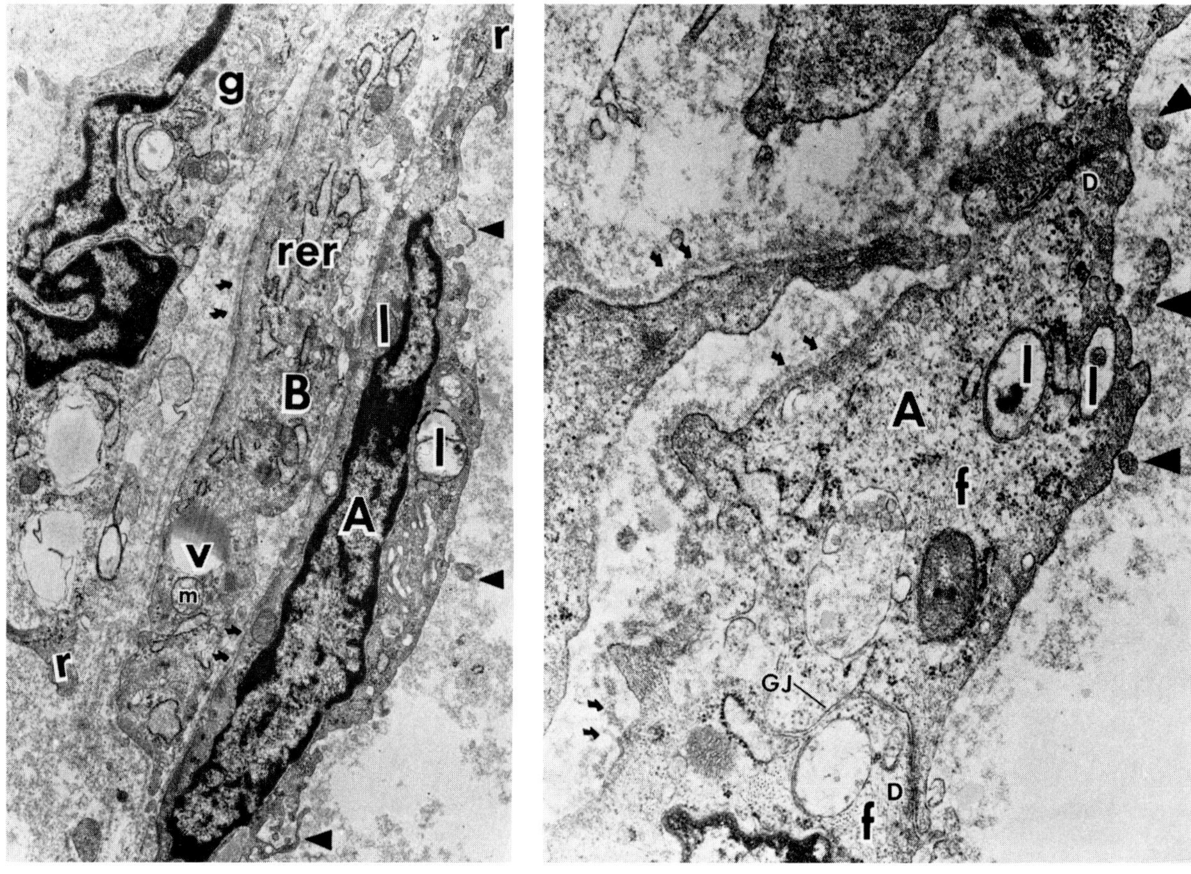

FIG. 13-26

FIG. 13-27

Possible Synovial Cell Origin to Bone Cyst Lining

FIG. 13-26. EM of the surface cells lining the cyst. Two types of cells were noted: an (*A*) cell and a (*B*) cell. Other features include filopodia (*arrows*), rough endoplasmic reticulum (*rer*), irregular basal lamina (*double arrows*), mitochondrion (*m*), Golgi apparatus (*g*), free ribosomes (*r*), vesicles (*V*), and lysosomes (*l*) (x8000).

FIG. 13-27. Portions of three luminal cystic lining cells. Lysosomes (*l*), irregular basal lamina (*double arrows*), microfilaments (*f*), filopodia (*arrows*), gap junction (GJ), desmosomes (D), and "A" cell (A) (x24000).

FIG. 13-28. "B" lining cell (*B*), filopodia (*arrows*), irregular basal lamina (*double arrows*), minimal intercellular contact (*apposed arrows*), and myofibroblast (MF) (x8000). The features of the lining cells of Figs. 13-27, 13-28, and 13-29 are most consistent with type "A" and "B" cells of synovial epithelial origin rather than endothelial origin.

FIG. 13-29. (*A*) Surface lining cells from a patient with SBC and cementoid production (*arrow*) (x300). (*B*) Surface lining of synovium from a patient with osteoarthritis (x400). Note the striking similarity of morphological features of the lining cells, suggesting that both may be of identical origin. Further corroboration with EM analysis of these cells is needed.

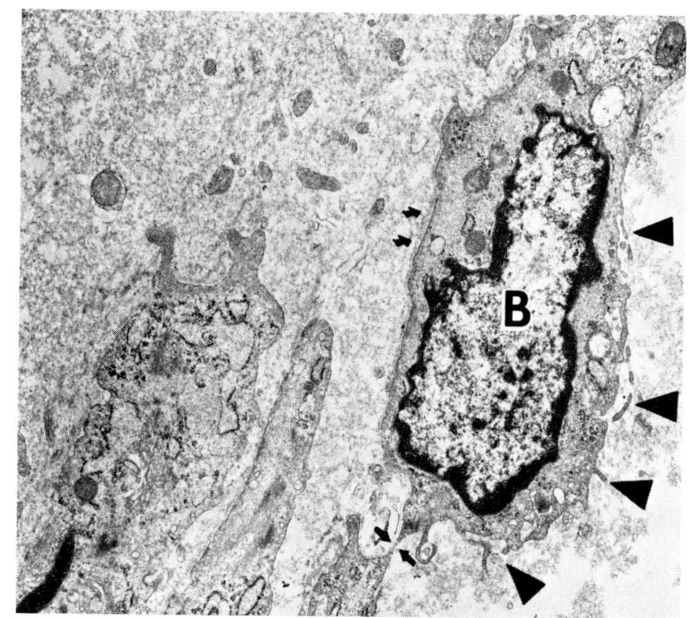

FIG. 13-28

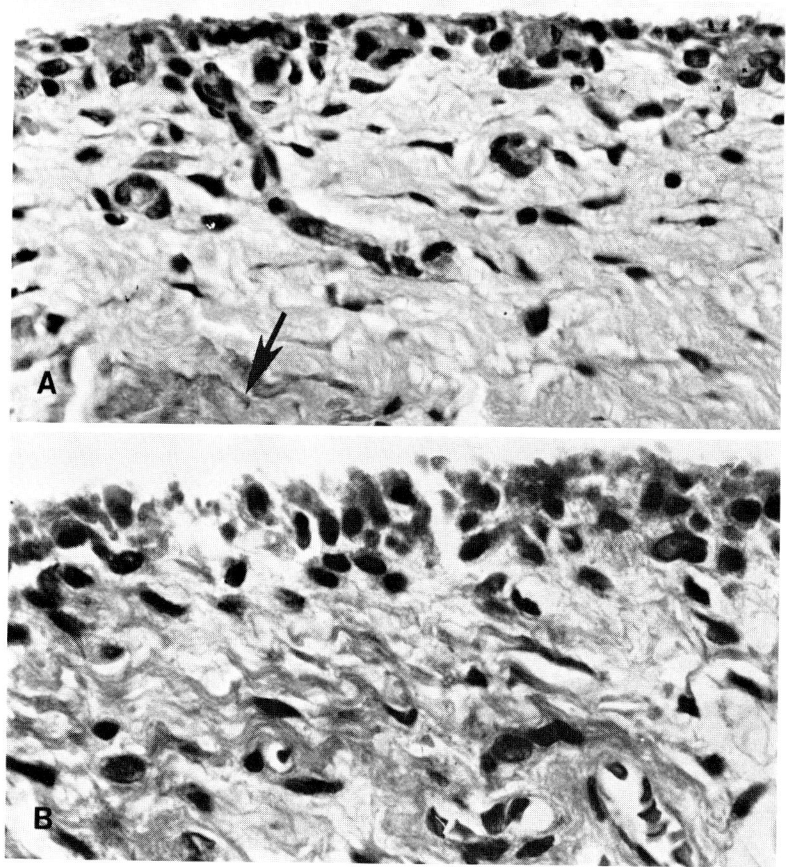

FIG. 13-29

Aneurysmal Bone Cyst (ABC)

Capsule Summary (Fig. 13-30)

Incidence. Approximately 1 per cent of biopsied primary bone tumors

Age. Approximately 70 per cent of patients between 5 and 20 years of age

Clinical Features. Swelling, pain, tenderness

Radiologic Features. Intramedullary lytic lesion often associated with a subperiosteal "blowout" appearance.

Gross Pathology. Dark reddish brown friable spongy tissue containing blood-filled cystlike spaces.

Histopathology. Usually nonendothelialized fibro-osseous septae filled with nonclotted blood. The walls may contain slivers of osteoid, woven bone, osteoclasts, and occasional inflammatory cells. There is no anaplasia.

Course. Benign. Recurrences quite common, but it is eventually controlled.

Treatment. Curettage and possibly cryosurgery.

Introduction and Theory of Pathogenesis

The so-called aneurysmal bone cyst (ABC) describes a radiologic-pathologic complex. Considerable controversy exists about whether the ABC represents a vascular response to an underlying primary tumorous process. Before Jaffe and Lichtenstein described the lesion, most often it was mistaken for a variant of the giant cell tumor or for the telangiectatic osteosarcoma (the so-called "malignant bone aneurysm"). The ABC is one of the most rapidly growing and destructive lesions of bone and it is not difficult to see why its growth behavior was equated with malignancy. Of all the theories relating to the aneurysmal bone cyst, the one that is rapidly gaining the widest acceptance is that stemming from Biesecker, *et al.*'s. article of a study of 66 cases.[38]

They made the following important observations:

1. Some 32 per cent of cases were associated with other apparently primary entities, such as the nonossifying fibroma, fibrous dysplasia, chondroblastoma, giant cell reparative granuloma, fibromyxoma, solitary bone cyst, and low-grade neoplastic giant cell tumor of epiphyses. These observations have been confirmed by others. This author has seen ABC in association with two chondroblastomas, one giant cell tumor, one nonossifying fibroma, one solitary bone cyst, and two cases of fracture, from a total of 12 aneurysmal bone cysts (personal observations). This represents an incidence of approximately 60 per cent associated with other lesions.

2. Significant vascular pressures were manometrically measured in several cases. These pressures were what would be expected to exist in arteriovenous fistulae.

As a result of these new observations, Biesecker, *et al.,* propose that the aneurysmal bone cyst is essentially an arteriovenous anomaly engrafted upon a precursor lesion.[38] This author would agree most emphatically with the conclusions of Biesecker, *et. al.* In essence, the ABC may not be a neoplasm at all but merely an arteriovenous or vascular anomaly induced by a benign or low-grade malignant precursor lesion. Apparently the tremendously rapid and destructive growth of this proposed anomaly can totally obliterate the precursor lesion in about half of the cases. If this hypothesis is correct the ABC could be a secondary entity, an arteriovenous malformation set into effect by a benign precursor lesion. This author has seen one case in which this hypothesis is very difficult to refute. The basic facts of this case, which were extremely complicated, are as follows.

At age 13 this female patient was irradiated for a lesion of the femur. All slides and records of the initial lesion were lost in a fire. At age 38 she developed a fracture through the radiated area of bone (radiation osteitis). At the age of 40, after several more fractures, she developed a slow-spreading lytic lesion which on histological examination proved to be an aneurysmal bone cyst (Fig. 13-31). Eight years later, the entire femur was replaced by the ABC (Fig. 13-32). Ambulation became impossible without crutches. At age 38 she also began to develop a large blastic lesion in the proximal femur area. Because the limb was useless and there was a blastic lesion present, a disarticulation was performed. The bone was cut into slabs and prominent arteriovenous malformation was noted (Figs. 13-33 and 13-35). Dissection revealed that the large artery branched into smaller arteries, which then opened into the large blood-filled to serosanguineous cyst-like cavities (Fig. 13-33, *B*). On histological section these were identical to those of an ABC. From the walls of the cystlike cavities emanated numerous tortuous veins by transmitted light (Fig 13-34). A thrombus was seen in a large branch of the artery feeding the malformation (Figs. 13-33, *B,* and 13-35). The blastic lesion represented either a massive hyperplastic callus due to multiple fracturing through the extremely attenuated cortex destroyed by the ABC or a very low-grade anaplastic radiation osteosarcoma. The patient is alive four years later without evidence of lung metastases, even though a residual bone-producing blastic lesion was present at the amputation margin. The remaining lesion has been extremely slow-growing and may represent a very low-grade form of osteosarcoma.

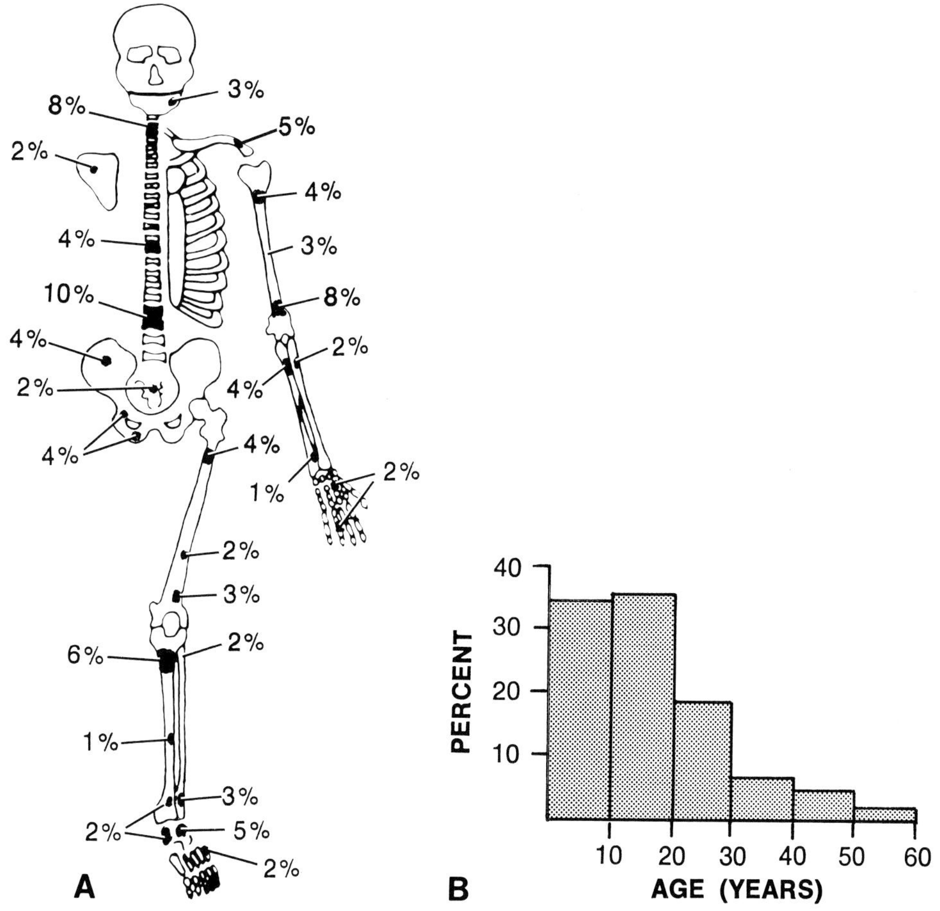

FIG. 13-30. Aneurysmal bone cyst. Frequency of areas of involvement in 129 cases. Male : female incidence, 1 : 1. (*B*) Age distribution of patients with the aneurysmal bone cyst. (Mirra, J., Bullough, P., and Freiberger, R.: Orthopedic Diseases, Part IV. New York, Famous Teachings in Modern Medicine, Med Com, Inc., © 1977).

In this author's estimation the case is explainable as follows: The patient was radiated for an unknown tumor. Many years later she sustained multiple fractures through a weakened and compromised area of radiation-damaged bone. As a result of multiple traumatic fracturing she developed hemorrhage and vascular trauma leading to the development of an arteriovenous malformation which completely replaced the bone within an 8- to 10-year period. It is well known that severe traumatic injuries may induce destructive arteriovenous malformations. This is particularly prone to occur in trauma to the hand, which leads to the development of an arteriovenous malformation of the soft tissue that may erode into the bones of the hand. Obliteration of such traumatically induced arteriovenous malformations is extremely difficult to achieve. Quite commonly the post-traumatic arteriovenous malformations of the hand may lead to local gangrene, necessitating amputation of fingers or even the whole hand. Several reports exist that attempt to relate trauma and fracture to the development of some examples of the ABC.[37,41,42] Ginsburg reported a case of a congenital fracture and ABC and believed that the intrauterine fracture could well have induced the ABC.

In summary, reported observations would favor the contention that the ABC is a rarely induced arteriovenous malformation secondary to trauma or the local destructive effects of benign or malignant neoplasms. The case we have presented (Figs. 13-31–13-35) shows a clear-cut arteriovenous malformation in association with an ABC. The reason for its demonstration may have been that the slow growth of the lesion so completely destroyed the bone

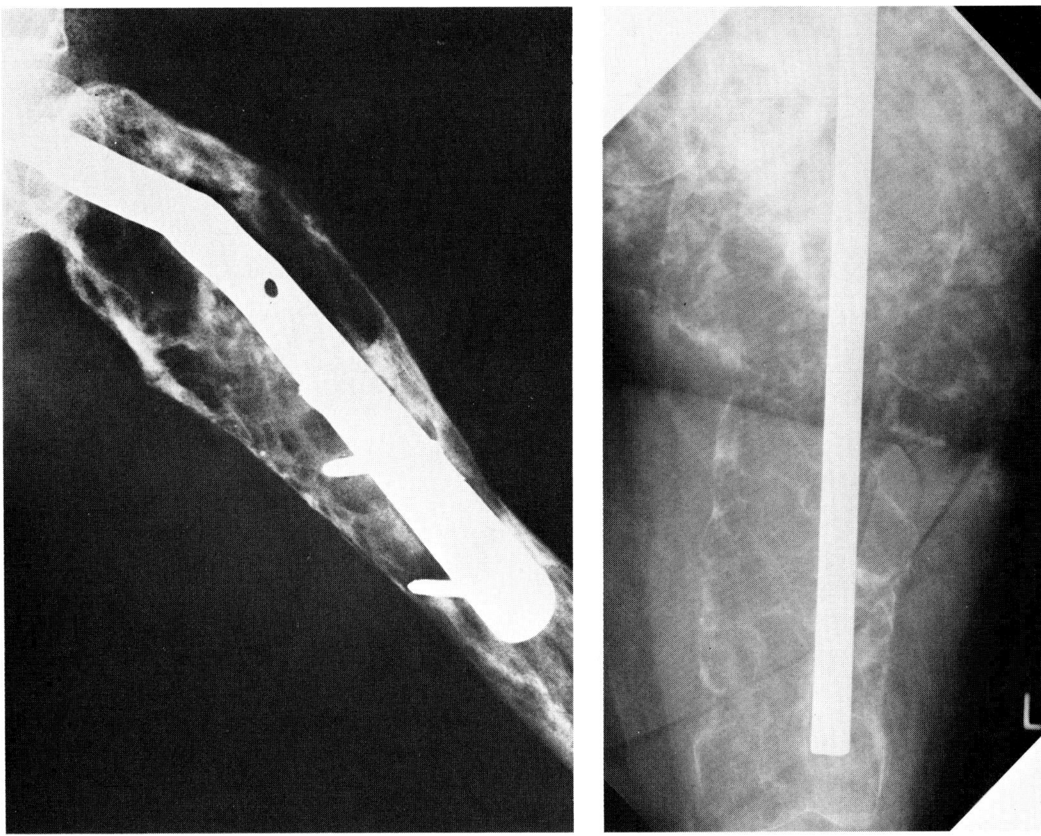

FIG. 13-31 FIG. 13-32

Aneurysmal Bone Cyst With Vascular Malformation

FIG. 13-31. A 40-year-old female showing a biopsy-proven lytic and expansive aneurysmal bone cyst that developed after multiple fracturing through an irradiated area of bone.

FIG. 13-32. Eight years later, the lesion extended to involve the entire femur. Note also the development of a new, ominous, proximal blastic lesion. Because of the patient's inability to use the leg and the blastic lesion, an amputation was performed.

that the malformation became easily recognizable on gross examination. ABC's are rarely examined intact and in the few cases where they have, the extreme degree of blood-filled cavities and residual bone may have obscured the underlying arteriovenous malformation. If other cases are to be reviewed intact, it would be important to wash away the blood and to slowly decalcify the specimen and to perform a very careful anatomic dissection to search for an arteriovenous malformation. If a feeder artery can be found, injection of a solidifying contrast material could facilitate demonstration.

Clinical Features

Approximately 85 per cent of patients present with swelling and/or pain before the age of 20. In most patients the first symptom reported is a bulge of the affected bone or a rapidly growing tumor. Pain is usually mild.[40] Lesions that involve the spine can lead to more serious symptoms such as paraplegia. Rapid growth usually lasts no more than several weeks. The duration of symptoms ranges from several months to several years. Approximately 80 per cent of the le-

(Text continues on p. 484.)

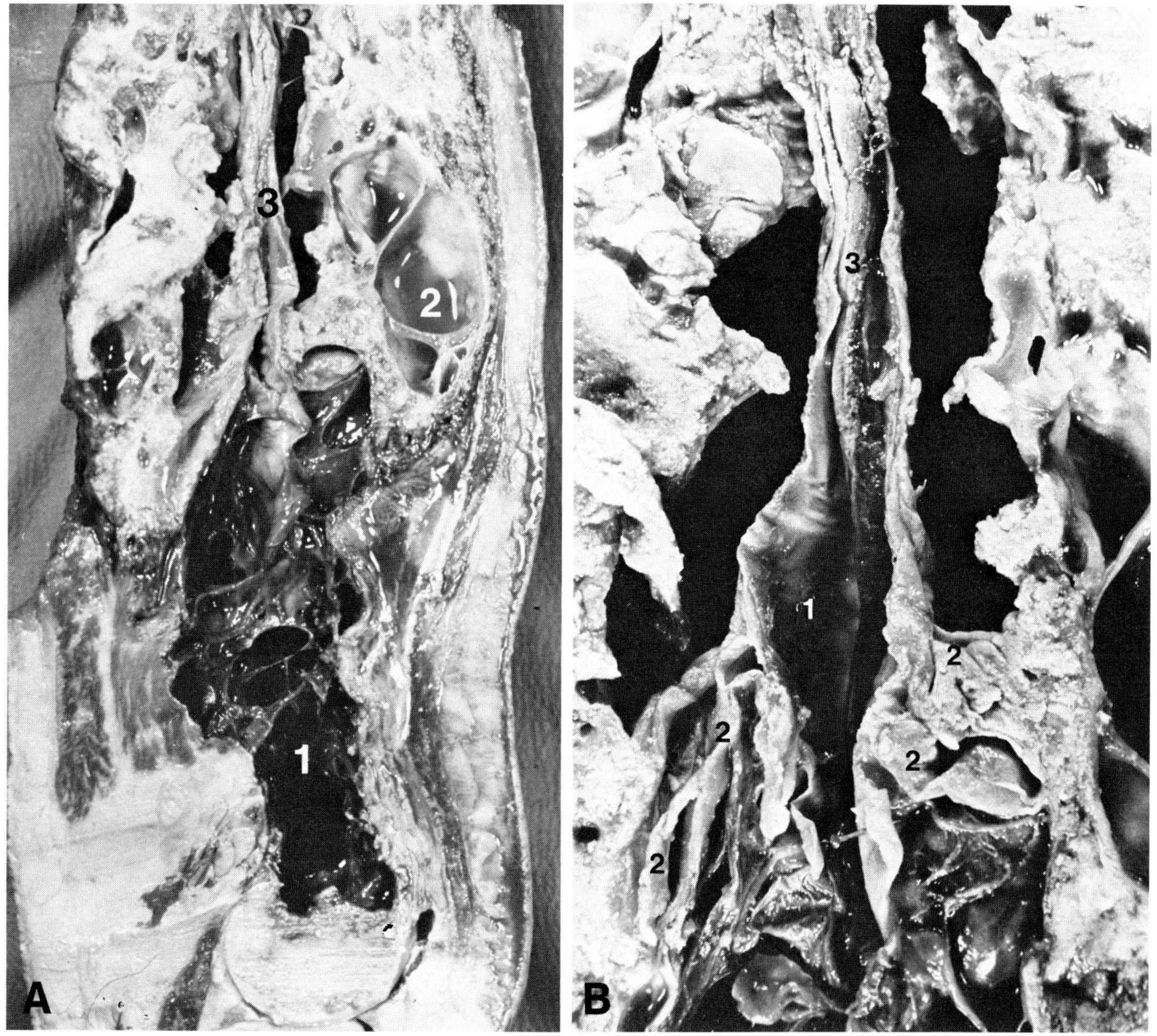

Aneurysmal Bone Cyst With Vascular Malformation

FIG. 13-33. The leg was frozen and cut into slabs. (**A**) The bulk of the lesion showed an expansive cystic aneurysmal bone cyst grossly and microscopically. The distal portion of the cyst lesion contained free-flowing blood (*1*), while the proximal portion showed clear fluid in the cysts (*2*) because of thrombus of the vessels (*3*) supplying this region. (*B*) Note the huge "feeder" vessel (*1*) that aborizes into smaller vessels (*2*) in the lower field and the large thrombus (*3*) it contains. The thrombus was attached to the proximal end, tapered, and placed free distally. The thrombus, therefore, is in the direction of arterial flow and identifies the vessel as a distended artery.

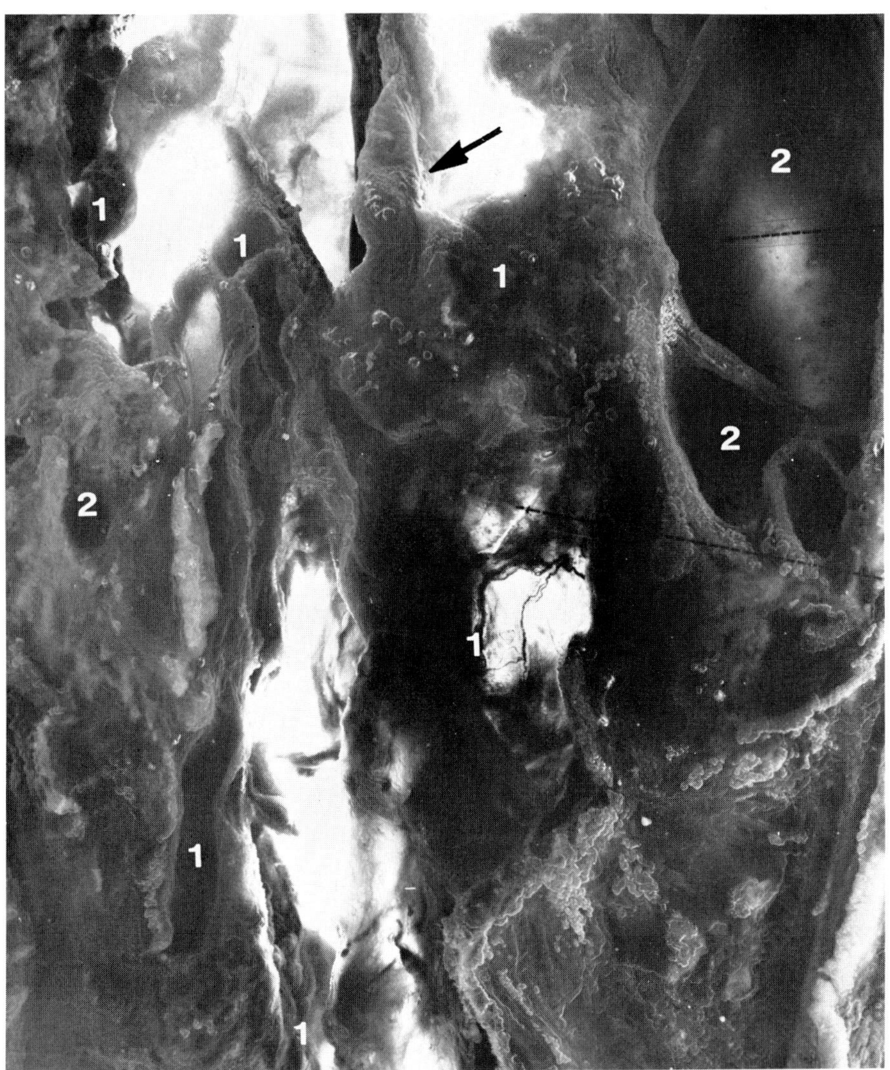

Aneurysmal Bone Cyst With Vascular Malformation

FIG. 13-34. Transillumination showed numerous fine vessels (capillaries and veins) (*1*) communicating with the cysts (*2*). The "feeder" artery is seen in the center (*arrow*). The anomaly is, therefore, a huge arteriovenous malformation associated with or actually giving rise to the entity known as aneurysmal bone cyst.

FIG. 13-35. In summary, the specimen showed the following: an arteriovenous malformation, a vascularized aneurysmal bone cyst, a large feeder artery with a thrombus, and in the upper portion of the leg, a large blastic lesion that, due to its persistant recurrence over 4 years, despite amputation, is apparently proving itself to be a low-grade, locally invasive, highly atypical variant of an osteosarcoma.

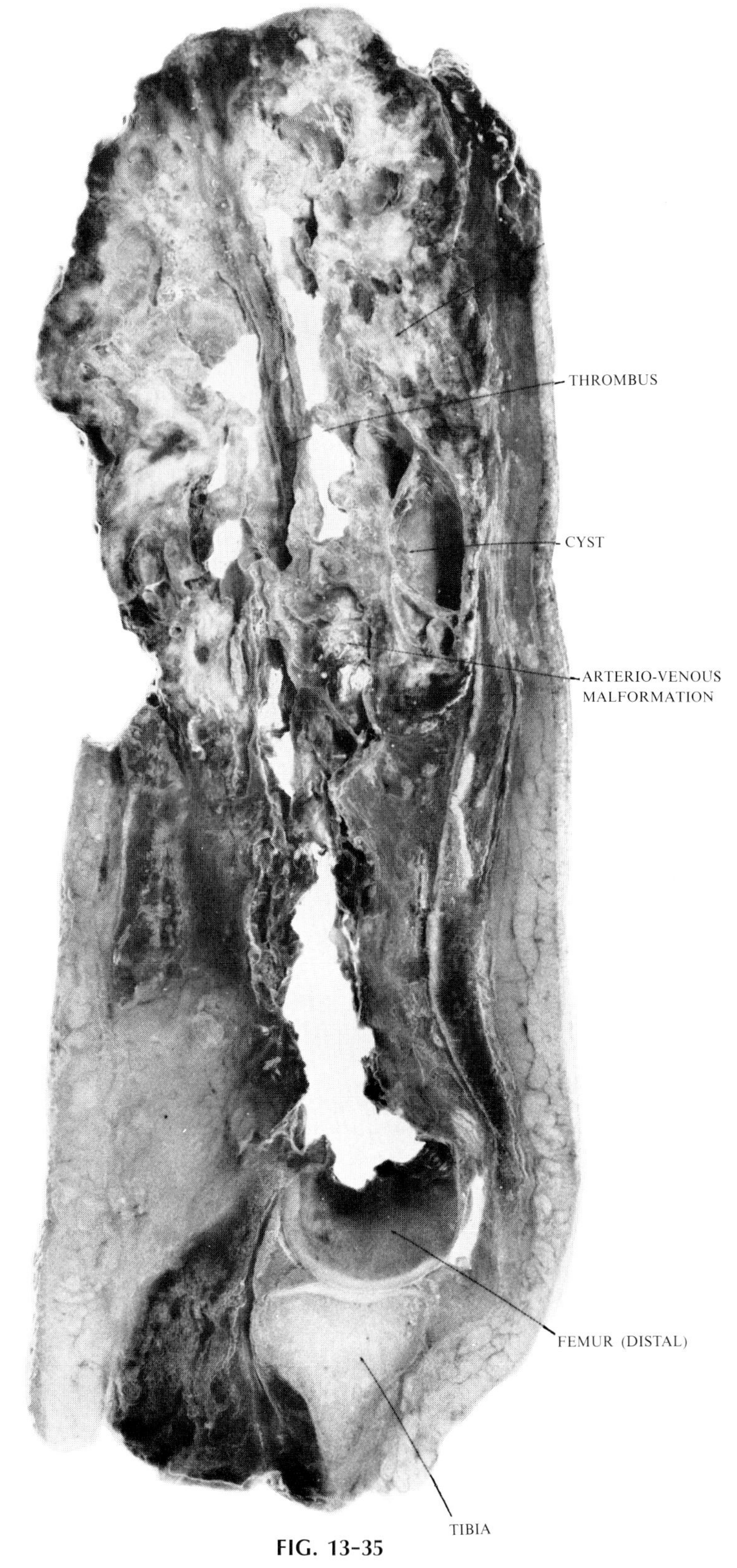
THROMBUS
CYST
ARTERIO-VENOUS
MALFORMATION
FEMUR (DISTAL)
TIBIA

FIG. 13-35

sions involve the long bones or posterior arch or transverse or spinous process of the spine. A solitary lytic lesion of a vertebral body is usually either a metastasis, infection, or giant cell tumor, not an ABC. The remainder affect the flat bones and jaw. Some patients may develop pathologic fracture, limitation of movement, or tenderness. Others may be associated with an unequivocal precursor lesion such as a nonossifying fibroma, simple bone cyst, chondroblastoma, traumatic fracture, or others.

Radiologic Features

The classic radiologic feature of the ABC has been described by Jaffe as a periosteal "blowout" lesion outlined by a paper thin shell of subperiosteal new bone (Figs. 13–38, 13–43).[44] However, although many cases may show the classical "blowout" lesions, not all do, and on rare occasion other entities may show a "blowout" lesion with no evidence of an ABC on biopsy (Fig. 13–46). In approximately 80 per cent of cases, the ABC involves the metaphyses of the long bones, the posterior arch, or the spinous or transverse process of the spine. The vertebral body is not often involved. The lesion may involve the bone centrally or subperiosteally or both in combination. Most cases eventually show both central and periosteal involvement.

The best method for understanding the radiologic features of an ABC is from those cases in which serial radiographs show the usual course of the disease. The ABC goes through phases that could be described as incipient, middle, and late radiological phases. Patients may present during any one of these phases but most present in the mid "blowout" (rapid growth) phase of development, when the tumor is usually approaching maximum size. At this time it would be most common for a small or gross pathologic fracture to develop or for gross swelling to prompt the patient to seek medical attention. In some cases the patients present with small, incipient lytic lesions or with advanced, large, well-circumscribed, bulging, late phase lesions. Both the incipient and late phases are often confused with other entities.

Phases of the ABC

INCIPIENT PHASE. The incipient phase of an ABC is characterized by either a small eccentric lytic lesion usually of a long bone metaphysis (Figs. 13–36 and 13–37, *A, B,* and *C*) or by a pure lifting off of the periosteum from the host bone without evidence of an intramedullary lesion (Fig. 13–43). Most cases show intramedullary involvement, but most patients do not present in the incipient phase. Except for focal cortical thinning the cortex may be otherwise preserved and the periosteum may show no reaction whatsoever (Fig. 13–37, *A, B* and *C*). In this phase of development the lesion will usually be mistaken for a simple bone cyst, nonossifying fibroma, or perhaps a lytic osteosarcoma. The pure intraperiosteal type may be due to blunt trauma leading to an intraperiosteal hematoma and arterio-venus malformation. This type may eventually erode into the medullary substance.

MIDPHASE. The midphase of development of an ABC represents its rapid destructive growth phase. It is characterized by extreme lysis of the bone, focal cortical destruction, and the development of one or more Codman's triangles (Figs. 13–37, *D–F,* 13–38, and 13–39).

The edges of the lesion as it abuts proximally or distally with the bone often show a "nibbling" destruction or ragged margin (Fig. 13–36, *F*). Nevertheless, the lesion is usually always fairly well circumscribed and does not show extensive permeative infiltration into the medullary substance beyond the area of "bulge" or focal destruction. An extensive permeative or moth-eaten pattern of destruction a considerable distance from the main lesion would be much more in keeping with a malignant tumor or osteomyelitis than would the ABC.

Within several more weeks the lesion tends to reach a maximal size and the classical "blowout" features are most evident. The bone is usually tremendously expanded, Codman's triangles may be prominent, and the periosteal region of the main tumor mass may show little to no bony circumscription at this time (Figs. 13–37, *D* and *E*. In other words the main tumor mass has a naked margin.

Because of the massive size, degree of bone destruction, and naked margins, the lesion can easily be mistaken for a malignant tumor in this phase. The "blowout" appearance is quite characteristic, however, of ABC. On occasion, myeloma, thyroid and kidney metastases, giant cell tumors, and the pseudotumor of hemophilia mimic this phase of ABC.

LATE HEALING OR STABILIZATION PHASE. Eventually the lesion grows much more slowly or may even cease growth entirely. When this occurs the periosteum has sufficient time to lay down a collar of periosteal new bone and the remaining intramedullary tissue and host bone surrounding the lesion forms new bone as a secondary or healing response. In this later phase of slow to absent growth the bone will show concentric (Figs. 13–40 and 13–45) or eccentric (Fig. 13–43) smooth-bordered, bone-collared expansion (Fig.

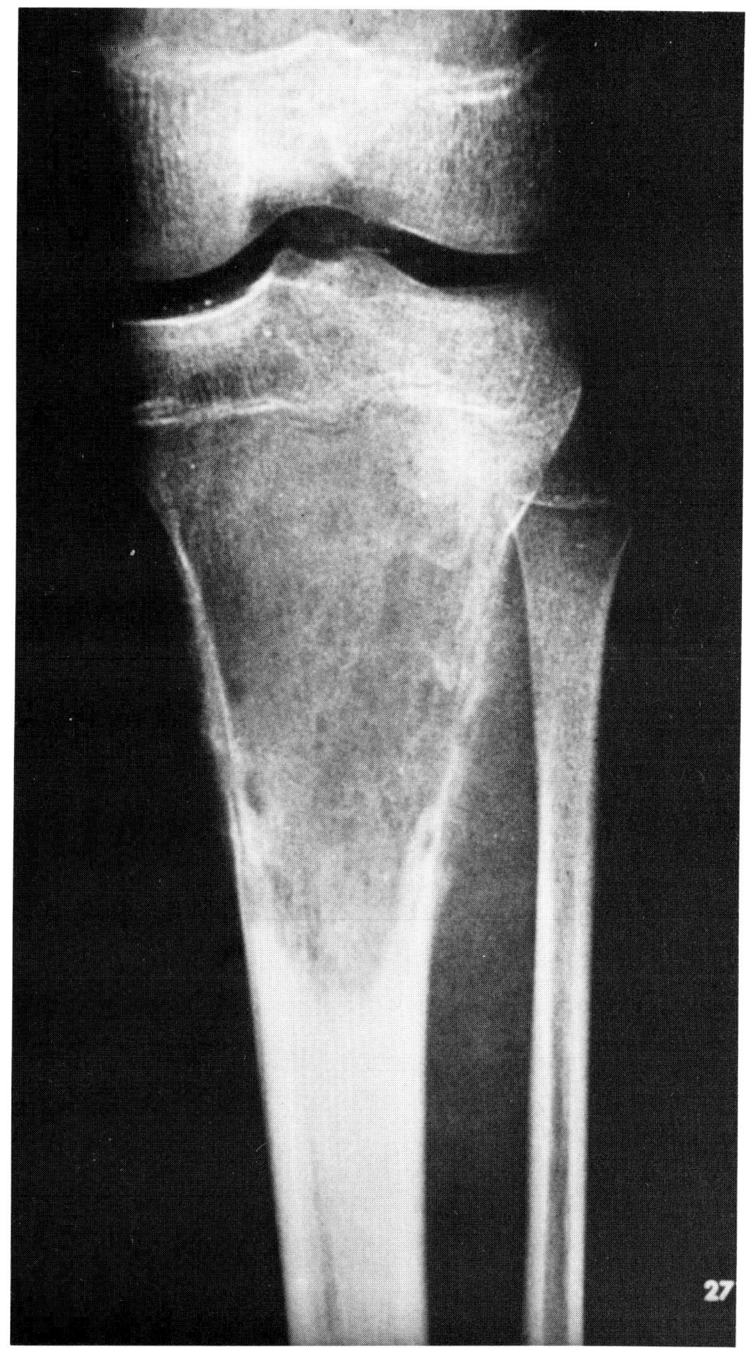

Aneurysmal Bone Cyst

FIG. 13-36. An example of the ABC in its incipient destructive phase with minimal periosteal new bone formation. The ragged edges of the lesion, extensive cortical destruction, and mild periosteal reaction are alarming and would ordinarily be signs pointing to malignancy.

13–43, *arrow*), a trabeculated to "bubbly" intramedullary appearance, and surrounding host bone sclerosis (Figs. 13–40 and 13–45). Codman's triangles disappear or merge into the expansile mass. All of these latter features now point to the benign nature of the process, which now become evident because its rapid growth and destructive phase has ended.

With these serially examined radiographic features in mind, several case examples will be shown in which patients have presented with the ABC in different phases of development. Figure 13–41 shows a large, expansive, poorly delineated lesion of the transverse process with a wisp of subperiosteal new bone (*arrows*). In essence, this is an ABC in midphase that is probably entering a phase of slower growth, evidenced by the presence of small amounts of periosteal new bone. In contrast, Figure 13–42 shows a late phase of an ABC in almost the exact same location as is the patient in the former illustration. Figure 13–43, left, shows an example of a late phase pure periosteal type of an ABC. Angiogram (right) shows the intense vascularity common to the ABC that supports the concept of an arteriovenous malformation. Figure 13–44 shows a relatively early phase of an ABC with extensive bone lysis, cortical destruction, and an absence of an obvious periosteal "blowout" or Codman's triangles. Figure 13–45 shows another example of a burnt-out phase of an ABC. It is symmetrically expansile, shows trabeculations, and a border of host bone sclerosis (Fig. 13–45, *arrows*). Other conditions that mimic this particular late example of ABC include fibrous dysplasia, osteoblastoma, and the giant cell tumor of hyperparathyroidism and epiphyses. The latter two could probably be eliminated on the basis of the fact that the radiograph shows a ground-glass appearance signifying significant amounts of spicular bone formation within the lesion. New bone formation of this degree could not be expected in giant cell tumor (GCT) of epiphyses unless they have been treated by radiation or in giant cell tumor of hyperparathyroidism, until after the adenoma has been removed. The border of host bone sclerosis is rarely seen in GCT of epiphyses unless it has been treated, or if the GCT has entered a phase of slow to absent growth. In addition the open epiphyseal plate virtually rules out the diagnosis of neoplastic giant cell tumor.

Figure 13–46 shows an example of severe hemorrhage into the bone and periosteal tissues in a patient with hemophilia. As can be seen from this illustration the "pseudotumor" of hemophilia may indeed closely mimic the classic features of the ABC, including the formation of Codman's triangles. Biopsy of the tissues from this particular patient showed severe hemorrhage, hemosiderin pigment, and evidence of new intramedullary and periosteal new bone formation. There were no blood-filled, fibrous, cystlike spaces indicative of an ABC component.

Gross Pathology

At surgery the ABC is characterized by disconcerting and persistent welling up of blood. Upon exposing the richly vascular lesion, the ABC appears as an expanded portion of bone showing a honeycomb of blood-filled lakes lined by fibro-osseous cystlike tissue (Fig. 13–47). The aneurysmal bone cyst is rarely resected en-bloc. In most cases the blood is dark red due to a slow but continuous circulation. If the circulation has been arrested to a portion of the ABC, the cysts are filled with a serous to serosanguineous fluid. Rarely, a grossly obvious arteriovenous malformation may be seen (Figs. 13–33, 13–34, and 13–35).

Histopathology

On low-power examination (Fig. 13–48) the ABC is composed of a honeycomb of large blood-filled

Aneurysmal Bone Cyst

FIG. 13–37. Six illustrations from the same patient showing the rather typical progression of an ABC. In *A, B,* and *C,* the lesion is lytic and eccentrically to centrally placed. There is no periosteal "blowout" at this particular incipient phase of development. The lesion at this time most closely resembles a simple bone cyst. *D* and *E,* however, are incompatible with a simple bone cyst and suggest either an ABC or lytic osteosarcoma. The bone is rapidly "expanding," the cortex is almost totally destroyed and ominous Codman's triangles are noted (*arrow*), a sign of rapid periosteal lifting. Further progression of the lesion is shown in *F* and *G.* Although a centrally expanding type of ABC, its "explosive" character would suggest malignancy to those not familiar with this lesion. The fine thin rim of periosteal new bone that is forming (*arrows*), in *F* and *G* is a sign that the lesion has finished its explosive growth phase and is now growing more slowly, because now the periosteum has time to lay down a smooth thin rim of containing bone. We would not expect to see this type of periosteal collar in a lytic osteosarcoma.

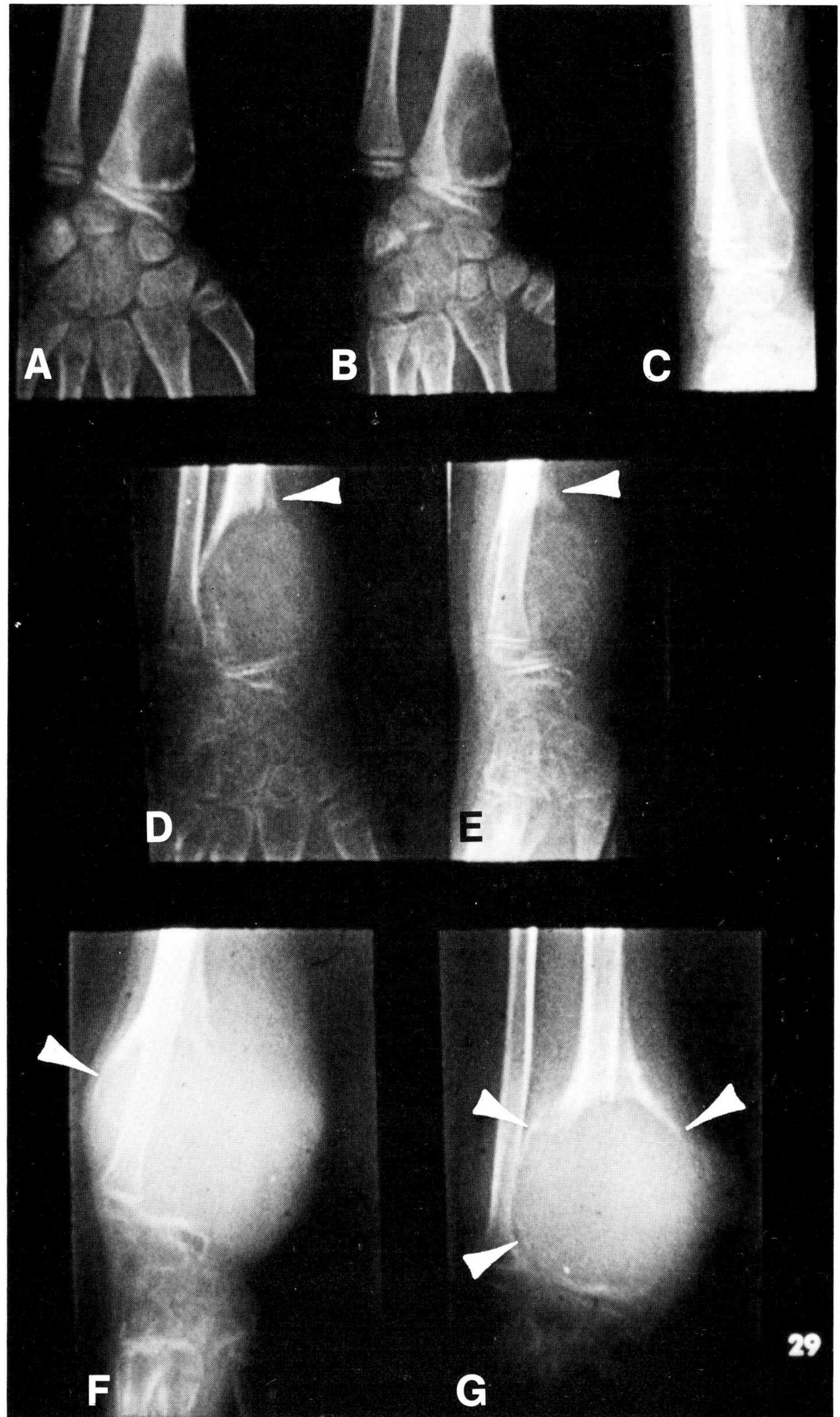

FIG. 13-37

spaces and numerous septae. On medium- and high-power examination (Figs. 13–49 and 13–50, *A*), the septae are composed of fibrous tissue through which endothelial lined capillaries may course. Variable numbers of chronic inflammatory cells, osteoclast-like giant cells, fibroblasts, and slivers of osteoid or woven bone are the other components usually present. The cells may be exuberant but do not show numerous mitoses, atypical mitoses, or other signs of anaplasia. The septae do not contain muscle. The presence of an endothelial layer of cells lining the septae is variable. The blood in the spaces usually shows that it was free flowing. Evidence of thrombosis or fibrin clots are unusual.

An occasional ABC is associated with extensive reparative fibro-osseous tissues, which may include a peculiar, primitive, chondroid matrix (Fig. 13–50, *B*). This chondroid tissue can be found in the cyst walls or in areas of fibro-osseous repair, which obliterate the former cystlike areas. The chondroid usually forms within or adjacent to pink ostoid or woven bone trabeculae. This chondroid (Fig. 13–50, *B*) is distinctly blue and roughly assumes a small, usually triangular shape. It has a latticework structure and the cells within it are small, flattened to ovoid, and innocuous in appearance. The chondroid islands are generally smaller than a mm. in greatest dimension and are haphazardly oriented. The characteristics of the matrix—sparseness, random distribution, typical association with osteoid, latticework, and hypocellularity—are such unusual features that the identification of this peculiar substance alone should alert the diagnostician to the possibility that the lesion in question is an ABC. It is especially important to realize that the exuberant fibro-osseous repair tissues of an ABC can occasionally be associated with small foci of chondroid matrix; otherwise, the lesion could be confused with the chondroblastoma, chondromyxoid fibroma, fibrous dysplasia with chondroid, or most seriously, with an osteosarcoma.

In order to identify possible benign precursor lesions, extensive sampling should be performed. Sections should be from any solid looking areas (i.e., those showing the fewest number of blood-filled spaces). In this way it may be possible to identify an area of fibrous dysplasia, osteoblastoma, nonossifying fibroma, giant cell tumor, chondroblastoma, or other lesions. Fibrous tissue, bone, and giant cells can be seen in the walls of ABC and are the usual elements seen in most other benign precursor lesions seen with the ABC. One should be particularly suspicious of any solid area 1 cm. or larger in size and should suspect that it represents another lesion. These areas should be carefully examined for the presence of another lesion. Its histology should be compared and contrasted to that of the tissues of the septae of the ABC. Usually they will contain features that are distinctly different in pattern from the ABC; this should permit their recognition.

Course and Treatment

The problem with the ABC is that although it is benign it is highly prone to local recurrence post-curettage. One or more recurrences post-curettage is in the range of 50 per cent. If the lesion is an arteriovenous malformation it is not difficult to understand the problem of its ablation by curettage. Some authors suggest radiotherapy to sclerose the vessels. The risk that must be weighed is the potential of radiation-induced sarcoma many years later. En-bloc resection has also been recommended but this procedure must also be weighed because of the extent of the loss of function that results from this procedure. Marcove has used cryosurgery to ablate the lesion[38]

(*Text continues on p. 492.*)

Aneurysmal Bone Cyst

FIG. 13-38. This example of an ABC shows extensive intramedullary involvement in addition to a small periosteal "blowout" lesion and a Codman's triangle. The thin collar of periosteal new bone (*arrow*) is again a strong clue that this is an ABC and not a malignant tumor. The following two illustrations are from the same patient.

FIG. 13-39. A few months later, the lesion is still expanding. The cortex is totally destroyed. The signs of ABC are the thin rim or collar of periosteal new bone (*white arrow*) and the fact that the bone protrudes into a lytic, blowout lesion in an unusual fashion. This latter appearance of ABC is referred to as the "finger-in-the-ballon" sign (*black arrow*).

FIG. 13-40. After surgical intervention, the lesion entered a healing phase. The lesion is trabeculated and the bone expanded because of new periosteal bone deposition. The new, smooth contours of the ridge of reactive host bone sclerosis (*arrows*) around the lesion clearly point to the ultimate benign nature of the ABC.

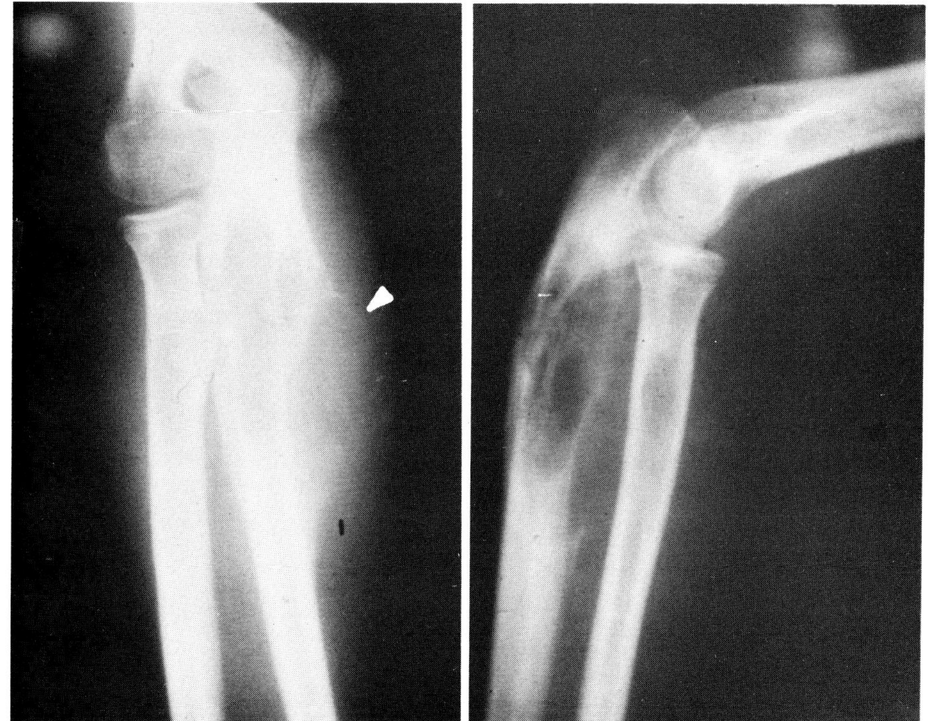

FIG. 13-38

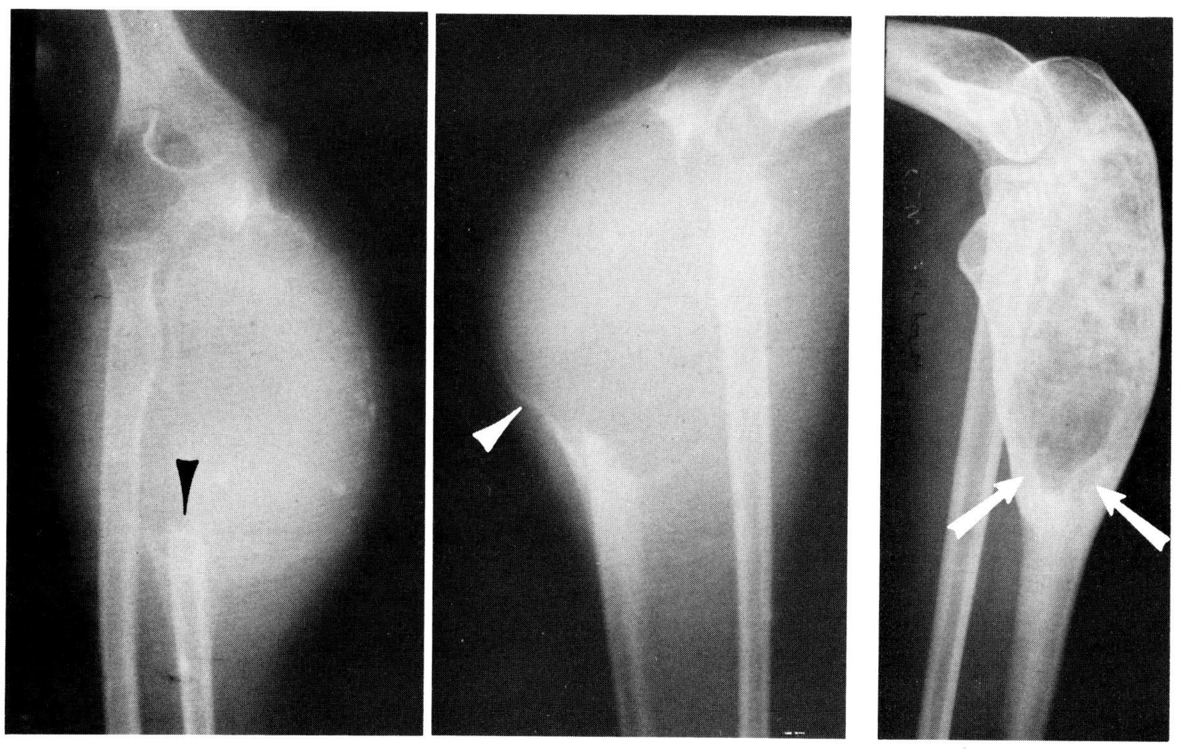

FIG. 13-39

FIG. 13-40

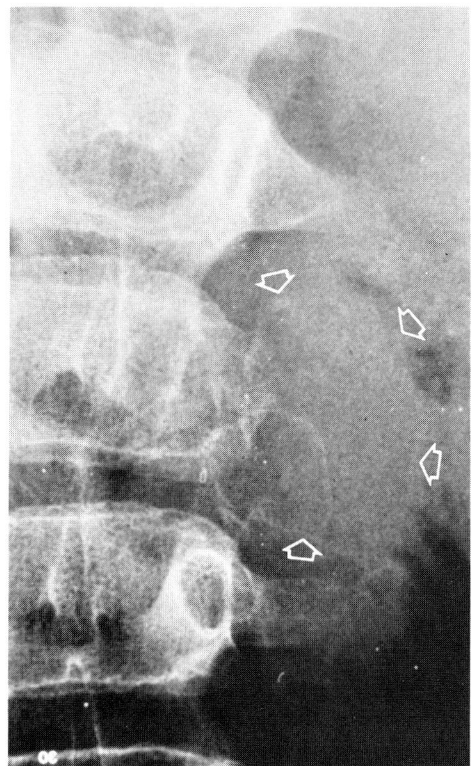

FIG. 13-41

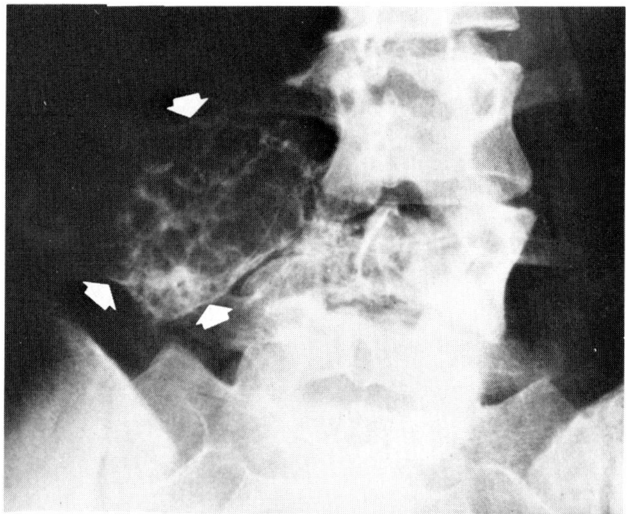

FIG. 13-42

Aneurysmal Bone Cyst

FIG. 13-41. The transverse process is blown out by an ABC in its incipient to midphase of growth. The presence of fine wisps of periosteal new bone (*arrows*) implies that its most rapid growth phase is over. Expansive lesions of the transverse process are usually either ABC's or osteoblastomas.

FIG. 13-42. This biopsy-proven ABC represents the lesion in its healing phase because of its extensive smooth-bordered periosteal new bone (*arrows*).

FIG. 13-43. On occasion, the ABC may appear to arise solely from an intraperiosteal position. As such, it will be clearly eccentric. The injection study shows its high degree of vascularity, as we would expect in an anomaly related to a probable arteriovenous malformation. Note the smooth, peripheral bony collar, a sign of its benignancy (*arrows*).

FIG. 13-44. This ABC is in a relatively early growth phase and shows extensive bone lysis, cortical destruction, and lack of a periosteal "blowout" or Codman's triangles.

FIG. 13-45. A healing to burnt-out phase of the ABC. The smooth border of periosteal new bone rules out malignancy and giant cell tumor (unless irradiated). Fibrous dysplasia and osteoblastoma could have a similar appearance, however. Note the rind of benign reactive host bone sclerosis (*arrows*).

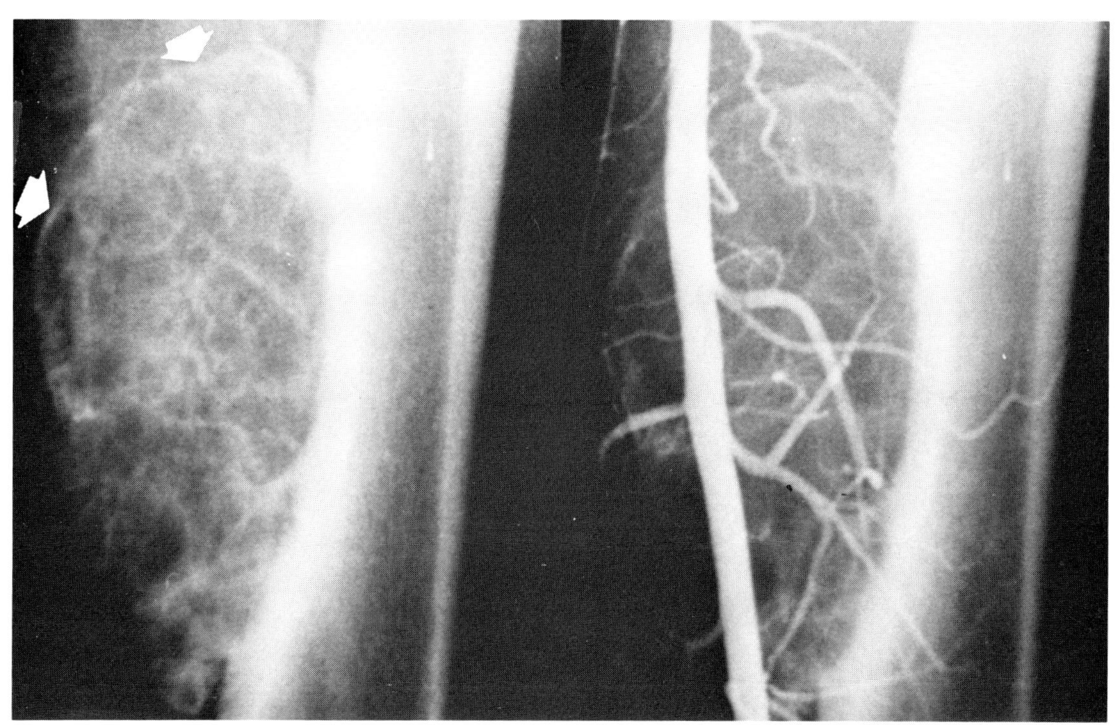

FIG. 13-43

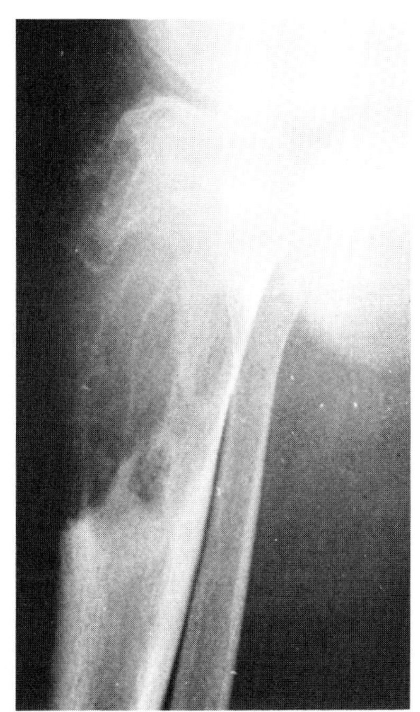

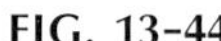

FIG. 13-44

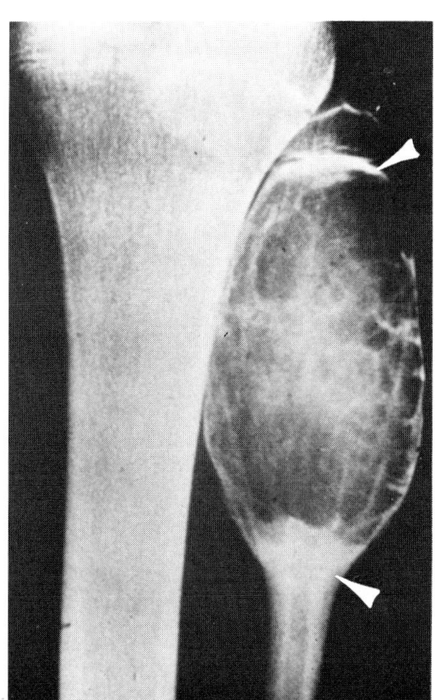

FIG. 13-45

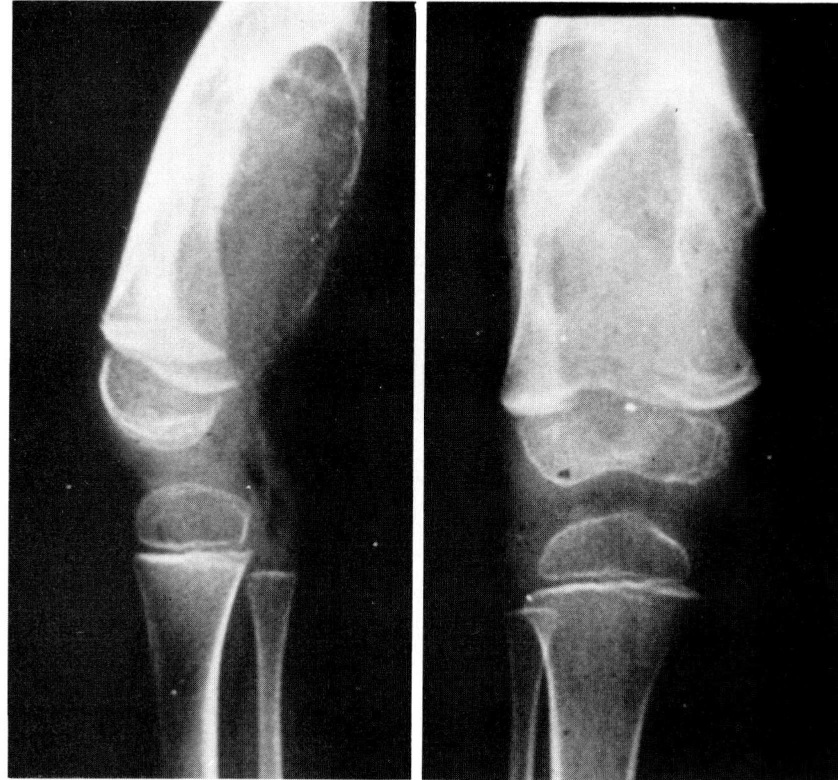

Pseudotumor of Hemophilia

FIG. 13-46. An example of the "pseudotumor" of hemophilia, which can mimic the ABC.

(see Fig. 15-14, *A-D*). There was only one recurrence in 13 patients so treated. Clough, in referring to Marcove's use of cryosurgery, states "certainly if the results of Biesecker and his colleagues can be repeated and it can be shown that there are no serious complications associated with its use, and here, harm to the growth plate or to nearby important structures seems a possibility, then the application of cryotherapy to those cysts which would otherwise be managed by curettage alone would seem a sound proposition."[39]

VASCULAR TUMORS: BENIGN

Solitary Hemangioma (Fig. 13-51)

Introduction

An hemangioma, whether of soft tissue or bone, is a benign, hamartomatous vascular malformation characterized by a proliferation of thin-walled capillary or larger, engorged vascular channels. Hemangiomas account for fewer than 1 per cent of clinically symptomatic primary bone tumors. Most hemangi-

---

Aneurysmal Bone Cyst

FIG. 13-47. Gross appearance of a typical ABC. Note the numerous dark, blood-filled cystlike cavities imparting a spongelike appearance.

FIG. 13-48. On low-power examination, the lesion is composed of numerous spongelike fibrous channels usually filled with unclotted blood (x40).

FIG. 13-49. Medium power of the cystlike wall and fresh blood (x125).

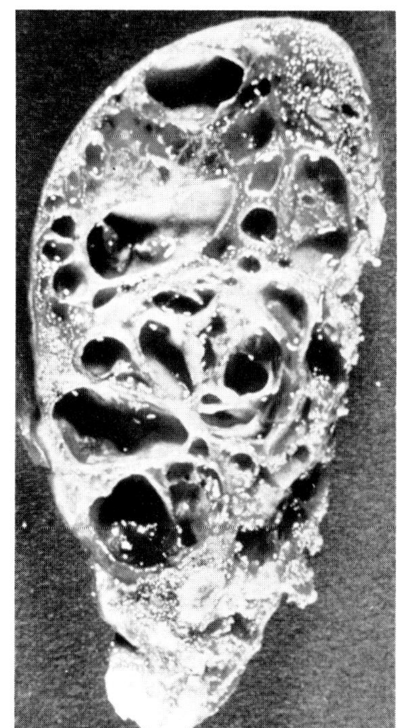

FIG. 13-47

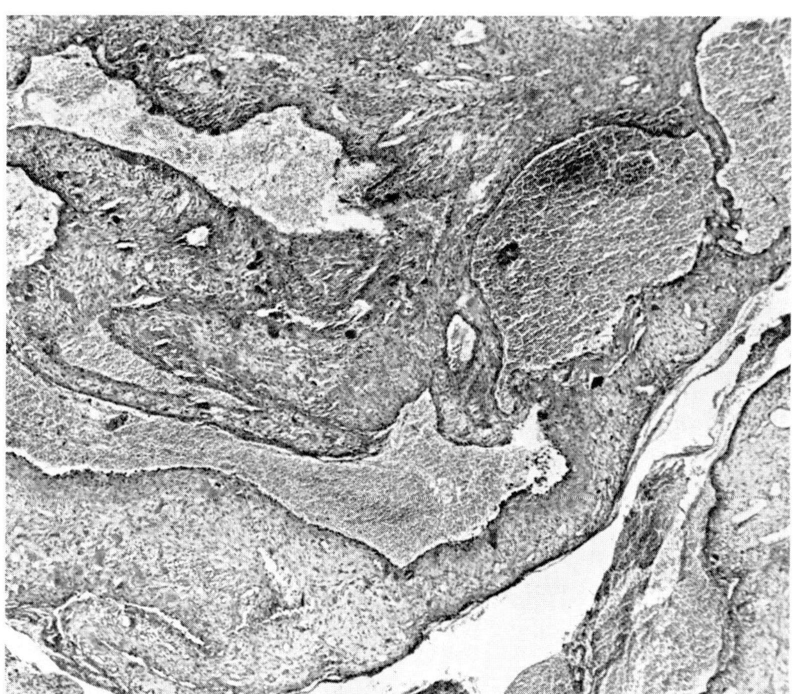

FIG. 13-48

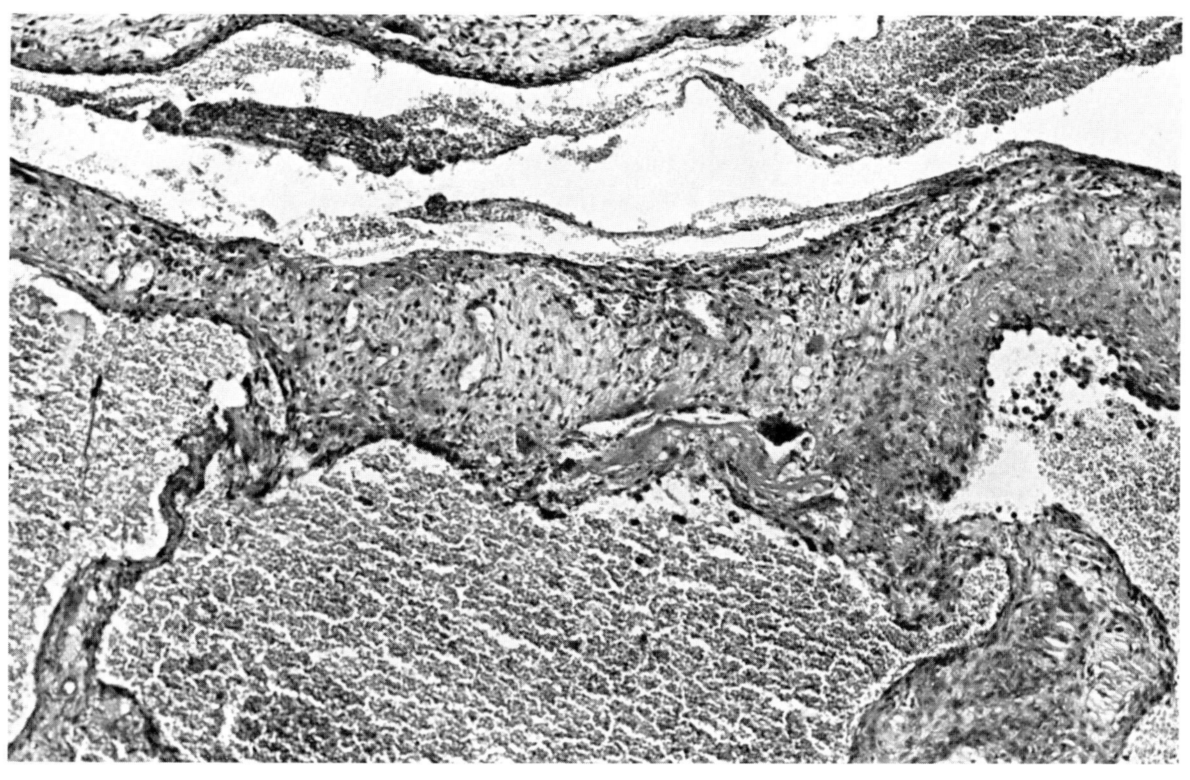

FIG. 13-49

omas are solitary lesions, although rarely multiple bones may be involved with or without soft-tissue hemangiomatosis. This is an expression of a multifocal abnormality of the vascoformative tissues.

The solitary hemangioma is most frequently observed in the vertebral column or skull. Schmorl found small, asymptomatic vascular lesions in 10.7 per cent of 3,829 consecutive vertebral columns removed at autopsy and serially sectioned. The great majority of these lesions consisted of large sinusoidal spaces filled with blood. There was mild destruction of the adjacent bone.[61] Although Schmorl called these lesions hemangiomas, it is much more likely that they represented local varicosities rather than hemangiomas in the strict sense of the term.

Clinical and Gross Features

An hemangioma of bone may assume large proportions and lead to clinical complaints, usually as the result of pathologic fracture. If the fracture is located in the spine, the patient usually complains of local pain and muscle spasm with rigidity. An hemangioma can extend through the vertebral body, compress the dura, and result in sensory disturbances, radicular pain, and even paraplegia. At gross examination an hemangioma stands out from the surrounding bone as a brownish-red or purple area. It may remain confined to the bone or extend into the soft tissue.

Radiologic Features

Approximately 50 per cent of solitary hemangiomas involve either the skull or spine. On radiologic examination an hemangioma of the spine usually involves the body alone, but occasionally a portion of the vertebral arch is involved as well. It usually results in a coarse, honeycomb pattern and marked accentuation of the vertical trabeculae (Fig. 13–52). A coarse, honeycomb pattern occurs in other conditions; therefore an hemangioma can easily be misconstrued as a solitary focus of Paget's disease or metastatic cancer. However, in cases of hemangioma, the pattern lacks the cortical thickening (Fig. 13–53) or "picture framing," which is characteristic of Paget's disease (Fig. 13–54). The hemangioma of spine can lead to compression of the spinal cord (Fig. 13–55).

An hemangioma that involves the skull, mandible, or flat bones of the pelvis or ribs may produce a characteristic pattern of bone spicules radiating from the center in a sunburst pattern. The intense nature of the radiating spicules of bone can mimic osteosarcoma.

An hemangioma of the long bones is usually characterized radiologically by fusiform expansion of the bony contour to a paperlike thinness and a "soap bubble" or coarsely loculated appearance in the shaft and even vertical striations (Fig. 13–68). The lesions generally involve the distal ends of the bones, sparing the epiphysis or those segments of the shaft in close proximity to the nutrient artery. Hemangiomas that are discovered as incidental findings are generally smaller than 1 to 2 cm. in size and do not alter the contour of the affected bone.

Histopathology

Microscopically, an hemangioma is composed of numerous capillary and/or larger vascular channels in a fibrous stroma (Fig. 13–56). The vessels are lined by flattened or slightly plump endothelial cells with benign nuclear characteristics. On occasion the hemangioma may be associated with more solid or sclerosing areas. If one is unfamiliar with these patterns the lesion can be mistaken for hemangiopericytoma, hemangioendothelioma, or angiosarcoma. In this author's estimation, if a vascular tumor of bone shows unequivocal benign hemangiomatous areas the entire lesion is probably an hemangioma. Great care must be exercised before concluding that the lesion is malignant or has transformed to a malignancy (See pp. 500–504).

(*Text continues on p. 498.*)

Aneurysmal Bone Cyst

FIG. 13-50. (*A*) The walls of the lesion consist of fibrous tissue, a sprinkling of chronic inflammatory cells, osteoclast-like giant cells, and occasional slivers of osteoid (*arrow*) or woven bone. Careful examination of the nuclei should be performed to rule out objective anaplasia, becuase the telangiectatic osteosarcoma can have a similar low-power appearance (x250). (*B*) The ABC may be associated with a peculiar, distinctly blue chondroid matrix usually oriented in triangular shapes (*1*). It is frequently associated with exuberant fibrous tissue and longitudinal slivers of pink osteoid to woven bone (*2*). This peculiar chondroid pattern is strongly suggestive, if not pathognomonic, of repair in an ABC (Dahlin, personal communication).

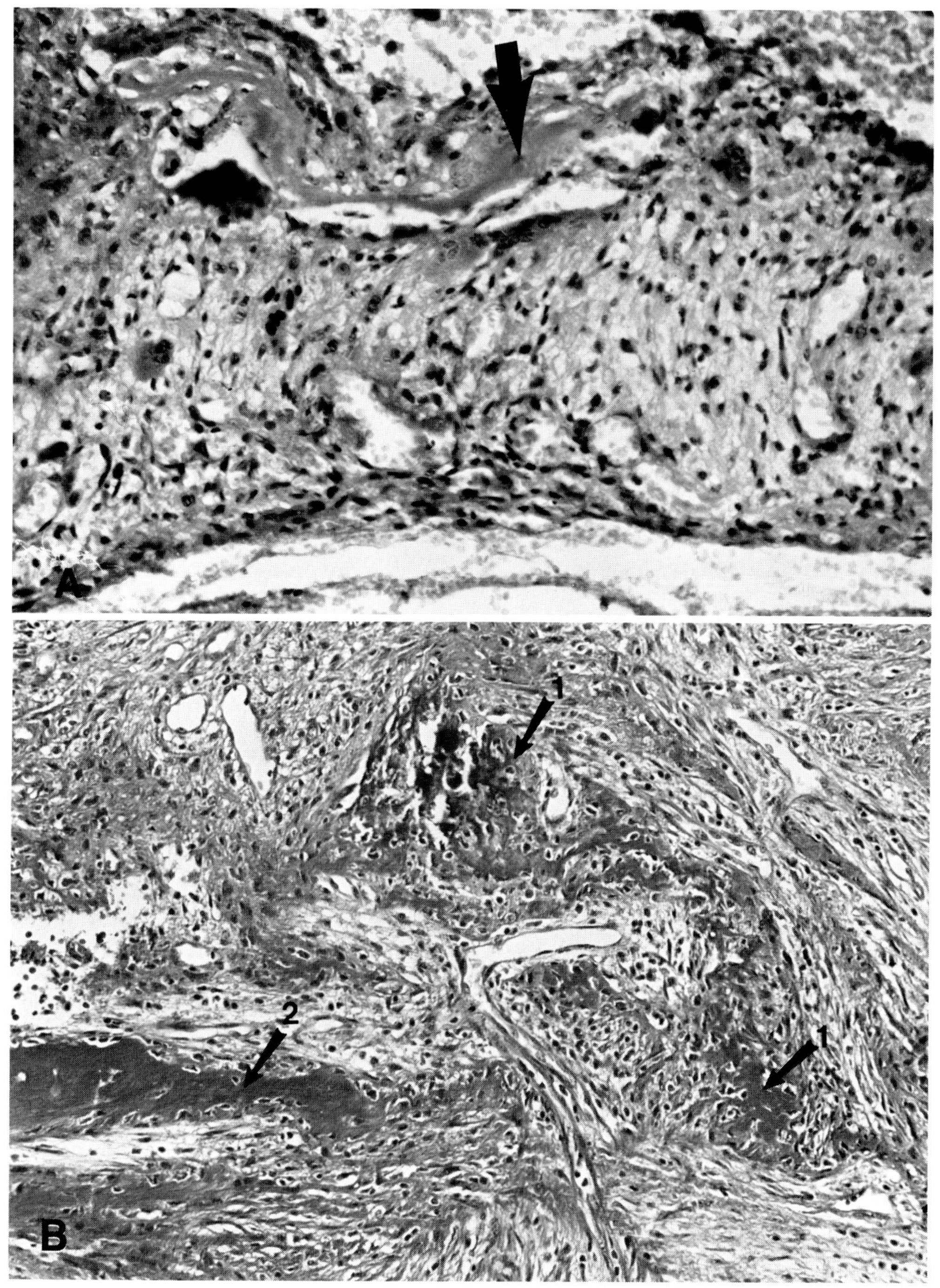

FIG. 13-50

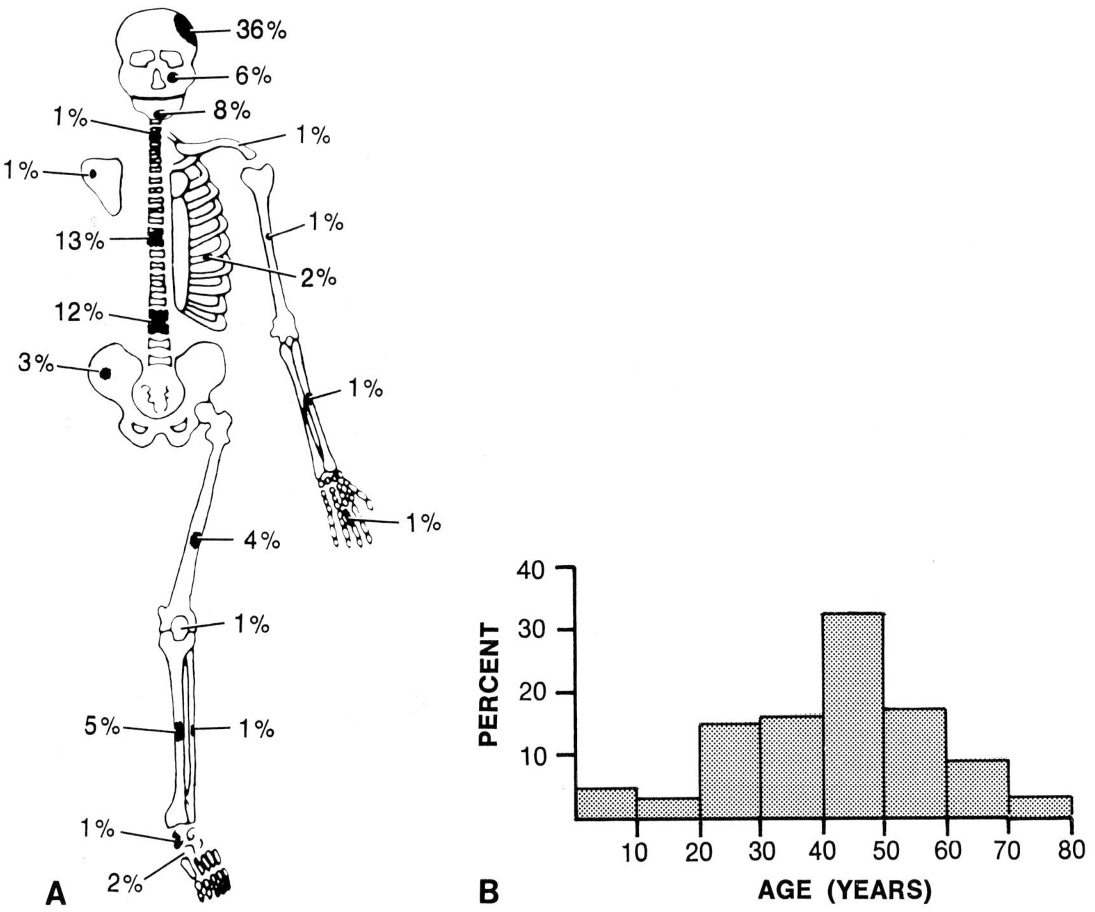

FIG. 13-51. (*A*) Solitary hemangioma of bone. Frequency of areas of involvement in 79 patients. Male:Female incidence, 1:1.5. (*B*) Age distribution of patients with solitary hemangioma of bone. (Mirra, J., Bullough, P., and Freiberger, R.: Orthopedic Diseases, Part IV. New York, Famous Teachings in Modern Medicine, MedCom, Inc., © 1977)

Hemangioma Versus Paget's Disease of Bone

FIG. 13-52. The solitary hemangioma is quite commonly found in vertebral bodies. The vertical striping and lack of enlargement of the body is virtually pathognomonic of hemangioma.

FIG. 13-53. Paget's disease for comparison. Although the accentuation of trabeculae mimic hemangioma, the cortical irregularity, the subchondral cortical sclerosis (*arrows*) and subtle enlargement of the bone subperiosteally indicate Paget's disease.

FIG. 13-54. (*A*) The vertebral body is obviously enlarged and the cortical thickening in a rim around the outer perimeter imparts the so-called "picture frame" effect pathognomonic of Paget's disease. (*B*) The gross of a vertebral body affected by Paget's disease in another patient. Note the accentuation of the vertical stress trabeculae that can be seen in both hemangioma and Paget's. The "picture frame" effect establishes the diagnosis with ease in either gross or radiologic examination.

FIG. 13-55. Hemangiomas of the vertebral body (*arrow*) can penetrate the cortex and compress the dura, leading to spinal cord compression and blockage of intraspinal contrast material, as seen here.

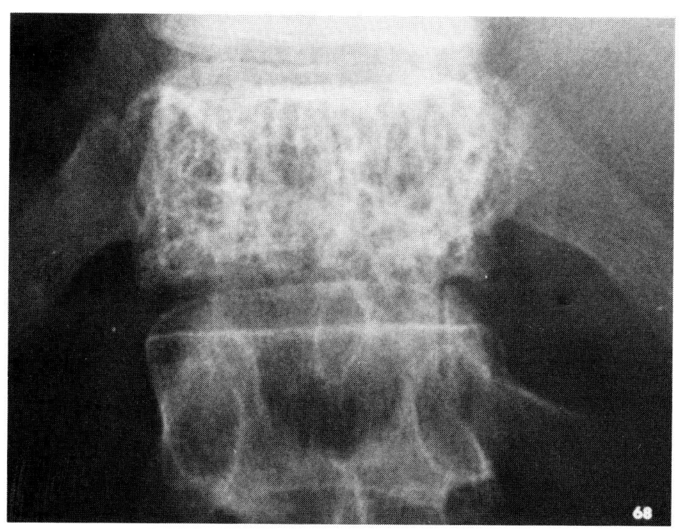

FIG. 13-52

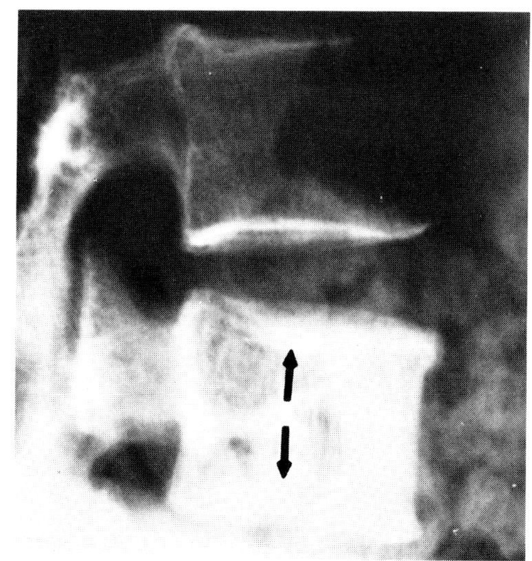

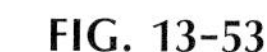

FIG. 13-53

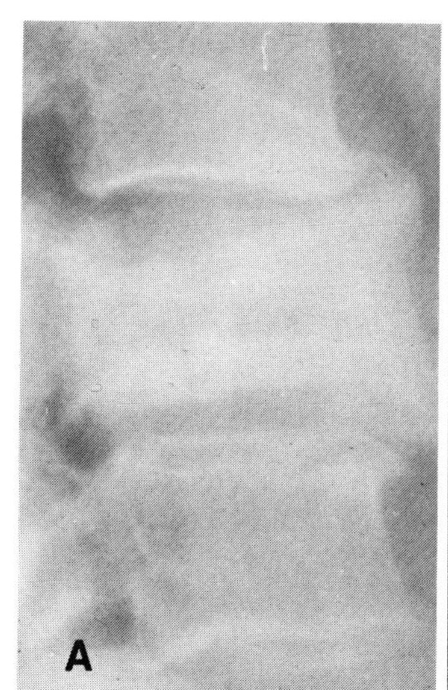

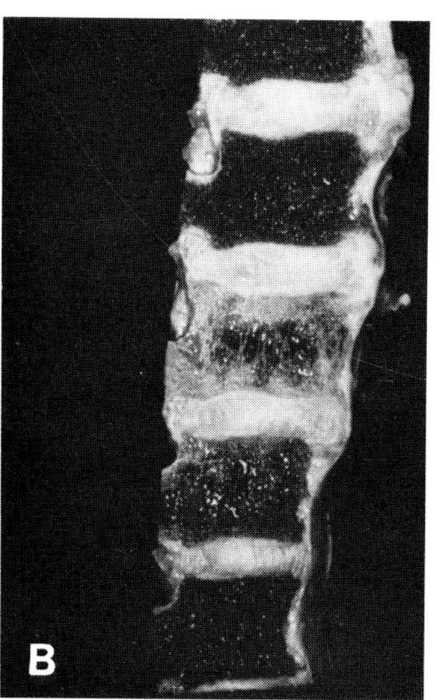

FIG. 13-54

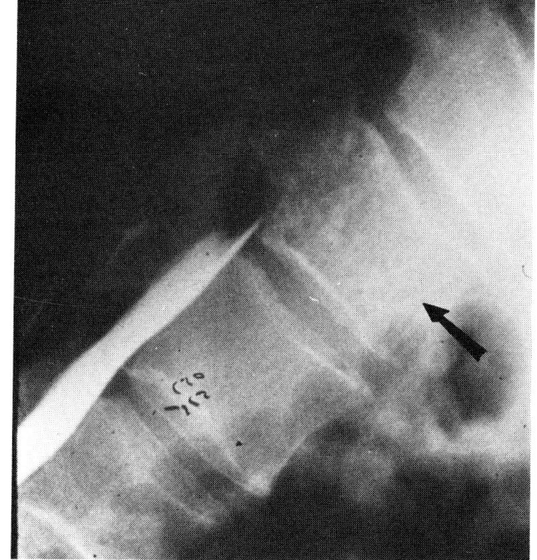

FIG. 13-55

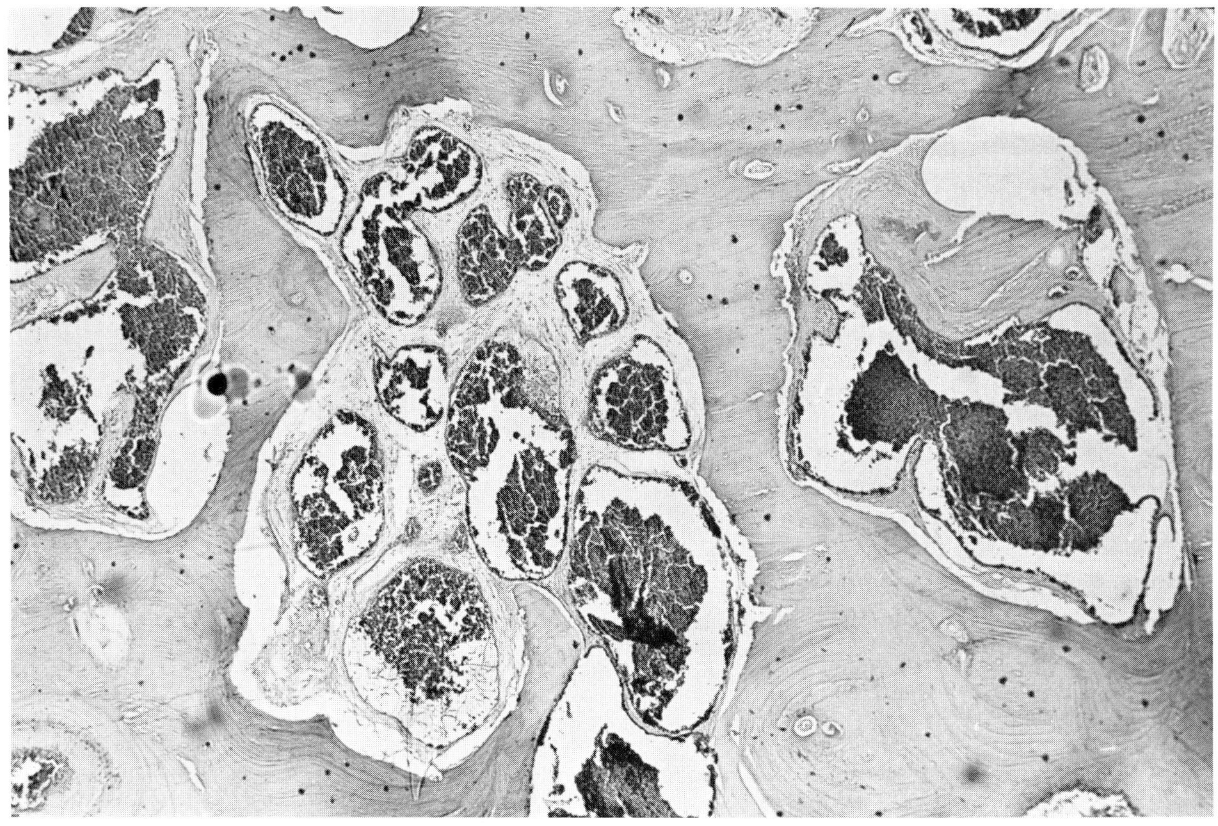

Hemangioma

FIG. 13-56. The hemangioma of bone is similar to soft tissue. It is either cavernous (this illustration), capillary, or mixed.

Course and Treatment

The majority of symptomatic cases of the spine respond well to irradiation or operation or both. Lesions in the skull or long bones are generally resected, curetted, or cauterized. The danger of severe hemorrhage must always be considered, particularly in lesions of the skull or spine. Mortality in spinal lesions is often due to overenthusiastic surgical efforts. Spinal cord compression should be relieved by removing only as much of the tumor mass as necessary to relieve pressure, and the dura should not be opened. Irradiation is recommended as an adjunct to surgery. In spinal lesions in which there is compression myelitis, irreparable damage to the cord may occur if high-dosage radiation is used alone.

Hypophosphatemic Rickets Induced by Sclerosing Hemangioma

FIG. 13-57. The severe osteomalacia consequent to the hypophosphatemic rickets induced by the distant soft-tissue tumor can lead to pathologic fracture.

FIG. 13-58. Pathologic fracture of the tibia and fibula in the same patient some 6 years before the last illustration.

FIG. 13-59. An example of a "Looser" zone (*arrow*) that is characteristically seen in osteomalacic bones. This patient had a number of such lesions.

FIG. 13-60. In this patient, the soft-tissue tumor that gave rise to the hypophosphatemic rickets penetrated the bone. Note the large, dilated vascular cavities (*a*), reactive bone and osteoid (*b*), and sheetlike areas of cells (*c*) (x40).

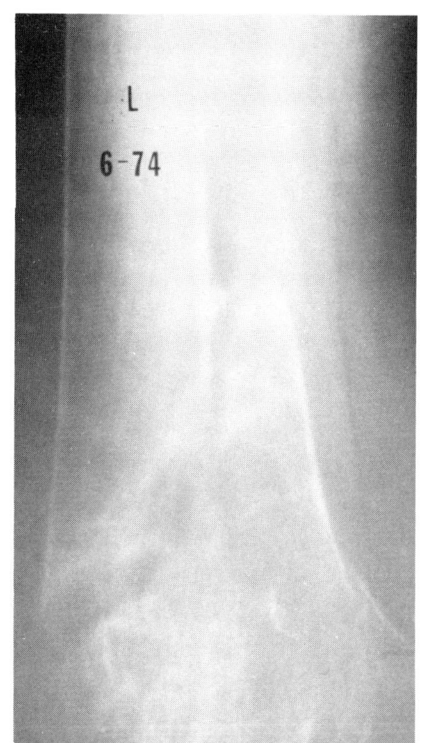

FIG. 13-57

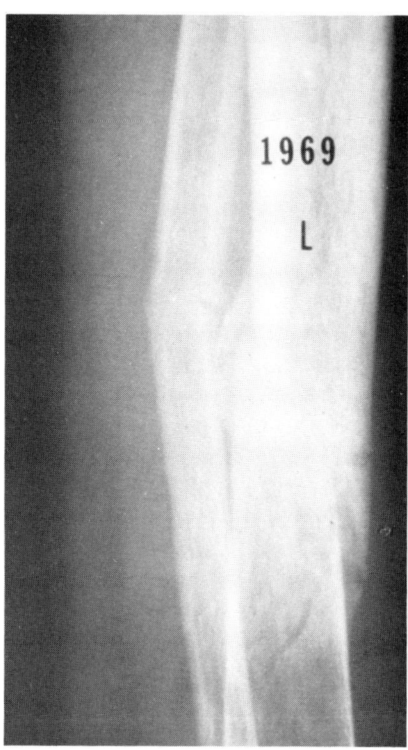

FIG. 13-58

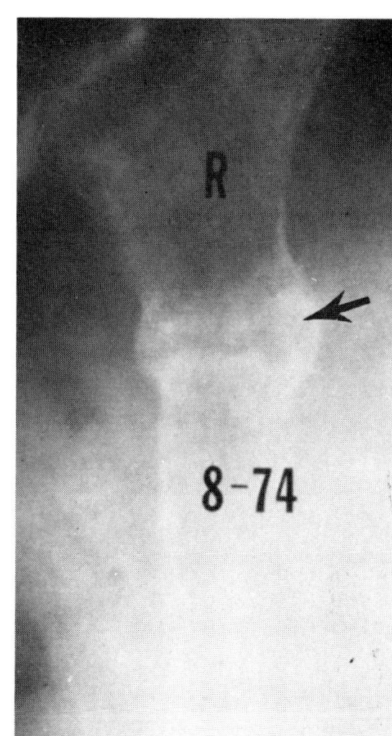

FIG. 13-59

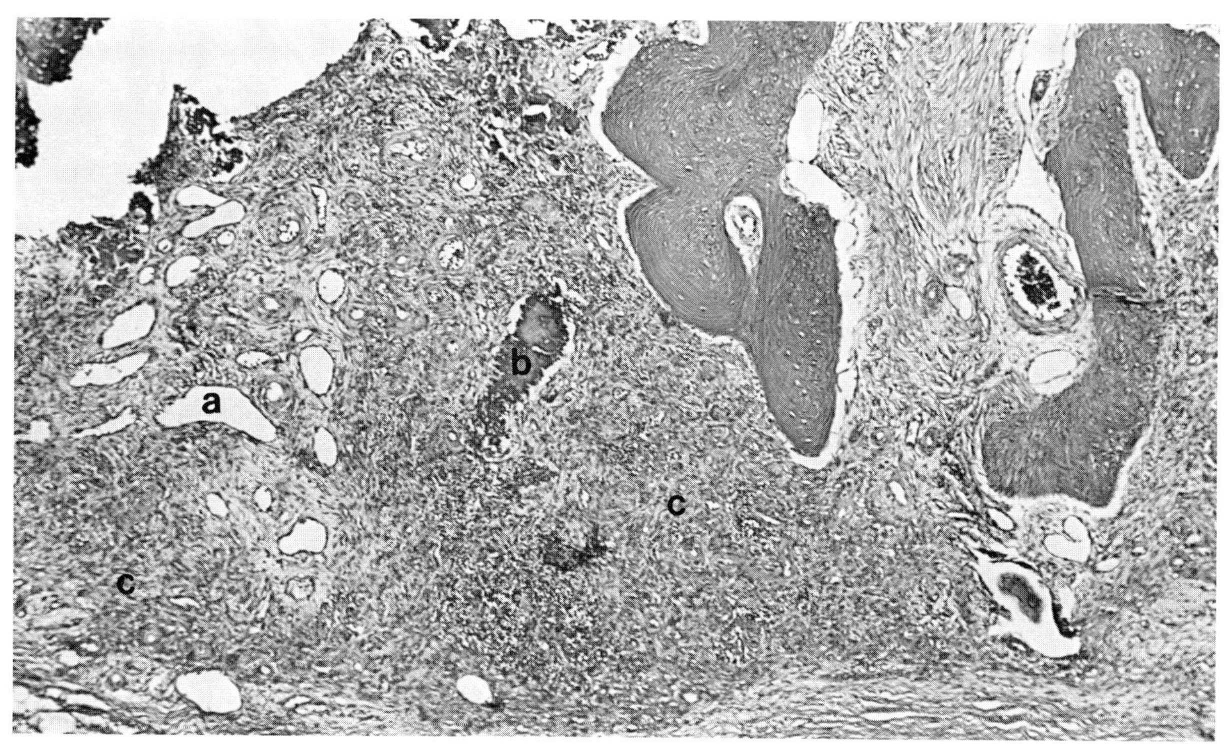

FIG. 13-60

Vascular Tumors of Soft Tissue and Bone That Induce Systemic Hypophosphatemic Osteomalacia

Introduction

This incredible, recently described syndrome is characterized by a solitary soft-tissue or bone tumor (usually vascular) that induces hypophosphatemic rickets by an unknown mechanism. Although several kinds of lesions have been reported this author suspects that all cases may represent one entity, namely, a sclerosing hemangioma that may mimic or be confused with hemangiopericytoma and angiosarcoma. This supposition will be carefully dealt with in the microscopic description of the tumor and the final summation.

Clinical Features

To date, 16 such patients have been reported.[62–73] The patients range in age from 7 to 54 years (average age at onset, 35 years). The male to female incidence is 1.3 to 1.

The usual presenting features are those of bone pain associated with pathologic fracture from severe osteoporosis and weakness. Laboratory examination shows marked hypophosphatemia. The serum calcium is generally normal to low. Parathormone assay is usually within normal limits. The tubular reabsorption of phosphates has been shown to be depressed, suggesting a possible action of the tumor on the renal tubules. It has also been suggested that the tumor may elaborate a vitamin D antagonist.[65] The patient's hypophosphatemic osteomalacia usually precedes the discovery of the tumor by months to several years. This would imply that all patients who present with hypophosphatemic osteomalacia should be carefully worked up for a relatively small to clinically inapparent soft-tissue or bone tumor.

At any rate, after discovery of the tumor, its removal results in reversal of the hypophosphatemia and clinical bone improvement in about 4 months to 2 years. If the tumor recurs, the serum phosphorus falls and the osteomalacia reexacerbates.

Radiologic Features

The most dramatic features are those associated with the effects of the tumor, namely, the osteomalacia. All of the bones become diffusely porotic and many show evidence of pathologic fracture and/or Looser's zones (Figs. 13–57, 13–58, and 13–59). The eventually discovered soft-tissue tumor may show a prominent mass on radiologic examination.

Histopathology

The tumors that have been described consist predominantly of abnormal vascular proliferations described as either hemangioma (1 case), sclerosing hemangioma (3 cases), hemangiopericytoma (3 cases) or sclerosing hemangioma converting to angiosarcoma (1 case). Other lesions were diagnosed as giant cell reparative granuloma (1 case), "degenerative osteoid tissue," giant cells and vascular tissue (1 case), ossifying mesenchymal tumors (3 cases), and nonossifying fibroma (1 case).

I have reviewed two of the reported cases (called angiosarcoma and hemangiopericytoma) and saw the following:

1. Unequivocal areas of cavernous hemangioma (Figs. 13–60 and 13–61).
2. Loosely sclerosing hemangiomatous areas that could be misconstrued as angiosarcoma (Fig. 13–62). The nuclei, however, were identical to those lining the obvious areas of hemangioma.
3. More solid areas of sclerosing hemangioma that mimic hemangiopericytoma to some extent (Fig. 13–63).
4. Focal destruction of bone by the tumorous process and extensive host woven-bone and osteoid reaction (Fig. 13–65).
5. Areas of intense hemosiderin pigment around dilated hemangiomatous spaces (Fig. 13–64).
6. Areas of fibrosis with occasional giant cells

In other words these fascinating cases show a variety of histological patterns mimicking hemangiopericytoma, angiosarcoma, and nonossifying fibroma. Their extensive reactive host bone repair has been

(*Text continues on p. 504.*)

Sclerosing Hemangioma That Induced Hypophosphatemic Rickets

FIG. 13–61. On high-power examination, fields can be found showing large, vascular, cavernous spaces lined by flattened to slightly plump endothelial cells lacking frank anaplasia (*a*). This clearly establishes the lesion as a form of hemangioma (sclerosing type). The sclerosing hemangioma portion to the right of field (*b*) mimics an hemangiopericytoma (x250).

FIG. 13–62. The reactive nature of the lesion can lead to plump endothelial cells that can be mistaken for hemangioendothelioma or angiosarcoma, as seen in this area (x400).

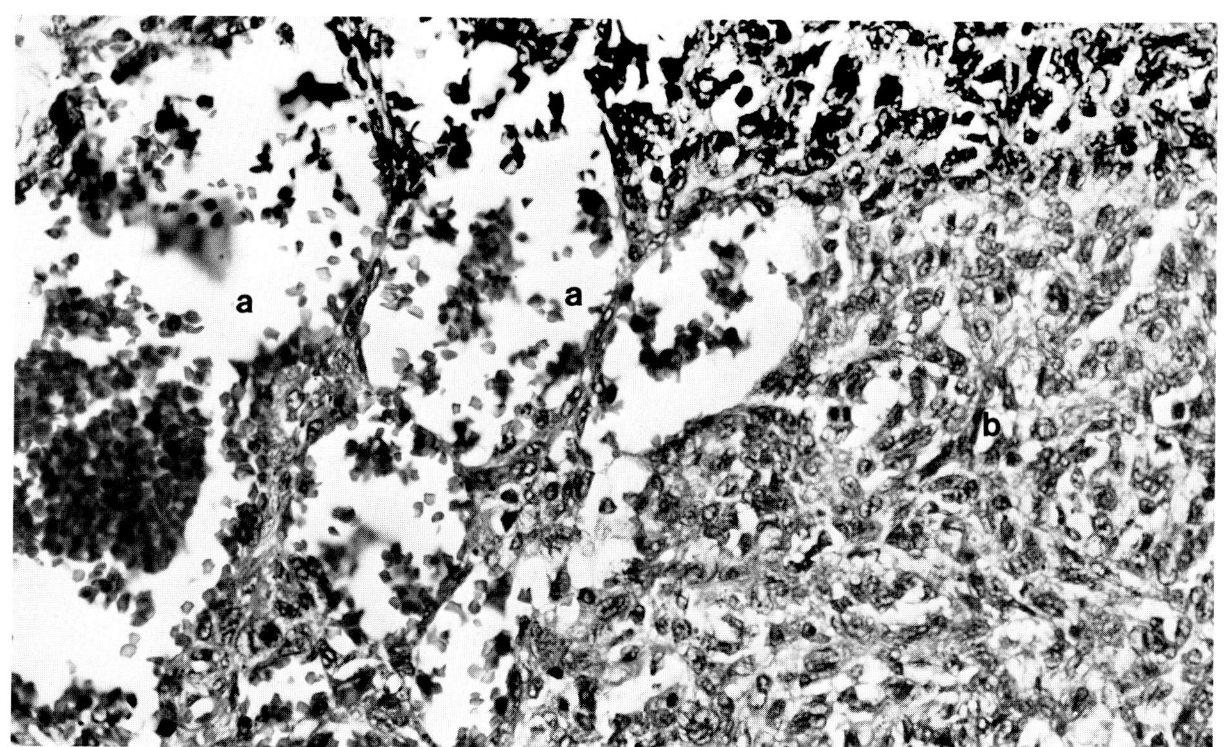

FIG. 13-61

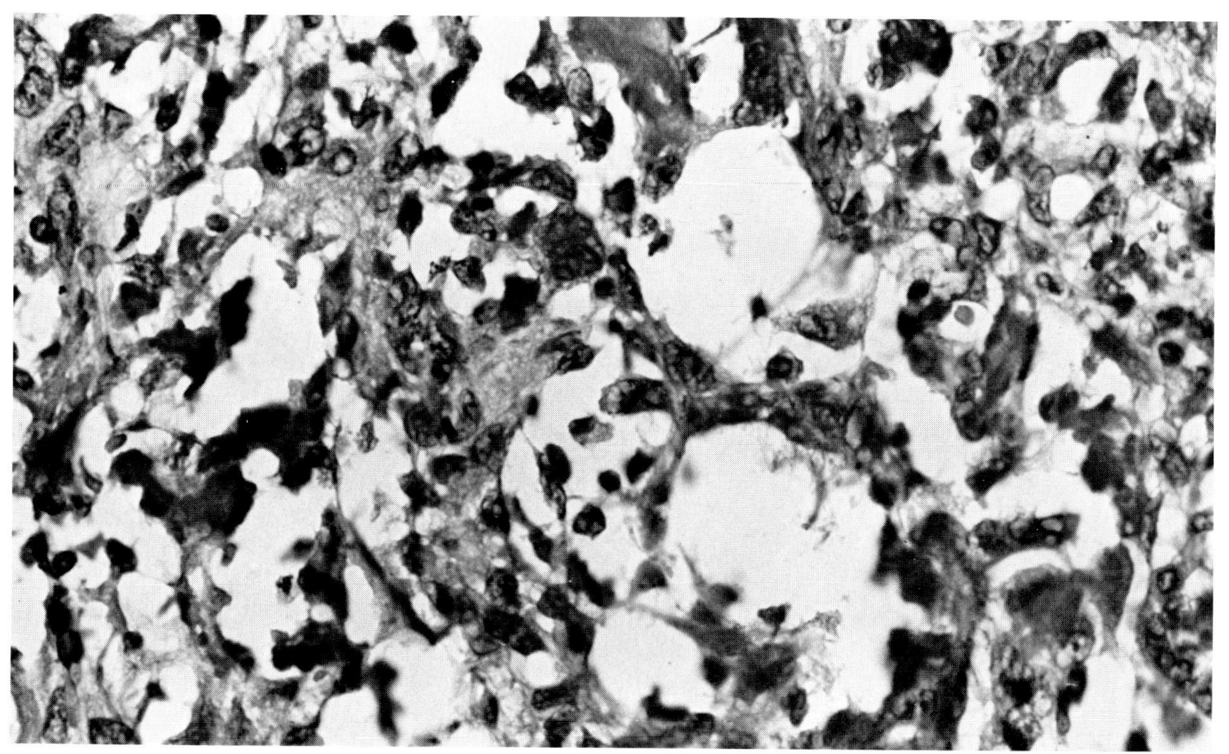

FIG. 13-62

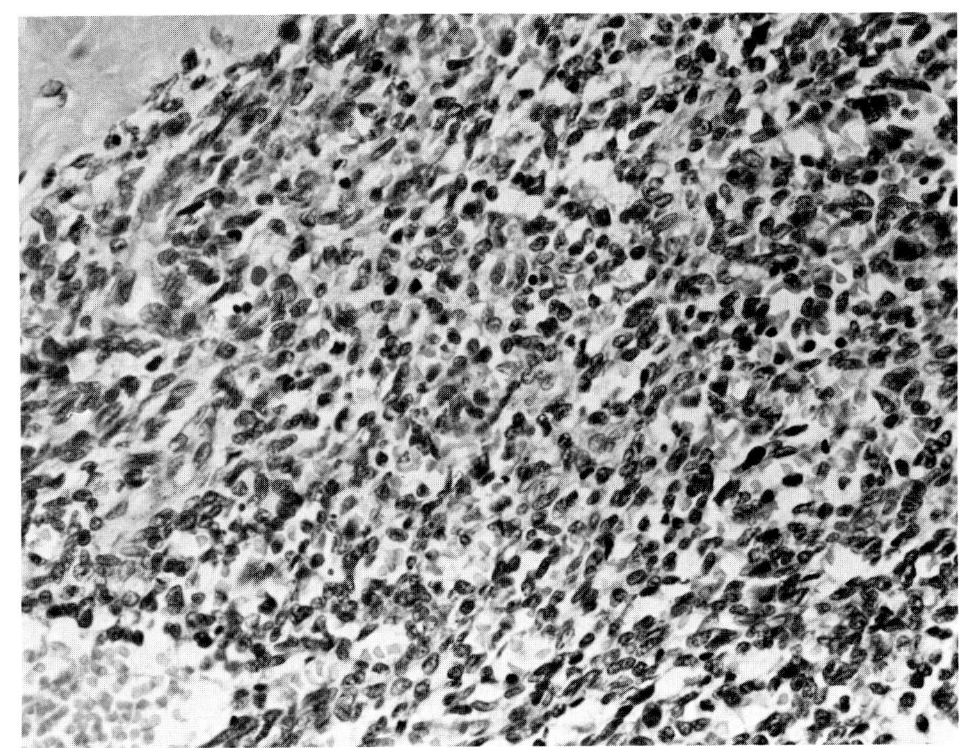

FIG. 13-63

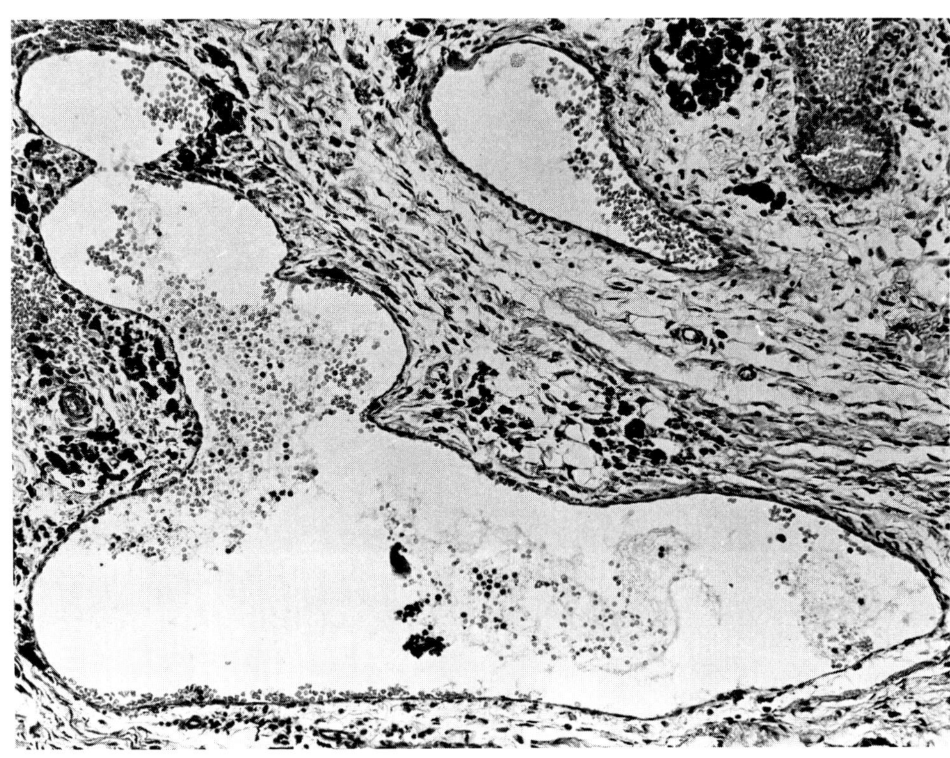

FIG. 13-64

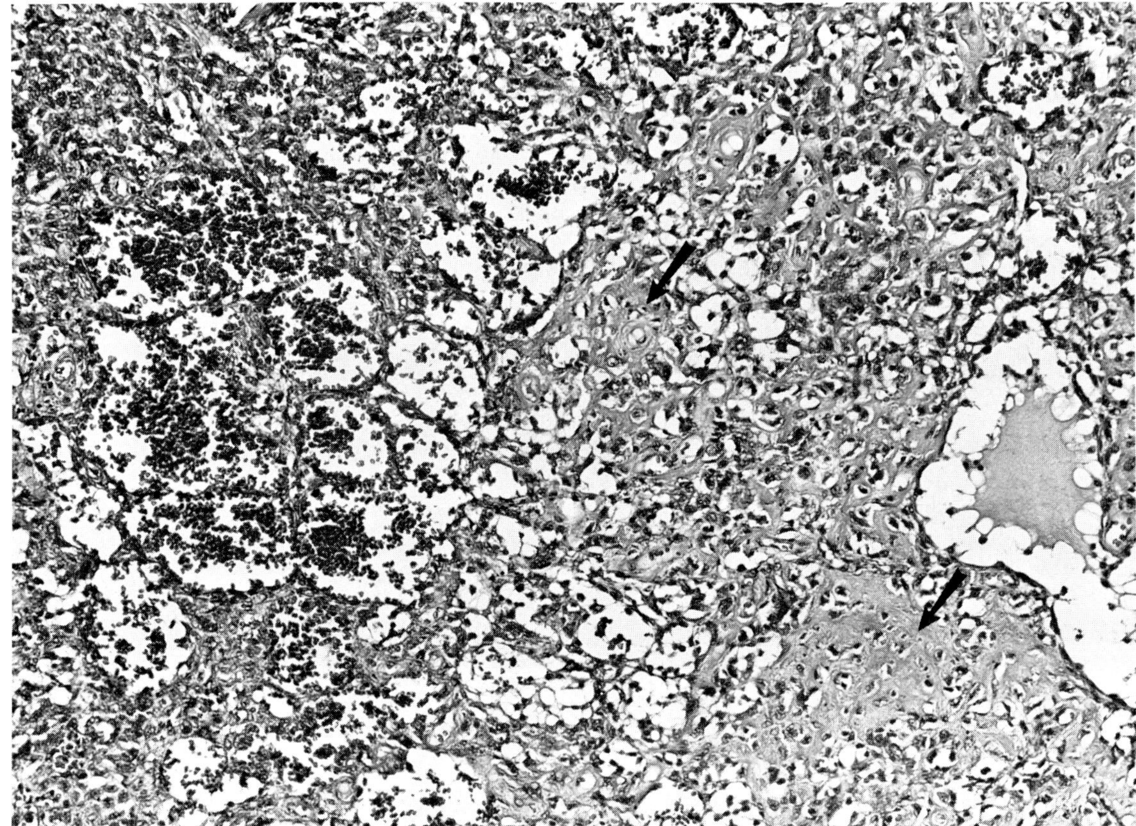

FIG. 13-65

Sclerosing Hemangioma That Induced Hypophosphatemic Rickets

FIG. 13-63. In other areas, the cells can form spindly sheets that can be confused with hemangiopericytoma or a spindle cell sarcoma. Note, however, the uniformly monotonous, although plump, nuclei. The nuclear chromatin is evenly distributed and no atypical mitoses are encountered (x25).

FIG. 13-64. In other areas, a much more benign appearance may be encountered. This area has large vascular lakes, few cells, and a stroma rich in dark hemosiderin-pigment-laden macrophages; these are all signs that the lesion is a sclerosing hemangioma (x125).

FIG. 13-65. Trapped bone mesenchyme within the proliferating lesion can lead to ominous masses of osteoid (*arrows*), further confusing the diagnosis in the direction of some form of primary ossifying tumor, including the osteosarcoma. Note the hemangiomatous vascular spaces to the left (x125).

misconstrued as an "ossifying mesenchymal tumor."[68] The crucial feature was the presence of unequivocal foci of hemangioma with various histological patterns, depending on its degree of sclerotic change and induction of host bone reaction.

Course

The osteomalacia is reversible upon discovery and removal of the tumor. Unfortunately, the tumor may recur in some of the patients. Most patients are eventually cured by local measures although those called malignant have been amputated. No metastases have been recorded even though follow-ups have been as long as 17 years. However, only four patients have had a follow-up of greater than 2 years.

Final Summation and Treatment

In this author's estimation this unique syndrome would be difficult to accept as being due to multiple kinds of tumors when the course, laboratory features, and histopathology show identical or marked similarities. This author has reviewed only two such cases in detail but the microscopic features of these cases certainly showed such a broad range of features that it would not be hard to understand why diagnoses such as hemangiopericytoma and angiosarcoma were considered. Large sclerosing hemangiomas of the soft tissues unassociated with hypophosphatemia are notorious for being misdiagnosed as angiosarcomas and other vascular tumors. The Armed Forces Institute of Pathology has a number of such cases (personal communication Dr. Phillip Cooper). Although this author cannot be absolutely sure at this time that this entity is due to one tumor and one tumor alone, namely, the sclerosing hemangioma, it certainly is odd that no metastases have been reported if malignant entities are also considered. Hemangiomas can be stubbornly recurrent tumors and have even been associated with penetration into bones by pressure erosion through either the soft tissues or joints. Pigmented villonodular synovitis is another primary extraosseous lesion that can penetrate the bones and be mistaken for malignant tumors (see p. 322 and Figs. 10–27 to 10–36). I think that before amputation is considered for this syndrome great care must be taken to establish an unequivocal diagnosis of malignancy. The diagnosis of sclerosing hemangioma must be most carefully ruled out. Until a definitely metastatic malignant case is shown, it might be wise to use locally ablative measures, including local or en-bloc resections and/or low- to moderate-dosage irradiation, to completely sclerose the tumor, particularly in stubbornly recurrent cases. Even if one case with unequivocal metastasis is someday reported the fact that a sclerosing hemangioma could be associated with malignant transformation would not be inconceivable. Obviously a much greater number of cases with long-term (5 or more years) follow-up are needed before a more adequate rationale of treatment can be formulated.

VASCULAR TUMORS: BENIGN AND MALIGNANT

Multiple Hemangiomatosis of Bone

Clinical Features (Fig. 13–66)

Clinically, multiple hemangiomatosis produces pain, pathologic fracture, and signs of cord compression. Angiomas of the skin may or may not be present. Skeletal hemangiomatosis is an extremely rare condition, accounting for less than 0.1 per cent of primary bone tumors. Approximately half of the reported cases also have associated extraosseous involvement. Extraosseous hemangiomas most frequently affect the liver, spleen, lungs, lymph nodes, kidneys, skin, and brain. The patients usually complain of recurrent fractures, the development of one or more masses, or pain. Patients with visceral involvement may also have hemorrhagic episodes, symptoms related to anemia, and respiratory insufficiency.

Patients with visceral involvement usually have a hypochromic anemia subsequent to multiple bleeding episodes and thrombocytopenia, in all probability the result of intravascular coagulation. Raised serum calcium and alkaline phosphatase levels have been reported in a few patients and have on occasion resulted in treatment for hyperparathyroidism. On rare occasion skeletal hemangiomatosis has been reported in association with Osler-Weber-Rendu disease, also known as hereditary hemorrhagic telangiectasia (Figs. 13–69, 13–70, and 13–71).[75,80]

Radiologic Features

In the early states of multiple hemangiomatosis, radiologic examination shows the lesion to be predominantly lytic (Fig. 13–69), the result of an active blood flow through the lesional tissue, which results in high local oxygen tension. In older patients, vascular stasis or thrombosis or both are believed to be the

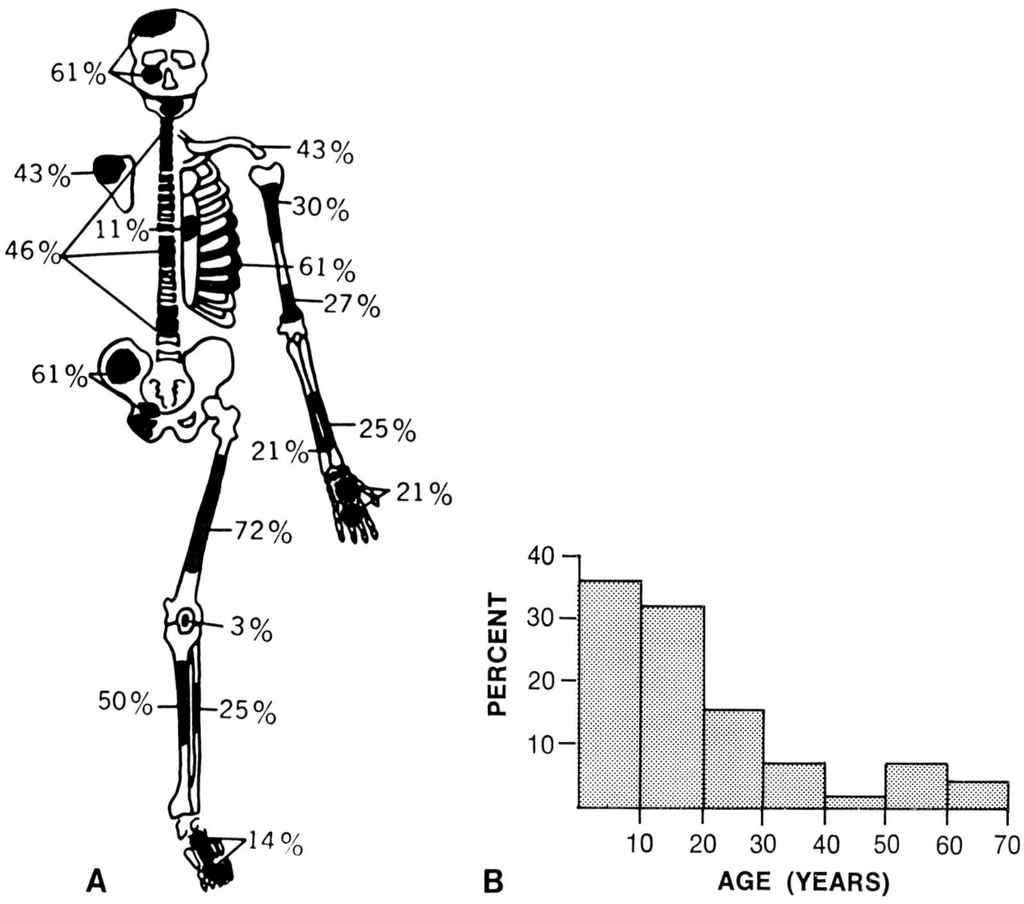

FIG. 13-66. (*A*) Multiple hemangiomatosis of bone. Frequency of areas of involvement in 28 patients. Male: female incidence, 1.1:1. (*B*) Age distribution of patients with multiple hemangiomatosis of bone. Male: female incidence, 1.1:1. (Mirra, J. Bullough, P., and Freiberger, R.: Orthopedic Diseases, Part IV. New York, Famous Teachings in Modern Medicine, MedCom, Inc., © 1977)

predominant factors causing lowered oxygen tension, which favors bone deposition (osteosclerosis).

The vertebrae usually show demineralization with one or more compression fractures. The long bones tend to show multiple foci of lysis with trabeculations or vertical striations (Fig. 13-67 and 13-68) similar to solitary hemangioma. With severe involvement the bones show "expansion" and a soap-bubble appearance. The epiphyses, metaphyses, or diaphyses may be involved. Most lesions involve the bone and often the lesions begin at the site where the nutrient artery enters the bone. The lesions are usually surrounded by a thin rim of periosteal new bone and host bone sclerosis, features of benignancy. Hemangiomatosis may be among the most coarsely loculated of all bone tumors. Often the multiple skeletal lesions are incorrectly diagnosed as other, more common lesions, such as metastastic malignancy, fibrous dysplasia, hyperparathyroidism, Hand-Schüller-Christian disease, and Ollier's disease. A diagnosis of multiple hemangiomatosis is, therefore, seldom considered until a biopsy is performed.

One of the features which, if present, should lead to the suspicion of either multiple hemangiomatosis or Ollier's disease is multiple soft-tissue phleboliths (Figs. 13-67 and 13-68). Both Maffucci's syndrome and the above entity may be associated with large soft-tissue hemangiomas and phleboliths. Both may also show similar radiologic features. The above en-

(*Text continues on p. 508.*)

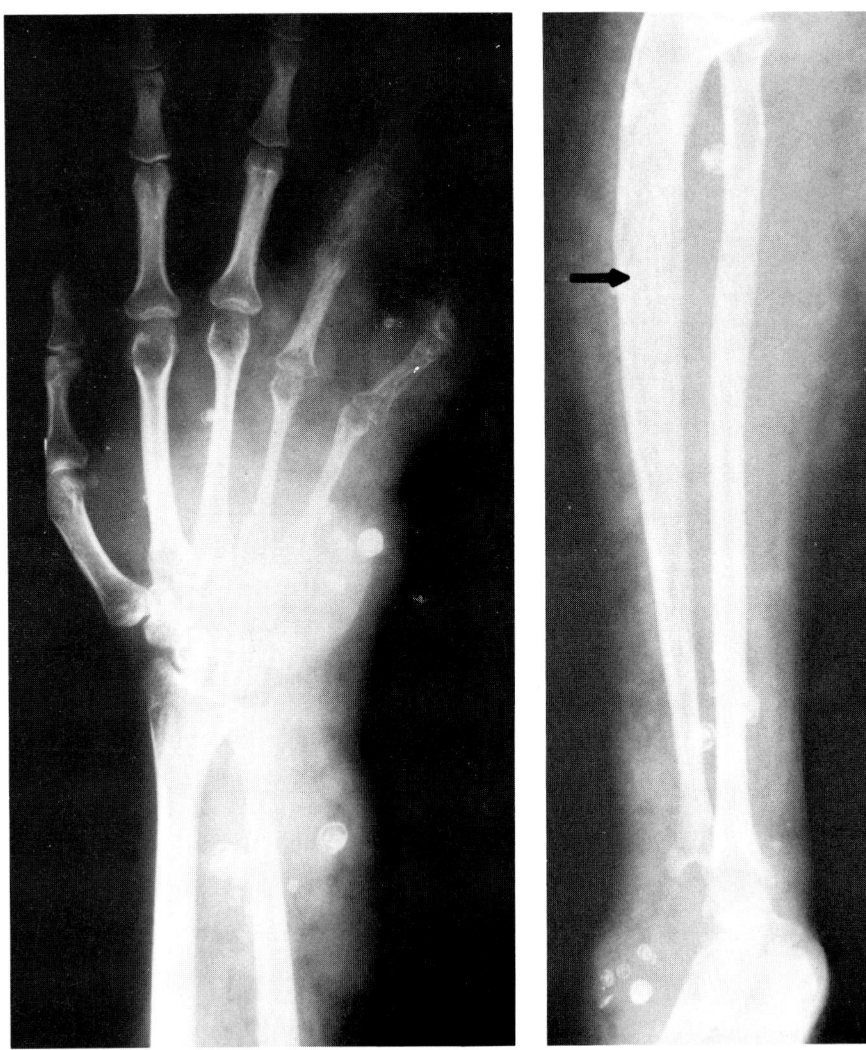

FIG. 13-67 FIG. 13-68

Multiple Hemangiomatosis

FIG. 13-67. Patient with diffuse hemangiomatosis. Note the obvious phleboliths, lytic destruction of many of the bones of the hand, and the vertical striations in some of the bones of the hand, radius, and ulna. The striations should immediately suggest hemangioma of bone.

FIG. 13-68. Same patient to show more clearly the vertical striations (*arrow*) of the affected long bones.

Osler-Weber-Rendu Disease With Multiple Hemangiomatosis

FIG. 13-69. Multiple lytic lesions (*arrows*) of the hands because of hemangiomatosis of the bones in association with hereditary hemorrhagic telangiectasia.

FIG. 13-70. Same patient showing the characteristic telangiectasias of the lips.

FIG. 13-71. Biopsy of the bone lesion showed an obvious hemangioma (*left*) and a much more closely packed hemangiomatous lesion (*right*), which could be misconstrued as hemangioendothelioma (benign or malignant). Before using the term *hemangioendothelioma,* one must be extremely careful to rule out the above peculiar form of cellular hemangioma or a well-differentiated angiosarcoma.

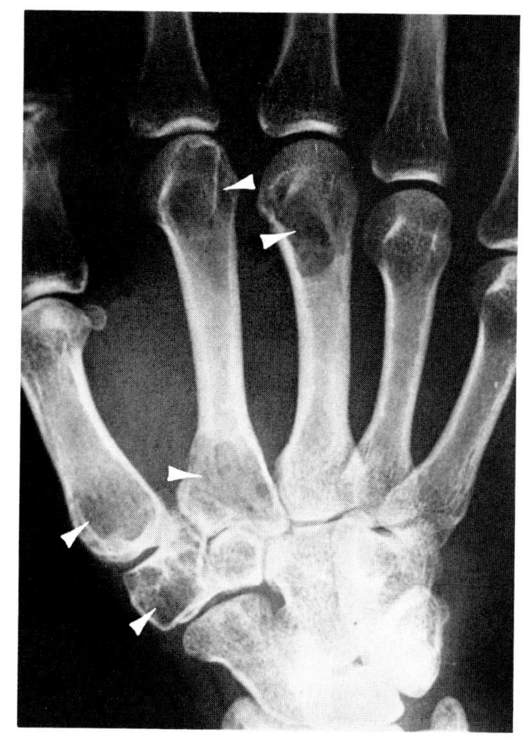

FIG. 13-69

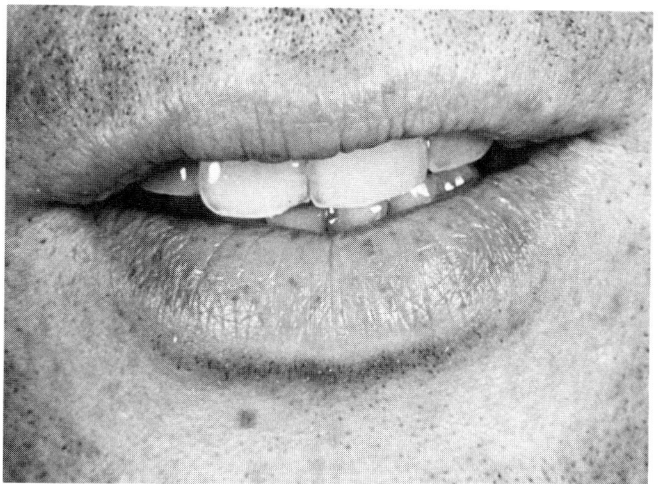

FIG. 13-70

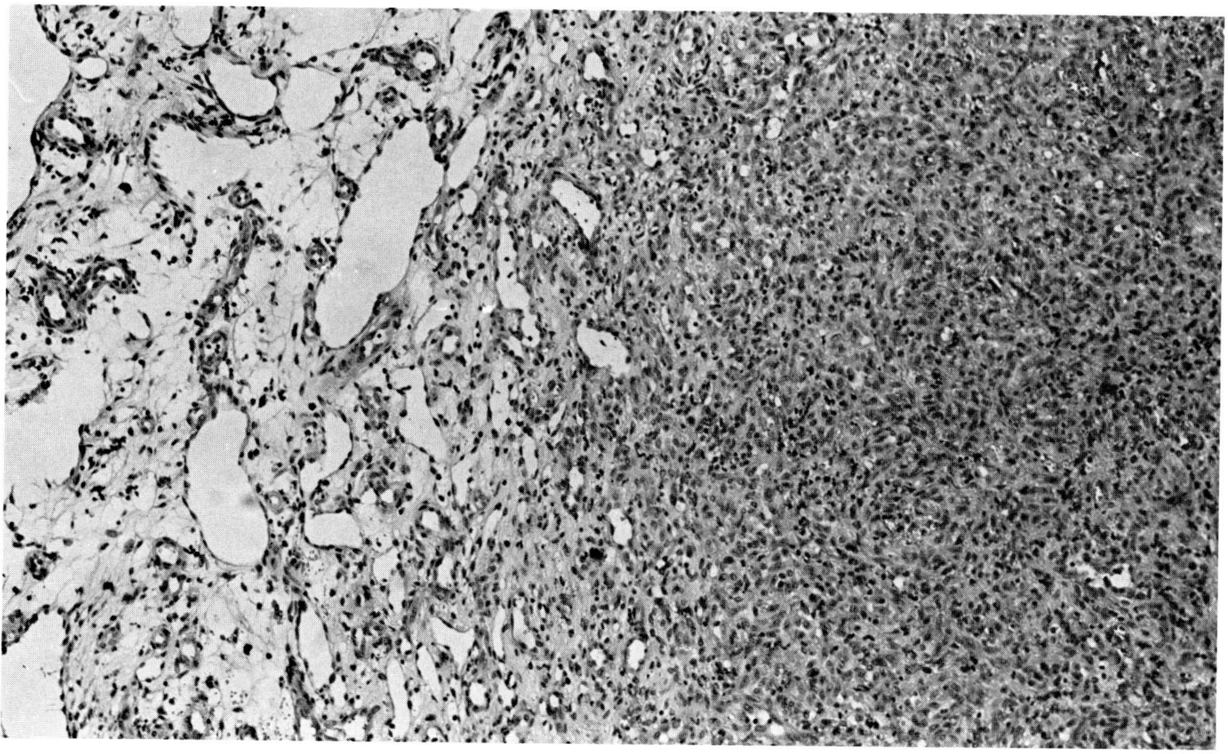

FIG. 13-71

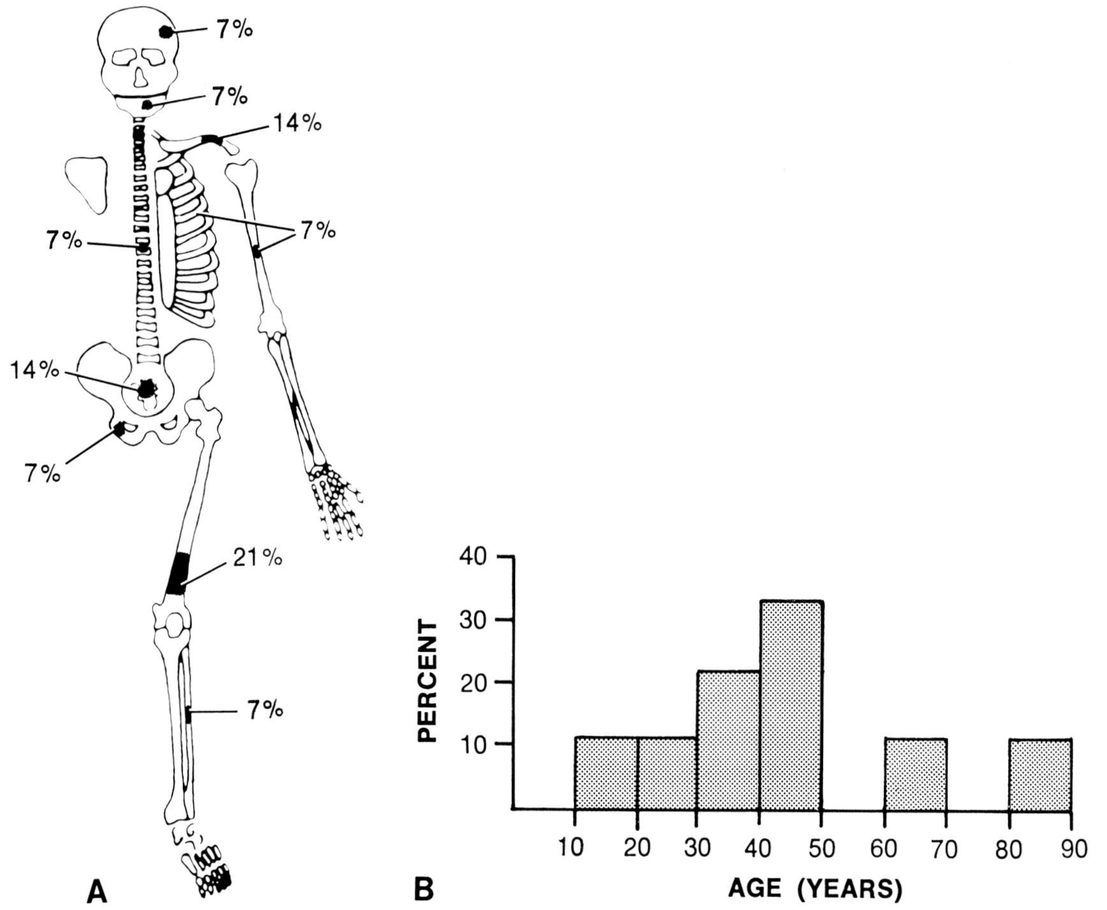

FIG. 13-72. (*A*) Primary hemangiopericytoma of bone. Frequency of areas of involvement in 14 patients. Male:Female incidence, 1.25:2. (*B*) Age distribution of patients with hemangiopericytoma of bone.

tity is, of course, never associated with enchondromatosis, which characterizes Maffucci's syndrome. Therefore, the distinction between Maffucci's syndrome versus the syndrome of multiple bone and soft-tissue hemangiomatosis depends on bone biopsy and radiological interpretation.

Gross Pathology

The gross appearance is that of a highly vascularized reddish to reddish blue lesions similar on appearance to the solitary hemangioma. The long bones and vertebral bodies can show very prominent vertical accentuations of the bone trabeculae.

Histopathology

The lesions are characterized by numerous capillary and/or cavernous vascular capillaries (Fig. 13-71). The capillaries may form quite solid-looking areas. If the lesion is composed mostly of these solid areas the tumor may be confused with an hemangioendothelioma or angiosarcoma. It is extremely important to search for unequivocal benign hemangiomatous areas. Even in the solid areas, the cell nuclei do not bud into the lumen significantly, and do not show abnormal chromatin clumping, a high mitotic rate, or atypical mitoses. Although angiosarcoma may involve two or even three continuous bones, it is

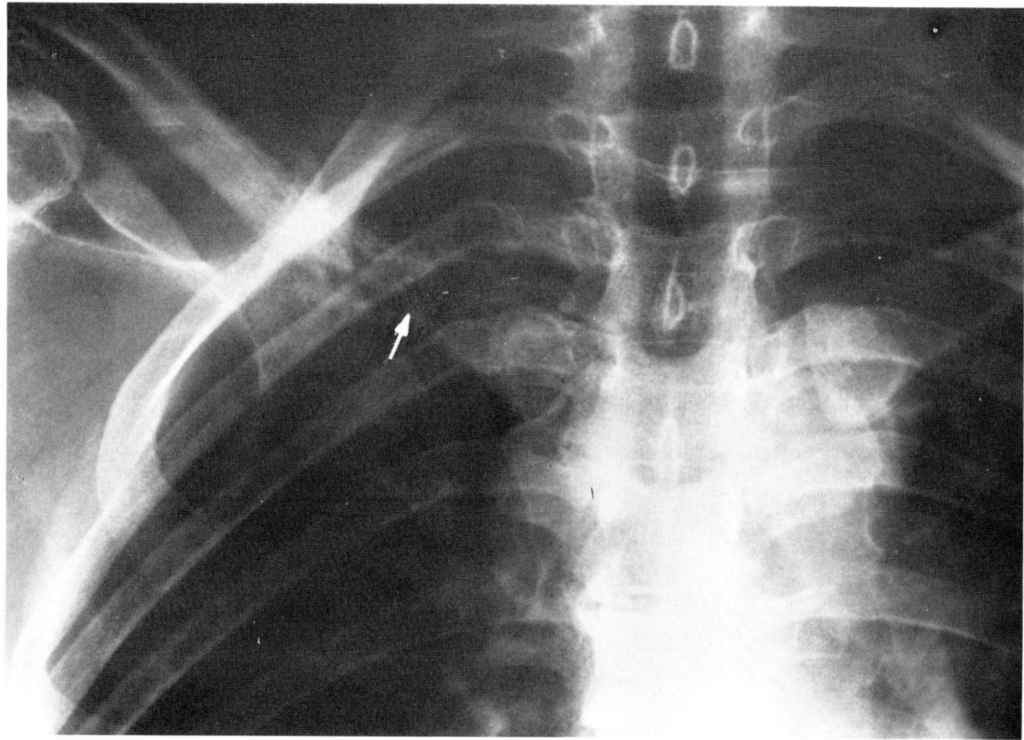

Hemangiopericytoma

FIG. 13-73. Note the destructive lesion of the clavicle (*arrow*), which, on biopsy (below), proved to be the rare primary hemangiopericytoma of bone.

hemangiomatosis that involves numerous distant bones.

A sprinkling of mononuclear chronic inflammatory cells may be seen in the stroma between the hamartomatous vessels.

Course and Treatment

Curettage, cauterization, and/or irradiation are the best forms of treatment. When there is no visceral involvement the prognosis is excellent. If, however, there is visceral involvement, the 5-year survival rate is approximately 50 per cent and the 10-year survival rate drops to 30 per cent. Death is usually associated with respiratory failure when there is thoracic involvement, massive hemorrhage, or heart failure. Many of these patients require multiple blood transfusions.

PRIMARY HEMANGIOPERICYTOMA

Introduction

The primary hemangiopericytoma is one of the rarest reported tumors of bone. To date approximately 13 cases have been reported. This author has seen only one such case. Its incidence is less than 0.1 per cent. The histological features of the tumor, of course, correspond to those of its soft-tissue counterpart (Fig.13-72).

Clinical Features

The most usual reported clinical signs and symptoms are pain associated with a mass or swelling. In one case there was pain in the knee for 20 years prior to the discovery of the tumor.[88] Usually, however, the pain is of much shorter duration. In one case of a sacral tumor the mass that broke out of the bone

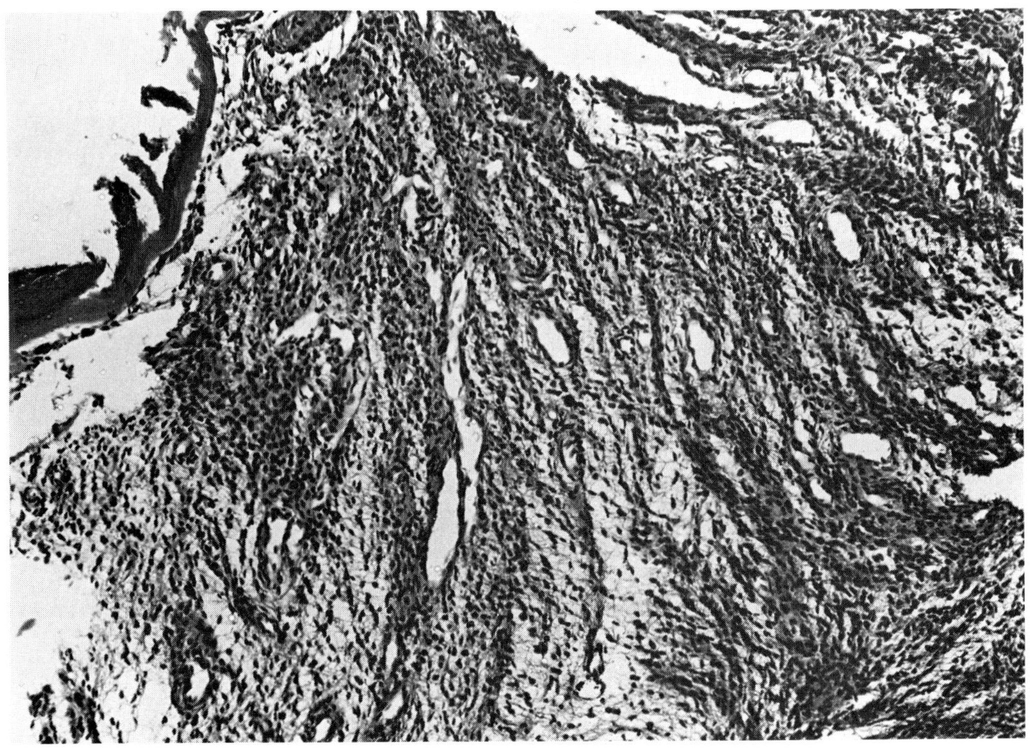

Hemangiopericytoma

FIG. 13-74. On low power, the tumor consists of numerous vessels surrounded by ovoid to spindly mesenchymal cells (x125).

resulted in bladder invasion with hematuria, nocturia, and a mass in the rectum.

Radiologic Features

The most consistent radiologic feature is lysis. The edges of the lesion are usually moth-eaten and have an aggressive-looking quality (Fig. 13-73). The lesions are usually poorly circumscribed and often show soft-tissue mass extension. Periosteal reaction with a Codman's triangle was described in only one case. The lesion does not show a benign border of host bone sclerosis. The lesion would almost never be considered in a radiological differential diagnosis because of its extreme rarity and the fact that it does not show any specific or highly characteristic radiologic features.

Gross Pathology

The tumors are described as firm and grayish white. The resected bone usually shows extension of the tumor into the surrounding soft tissues.

(*Text continues on p. 516.*)

Hemangiopericytoma

FIG. 13-75. On high power, the neoplastic cells lie outside the capillaries, as shown here. The nuclei are oval and usually quite monotonous in size and shape. They do not appear frankly malignant. Mitoses are variable, depending on the degree of malignancy of the tumor. The lesion would best be recognized by having firsthand knowledge of the appearance of its much more common soft-tissue counterpart (x400).

FIG. 13-76. Only if the diagnosis is suspected should the corroborative reticulin stains be ordered. Note the great mass of fine reticulin fibers that surrounds each tumor cell. The cells lie outside of the nutritive blood vessels (*arrows*) (x125).

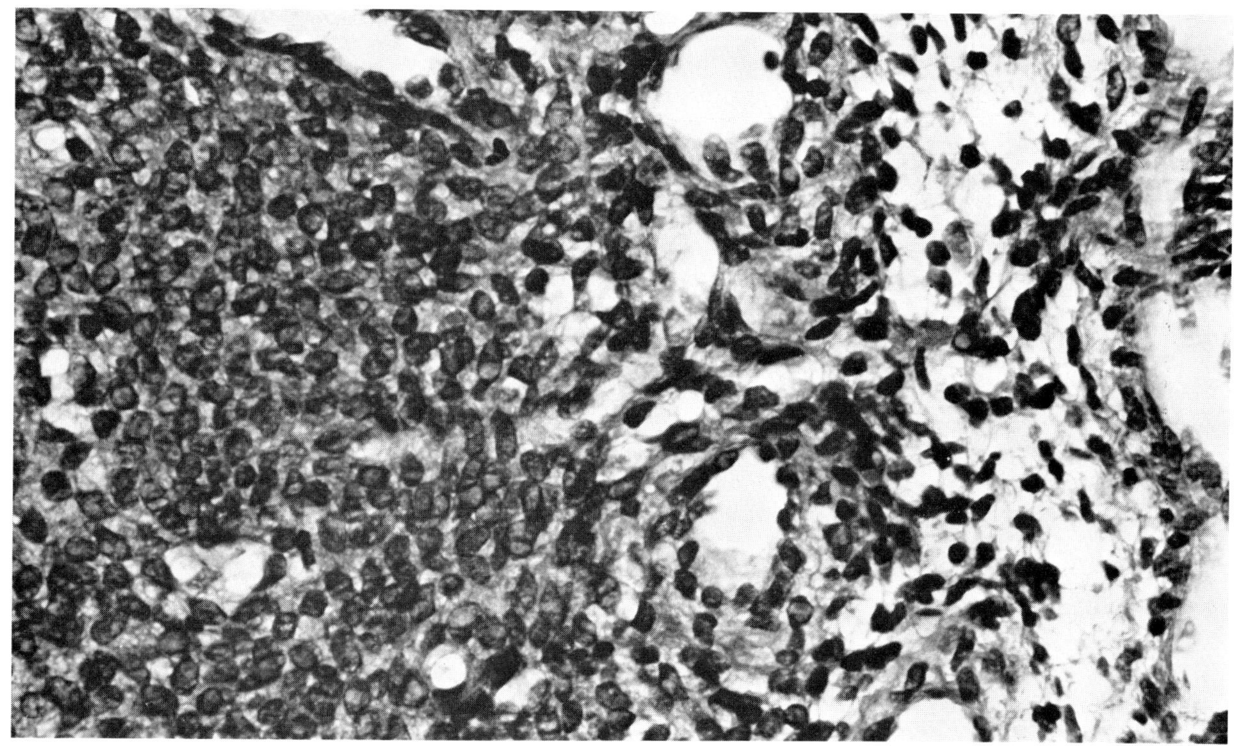

FIG. 13-75

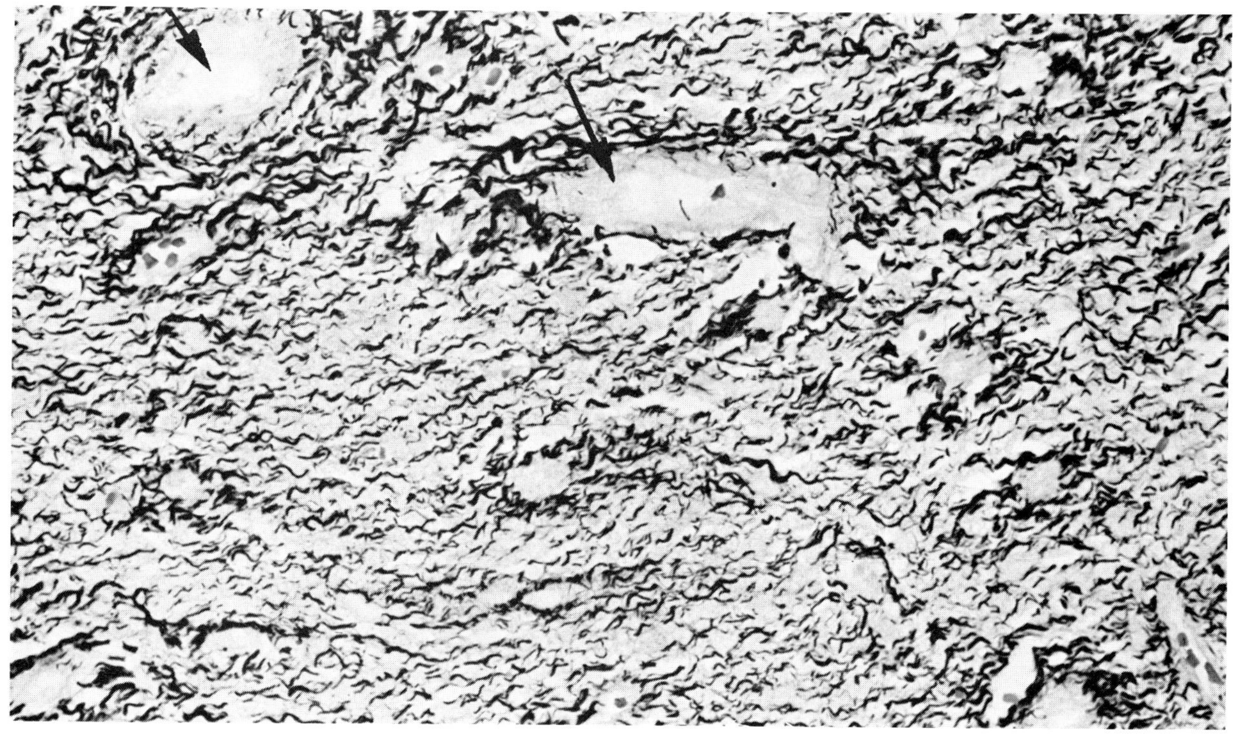

FIG. 13-76

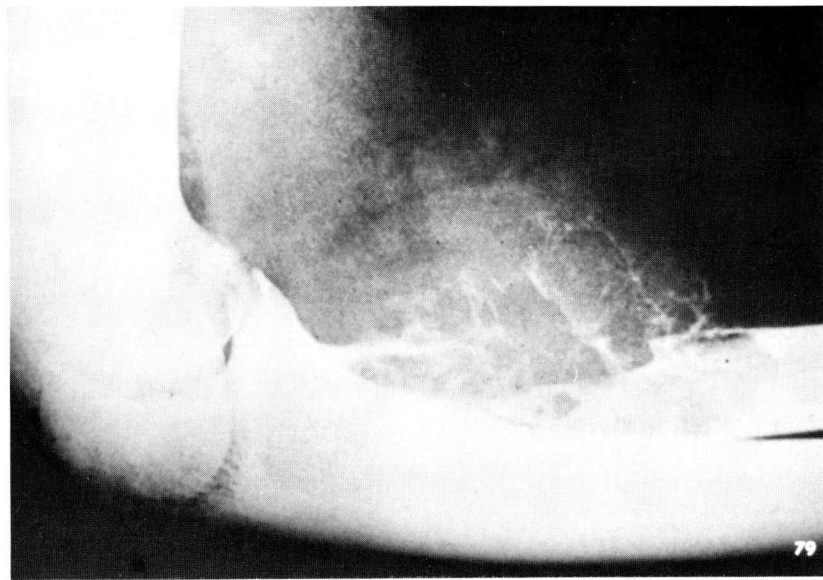

FIG. 13-77

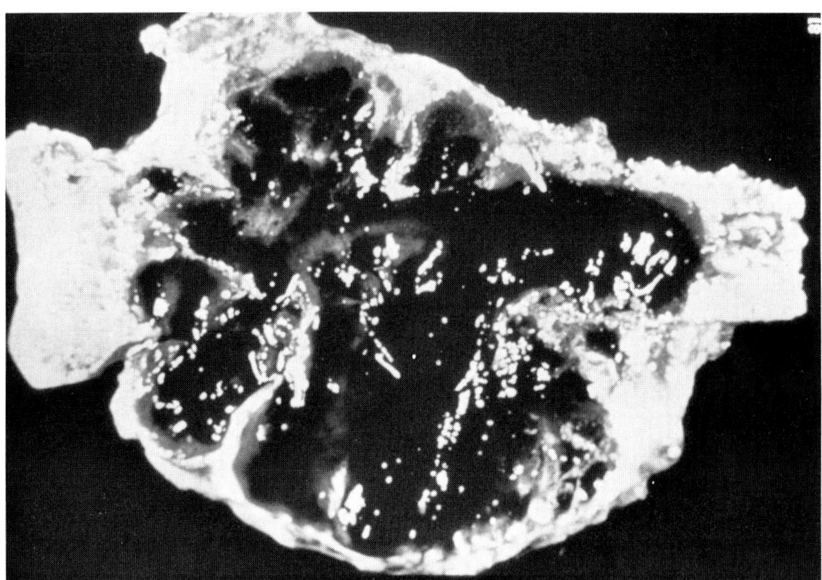

FIG. 13-78

Angiosarcoma

FIG. 13-77. Example of an angiosarcoma of bone. (Grateful courtesy of Drs. G. Steiner and H. Dorfman)

FIG. 13-78. The gross specimen from the above patient showed a large, almost cystic, destructive, obviously bloody tumor. (Grateful courtesy of Drs. G. Steiner and H. Dorfman)

FIG. 13-79. Specimen radiograph to show the permeative lytic destruction of an angiosarcoma of the sternum.

FIG. 13-80. Gross appearance.

FIG. 13-81. The tumor is composed of anaplastic cells lining vascular structures. The reticulin stain will corroborate that the neoplastic cells lie internal to the reticulin of the vascular structures and the perivascular stroma. (Grateful courtesy of Drs. G. Steiner and H. Dorfman)

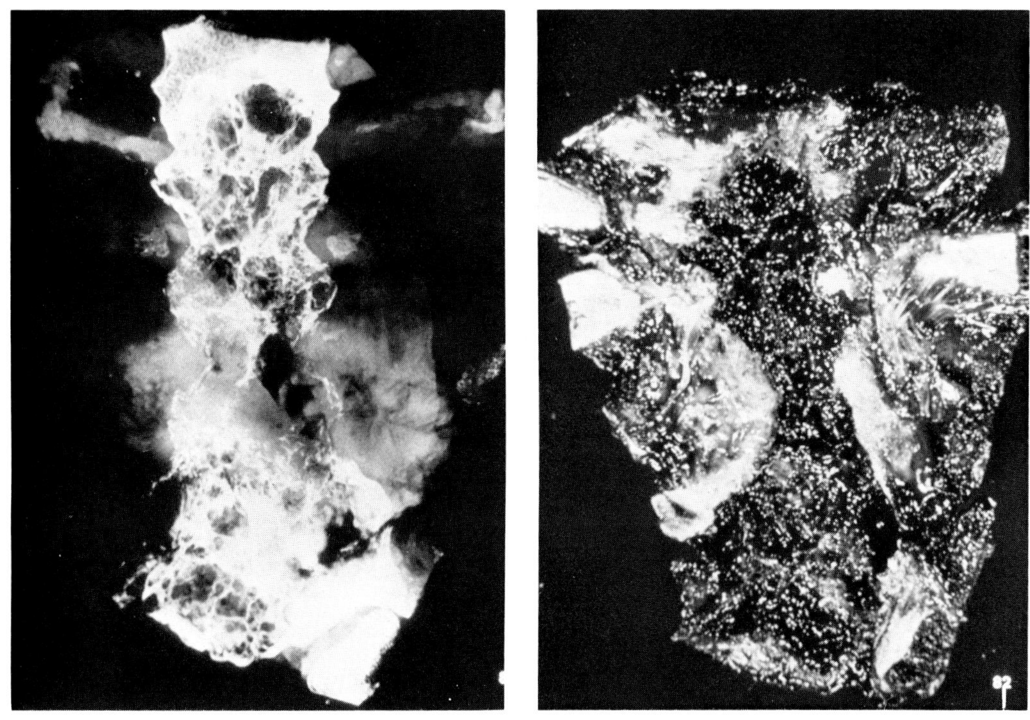

FIG. 13-79

FIG. 13-80

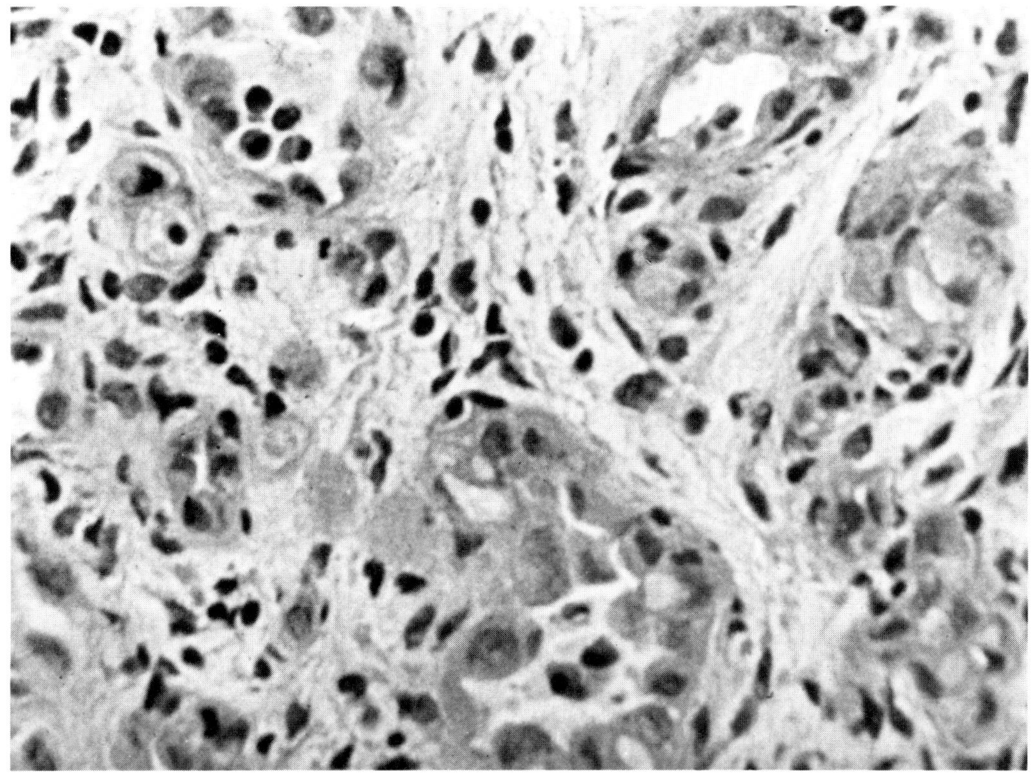

FIG. 13-81

Table 13-1. Patient Data Relating to

Case Number	*Author(s) (Year of Publication)*	*Age*	*Sex*	*Location*	*Symptoms*
1	Marcial-Rojas (1960)	83	F	Clavicle, middle third	Pain, mass
2	Stout (1956)	29	M	Femur	N.S.
3	Stout (1956)	32	M	Fibula	N.S.
4	Stout (1956)	N.S.	N.S.	Skull (may be extension from meningeal tumor)	N.S.
5,6,7,8	Dahlin (1957)	N.S.	N.S.	Vertebra, rib, ischium, and sacrum	N.S.
9	McCormack Gallivan (1954)	40	F	Femur, lower (periosteal in origin)	Swelling, pain, tenderness in back of knee-20 years. 18 years later, increasing stiffness, pain, and mass
10	Gutierrez et al (1976)	45	M	Sacrum	Hematuria, nocturia, mass in rectum
11	Dunlop (1973)	41	F	Mid-humerus, eccentric (periosteal in origin?)	Itching hand, pain on shoulder abduction, mass
12	Dunlop (1973)	37	M	Femur, distal diaphysis	Pain and mass
13	Sage and Salman (1968)	16	M	Mandible	Facial swelling, mass
14	Mirra et al (submitted for publication)	60	F	Clavicle, anterior third	Pain, mass

N.S. = Not stated

Radiographic Features	*Diagnosis*	*Therapy*	*Course*
Lytic destruction with soft-tissue extension	Hemangiopericytoma with good differentiation. Occasional mitoses.	En-bloc resection	11 months, recurrence and lung mets. 17 mos., died with lung mets.
N.S.	Hemangiopericytoma	Radiotherapy	N.S.
N.S.	Hemangiopericytoma	Resection	N.S.
N.S.	Hemangiopericytoma	N.S.	N.S.
N.S.	Hemangiopericytoma	N.S.	N.S.
N.S.	Hemangiopericytoma	Amputation	20-year history of pain 18 years, later biopsy of neoplasm. Three mos later, fracture and amputation. Seven mos later, solitary 2.5 cm. lung mets. removed. No further follow-up
"Aggressive" lytic lesion	"Malignant" hemangiopericytoma- Enzinger & Johnson (AFIP)	Resection	2 year follow-up. Free of disease
Lytic erosion with periosteal reaction and Codman's triangle	Malignant hemangiocytoma	Amputation	1 year follow-up. Free of disease
Circumscribed lysis with moth-eaten borders and no "reactive" sclerosis	Hemangiopericytoma	Cobalt irradiation to 6250 R.	8 year follow-up. Free of disease
Lytic destruction, multilocular	Ameloblastoma 4 yrs later "malignant" hemangiopericytoma	Resection of ameloblastoma & hemangiopericytoma	Ameloblastoma removed. 4 yrs later developed hemangiopericytoma. Same region resected. Died 4 yrs later with massive pleural effusion
Lytic destruction Poorly circumscribed soft tissue extension	Borderline malignant hemangiopericytoma Less than 1 mitosis/ 50 HPF. Moderate cellularity. No necrosis or hemorrhage.	Resection 5500 R.	Well with no evidence of recurrence or metastasis, $2\frac{1}{2}$ year follow-up.

Histopathology

The hemangiopericytoma is characterized by the following:

1. Sheets of spindly cells surrounding numerous capillaries (Fig. 13–74)
2. Monotonous oval nuclei usually lacking frank anaplasia (Fig. 13–75)
3. Indistinct cytoplasmic borders
4. Silver stains show that each cell is surrounded by a reticulin sheath that lays outside of the capillary walls (Fig. 13–76).

Course Related to Pathology

Enzinger and Smith studied 106 hemangiopericytomas from various sites but none were primary in the bone. They were able to relate prognosis very closely to mitotic count, cellularity of the tumor, degree of necrosis, and size of the tumor. Of 16 cases that metastasized, eight averaged more than 32 mitoses/50 HPF's. In the remaining eight cases fewer figures were counted but all showed a significant increase in cellularity, often combined with foci of necrosis and hemorrhage. In 46 of 66 cases without recurrence or metastasis not a single mitotic figure was detected in a count of 30 HPF's. The 10-year survival was 77 per cent for tumors with 1 to 15 mitoses, and 29 per cent for tumors with 20 or more mitotic figures per 50 HPF's. Necrosis and hemorrhage were twice as common in hemangiopericytomas that later recurred or metastasized as they were for those with a benign course. The 10-year survival for patients with tumors larger than 6.5 cm. was 65 per cent, and 92 per cent for those smaller than 6.5 cm. Circumscription versus its lack did not correlate to survival. Recurrence was an ominous sign, because 11 of 16 tumors that recurred eventually metastasized.

Although the hemangiopericytoma of bone may not behave identically to those of soft tissue it would be appropriate in future cases to report mitotic count, degree of cellularity, necrosis, and tumor size to see if similar pathological to clinical course correlations are possible. This may help to determine the type of therapy used. Also it would be of interest to correlate circumscription of the bone tumor versus its look to whether the tumor is confined to the bone or broken out of the bone to course. Of the 14 reported cases of bone, only five had recurrent or metastatic hemangiopericytoma after more than 2 years of follow-up. Of these five cases two developed lethal lung metastases within less than 5 years time. Four patients were free of disease at 1, 2, 2, and 8 years, respectively. One patient had a solitary lung metastasis removed 7 months post-amputation but then he was not followed.

Treatment

The most appropriate form of therapy would probably be en-bloc resection with a complete margin of healthy uninvolved tissue. Hemangiopericytomas that are inoperable may be quite responsive to irradiation. Soft-tissue hemangiopericytoma has not been particularly responsive to chemotherapy.

Refer to Table 13–1 for a summary of the reported cases.

HEMANGIOSARCOMA

CAPSULE SUMMARY

Incidence. 0.1 per cent of primary bone tumors. Male to female incidence is 1.5 to 1.

Age. Rare before age 10. 10 to 30 years (38%), 31 to 40 years (32%), 40–60 years (22%).

Sites of Involvement. Any bone. Femur (24%), tibia (14%), pelvis (12%), humerus (10%), fibula (6%), spine (6%), skull (4%), ribs (4%).

Signs and Symptoms. Pain and/or swelling.

Radiologic Findings. Cystic, coarsely loculated, trabeculated, or bubbly radiolucent lesions (Figs. 13–77 and 13–79).

The hemangiosarcoma (malignant hemangioendothelioma) of bone is a very rare malignant lesion derived from vascular mesenchyme. On gross examination the lesions are dark red and diffusely permeative to cystlike (Figs. 13–77 and 13–80).

Diagnosis depends upon the demonstration of vessels lined by plump endothelial cells that display features of anaplasia (Fig. 13–81). The cells may form papillary projections and "bud" off and lie free in the vascular spaces. This is seen uncommonly in benign vascular processes. The tumor may form solid sheets and be confused with a type of spindle cell sarcoma. Benign hemangiomatous-looking areas should make one suspicious of a sclerosing hemangioma mimicking an angiosarcoma. Reticulin stains of the angiosarcoma show that the neoplastic cells are contained within the luminal side of the basement membrane of the blood vessel.

These are highly malignant tumors and must be treated by radical methods.

REFERENCES

Myxoma of Jaws and Skull

1. Bauer, W.H., and Harell, A.: Myxoma of bone. J. Bone Joint Surg., *36A:*263, 1954.
2. Dutz, W., and Stout, A.P.: The myxoma in childhood. Cancer, *14:*629, 1961.
2. Enzinger, F.M.: Intramuscular Myxoma. A review and follow-up study of 34 cases. Am. J. Clin. Pathol., *43:*104, 1965.
4. Fu, Y.S., and Perzin, K.H.: Non-epithelial tumors of the nasal cavity, paranasal sinuses and nasopharynx. A clinico-pathologic study. VII myxomas. Cancer, *39:*195, 1977.
5. Ghosh, B.C., Huvos, A.G., Gerold, F., and Miller, T.R.: Myxoma of the jaw bones. Cancer, *31:*237, 1973.
6. Harrison, J.D.: Odontogenic myxoma. Ultrastructural and histochemical studies. J. Clin. Pathol., *26:*570, 1973.
7. Kangur, T.T., Dahlin, D.C., and Turlington, E.G.: Myxomatous tumors of the jaws. J. Oral Surg., *31:*523, 1975.

7a. Jaffe, H.L., and Lichtenstein, L.: Chondromyxoid fibroma of bone. A distinctive benign tumor likely to be mistaken for chondrosarcoma. Arch. Pathol., *45:*541, 1948.

8. Marcove, R.C., Kambolis, C., Bullough, P.G., and Jaffe, H.L.: Fibromyxoma of bone. Report of 3 cases. Cancer, *17:*1209, 1964.
9. Mori, M., Murakami, M., Hirose, I., and Shimozato, T.: Histochemical studies of myxoma of the jaws. J. Oral Surg., *33:*529, 1976.
10. Scaglietti, O., and Stringa, G.: Myxoma of bone in childhood. J. Bone Joint Surg., *43A:*67, 1961.
11. White, D.K., Chin, S.Y., Mohnac, A.M., and Miller, A.S.: Odontogenic myxoma, a clinical and ultrastructural study. Oral Surg., *39:*901, 1975.
12. Wirth, W.A., Leavitt, D., and Enzinger, F.M.: Multiple intramuscular myxomas. Another extraskeletal manifestation of fibrous dysplasia. Cancer, *27:*1167, 1971.
13. Zimmerman, D.C., and Dahlin, D.C.: Myxomatous tumors of the jaws. Oral Surg., *11:*1069, 1958.

Solitary or Unicameral Bone Cysts

14. Baker, D.M.: Benign unicameral bone cyst. A study of 45 cases. Clin. Orthop., *71:*140, 1970.
15. Barland, P., Norikoff, A., and Hammerman, P.: Electron microscopy of human synovial membrane. J. Cell Biol., *14:*207, 1962.
16. Boseker, E., Bickel, W., and Dahlin, D.: A clinipathologic study of simple unicameral bone cysts. Surg. Gynecol. Obstet., *127:*550, 1968.
17. Broder, H.M.: Possible precursor of unicameral bone cysts. J. Bone Joint Surg., *50A:*503, 1968.

17a. Campanacci, M., De Sessa, L., and Trentani, C.: Scaglietti's method for conservative treatment of simple bone cysts with local injections of methylprednisolone acetate. Ital. J. Orthop. Traumatol., *3:*27, 1977.

18. Cohen, J.: Simple bone cysts. Studies of cyst fluid in 6 cases with a theory of pathogenesis. J. Bone Joint Surg., *42A:*609, 1960.
19. Cohen, J.: Etiology of simple bone cyst. J. Bone Joint Surg., *52A:*1493, 1970.
20. Clark, L.: The influence of trauma on unicameral bone cysts. Clin. Orthop., *22:*209, 1962.
21. Coley, B., and Higinbotham, N.L.: Solitary bone cyst. Ann. Surg., *99:*432, 1934.
22. D'Ambrosia, R., and Ferguson, A.: The formation of osteochondroma by epiphyseal cartilage transplantation. Clin. Orthop., *61:*103, 1968.
23. Friedman, N., and Goldman, R.C.: Cementoma of long bones. Clin. Orthop., *67:*243, 1969.
24. Gabbiani, G., Kay, G., Lattes, R., and Majuo, G.: Synovial sarcoma—E-M study of a typical case. Cancer, *28:*1031, 1971.
25. Galasko, C.: The fate of simple bone cysts which fracture, Clin. Orthop., *101:*302, 1974.
26. Groth, H.: Cellular contacts in the synovial membrane of the cat and rat. An ultrastructural study. Cell Tissue Res., *165:*525, 1975.
27. Hagberg, S., and Mansfeld, L.: The solitary bone cyst. Acta Chir. Scand., *133:*25, 1967.
28. Jaffe, H.L.: Tumors and Tumorous Conditions of the Bones and Joints. Philadelphia, Lea & Febiger, 1958.
29. James, A., Coley, B., and Higinbotham, N.L.: Solitary (unicameral) bone cyst. Ann. Surg., *57:*137, 1948.
30. Lodwick, G.S.: Juvenile unicameral bone cyst. A roentgen reappraisal. Am. J. Roentgenol. Radium Ther. Nucl. Med., *80:*495, 1958.
31. Mirra, J.M., *et. al.:* Cementum-like bone production in solitary bone cysts (so-called "cementoma" of long bones). Report of 3 cases. Electron-microscopic observations supporting a synovial origin to the simple bone cyst. Clin. Orthop., *135:*295, 1978.
32. Neer, C., Francis, K., Johnston, A., and Kiernan, H.A.: Current concepts on the treatment of solitary unicameral bone cyst. Clin. Orthop., *97:*40, 1973.
33. Neer, C., *et. al.:* Treatment of unicameral bone cyst. J. Bone Joint Surg., *48A:*731, 1966.
34. Porat, S., Lowe, J., and Rousso, M.: Solitary bone cyst in the infant radius. Clin. Orthop., in press 1978.
35. Spence, K., Sell, K., and Brown, R.: Solitary bone cyst: treatment with freeze-dried cancellous bone allograft. J. Bone Joint Surg., *51A:*87, 1969.
36. Virchow, R.: Ueber multiple exostosen, mit. vorlegung von preparaten berl. klin. Wochnschr., *28:*1082, 1891.

Aneurysmal Bone Cyst (ABC)

37. Barnes, R.: Aneurysmal bone cyst. J. Bone Joint Surg., *38B:*301, 1956.
38. Biesecker, J.L., Marcove, R.C., Huvos, A.G., and Mike, V.: Aneurysmal bone cyst. A clinico-pathologic study of 66 cases. Cancer, *26:*615, 1970.

39. Clough, J.R., and Price, C.H.G.: Aneurysmal bone cyst: pathogenesis and long term results of treatment. Clin. Orthop., *97:*53, 1973.
40. Dabska, M., and Buraczewski, J.: Aneurysmal bone cyst. Pathology, clinical course and radiologic appearance. Cancer, *23:*371, 1969.
41. Donaldson, W.F.: Aneurysmal bone cyst. J. Bone Joint Surg., *44A:*25, 1962.
42. Ginsburg, L.D.: Congenital aneurysmal bone cyst. Radiology, *110:*175, 1974.
43. Howard, R.C.: A case of congenital aneurysm involving the femur. J. Bone Joint Surg., *41B:*358, 1959.
44. Jaffe, H.L.: Aneurysmal bone cyst. Bull. Hosp. Joint Dis., *11:*3, 1950.
45. Jaffe, H.L., and Lichtenstein, L.: Solitary unicameral bone cyst with emphasis on the roentgen picture, the pathologic appearance and the pathogenesis. J.A.M.A., *83:*1224, 1924.
46. Levy, N., Miller, A., Bonakdapur, A., and Aegertar, E.: Aneurysmal bone cyst secondary to other osseous lesions. Report of 57 cases. Am. J. Clin. Pathol., *63:*1, 1975.
47. Lichtenstein, L.: Aneurysmal bone cyst. Cancer, *3:*279, 1950.
48. Lichtenstein, L.: Aneurysmal bone cyst. Observation 50 cases. J. Bone Joint Surg., *39A:*873, 1957.
49. Lindbom, A., Soderberg, G., and Spjut, H.J.: Angiography of aneurysmal bone cyst. Acta Radiol., *55:*12, 1961.
50. Marcove, R.C., and Miller, T.R.: The treatment of primary and metastatic bone localized bone tumors by cryosurgery. Surg. Clin. North Am., *49:*421, 1969.
51. Nobler, M.P., Higinbotham, N.L., and Phillips, R.F.: The cure of the aneurysmal bone cyst. Radiology, *90:*1185, 1968.
52. Ring, S.M., Baranbaum, E.R., and Madayag, M.A.: Angiography of aneurysmal bone cyst. Bull. Hosp. Joint Dis., *33:*1, 1972.
53. Schenk, W.G., Bahee, R.A., Cordell, A.R., and Hephans, J.G.: The regional hemodynamics of experimental acute arterio-venous fistulas. Surg. Gynecol. Obstet., *105:*733, 1957.
54. Sherman, R.S., and Soong, K.Y.: Aneurysmal bone cyst: its roentgen diagnosis. Radiology, *68:*54, 1957.
55. Slowick, F., Cambell, C., and Kettlekamp, D.: Aneurysmal bone cyst. An analysis of 13 cases. J. Bone Joint Surg., *50A:*1142, 1968.
56. Tillman, B.P., Dahlin, D.C., and Lipscomb, P.R.: Aneurysmal bone cyst: An analysis of 95 cases. Mayo Clin. Proc., *43:*478, 1968.

Solitary Hemangioma

57. Anspach, W.: Sunray hemangioma of bone: With special reference to roentgen signs. J.A.M.A., *108:*617, 1937.
58. Farber, L., and Lampe, I.: Hemangioma of vertebra associated with compression of the cord. Arch. Neurol. and Psychiatry, *47:*19, 1942.
59. Jaffe, H.L.: *Tumors and Tumorous Conditions of the Bones and Joints.* chap. 15. Philadelphia, Lea & Febiger, 1958.
60. Sherman, R.S., and Wilner, D.: The roentgen diagnosis of hemangioma of bone. Am. J. Roentgenol. Radium Ther. Nucl. Med., *86:*1146, 1961.
61. Schmorl, G.: Die pathologische anatomie der wirbelsaule. Verhandl diDeutsch Orthop. Gesellsch. Kong, *21:*3, 1927.

Vascular Tumors of Soft Tissue and Bone That Induce Systemic Hypophosphatemic Osteomalacia

62. Case Records of the Massachusetts General Hospital: case 38–1965. New Engl. J. Med., *273:*494, 1965.
63. Dent, C.E., and Freidman, M.: Hypophosphatemic osteomalacia with complete recovery. Br. J. Med., *1:*1676, 1964.
64. Evans, D.J., and Azzopardi, J.G.: Distinctive Tumors of bone and soft tissue causing acquired Vt. D-resistant osteomalacia. Lancet, *1:*353, 1972.
65. Linovitz, R., *et. al.:* Tumor induced osteomalacia and rickets: a surgically curable syndrome. J. Bone Joint Surg., *58A:*419, 1976.
66. McCance, R.A.: Osteomalacia with Looser's zones due to a raised resistance to vt. D. acquired about the age of 15 years. Qu. J. Med., *16:*33, 1947.
67. Moser, C.R., and Fessel, W.J.: Rheumatic manifestations of hypophosphatemia. Arch. Intern. Med., *134:*674, 1974.
68. Olefsky, J., Kempson, R., Jones, H., and Reaven, G.: "Tertiary" hyperparathyroidism and apparent "cure" of Vt-D resistant rickets after removal of an ossifying mesenchymal tumor of the pharynx. New Engl. J. Med., *286:*740, 1972.
69. Pollack, A., Illig, R., Eublinger, R., and Stalder, G.: Rachitis infolge knochentumors. Helvetica Paediatr. Acta, *14:*554, 1959.
70. Renton, P., and Shaw, D.G.: Hypophosphatemic osteomalacia secondary to vascular tumors of bone and soft tissue. Skeletal Radiol., *1:*21, 1976.
71. Salassa, R., Jowsey, J., and Arnaude, C.D.: Hypophosphatemic osteomalacia associated with "nonendocrine" tumors. New Engl. J. Med., *283:*65, 1970.
72. Wilboite, D.R.: Acquired rickets and solitary bone tumor. Proceeding of the Clinical Orthopedic Society. Clin. Orthop., *109:*210, 1975.
73. Yochikawa, S., *et. al.:* Atypical Vt. D. resistant osteomalacia. J. Bone Joint Surg., *46A:*998, 1964.

Multiple Hemangiomatosis of Bone

74. Ackerman, A., and Hart, M.: Multiple primary hemangioma of the bones of the extremity. Am. J. Roent. *48:*47, 1942.

75. Czerniak, P., and Schorr, S.: Hereditary Hemorrhagic Telangiectasis with Involvement of Bone. Am. J. Roentgenol. Radium Ther. Nucl. Med., *74:*299, 1955.
76. Dorfman, H.D., Steiner, G.C., and Jaffe, H.L.: Vascular tumors of bone. Human Pathol., *2:*349, 1971.
77. Geshickter, C., and Maseritz, E.: Primary hemangioma involving bones of the extremities. J. Bone Joint Surg., *20:*888, 1938.
78. Gutierrez, R., and Spjut, H.: Skeletal angiomatosis. Report of 3 cases and revies of the literature. Clin. Orthop., *85:*82, 1972.
79. Jacobs, J., and Kimmelstiel, P.: Cystic angiomatosis of the skeleton. J. Bone Joint Surg., *35A:*409, 1953.
80. Mirra, J.M., and Arnold, W.D.: Skeletal hemangiomatosis in association with hereditary hemorrhagic telangiectasia. J. Bone and Joint Surg., *55A:*850, 1973.
81. Moseley, J., and Starobin, S.G.: Cystic angiomatosis of bone. Manifestation of a hamartomatous disease entity. Am. J. Roentgenol. Radium Ther. Nucl. Med., *91:*1114, 1964.
82. Ritchie, G., and Zeier, F.: Hemangiomatosis of the skeleton and spleen. J. Bone Joint Surg., *33A:*115, 1956.
83. Spjut, H., and Lindobom, A.: Skeletal angiomatosis. Acta Pathol., *55:*49, 1962.

Primary Hemangiopericytoma

84. Dahlin, D.C.: Bone Tumors. pp. 100, 105. Springfield, Charles C Thomas, 1967.
85. Dunlop, J.: Primary hemangiopericytoma of bone. J. Bone Joint Surg., *55B:*854, 1973.
86. Gutierrez, J.R., Azar, H., and Bolivar, J.: Low grade hemangiopericytoma of the sacrum. *In* Regato, Juan (ed): Cancer Seminar, second series. vol. 7, Juan Regato, pp. 42–46, 1976.
87. Marcial-Rojas, R.A.: Primary hemangiopericytoma of bone. Cancer, *2:*308, 1960.
88. McCormack, L.J., and Gallivan, W.F.: Hemangiopericytoma. Cancer, *7:*595, 1954.
89. Sage, H., and Salman, O.: Malignant hemangiopericytoma in the area of a previous ameloblastoma of the mandible. Oral Surg., *26:*275, 1968.
90. Stout, A.P.: Tumors featuring pericytes; glomus tumor and hemangiopericytoma. Lab. Invest., *5:*217, 1956.

Hemangiosarcoma

91. Dorfman, H.D., Steiner, G.C., and Jaffe, H.L.: Vascular tumors of bone. J. Bone Joint Surg., *48A:*528, 1966.

PERIOSTEAL AND OSSEOUS SOFT-TISSUE TUMORS

14

INTRODUCTION

This chapter concerns the juxtacortical (periosteal and intracortical) tumorous lesions and true neoplasms. Also included are osseous-producing soft-tissue tumors, both benign and malignant, some of which can be associated with a periosteal component as well, such as in combined myositis ossificans and traumatic periostitis. The benign lesions of the juxtacortical region include the following: the osteochondroma (a developmental error), parosteal chondroma, traumatic periostitis, parosteal osteomatosis (very rare), and the parosteal fibroma (rare). The malignant juxtacortical lesions include the low-grade malignant parosteal osteosarcoma (Grades I and II), and the higher-grade malignant periosteal fibrosarcoma, chondrosarcoma, Grade III parosteal osteosarcoma, and the periosteal osteosarcoma.

The soft-tissue ossifying lesions that are compared and contrasted are myositis ossificans and the low- and high-grade soft-tissue osteosarcoma.

Avulsive or tearing injuries of ligaments and tendons or muscle insertions can lead to ominous radiologic and morphologic changes that can be mistaken for sarcoma. The author prefers to group these lesions as "avulsive ligamento-tendinitis ossificans." The entities that are included in this group include the so-called "cortical irregularity syndrome," Osgood-Schlatter disease (avulsion of the tibial tubercle), and others, some of which have syndrome names and others not. In essence these lesions are the dense, fibrous connective tissue injuries that are counterpart of myositis ossificans and traumatic periostitis. In fact, it is not uncommon in the injuries of musculotendinous ligamentous soft tissue and periosteum for more than one component to be involved in the process. This can lead to various confusing combinations such as myositis ossificans and traumatic periostitis, avulsive ligamentitis ossificans and traumatic periostitis with or without myositis ossificans, and others. This chapter stresses how these benign injury reparative pseudosarcomas can be separated from the parosteal or other soft-tissue sarcomas. If they are mistaken for sarcomas the outcome is, of course, disastrous to the patients. Similarly, mistaking a low-grade sarcoma for any of these entities usually results in multiple recurrence and eventual metastases because of inadequate treatment. These benign and malignant lesions may be virtually indistinguishable histologically, and clinical behavior such as recurrence and continuous growth may be crucial to proper interpretation.

THE OSTEOCHONDROMA, SOLITARY AND MULTIPLE

Capsule Summary (Fig. 14-1)

Incidence. Solitary and multiple osteochondromas represent approximately 11 per cent of biopsied primary bone tumors. Male to female incidence is 1.4 to 1.

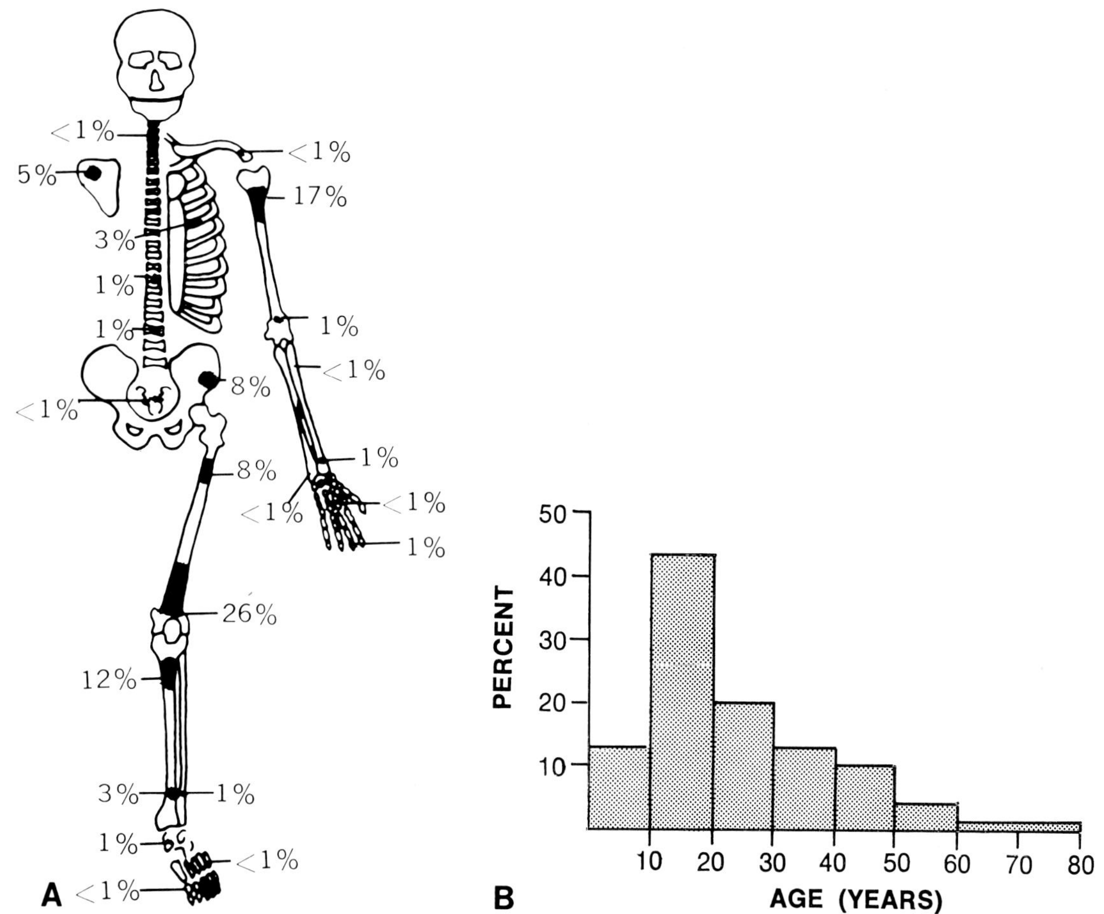

FIG. 14-1. (*A*) Solitary osteochondroma. Frequency of areas of involvement in 464 patients. Male:female incidence, 1.4:1. (*B*) Age distribution of patients with solitary osteochondroma. (Mirra, J., Bullough, P., and Freiberger, R.: Orthopedic Diseases, Part II. New York, Famous Teachings in Modern Medicine, MedCom, Inc., © 1972)

Age. Two to 10 years (12%), 11–30 (63%), 30–60 (22%).

Areas of Involvement. Femur (34%), humerus (18%), tibia (15%), pelvis (8%), scapula (5%), ribs (3%), rare in other bones.

Symptoms and Signs. Bony protuberances with or without pain.

Radiologic Features. Refer to discussion.

Gross Pathology. Cartilage-capped bony protuberance.

Histologic Features. Benign cartilage cap, spongy and cortical lamellar and/or woven bone.

Treatment. Local excision, if indicated.

Course. Benign, rarely, malignant chondrosarcomatous degeneration. Sudden increase in pain or size of the lesion may be due to fracture through the stalk, development of an extensive bursa in the soft tissues, nerve compression, degeneration of the cartilage cap with imbibition of water, or sarcomatous degeneration.

Definition. An osteochondroma is a benign, developmental growth defect in which experimental evidence strongly supports the contention that it is pathogenetically related to a focal herniation of the lateral component of the epiphyseal plate, resulting in the formation of an aberrant cartilage-capped eccentric "little bone."

Importance. May rarely undergo sarcomatous transformation. Must be distinguished from the much more rare rounded form of parosteal osteosarcoma.

Pathogenesis of the Osteochondroma

Benign cartilage-capped bony lesions of the lateral epiphyseal margins are referred to as *marginal osteophytes* and form as a consequence of degenerative joint disease. They are not at all related to the pathogenesis of the osteochondroma. However, because resected osteochondromas and marginal osteophytes may look histologically identical when removed from their site of origin, they have both been called exostoses. Because these two lesions occur in different areas of the bone and result from differing pathogenetic mechanisms, the term *exostosis* should perhaps be used for only the marginal osteophyte or marginal exostosis, and not the osteochondroma. This would avoid unnecessary confusion.

Virchow, in 1891, was the first to suggest that the osteochondroma may be related to epiphyseal cartilage that somehow separated from the parent tissue.[10] Müller, on the other hand, believed that osteochondromas form by cartilaginous metaplasia of the periosteum.[6] We now know that Virchow was correct. The lesion about which Müller hypothesized is the periosteal chondroma, whose features are clearly distinguishable from the osteochondroma (pg. 532 and Figs. 14-25–14-31).

Keith, in 1920, sought to explain the osteochondroma as resulting from a defect in the periosteal cuff of bone that normally surrounds the lower end (the vacuolating zone) of the epiphyseal plate cartilage during embryogenesis (Fig. 14-2).[4] Herniation of epiphyseal plate cartilage through this defect would presumably set up the circumstances that result in the gradual evolution of the osteochondroma. The larger the defect, the larger the osteochondroma. A single defect presumably would explain a solitary osteochondroma, and multiple defects in several or more bones would presumably explain the disease of hereditary multiple osteochondromatosis. Although this refinement of Virchow's hypothesis has not been proven, an elegant series of experiments by D'Ambrosia and Ferguson proves that osteochondromas can form from epiphyseal plate cartilage and that Keith's hypothesis may well explain how this cartilage ends up in an aberrant position.[1] In their experiment they transplanted small portions of rabbit epiphyseal plate cartilage under the periosteum (Fig. 14-3). After several weeks classic osteochondromas developed (Figs. 14-4, 14-5, and 14-6), provided that the following conditions were met:

1. The epiphyseal plate cartilage was placed in the metaphysis. If this was not done, the production of osteochondroma dropped precipitously and only small protuberances formed.
2. All zones of the plate were necessary to transplant in order to produce distinct osteochondromas. Smaller portions produced only small protuberances.
3. Articular cartilage did not work.
4. The epiphyseal plate had to face with the proliferating zone most distal to and parallel to the cortical surface. If the cartilage were rotated 180° or 270°, an osteochondroma did not form. These latter results also supported Virchow's theories, which assumed that the detached epiphyseal cartilage had to undergo a medial rotation of 90° for the osteochondroma to develop. This was in the exact position in which osteochondroma developed in the D'Ambrosia and Ferguson experiments.

Because the aberrant epiphyseal plate cartilage is under the same influences as its parent organ, it undergoes the same processes of growth, except that it is lateral to or grows out from the normal host bone. In a sense, the osteochondroma is nothing more than a small, aberrant, extraneous enchondral bone that forms from a herniation of epiphyseal plate cartilage. Since the osteochondroma is a slow-growing developmental anomaly, it is not difficult to understand

---

Pathogenesis of Osteochondroma

FIG. 14-2. The arrow points to the fine periosteal cuff of bone that surrounds the vacuolating zone of epiphyseal plate cartilage. Focal loss of this containing collar could theoretically result in a focal herniation of epiphyseal plate cartilage.

FIG. 14-3. Experimental production of osteochondroma by removal of a portion of epiphyseal plate cartilage of rabbits. (D'Ambrosia, R., and Ferguson, A.: Clin. Orthop., *61*:103, 1968)

FIG. 14-4. Radiographic demonstration of the osteochondroma (*arrow*) produced by placing the epiphyseal plate cartilage in a subperiosteal-metaphyseal position. In order for an osteochondroma to develop, the cartilage must be rotated 90° from its normal anatomic position. (D'Ambrosia, R., and Ferguson, A.: Clin. Orthop., *61*:103, 1968)

FIG. 14-5. Low-power histology of the osteochondroma (*arrow*) produced. (D'Ambrosia, R., and Ferguson, A.: Clin. Orthop., *61*:103, 1968)

FIG. 14-6. Typical microscopic features of an experimentally produced osteochondroma. (D'Ambrosia, R., and Ferguson, A.: Clin. Orthop., *61*:103, 1968)

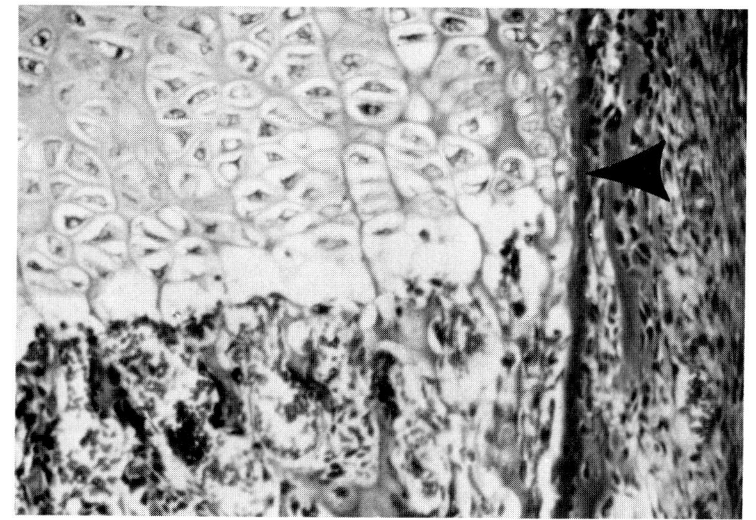

FIG. 14-2

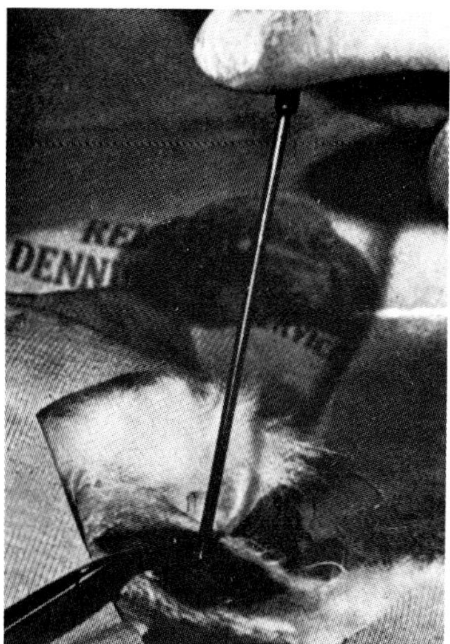

FIG. 14-3

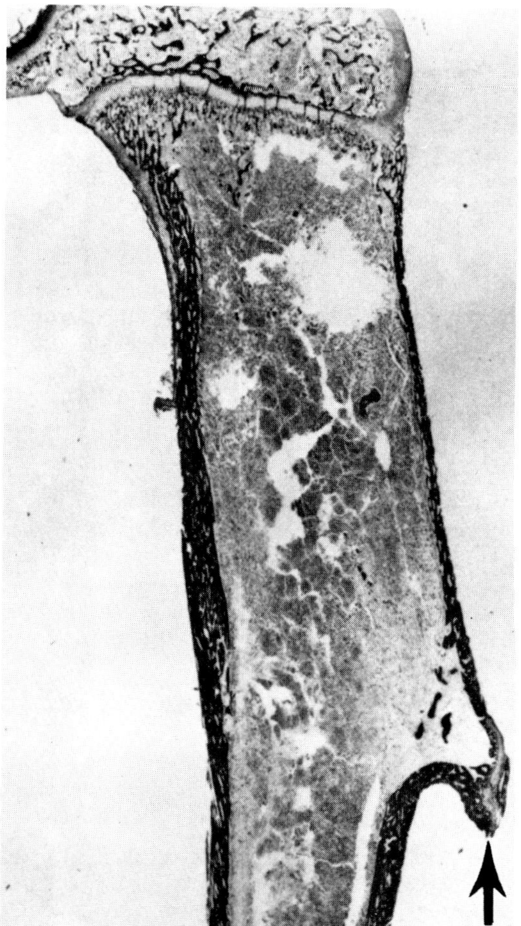

FIG. 14-5

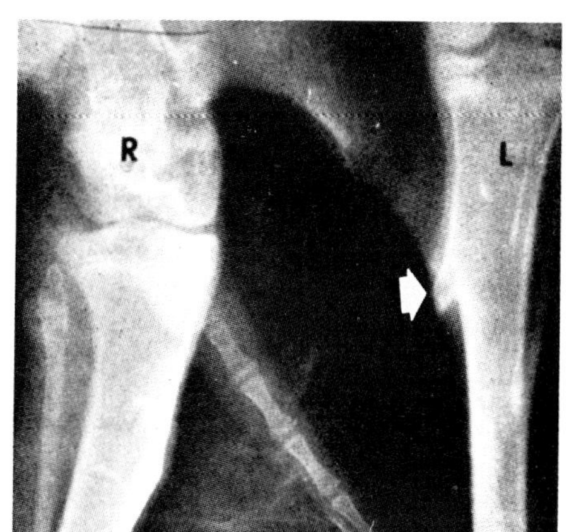

FIG. 14-4

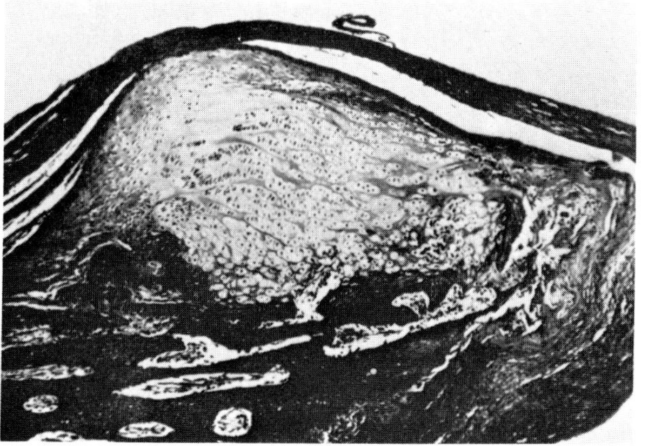

FIG. 14-6

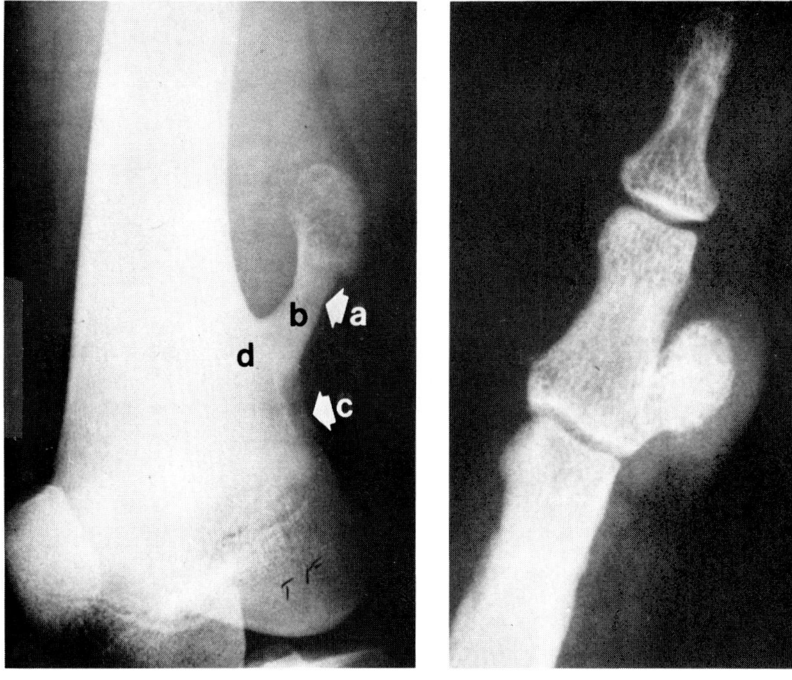

FIG. 14-7

FIG. 14-8

Osteochondroma

FIG. 14-7. Classic and pathognomonic radiologic features of an osteochondroma. The lesion points away from the joint. The cortex (*a*) and spongiosa (*b*) of the lesion blends imperceptibly with the bone cortex (*c*) and spongiosa (*d*) of the host bone.

FIG. 14-8. Although this figure shows an unequivocal osteochondroma, osteochondroma arising in relation to phalanges is unusual.

why it is first noted in childhood and why it stops growing at about the same time that the parent epiphysis closes. Significant growth of the lesion after plate closure usually signifies chondrosarcomatous change. Its pathogenesis also beautifully explains why the cortex and spongiosa of the osteochondroma blends imperceptibly with the cortex and spongiosa of the host bone; this gives the lesion a pathognomonic radiographic appearance. Any deviation from these pathognomonic features means that the lesion is not an osteochondroma. Examples of lesions that may be confused with osteochondroma if the pathogenesis and pathognomonic features are not clearly understood are given later in the section on differential diagnosis.

Pathognomonic Features of Osteochondroma

RADIOLOGIC FEATURES. The pathognomonic radiologic features of osteochondroma(s) are as follows:

1. The lesion protrudes from the host bone on a sessile or pedunculated bony stalk. It occurs either in the metaphysis or, as the parent epiphysis grow away from the lesion, in the diaphysis. *It is never found in the epiphyseal end of the bone.*
2. *The cortex and spongiosa of the osteochondroma blend imperceptibly with the cortex and spongiosa of the host bone* (Figs. 14-7, 14-8, 14-9, 14-10, and 14-12). This is its key radiologic feature. Any deviation should make the pathologist suspect either some other lesions or possibly malignant degeneration.
3. The outer surface is rounded (Figs. 14-7 and 14-8), bosselated (Fig. 14-11), or plateau-like (Fig. 14-9).
4. Size range is from 2 to 12 cm.

GROSS FEATURES. The distal end is composed of a complete cap of glistening, bluish translucent cartilage, provided that the patient's epiphysis has not

(*Text continues on p. 528.*)

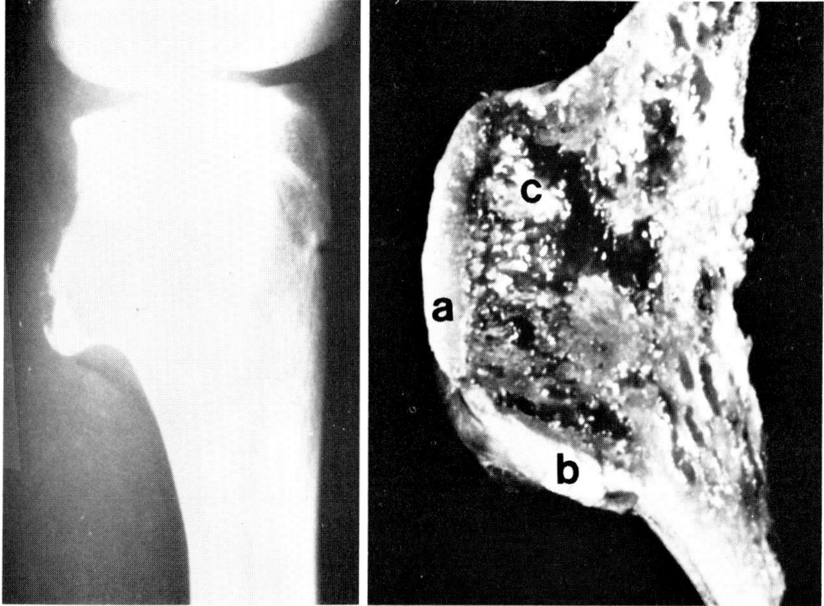

FIG. 14-9

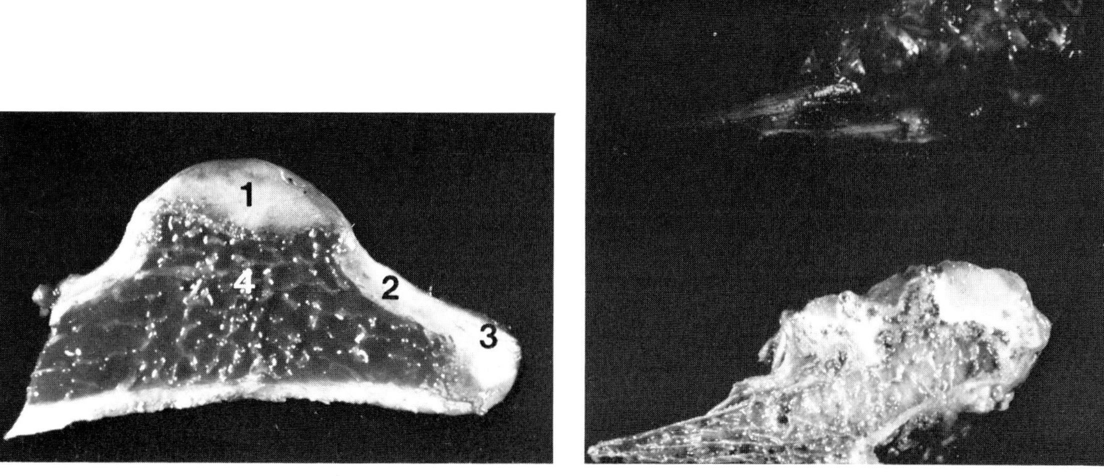

FIG. 14-10

FIG. 14-11

Osteochondroma

FIG. 14-9. *Left:* This osteochondroma has a sessile rather than pedunculated base. (*Right*) This lesion was removed and shows the typical gross features of an osteochondroma; namely, a bland cartilage cap (*a*), cortex (*b*), and spongiosa (*c*).

FIG. 14-10. Osteochondroma of the rib. Cartilage cap (*1*), cortex of osteochondroma (*2*), cortex of host bone (*3*), and imperceptible blending of the medulla of the osteochondroma with the host medullary bone at (*4*).

FIG. 14-11. *Top:* An example of an osteochondroma with a bosselated surface. *Bottom:* Portions of the cartilage cap are being replaced by bone, a sign that the patient's epiphyses have closed. Senescent osteochondromas, on rare occasion, may have the cartilage cap completely replaced by bone.

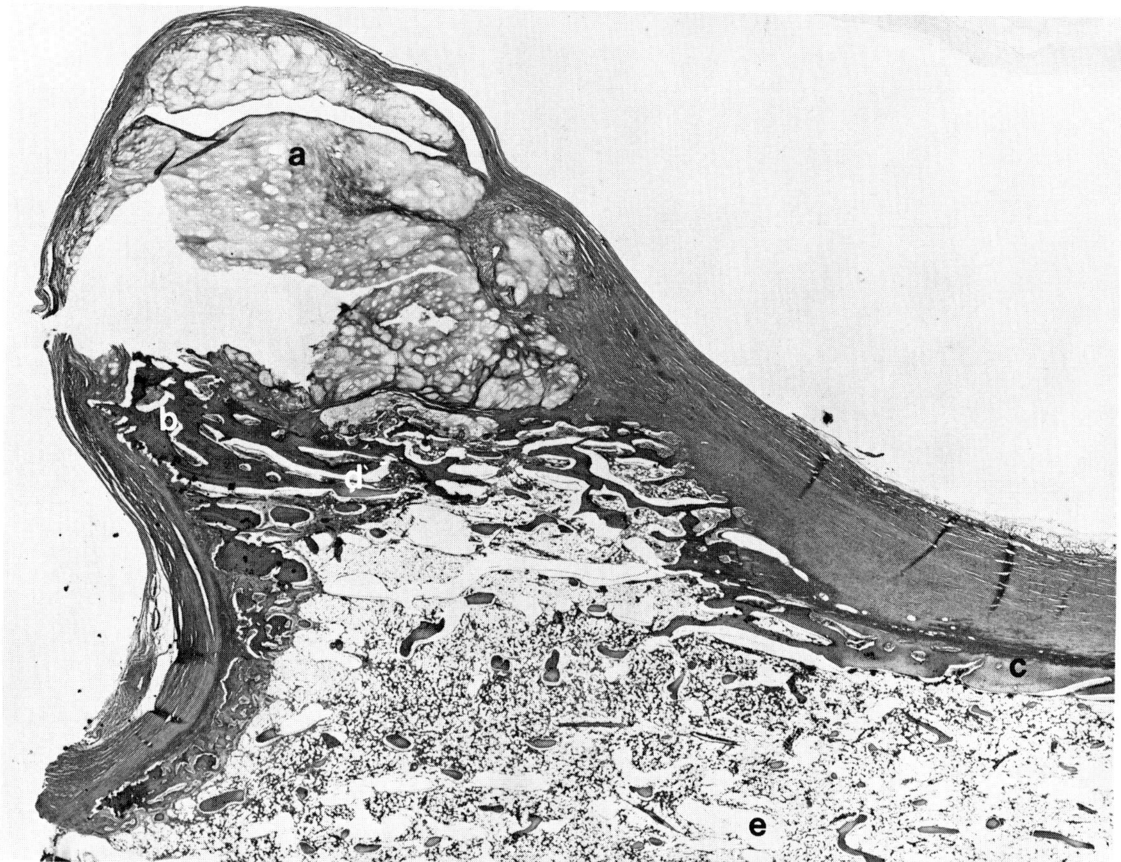

FIG. 14-12

Osteochondroma

FIG. 14-12. Typical low-power features. Cartilage cap (*a*), cortex of osteochondroma (*b*), cortex of host bone (*c*), spongiosa of osteochondroma (*d*), spongiosa of host bone (*e*) (x10). (Coulson, W.: Surgical Pathology. Philadelphia, J.B. Lippincott Company, 1978)

FIG. 14-13. This osteochondroma cap shows distinct endochondral ossification at its base (*1*). The host bone epiphysis would also be open and in its growth phase. (x40).

FIG. 14-14. In this example, the cartilage cap no longer shows endochondral ossification. The host bone epiphysis would also be closed, since the two are related pathogenetically (x60).

FIG. 14-15. The processes of endochondral ossification of the osteochondroma cap may not proceed normally, however. It is not uncommon for islands of poorly calcified cartilage to be trapped in the spongious portion of the lesion (*1*). Note the plates of bland lamellar bone (*2*) that surround these trapped intraosseous islands of cartilage, similar to that observed in benign enchondroma and parosteal chondroma (x125).

FIG. 14-16. Osteochondromatous lesions seen as wavy lytic undulations of both femoral metaphyses (*arrows*). These represent an incipient phase of cartilage growth before endochondral ossification has begun in a child with multiple osteochondromatosis.

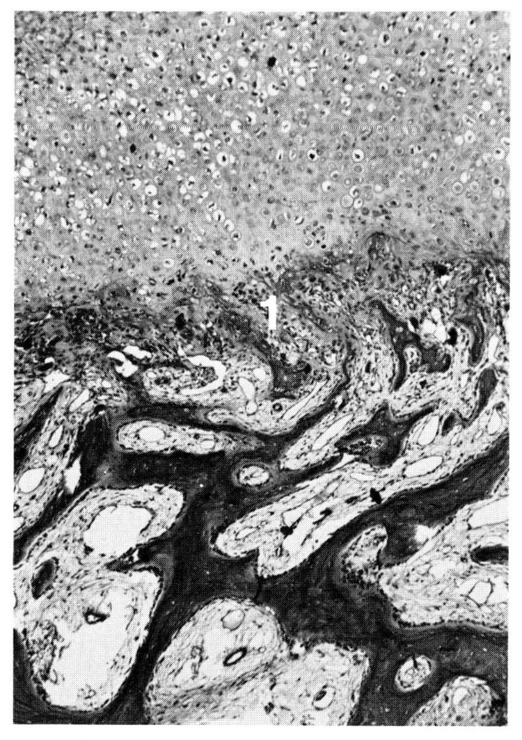

FIG. 14-13

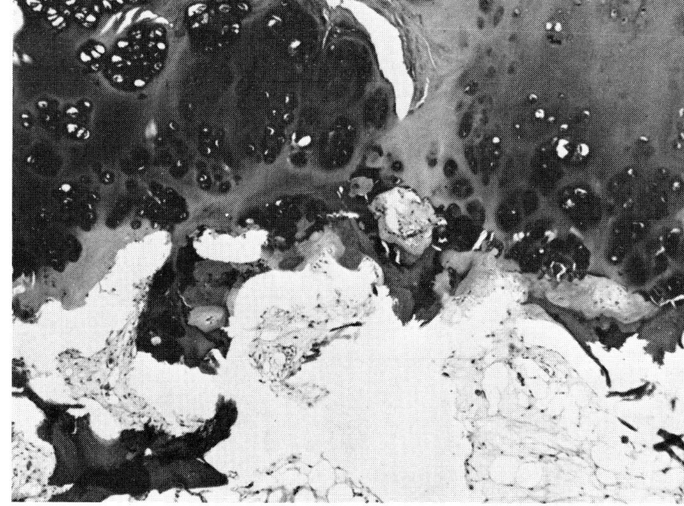

FIG. 14-14

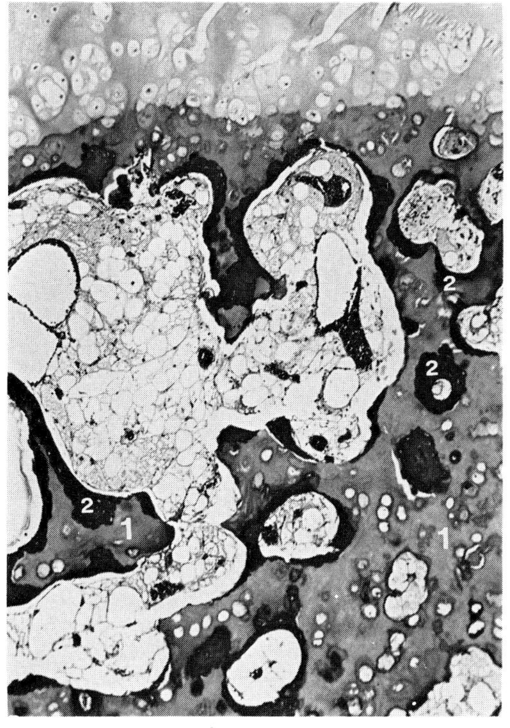

FIG. 14-15

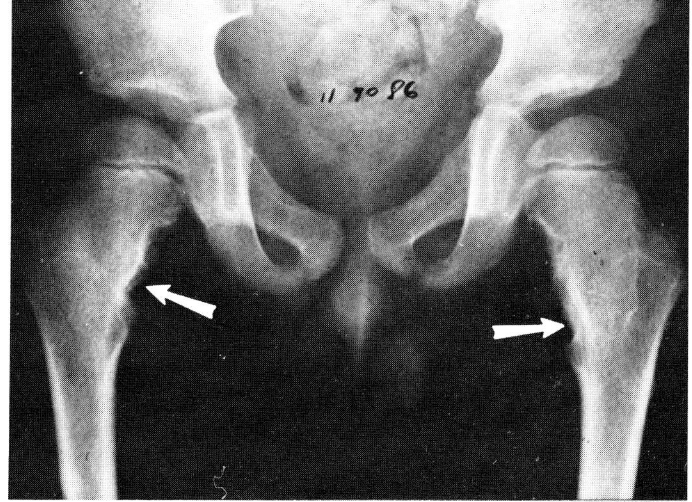

FIG. 14-16

closed (Figs. 14–9 and 14–10). When the epiphysis of the host bone fuses, the cartilage cap may eventually be partially or completely replaced by bony tissue (Fig. 14–11).

The bone of the osteochondroma is mature and blends imperceptibly with the cortex and spongiosa of the underlying host bone (Figs. 14–9 and 14–10).

HISTOLOGY. The cap is composed of bland hyalin cartilage. Variable degrees of cellularity are permissible but anaplasia is not. If the epiphyses are not closed, typical endochondral ossification with columnization and vacuolization of the chondrocytes is noted (Fig. 14–13). If the parent epiphysis is closed, no enchondral ossification is noted in the osteochondroma (Fig. 14–14).

Huge Solitary Osteochondroma Versus Chondrosarcomatous Degeneration

On occasion an osteochondroma may attain huge size (10–12 cm.) and yet still be benign (Figs. 14–18 and 14–19). What are the features that distinguish this ominous radiologic lesion from an osteochondroma with chondrosarcomatous transformation?

1. The benign lesion may be quite lobulated but radiographs and tomograms from different views should show smooth borders on all aspects (Figs. 14–18 and 14–19).
2. The base of the lesion should be smooth-bordered and blend imperceptibly with the host bone (Fig. 14–19). Fluffs of calcification with indistinct borders or soft-tissue swelling with obscuration of muscle planes is usually a sign of malignancy.
3. Rapid growth and pain after closure of the host bone epiphysis is usually a sign of malignant change.

Cartilage-Cap Infarction Resulting in Rapid Growth and Pain That Simulates Chondrosarcoma

This author has twice seen in consultation benign osteochondromas that were thought to have chondrosarcomatous degeneration because of rapid growth, pain, and thick cartilage caps. These two lesions were remarkable in that the cartilage was edematous and contained very large and swollen lacunae (Fig. 14–21). Close inspection revealed absence or degenerating ghosts of former chondrocyte nuclei (Fig. 14–21). In none of the sections was invasion of soft tissue or viable neoplastic cartilage noted. The underlying bone and marrow fat was, however, viable (Fig. 14–22). The diagnosis was infarction of the osteochondroma cartilage cap with cellular necrosis. As a result of focal hemorrhages and the cellular breakdown products, fluid was probably absorbed into the dead cartilage, which could well explain the lesion's rapid growth in size and consequent pain. The bone was alive so that its vascular supply was not interrupted. Cartilage normally receives its nutrition from synovial or bursal fluid. Infarction of cartilage would imply that there was significant compromise of the fluid that supply the cartilage cap through the aberrant fibrous bursal or capsulelike tissues that usually surround these protuberances and was not due to a fracture at the base of the lesion, which would have resulted in ischemic necrosis of the bone elements as well. Even with fracture of the base of an osteochondroma the cartilage would not be expected to undergo necrosis, because it receives its supply of nutrients from the bursal or synovial recess in which it is contained.

Osteochondroma

FIG. 14–17. Compared to the previous figure, this metaphyseal lesion shows bone formation that blends imperceptibly with the underlying host bone, clearly establishing it as an osteochondroma.

FIG. 14–18. An example of a very large, yet benign, osteochondroma. Note the smooth outer contours and the absence of poorly defined soft tissue calcifications along the periphery of the lesion or signs of an ominous, noncalcified, soft-tissue mass.

FIG. 14–19. Another example of a large, well-circumscribed osteochondroma. There is no radiographic evidence of malignant degeneration; the osteochondroma has sharp outer contours and does not have a soft-tissue mass.

FIG. 14–20. The presence of a soft tissue mass (*arrows*) is strong evidence in favor of malignant degeneration in a formerly benign osteochondroma (*a*).

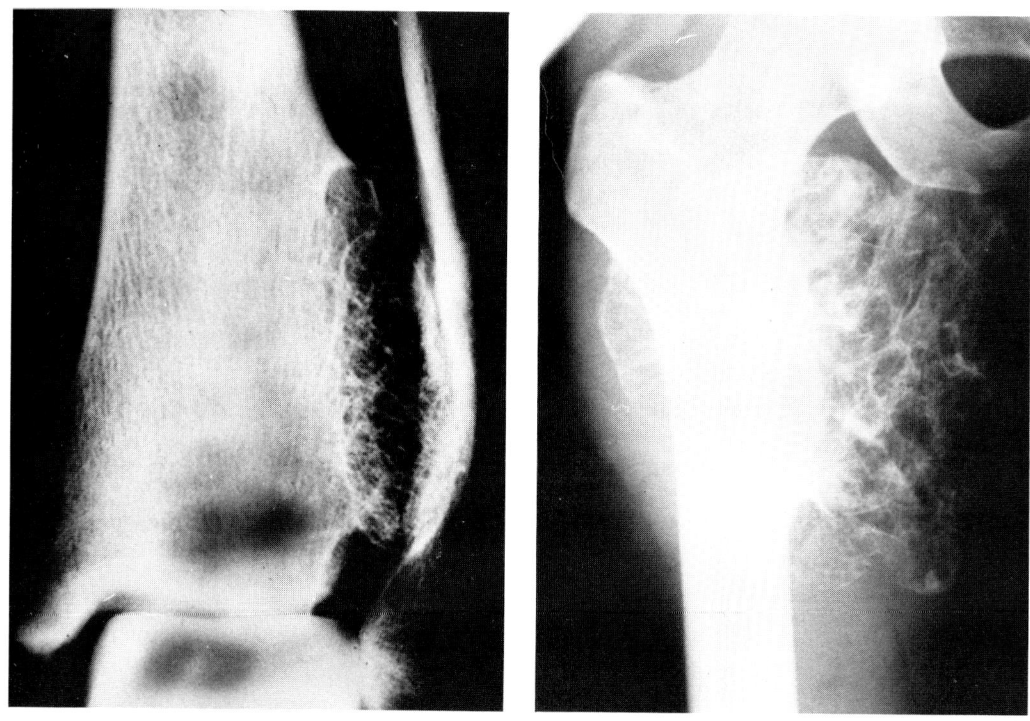

FIG. 14-17

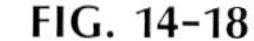

FIG. 14-18

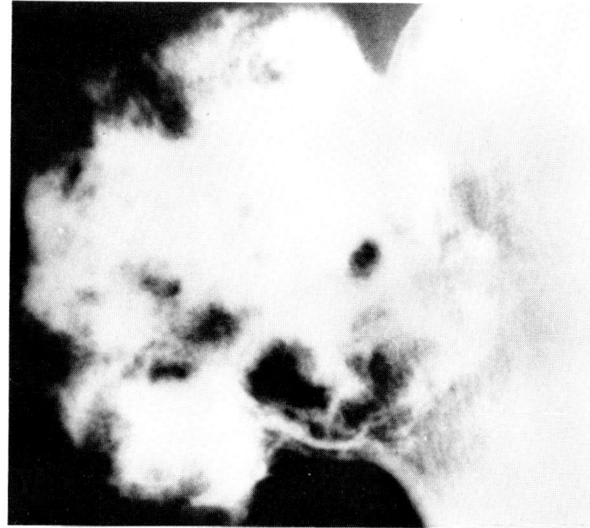

FIG. 14-19

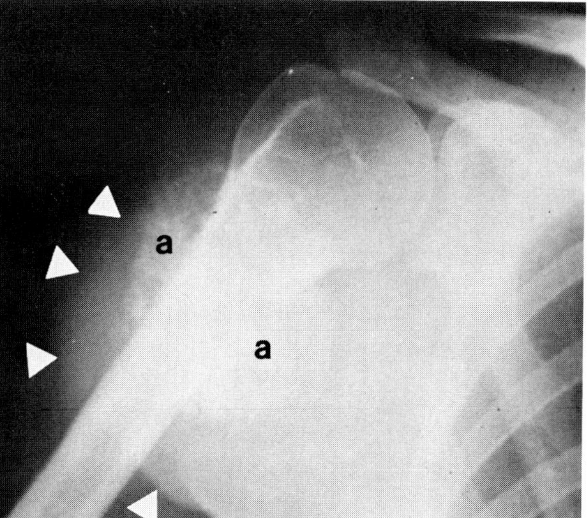

FIG. 14-20

Fracture of the Base of an Osteochondroma

Osteochondromas with thin stalks may on occasion undergo fracture. This would, of course, result in pain and fracture callus. This could then lead to ominous fluffs of ossification at the base, and pathologic analysis could lead to a mistaken diagnosis of osteogenic sarcoma arising in an osteochondroma if the diagnosis of stalk fracture is not made clear to the pathologist by the clinician. Tomograms should show a fracture line and histology would show osteoid, woven bone, and/or cartilage with varying degrees of atypia depending of course on the age of the callus. If the blood supply to the osteochondroma is compromised the bone and marrow fat will show evidence of ischemic necrosis. The cartilage cap should remain viable.

Chondrosarcomatous Degeneration of Osteochondroma

Chondrosarcomatous change in a solitary osteochondroma is a rare occurrence (around 1% or less). However, in patients with multiple osteochondromas the incidence naturally rises and is estimated by Jaffe to be in the range of 10 to 20 per cent.

The typical history of a patient with a solitary osteochondroma undergoing malignant change is that of an over 50-year-old patient who notices rapid growth and pain in a bony protuberance that had remained stable in size for many years. Patients with multiple osteochondromatosis may present 10 to 20 years earlier with this change. The radiograph will usually show an osteochondroma and an area of eccentric, fluffy, irregular density anywhere along the benign lesion but usually at its periphery. There may be soft-tissue swelling (Figs. 3–28, 14–20) and loss of overlying muscle planes. For most cases the area of malignant change is obvious on the gross and microscopic examination. In some cases, however, the focus of malignant change may be small and many sections must be taken if it is to be found. The chondrosarcoma will usually have invaded the soft tissues and its underlying bone and usually show signs of Grade II or III chondrosarcoma. If the lesion is Grade I, more reliance must be placed on radiographic and clinical features and evidence of invasion than by cytologic features alone, because some osteochondromas may be quite cellular and overlap those of Grade I chondrosarcoma. These difficult cases fortunately are very rare.

Differential Diagnosis of Osteochondroma

1. Chondrosarcoma arising in an osteochondroma.
2. Rounded form of parosteal osteogenic sarcoma (see Figs. 14–42, 14–43, and 14–44).
3. Juxtacortical chondroma (Figs. 14–25–14–31).
4. Ollier's disease with prominant periosteal component (Figs. 14–32, 14–33, and 14–34).
5. Myositis ossificans with cartilage cap ("traumatic osteochondroma"). In this entity the lesion does not blend imperceptibly with the cortex and spongiosa of the host bone, even though it may be attached to the periosteum. It basically results as a consequence to injury to the soft tissues and/or periosteum. The radiographic features are thus crucial to separating a long-standing, matured myositis ossificans from osteochondroma (Fig. 14–62), because the two lesions may otherwise appear identical by histology alone.

Osteochondroma

FIG. 14–21. Rapid swelling of an osteochondroma is usually a sign of malignant degeneration. However, it can be due to sudden infarction of the cartilage cap, with total loss of cartilage nuclei, as shown here (x125).

FIG. 14–22. Note the necrosis of the chondrocytes. The bone cells and osteoblasts are, however, still viable (*arrows*). This is because the cartilage receives its nutrients from synovial or bursal fluid while the bone receive its nutrients from blood vessels. Therefore, the necrosis of the cap must have been related to interference of synovial or bursal fluid bathing the cartilage rather than because of an interference with the vascular supply to the bony portion of the osteochondroma.

FIG. 14–23. An example of the multiplicity of lesions seen in a patient with multiple osteochondromatosis. The patient was an adult, which explains the lesion's diaphyseal position. Although the osteochondroma begins in the metaphyseal region immediately beneath or adjacent to the epiphyseal plate, the normal plate eventually grows away from the osteochondroma(s) as the patient matures.

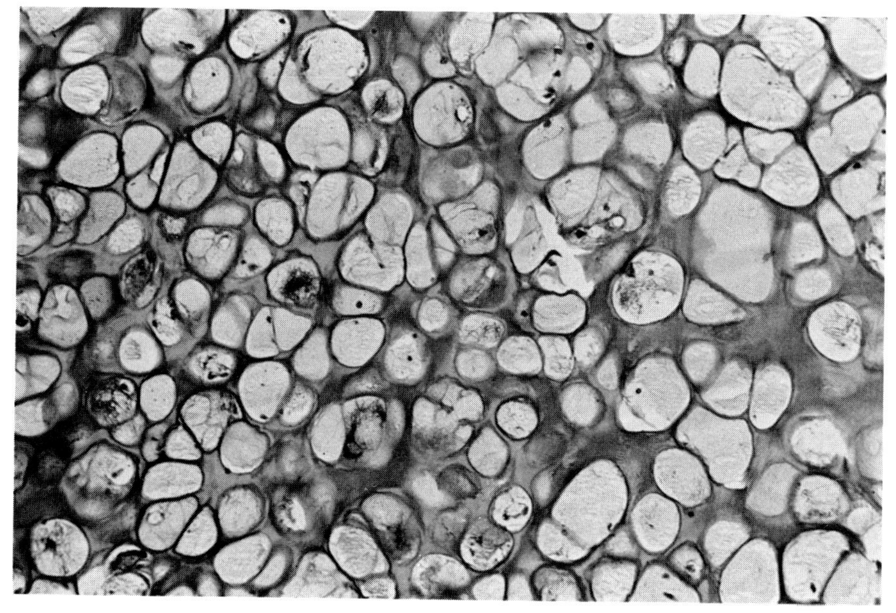

FIG. 14-21

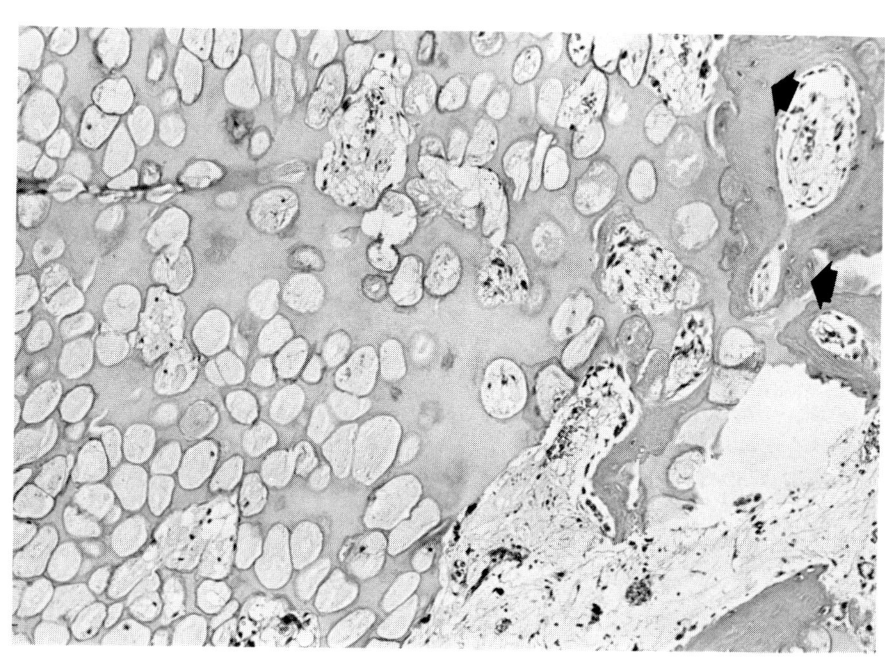

FIG. 14-22

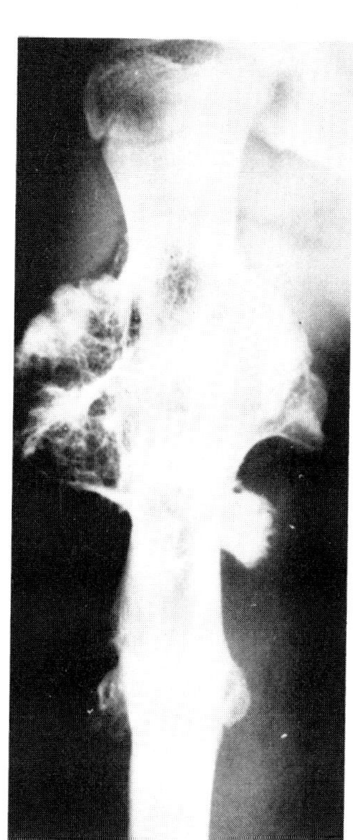

FIG. 14-23

MULTIPLE OSTEOCHONDROMAS (HEREDITARY MULTIPLE EXOSTOSES)

CAPSULE SUMMARY

Incidence. An uncommon dominantly inherited disorder.

Age. Patients usually present in childhood or young adolescence.

Clinical Features. Development of multiple protuberances at the ends of enchondrally formed bones; associated with some shortening and other bony abnormalities.

Radiologic Features. Juxtacortical bony growths that usually involve a greater circumference of the bone than do solitary lesions.

Pathology. Irregular, cartilage-capped protuberances.

Treatment. Local excision, if indicated. Radical surgery for chondrosarcomatous transformation.

Course. A number of patients with this condition may develop chondrosarcoma in one or more of these lesions (in the range of 10–20%).

Pathogenesis. Hereditary multiple exostoses is an autosomal, dominant-inherited condition characterized by multiple, cartilage-capped bony protuberances of enchondrally formed bones.

Signs and Symptoms. Signs and symptoms of this disease do not usually manifest themselves before the patient reaches the age of 2. The signs may be so striking that they will lead to the correct diagnosis by mere inspection. The most characteristic sign is multiple knobby, bony, hard, protuberances under the skin. Eventually these patients usually manifest shortening of the limbs, bony curvature, and other deformities. These deformities are directly related to the extent and severity of involvement of the affected bones. They may be due to dissipation of the longitudinal growth forces in the lateral direction at the metaphyses.

As the lesions enlarge, they may cause pain by pressure on neighboring tissue and nerves and may hinder normal joint mobility. Deformity of the forearm with ulnar deviation of the hand is seen in approximately 30 per cent of cases. If both the ulna and radius are involved by multiple osteochondromatosis, the ulna grows disproportionately less than the radius, thereby accounting for the ulnar deviation.

Radiologically, in contrast to solitary osteochondromas, these lesions generally involve a much larger portion of the metaphysis or shaft and are generally more irregular (Figs. 14–16 and 14–23). Eventually lesions that originated in the metaphyseal ends of the bones may be incorporated into the shaft (Fig. 14–23). Incipient osteochondromas are composed almost entirely of cartilage with little or no underlying bone formation, resulting in cortical irregularities on radiograph (Fig. 14–16). This radiographic picture can be confusing to those who have not had experience analyzing this appearance. In later stages affected bones show large, roundish, or cauliflower-like lesions and/or small, warty, pea-sized excrescences on the surface of the metaphysis and/or shaft. All of the lesions are cartilage-capped, and the cortex and spongiosa of the lesions blend with the involved bone at the affected sites as they do in solitary osteochondromas.

Microscopically the cartilage cap is seen to be composed of hyalin cartilage and may vary considerably in thickness. In the child, considerable growth activity is seen in the form of active enchondral ossification.

The cellularity of the cartilage is generally more pronounced than in solitary osteochondromas. This is true in larger lesions, where the nuclei may show greater degrees of atypism or dysplasia.

One may find nests of calcified cartilage in the spongiosa of the lesion, representing portions of the cap that have not been replaced by normal ossification (Fig. 14–15). The lobules of cartilage in the spongious portion of the bone may be partially to completely surrounded by plates of lamellar bone (a sign of benignancy in relation to cartilage-productive lesions) similar to that seen in enchondroma and parosteal chondroma. Removal of these lesions may be for cosmetic purposes or to alleviate local pain.

Jaffe has stated that in approximately 10 to 20 per cent of these patients, one or more of these lesions undergo chondrosarcomatous change.[3] Where feasible, radical resection above the level of the tumor is indicated. In sites such as the pelvis, thorough eradication may not be feasible, and the surgeon may have to be content with resection. Irradiation does not significantly alter the course.

PAROSTEAL CHONDROMA

CAPSULE SUMMARY (FIG. 14–24)

Definition. A rare to uncommon benign cartilagenous tumor that arises from the periosteum.

Age. 75 per cent of patients are younger than 30 years old at presentation.

Sites of Involvement. Most lesions are located in the hands, feet, humerus, tibia, and femur. Males rarely have hand involvement.

Importance. Because of its high degree of cellularity in some cases, the lesion may resemble a Grade I chondrosarcoma. It must be distinguished from the very rare true periosteal chondrosarcoma (Figs. 14–35 and 14–36), Ollier's disease with a predominant periosteal component (Figs. 14–32, 14–33, and 14–34) and cartilage-containing

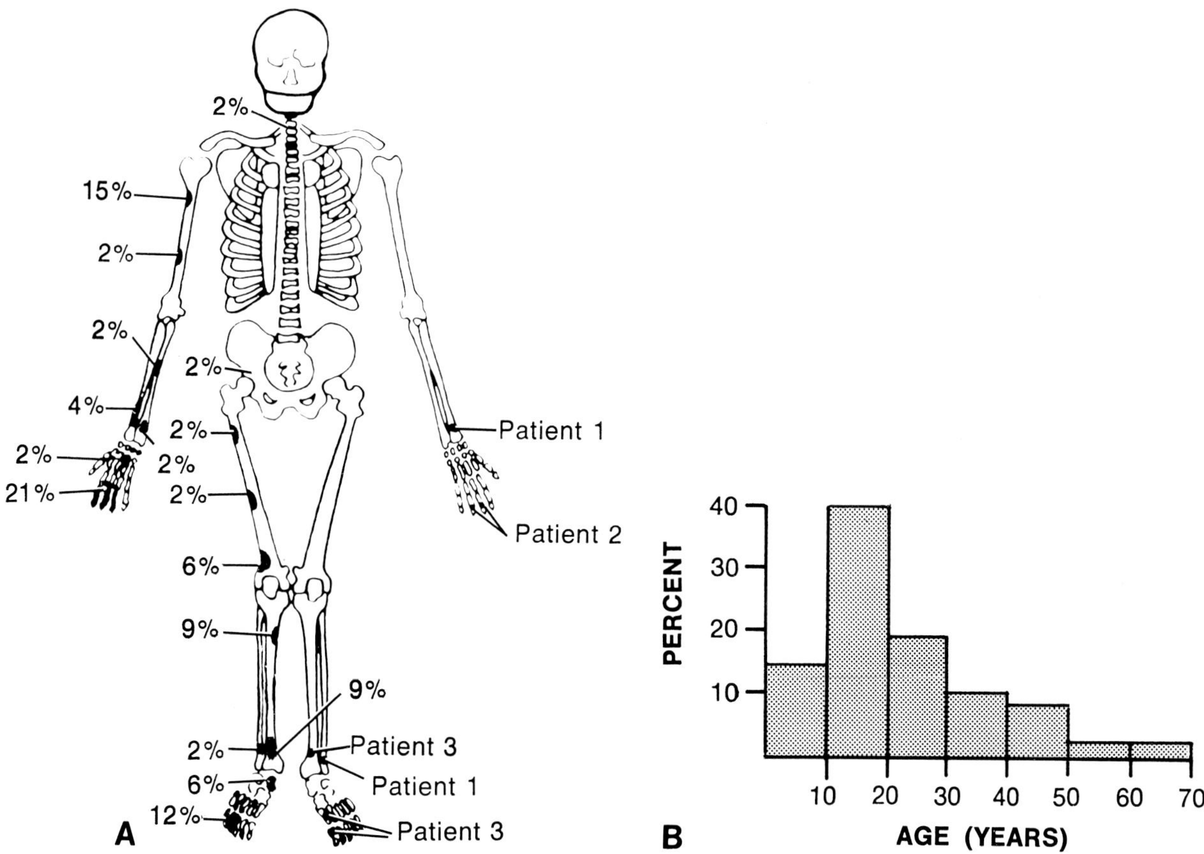

FIG. 14-24. (*A*) Parosteal Chondroma. Frequency of involvement in 55 patients with parosteal chondroma (*left*) and in 3 patients with multiple parosteal chondromatosis. Male: female incidence, 1.2:1. (*B*) Age distribution of patients with parosteal chondroma. (Mirra, J., Bullough, P., and Freiberger, R.: Orthopedic Diseases, Part II. New York, Famous Teachings in Modern Medicine, MedCom, Inc., © 1972)

reparative processes such as the cortical irregularity syndrome (Figs. 14-74–14-77). It is benign but may rarely undergo sarcomatous transformation.

Diagnostic Radiologic, Gross, and Histopathologic Features

Radiologic Features

1. The lesion may range in size from a few millimeters to as much as 8 to 10 cm. (Figs. 14-25 and 14-26).
2. It is eccentrically located and may jut into the soft tissues (Figs. 14-25 and 14-26), burrow into the cortical and subcortical osseous tissues, or both (Figs. 14-25 and 14-26).
3. Its main feature of benignancy, which is of extreme importance in distinguishing it from a low-grade chondrosarcoma in which histology may be identical, is the presence of sclerotic border about its edges (Figs. 14-25, 14-26, 14-27, and 14-28). This is a sign of "encapsulation" of the tumor or containment by the host bone seen in very slow growing, usually benign tumors.
4. In most cases if the lesion extends into the soft tissue, the periosteal borders are lifted and ossified but run smoothly into the adjacent normal cortex. Small densifications can be seen in the soft tissues but are generally rounded and innocent-looking (Fig. 14-25, *B*). If the lesion has a more ominous periosteal reaction such as fluffs or sunburst-type reaction and is purely cartilagenous in nature histologically, then parosteal chondroma is not the most likely diagnosis. More probable diagnoses are either a chondrosarcoma, periosteal or parosteal osteosarcoma,

or an early reparative traumatic lesion such as is seen in traumatic periostitis or the cortical irregularity syndrome. Extra care must be given to performing adequate en-bloc excision in those cases in which the distinction between malignant or early pseudosarcomatous reparative lesions is not clear.

Gross Pathology

The parosteal chondroma is composed of lobules of cartilage that arise from the periosteum and may be found eccentrically within the medulla of the bone surrounded by a rim of dense sclerotic host bone. Rarely does the parosteal chondroma extend deeper than one-third of the width of a long bone.

Histopathology

If the lesion is en-blocked, the lesion will be seen to involve the periosteum and either jut from the surface or erode through the cortex into a variable portion of the medulla (Fig. 14–27). The interior edge of the lesion is often walled off by host reactive lamellar bone that in some instances may even resemble a new cortex (Figs. 14-27 and 14-28).

On low-power examination this lesion is usually composed of distinct lobules of cartilage that blend imperceptibly into the periosteum (Fig. 14–29).

The size of the nuclei (7–12 microns) and cellularity (Fig. 14–31) may overlap with that of Grade I chondrosarcoma. The distinct lobularity; the placement of chondrocytes into well-defined lacunae (Fig. 14–30) or those evenly disposed (Fig. 14–31); the border of host bone sclerosis; the absence of invasion between fat septae, mitoses, and frank anaplasia are all features that support the diagnosis of parosteal chondroma. The presence or absence of double nuclei serve no useful purpose in distinguishing this lesion from a chondrosarcoma.

DIFFERENTIAL DIAGNOSIS

OSTEOCHONDROMA. The cortex and medulla of the lesion blend imperceptibly with the host bone and is easily distinguished from parosteal chondroma (Figs. 14–7, 14–8, 14–9, and 14–12). The very earliest stages of osteochondroma can be confused with parosteal chondroma (Fig. 14–16), however, these lesions will usually be multiple and eventually develop the typical radiologic features of osteochondroma (Fig. 14–17). The parosteal chondroma is very rarely multiple.

OLLIER'S DISEASE. Ollier's disease can affect any part of the mesenchyme of the bone periosteum, medulla, articular cartilage, and epiphyseal plate (See Figs. 8–59, 14–32, 14–33, and 14–34). If the lesions are predominantly periosteal, confusion with multiple parosteal chondromas is possible. The key feature is finding enchondromatons tissues deep within the medullary cavity of more than one bone (Figs. 8–59, 14–32, 14–33, and 14–34).

PAROSTEAL CHONDROSARCOMA (FIG. 14–35). These are vary rare tumors. Parosteal chondromas outnumber their malignant counterparts at least 8 to 1. The parosteal chondrosarcoma is usually larger than 5 cm., usually shows frank anaplasia (large nuclei over 12 microns with an open chromatic pattern), large nucleoli, and mitoses (Fig. 14–36), and may show frank invasion of soft tissues and invade between marrow fat septae. The lesion on radiograph does not show a border of host bone sclerosis, although not all parosteal chondromas do either. Certainly if this radiologic feature is present, it is much more likely to be benign.

TREATMENT AND WORKUP OF SPECIMEN

The procedure of choice is an adequate en-bloc excision. By adequate it is meant the removal of all of

---

Parosteal Chondroma

FIG. 14–25. The variable radiographic appearances of a parosteal chondroma are represented in these three illustrations. Note that all are eccentric lesions; the main clue to their periosteal origin. (*A*) Eccentric rounded lytic tumor with a dense border of benign host bone sclerosis (*arrow*). (*B*) Periosteal chondroma jutting into the soft tissue (*arrow*). Note the nodular calcifications, a common accompaniment to cartilage tumors. (*C*) A very large, ominous, lytic, obviously periosteal tumor. This lesion is so large and irregular in appearance that it could easily be confused with a malignant lesion by radiographic analysis alone. Biopsy and local excision demonstrated an ordinary parosteal chondroma, however. Follow-up has been uneventful.

FIG. 14–26. Another example of a large periosteal chondroma. There is considerable reactive host bone sclerosis containing the tumor. The relatively smooth outlines are more in keeping with its benign nature than the last example shown.

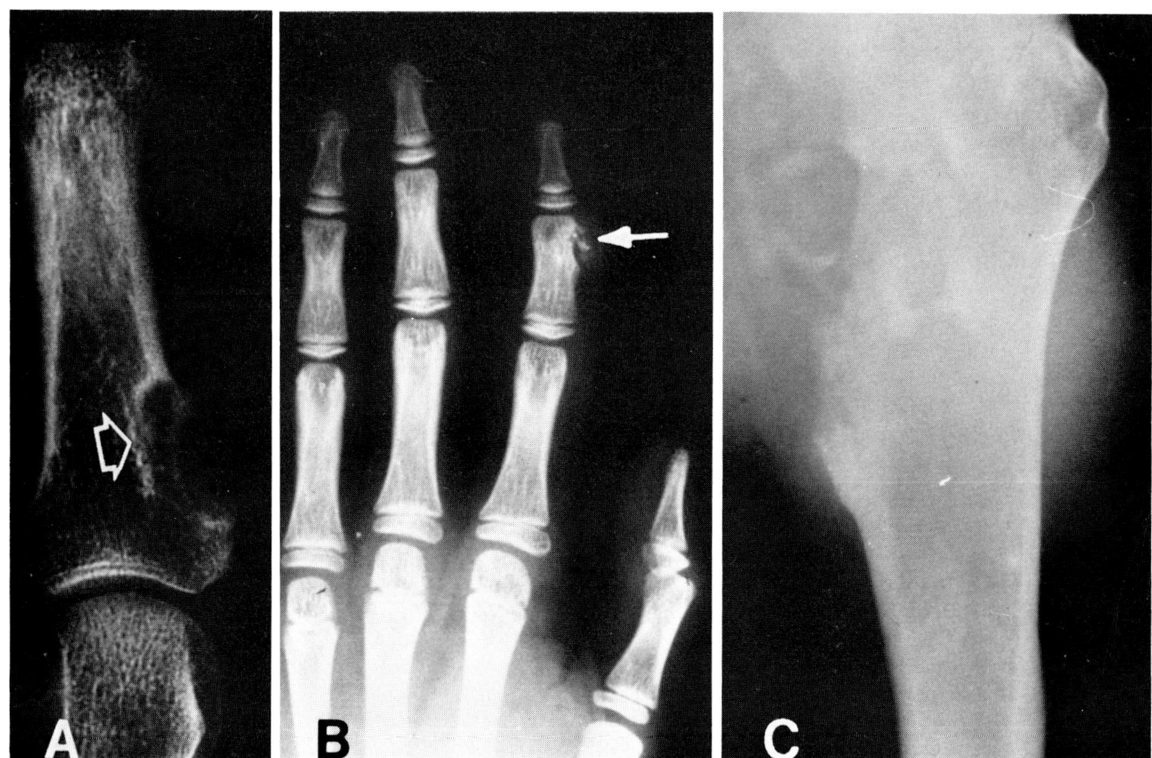

FIG. 14-25

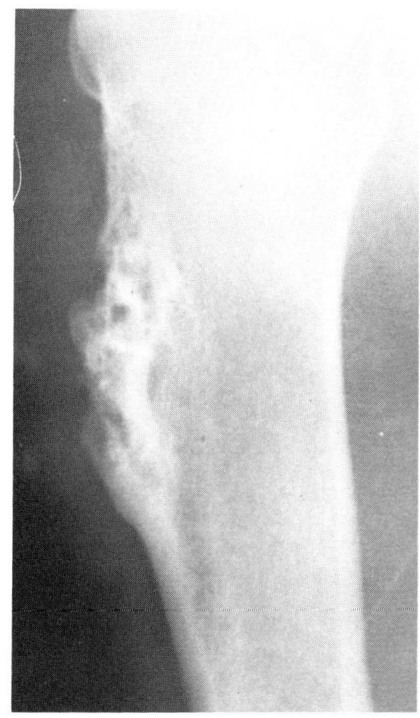

FIG. 14-26

the lesional cartilage, since the tumor has been reported to recur and to undergo malignant transformation on occasion, as does the enchondroma (Dr. Lent Johnson, personal communication). Since the cartilage may be found in the sclerotic border and may be present for several millimeters beyond what is obvious on radiograph, the lesion should be removed with knowledge of these facts taken into consideration. Perhaps 1 to 2 cm. of the periosteum should also be stripped and removed in the areas surrounding the en-bloc excision in an attempt to ensure that there are no cartilage rests left behind. This extra insurance against recurrence should not seriously hamper bone repair. A large cortical window can, of course, result in pathologic fracture but these are problems the orthopaedic surgeon is well aware of and he will most assuredly employ those techniques that will best reduce the chances of the occurrence of this mishap.

If the periosteal tumor strays from the classic range of periosteal chondroma, such as having ominous fluffs or spiculations of periosteal new bone and a faint to absent sclerotic border, it is even more important that the surgeon perform an "adequate" en-bloc excision and make all attempts not to seed possibly malignant tissue into the wound. But he must also take care not to seriously impair function until the benignancy or malignancy of the lesion is firmly established.

PERIOSTEAL CHONDROSARCOMA

The periosteal chondrosarcoma is an extremely rare tumor. The lesions are generally quite large and have ominous fluffy to windblown calcification, but smaller, more innocent forms are possible (Fig. 14–35). There is no border of host bone sclerosis. The diagnosis depends most upon finding Grade II to III anaplasia (Fig. 14–36). This consists of foci of round nuclei larger than 12 microns, with distinct open chromatin network, nucleoli, and even mitoses. If the lesion is removed en-bloc, it is possible to see soft-tissue invasion beyond the periosteum and occasionally, invasion between the host marrow septae. Grade I periosteal chondrosarcomas might be impossible to distinguish from the perosteal chondroma. Recurrence of any "parosteal chondroma" should be considered an ominous sign and the lesion treated, perhaps, as a low-grade neoplasm and a generous en-bloc resection or cryosurgery applied.

JUXTACORTICAL OSTEOSARCOMA (PAROSTEAL AND PERIOSTEAL TYPES)

Capsule Summary

Incidence. 0.6 per cent of primary bone tumors. Male to female incidence, 1 to 2.5.

Age. 10–20 (12%), 20–50 (80%).

Areas of Involvement. Distal femur and proximal tibia (72%), proximal and distal humerus (14%), proximal femur and distal tibia (9%), rare in other long bone sites.

Clinical Features. Swelling, slow growth, no history of significant trauma.

Radiologic Features. Juxtacortical ossifying mass, no medullary involvement, continuous growth.

Gross Pathology. Lobulated, bony mass attached to cortex.

Histopathology. Parosteal type: well-formed osseous trabeculae, usually minimal anaplasia of stroma with the appearance of a well-differentiated fibrosarcoma. Some cases may show moderate to severe anaplasia. Periosteal type: similar in appearance to an intramedullary type osteosarcoma.

Treatment. Refer to discussion.

Course. Will recur if not completely excised. Metastasizes late. Five-year survival rate, approximately 95 per cent, 10-year rate, 90 per cent, for the usual, well-differentiated tumor. Grade III tumors appear to be associated with poor 5-year survival statistics.

Definition. The ordinary parosteal osteosarcoma is a low-grade malignant tumor that arises in the periosteum of long bones and is characterized by trabeculae of woven and possibly fine lamellar bone and a fibrous stroma likened to low-grade fibrosarcoma. Cartilage may also be produced. The less common Grade III variant is a highly malignant neoplasm.

Importance. The parosteal osteogenic sarcoma, unlike intramedullary osteogenic sarcoma, is most often neoplasm of low-grade malignancy. It grows slowly, recurs if not

---

Parosteal Chondroma

FIG. 14–27. Low-power view of a complete intact parosteal chondroma of a rib. Chondroma (*1*), reactive endosteal bone forming a new cortex replete with haversian systems (*2*). On radiograph this lower border (*2*) would appear as a dense benign sclerotic line not dissimilar to that seen in Figure 14–25, *A* (*arrow*) (x5).

FIG. 14–28. High-power view of above case. Note the formation of the new subchondral cortical bone (*2*) containing the chondroma (*1*). The opposite uninvolved cortex is also seen (*3*) (x40).

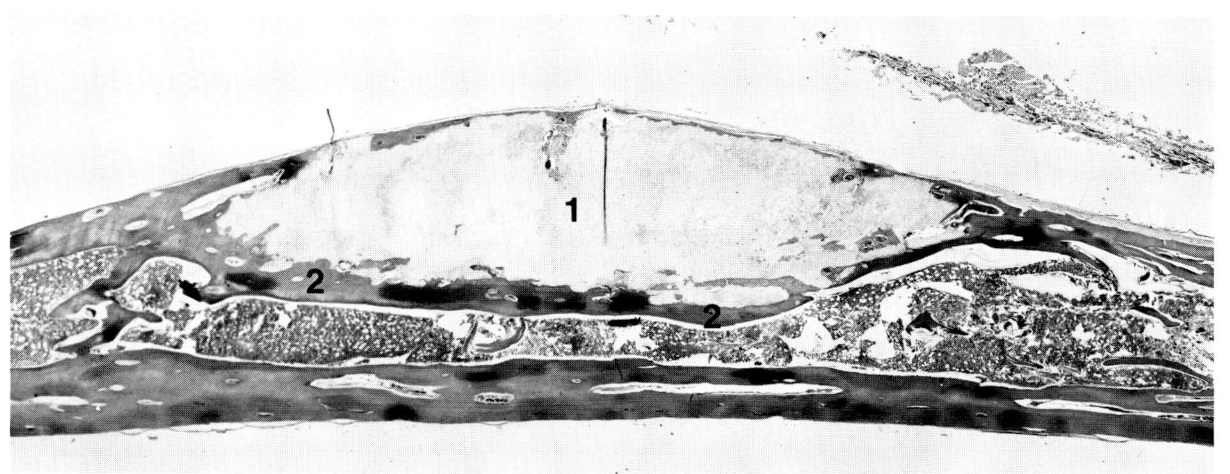

FIG. 14-27

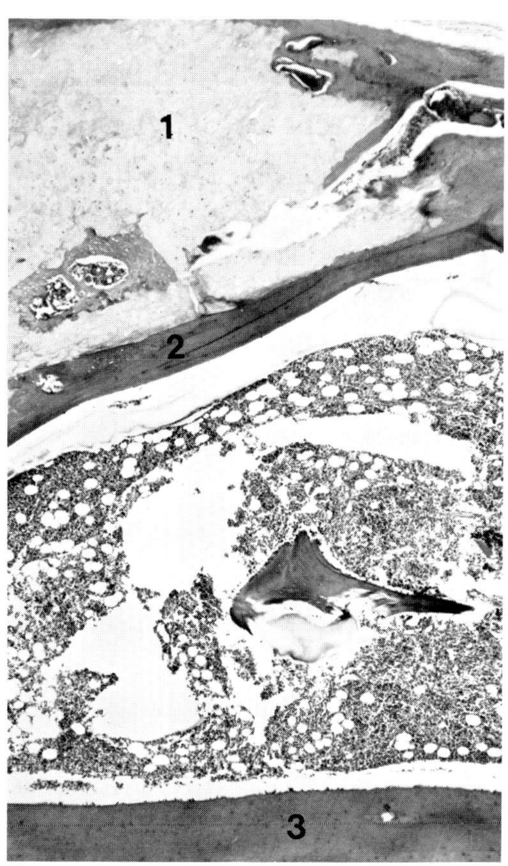

FIG. 14-28

completely excised, and attains a more malignant appearance with each recurrence. Metastases, if they occur, do so only after many years. Even then, the metastases of parosteal osteogenic sarcoma do not portend the same dismal course as those of intramedullary osteogenic sarcoma, unless it is a Grade III tumor. Survival and cure should perhaps be measured in intervals of 10 to 15 years or longer, since a number of patients have manifested metastasis 10 years or more after tissue diagnosis.

On occasion the tumor may attain a rounded appearance and can superficially resemble an osteochondroma by radiograph. It must always be distinguished from benign traumatic periostitis.

The periosteal OS is a recently described type with characteristic radiologic and histologic features.[42] Even though it may demonstrate significant anaplasia, the course is generally quite good provided that it is completely extirpated and shows no evidence of intramedullary involvement.

Characteristic Radiologic, Gross, and Microscopic Features

The characteristic but not necessarily pathognomonic radiologic features of a *parosteal osteosarcoma* are listed below (Figs. 14–38 and 14–39).

1. An irregular, fluffy, densely calcified mass attached to the periosteal surface, extending away from the cortex on a sessile base.
2. The mass is denser near the cortex than at the periphery (Fig. 14–38).
3. A fine radiolucent line on either side of the growing tumor may be seen separating tumor bone from the cortex. This line represents a thickened periosteal cuff lying between bone cortex and the tumor (Fig. 14–39, *A*). This is not a pathognomonic sign, because it may also be seen in traumatic periostitis (Fig. 14–62).

The characteristic, if not pathognomonic, specimen radiologic features of the low-grade parosteal osteosarcoma is very fine lamellae of bone ("steel wool" appearance), which takes origin from a juxtacortical position (Fig. 14–43). The author has seen this pattern in no other tumor, not even benign traumatic periostitis. This very fine steel wool pattern corresponds histologically to very long, thin, fine lamellar to woven tumor bone trabeculae (Figs. 14-44 and 14-45). Unfortunately, this pattern usually cannot be appreciated by standard radiographic analysis. The less well differentiated higher Grade II to III tumors show a much fluffier or irregular pattern of ossification.

The characteristic gross features are listed below (Figs. 14–39 and 14–40).

1. A whitish mass streaked with yellowish flecks of bone can be capped with translucent cartilage arising from the periosteum or cortex.
2. Extension into the bone medulla is often not present (Figs. 14–39 and 14–40) or minimal (Fig. 14–42). In rare cases invasion of the shaft may be extensive, making the differentiation from an intramedullary osteosarcoma that broke out of the bone a complex and sometimes an impossible task.

The characteristic microscopic features of the usual grade I variety include:

1. Long, flowing traeculae of predominantly woven bone separated by a fibrous stroma (Fig. 14–44). Some trabeculae may show a fine lamellar pattern by polarized light (Fig. 14–45). In some areas islands of osteoid and woven bone form primarily by a fibro-osseous metaplasia, similar to fibrous dysplasia. Plump osteoblast rimming is usually inconspicuous.
2. On high power the stroma contains cells with

Parosteal Chondroma

FIG. 14–29. On low-power examination, the parosteal chondroma is usually distinctly lobular. The fibrous perichondrium is seen to the left. The parosteal chondroma is basically formed consequent to intraperiosteal chondromatous metaplasia (x40).

FIG. 14–30. The nuclei of the parosteal chondroma can be moderately enlarged. Purely intraosseous cartilage lesions of the long bones with this degree of enlargement and cellularity are quite often low-grade chondrosarcomas. Note, however, that despite their enlarged nuclei, the cells are disposed in regular nests, an infrequent finding in all but the most extremely well-differentiated chondrosarcomas (x125).

FIG. 14–31. A very cellular example of a parosteal chondroma with small, innocent nuclei. Periosteal cartilage lesions should not be diagnosed as malignant unless there is frank anaplasia of chondrocytes or definite soft-tissue invasion. (x125)

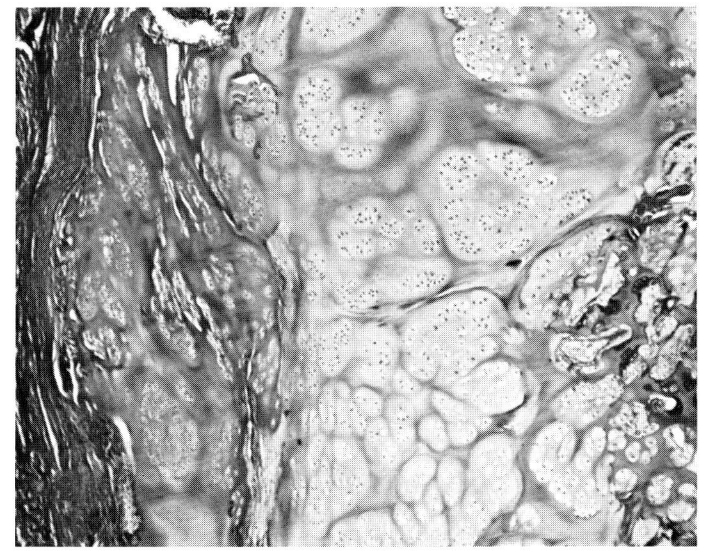

FIG. 14-29

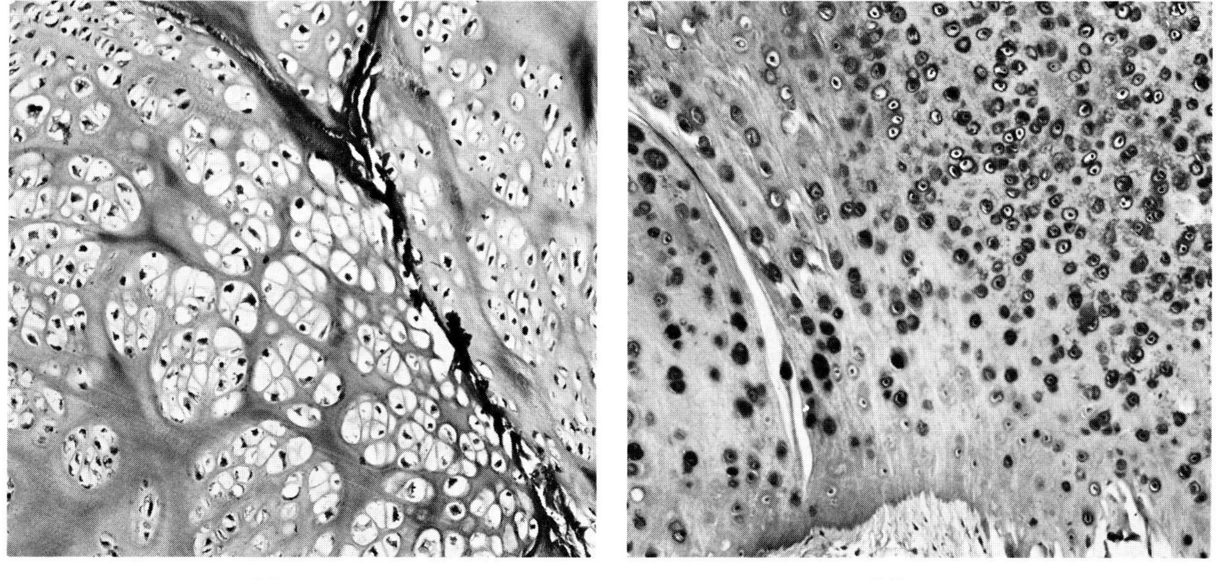

FIG. 14-30

FIG. 14-31

slightly plump nuclei (Figs. 14–46 and 14–47) and occasional mitotic figures. The appearances of this stroma have been likened to a Grade I fibrosarcoma.

3. Islands of cellular hyalin cartilage are not uncommonly present. The cartilage is usually not clearly malignant. The features are usually borderline between those which would be seen in an atypically cellular enchondroma versus a well-differentiated (Grade I) chondrosarcoma. Occasionally, the chondrosarcomatous cartilage rims the periphery of the neoplasm. This feature must not be confused with the cartilage cap of an osteochondroma. The differentiation depends on the demonstration of a fibrosarcoma-like stroma and woven to primitive lamellar bone production. The stroma of an osteochondroma is bland marrow fat and usually mature lamellar bone.
4. *Maturation to completely mature lamellar bone and distinct marrow fat is not seen.*
5. Uniform appearance throughout the lesion.

The morphologic uniformity of most parosteal osteosarcomas is in striking contrast to the much more aggressive and rapidly lethal intramedullary type of osteosarcoma or the Grade III variant of parosteal osteosarcoma. These latter osteosarcomas show much greater variation in the type of osteoid, woven bone, and cytologic characteristics from field to field (see Plates 4, B, C, F, G, K; 5C, F, G, H). Cartilage, if present, is usually clearly chondrosarcomatous.

The only lesion that can simulate the low-grade malignant parosteal osteosarcoma with exactitude both radiologically and microscopically is an early "ripening" traumatic periostitis or myositis ossificans associated with traumatic periostitis. The distinguishing features of these benign, mimicking entities will be discussed in the next section.

Ahujia, *et al.*,[34] have reported that grading of the parosteal osteosarcoma correlates well to prognosis. They describe three grades. Of 27 patients, eight had Grade I tumors, ten, Grade II tumors, and six, Grade III. Grade I tumors are defined as those in which the fibrous stroma is composed of cells with minimal anaplasia and occasional mitoses. The fibrous stroma tends to be heavily collagenized. The trabecular bone is well organized and has mostly a lamellar or woven pattern with occasional rimming of osteoblasts. Grade II tumors have a more fibrocellular stroma with plumper nuclei (Fig. 14–48), moderate anaplasia, and more than occasional to rare mitoses. The bone is usually of the pure woven type and could be rimmed by osteoblasts. Although osteoblastic rimming is rarely, if ever, seen in ordinary intramedullary osteosarcomas, it can be seen in parosteal osteosarcomas. Therefore, this feature cannot be used to assess benignancy or malignancy when dealing with periosteal tumors.

Grade III parosteal osteosarcomas behave with full

Ollier's Disease Mimicking Multiple Parosteal Chondromas

FIG. 14–32. Note the periosteal lesions (*arrows*), which mimic parosteal chondromas of multiple bones.

FIG. 14–33. Because of a mistaken diagnosis of chondrosarcoma in the above patient, the toes were amputated. They showed, in addition to periosteal cartilage, intraosseous cartilage islands (*arrows*).

FIG. 14–34. The above patient also had a fairly large intraosseous cartilage tumor of the distal tibia. The full extent of the lesion is outlined by arrows, although a more prominent focus of lysis is seen at *1*. Thorough review of this patient's outside slides and radiographs led me to the conclusion that this patient simply had Ollier's disease with a prominent periosteal component. This disease can affect any portion of the bone in variable proportion, including articular cartilage, epiphyseal plate, periosteum, or host medullary bone (see Fig. 8–59). The clinical course of this patient has been benign despite simple curettage of the tibial lesion. This case points out the fact that in any patient with multiple "periosteal" chondromatous lesions, the entity of Ollier's disease must be strongly considered. Special precautions should be taken not to confuse this entity with multiple periosteal chondroma or with periosteal chondrosarcoma.

Periosteal Chondrosarcoma

FIG. 14–35. Note the relatively small, fluffy periosteal tumor. The boxlike hole seen in this figure is secondary to a biopsy of the lesion and cortex. There is nothing diagnostic about this radiograph.

FIG. 14–36. Biopsy of the above lesion showed a pure cartilage tumor with unequivocal malignant nuclei. Many of the nuclei are greater than 13 microns in size, with a distinct open chromatin network, abundant double nuclei, and even mitoses (*arrows*). The tumor was not seen to involve the medulla. Therefore, this lesion qualifies as a periosteal chondrosarcoma (x300).

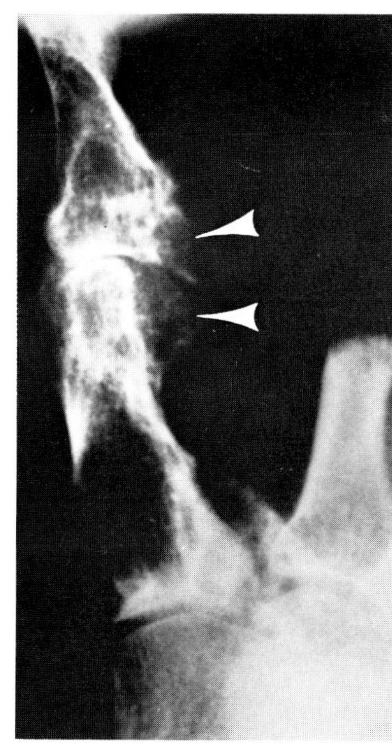

FIG. 14-32

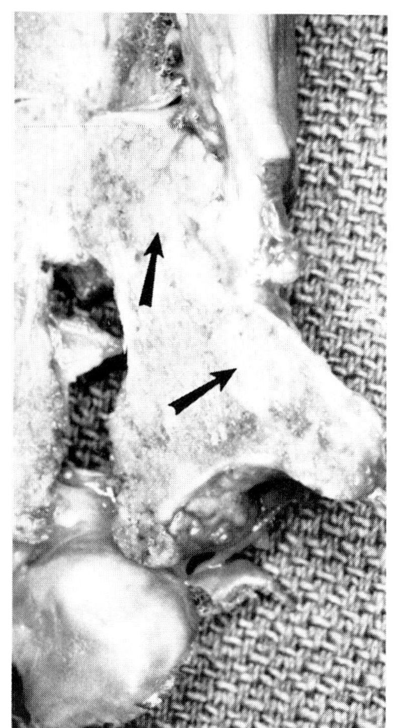

FIG. 14-33

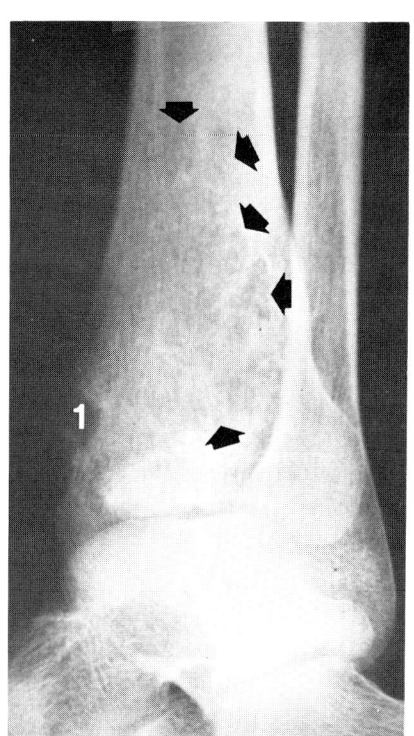

FIG. 14-34

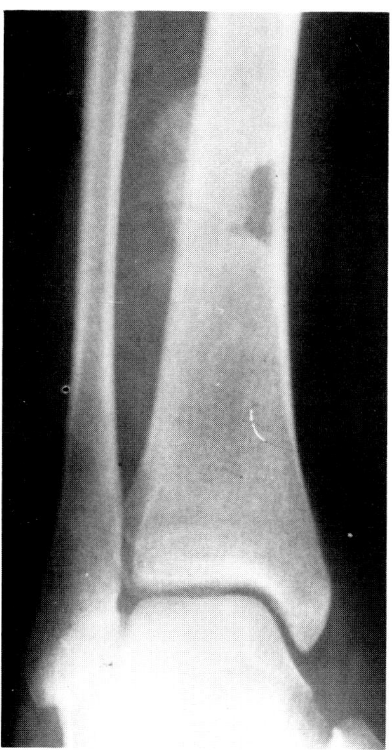

FIG. 14-35

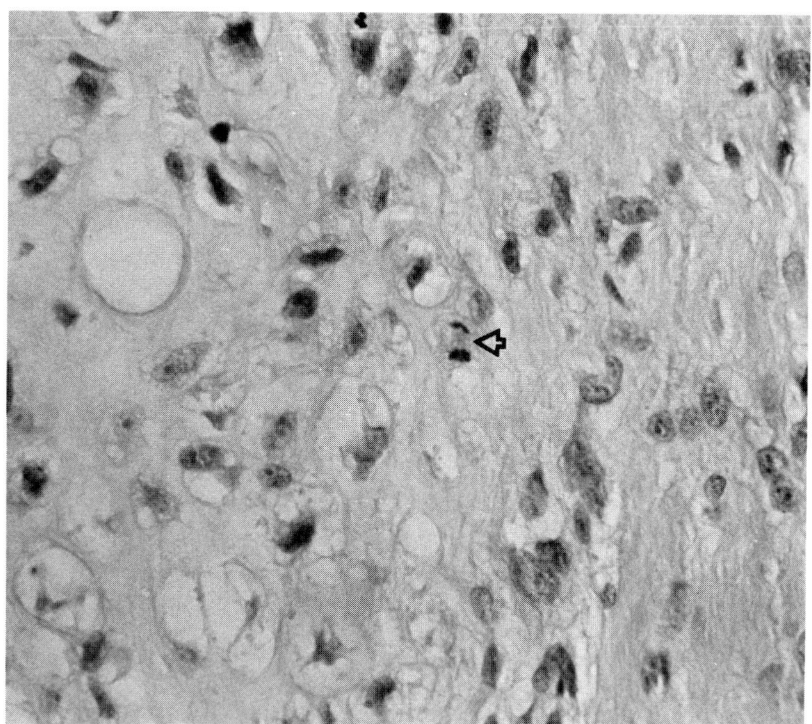

FIG. 14-36

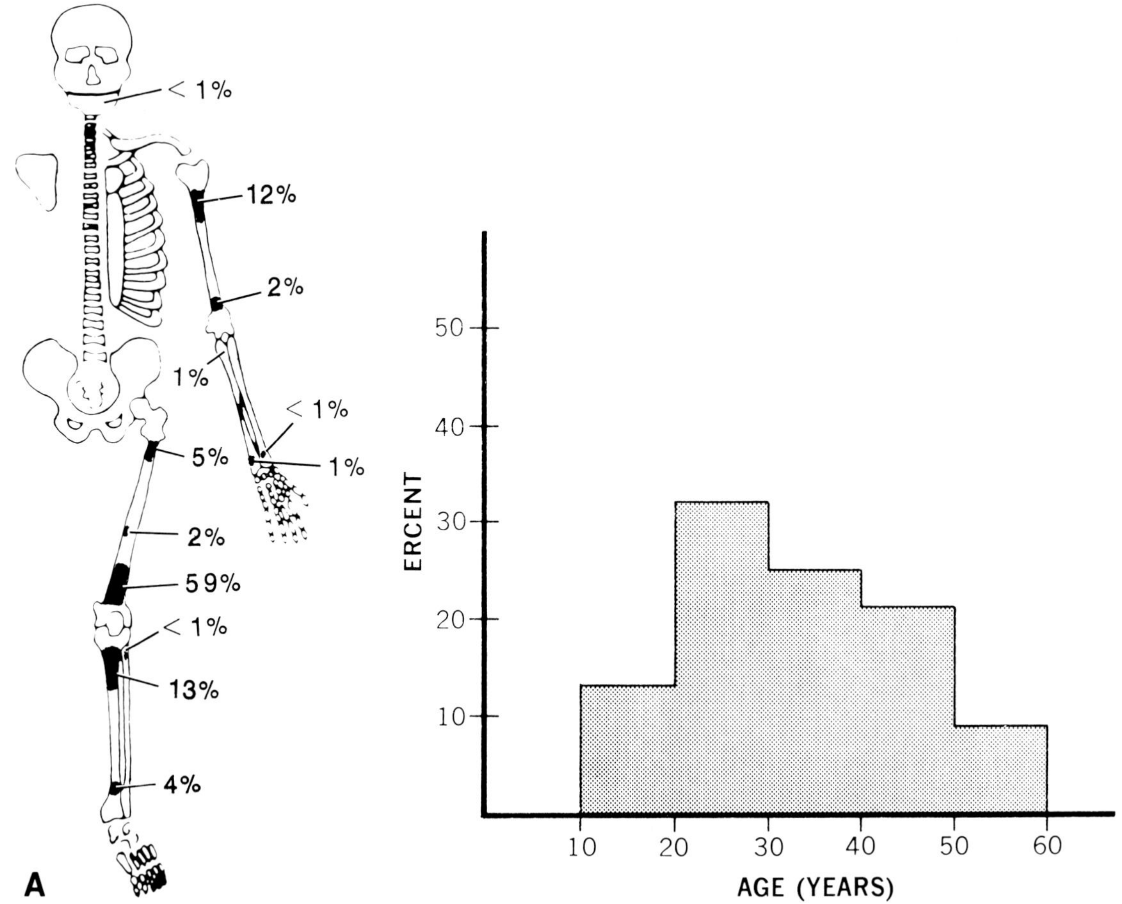

FIG. 14-37. (*A*) Juxtacortical osteogenic sarcoma. Frequency of areas of involvement in 164 patients. Male: female incidence, 1:1.5. (*B*) Age distribution of patients with juxtacortical osteogenic sarcoma. (Mirra, J., Bullough, P., and Freiberger, R.: Orthopedic Diseases, Part I: Bone Tumors. New York, Famous Teachings in Modern Medicine, MedCom, Inc., © 1971)

virulence and in essence, could not be distinguished from ordinary intramedullary osteosarcomas by histology alone. The fibrous, osseous, and even cartilagenous components were graded individually in these studies and the overall grade assigned to the tumor is the highest grade assigned to any one component. Generally, however, most tumors have similar grading for each component.

Unni, *et al.*,[43] have reported what is called the *"periosteal osteosarcoma."* From a series of juxtacortical osteosarcomas, they deemed 79 juxtacortical or parosteal tumors as ordinary and 23 as "periosteal." The periosteal osteosarcoma showed high-grade anaplasia. If there was any involvement of the medullary portion of the bone at all, the designation of periosteal osteosarcoma was dropped and the lesion defined as an intramedullary osteosarcoma with periosteal involvement. The radiographic features of the lesion are perhaps the most specific feature of this newly described entity. The tumor was always located superficially in the bone cortex. There was densification of part of the tumor mass and, on occasion, radiating spicules of bone perpendicular to the long axis of the bone. The overall appearance was "saucer shaped," usually with Codman's triangles at the edges of the lesion. They most frequently involve the external shaft of the tibia. Almost all cases look alike and are quite distinctive radiologic lesions. Dr. Dahlin is studying whether or not lesions with the overall configuration of periosteal osteosarcoma, but with some marrow in infiltration, have survival statistics different from those without marrow infiltration (personal communication). However, whether the tumor was a so-called parosteal or "periosteal" osteosarcoma, the overall survival was generally favorable for both.

Periosteal tumors without evidence of intramedullary involvement have overall better prognosis than their medullary counterpart, no matter what histologic grade (Dahlin, personal communication). Perhaps this is related to the different or less dangerous vascular supply of a pure periosteal tumor. As was stated above, in Ahujia's series those Grade III tumors with medullary involvement did lead to metastases and death. But other patients in their series also succumbed to metastases even though medullary involvement was not described. In fact, five of six of their patients with Grade III tumors died of their tumor. Therefore the important thing to remember is that apparently high-grade osseous sarcomas of the periosteum exist, and that if there is intramedullary extension (which could be an intramedullary tumor extending to periosteum), the prognosis is poor and the tumor should be treated more radically than Grade I to possibly Grade II parosteal osteosarcomas or the newly described periosteal osteosarcoma.

In order to grade the parosteal osteosarcoma, the pathologist should compare the illustrations of Grade I to II parosteal osteosarcoma (Figs. 14–46, 14–47, and 14–48) to those given for the ordinary intramedullary osteosarcoma (See Plate 4, inclusive). The differences are substantial: a low-grade parosteal osteosarcoma has quite distinctive low- and high-power histologic characteristics, compared to the intramedullary osteosarcoma, which has basically identical histological characteristics to the so-called Grade III parosteal osteosarcoma.

Less Common, Possibly Confusing Radiologic Appearances of Parosteal Osteosarcoma

Location Around the Affected Bone

On occasion the parosteal osteosarcoma may completely encircle the bone (Fig. 14–40). In such instances it may be impossible by ordinary radiologic analysis to determine whether the lesion in question is truly periosteal in origin or if it is an intramedullary tumor that has broken through the cortex at multiple sites. The reason this may be difficult is that the density of the tumor may obscure the medulla. However, before biopsy is obtained, high, penetrating tomograms or computerized axial tomography (CAT) would be of great benefit to determine whether there is medullary involvement. If a lucent line is seen in the center of the lesion, the most obvious cause of the periosteal new bone is stress fracture (see Fig. 7–16). If the osseous network of the medulla is involved in the absence of a central fracture line, the usual cause is a primary intramedullary malignant bone tumor that has broken out of the bone or an unusual, almost fully healed stress fracture. If the medullary bone appears intact, a parosteal or periosteal osteosarcoma is the probable diagnosis. Traumatic periostitis is almost always consequent to a severe trauma, and the new bone formation may be extensive but is almost always eccentric and does not wrap entirely around the bone. This benign lesion should not invade the medullary bone, although on very rare occasion an associated myositis ossificans component may erode into the bone as a rounded mass (Fig. 14–66, *B*) (personal observations).

Appearance as a Spherical Mass

Approximately one in ten parosteal osteosarcoma present as a spherical or rounded lesion of the metaphysis (Figs. 14–41, 14–42, and 14–43), which can result in an erroneous radiologic diagnosis of osteochondroma. The differential radiologic features are presented in Figures 14–7 and 14–42 and Table 14–1. Microscopically, the two are easily distinguishable: an osteochondroma is composed of benign hyalin cartilage capping woven to mature lamellar bone and marrow fat and though a parosteal osteosarcoma may contain a cap of cartilage, the subchondral tissues are woven to fine lamellar bone type, and most, importantly the stroma is fibrosarcoma-like and not fatty marrow. An osteochondroma never contains fibrosarcoma-like intertrabecular tissue, unless, of course, it has undergone fibrosarcomatous degeneration, which is very rare. There are only one or two such reported cases.

Course

The Grade I parosteal OS has excellent 5- to 10-year survival statistics (90–95%). The main threat is inadequate extirpation of the tumor, which results in increasing chances of more malignant transformation and increased metastatic potential with each recurrence. Of the 10 Grade II tumors of Ahujia, *et. al.*,[34] three were associated with metastases. Two of these patients are now dead of this disease. Of the six

(*Text continues on p. 548.*)

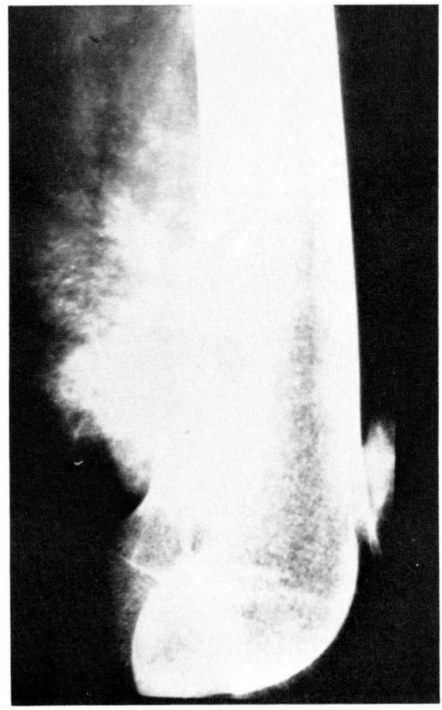

FIG. 14-38

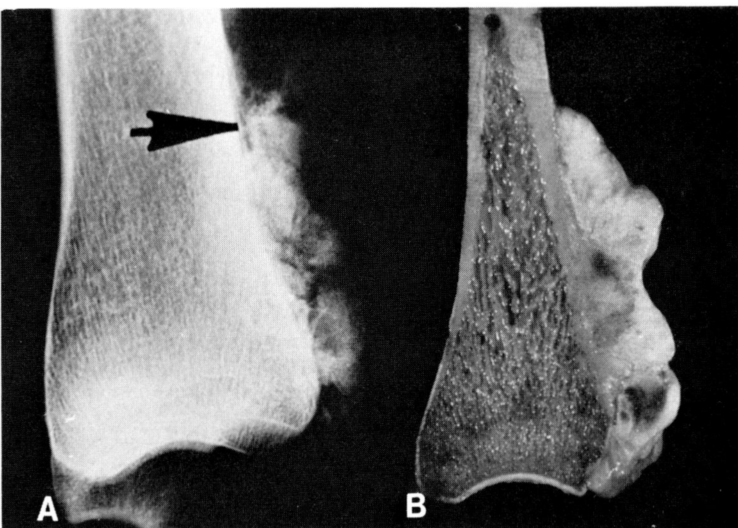

FIG. 14-39

Parosteal Osteosarcoma

FIG. 14-38. Typical appearance of a rather large parosteal osteosarcoma of the distal femur. Note the "pasted-on" appearance, signifying its origin from periosteum, lack of significant intramedullary involvement, and ominous radiating deposits of bone. The lesion gets denser as the cortex is approached.

FIG. 14-39. (*A*) Specimen radiograph of another typical parosteal osteosarcoma of the distal tibia. The arrow points to the hyperplastic thickened periosteum stimulated by the tumor extending over it. The intramedullary bone is uninvolved. (*B*) Gross of the same specimen. On close examination, the tumor is whitish in color and will contain gritty streaks of bone.

FIG. 14-40. An example of a large parosteal osteosarcoma that has enveloped the entire bone. The shaft is uninvolved. The lesion also produced significant amounts of glistening cartilage (*1*).

FIG. 14-41. Gross view of an innocent-looking bony, hard, rounded lesion of the distal femur.

FIG. 14-42. Although the above lesion resembles an osteochondroma, the following features distinguish it as a parosteal osteosarcoma: (*A*) The lesion is "pasted on" the bone. The cortex and spongiosa of the lesion do not blend imperceptibly with the host bone, as does an osteochondroma (refer back to Fig. 14-7 and 14-10). Note also the ominous fluffs at the base of the lesions (*arrows*); this is never seen in osteochondroma unless it has undergone malignant degeneration. (*B*) The lesion in cut section is a "pasted on," greyish pink, gritty, bone-producing lesion. It has destroyed the cortex focally and encroached upon a small portion of the medullary bone.

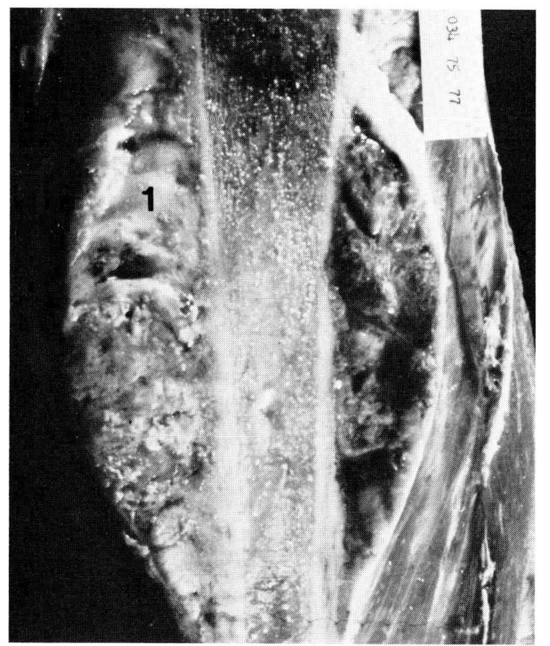

FIG. 14-40

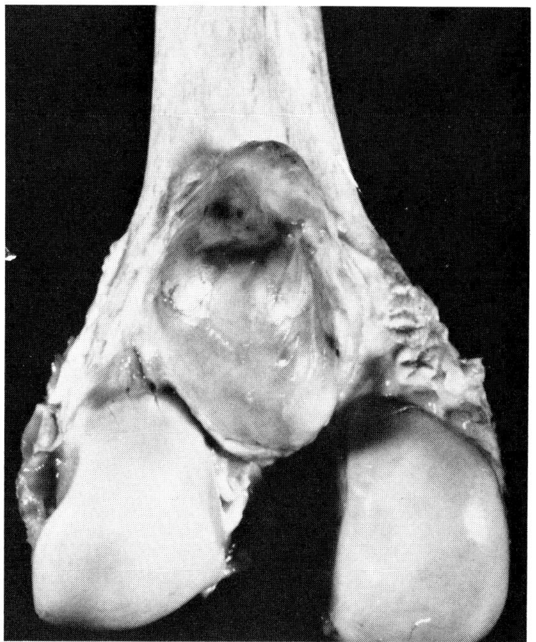

FIG. 14-41

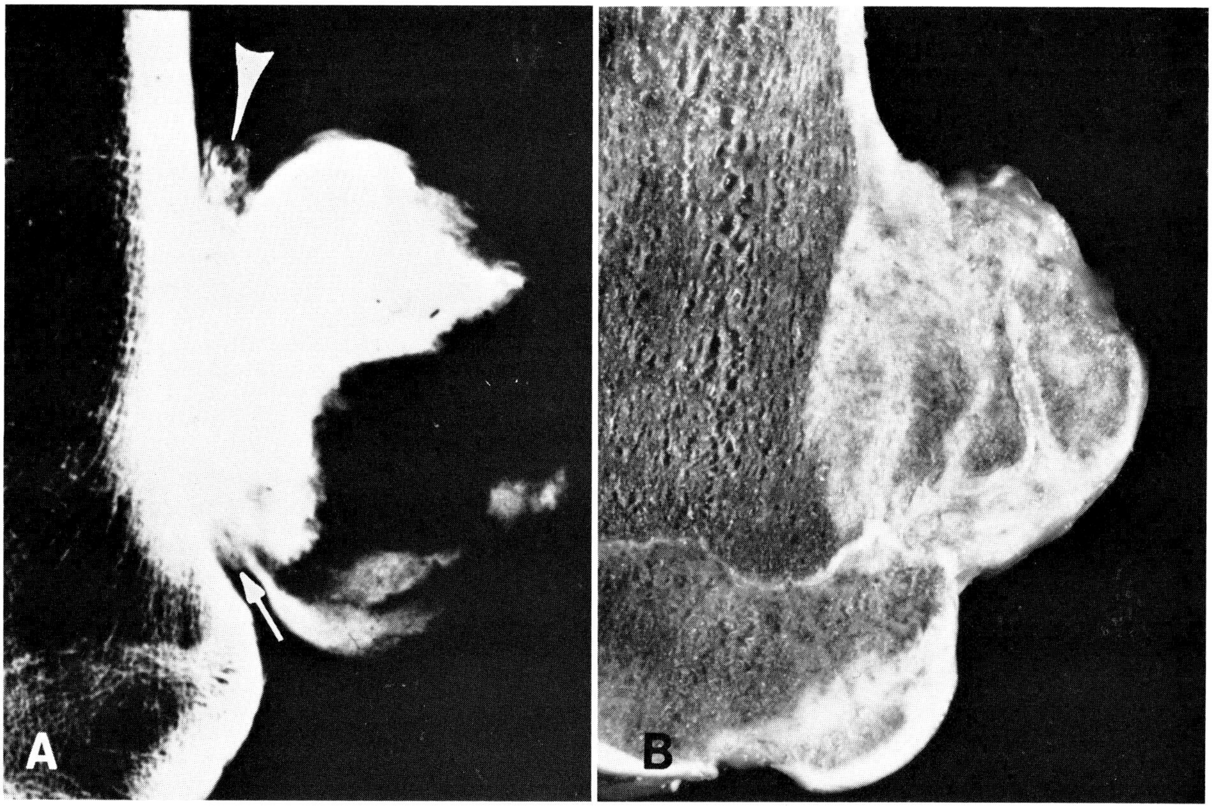

A

B

FIG. 14-42

Table 14-1. Differential Features of Parosteal Osteosarcoma, Traumatic Periostitis, Stress Fracture and Intramedullary Osteosarcoma

	Parosteal Osteosarcoma	*Traumatic Periostitis*	*Stress Fracture*	*Intramedullary Osteosarcoma With Extensive Periosteal Component*
History	Pain and/or swelling. Growth is continuous.	Pain and/or swelling. Usually history of significant trauma.	Pain. Usually history of repetitive or blunt trauma.	Pain and/or swelling.
Radiology	Fluffy, blastic, growth. May be eccentric ("pasted-on" look), surround the bone, or have a rounded osteochondroma-like appearance. Tomograms should show little to no intramedullary involvement and no fracture lines.	Incipient phase may be similar to the parosteal osteosarcoma (OS). Older lesions have a "dotted-veil," lamellated appearance due to deposition of fully mature bone and marrow fat. Tomograms will show no fracture line and CAT scans no intramedullary involvement.	Usually a rectangularly shaped blastic lesion of diaphysis. Tomograms usually, but not always, show fracture line lucency. Will have homogeneous to fluffy intramedullary involvement indistinguishable from an intramedullary osteosarcoma.	Tomogram should show extensive intramedullary involvement. Lesions usually larger than most stress fractures. Most often metaphyseal.
Behavior	Lesions will continue to grow beyond 8–10 week period by serial x-rays.	Lesion will cease growth and mature by 8–10 weeks from inception. May be associated with myositis ossificans.	Will cease growth and mature at 8–10 weeks post-inception with good immobilization.	Lesion will grow rapidly and ceaselessly. Fully malignant with high metastatic rate.
Histology	Grade I to II tumors show long trabeculae of bone between which is low-grade fibrosarcoma-like stroma. Cartilage may be present. Intramedullary involvement, if present, is usually minimal and distinctly eccentric. Grade III tumors identical to the intramedullary OS.	Incipient phases similar to stress fracture callus. Midphase shows tissues similar to low-grade parosteal OS. No unequivocal anaplasia. Medulla uninvolved. Exuberant cartilage may be present.	Incipient phases may mimic a sarcoma. Later phases show osteoblastic rimming and the formation of lamellar bone and marrow fat. Intramedullary extension of the process through marrow is generally not extensive. Exuberant cartilage may be present. No unequivocal anaplasia is ever seen.	Extremely variable. Most cases do show unequivocal anaplasia, however. Tumor infiltrates extensively through host marrow spaces. Benign osteoblastic rimming and maturation to lamellar bone and marrow fat not seen in the neoplastic tissues. Cartilage, if present, is usually obviously malignant.

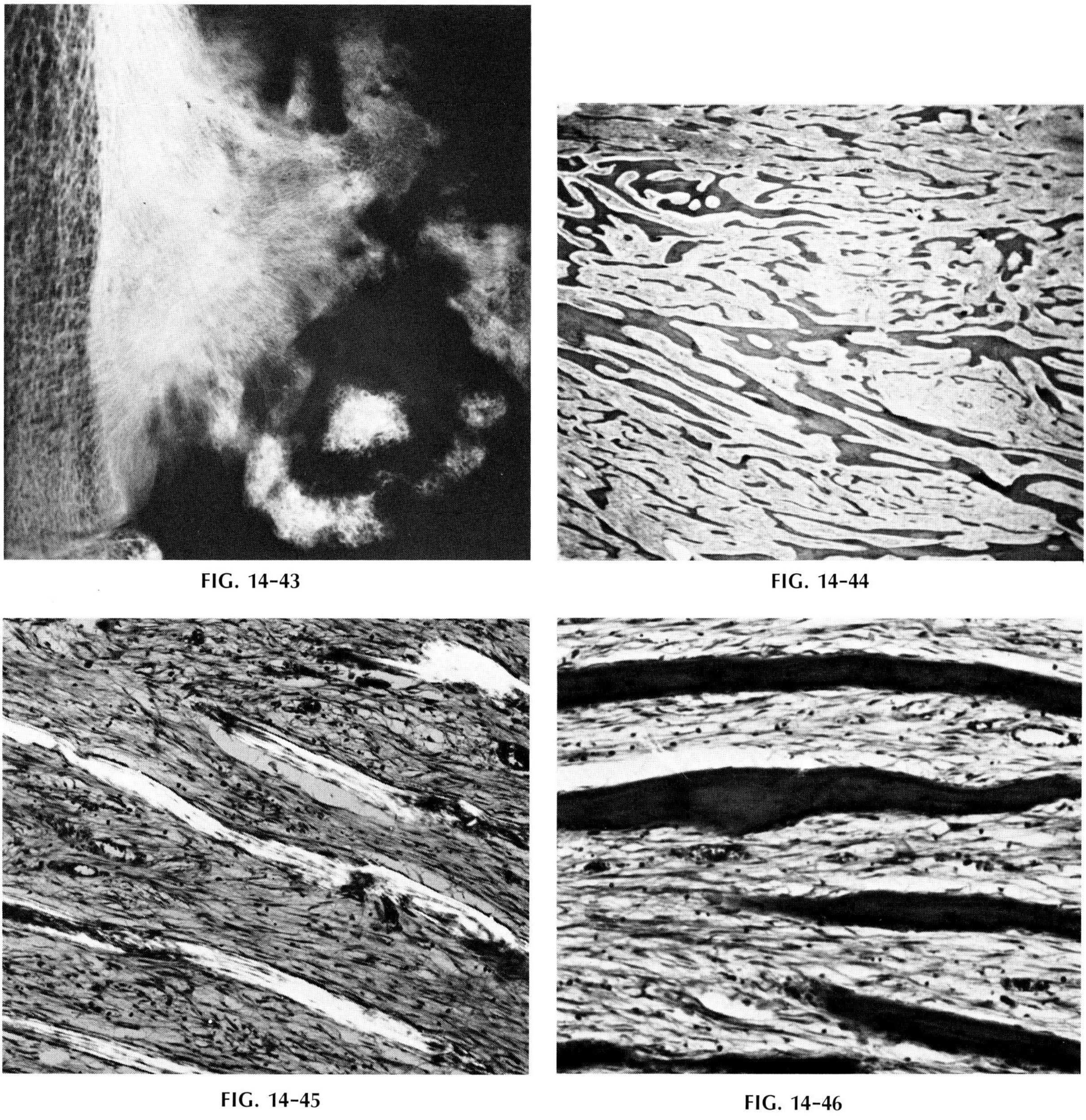

FIG. 14-43

FIG. 14-44

FIG. 14-45

FIG. 14-46

Parosteal Osteosarcoma

FIG. 14-43. Specimen radiograph of a similar rounded form of a parosteal osteosarcoma of the distal femur. This shows the "steel wool-like" appearance from deposits of long slivers of woven to lamellar bone characteristically seen in Grade I parosteal osteosarcoma. Note again the distinctive "pasted on" appearance.

FIG. 14-44. Note the extremely long trabeculae of woven bone between which is a fibrous stroma. This histologic section was taken from the above specimen and easily explains the "steel wool" pattern seen on the radiograph (x10).

FIG. 14-45. Polarized light of the bone spicules may show, in addition to woven bone, a fine lamellar bone pattern usually, but not always associated with benign bone-producing lesions. The well-differentiated parosteal osteosarcoma is an exception to this rule (x40).

FIG. 14-46. Grade I parosteal osteosarcoma. Note the relative sparseness of the nuclei and prominent stromal fibrous pattern (x125).

Grade III tumors, five patients died of disease in less than 1 to 6 years. Of the 23 patients in Unni, *et. al.*'s series with periosteal osteosarcoma,[42] five died with pulmonary metastases and one is alive with metastases. Most of the patients in Ahujia's or Unni's series who died did so in less than 2 years time.

Treatment

The Grade I to low Grade II parosteal osteosarcomas and the periosteal osteosarcoma should be treated by either a radical and adequate en-bloc resection or cryosurgery combined with en-bloc resection. If the tumor seems too large to locally extirpate, radical modalities such as amputation are required. Involvement of neurovascular bundles by the tumor need not necessarily require amputation if it is possible to freeze the area and to free the neurovascular bundle prior to resection. This assumes that freezing and resection can be adequately performed without violating the principle of "tumor sterility" (see Chap. 15, p. 579). The high Grade II or III tumors are more aggressive to highly dangerous lethal tumors that require forms of therapy basically equivalent to that used for intramedullary osteosarcoma. Perhaps chemotherapy with radiation or chemotherapy with freezing and/or en-bloc resection can be used to salvage limbs and life with even these more lethal grades.

Differential Diagnoses

INTRAMEDULLARY OSTEOSARCOMA. The Grade I to low Grade II parosteal osteosarcoma is distinctly different by histologic, radiologic, and gross parameters from the intramedullary osteosarcoma. But high Grade II and III tumors and the periosteal OS are not distinguishable from intramedullary osteosarcomas on purely histological grounds. Radiologic and gross examination are both necessary. Pure periosteal to intracortical tumors should be designated as parosteal or periosteal osteosarcomas, and graded as to degree of anaplasia.

Grade II to III tumors that also show intramedullary involvement present a dilemma. With our present knowledge, it is perhaps impossible to be able to distinguish a Grade III parosteal or a periosteal osteosarcoma that is invading bone from an intramedullary osteosarcoma that is involving periosteum. In either case the treatment should probably be the same and should be the more radical forms of alternatives.

OSTEOCHONDROMA. See Figures 14–6 through 14–18.

TRAUMATIC PERIOSTITIS AND AVULSIVE LIGAMENTO-TENDINITIS OSSIFICANS. (See Figs. 14–64 and 14–67–14–77.) Basically these lesions may very closely resemble the parosteal osteosarcoma in all histologic and radiologic parameters. The former, however, are benign, self-limited diseases and the latter, a sarcoma with unlimited growth and even metastatic potential. After 10 to 12 weeks, the above benign entities will begin to show signs that mature lamellar bone and marrow fat is being deposited. Eventually, the characteristic radiologic feature of benignancy, the "dotted veil" appearance, becomes evident (see Figs. 14–67 and 14–68).

However, before the 8- to 10-week period post-trauma, the radiological and pathological features may exactly mimic an ominous parosteal osteosarcoma. Both entities are about equally as rare, so probabilities cannot be used as a distinguishing factor. It is quite important to ask the patient if he sustained a severe injury or a blunt trauma to the area in recent weeks. Trauma must be suspected in all children and athletes with soft-tissue, periosteal, or ligamentous ossifications. But, the most crucial aid to diagnosis in equivocal cases may be patience. Traumatic periostitis and avulsive injuries to tendons and ligaments are reactions to injury and are, therefore, reparative processes. They will reach maximum size in 8 to 10 weeks and begin to involute some by 12 weeks and in a period of a year may actually disappear. In addition, within 10 to 12 weeks, mature lamellar bone and marrow fat will begin to be laid down, first at the periphery of the lesion; in time, it will extend toward the center. The radiograph will, therefore, begin to show signs of organization into

---

Parosteal Osteosarcoma

FIG. 14–47. Grade I tumor. The nuclei most resemble those seen in a very low-grade fibrosarcoma. The Grade I tumor is deceptively innocent-looking, however, and diagnosis depends on radiologic and clinical correlation (x400).

FIG. 14–48. Grade II tumor. There is increased cellularity and the nuclei and nucleoli are plumper and more obviously anaplastic. Extreme anaplasia is not present, however (x400).

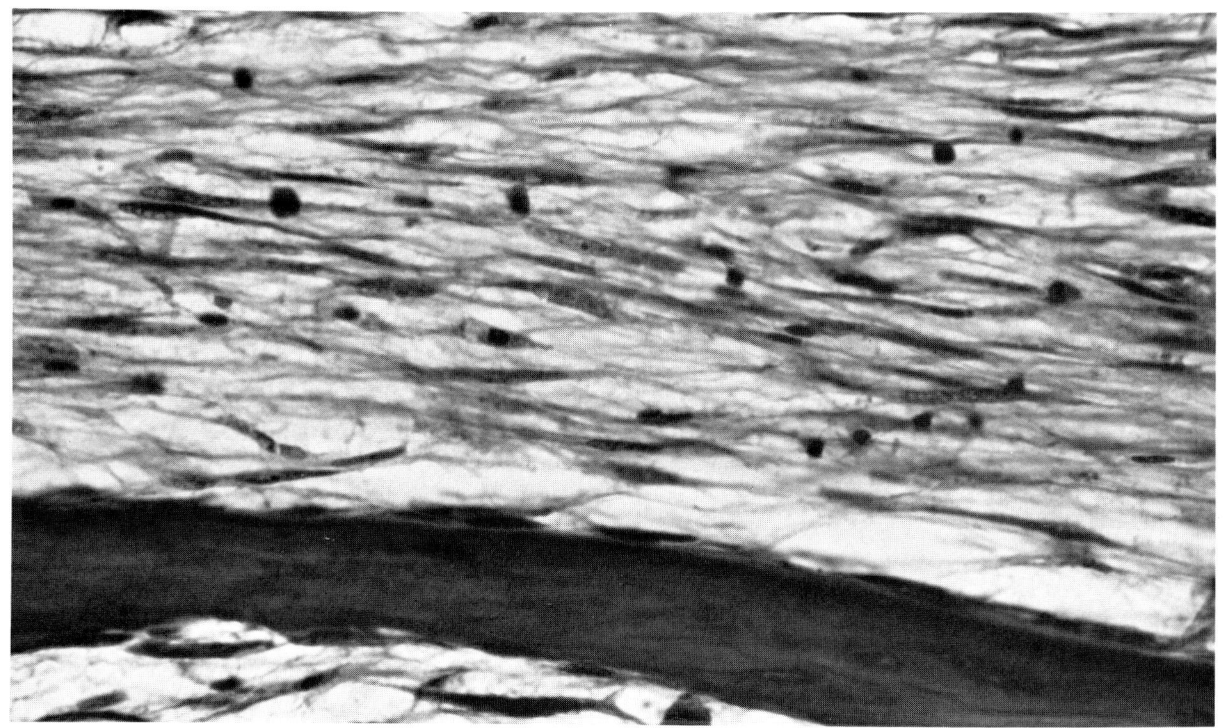

FIG. 14-47

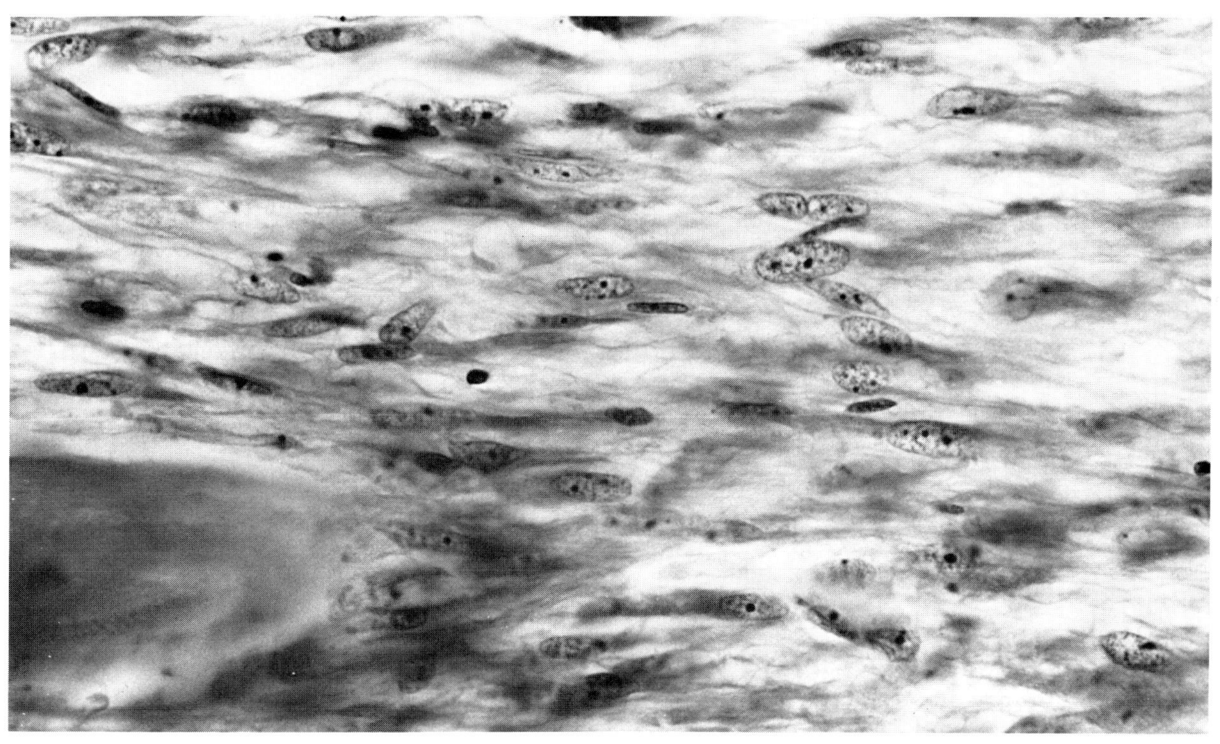

FIG. 14-48

lamellar bone and in time, the benign "dotted veil" or stratified appearance becomes evident. Biopsy of the peripheral and central portions of the lesion of the benign entity can show, after 10 weeks, definite mature lamellar bone and marrow fat maturation. It is not terribly unusual to see myositis ossificans and traumatic periostitis superimposed, because both the extraosseous mesenchyme and periosteum can respond similarly to the inciting injury (see Figs. 14-62-14-66).

On the other hand, within 10 to 12 weeks after the patient notices a lump secondary to the development of a parosteal osteosarcoma, the lump will continue to enlarge and show few to no signs radiologically or pathologically of fully benign maturation. Biopsy of the periphery, if anything, will contain more spindle cells and less mature woven bone than its more central portions, the opposite of a reparative process. This is because it is a true neoplasm expanding ever outwardly; the "older" and more mature tissue will be centrally placed and the "younger," more immature tissue, peripheral. Therefore, in equivocal cases it may be justified to follow the lesion for several weeks, taking radiographs every 2 or 3 weeks and measuring whether the lesion progresses steadily in size and whether or not it shows increasing signs of maturation. If, after 12 weeks from inception of the "lump," the lesion shows none of these features, a biopsy or wedge excision from the peripheral and central portion should confirm the diagnosis of parosteal osteosarcoma. At that juncture the proper surgery should be performed, either radical en-bloc excision, if feasible, or amputation. The usual parosteal osteosarcoma is slow growing and usually only metastasizes after one or more recurrences; therefore, a few weeks delay should not significantly interfere with good long-term results. The benefits are obvious, because patients with traumatic periostitis or avulsive injuries will not then be subjected to loss of bone and joint structures by unnecessary surgery. Instead, a simple excision of the reparative osseous tissue should be sufficient to protect against the rare possibility of malignant transformation of the abnormal tissues many years later.

TRAUMATIC MESENCHYMAL FIBRO-CHONDRO-OSSIFYING LESIONS VERSUS SOFT-TISSUE AND PAROSTEAL OSTEOSARCOMAS

Significant trauma to the mesenchymal tissues may lead to hyperplastic reparative tumorous lesions that can be mistaken for sarcoma. These lesions can be designated as pseudosarcomas. A definition and discussion of sarcomas and pseudosarcomatous lesions are given in Chapter 4.

In the above chapter, "the injury type" of lesion is referred to as hyperplastic or reparative pseudosarcomas. These lesions may be replete with ominous cellularity and even numerous typical mitotic figures. The reparative pseudosarcomas have their most malignant aura in the first 2 to 3 weeks from the inception of injury, show signs of reasonable maturity by 7 to 8 weeks, and are quite mature or benign looking by 10 to 12 weeks post-inception. However, this author has seen such lesions mistaken for sarcoma even when they are in the stage of producing mature, benign-looking matrices, either because the history of significant trauma was not obtained by the clinician and given to the pathologist, or remembered by the patient. Without the positive trauma history, the presence of an apparent *de novo* chondro-ossifying mass can be alarming and misdiagnosed.

Another point to remember is that the tumor provoking injury need not be blunt trauma, which is what most clinicians think of when they think of the term *trauma*. The injury can often be consequent to a tearing, torsional, or repetitive stress. For example, most children, as we well know, run, which on rare occasion can lead to the child avulsing a musculoligamentous insertion from the linea aspera of one or both femora. A few weeks later the initial episode may be forgotten but it may have given rise to the so called tumorous "cortical irregularity syndrome." The clinician and pathologist may be faced with an ominous chondro-ossifying mass in this region and have not obtained a history of trauma, because the child may not have remembered the initial episode or may not have been specifically asked whether he felt a sharp pain while running a few weeks before the mass was felt or before it became even more painful. They may thus be confronted with an apparent alarming ossifying radiological mass for which no history of trauma was gleaned.

Many other such examples can be given. In another case this author has seen a patient with a most alarming appearing ossifying soft-tissue and periosteal 5-cm. mass over the anterior aspect of his left femur (Fig. 14-63). Biopsy showed a very ominous chondro-ossifying mass replete with mitoses. It was not inconsistent with a soft-tissue osteosarcoma or with a traumatic lesion either. No atypical mitoses were seen. This young adult's lesion was diagnosed as an osteosarcoma and he was sent to UCLA for treatment. Although no history of trauma was obtained, the histology showed very prominent rimming of osteoblasts (a clue to benignancy) and the radiologic periosteal reaction was highly suggestive of traumatic periostitis (Fig. 14–63). However, upon personally questioning the patient crucial history was obtained. He had been working in a tank factory and his job was to move 200-pound aluminum slabs onto a table. He often did this by shoving or kicking them onto the table with his shin exactly over the spot where the lesion developed. In fact, he sought medical advice because the pain became so great over the area he could no longer perform his job. Because of this history we decided to watch the lesions for a few weeks. It reached a maximum size in 8 to 10 weeks in the area where he had first experienced the pain. The soft-tissue and periosteal mass became more mature-looking on radiograph, an occurrence that is also in keeping with a benign lesion (myositis ossificans combined with traumatic periostitis). The lesion was then simply excised and the patient remains absolutely disease-free. These two examples show how aggressive one must be in order to obtain the history of trauma, which may be very important to diagnosis and therapy when dealing with fibro-osseous lesions of the soft tissues and/or periosteum.

Some of the lesions will, even with a positive trauma history be malignant. The following discussion will attempt to show how benign pseudosarcomas can be distinguished from true sarcomas in the vast majority of cases.

There are several kinds of osseous-provoking traumatic lesions that can be confused with malignancy. They include stress fracture, myositis ossificans, traumatic periostitis, and avulsive musculo-tendino-ligamentous injuries. One of the main clues to these lesions is that the patient is usually either a child, an athlete, or is engaged in a heavy manual work occupation.

Stress Fracture Compared to the Osteogenic Sarcoma

Usually it is possible to obtain a history of repetitive injury or blunt trauma to the area where the lesion has developed. One may have to seek out the history, because many patients will not specifically recall the traumatic incident that may antedate by several weeks their tumor mass or severe pain.

For example, in "honeymoon" stress fractures the woman may not remember until specifically asked whether she first experienced rib pain during her recent honeymoon or during vigorous lovemaking. Most other stress fractures are usually either diaphyseal or metaphyseal lesions, rectangular in shape, and show periosteal new bone and intramedullary sclerosis (callus) (Figs. 7–15 and 7–16). Tomograms may have to be ordered to visualize the important hairline impacted fracture (Fig. 7–16). However, in rare cases the stress fracture line cannot be visualized. In other cases, cumulus cloudlike fluffs can be seen. These cases may be impossible to differentiate from incipient osteosarcomas (Figs. 7–85 and 7–86), and great care must be given to history and if biopsy is performed, to cytological details and patterns of involvement. Stress fractures can also be due to Charcot joint disease, congenital insensitivity to pain, osteomalacia, and others. The reader is referred to pages 86–97 and Figures 7–15 and 7–16 for more specific clinical radiologic and pathologic details relating to the stress fracture, and to page 141 and Figures 7–43, 7–44, 7–45, 7–46, 7–85, and 7–86 for the specific details of the small, incipient blastic osteosarcoma that can on occasion be confused with stress fracture, and vice versa.

Myositis Ossificans Versus Soft-Tissue Osteosarcoma

Myositis Ossificans

CLINICAL FEATURES. In 40 to 60 per cent of patients, a history of significant blunt trauma is obtained. However, even a physiologic process such as giving birth can rarely give rise to a pelvic myositis ossificans. Usually myositis ossificans is heralded by rather severe muscle pain and limitation of movement during the first few weeks following onset. It does not present as a protruding lump. Malignant soft-tissue tumors are usually painless and they usually present as a lump.

An extremely important differential clinical feature is that myositis ossificans will reach maximum size by 8 to 10 weeks after its inception and may shrink in size after 12 weeks and can even totally disappear. In those cases in which the lesion is surgically removed before full maturation, recurrence is possible.

RADIOLOGIC FEATURES. For 3 to 4 weeks following inception, no ossification will be seen. The appearance of the lesion will be merely an ill-defined, soft-tissue, rounded density.

The main clue to diagnosis is that at about 4 weeks (Fig. 14–49), the lesion begins to ossify from the periphery toward the center. This is its most important parameter and is reflected histologically as well. The lesions are usually quite dense along the periphery by 12 weeks (Fig. 14–50).

(Text continues on p. 554.)

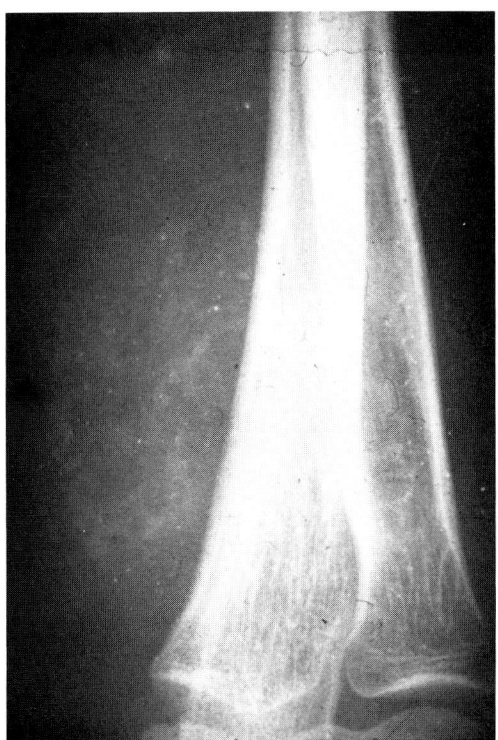

FIG. 14-49

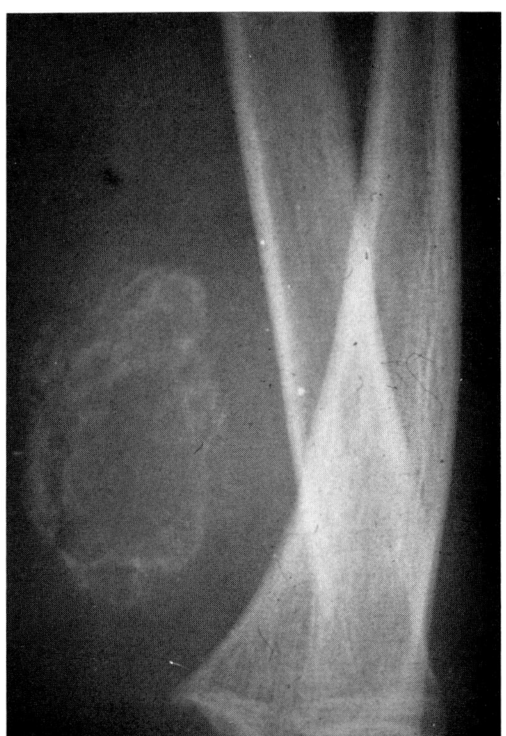

FIG. 14-50

Myositis Ossificans

FIG. 14-49. Myositis ossificans 4 weeks post-trauma. There is beginning ossification of the soft-tissue mass. It is difficult to tell at this time whether there is peripheral localization, however.

FIG. 14-50. At 12 weeks post-trauma the lesion is distinctly round, and peripheral ossification is clear-cut, establishing the diagnosis of myositis ossificans by radiology alone.

FIG. 14-51. Entire slab section of myositis ossificans. Note the formation of bone spicules peripherally and the pure spindle cell stroma centrally (*arrow*). This zonation phenomenon is pathognomonic of the lesion.

FIG. 14-52. The width of the peripheral ossification depends, of course, on the age of the lesion. This lesion was only 5-weeks old and the width of ossification (*arrows*) was, therefore, narrow (x10).

FIG. 14-53. Note the striking contrast between the bone at the periphery (*1*) and the ominous spindly stroma in the center of the lesion (*2*) (x40).

FIG. 14-54. A higher-power view of the peripheral bone production. Note also the rather benign osteoblastic rimming (*arrows*) (x125).

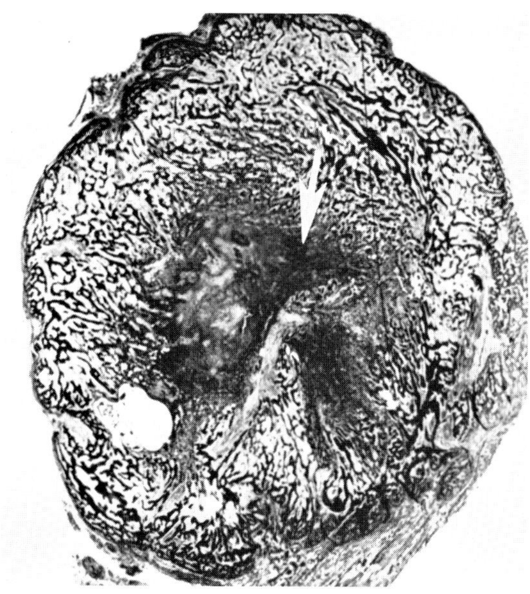

FIG. 14-51

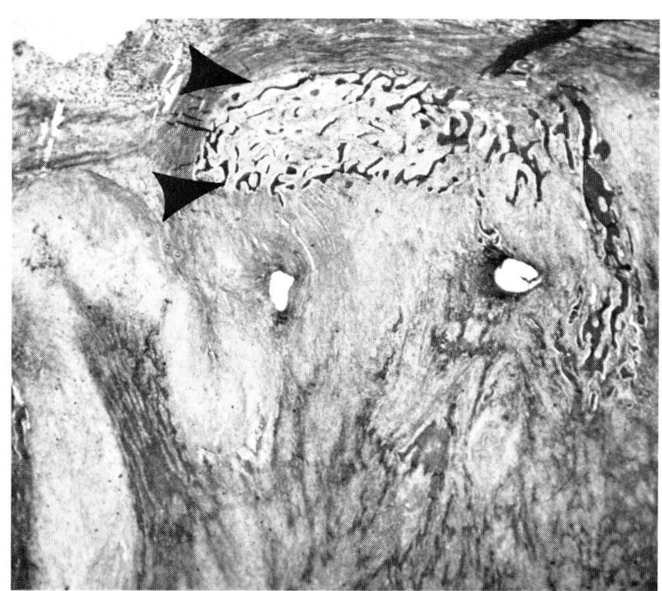

FIG. 14-52

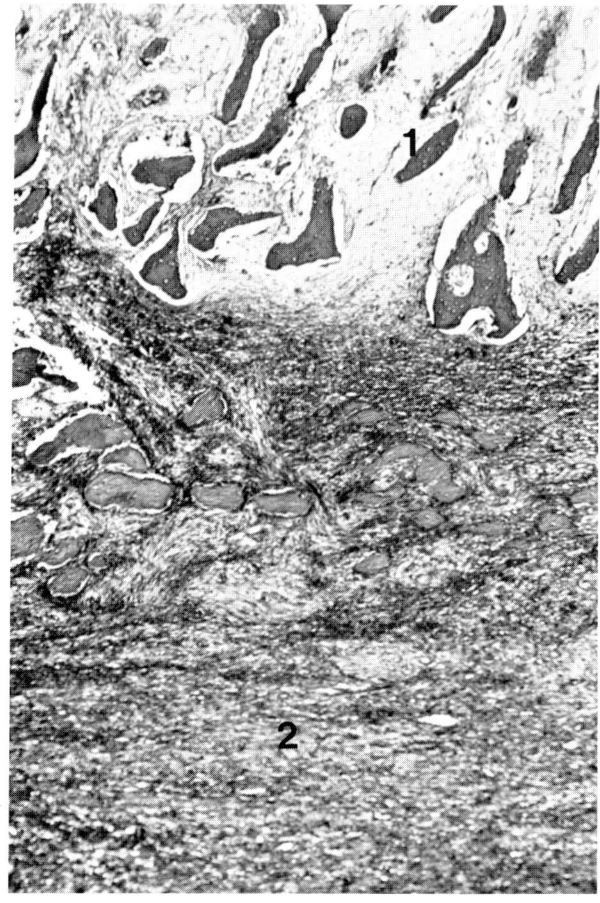

FIG. 14-53

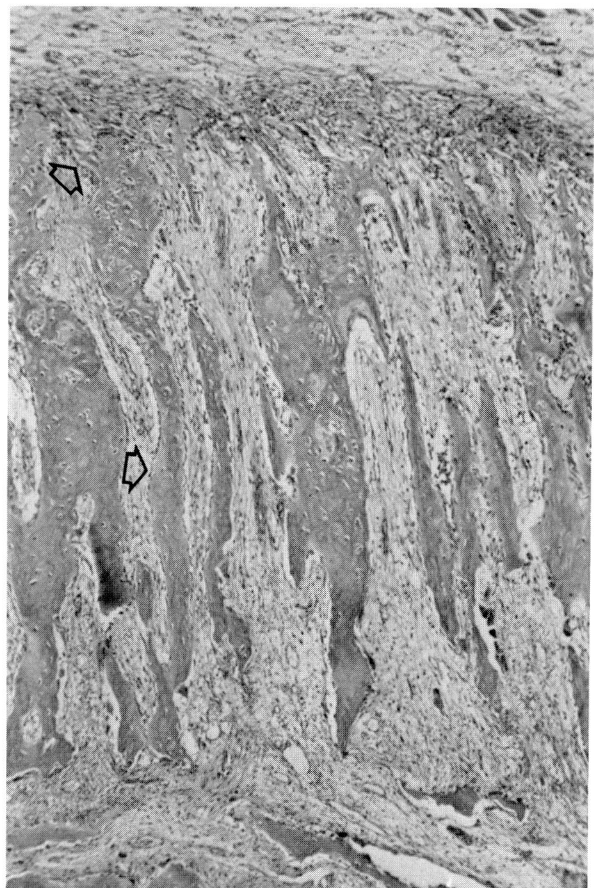

FIG. 14-54

PATHOLOGY

EARLY PHASE (1 TO 3 WEEKS). The early phase is characterized by a massive proliferation of tissue culturelike to spindly fibrosarcoma-like cells (Fig. 14–55). All of the nuclei seem to be in about the same phase (see pp. 49–50) and although mitoses may be abundant, they are typical. This is the most difficult period in which to diagnose myositis ossificans with certainty, because there is no osteoid, chondroid, or bone production. Without these tissues it is impossible to identify the characteristic myositis ossificans zonation phenomenon. This is why it is recommended thay if myositis ossificans is suspected from the history, the lesion should not be removed until definite peripheral localization of bone can be seen radiologically. If the early lesion (less than 6–8 weeks) is simply excised, there is a reasonable chance of recurrence, since the lesion has been removed before complete "ripening," and the residual cells remaining could lead to recurrence. If this occurs and if the lesion does not show unequivocal or frank anaplasia, it would be wise to wait 4 to 5 weeks more and to repeat the radiologic examination. If no peripheral ossification is yet occurring, the probability of a spindle cell sarcoma is high. If the lesion that is being observed clinically continues to grow rapidly or does not reach a maximum size within 8 to 10 weeks, it is probably not a reparative lesion but a sarcoma. If, after 8 to 10 weeks, the cells look no more mature than they did at the time of the original excision or biopsy and no zonation phenomenon is seen, it is almost surely malignant and should be appropriately diagnosed and treated.

MIDPHASE (4–8 WEEKS). It is possible to obtain a firm diagnosis of myositis ossificans after 3 to 4 weeks from its inception. The decisive zonation phenomenon was first recognized by Ackerman.[44] The zonation phenomenon of myositis ossificans consists of unequivocal peripheral maturation of the lesion prior to its central maturation. In other words, the periphery of the lesion is the first to demonstrate osteoid and woven bone and/or cartilage (Fig. 14–56), and the center of the lesion mimics well differentiated cellular fibrosarcoma (Fig. 14–55).

The opposite zonation is true of an osteosarcoma. The periphery is poorly differentiated and the center of the lesion contains more mature tissue (Fig. 14–59). What seems to be happening to explain this difference is the following: myositis ossificans appears to be due to a mesenchymal muscle injury in which a nodule of damaged tissue forms. Undifferentiated mesenchymal cells apparently invade from the periphery of the injured mass to its center. The older cells are thereby peripherally placed and would be expected to be the first to produce an osseous matrix.

Mesenchymal cells require at least 3 to 4 weeks to produce woven bone. The center of the lesion contains "younger" migratory cells and will not have produced an osseous matrix unless they are at least 3 to 4 weeks old. On the other hand, an osteosarcoma is an ever expanding neoplasm with the "younger" cells peripheral and the "older" central. Ossification will, therefore, first proceed in its center while the peripheral cells will be undifferentiated. However, the so-called periphery may be less than 1 mm. in thickness. In myositis ossificans it is sometimes possible to see about four to five layers of spindle cells at the periphery producing bone beneath them. If the external layer is 10 to 20 cells thick before bone is seen, the lesion usually, but not always, is an osteosarcoma. The importance of properly sampling the periphery and center of soft-tissue ossifying tumors cannot be overstressed. If only a biopsy is performed, the surgeon must properly identify the tissue removed as either peripherally or centrally located.

LATE PHASE (8–12+ WEEKS). By 8 to 12 weeks the peripheral woven bone becomes replaced by bland lamellar bone and marrow fat (Fig. 14–57). The center of the lesion may still contain fibrosarcoma-like cells or osteoid and/or woven bone, depending upon the size of the lesion. After many weeks the entire lesion will be converted to bland lamellar bone and marrow fat. Foci of cartilage can be seen, of course, in the mid- or late phases. In fact, a benign cartilage cap may rim the fully ripened lesion. A myositis ossificans

---

Myositis Ossificans

FIG. 14–55. The center of the lesion, if nonossified, mimics a Grade I to II fibrosarcoma replete with mitoses (*arrow*) (x400).

FIG. 14–56. Ominous-appearing osteoid (*1*) can be seen for many weeks. This tissue is usually seen at the interface of the bone with the central fibrosarcoma-like component (x125).

FIG. 14–57. Fully mature (several months to years old) lesions become converted to completely innocent-looking lamellar bone and marrow fat (partial polarized light, x40).

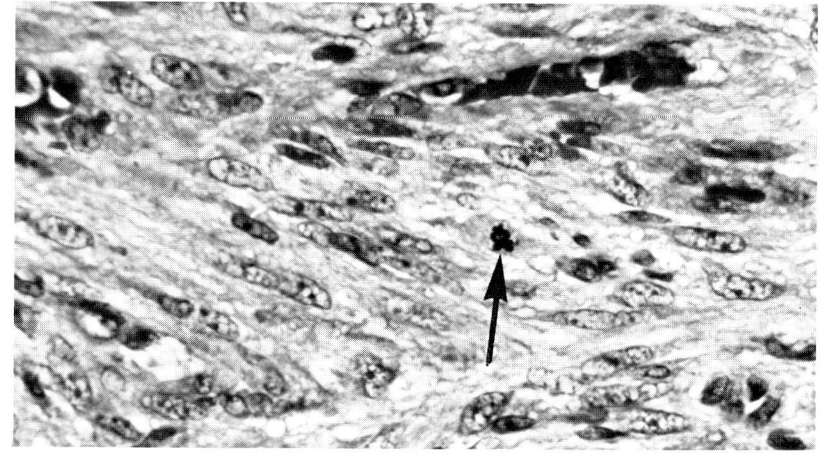

FIG. 14-55

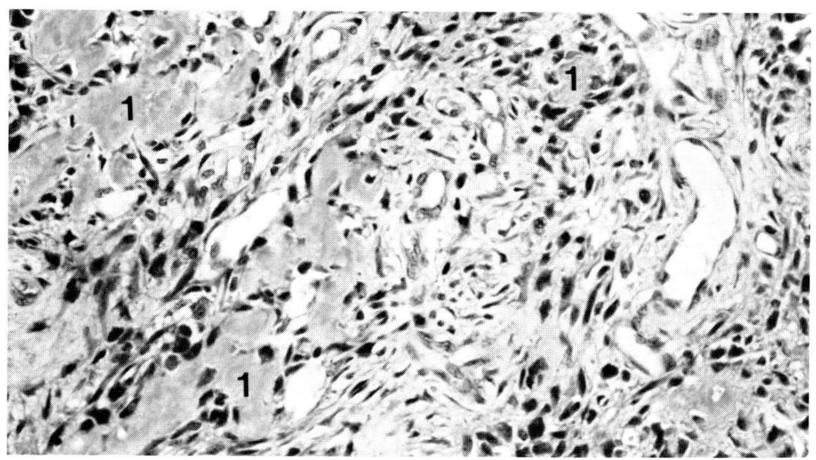

FIG. 14-56

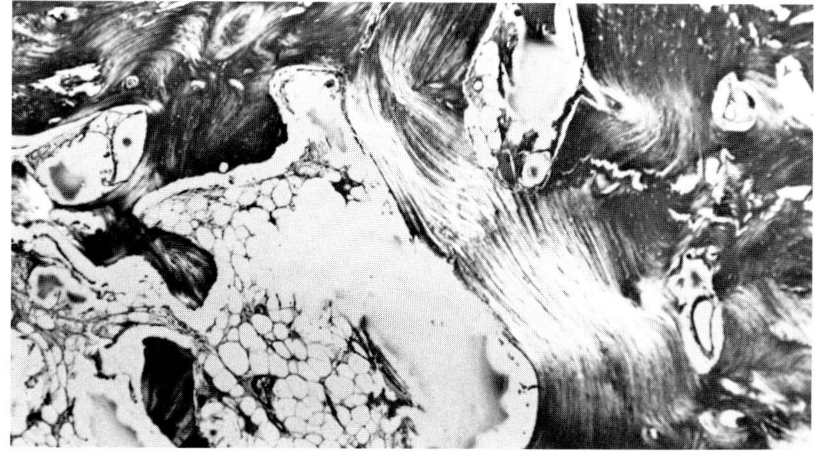

FIG. 14-57

with this feature has even been called post-traumatic osteochondroma (a misnomer, of course).

COURSE BENIGN. Approximately 1 per cent of all myositis ossificans lesions may undergo transformation to a true sarcoma. One should not accept such cases as valid transformations unless the myositis ossificans nodule has remained static in size and appearance for at least 5 years. Malignant transformation is heralded by a sudden increase in size and perhaps pain. The reader must be warned against a diagnosis of so-called "atypical" myositis ossificans. By "atypical" I mean any case that does not show unequivocally the typical myositis ossificans pattern of zonation or any lesion that recurs after the lesion supposedly is in its peripherally ripened stage (8–10 weeks post-inception), no matter how innocent the nuclei of the osseous-producing lesion may be. Of two cases of so-called "atypical" myositis ossificans that I have seen with the above features, multiple recurrences occurred over a 3- to 5-year period preceding distant metastases. This author deems these cases to be Grade I or low-grade anaplastic soft-tissue osteosarcomas. This rare entity will be discussed in greater detail in the next section.

Soft-Tissue Osteosarcoma

HIGH-GRADE ANAPLASTIC TYPE (TYPICAL FORM). Although soft-tissue osteosarcomas are rare, the majority of them show frank anaplasia and are not difficult to diagnose. These tumors may show identical histologic characteristics as those described for the intramedullary osteosarcoma. Besides frank anaplasia, the zonation phenomenon is reversed, woven bone and osteoid is centrally placed, and ominous spindly cells invade out from the periphery of the lesion (Fig. 14–59). The high-grade anaplastic soft-tissue osteosarcoma does not show prominent osteoblastic rimming similar to the intramedullary osteosarcoma. Myositis ossificans often shows prominent osteoblastic rimming.

LOW-GRADE (I) SOFT-TISSUE OSTEOSARCOMA. This author has seen at least two treacherous cases of extremely innocent-looking osseous lesions that were originally called atypical myositis ossificans and certainly looked no worse than some of the so-called pseudomalignant osseous tumors of soft tissue. Both cases eventually proved to be malignant and had little to no essential change in histology through their course.

The essential findings were:

1. Both patients were 55 years old and both noted a gradually enlarging mass; the first, within 6 months, and the second in $1\frac{1}{2}$ years. There was no history of significant trauma. One mass was located in the biceps, and the other, in the thigh.

2. Excisional biopsy showed foci of osteoid, woven, and lamellar bone with some degree of osteoblastic rimming in both. The bone was in various phases of maturation. The maturation was haphazard, that is, the most mature looking woven or lamellar bone could be found either centrally or peripherally (Fig. 14–60). In both cases small foci of slightly plump spindle cells scattered haphazardly throughout the tumor were noted (Fig. 14–61). In the patient with the thigh lesion, abundant hemorrhage and aneurysmal bone cystlike spaces were seen. No marrow fat was observed.

3. Multiple recurrences (3 in one and 4 in the other) were noted over a 3- and 4-year period.

4. Both patients developed multiple lung metastases 4 years after the original excision. The patient with the biceps tumor died shortly thereafter.

5. The lung metastases showed little to no

Soft-Tissue Osteosarcoma

FIG. 14-58. Although this lesion resembles a myositis ossificans by cursory examination, the presence of a nonossified mass (*arrows*) peripheral to the bone production almost always signifies a malignant tumor; in this case, a soft-tissue osteosarcoma.

FIG. 14-59. Soft-tissue osteosarcoma show a zonation phenomenon opposite to myositis ossificans. The periphery of the tumor shows undifferentiated cells (*1*). The center of the lesion contains the osseous elements; in this figure, malignant osteoid and chondrosarcoma (*2*).

FIG. 14-60. Rare, soft-tissue, low-grade anaplastic osteosarcoma can show deceptively benign-appearing bone production (x40).

FIG. 14-61. They usually are also associated with a spindly stroma very subtly anaplastic, particularly when compared to the stroma of a myositis ossificans. The chief differentiating features, however, are the lack of a distinct zonation phenomenon and one or more recurrences if treated as a benign tumor (x125).

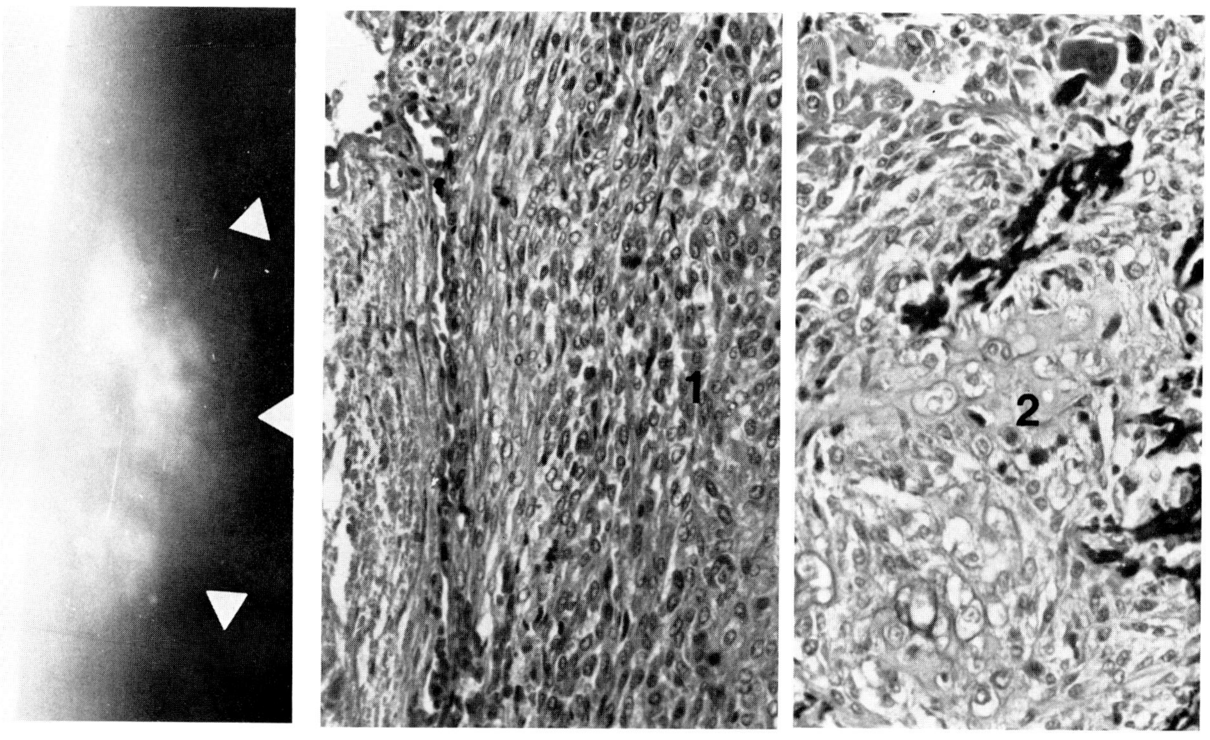

FIG. 14-58

FIG. 14-59

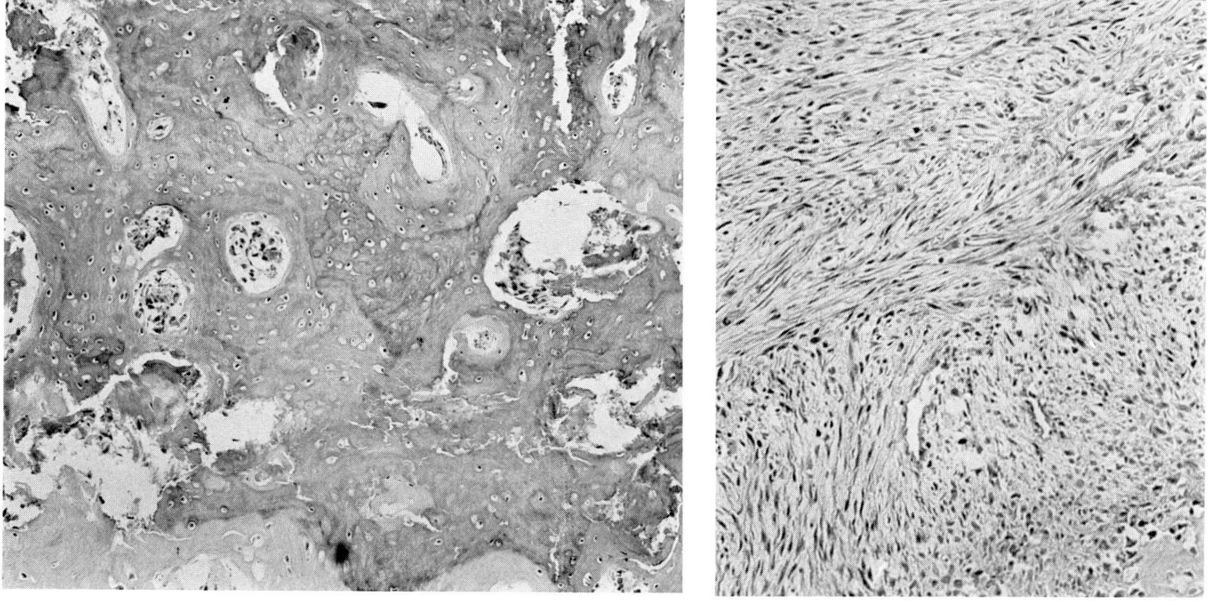

FIG. 14-60

FIG. 14-61

cytologic changes, compared to the primary lesion. Both patients produced bone in the lung metastases. One of the patients had, in addition to the low-grade osteosarcoma in the lung metastases, large foci of histiocytes and cholesterol clefts.

In summary, these two cases are unequivocally malignant by behavior, but they showed little histologic evidence of their true nature either in the primary lesion or in their metastases. The most significant parameters to distinguish them are the following:

a. Evidence of quite slow growth without a history of trauma. Myositis ossificans grows quickly and reaches maximum size in 10 to 12 weeks.
b. No typical myositis ossificans zonation phenomenon.
c. Evidence of relatively bland osteoid and bone production in various phases of maturation haphazardly scattered throughout the stroma.
d. Absence of benign marrow fat.
e. Multiple recurrences.

The case reported by Umiker and Jaffe[61] is identical to the two cases described above. The lesion mistaken for benign myositis ossificans recurred and lead to distant metastases and death within $4\frac{1}{2}$ years. The degree of pleomorphism did increase with the recurrence. However, the lesion was not substantially different from the primary very low-grade anaplastic neoplasm. Perhaps all slow growing unifocal osseous-producing tumors of the soft tissues that do not show absolutely typical features of myositis ossificans (uniform peripheral bone maturation, compared to less mature central ossification or fibrosarcoma-like tissue) and an haphazard arrangement of osseous-forming tissue should be initially en-blocked with a margin of healthy tissue, despite apparent cytologic innocence. Although some cases with the above features could perhaps represent peculiar rare forms of recurrent myositis ossificans or a benign pseudomalignant osseous tumor of soft tissue, I know of no particular way to distinguish these possible entities from the low-grade osteosarcoma. Certainly, if there is recurrence after 6 or more months, more aggressive surgical treatment would appear warranted, particularly if the original lesion was simply excised without a margin of healthy tissue.

Pseudomalignant Osseous Tumor of Soft Tissues

This lesion does not lend itself to easy summary, because the literature is both contradictory and is ambiguous about its definition. Fine and Stout were the first authors to coin the term *pseudomalignant osseous tumor of soft tissues.*[48] They reported four cases of their own and four cases from the literature they believe to be similar examples. In distinction to soft-tissue osteosarcoma, they mentioned that this entity occurs in a younger age group (6 patients were younger than 30 years of age). Three had a history of previous trauma. Mitoses, cellular pleomorphism, and giant cells were infrequent. The lesions were circumscribed and the periphery of the tumors was poorly to moderately cellular and showed fibrous tissue or well-formed spicules of bone that sometimes produced a definite shell. Attachment to bone was not present. All of the patients remained well without recurrence or metastasis for a period of 2 to 29 years. Unfortunately, no mention is made about whether zonation was present, if the bone was pure woven or a mixture of woven and lamellar, or if there was marrow fat present. In essence no mention is made of features that probably made them consider this entity

---

Traumatic Periostitis and Myositis Ossificans

FIG. 14-62. Injury to the soft tissue may also result in injury to the periosteum. The result can be a combination of myositis ossificans (*A*) and periosteal new bone formation, called *traumatic periostitis* (*B*). (*A*) This was taken only 2 weeks post-injury, at which time visible osseous production could not be evident. However, a soft-tissue mass is evident (*arrow*). (*B*) This is of the same lesion at 20 weeks. It shows the characteristic mature, "dotted veil" appearance (*arrow*) of traumatic periostitis and the combined myositis ossificans (*1*) with peripheral ossification. Note, however, the fine line separating the traumatic periosteal new bone from the bone cortex. This sign may also be seen in parosteal osteosarcoma. Therefore, this sign should not be taken as conclusive or pathognomonic evidence of a parosteal osteosarcoma.

FIG. 14-63. Although the histology of this lesion was interpreted as an osteosarcoma, review of the radiographs and history were conclusive of myositis ossificans in association with traumatic periostitis. The conclusive radiographic findings were a rounded, pedunculated, ossifying soft-tissue mass (*a*) in association with a fine strand of layered periosteal new bone on either side of the lesion (*arrows*). Neither a soft-tissue osteosarcoma nor a parosteal osteosarcoma shows this unusual combination. When the patient was requestioned, an obvious occupational history of trauma to the area was revealed.

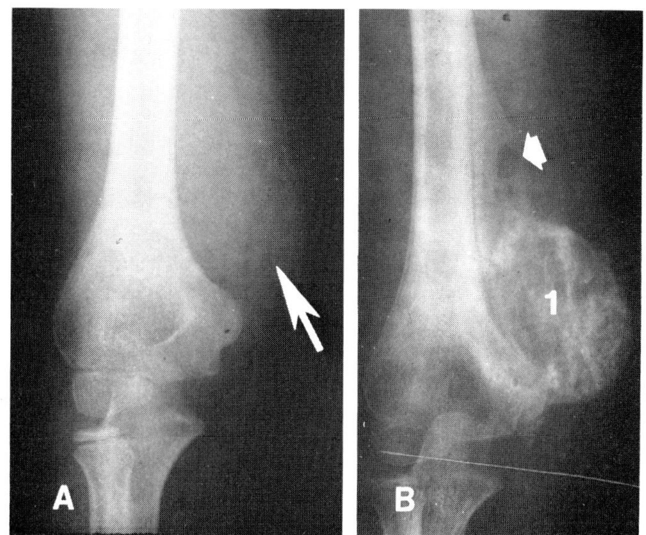

FIG. 14-62

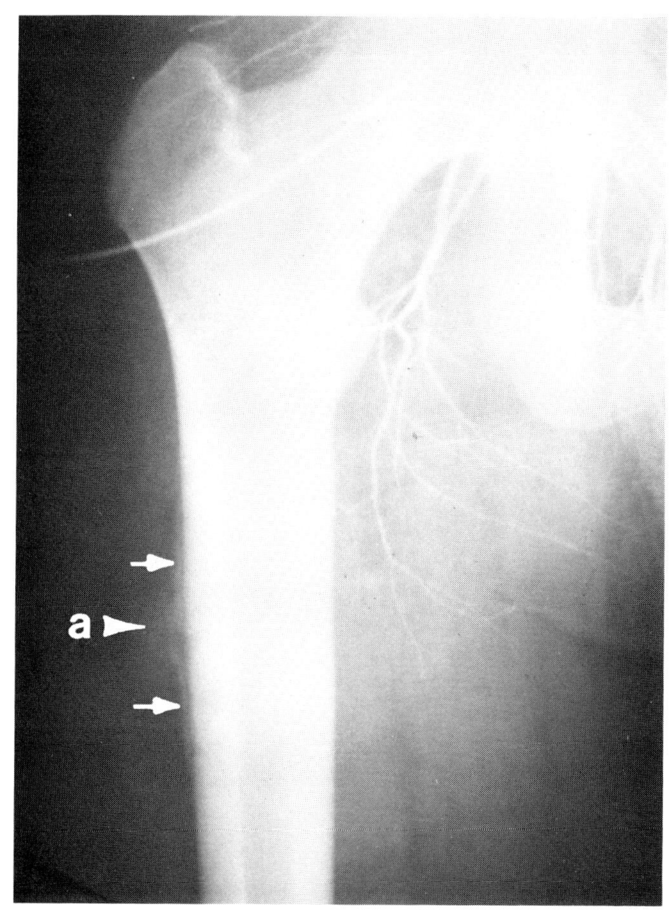

FIG. 14-63

distinct from ordinary myositis ossificans. Subsequently there have been sporadic reports of the so-called pseudomalignant osseous tumor of soft tissue that describe eight more cases, all of which have the typical zonation or myositis ossificans as described by Ackerman.[45,46,52] Similarly, all of these lesions were characterized by lack of recurrence following simple excision. None of these eight cases had an antecedant history of trauma.

Angervall makes a case based on five of these patients that these lesions are possibly post-inflammatory in nature, because two patients had history of antecedant respiratory infections, four had high temperatures, all five patients had elevated erythrocyte sedimentation rate (ESR), and four had elevated antistreptolysin-O titers. Except for these latter findings, the lesion is clinically and pathologically identical to myositis ossificans circumscripta. To my knowledge, similar studies relating to ESR's, body temperature, and antistreptolysin-O titers have not been reported in association with ordinary post-traumatic myositis ossificans, so it it hard to know if the entity described by Angervall and others is clearly separable from myositis ossificans by clinical criteria.

To confuse the issue even further, Jaffe, in a short paragraph on this "entity," described it as one which is not associated with trauma, may be virtually indistinguishable from soft-tissue osteosarcoma except "for the presence of trabeculae of well-formed osseous tissue here and there at its periphery" and the absence of marked atypism of "its stromal cells or the presence of sarcoma giant cells. . . The pseudomalignant tumor grows rather slowly. However, in contrast to a focus of post-traumatic myositis ossificans, it does not reach maturity and stop growing. It is true that the lesion does not metastasize and will not recur if completely excised."[51] However, Jaffe is inclined to think that if not excised and it continues to grow it may eventually undergo malignant transformation. Dr. Jaffe does not show any illustrations of the entity he is describing nor does he mention whether or not lamellar bone and marrow fat was present in the lesion, as marrow fat is rarely associated with malignant soft-tissue osseous tumors.

Are the cases Dr. Jaffe is describing very low-grade osteosarcomas that were adequately excised before they displayed metastasis, as occurred in the two cases presented here (Figs. 14–60 and 14–61)? Is the reported pseudomalignant osseous tumor of soft tissue a distinct entity or could it be a syndrome complex composed of a self-limited form of myositis ossificans in which a history of trauma is not usually elicted and a rarer continuously growing and if inadequately excised, recurrent, potentially metastatic low-grade osteosarcoma? Do so-called recurrent "pseudomalignant osseous tumors" of soft tissues that metastasize simply become reclassified as osteosarcoma? If so, it would not be difficult to understand why they are not reported. However, if such cases exist and are not being reported, then the diagnosis of recurrent pseudomalignant osseous tumor of soft tissues or "atypical" recurrent myositis ossificans must certainly be a dangerous one. Obviously there is a great need to study "atypical" ossifying lesions of the soft tissue in great depth and to develop better criteria of benignancy and malignancy.

Traumatic Ossifying Periostitis

Injury to the periosteum may result in a very ominous chondro-osseous repair that may in its early phases mimic the parosteal osteosarcoma both radiologically and pathologically. Injuries to the periosteum can be from either blunt trauma or tearing of ligaments or muscle attachments. With the latter injuries, the history of trauma is usually more difficult to obtain, because it is not so distinctly a remembered blunt trauma. More often it is as a torsional trauma received during strenuous physical exercise (running, wrestling, *etc.*).

Traumatic Periostitis and Myositis Ossificans With Erosion Into Bone

FIG. 14-64. After a significant twisting trauma this young boy complained of pain in his distal arm. A radiograph at 4 weeks shows an ossific mass forming, perhaps in the interosseous ligament.

FIG. 14-65. A lateral view clearly shows concomitant traumatic periostitis 3 weeks later.

FIG. 14-66. *Left:* Two weeks later, another radiograph shows not only traumatic periostitis (*arrows*) but also myositis ossificans (*1*). *Right:* Several months later, the mass of myositis ossificans was found within the ulna. This presumably was consequent to pressure erosion from repeated supination and pronation. This latter phenomenon of pressure erosion of myositis ossificans into a contiguous bone is rare.

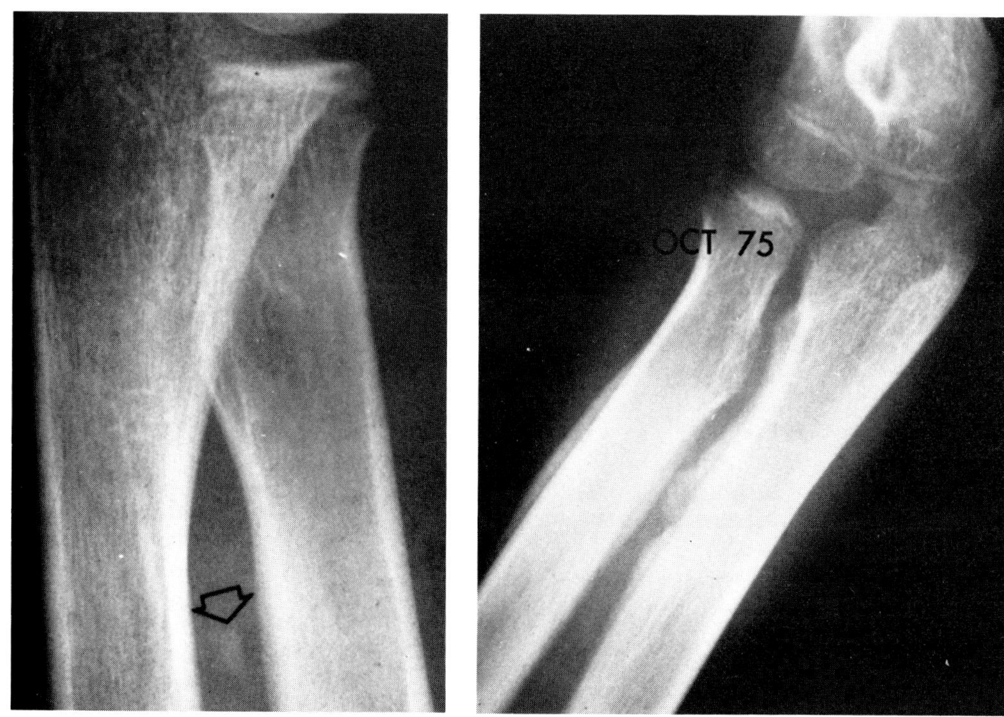

FIG. 14-64

FIG. 14-65

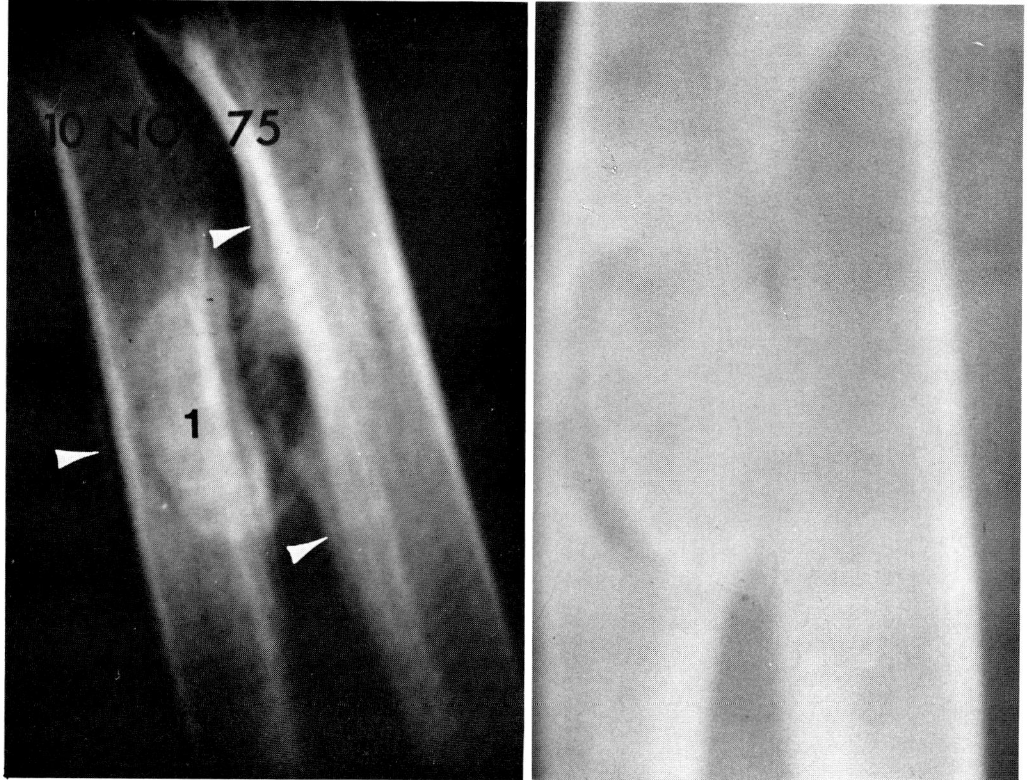

FIG. 14-66

The features this author uses to recognize this difficult benign lesion are the following:

1. Associated concommittant myositis ossificans. On occasion the blunt trauma that leads to the traumatic ossifying periostitis also leads to typical myositis ossificans (Figs. 14–62, 14–63, 14–64, 14–65, and 14–66). The presence of the typical features of myositis ossificans virtually establishes the periosteal reaction as benign.
2. A "dotted veil," lamellated periosteal bone appearance (Figs. 14–67 and 14–68). The dotted veil appearance corresponds histologically to well-differentiated lamellar bone and marrow fat (Fig. 14–70). There are apparently old, fully ripened examples of traumatic periostitis that are easy to recognize as benign by the completely bland appearance of the histology. However, such cases may not even need biopsy or excision if they show the absolutely classic radiologic features. They should perhaps be followed for months to ascertain complete absence of growth.
3. In lesions that are radiologically borderline between traumatic periostitis and parosteal osteosarcoma, the lesions can be followed for several weeks by radiologic examination. If the lesion continues to grow after 8 to 10 weeks from inception, during which it shows no signs of maturation to lamellar bone, the lesion is likely a parosteal osteosarcoma. Biopsy taken at this point should show the typical features of parosteal osteosarcoma (see Figs. 14–44–14–48).

   By 8 to 10 weeks time, if the lesion is benign, a biopsy of the periphery and center of the benign lesion should show the formation of bland lamellar bone, conversion of the intertrabecular stroma to marrow fat, and perhaps very prominent, bland osteoblastic rimming, although this latter feature has on occasion been reported in the parosteal osteosarcoma.[34] I have not seen prominent, bland, osteoblastic rimming in the unequivocally tumorous portions of the parosteal osteosarcoma, however.
4. Absence of an intramedullary lesion. Traumatic periostitis does not invade the bone. If a sclerosing periosteal lesion also involves the medulla, it is either a juxtacortical osteosarcoma invading bone; an intramedullary osteosarcoma breaking out and involving periosteum; or a stress fracture. Tomograms usually, but not always, show a fracture line.

In my experience I have seen approximately 10 parosteal osteosarcomas for every four traumatic periostitis lesions. Two of the four traumatic periostitis lesions were clear-cut (dotted veil appearance) or associated with myositis ossificans. The diagnosis of the other two depended on benign clinical course, namely, the absence of growth beyond a period of several weeks of observation or 8 to 10 weeks from the inception of the patient's symptoms.

AVULSIVE MUSCULO-TENDINO-LIGAMENTITIS OSSIFICANS (AN ENTITY THAT CAN BE CONFUSED WITH FIBRO-, CHONDRO-, OR OSTEOSARCOMA)

Blunt and tearing injuries to mesenchymal muscle and tendon and ligament attachments to bone can give rise to fibrous and/or chondromatous and/or bony repair tissues identical to those described for myositis ossificans or traumatic periostitis. Usually, however, a distinct zonation phenomenon is difficult to observe. Apparently the tearing injuries lead to a reparative response that may not have a zonation phenomenon identical to myositis ossificans circumscripta. Therefore, this feature may not be present to determine its benignancy. The other principles seen with myositis ossificans apply to these injuries, however. In the first few weeks post-injury the tissues are

---

Traumatic Periostitis-Ligamentitis Ossificans

FIG. 14-67. Note the fairly distinct, lamellated, "dotted veil" (*arrows*) appearance of this bony lesion arising in the interosseous ligament between the tibia and fibula. Even though it was called benign radiologically, the surgeon decided to remove it. (Figs. 14-67 to 14-70 are all from the same patient).

FIG. 14-68. A specimen radiograph clearly shows the lamellated, dotted veil appearance, a sign of completely benign lamellar bone and marrow fat production.

FIG. 14-69. In the gross, the lesion formed a ridge of bone in the interosseous ligament, seen as a small nubbin in cross section (*arrow*).

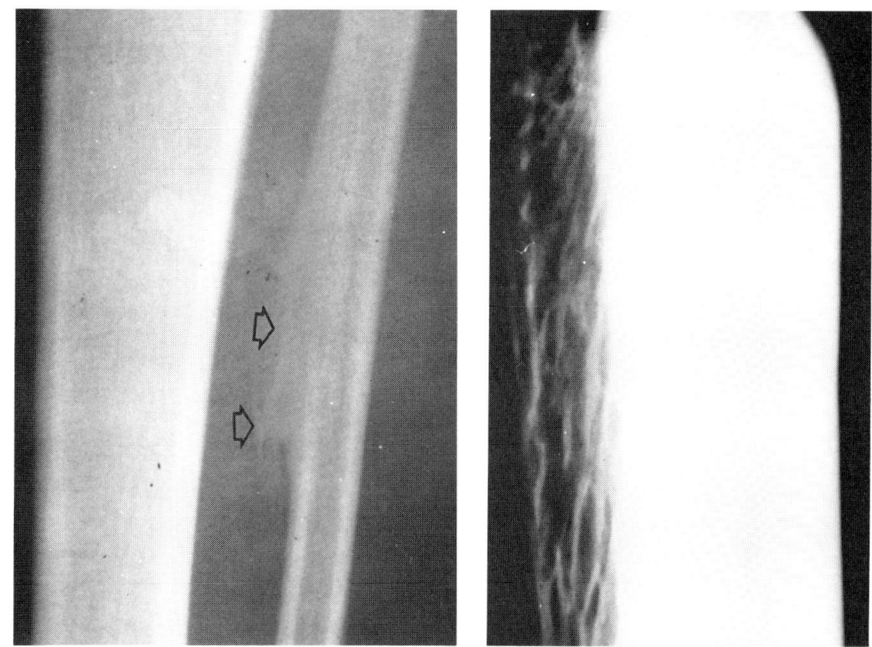

FIG. 14-67

FIG. 14-68

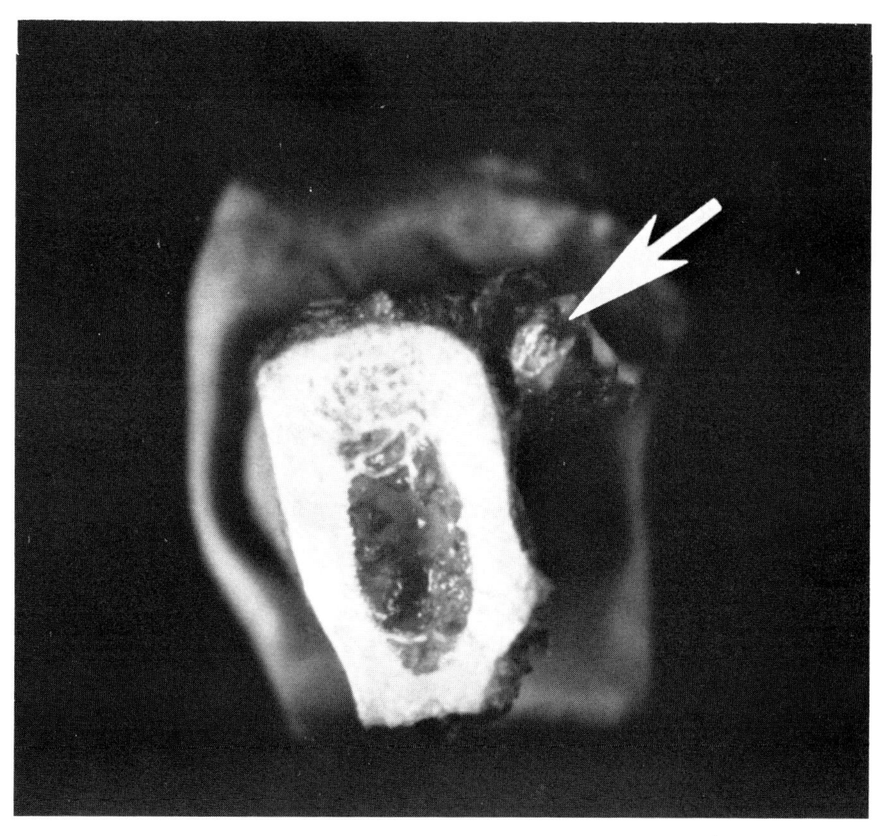

FIG. 14-69

most sarcomatous appearing. Within 8 to 10 weeks, the histology is quite innocent. Because of the admixture of variably exuberant fibrous and/or osseous tissue, the lesions can and have been mistaken for fibro-, chondro-, and osteosarcomas.

This author has seen this disease manifest itself in innumerable clinical and radiologic ways, but the unifying threads are the following:

1. Most patients are either children or physically active adults. The lesions usually occur due to vigorous activity, such as running, jumping, or wrestling.
2. The lesions are usually smaller than 3 to 4 cm. in size.
3. At the time of biopsy most of the lesions usually show a mixture of fairly bland fibrous tissue and/or cartilage, osteoid, woven, and/or lamellar bone.
4. If searched for radiologically, not uncommonly the opposite bone shows a similar lesion (Fig. 14–73). For example, a lesion of the right distal femur may, upon examination of the left femur, show a similar lesion.
5. The lesions do not grow beyond an 8- to 10-week observation period.
6. They are not associated with recurrence unless the vigorous physical activity that gave rise to them is repeated or the lesion is excised before fully ripened.
7. Examples of this lesional complex include the following syndromes:
   a. "Cortical irregularity syndrome" or "periosteal desmoid"
   b. Osgood Schlatter's disease (chronic avulsion injury of the tibial tuberosity, Fig. 14–71).
   c. Larsen-Johansson disease (patellar-ligament avulsion injury, Fig. 14–72).

The most common avulsion injuries that may give rise to ossifying tumors include the following areas. There may be no given syndrome names for these conditions.[71]

1. *Anterior inferior spine of the ilium* at the origin of the rectus femoris muscle. Usually due to kicking a football or cricket bowling.
2. *Ischial apophysis* at the origin of the adductor muscles. Can be seen in hurdlers, fencers, footballers, ballet, and acrobatic dancers.
3. *Lesser trochanter of the femur*
4. *Anterior superior spine of ilium*
5. *Clavico-sternal junction,* seen in wrestlers and weight lifters (Figs. 14–73 and 14–74).

CORTICAL IRREGULARITY SYNDROME

Patients with the "cortical irregularity syndrome" are usually young children or adults who complain of pain in the knee. Radiographs will usually show a distal cortical scalloping irregularity that may or may not be associated with an ossifying mass (Fig. 14–74). Examination of the other knee, if performed, may show a similar lesion. Biopsy can show either pure fibrous tissue or a mixture of fibrous tissue, woven to lamellar bone, cartilage, and, frequently, prominent organized "injury" capillaries (Fig. 14–73, *D*). The surrounding ligamentous or periosteal tissue may show evidence of tearing injury, that is, a reparative fibroplasia. It has also been called the cortical desmoid tumor. This lesion is almost surely due to a tearing of the musculo-ligamentous attachments along the distal linea aspera of the femur, and as such should be classified as an avulsion reparative injury and not as a neoplasm, which the term *periosteal desmoid* implies.

This author has seen truly recurrent large fibrous tumors of the periosteum that are best called desmoid tumors. However, these act and appear to be true neoplasms related to their soft-tissue counterpart,

Traumatic Tendinitis-Ligamentitis Ossificans

FIG. 14–70. Histology confirmed the radiographic appearance that the lesion (*arrow*) was composed of pure lamellar bone and marrow fat. Such lesions represent old injuries: in this case, tearing of the interosseous ligament with reparative ossification (ligamentitis ossificans) (x10).

FIG. 14–71. Note the presence of a triangular ossific mass anterior to the anterior tibial tubercle (*arrow*). This injury lesion is common to basketball players and represents a tearing injury to the ligament inserting into the tibial tubercle. Post-injury ossification may then proceed. A portion of the tibial bone is usually avulsed too, resulting in its necrosis. Until recently, this lesion was mistaken for a primary avascular necrosis of bone.

FIG. 14–72. Note the ossific mass (*arrow*). This is another example of tendinitis ossificans consequent to traumatic tearing of the infrapatellar tendon.

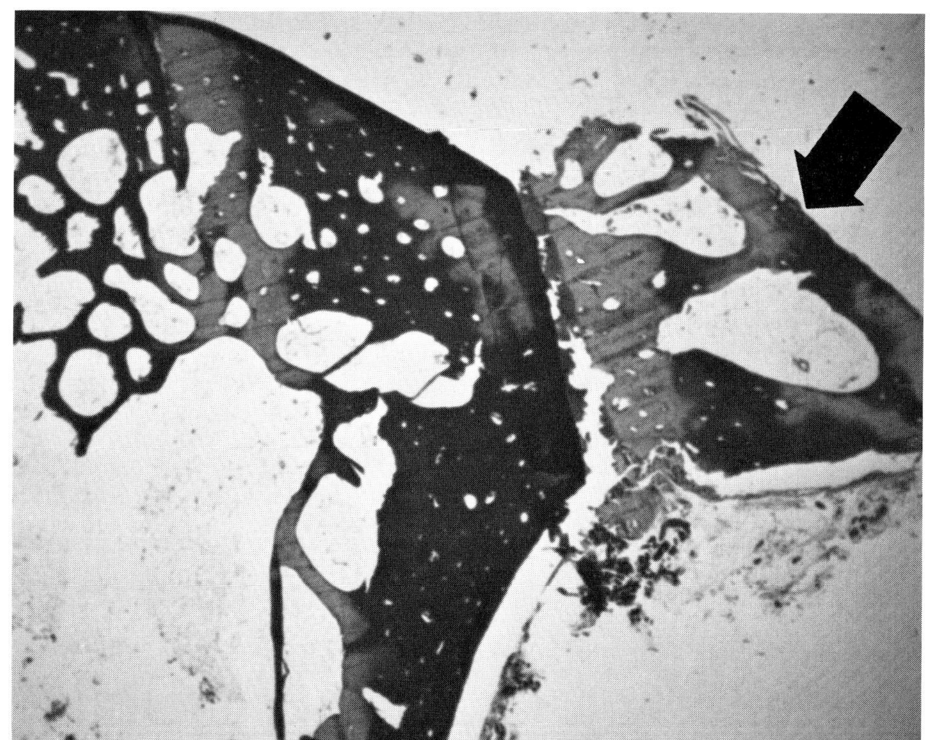

FIG. 14-70

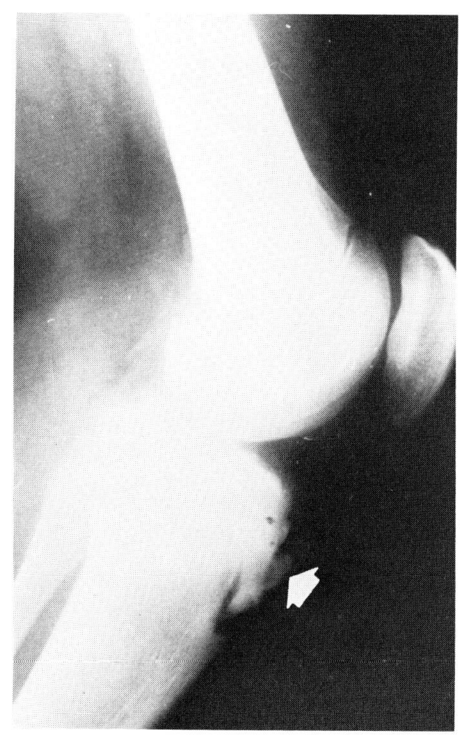

FIG. 14-71

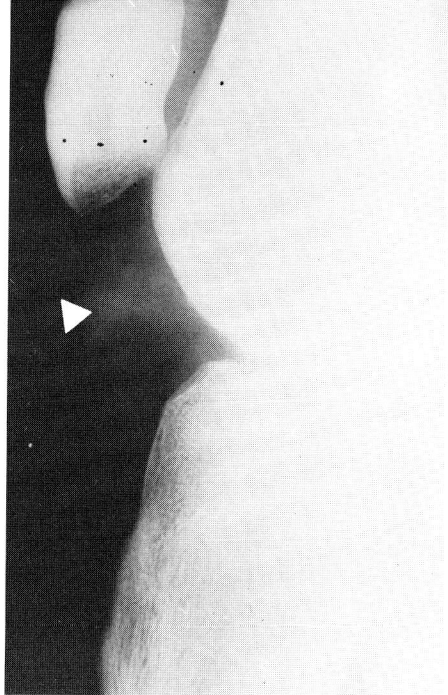

FIG. 14-72

aggressive fibromatosis, and appear to have nothing to do with an injury repair. The neoplastic periosteal desmoid does not produce metaplastic bone or cartilage either (see p. 572 and Figs. 14–86, 14–87, and 14–88 for more detailed discussion). In essence, the term *periosteal desmoid* should be dropped from the literature, if the lesion is ascertained to be due to an avulsion injury. This term should be used only for low-grade neoplastic, continuously growing, possibly very low-grade fibrosarcomatous lesions.

Most of the reported cases of cortical irregularity syndrome pertain to the distal femur (Fig. 14–74); however, this author has seen for consultation an identical avulsion syndrome in a wrestler's clavicle (Fig. 14–73) that was thought to be a possible chondrosarcoma. There is little doubt that the cortical irregularity syndrome is a fibro-osseous response to a ligamentous or tendinous periosteal avulsion injury that should occur in numerous bony sites, of which the distal femur may be the most common, but certainly not the exclusive site.

PERIOSTEAL FIBROMA

This author has seen two cases of a peculiar benign periosteal nodule composed almost purely of fibrous tissue. One patient was a 2-year-old female with a 6-mm. nodule centrally placed in the parietal bone (Figs. 14–78 and 14–79). The histology of the lesion showed a fibrous tissue lesion with some peripheral reactive bone ossification (Figs. 14–80 and 14–81). The child's parents could give no history of trauma. The author diagnosed the lesion as a benign fibroma but could not rule out for certain a small neoplastic desmoid or very low-grade fibrosarcoma. The lesion was sent to the AFIP. Dr. Enzinger has seen eleven similar benign cases, mostly in young children and some with a positive history of trauma (personal communication, observations to be published).

I saw a second, almost identical (4 mm.) lesion 1 month later arising from the internal aspect of the angle of the mandible of an adult female. Suspicious of trauma, the patient was questioned about injury. Two months before she had had a hysterectomy and had developed intense laryngeal spasm when the endotracheal tube had been inserted. Trauma to the internal area of the angle of the mandible could certainly have happened at this time.

Despite simple curettage, both lesions have not recurred with a 2-year follow-up in both cases.

In summary, the characteristics of this lesion are:

1. A small, less than 1 cm. round nodule on radiograph, usually found in a skull bone
2. The nodule may show radiologic or pathologic evidence of a fine rim of peripheral ossification.
3. A history of significant trauma in some cases.
4. Most cases occur in children.
5. Minimal extension into the diploe.
6. No evidence of recurrence despite simple procedures.

I would suspect that exuberant but not frankly anaplastic fibrous lesions greater than 2 cm. in size, with extensive involvement of the diploe space, would more likely be either neoplastic desmoid tumors or low-grade fibrosarcomas. Such lesions should probably be treated by an adequate en-bloc excision. If curetted, they should be followed closely for recurrence. Recurrence most likely proves that in spite of relative histologic innocence, the lesion is a neoplasm and that the appropriate surgical procedure be undertaken.

Traumatic Periostitis-Ligamentitis Ossificans

FIG. 14–73. This patient was referred to me to rule out chondrosarcoma of the right clavicle. (*A*) Note the ominous destructive lesion of the clavicle (*arrow*) and periosteal new bone. Review of the slides showed the following. (*B*) Fibrocartilaginous tissue (*arrow*) and vessels. (*C*) On high-power examination the cartilage was quite cellular (*left*). But note its imperceptible blending with the fibrous tissue to the right, most suggestive of chondroid metaplasia of stimulated or injured mesenchymal fibrous tissue. (*D*) Also suggestive of injury to the capsular tissues was numerous small capillary structures in the fragmented and fibrillated fibrous tissue. These tissues are usually avascular unless torn. (*E*) The remainder of the fibrous tissue showed fibrillation cracks (*arrows*) very similar to degenerated spinal disk tissue; another sign of degenerated or injured fibrocartilaginous tissues. (*F*) The ultimate radiologic clue to the diagnosis of benignancy was found upon reviewing the tomograms. Note that the opposite clavicle also shows a periostitis (*arrows*). The bilateral symmetricity completely negates the possibility of two concomitantly arising chondrosarcomas. Bilateral lesions are not uncommon with twisting injuries, however. This radiologic observation was confirmed by the histologic findings of cartilage metaplasia within injured mesenchyme. Further history was obtained about the patient. He was an active college wrestler!

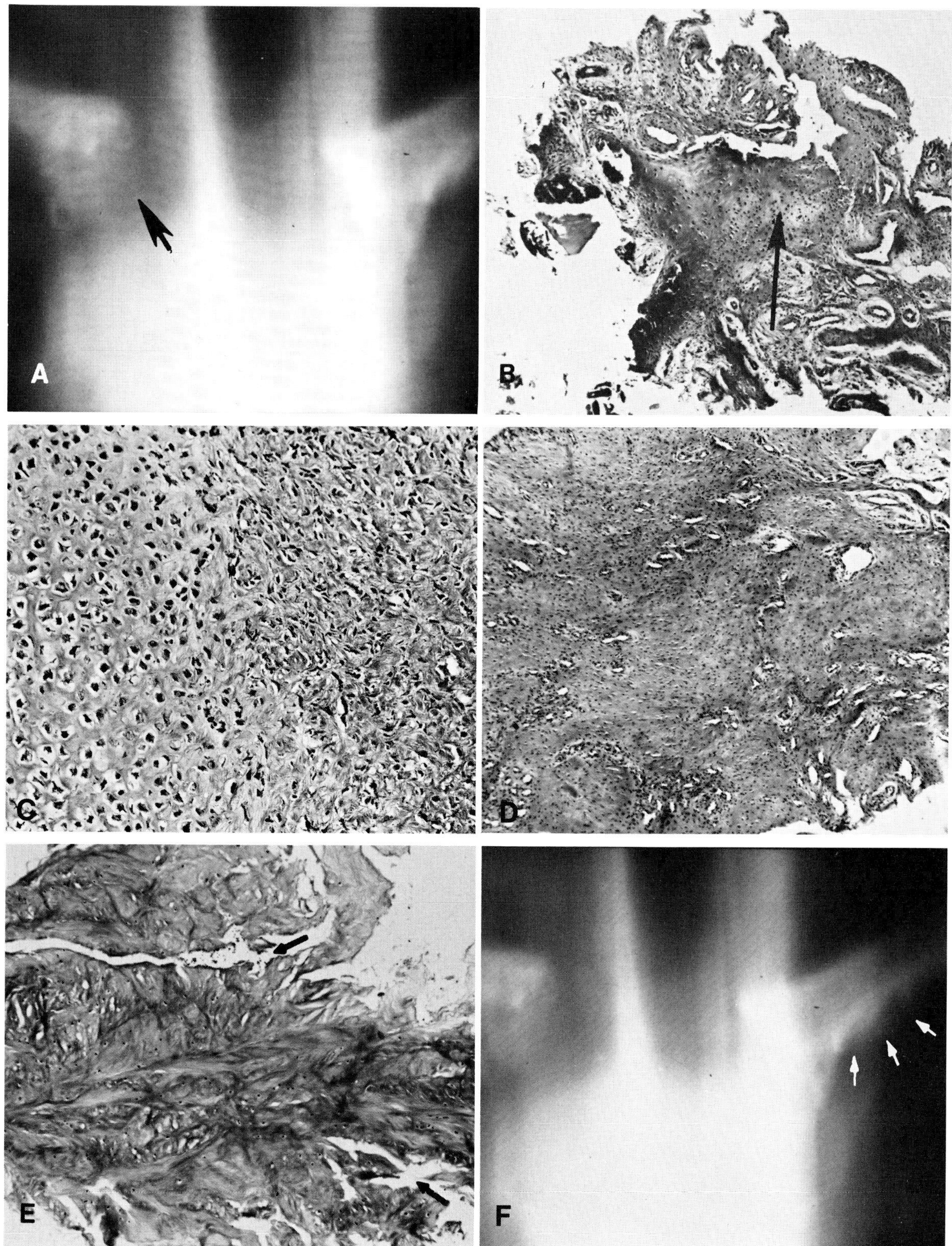

FIG. 14-73

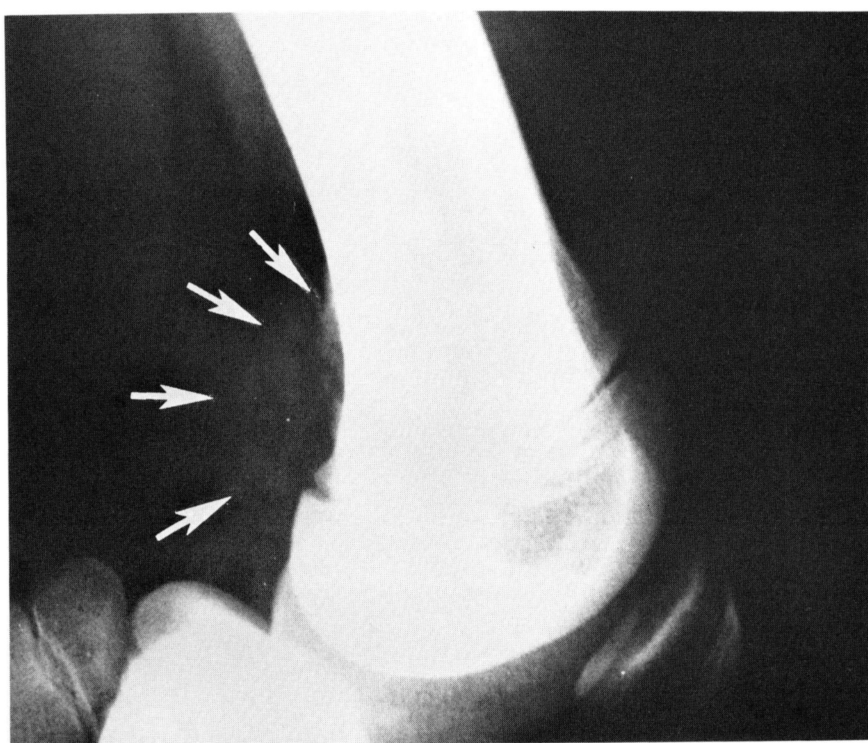

Traumatic Ligamentitis Ossificans (Cortical Irregularity Syndrome)

FIG. 14-74. Note the presence of a posterior femoral ossifying mass (*arrows*). Figs. 14–74 to 14–77 are all from the same patient.)

The fibroma of periosteum may be associated with significant ossification peripherally. As such, it might, perhaps, be called by some an "ossifying fibroma," but, I believe the lesion is basically a fibromatous hyperplasia with secondary reactive, reparative, ossification. The presence of ossification and exuberant fibrous tissue could be mistaken for fibrous dysplasia or parosteal osteosarcoma. However, of the few lesions seen by Dr. Enzinger and myself, they are distinguished by their small size, distinct nodular shape, shallow cortical erosion, relative youth of most patients, and their location in the skull. Perhaps this is so because such small lesions would not be palpable except when they are close to the skin as the skull bones. If it can be shown (as I suspect) that the lesions are consequent to trauma, this entity could represent merely another form of quite localized nodular "traumatic periostitis" with fibrous or fibro-osseous hyperplasia.

PERIOSTEAL OSTEOMATOSIS

This author has seen only one case of a peculiar benign ossifying lesion of the periosteum which could be designated periosteal osteomatosis.

(*Text continues on p. 572.*)

Traumatic Ligamentitis Ossificans (Cortical Irregularity Syndrome)

FIG. 14-75. It was excised and showed a mixture of fibro-osseous and cartilage tissue (x10).

Cortical Irregularity Syndrome

FIG. 14-76. (*A*) Bone is seen at (*1*), cartilage at (*2*), and fibrous tissue at (*3*), (x40). (*B*) Careful examination of the fibrous tissue cartilage junction is highly suggestive of benign chondromatous metaplasia (*1*) of injured fibrous tissue (*2*) (x125).

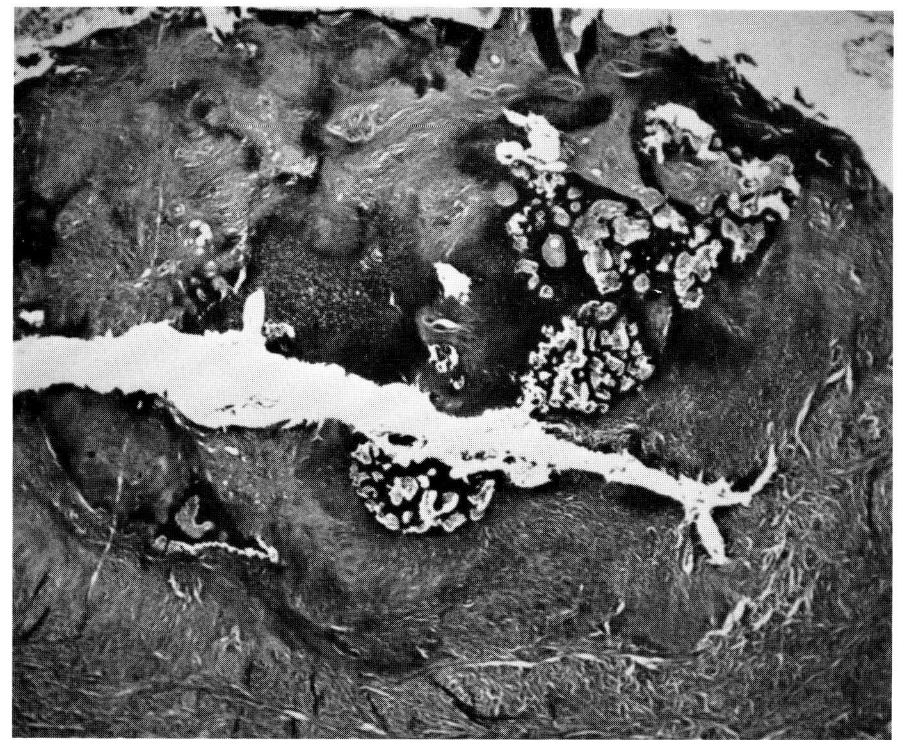

FIG. 14-75

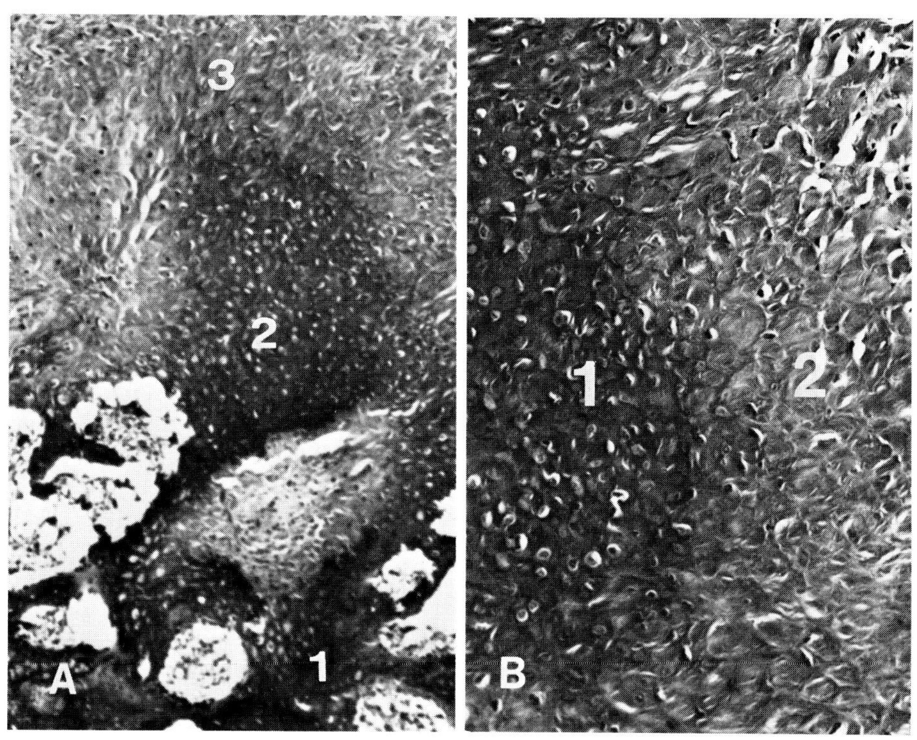

FIG. 14-76

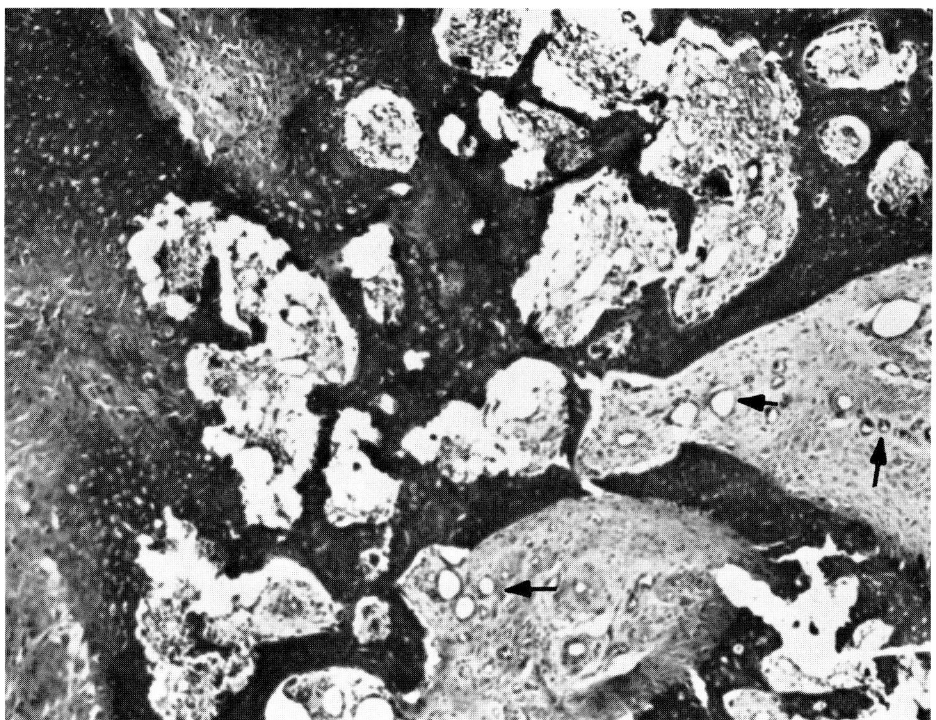

FIG. 14-77

Cortical Irregularity Syndrome

FIG. 14-77. In focal bone areas, numerous small distinct capillaries were seen (*arrows*), again suggestive of injury. The features, therefore, are all consistent with an injury lesion and the diagnosis of posterior cortical irregularity syndrome was then made. In essence, this lesion is the result of tearing of ligaments from the linea aspera, the consequence of which can be fibro-osseous repair. This lesion is, therefore, but another variant of ligamentitis-periostitis ossificans. This injury–repair syndrome is usually seen in runners and children (x40).

Periosteal Fibroma

FIG. 14-78. A 5-year-old child with a single, small, round, lucent lesion in the skull (*arrows*).

FIG. 14-79. Lateral of the skull shows some degree of cortical nibbling, lucency, and a very faint soft-tissue shadow (*arrows*).

FIG. 14-80. The entire lesion was curetted. It was only 6 mm. in its greatest dimension. It arose from within the periosteum and was composed of a mixture of fibrous tissue with numerous long vascular slits (left of field). Surrounding the lesion was reparative fibro-osseous tissue (*arrows*).

FIG. 14-81. On high-power examination, the fibrous tissue was moderately cellular and showed rare mitoses, but no evidence of obvious anaplasia. The diagnosis was periosteal fibroma with reactive osseous metaplasia. Because of the unusual nature of the lesion and the difficulty in excluding a periosteal desmoid neoplasm, it was sent to the A.F.I.P. Dr. Enzinger has seen at least 11 such cases of the skull, all of which have behaved in a benign fashion. Most of his cases were seen in children (personal communication). Two-year follow-up in this patient has been uneventful. The only features that may distinguish this benign lesion from a low-grade fibrous neoplasm may be the peculiar elongated vessels and the small size of the lesion at presentation. I would suspect that the periosteal fibroma is a form of localized injury lesion that results in periosteal fibrous hyperplasia with or without concomitant osseous metaplasia (x250).

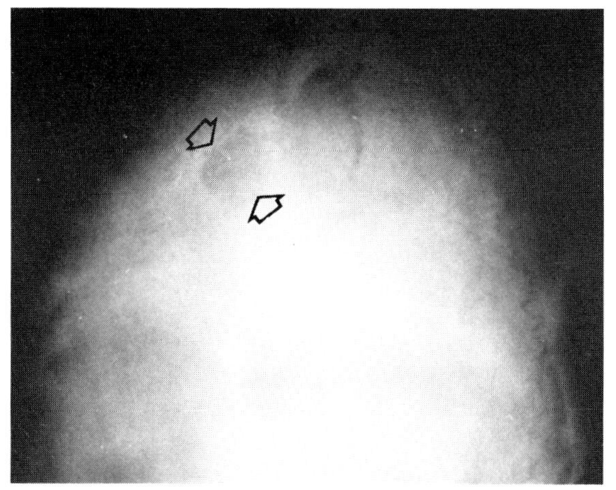

FIG. 14-78

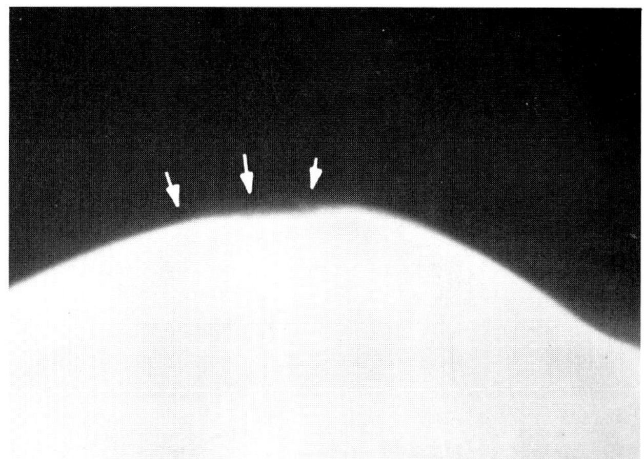

FIG. 14-79

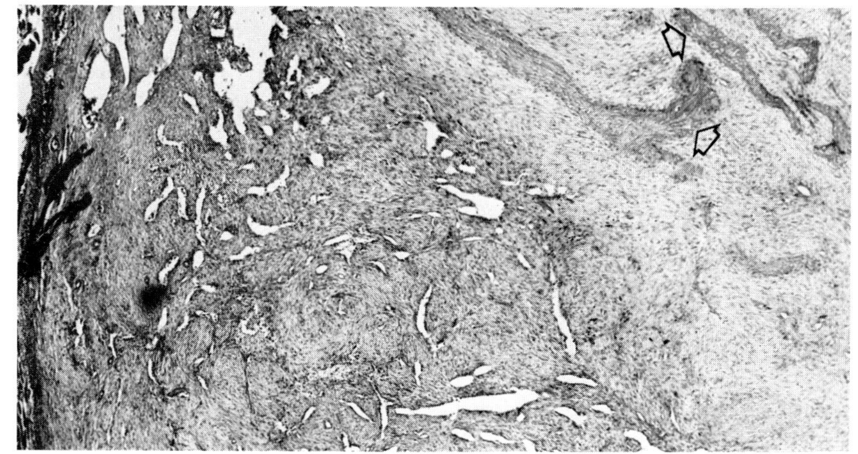

FIG. 14-80

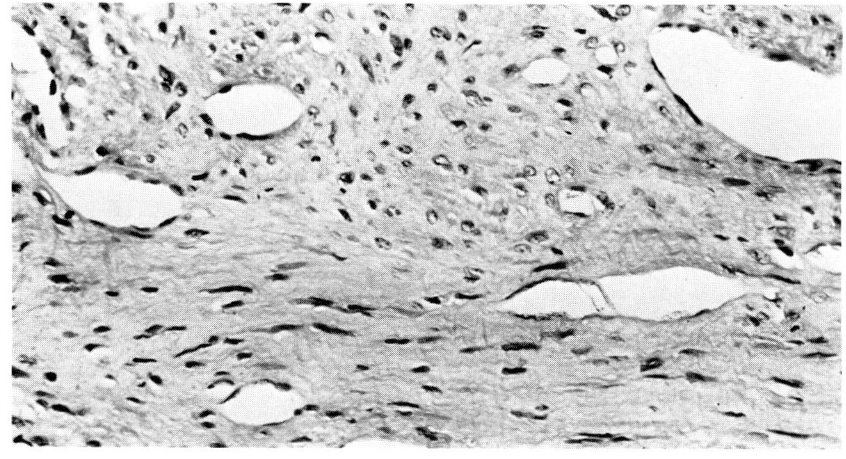

FIG. 14-81

The patient was a young male child who presented with a "lump" on his skull. Radiologically the lesion consisted of an intradermal ossifying mass in juxtaposition to warty, ossifying excrescences of the outer table of the skull (Fig. 14–82). The lesion was excised. A sac of fibrous tissue with numerous fragments of benign lamellar bone was found that corresponded to the intradermal mass. The portion of the skull that was removed showed several benign osteomatous excrescences budding from the periosteal surface of the skull (Fig. 14–83). Specimen radiographs and histology showed them to be composed of completely benign lamellar bone with marrow spaces (Figs. 14–84 and 14–85). The fragments of bone contained within the dermal tissues obviously reached their extraosseous position by fracture of some of the warty skull growths associated with this peculiar entity. These loose fragments eventually became surrounded by fibrous tissue, giving rise to the ominous "lump" seen clinically.

The patient has had no recurrence with 3-year follow-up. In addition, there has been no evidence of Gardner's syndrome (pg. 86) which can be associated with periosteal osteomas.

PERIOSTEAL DESMOID (AGGRESSIVE FIBROMATOSIS)

The term *periosteal desmoid* should be restricted to those rare, periosteal, low-grade neoplasms of nontraumatic origin, characterized histologically by features equivalent to the intramedullary desmoid tumor (Figs. 9–27, 9–28, and 9–29) or to the soft-tissue entity known as aggressive fibromatosis (extra-abdominal desmoid). Radiologically, the periosteal desmoid shows a periosteal or juxtacortical lytic bulge with focal cortical erosion (Fig. 14–86). Grossly, they are very firm and white and have a whorled appearance (Figs. 14–87 and 14–88).

These tumors are characterized by slow but continuous growth and will recur unless resected with a margin of uninvolved tissue. They do not metastasize. This entity must be distinguished from the benign, trauma-related cortical irregularity syndrome, erroneously also called the periosteal desmoid (Figs. 14–72–14–74). The periosteal fibrosarcoma will usually show features of anaplasia and does have the capacity to metastasize.

PERIOSTEAL FIBROSARCOMA AND CHONDROSARCOMAS

The only sure method to diagnose a periosteal fibrosarcoma or chondrosarcoma are those cases that show unequivocal Grade II to III anaplasia (Fig. 14–36). The parosteal chondroma, for example, can show ominous cytology that overlaps with those of Grade I chondrosarcoma (Figs. 14–30 and 14–31). However, these benign lesions will usually be surrounded by a border of reactive host bone sclerosis, the chondrosarcoma will usually not, because it is a progressively growing and destructive tumor.

True neoplastic periosteal desmoids and low-grade fibrosarcomas can be extremely difficult if not impossible to distinguish from the benign periosteal fibroma. All of these lesions bulge from the cortex. The nonossifying fibroma and fibrous cortical defect do not. One must be extremely suspicious of malignancy in any periosteal fibrous tumor that is:

1. Over 2 to 3 cm. in size and bulges from the cortex

Periosteal Osteomatosis

FIG. 14–82. This lesion of skull contained ossified fragments in the dermis and warty excrescences arising from the outer table. Careful radiologic analysis of the bone produced (*A*) shows a definite trabecular pattern consistent with benign lamellar bone. However, because of the ominous appearance of the soft-tissue mass (*B*), the lesion was excised.

FIG. 14–83. Cut section of the skull showing nubbins of benign-looking bone along its surface (*arrows*).

FIG. 14–84. Specimen radiograph clearly shows the benign, trabecular, lamellar bone pattern of the excrescences (*arrow*).

FIG. 14–85. Histology confirmed that the above lesion was composed of mature bony elements (*arrows*) with haversian systems and marrow fat. The position of the lesion is consistent with a primary periosteal lesion, since the diploe were normal. Because of these facts, it was diagnosed as focal periosteal osteomatosis. Some of the bone nubbins apparently fractured away from the main skull lesion and were deposited in the dermal soft tissue, forming the clinically ominous mass at initial presentation. Three years of follow-up has been completely uneventful (x40).

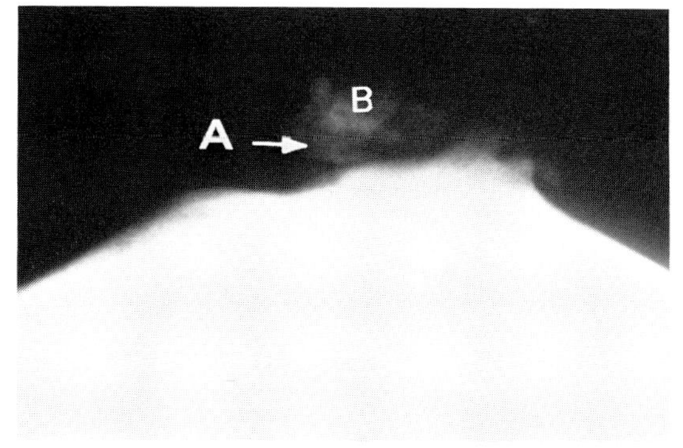

FIG. 14-82

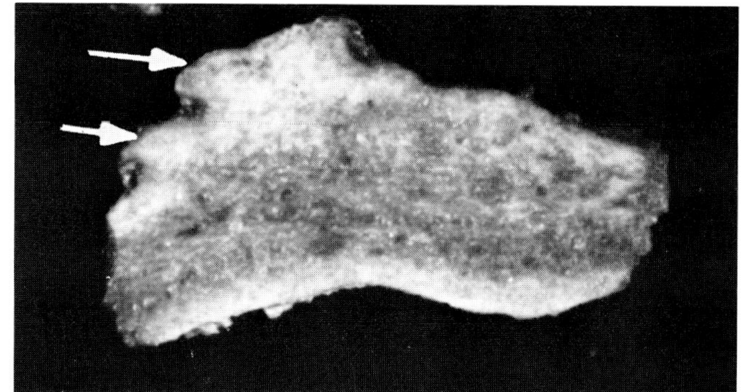

FIG. 14-83

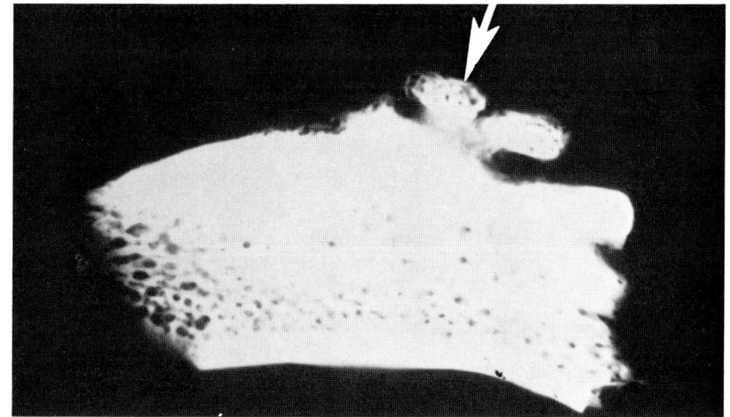

FIG. 14-84

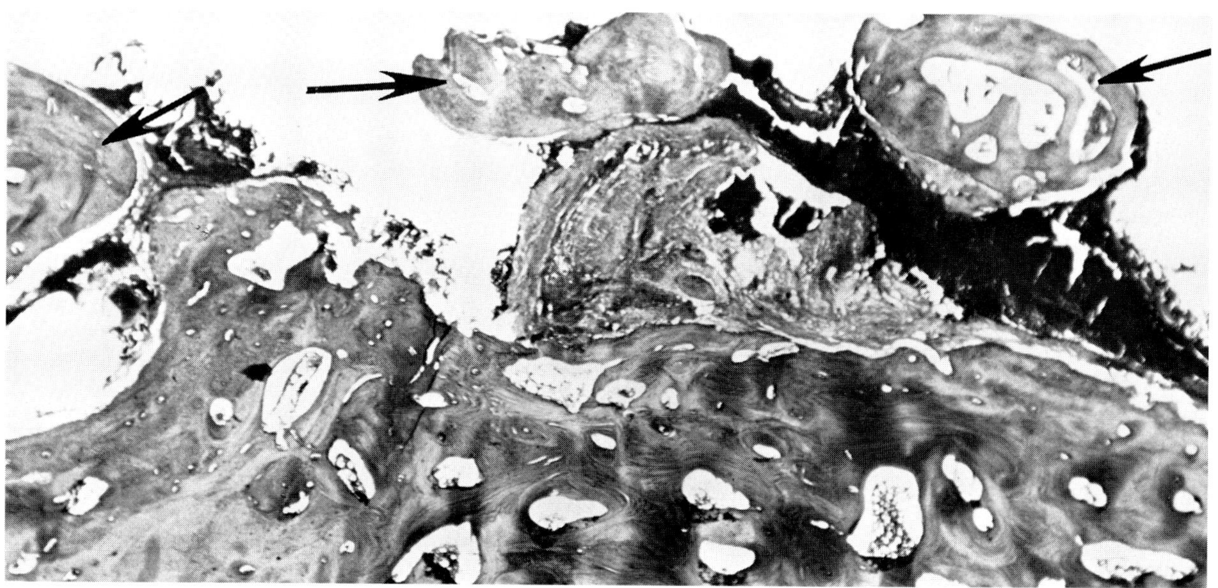

FIG. 14-85

2. Invades the medullary space or extensively into the diploe
3. Has plump nuclei with open chromatin pattern, nucleoli, more than occasional mitoses, and any atypical mitoses
4. Recurs if treated as a benign lesion.

Cases with the above features are probably low-grade malignant growths that should be diagnosed and treated appropriately. For this author, low-grade periosteal fibrosarcomas have been the most difficult of all bone tumors to recognize for what they are. On two occasions I misjudged them as either reparative lesions or aggressive fibromatoses. In both instances the lesions recurred, developing unequivocal and increasing anaplasia with each recurrence and both eventually metastasized and destroyed the patients.

REFERENCES

Osteochondroma

1. D'Ambrosia, R., and Ferguson, A.: The formation of osteochondroma by epiphyseal cartilage transplantation. Clin. Orthop., *61:* 103, 1968.
2. Fairbank, H.: Diaphysial aclasis. J. Bone Joint Surg., *31B:* 105, 1949.
3. Jaffe, H.L.: *Tumors and Tumorous Conditions of the Bones and Joints.* chap. 10. Philadelphia, Lea & Febiger, 1958.
4. Keith, A.: Studies on the anatomical changes which accompany certain growth disorders of the human body. J. Anat., *54:* 101, 1920.
5. Katzman, H., Waugh, T., and Bendon, W.: Skeletal changes following irradiation of childhood tumors. J. Bone Joint Surg., *51A:* 825, 1969.
6. Müller, E.: Uber hereditare multiple cartilagenare exostosen und ecchondrosem. Beitr. 2. Path. Anat. U.Z. Allg. Path., *57:* 232, 1913.
7. Murphy, F.D., Jr., and Blount, W.P.: Cartilagenous exostoses following irradiation. J. Bone Joint Surg., *44A:* 662, 1962.
8. Ollier, L.: Exostoses osteogeniques multiple. Lyon Med., *88:* 484, 1898.
9. Solomon, L.: Hereditary multiple exostosis. Am. J. Hum. Genet., *16:* 351, 1964.
10. Virchow, R.: Ueber multiple exostosen mit. vorlegung von Praparaten. Berl. Klin. Wsch., *28:* 1082, 1891.

10a. von Recklinghausen, F.: Ein fall von multiple exostosen. Virchows Arch., *35:* 203, 1866.

Parosteal Chondroma

11. Adcott, D.L., and Dubsansky, Marvin: Periosteal chondroma. Report of a case. Am. J. Clin. Pathol., *26:* 394, 1956.
12. Cary, G.R.: Juxtacortical chondroma. A case report. J. Bone Joint Surg., *47A:* 1405, 1965.
13. Carroll, R.E.: Glomus tumours of the hand. J. Bone Joint Surg., *54A:* 691, 1972.
14. Feinberg, S.B., and Wilber, M.D.: Periosteal chondroma. Report of two cases. Radiology, *66:* 383, 1956.
15. Cooper, R.R.: Juxtacortical chondrosarcoma. A case report. J. Bone Joint Surg., *47A:* 524, 1965.
16. Fornasier, V.L., and McGonigal, D.: Periosteal chondroma. Clin. Orthop., *124:* 233, 1977.
17. Grayson, A., and Bain, M.: Juxtocortical chondroma of the hyoid arch. Otolaryngol., *86:* 679, 1967.
18. Jaffe, H.L.: Juxtacortical chondroma. Bull. Hosp. Joint Dis., *17:* 20, 1956.
19. Jaffe, H.L.: Tumours and Tumorous Conditions of the Bones and Joints. p. 196. Philadelphia, Lea & Febiger, 1958.
20. Keiller, V. H.: Cartilagenous tumours of bone. Surg. Gynecol. Obstet., *40:* 512, 1925.
21. Kimmelstiel, P.: Cortical defect due to periosteal desmoid. Bull. Hosp. Joint Dis., *12:* 286, 1951.
22. Lichtenstein, Louis: Tumours of periosteal origin. Cancer, *8:* 1060, 1955.
23. Lichtenstein, Louis: Bone Tumours. ed. 2, p. 345. St. Louis, C.V. Mosby, 1965.
24. Lichtenstein, Louis, and Hall, J.: Periosteal chondroma. A distinctive benign cartilage tumour. J. Bone Joint Surg., *34:* 691, 1952.
25. Marmor, L.: Periosteal chondroma. Clin. Orthop., *37:* 150, 1965.
26. Mason, M.L.: Tumours of the hand. Surg. Gynecol. Obstet., *64:* 129, 1937.
27. McWorter, G.L.: Chondromata of the thumb. Surg. Clin. North Am., *4:* 629, 1920.
28. Merlino, A.F., and Nixon, J.E.: Periosteal chondroma. Report of an atypical case and review of the literature. Am. J. Surg., *107:* 773, 1964.

Periosteal Desmoid Tumor

FIG. 14-86. Note the lytic periosteal tumor characterized by a saucer shape.

FIG. 14-87. The tumor was, unfortunately, amputated because of recurrence, despite the diagnosis of periosteal desmoid (aggressive fibromatosis). The lesion is oval and bulges from the cortex.

FIG. 14-88. On cut section, the tumor was very firm, tough, and white, with a distinct, whorled appearance.

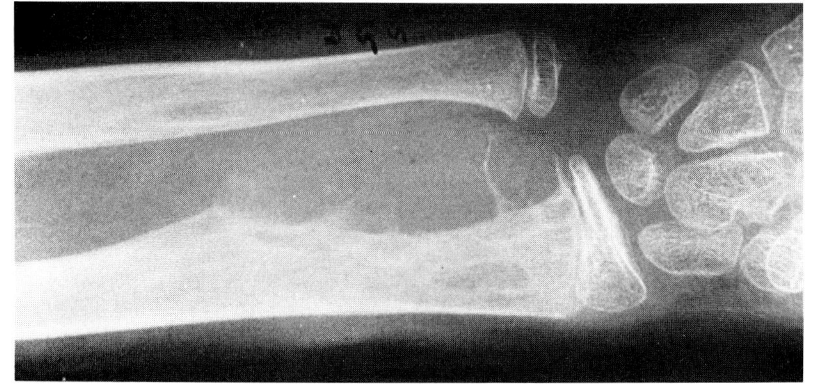

FIG. 14-86

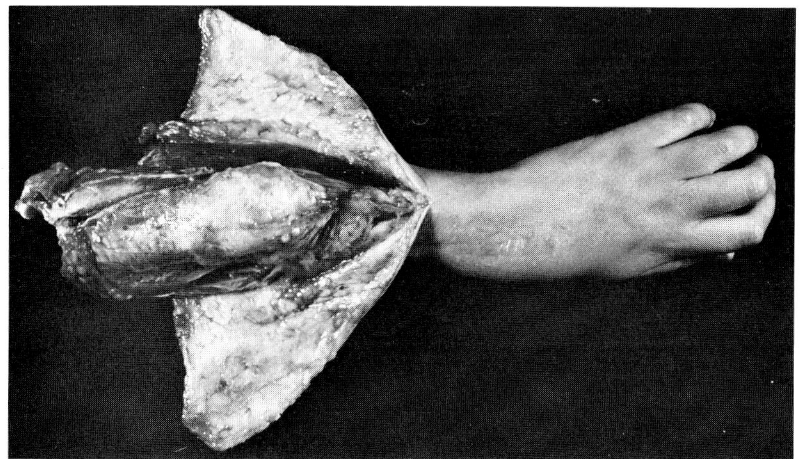

FIG. 14-87

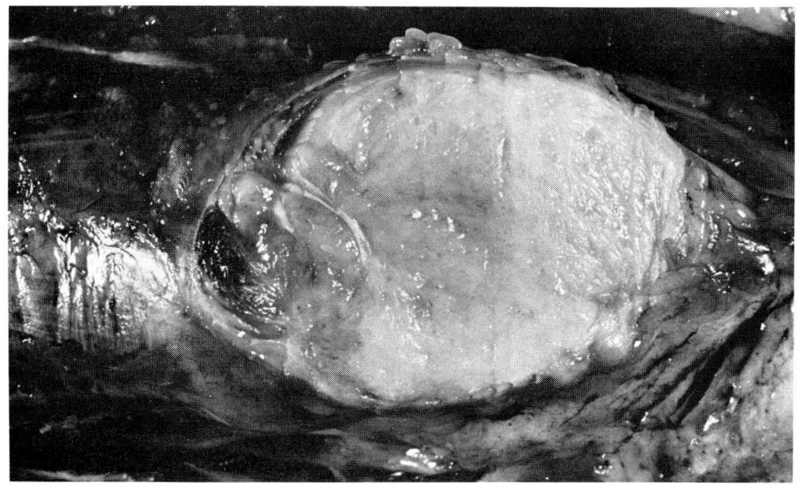

FIG. 14-88

29. Myer, R.: Juxtacortical chondroma. Br. J. Radiol., *31:* 106, 1958.
30. Nosanchuk, J.S., and Kaufer, H.: Recurrent periosteal chondroma. Report of two cases and a review of the literature. J. Bone Joint Surg., *51A:* 375, 1969.
31. Roberts, R.E.: Some observations on osteochondromata. Chondromata and cystic diseases of bone. Br. J. Radiol., *10:* 196, 1937.
32. Rockwell, M.A., *et. al.:* Periosteal chondroma. J. Bone Joint Surg., *54A:* 102, 1972.
33. Scaglietti, O., and Stringa, G.: Periosteal myxoma of infancy and periosteal chondroma of adolescence with local malignancy. Clin. Orthop., *9:* 147, 1957.

Parosteal and Periosteal Osteosarcoma

34. Ahujia, S.C., *et. al.:* Juxtacortical (parosteal) osteogenic sarcoma. J. Bone Joint Surg., *59A:* 632, 1977.
35 Copeland, M.M., and Geschickter, C.F.: The treatment of parosteal osteoma of bone. Surg. Gynecol. Obstet., *108:* 537, 1959.
36. Dwinnel, L.A., Dahlin, D.C., and Ghormley, P.: Parosteal (juxtacortical) osteogenic sarcoma. Am. J. Roentgenol. Radium Ther. Nucl. Med., *111:* 579, 1971.
37. Jacobson, S.A.: Early juxtacortical osteosarcoma (parosteal osteoma). J. Bone Joint Surg., *40A:* 1310, 1958.
38. Jaffe, H.L.: Tumors and Tumorous Conditions of the Bones and Joints. chap. 18. Philadelphia, Lea & Febiger, 1958.
39. Roca, A.N., Smith, J.L., and Jing, B.S.: Osteosarcoma and parosteal osteogenic sarcoma of the maxilla and mandible: study of 20 cases. Am. J. Clin. Pathol., *54:* 625, 1970.
40. Scaglietti, O., and Colandriello, B.: Ossifying parosteal sarcoma. Parosteal osteoma (juxtacortical osteogenic sarcoma). J. Bone Joint Surg., *44A:* 635, 1962.
41. Stevens, G.M., Pugh, D.G., and Dahlin D.C.: Roentgenographic recognition and differentiation of parosteal osteogenic sarcoma. Am. J. Roentgenol. Radium Ther. Nucl. Med., *78:* 1, 1957.
42. Unni, K., Dahlin, D.C., Beabout, J.W., and Ivins, J.C.: Periosteal osteogenic sarcoma. Cancer, *37:* 2476, 1976.
43. Unni, K., *et. al.:* Parosteal osteogenic sarcoma. Cancer, *37:* 2466, 1976.

Ossifying Tumors of the Soft Tissues

44. Ackerman, L.V.: Extraosseous localized non-neoplastic bone and cartilage formation (so-called myositis ossificans). J. Bone Joint Surg., *40A:* 279, 1958.
45. Angervall, L., Stener, B., Stener, I., and Ahren, C.: Pseudomalignant osseous tumor of soft tissue. J. Bone Joint Surg., *51B:* 654, 1969.
46. Chaplin, D.M., and Harrison, M.: Pseudomalignant soft tissue osseous tumor. J. Bone Joint Surg., *54B:* 334, 1972.
47. Coley, W.B.: Myositis ossificans traumatica. *57:* 305, 1913.
48. Fine, G., and Stout, A.P.: Osteogenic sarcoma of the extraskeletal soft tissues. Cancer, *9:* 1027, 1956.
49. Geshickter, C.F., and Maseritz, I.H.: Myositis ossificans. J. Bone Joint Surg., *20:* 661, 1938.
50. Gupta, T., Hajdu, S., and Foote, S.: Extraosseous osteogenic sarcoma. Ann. Surg., *168:* 1011, 1068.
51. Jaffe, H.L.: Tumors and Tumorous Conditions of the Bones and Joints. pp. 521–527. Philadelphia, Lea & Febiger, 1958.
52. Jeffreys, T.E., and Stiles, P.J.: Pseudomalignant osseous tumor of the soft tissue. J. Bone Joint Surg., *48B:* 488, 1966.
53. Kauffman, S.L., and Stout, A.P.: Extraskeletal osteogenic sarcoma and chondrosarcomas in children. Cancer, *16:* 432, 1969.
54. Lagier, R., and Cox, J.: Pseudomalignant myositis ossificans. A pathologic study of 8 cases. Human Pathol., *6:* 653, 1975.
55. Lieberman, U., Barzel, U., and DeVries, A.: Myositis ossificans traumatica with unusual course effect of EDTA on calcium, phosphorous and manganese excretion. Am. J. Med. Sci., *254:* 25, 1967.
56. Pack, G.T., and Braund, R.: The development of sarcoma in myositis ossificans. J.A.M.A., *119:* 776, 1942.
57. Paterson, D.C.: Myositis ossificans circumscripta. Report of 4 cases without history of injury. J. Bone Joint Surg., *52B:* 296, 1976.
58. Ryan, A.J.: Quadriceps strains, rupture and charlie horse. Med. Sci. Sports, *1:* 106, 1969.
59. Shanoff, L.B., Spira, M., and Hardy, S.: Myositis ossificans: evolution to osteosarcoma. Report of a histologically verified case. Am. J. Surg., *113:* 537, 1967.
60. Spjut, H.J., Dorfman, H.D, Fechner, R.E., and Ackerman, L.V.: Tumors of Bone and Cartilage. *In* Atlas of Tumor Pathology. Washington, D.C., A.F.I.P., second series, Fasc. 5., 1971.
61. Umiker, W., and Jaffe, H.L.: Ossifying fibrosarcoma (extraskeletal osteogenic sarcoma) of thigh muscle. Ann. Surg., *124:* 795, 1953.
62. Wilson, H.: Extraskeletal ossifying tumors. Ann. Surg., *113:* 95, 1941.

Avulsive Ligamentous and Tendinous Ossifying Injury Lesions

63. Barnes, G., and Gwinn, J.: Distal irregularities of the femur simulating malignancy. Am. J. Roentgenol. Radium Ther. Nucl. Med., *122:* 180, 1974.
64. Bufkin, W.J.: The avulsive cortical irregularity. Am. J. Roentgenol. Ther. Nucl. Med., *112:* 487, 1971.
65. Codman, E.A.: The Shoulder. Brooklyn, G. Miller and Co. Medical Publishers, Inc., 1934.
66. Codman, E.A.: Rupture of the supraspinatus. Am. J. Surg., *42:* 603, 1938.
67. Hirsh, E.F., and Morgan, R.H.: Causal significance to traumatic ossification of the fibrocartilage in tendon insertions. Arch. Surg., *39:* 824, 1939.

68. Jaffe, H.L.: Tumors and Tumorous Conditions of the Bones and Joints. Philadelphia, Lea & Febiger, 1958.
69. Kimmelstiel, P., and Rapp, K.: Cortical defect due to periosteal desmoids. Bull. Hosp. Joint. Dis., *12:*286, 1951.
70. Levinthal, D.H., and Kaplan, L.: Post-traumatic ossifying, hematoma of the interosseous tibiofibular ligament in the lower leg. Clin. Orthop., *23:*171, 1962.
71. Murray, R.O., and Jacobson, H.G.: The Radiology of Skeletal Disorders. pp. 272–280. Edinburgh, London and New York, J & A Churchill, 1977.
72. Norman, A., and Dorfman, H.D.: Juxtacortical circumscribed myositis ossificans: evolution and radiographic features. Radiology, *2:*301, 1970.
73. Unthoff, H.K.: Calcifying tendinitis: an active cell mediated calcification. Virchows Arch., *366:*51, 1975.

PRINCIPLES AND TECHNIQUES OF TREATMENT

Ralph C. Marcove, M.D., and
Joseph M. Mirra, M.D.

15

INTRODUCTION

Most of the benign tumors are adequately treated by standard and well-known procedures, such as curettage and packing with bone chips, small en-bloc excisions, low-dosage irradiation, and occasionally mild forms of chemotherapy, employing such agents as steroids, antibiotics, and methotrexate. The standard treatments for particular lesions have been alluded to in previous chapters.

In this chapter principles and newer techniques applicable to therapy of primarily the aggressive tumors are discussed. Although some of the techniques discussed in this chapter began two decades ago, many of the major innovations or refinements of technique are less than five years old. The three areas of major technical advance are chemotherapy, cryosurgery, and radical en-bloc resection. For example, the standard treatment of a decade ago resulted in 5-year cure rates of 15 to 20 per cent of patients with osteogenic sarcoma and 5 to 15 per cent for patients with Ewing's sarcoma, despite amputation or high-dosage irradiation. Today these figures are radically different. Some 60 to 75 per cent of patients with these highly malignant tumors now have 5-year actual or projected survival rates from some centers.[55a] It also is becoming increasingly clear that not only do these figures represent a marked increase in survival time, but in apparent complete cure as well. Even if the cure rates for these tumors are shown to be in the range of 50 per cent, this represents a major advance in therapy of malignant bone tumors.

As stated in the introductory chapter, the most important initial step in the treatment of the tumor of the bone is accurate diagnosis. No longer is it just a question of distinguishing benign from malignant: in the light of today's dramatic newer therapies, each tumor type and each patient, for that matter, may require a different approach. No longer are we in the era of "one tumor, one treatment" (usually amputation).

There is no doubt that the principal service-related role of the tumor pathologist should be to correlate the clinical and pathologic findings and arrive at a diagnosis. But should this or must this be his only role? A pathologist can have other service-related roles of importance. The pathologist is, after all, in the best position to analyze the results of therapy on the basis of the adequacy of the margin of safety on radical en-bloc excisions, or amputations. No one is in a better position than he to determine, by documenting the absence of tumor in the margin, whether an en-bloc excision was performed adequately. This, of course, requires considerable care in dissection; techniques of pathological examination has been treated in detail in Chapter 2.

The pathologist is also in the best position to monitor the effects of chemotherapy and/or radiotherapy in order to verify the extent of tumor necrosis. The degree of tumor necrosis may provide extremely important information to the therapists who may wish to base their treatment modalities on this information. Massive necrosis of the tumor prior to surgery appears to be due to the newer therapies. Preliminary studies at this time seem to indicate that such patients may have better survival rates than those with lesser degrees of necrosis. The clinical specialists and pathologist should go over the findings together whenever possible to help determine the treatment plan. It is imperative that the various specialists keep in close communication with one another.

We have now entered a remarkable era in the treatment of bone sarcomas in that increasing numbers of these tumors are being successfully treated without amputation. The number of formerly "inoperable" and so-called "incurable" cases are being reduced by the latest treatments. Not only are survival rates much improved but the quality of life for many survivors is becoming better. However, if these modalities are not performed expertly there could be a return to amputation and a gradual decline in cure rates. A preliminary arteriogram done in two planes (anterior-posterio [AP] lateral) is often helpful in planning the feasibility of an en-bloc resection. Cat scans, too, may be helpful. An arteriogram done several months after en-bloc resection may be the first detectable indication of a local recurrence.

The patient must be told realistically and appreciate that the en-bloc radically resected limb will have certain weaknesses and need bracing; therefore, the pathologist and surgeon must use judgment in deciding how to proceed and whether a resected or artificial limb will function better.

Cryosurgery may also lead to post-operative weaknesses and the need for bracing for several years until the bone regenerates. These facts must be discussed realistically with the patient. It is helpful if the patient can see others with alternative therapy, such as fixed knees or Geupar joints. After performing a biopsy, the clinician should have in mind the definitive future operation as well as an idea of how best to prove the presumptive clinical diagnosis.

A poorly planned surgical incision may make a future en-bloc radical resection impossible, because further surgery may not be able to remove biopsy-contaminated tissue. A biopsy of the upper humerus, for example, may contaminate the neurovascular bundle area (if it is too close) and make an arm-saving Tikhoff-Linberg resection impossible.

Cryosurgery as a preliminary procedure to en-bloc radical resection for an upper femoral lesion may make the latter procedure feasible. Otherwise the tumor may be too close to the hip joint, necessitating hemipelvectomy.

PRINCIPLE OF "TUMOR STERILITY"

In our experience the main cause of short-term failure in local attempts to remove malignant tumors is an inadequate en-bloc margin of excision that allows viable tumor to be spilled into the wound. Deposits of malignant cells in the wound are likely to initiate a recurrence of the tumor. This usually occurs shortly before or after the full course of chemotherapy is completed. Such recurrences can even show greater anaplasia than the original tumor.

Therefore, "sterile" procedures in tumor treatment are essential. We define "tumor sterility" as a condition in which the tumor remains inviolate and untouched, surrounded by a margin of healthy tissue. We must avoid ever entering viable tumor during a local ablative procedure. If the tumor cells spill into the wound, the wound becomes contaminated. If this occurs immediate amputation is our suggested procedure of choice. Any attempt to salvage the limb at this point is likely to fail. Joseph M. Mirra has reviewed four recent cases of so-called benign "enchondromas" of long bones, which in actuality were Grade I chondrosarcomas arising in enchondromas, and has read of a reported patient with a "benign" cyst of the distal radius. The latter, upon analysis of the biopsy material, proved to be a lytic osteosarcoma. The surgeons in these five cases curetted the lesions and, without changing their instruments, removed bone chips from the pelvis for packing. In four of these five cases inoperable sarcomas developed in the very area from which the bone chips were removed. In one of the low-grade chondrosarcoma cases the elapsed time since treatment has only been 2 months, too early to tell whether or not transplant recurrence will take place. Because of the history of probable contamination and likelihood of recurrence in the pelvic area, where the chips were taken from, the area was frozen and the wound tissue removed en-bloc. The principle is therefore clear: violation of tumor sterility may be disastrous.

In order to achieve tumor sterility we would suggest the following:

1. *Obtain the bone chips or host donor graft bone prior to treating a "benign" lesion or use a totally different set of instruments. Do not assume, without pathological confirmation, that a "benign" clinical lesion is indeed benign. Occasionally one*

is malignant or is a benign lesion with a focus of malignant transformation. The surgeon should, therefore, be prepared to use proper surgical technique at all times.

2. *If an en-bloc resection is to be performed for a malignant tumor, the previous biopsy site and surrounding wound tissue should be removed as well since these sites can contain microfoci of viable tumor cells.*
3. *Great care must be taken in planning the extent of resection to obtain a truly adequate procedure.*

The following suggestions should help minimize the dangers of an inadequate resection:

1. Obtain tomograms, bone scans, CAT scans, and AP and lateral arteriograms to best visualize the actual extent of the tumor. Standard radiographs used alone to determine the extent of the cut can be deceptive.
2. Palpate for the tumor. Do not approach the tumor too closely with your instruments.
3. If one is not sure whether the soft tissue adjacent to a vital nerve and/or vascular structure contains viable tumor tissue, the local site can be frozen first. After thawing, the neurovascular bundle can be freed and the suspicious tissue then safely cut with the scalpel and removed en-bloc. In Dr. Marcove's experience the frozen nerve will eventually regain function, although it may take as long as 2 years in very long nerves such as the sciatic. The vessels will thaw within minutes after freezing, circulation will be restored, and later they will become reendothelialized. In over 800 cryosurgery operations, Dr. Marcove has never encountered a permanent nerve palsy, gangrene due to vessel thrombosus, or a rupture of a major vessel either during the operation or after.

FACTORS THAT DETERMINE THE MODE(S) OF TREATMENT

In the past decade, advances in the treatment of malignancies in many organ systems, including bone, have been significant. Although combined multimodality therapy (chemotherapy, radiotherapy, en-bloc excision, cryosurgery) is still in the formative stage and to some extent still experimental, they appear to hold great promise for the future. In many large tumor treatment centers amputation and/or high-dosage irradiation alone is no longer the desirable initial form of therapy. The factors that determine the mode(s) of therapy or the tailoring of treatment to individual patient needs include the following:

The Known Biological Behavior of the Tumor

Benign, low-grade, highly malignant tumors all require radically different therapeutic approaches.

BENIGN. They may be treated by curettage with or without packing, small en-bloc excisions, cryosurgery, and low-dosage irradiation.

LOW-GRADE MALIGNANCIES. These are treated either by more extensive en-bloc excisions, including a margin of healthy tissue, higher doses of radiation, or cryosurgery. Amputation is usually avoided.

HIGH-GRADE MALIGNANCIES. These may be treated by chemotherapy, high-dose irradiation, radical en-bloc excision or a combination of these techniques versus amputation.

The Specific Histogenetic Tumor Type

Each tumor type responds with variable sensitivity to chemo- and/or radiotherapy. The known differences in spread of a particular tumor will also modify the treatment approach used. For example, osteosarcoma almost always spreads in the bone along a fairly well-defined front, while Ewing's and other round cell sarcomas spread through the bone more diffusely. If local ablative procedures are to be used, these factors must be taken into account. The science of chemotherapy concerns itself with that agent or combination of agents that will produce the greatest destruction or tumor cells without seriously affecting the normal tissues. These effects depend upon such differences as those in metabolism and division rates between the tumor and normal cells.

The Size and Extent of the Tumor

If local ablation is contemplated, large, malignant intraosseous tumors or tumors with soft-tissue extension and nerve and/or vascular involvement require more highly specialized procedures compared to smaller tumors confined to bone. If too extensive, amputation may be unavoidable. On the other hand, even certain, very extensive malignancies can today be treated by removal of the entire bone and a block of surrounding soft tissues, provided that the tumor can be completely contained by such a procedure. The removed host tissues can be replaced by man-made appliances such as the total metal femur and the total knee.

The Effect of Preoperative Chemotherapy and/or Radiotherapy Upon the Tumor

On an experimental basis, several large centers are now employing these therapies to shrink and necrose malignancies, to salvage limbs, improve survival, and hopefully effect complete long-term cure. Obviously these effects depend upon the sensitivity of the neoplasm to these tumorstatic and tumoricidal therapies. The long-term success of these procedures will depend on the expertise with which the chemotherapy, excision and/or cryosurgery is performed. If an en-bloc resection is performed in which viable malignant tumor is transected, the wound will become contaminated.

Specific Location of the Tumor

Localized diaphyseal tumors may be easier to ablate and still preserve good function, compared to those that involve the metaphysis or epiphysis. Lesions of the skull, spine, sacrum, and pelvis are the most difficult to cure because of their proximity to vital neural structures.

Demonstrable Metastases

The demonstration of metastases prior to or after therapy usually modifies the therapist's approach to the tumor. However, pulmonary-wedge resections, preceded and followed by chemo- and/or radiotherapy, in combination with total ablation of the local bone tumor has resulted in cure.

Particular Preferences of the Therapists

Unless a specific method of treatment can be shown to be clearly or statistically superior to all others, it is obvious that a particular mode of therapy will often depend upon the individual preferences of the therapists involved.

EN-BLOC RESECTION

DEFINITION. An en-bloc resection refers to the removal of a complete bloc of tissue from the host. For malignant tumors of the bone, the entire tumor, a cuff of surrounding muscle, fascia, and, if necessary, nerves and vessels are removed. Viable tumor must not be transected during the procedure. Since tumor cells frequently penetrate the pseudocapsule, it should never be visible or penetrated at any time during the procedure.

AIMS OF PROCEDURE. The aim of the procedure is to remove the entire malignancy without violating the principle of tumor sterility. If this principle is adhered to, the en-bloc resection can be said to be "adequate;" if not, it is an "inadequate" procedure. In special instances the tumor is too large to be removed en-bloc. However, preliminary chemo- and/or radiotherapy can sufficiently shrink and necrose the tumor to permit an adequate resection. Such operations have been successful with Ewing's tumor, for example. Much is to be learned about en-bloc resections from cases of Grade I to Grade II juxtacortical osteosarcomas from Memorial Hospital over the past 30 years. Even after multiple recurrences and finally amputation, the cure rate was still 95 per cent, including those years in which no pulmonary-wedge resections were done for metastasis. Perhaps even a higher cure rate would have resulted had pulmonary-wedge resections been performed. However, even in this low-grade neoplastic situation the rate of cure at the local site without amputation was very low. Only 7 per cent of en-bloc resections resulted in permanent local cure. This proves that if en-bloc resections are to be of value, they must never violate the tumor, that is, they must be performed without exposing the pseudocapsule, even in the most low-grade malignancies. Certainly, if such a low-grade malignancy cannot be cured by "en-bloc" surgery (conservative surgery), how can much more anaplastic lesions be cured? En-bloc surgery should not be undertaken by a relatively inexperienced surgeon. If the decision is to perform an en-bloc excision, it must be more radical than previously practiced. *Radical en-bloc excision means staying away from the tumor and cutting only through normal, healthy, or adequately cryonecrosed tissue at all times. Mistakes in technique can be fatal. The surgeon should never expose the pseudocapsule of the tumor.*

A thorough pathologic study of the specimen is mandatory (see Chap. 2). If viable or unfrozen tumor is detected in a surgical margin in a malignant situation, the limb should probably be amputated as soon as possible. At this point washing off the wound to remove tumor cells will probably be insufficient to prevent recurrence.

ADVANTAGES. En-bloc excisions allow the surgeon to completely ablate low- and high-grade malignant neoplasms in order to salvage limb; to remove aggressive benign bone tumors if the involved bone is not of particular structural importance, such as portions of rib or fibula; and to remove particularly bulky or locally aggressive benign tumors.

DISADVANTAGES. Removal of block segments of bone and/or muscle tissue can result in obvious decrease of function, particularly if large nerves and vascular structures of large masses of muscle have to be sacrificed. Lesions of distal bone ends usually require the insertion of metal prostheses, cadaver grafts, or fusion across joints using long bone stuts with or without long nails. Their obvious consequences include stiffness, fracture, possible permanent nerve damage, and infection. These complications may eventually result in amputation because the limb becomes more of a disadvantage to the patient than an advantage. Also, viable tumor cells can spill into the wound.

Specific Applications of En-Bloc Resection

Giant Cell Tumor

Although curettage is occasionally advocated as a definitive treatment, the success rate in any well studied large series is only about 50 per cent. This is because of the extreme penetration of the tumor cells to the articular cartilage as well as to subperiosteal infiltration. En-bloc resections with either a fusion or prosthetic replacement results in an abnormal gait and difficulties with either flexibility or stability, the latter necessitating permanent bracing. En-bloc resections, if performed inadequately, can lead to recurrence. Cryosurgery, on the other hand, necessitates only temporary bracing during the healing phase because it preserves joint function and is therefore our preferred method. Both the local recurrence rate, the malignant transformation rate, and the metastatic rate are all favorably influenced by this procedure. Cryotherapy, properly performed, is the most curative and least debilitating procedure. Occasionally, however, amputation may become a necessity. Jaffe's metastatic rate of 15 per cent in a large number of his cases studied over a period of years was reduced to fewer than 1.5 per cent in Marcove's long-term study of 52 consecutive cases.[72]

Cartilaginous Tumors of the Ribs

From 335 malignant and 94 benign cartilage tumors, 27 were chondrosarcomas of the ribs and eight were benign osteochondromas, enchondromas, or parosteal chondromas.[33a] The average age of the patients with chondrosarcoma of the ribs was 42, and those with benign lesions, 25. From this study it was ascertained that patients with chondrosarcoma of the ribs require local excision that includes an en-bloc resection of at least one normal rib above and below the tumor and adjacent pleura. In four cases where the lesions were greater than 4 cm., even when malignancy was not confirmed by the pathologist, all eventually resulted in prompt local recurrence and even death where local surgery was performed without adequate margin. Therefore, in all cases of central cartilaginous tumors of the ribs that are over 4 cm. in size should be treated as malignant since the histologic criteria of malignancy may be too subtle to identify.

All cases smaller than 4 cm. in size were cured by simple local excision. The affected portion of the rib was removed and the pleura simply stripped. In these cases this procedure was an effective cure, even though it would be insufficient for a true malignancy. Therefore, we feel justified in designating lesions larger than 4 cm. even with "benign" histology as borderline or probable chondrosarcoma. Another diagnostic aid was the presence of pain or tenderness in $\frac{1}{3}$ of the chondrosarcoma patients. These signs were not present in the benign lesions.

Osteogenic Sarcoma

The following principles of en-bloc resection for osteosarcoma in different sites are abstracted from an article by Marcove, *et al.*[33]

Preservation of a limb without sacrificing the principle of tumor sterility is a desirable goal when working with young people with osteosarcoma. Usually, for a tumor close to a joint (a metaphyseal lesion that has broken through at the cortex), en-bloc resection should include excision of a part of the adjacent bone as well as wide removal of the joint itself to encompass potential capsular and intrasynovial spread. Preliminary observations on metaphyseal osteosarcomas show spread to capsule and joint in about 30 per cent of cases (direct observation of Dr. Mirra). The distal femur lesion, which has the lowest cure rates, may require removal of the entire bone.

MATERIALS AND METHODS. All patients had a complete history, physical, and laboratory examination. Standard AP and lateral radiographs of the involved bone, skeletal survey, biplane arteriography of the lesion, and chest tomography are performed prior to surgery. The data were used to evaluate size, location, and resectability of the tumor and soft-tissue components as well as the presence of clinically evident metastatic disease or "skip" areas. The objectives and potential risks of the protocol were carefully explained to the patients and their parents. The presence of lung metastases was not a contraindication to local bone tumor en-bloc excision, provided that the lung metastases appeared surgically resectable.

Distal Femur Lesions (Marcove Total Femur Operation)

After the initial workup is completed, construction of the total metal femur with total knee prosthesis begins (Fig. 15–1, *A* and *C*). This takes about 8 weeks to manufacture.[35] During this time the patient is maintained on the chemotherapeutic regimen considered most effective at the time. After the prosthesis is ready, the patient is reevaluated and if the protocol criteria are still valid, the replacement is performed. After sufficient post-operative wound healing, systemic chemotherapy is restarted for several cycles. Immediately after surgery the patient is placed in a long-leg ischial weight-bearing brace with a pelvic band and started on active range-of-motion and ambulation, as the clinical situation allows. The band is removed in about 6 weeks.

OPERATIVE TECHNIQUE. A lateral biopsy is used in previously untreated cases and usually becomes the proposed site of surgical incision. Through a long Gibson skin incision, posterior and anterior approaches are made into the hip on the affected side. The incision is carried along the greater trochanter to the lateral aspect of the femur distal to the knee and then curved slightly anteriorly over the proximal lateral tibia. It extends to 4 cm. distal to the tibial tubercle. The previous biopsy scar and tract are included in the surgical resection. The incision is carried through layers and as the resection approaches tumor, ample margin is left on the femur so that neither the tumor nor its pseudocapsule is seen. Careful palpation for tumor through the uninvolved layers is continued throughout this procedure. If pseudocapsule is seen, the principle of tumor sterility has been violated and an amputation is performed, taking care not to spread tumor cells to the amputation stump site by stopping the operation and sterilizing the proposed amputation site and, of course, by changing to a completely new set of instruments. (This had to be done in one case.)

If the principle of tumor sterility has not been violated, the operation proceeds as planned. The knee is removed en-bloc with the distal femur. The patella tendon is maintained intact and the patella is split in a coronal plane so that its inner half stays with the specimen and the outer half maintains its continuity with the remaining quadriceps mechanism. The tibia is reamed to accept the stem of the total knee prosthesis, and acrylic is placed in the tibia after trial reduction of the prosthesis. The glutei are attached with heavy silk through preformed holes in the prosthetic shaft proximally, and the medial and lateral thigh musculature are attached to each other (Fig. 15–1, *C*). We often transfer the distal hamstrings anteriorly to act as knee extensors and to help form a decent layer of tissue below the skin incision. The wound is checked for hemostasis and closure with hemovacs is performed. The patients receive prophylactic antibiotics preoperatively and postoperatively. The wound is also flushed with antibiotics during and immediately following surgery. The legs are elevated postoperatively. The en-bloc resection specimen is examined by the pathologist to ensure that no viable tumor extended the margins (Fig. 15–1, *D*).

RESULTS. Of 26 patients who started on the protocol, five had to undergo amputations because of excessive tumor size, which was based on the analysis of the preoperative workup. Only one patient required amputation at the time of the planned en-bloc total femur replacement procedure because of visualization of the tumor pseudocapsule.

Of the remaining 20 patients followed from 2 to 35 months, 65 per cent are alive and disease-free and one is alive with disease. Of three patients admitted with pulmonary lesions, one is alive and without disease 2 years after the replacement. The other two died between 21 and 30 months later. Of six patients who received therapy for the development of metastases postoperatively, 50 per cent are alive without disease. Seven patients required amputation: three for infection, two for local recurrence, one for prosthesis breakage, and one for radiation necrosis. These results compared most favorably against the 2 year survival rates (20%) of osteogenic sarcoma of the distal femur, in which the whole bone is removed, versus the subtrochanteric amputation (8% survivors) without other therapy.[35]

Shoulder Girdle Lesions (Tikhoff-Linberg Procedure)

The Tikhoff-Linberg procedure (en-bloc upper humeral interscapulo-thoracic resection) is an alternative to amputation for neoplasms of the shoulder girdle.[4,13,26,30,31,33,44,55]

OPERATIVE TECHNIQUE. The initial incision is made over the two-thirds of the clavicle and then extended from the region of the coracoid distally along the medial side of the arm overlying the neurovascular bundle. Posteriorly the incision is extended longitudinally in the mid-scapular region. The incision is altered so that the biopsy scar and tract are taken along with the specimen. If the neurovascular bundle appears clearly free of tumor, then the mobilization of the bundles can proceed. The musculocutaneous and radial nerves are identified and usually preserved. However, if the tumor is in dangerous proximity to important nerve and vascular structures, they may have to be sacrificed unless cryosurgery of the area can be used to salvage them. The posterior skin incision originates over the lateral one-third of the clavicle line and is carried posteriorly and longitudinally along the midscapula to the angle of the scapula. The inferior angle of the scapula is mobilized and the entire vertebral border is resected from the chest wall much the same as the plane developed in the forequarter amputation.

For tumors of the scapula care must be taken to maintain an adequately wide soft-tissue margin. In upper humeral lesions, the skin flap from the initial incision is raised over the proximal humerus, leaving the deltoid intact with the specimen. When a large bloc of humerus is removed, excessive shortening can be avoided and better flexor elbow power provided by a humeral prothesis or Küntscher nail replacement fixated into the proximal soft tissue or clavicle stump. Some patients are more comfortable if a greater residual amount of clavicle is removed and if nail fixation is into the soft tissue. Hemovacs are then placed and the wound is closed. A postoperative sling and swathe or Velpeau dressing is applied. Hand and elbow motion is encouraged postoperatively.

RESULTS (SEE FIGS. 15-2 AND 15-3). Of the 37 Tikhoff-Linberg procedures performed by this author, eleven were for osteosarcoma. The other cases included chondrosarcomas, renal cell carcinoma, fibrosarcoma, and malignant fibrous histiocytoma. Follow-up has been from 2 to 37 months. Some 63 per cent of the patients are alive and well and show no evidence of disease. Only five patients in this group had chemotherapy and all are free of disease, including one patient who had three thoracotomies for lung metastases.

The wrist and hand functions were normal in this group. In those with radial nerve palsy, a cock-up splint was used and tendon transfers were done 2 years later. A small amount of shoulder padding usually corrects the surgical deformity when wearing clothes.

Proximal Tibia Lesions[33]

The initial workup to determine resectability is similar to that described for en-bloc resection protocol of the distal femur. After the en-bloc resection and total long-stem knee replacement, patients begin receiving chemotherapy.[21,33,50,51]

OPERATIVE TECHNIQUE. A posterior medial incision is made and the neurovascular bundle identified. The anterior tibial artery as well as the interosseous perforating vessels are ligated at the posterior tibial vessel. The popliteal fossa vessels are also ligated, preserving the main stem. The fibula is removed en-bloc with the upper tibia (for tumor in the latter) because of its proximity. The total proximal tibia and distal femur is also removed en-bloc, keeping a margin of normal tissue planes around the tumor. Care is taken to preserve cutaneous nerves. If tumor has grown into the skin or subcutaneous tissue, it must, of course, also be taken. The long-term Guepar knee (with solid shafts) is cemented into the residual distal tibia and proximal femur (Fig. 15–4).

RESULTS. Eleven patients were treated with a follow-up of 4 to 23 months. Some 72 per cent never showed evidence of distant disease. Two are alive with disease and one has died. One patient requested amputation because of excessive foot numbness (too many cutaneous nerves had been sacrificed).

Fibula Lesion

HISTORY. A 15-year-old girl showed radiographic evidence consistent with an osteogenic sarcoma of the

(*Text continues on p. 588.*)

Marcove Total Femur Operation for Osteosarcoma

FIG. 15-1. *A–D.* The Total femur operation. (*A*) The Marcove total metal femur with Guepar total hinge knee prosthesis. (*B*) An extensive osteosarcoma of the distal femur for which a total femur operation was considered necessary. (*C*) Operative view post-en-bloc resection of entire femur and upper tibia with a cuff of normal tissue. The total femur is in place. (*D*) View of the cut section of en-bloc resection. Note that the distal tibia, joint, and the mass of muscle that forms a cuff of normal tissue are taken en-bloc. For an en-bloc resection to be adequate for a malignant tumor, it must be so radical that tumor is never seen during operation or by pathologic examination at any margin. Perhaps in the future the en-bloc excision can be combined with cryosurgery to kill tumor at particularly hazardous margins.

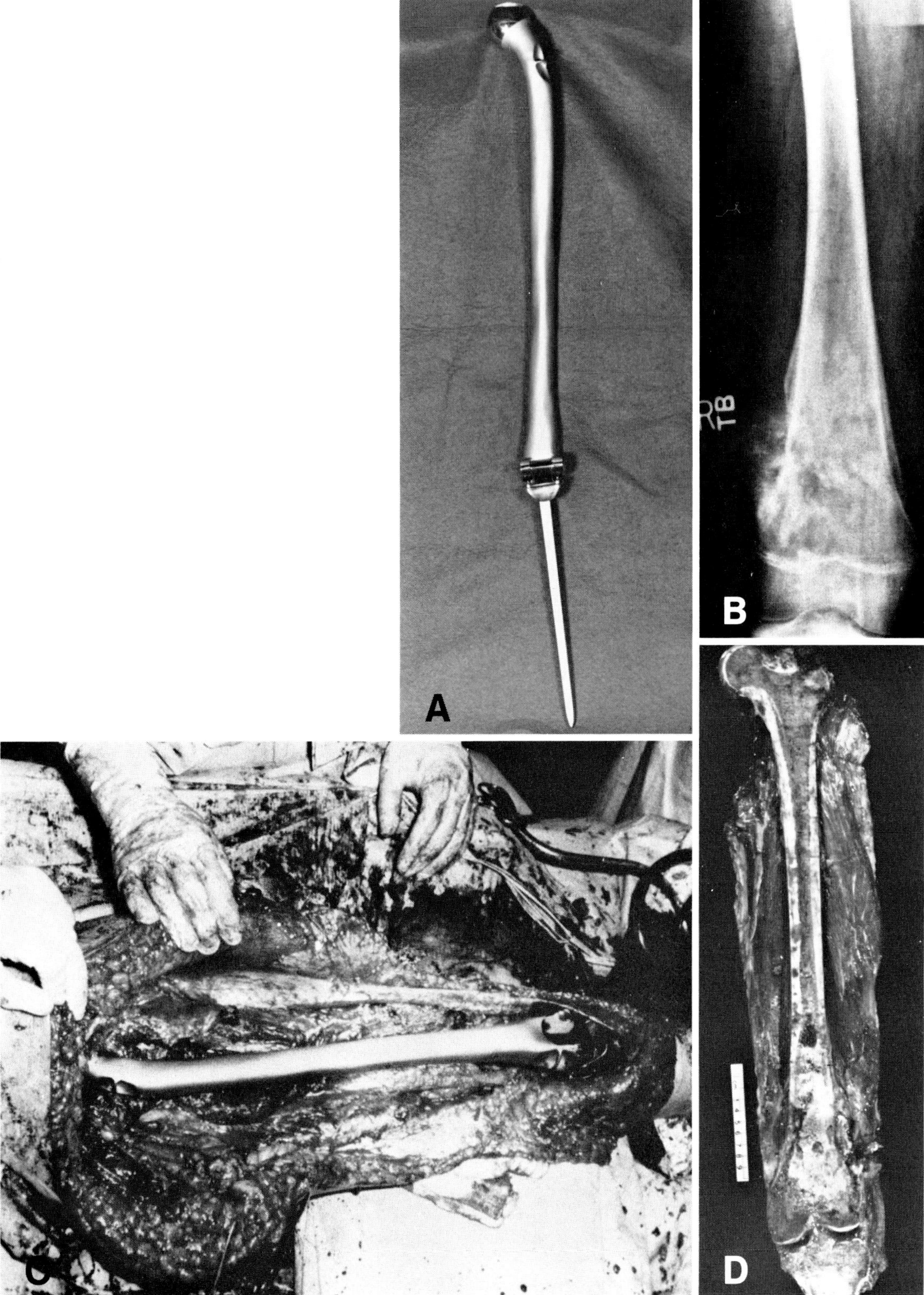

FIG. 15-1

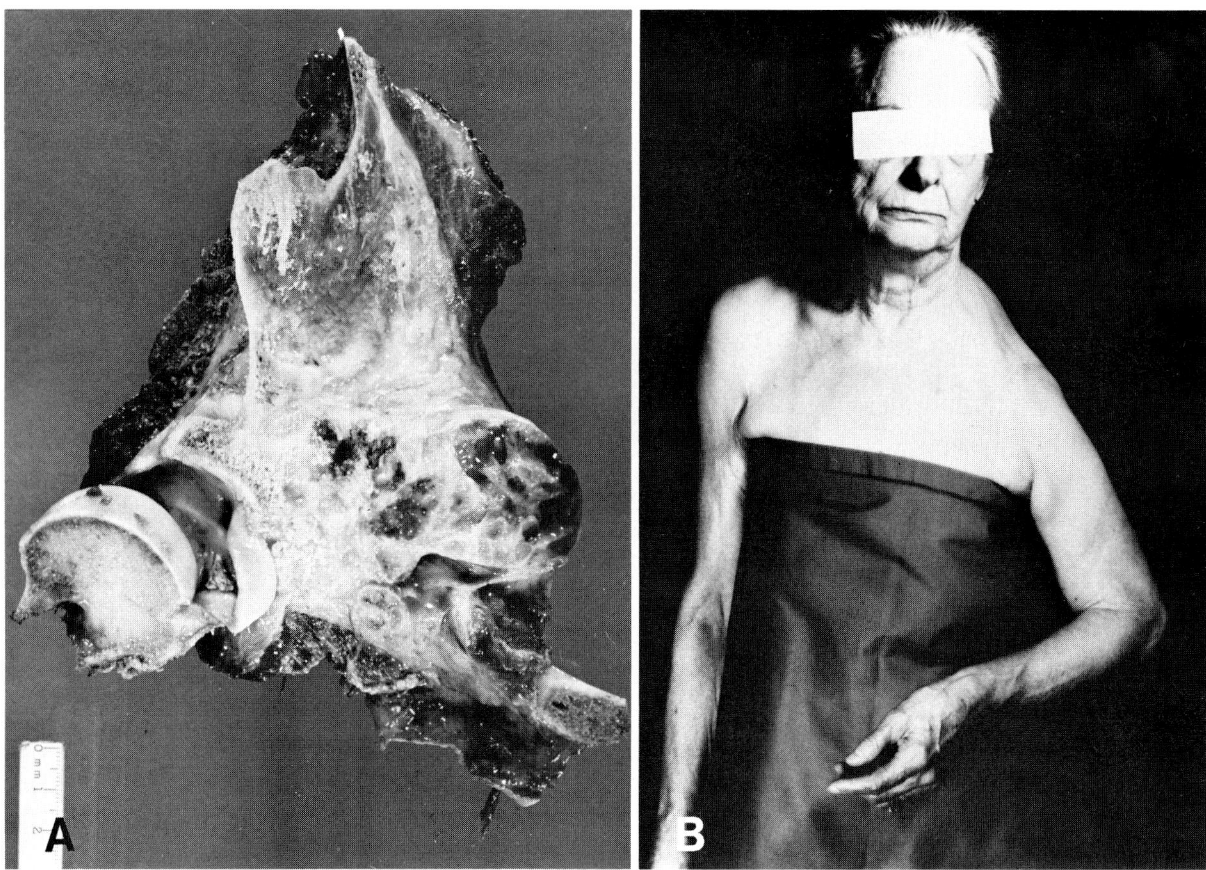

FIG. 15-2

Tikhoff-Lindberg Resection for Chondrosarcoma

FIG. 15-2. The Tikhoff-Linberg procedure (interscapulo-humeral resection) for resectable malignant tumors of the shoulder girdle. (*A*) Cross section of the specimen. Note the chondrosarcoma of the scapula, the humeral head, and complete joint to the left. (*B*) The patient retains excellent function but cannot lift her arm over her head. She has been disease free for 5 years.

FIG. 15-3. Tikhoff-Linberg procedure for osteosarcoma. (*A*) Note the large blastic osteosarcoma of the proximal humerus in this young boy. (*B*) Post chemo- and radiotherapy the en-bloc excision was performed. In this case the tumor can be seen close to the lateral margins. Microscopy did not show invasion beyond the small cuff of muscle over it. However, in such cases the soft-tissue component could be frozen first to reduce the risk of viable tumor spillage before proceeding to resection. (*C*) Postoperative radiograph. Note a small hole (*arrow*) at the top of the remaining humerus. Through this site, muscle and ligament is placed to give proximal support to the bone. (*D*) Note the excellent functional result. This patient is now free of disease with a 5-year follow up.

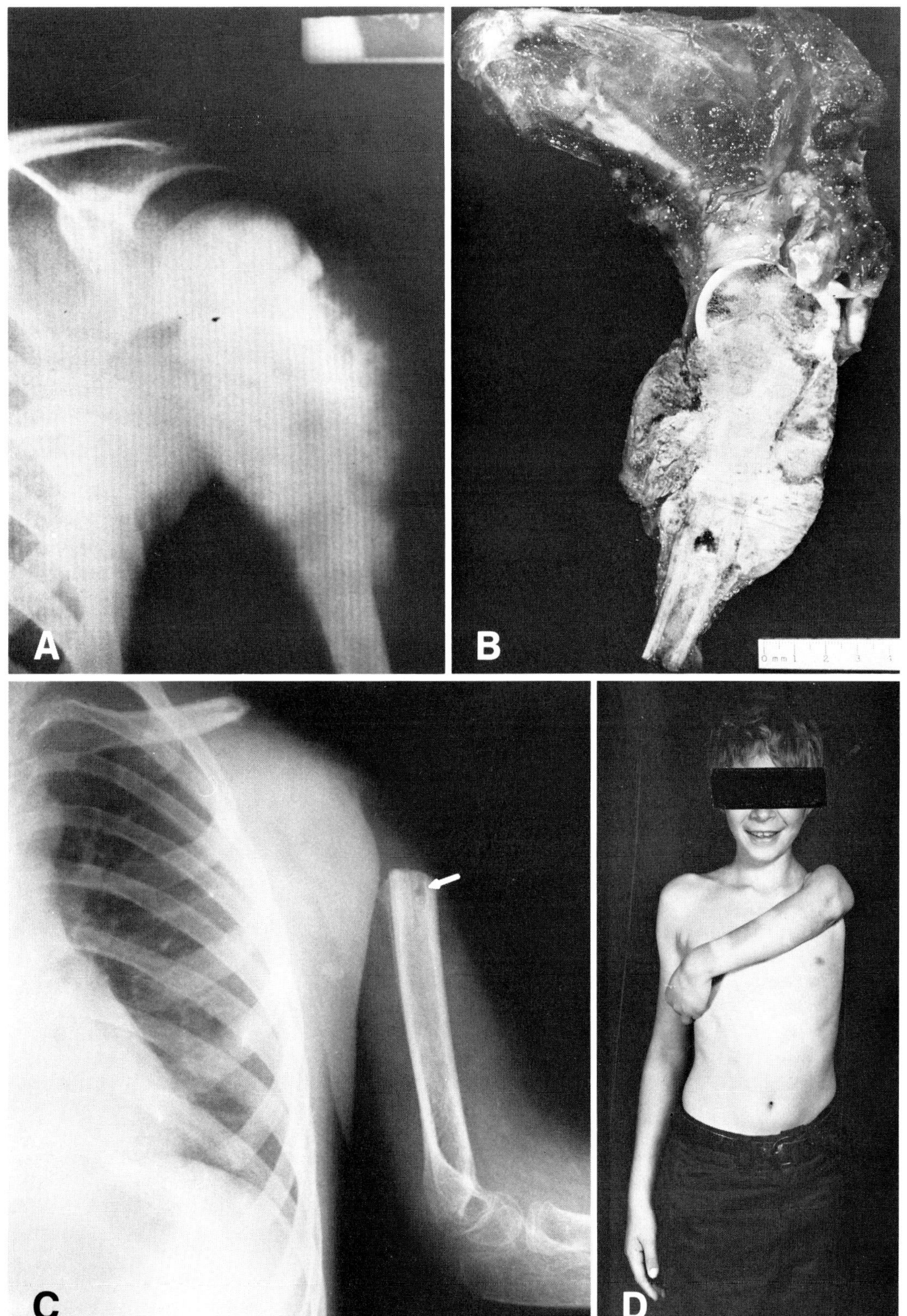

FIG. 15-3

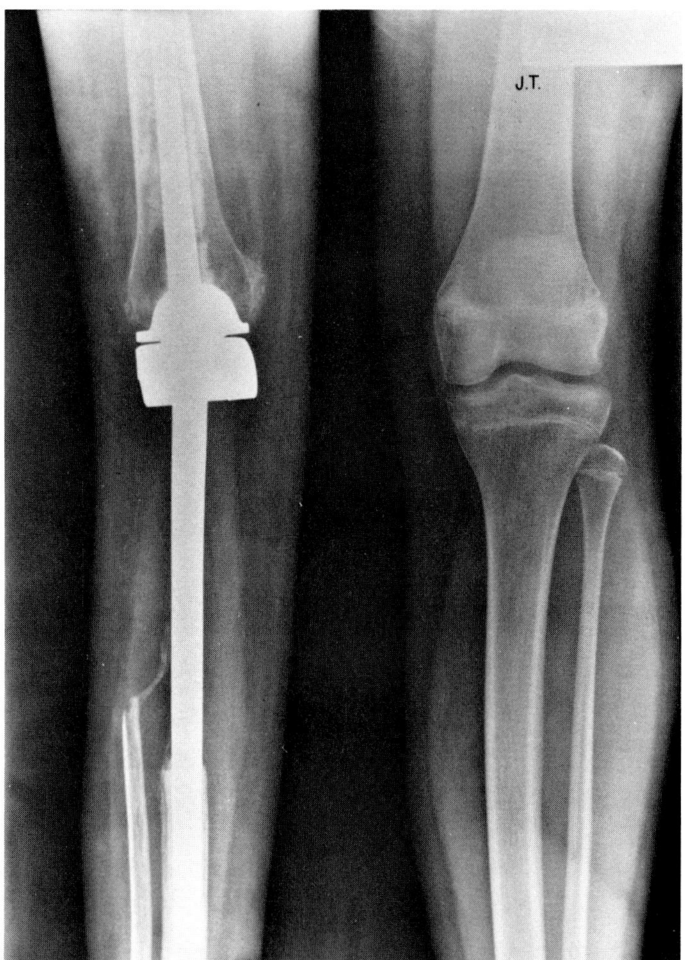

Prosthesis Replacement for Osteosarcoma of Tibia

FIG. 15-4. Long-stem total Guepar knee endoprosthesis post-en-bloc resection of an osteosarcoma of the proximal tibia. Note that a portion of the distal femur, joint, and a large block of tibia and fibula were removed along, of course, with an adequate soft-tissue margin.

right fibula. Further workup and arteriograms showed that resectability of the tumor was possible (Fig. 15-5, *A*). She was given the chemotherapy regimen and had surgery performed after a frozen section biopsy.[34]

OPERATIVE TECHNIQUE. A long-skin incision was made from above the knee joint to the ankle, leaving a segment of skin directly overlying the tumor. Skin flaps were developed anteriorly and posteriorly. Dissection was deepened. Again, the tumor was never encountered, and a 2-cm. normal margin was left over the tumor. The lower fibula was diarticulated at the ankle mortise. Using an osteome, a rim of tibia above and medial to the tibio-fibula joint, including part of the lateral tibial condyles, was removed en-bloc with the specimen. Thus, an "en-bloc" of the whole of the fibula was removed with the tumor, tibio-fibula joint, and a wide surrounding margin of muscles; the common peroneal nerve and two of three lower limb arteries were ligated. A long-leg plaster-of-paris cast was applied with the ankle in the neutral position and was kept on for 6 weeks. Later stress views showed no instability.

RESULTS. Because of persistent fluid collection, chemotherapy was delayed for 2 months postoperatively. Vincristine, methotrexate, and citrovorum fac-

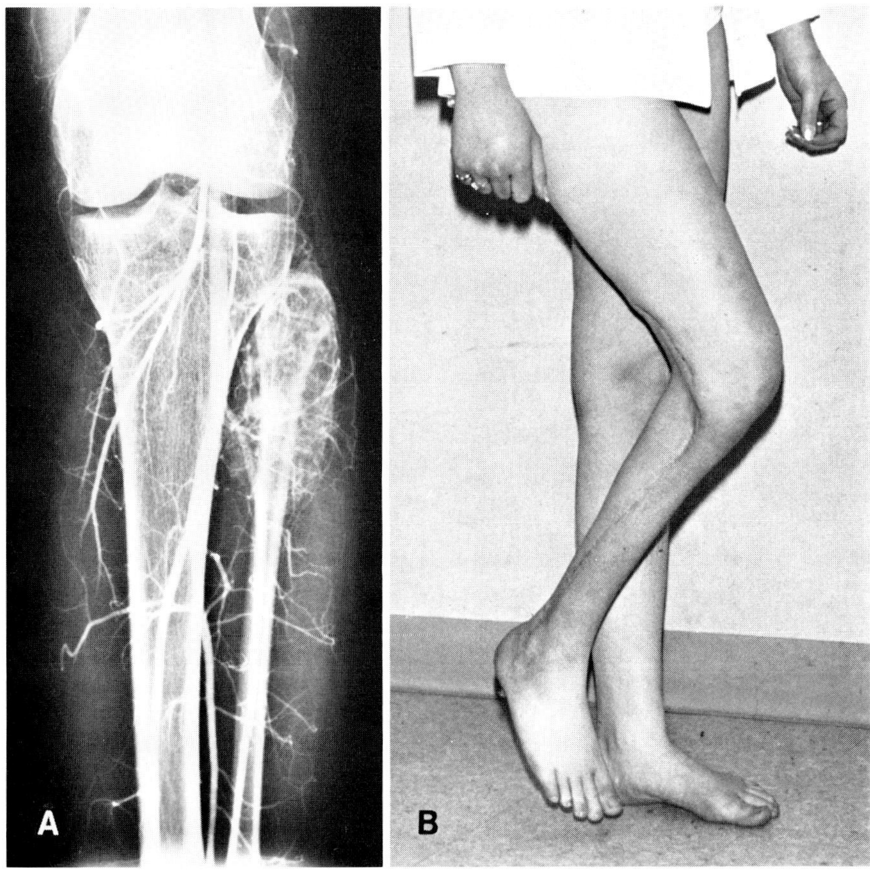

Resection for Osteosarcoma of Fibula

FIG. 15-5. Osteosarcoma of fibula. (*A*) An arteriogram more clearly shows the extent of the lesion. Surgically it appeared resectable. (*B*) Note the excellent result. This patient subsequently required a total knee operation for a small nodule seen in the tibia. The results were still excellent and she has been free of disease for 5 years.

tor was given according to our protocol for 1 year.[51,52,53] A nodule did, however, develop inside the upper tibia; the upper tibia was then removed en-bloc and a Guepar total knee with long-stem prosthesis was inserted. She is doing well almost 5 years since the original operation and has good stability of the ankle joint. The residual capsule as well as the lateral ligaments contribute to the lateral stability of the ankle joint (Fig. 15-5, *B*).

The Treatment of Pulmonary Metastasis in Intermedullary Osteosarcoma

Since 1969 the bone service at Memorial Hospital has encouraged the thoracic service to resect solitary or multiple pulmonary nodules after amputation, provided that no other bones were involved, no other organ systems other than the lungs were involved, and the resections appeared possible.[39,36] Other authors who have studied the effect of resection of pulmonary metastases under special circumstances include Gleidman, *et al.*, and Higginson.[15,19]

By aggressive wedge resections it is meant that all visible lung metastases are removed with as sufficient an amount of healthy tissue around it as possible to contain the tumor. At the same time, however, it is important to also conserve as much healthy lung tissue as possible, for obvious reasons.

It was found that after primary amputation, of those patients who developed pulmonary metastases and were left untreated, only 5 per cent survived for 5 years pre- or postoperative lung metastases. After 5 years, however, 31 per cent of patients treated with aggressive wedge resections are still alive.[39] Of those who died, 80 per cent developed disease in sites other than the lung. This appears to be the single largest factor in lung resection failure. Some 18 per cent of the patients with 5-year follow-ups appear free of disease; almost all of these patients would have died had not these procedures been performed. (In the light of previous studies only 2% would have been expected to survive.) With the advent of chemotherapy these statistics are improving even more dramatically (Dr. Marcove, unpublished observations). This is because chemotherapy kills the local tumor and shrinks nodules, which permits greater conservation of lung tissue mass.

Our present attitude in the treatment of pulmonary metastases is that the local lesion should be first brought under control; then bilateral thoractomies should be staged and, if possible, multiple wedge resections performed, unless there are signs of inoperability, such as involvement of the primary bronchial tree, myocardium, diffuse pleural involvement, positive pleural cytology, or distant metastases to other organs.

The largest number of nodules yet removed in a surviving patient was 11, although one patient who had 21 nodules removed died of a pulmonary embolus and at autopsy no residual tumor was found anywhere.

CRYOSURGERY

DEFINITION. Cryosurgery is defined as the use of repetitive freezing of lesional tissues to at least $-20°C$ during surgery. It is usually applied directly to a neoplasm to cause its complete necrosis.

HISTORY AND THEORY. In 1964, Marcove, *et al.*, treated the first bone tumor patient by cryosurgery. The patient had painful metastatic lung carcinoma that spread to his humerus. After two courses of x-ray therapy his pain was unrelieved. Post-cryosurgery relief of pain was complete. In 1966 Gage published a study of cryosurgery in laboratory animals in which the freezing was accomplished by wrapping a tube in a coil-like fashion around a bone.[62] Through this tube, liquid nitrogen was circulated at $-196°C$. He demonstrated bone necrosis and subsequent bone regeneration periosteally and endosteally. Marcove and Miller were able to demonstrate similar bone necrosis and subsequent bone regeneration in the dog as well as the human.[68] Bone necrosis occurs at $-20°C$ or colder.[63] In Marcove's and Miller's experience the region of bone necrosis includes not the 81 per cent of the radius of ice from the "heat sink" predicted by Jennings, but only 50 per cent of the radius of ice from the "heat sink."[68] The heat sink refers to the area immediately surrounding the liquid nitrogen, which may be in a coil, spray tip device, or funnel.

Factors involved in the spread and freezing of the bone are vascularity, density of the bone, presence or absence of a tourniquet, size and temperature of the heat sink, rate and duration of freezing, as well as thawing, and the presence of cryoprotective molecules.

The plan of treatment is to reduce the temperature of the tumor to at least $-20°C$.[63,73] Freezing and thawing is done at least three times to ensure necrosis. This is best monitored by thermocouples. Tumor recurrences are due to incomplete exposure to liquid nitrogen. One can necrose tumor cells as deep as 2.5 cm. from the cavity wall, which leaves the surrounding bone *in situ* attached as on autograft. This method kills cells beyond the limits of usual surgical curettage. To achieve a similar extent of tumor destruction without cryosurgery one would have to remove the neoplasm en-bloc or amputate.

Originally, a double lumen probe was used. Recent instrumentation includes the open funnel technique or a tube with holes (spray technique) since a deeper freeze results with direct nitrogen contact.

The technique of cryosurgery in bone disease was originally applied to metastatic tumors with excellent local palliative results.[68] Cures could be obtained for solitary metastases such as the renal cell carcinoma. Eventually it became clear that the technique was also highly useful for many primary bone tumors, including the giant cell tumor, borderline enchondroma-chondrosarcoma, chondrosarcomas, Grades I and II, aneurysmal bone cyst, simple bone cyst, and others.

INDICATIONS. Marcove has used cryosurgery with excellent results in the following instances:

1. Large, recurrent, or stubborn locally aggressive benign tumors such as the aneurysmal bone cyst, simple bone cyst, and fibrous dysplasia.
2. All borderline or low-grade malignant lesions, Grade I sarcomas in which local cure is considered feasible (i.e., the tumors are small enough to be locally ablated by the cryosurgical procedure). These tumors include the giant cell tumor, juxtacortical osteogenic sarcoma, borderline or atypical enchondroma, chondrosarcoma, Grades I to II, and low-grade fibrosarcoma.
3. Solitary metastases in which clinical evidence of

dissemination is ruled out, such as in renal cell carcinoma and thyroid carcinoma.

4. Metastatic lesions for relief of pain (often when internal fixation is needed anyway). Since tumor cells frequently penetrate the pseudocapsule, it should never be visible or transected at any time during the procedure.

5. To "sterilize" those areas of the bone and soft tissue in which the potential for cutting through viable tumor is significant. It may be used before en-bloc excision if that is to be performed as an alternative to a major ablative procedure. If frozen tumor is found at the margin at the time of cryosurgery, continue refreezing the area until a pathologically tumor-free site is obtained. When this is achieved, the full extent of the en-bloc excision is determinable without violating the principle of tumor sterility. The odds of spreading viable tumor in the wound tissue are greatly minimized by this combination of a cryosurgical en-bloc resection approach. In other words, freezing at the proposed margin cut sites could provide the surgeon with a frozen area of safety, which can be extended if found to be tumor-infested.

Methods

CLOSED TUBE TECHNIQUE (FIGS. 15-6 AND 15-7). Although the authors' experience with the closed-tube liquid nitrogen cryosurgical technique is not extensive (14 cases), over 800 operations have been performed by the spray and open-funnel technique. It has been Marcove's observation that the extent of freeze and the degree of necrosis is less with the closed-tube technique compared to the two others. This is probably a result of layers of insulation that develop between liquid nitrogen and tumor such as the intervening metal and any layers of water and ice that form on the metal surface.

There are, however, certain situations where a probe may be ideal, such as when the extent of tumor is limited, the tumor in a limited (phalanx) or dangerous site (cervical vertebrae and other spinal bones), and when local control of the freeze is essential. Dr. Mirra, upon seeing a hazardous giant cell tumor of a C–2 vertebral body, suggested this limited technique to a neurosurgeon (Dr. R. Rand), who had experience with this technique in the treatment of brain tumors. The lesion was entered through a pharyngeal approach and frozen three times at multiple sites. In order to ensure adequacy of treatment, the patient was also treated with 4500 R. Three years later healing is excellent. A similar patient with a C–2 GCT treated by 6000 R alone has had a continuously destructive, recurrent and life-threatening lesion after 3 years follow-up. She has to be supported continuously with a neck brace in order to prevent transection of the spinal cord. The spinal cord of the first patient was protected against the dangers of freezing by placing thermocouples in the region of the cord. (These observations have been submitted for publication.) To our knowledge this case represents the first time cryosurgery has ever been applied to the spine area (excluding the sacrum).

SPRAY TECHNIQUE. In this technique liquid nitrogen is sprayed from holes at the end of a probe. Its particular advantage is that the temperature of the local area drops quickly and the spray blows any liquid or blood from the area, reducing their warming effect. Some therapists prefer this method of cryosurgery and claim to have good success.

FUNNEL TECHNIQUE (FIG. 15-8). This is the preferred method of the author. All available radiographs, tomograms, biplanar arteriography, CAT scans, and bone scans, if deemed necessary, should be reviewed prior to operation. The skin and subcutaneous tissue is then incised for as long as considered necessary and retracted widely to protect them from the effects of freezing necrosis. Normal, healthy tissues such as muscle, fascia, nerves, and vessels should be retracted until the surgeon approaches close to the pseudocapsule of the tumor. The surgeon should never dissect down to the pseudocapsule of a malignant lesion because the danger of tumor spillage into the wound is too great. This is avoided by careful palpation and experience. Following the incision spreaders are used to retract the normal tissues widely, and the funnel is placed over the center of the tumorous area. Test with water to see if there is leakage at the funnel-bone contact area. If not, continue the operation with the pouring of the liquid nitrogen. If it does leak, seal the funnel end with a moistened gelfoam sponge in which a hole has first been cut out slightly smaller than that of the funnel tip opening. Pour the liquid nitrogen slowly into the area to see if there are any leaks (Fig. 15–9). If there are none add the liquid nitrogen slowly until all the gelfoam, funnel, and tumor area form a solid block of ice. One can then let go of the funnel and it will not move (Fig. 15–10). At that point, liquid nitrogen can be poured one-half the way up funnel. This will result in a gradually advancing frozen area. One can then follow the extent of freeze by observing the extent of ice forming beyond the rim of the funnel (Fig. 15–11). If no ice is seen, then freezing has not occurred. Thermocouple application can be used to aid or monitor the extent and depth of the freeze. One can either aim

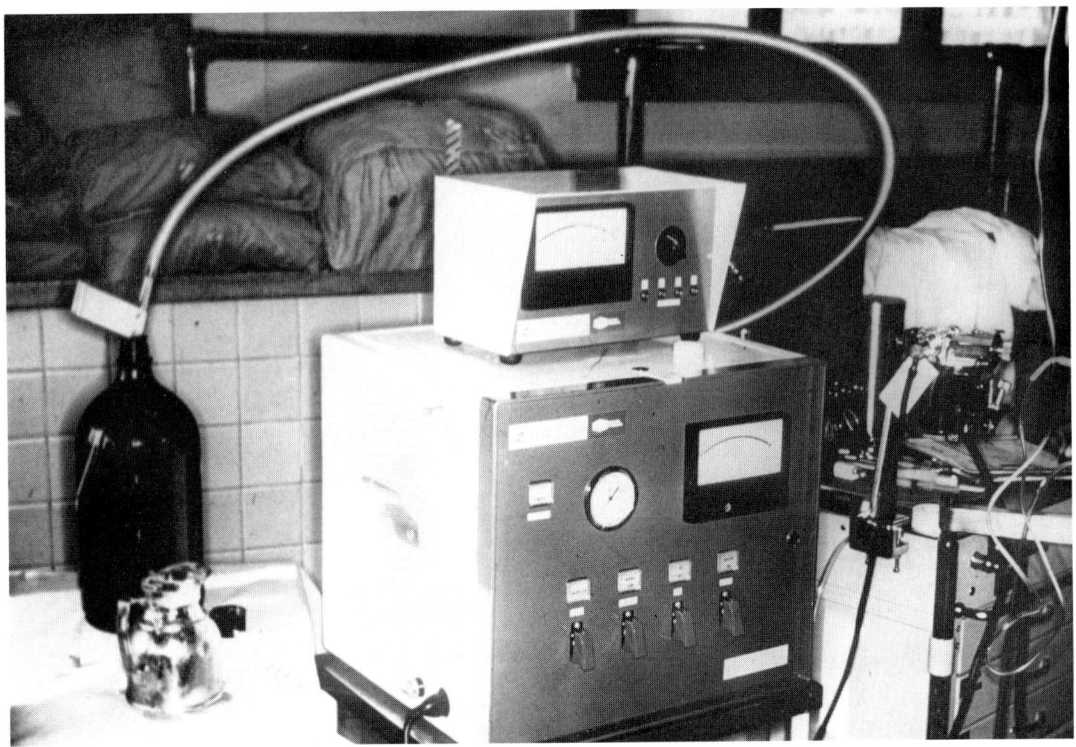

Cryosurgery

FIG. 15-6. Cryosurgical probe instrument that is supplied with thermocouples (Linde Corporation). This instrument is particularly useful for smaller tumors (smaller than 2–3 inches) and may be useful for tumors in inaccessible sites, such as cervical vertebral body lesions. If a cervical body is to be frozen, the cord must be protected against freezing by using appropriately placed thermocouples.

for a single freeze at $-60°C$ (usually applicable to only limited areas) or for three freeze cycles at $-20°C$. This method can freeze an area up to 6 inches in diameter, depending on the size of the heat sink (funnel size). Both methods have been shown to completely necrose tumors. A biopsy can then be obtained by chipping through the block of ice. The biopsy will usually show only minimal cytologic distortion. This method of freezing is particularly useful for seedable tumors (any sarcoma) and for highly vascular tumors, such as the aneurysmal bone cyst or metastatic renal cell carcinoma.

Giant Cell Tumor: Case Example

A specific example will illustrate as fully as possible the technique of cryosurgery. Again it is stressed that each case may need various modifications, depending on the size of the tumor, type of tumor, grade, location, and other factors. Most of the modifications

(*Text continues on p. 596.*)

Cryosurgery

FIG. 15-7. Surgical drawing illustrating the use of the cryoprobe. Liquid nitrogen circulates through it at $-196°C$.

FIG. 15-8. Marcove's application of the use of cryosurgery for the treatment of bone tumors using the funnel technique, through which is poured liquid nitrogen. For benign lesions, the tumor can be curetted first and then frozen, as shown here. For malignant neoplasms, the tumor should never be exposed until after freezing to prevent viable tumor spillage into the wound and contamination of instruments.

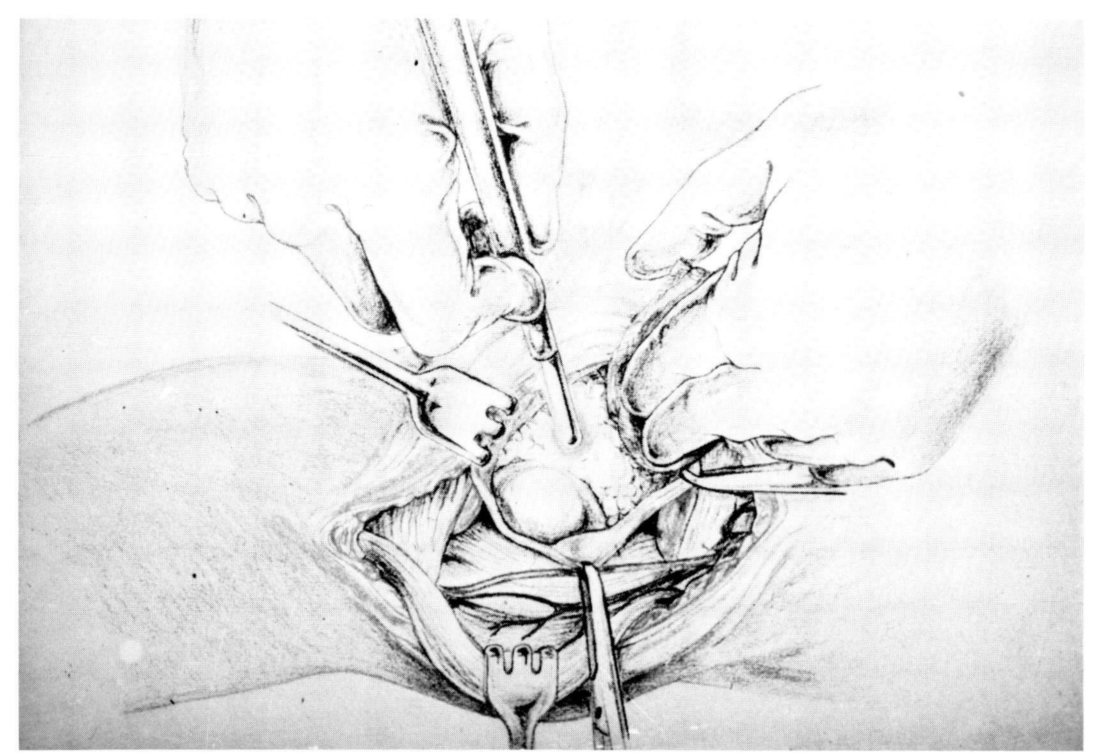

FIG. 15-7

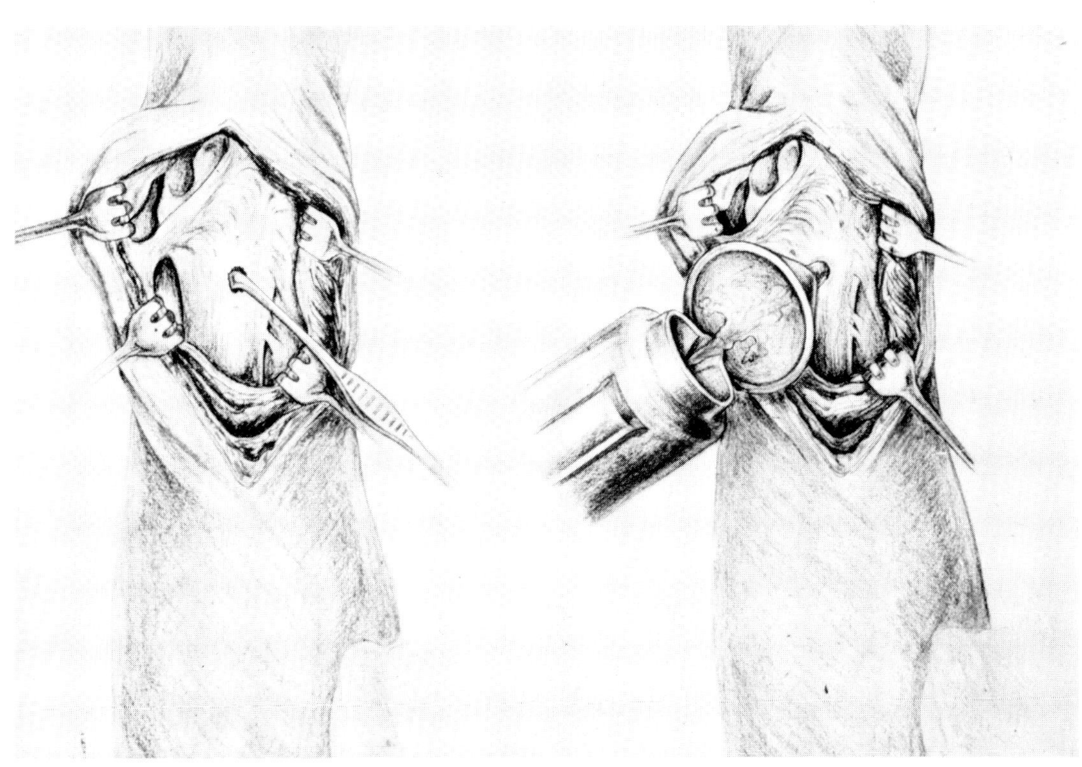

FIG. 15-8

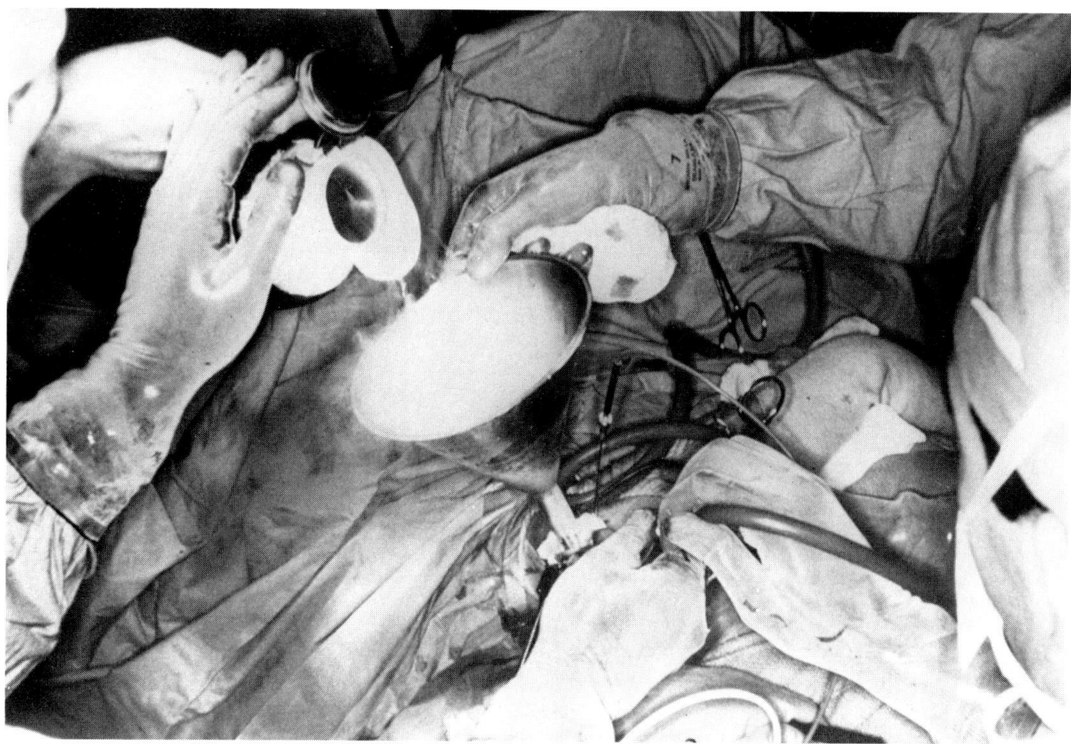

FIG. 15-9

Cryosurgery

FIG. 15-9. The funnel has been placed over a piece of moistened gelfoam with a hole slightly smaller than the funnel. Marcove now uses wider funnel mouths to increase the size of the "heat sink," which increases the size of the initial "ice ball" for larger tumors (over 3–4 inches). After the seal is tested for leakage, more liquid nitrogen is poured in while the assistant holds the funnel (shown here). Within a couple of minutes, a small ice ball will form; the assistant then releases his hands. The funnel should stay in place. It should not be touched again during freezing in order not to break the seal. (If that occurs, liquid nitrogen would spill into the wound and freeze normal tissues.) The tip of the suction catheter used later to aspirate the frozen tumor can be dipped into the liquid nitrogen in the funnel to ensure tumor sterility.

FIG. 15-10. Note the newer wide-mouth funnel, gelfoam seal, and underlying bulging muscle mass. In this case, a rim of benign muscle was left, because a highly malignant tumor is underneath it. In this way, the tumor is frozen and killed without viable spillage into the wound. Note also the massive swelling of the muscle from the beginning effects of freezing.

FIG. 15-11. Note the large size and obvious nature of the ice ball. It is through the 1 inch hole that the curettage of the tumor will be performed. One should not curet beyond 50 per cent of the diameter of the ice ball (approximately −20°C at this region), or one may enter into frozen but possibly viable tumor. After curettage, the technique can be repeated, extending the size of the ice ball and tumor kill. The process is usually done at least three times. The edge of the ice ball is only 0°C. Thermocouples can be used to monitor temperature. Concomitant with freezing, the tourniquet is applied to reduce the warming effects of blood flow. The surrounding normal soft tissues are constantly bathed in room temperature fluid to avoid unnecessary damage from the freezing. The fluid is frequently aspirated by a suction probe and repeated as necessary during the freezing procedures.

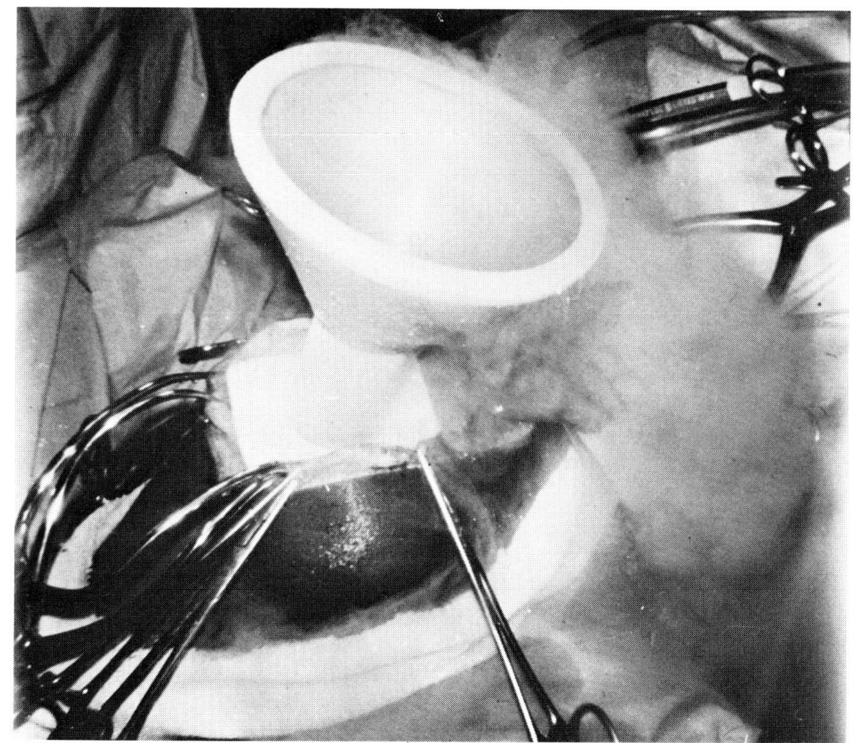
FIG. 15-10

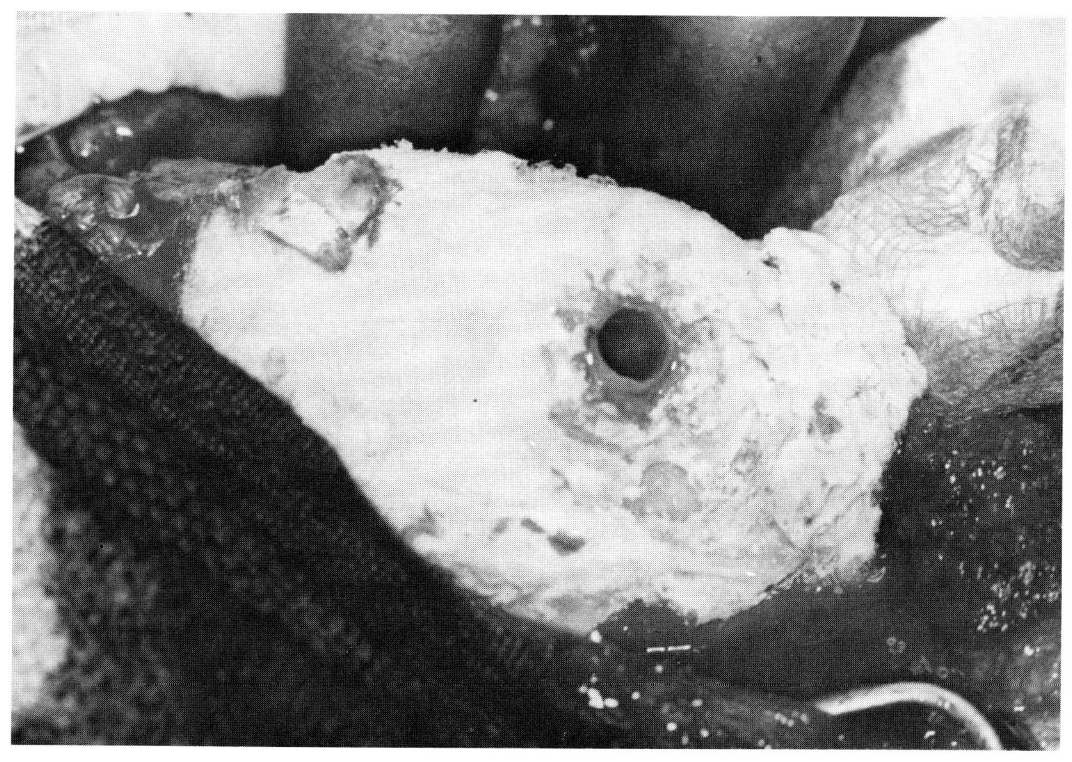
FIG. 15-11

relate to support of the area after freezing and curettage. In some cases bone struts, which are obtained from the fibula or pelvis, are put into place; in others, rush pins with methylmethycrylate. Also the patient's radiographs, biopsy diagnosis, age, and other factors go into the final decision-making process.

A 30-year-old female with an ordinary giant cell tumor of the proximal tibia was curetted 6 months previously. After the curettage the pain persisted (a good sign of recurrence). Serial radiographs showed unequivocal increasing destruction, and the patient was referred to Marcove. The lesion was at least 4 cm. in size. The patient was taken to the operating room, prepared, and a tourniquet placed on her leg above the lesion. Through a 20-cm. lateral incision, the muscles were split or freed and retracted widely. The region of the proximal tumor was carefully palpated for tumor and none was felt, although portions of the cortex of the tibia felt weak through the periosteum. Since the GCT rarely penetrates through the periosteum, it is safe to free the tissues, nerves, and vessels as much as possible and expose the periosteal surface of the bone area to be frozen without fear of entering the tumor. After following these steps, freezing was ready to begin. A large funnel with a 2 inch wide tip was decided to be used in this case (Fig. 15–10). The funnel tip was pressed over dry gelfoam to get its impression. The gelfoam was then cut about $\frac{1}{4}$ of an inch larger around this impression. The center hole was cut about 1 mm. smaller in diameter than the impression. The gelfoam was then moistened and placed over the central portion of the tumor (obtained by radiologic analysis, palpation, and bone percussion), where the cortex felt thinnest. The funnel was placed on top carefully. A small portion of saline, then liquid nitrogen was poured into the funnel to test for leaks. Leaks under the funnel or gelfoam will spill into the surrounding soft tissues and cause unnecessary excess freezing of these uninvolved tissues. The seal was good so that more liquid nitrogen was poured while holding the funnel steady. In 30 seconds or so the funnel and gelfoam was frozen to the surface and remained solid, no longer needing hand-held support. The funnel was kept $\frac{1}{2}$ full of liquid nitrogen. After 10 minutes or so an "ice ball" of 3 to 6 inches was seen. In the meantime and throughout all of the freezing periods, room temperature isotonic fluid was used to flood the surrounding soft tissues to reduce the degree of cooling. This fluid was removed by a suction tip device but prior to using it the device was "sterilized" by dipping it into the boiling liquid nitrogen in the funnel. Care was taken not to touch or jar the funnel, because the frozen seal is fragile and can be broken. After the visible ice ball formed, the pouring of liquid nitrogen was stopped. When it was fully evaporated the funnel was removed and the gelfoam scraped and washed away. One half of the diameter of the ice ball was then chiseled and curetted thoroughly. A portion of the frozen tumor was seen and sent to pathology for confirmation. After the frozen and thawed tumor was curetted, a new piece of gelfoam was cut, the funnel replaced on the moistened gelfoam, and the procedure repeated. The procedure is done two or three more times; malignant tumors should always remain within the confines of the previously attained ice ball until the curettage is found to enter normal fatty (yellow) bone marrow. Between each procedure the hole was flooded with room temperature isotonic fluid and suctioned out. The curettage was performed until the walls of the lesion were up to smooth cortical bone. All instruments used during curettage of the tumor were discarded to reduce risk of contamination. A 4- to 5-inch GCT will take approximately 1 to $1\frac{1}{2}$ hours to complete the freeze-thaw-curetting cycles.

As thawing continues observation was important, because all bleeders that had become evident were tied or cauterized. The degree of blood oozing can be reduced by the tourniquet and this is most helpful in obtaining a good freeze. Any large bleeding points in the bone are cauterized.

After the cryosurgery the lesion must now be strengthened to prevent collapse with stress. In this particular case Rush pins and acrylic were used instead of bone struts. Three holes were drilled in the strong part of the cortex and Rush pins inserted through the lesion to give added strength to the methylmethycrylate, which was subsequently packed into the defect. The tourniquet was released to be sure most of the bleeding had stopped. (Do not close the wound or proceed until the tissues are completely thawed or bloodless or leakage of blood into the wound will be a problem.) After the Rush pins were inserted, the methylmethycrylate was mixed and thoroughly placed into the hole. Small vent holes above and/or below the lesion makes packing easier. The wound was then closed after a final washing of the areas.

Advantages

The advantages of cryosurgery are as follows:

1. In a situation where cryosurgery is feasible one can leave anatomic structures intact which, of course,

is more favorable for the preservation of near normal function than tissue sacrificed in an en-bloc excision (Figs. 15–12, 15–13, and 15–14). The normal gait witnessed after cryosurgery for a primary giant cell tumor around the knee joint area, for example, compared to the klunky metallic clicking gait using a Guepar knee substitute or the obvious disability of a knee fusion, is indisputable.

2. There is less chance for violating the principle of tumor sterility or producing secondary tumor implants by using cryosurgery (where it is technically feasible), compared to en-bloc excision. In fact, the former method may make the latter possible. The author has treated a few local recurrences of GCT after previous bloc excision with total cure after a single cryosurgical procedure (obviously the function lost on the prior bloc excision persisted). In a large series of bloc excisions for GCT,[74,75] approximately 30 per cent eventually recurred or were advised to have later amputation because of various factors such as fracturing of graft or prosthesis, sepsis, or recurrence.

3. Blood loss with the use of cryosurgery can be minimized. For example, in a renal cell carcinoma metastatic to bone a bloc excision can lead to devastating hemorrhage. Renal cell carcinoma can be so highly vascularized that high output cardiac failure has been reported. After removal cardiac output returns to normal. In cryosurgery if the renal cell tumor is not entered until it is already a ball of ice, the blood loss is minimized. Acrylic packing afterward keeps the loss minimal.

4. The patient's bone is as an *in-situ* homologous bone graft when after 8 to 12 weeks new periosteal and endosteal bone growth ensues, which in time leads to excellent viable bone reconstitution (Figs. 15–12, and 15–13).

5. This procedure can be used as an adjunct to en-bloc excision if that approach is considered best applied over the most "dangerous" (possibly tumor-ridden) margin areas. For example, suppose an osteosarcoma is to be removed en-bloc post-chemotherapy and/or radiotherapy. If the saw cut goes through an unsuspected viable tumor-positive area of the bone, the principle of tumor sterility is abrogated and the limb should be amputated. However, if the area was first protected by freezing to −60°C, then even if one cuts through tumor the limb can still be salvaged, because nonviable tumor cells will have been broached. By repeating this procedure with an on-the-spot pathological backup until tumor-free margins are demonstrated, the excision can be performed adequately with minimum risk. (Of course, it's best to transect farther away in the first place.)

6. As previously mentioned, it can also be used for the treatment of solitary carcinomas and other tumors.

7. This reduces the hazards associated with high-dosage irradiation for control of a renal or thyroid carcinoma.

Dangers and How to Avoid Them

SPREADING VIABLE TUMOR IN THE WOUND PRIOR TO FREEZING. If the malignant tumor has broken out of the bone, freezing is started before one enters the pseudocapsular tumor area. Before freezing first palpate the tumor. Then take the spreaders and retract the normal tissue and place the funnel down on gelfoam, as discussed previously. Start the freezing. Observe the extent of freeze by the ice ball that forms (Fig. 15–11). If no ice ball is seen, inadequate "freezing" has occurred. Thermocouple monitoring may give further aid to the extent of the freeze. Aim for either one freeze at −60°C or three freeze cycles at −20°C. This method of freezing is particularly useful for seedable tumors (any sarcoma) and for very vascular tumors such as the renal cell carcinoma. In general, use the biggest size funnel hole to obtain the biggest heat sink that is feasible. The warming effect against the heat sink by oozing blood is reduced by using the tourniquet or local packing. If a 2-inch funnel hole is used, the diameter of the freeze zone can eventually be extended to a diameter of 6 to 7 inches and to a similar depth. The necrosis zone will be up to 3 to 4 inches.

FAILURE TO KILL ALL OF THE LOCAL TUMOR

LACK OF ADEQUATE FREEZING. For tumor cells to be killed in total, it is recommended that either three freeze and thaws at about −20°C or a single one at −60°C be performed. This area of kill based on these temperatures can be monitored by thermocouples. If thermocouples are not used, one must watch for an ice ball that forms a block of solid ice. The kill zone is within 50 per cent of the inside diameter of the visible ice ball. The edge of the ice ball will be 0°C and is often not a kill zone.

WARMING EFFECT OF BLOOD. Excessive bleeding will retard adequate freezing. During freezing the amount of blood to the tumor can be diminished by the use of a pneumatic tourniquet. Do not forget to release the tourniquet between freezes. Blood must be suctioned from the cavity as completely as possible after each curettage to avoid blocking off a portion of the space from contact with the liquid nitrogen. If blood clot is allowed to accumulate, a deep uniform freeze is not possible.

INADEQUATE AREA OF FREEZE. A good freeze will kill cells about 2 to 2.5 cm. from the curettage cavity. The best method to ensure that the tumor has been completely destroyed is when one reaches normal nontumorous marrow or other tumor-free margins such as articular cartilage. One can check for tumor-free margins by requesting frozen sections and/or imprint analysis of the thawed margin tissues looking for tumor.

NITROGEN EMBOLISM. *Danger:* Never occlude the egress of the liquid nitrogen from the hole in the bone. Do not place an obstructing object over the hole, such as a finger during freezing. If this is done lethal nitrogen gas embolism may be the result. In over 800 cases of freezing performed by Marcove where free gas outlet was permitted, there were no clinical symptoms of embolism or shock. In one case, obstruction of the exit of nitrogen converting to gas lead to lethal embolization.

SKIN NECROSIS. Long-skin incisions, wide retraction, and warming with physiological fluids around the wound and aspirating such fluid continuously protects against this hazard.

NERVE PALSY. Nerves may be frozen in the procedure. In treating malignant lesions major nerves may be too close to the tumor to risk the spill of tumor in order to retract them. The resultant palsy that develops has not been a major permanent disability, only a temporary one. The portion of the nerve that is frozen probably undergoes necrosis, but the nerve sheath remains intact. Since the nerve cell bodies are not destroyed the axons will regenerate and grow down the intact nerve sheath. Long nerves such as the sciatic may take up to $2\frac{1}{2}$ years before complete restoration of function. Shorter nerves may return to full formation in several months. Marcove has seen no permanent nerve palsy from among his 800 cryosurgical cases. Therefore, if there is a possible chance of entering and, therefore, spreading the tumor, do not dissect to retract the nerve.

POST-CRYOSURGICAL LOCAL HEMORRHAGE. The wound tissue must be observed after *complete thawing* to see if an arterial "pumper" has entered the tumor area. This will not be the case if the wound area is closed prematurely while the area is still frozen.

FRACTURE. In any tumor where the bone has undergone significant tumor destruction, the bone is prone to fracture. The cortical bone window through which cryosurgery is performed also increases bone fragility. The addition of cryonecrosis of bone further increases the risk. Therefore, it is important after surgery to avoid overly stressing the affected area. In order to prevent post-surgical fracture complication, the treated site may need local bone struts, internal fixation with or without pins, and methylmethacrylate, reinforcement. External supports are advised as well, including braces or cylinder casts and ischial weight-bearing braces. The external braces can be discarded after adequate radiologic evidence of healing. In contrast, in the author's opinion a Guepar knee prosthesis following en-bloc excision should have an ischial weight-bearing brace used permanently during ambulation.

Fibular struts used instead of bone chips are particularly helpful in preventing late fractures and their sequelae and to fixate fractures when they do occur (Figs. 15-12, *B*, and 15-13). Dr. V. Luck has illustrated the benefit of such struts many years ago! After cryosurgery it has been shown by histologic studies that new bone first develops along the periphery of the frozen residual bone.[68] This is seen as a sclerotic rind (Fig. 15-13, *A*) growing around the area previously treated. Weight-bearing should not be attempted before an adequate peripheral rind of bone development occurs.

INFECTION. In the early series of Marcove in 1973 (25 giant cell tumors), infections (up to 10%) were a problem. Since that time the infection rate has been

---

Cryosurgery for and Bone Grafting for Giant Cell Tumor

FIG. 15-12. (*A*) Recurrent giant cell tumor of distal femur (1969). (*B*) Three years post-freezing, the patient ambulates perfectly. Note the fibula strut to give support and the excellent rind or ring of host bone sclerosis, which gives additional corticomedullary support against fracture. The patient is still doing excellently 9 years post-surgery.

FIG. 15-13. Giant cell tumor (GCT). This patient had an extensive GCT of the ilium and acetabulum. Nine years postoperatively he is functioning excellently. Note the fibular strut (*arrows*) to give acetabular support to prevent protrusio acetabuli and the excellent bone healing, which forms a dense ring or collar of sclerosis around the former lytic lesional area.

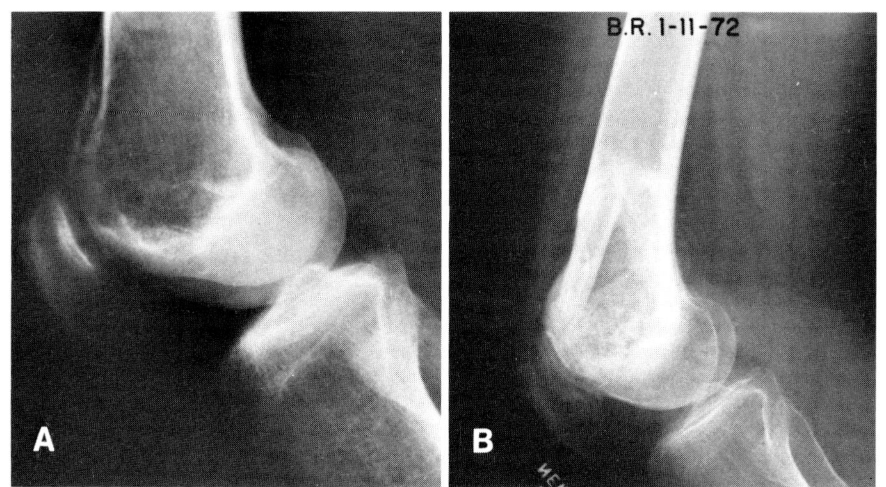

FIG. 15-12

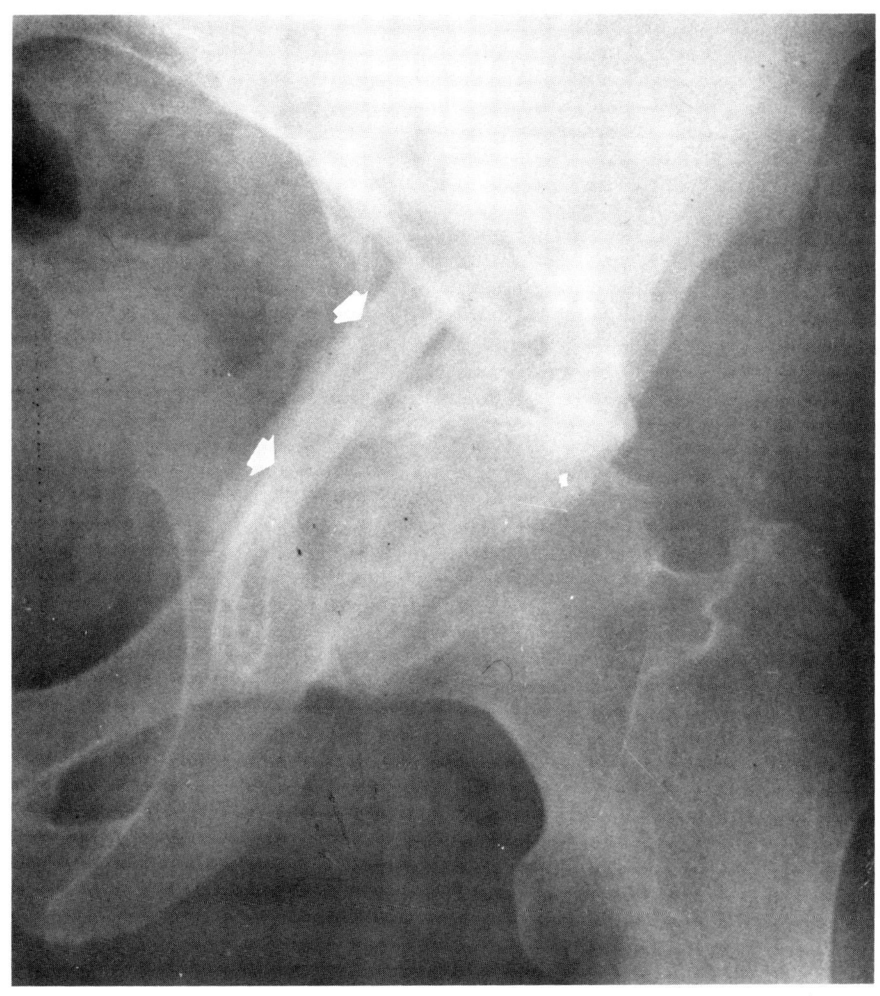

FIG. 15-13

reduced to less than 2 per cent. The explanation is not completely understood except for the fact that vigorous local and systemic prophylactic antibiotic therapy is started at onset of anesthesia and continued for 10 postoperative days in proper therapeutic doses. Also protection of the wound against necrosis by wide-skin retraction and flooding with room temperature isotonic fluids during cryosurgery may be another factor that reduces bacterial contamination.

Second Look Procedure

The "second look" post-freezing concept would apply to locally aggressive, borderline, and malignant tumors. In a benign tumor such as aneurysmal bone cyst, simple bone cyst, or fibrous dysplasia, a second look procedure is unnecessary. However, in all low-grade to borderline malignancies where cryosurgery is utilized, a second look can be extremely useful to ensure that cure has been complete. Waiting for gross radiologic or clinical signs of recurrence may increase the chances for residual tumor to grow, transform to a higher-grade malignancy, or to develop metastases. A second look procedure can show up any cases inadequately frozen at an earlier stage of development. Of course, if there are any signs of recurrence before the planned delayed second look procedure was contemplated, an immediate relook procedure is required anyway.

The planned second look timing is variable and depends on many factors but in general one should allow a minimum of at least 1 to 2 months for viable tumor foci to manifest themselves, contrasted to necrotic or healing foci. In the more slowly growing tumors such as GCT and Grade I chondrosarcoma a several month wait may be indicated before one could hope to grossly visualize recurrent tumor.

The factors that Marcove uses to guide his second look timing are as follows:

1. The pathologist's prediction of the rate of growth and metastatic potential of the tumor.
2. Bone sclerosis around the treated area usually follows healing based upon the development of reactive host bone sclerosis (2 to 6 months). If one sees early, rapid bone healing and the patient has no evidence of pain or tenderness, one may not want to do the second look at all.
3. Worrisome clinical setting: If there is continued, increasing or sudden development of pain and tenderness or lytic lesions developing on radiograph, one may elect to do an immediate second look procedure based upon the strong circumstantial evidence of recurrence.

Contraindications to the Use of Cryosurgery

1. Area too large to freeze: In Marcove's experience this would be an area of tumor 6 inches or larger using the present largest heat sink available. A giant funnel (heat sink) could be tried.
2. Substantial hazard of a poor functional result: On occasion en-bloc excision with prosthesis implant is more favorable than cryosurgery alone. This would apply to those cases in which the lesion is so large that there is too little normal residual bone left to expect a good functional result upon weight bearing. In these instances, en-bloc excision followed by large prosthesis insertion would be more advantageous. An exception to this rule would be where cryosurgery is used as an adjunct to en-bloc resection, because at times freezing allows the surgeon to come closer on resection to one particular area without fear of tumor implant. One can also, by this combined technique, save vital nerve and vascular structures that would be jeopardized by the extent of the en-bloc resection needed because of the large size of the malignant soft-tissue mass.
3. Inaccessible sites: Certain tumors may be inaccessible to cryosurgery because of their proximity to absolutely vital structures, as, for example, in the case of large cervicothoracic and upper lumbar epidural masses in which the danger of destruction of the spinal cord post-cryosurgery may be too great to risk.

Cryosurgery for Aneurysmal Bone Cyst

FIG. 15-14. *A–D* Aneurysmal bone cyst (ABC). (*A*) Massive ABC lesion. (*B*) One month post-freezing, note the organizing benign sclerosis of lesion. (*C*) Two years later, it is almost completely healed. (*D*) Five years later, very little residua is noted. The patient's hand functions normally.

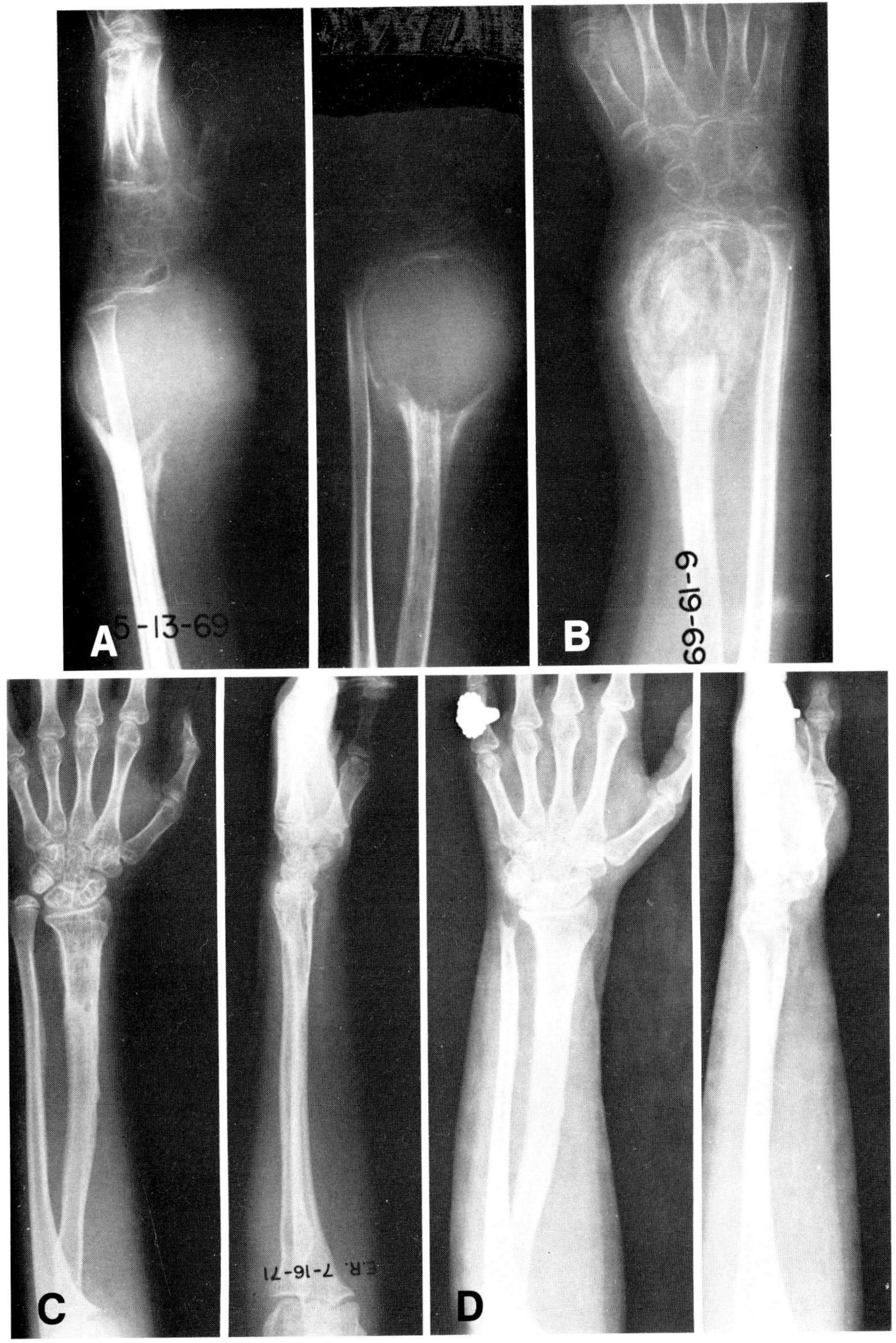

FIG. 15-14

Application of Cryosurgery to Specific Tumors

Giant Cell Tumor

Giant cell tumor is a highly recurrent lesion following curettage alone (over 55%). The local recurrences can cause so much local tissue destruction that amputation eventually becomes necessary in a significant proportion of cases (approximately 33%). Also with increasing numbers of recurrences the risk of a transformation into a more highly or fully malignant lethally metastatic tumor rises. Because of the very high recurrence rate and its associated dangers, Jaffe[77,78] concluded that a large en-bloc excision should be the initial therapy. Jaffe reversed himself following his personal study of cryosurgical case results (personal communication and speech to the American Academy of Orthopedics, 1968). Further experience has not only lead to the conclusion that 90 to 95 per cent or greater curability[72] with the usual preservation of good joint function (Figs. 15–12 and 15–13) is possible, but has also shown a marked decrease in the metastatic rate. Only one case of overt malignancy had been found from 52 GCT's treated by cryosurgery.[72] This number is about three standard deviations different from Jaffe's approximation of the metastatic rate for giant cell tumors of 15%, when they were treated by various modalities other than cryosurgery. A GCT in which the tumor has already fractured or has spilled into the joint cavity and soft tissues should be treated by en-bloc excision. Uncommonly, in highly exceptional cases when one encounters a giant cell tumor with a huge soft-tissue mass, certainly the quickest rehabilitation of that patient may be amputation.

Most patients who have a resection prefer to have a mechanical knee instead of knee fusion because most patients do not like to sit with their leg stuck out straight. In fact, on questioning patients with the Guepar in place and walking with a supportive ischial weight-bearing brace, no one has ever elected to have their knee fused, although there are orthopaedists who feel a knee fusion is preferable. If a knee fusion is planned, a straight, long Küntschner nail driven from the greater trochanter down to just above the ankle is an excellent method and has given quite successful fixation.

Results

The results obtained in the treatment of 52 cases of GCT by Marcove, *et al.*, are as follows:

RESIDUA AND RECURRENCES. Of the first 25 cases there were nine instances of residual tumor at the second look procedure.[72] In the subsequent 27 cases only three showed residua of viable tumor. In one of these cases there was a solitary lung metastasis. Six years following pulmonary-wedge resection the patient is alive and free of disease.

INFECTIONS. There was a sharp decline in the infection rate of the second series, compared to the first.[72] There was only one infection in this second group of 27 cases.

NERVE PROBLEMS. Temporary nerve palsies occurred in only four patients but there was eventual complete resolution and return of function.

SKIN PROBLEMS. Only one significant case of local skin necrosis, which delayed wound healing occurred in the second series of patients.

FRACTURES. There were five patients in the second series who developed fractures post-cryosurgery. One healed spontaneously, two required bone grafting, one needed internal fixation, and one infected fracture required bloc resection and knee fusion. Only one patient needed an amputation. This patient developed infection with pathologic fracture and single lung metastasis.

JOINT MOTION. In the second series, 81 per cent (17 cases) of the patients were salvaged without arthrodesis or prosthetic arthroplasty, although six cases did require additional bone grafting. The other four cases required one femoral head prosthesis replacement, one distal tibial endoprosthesis for joint deformity, one en-bloc resection and knee fusion for pathologic fracture and lung metastasis, and one total knee arthroplasty for pathologic fracture.

Summary

In evaluating the complications in these 52 patients, it is important to note that many of the cases were referred after other procedures had failed. Fifty per cent of the patients had undergone at least one unsuccessful previous surgical attempt at treatment and nine were subjected to multiple procedures. Most of the lesions were quite large GCT's, and 70 per cent involved the major weight-bearing bones of the knee. Because of these stresses the knee is an especially difficult area to eradicate the tumor while preserving function. The time needed for the bone to heal after cryosurgery is prolonged, because the tumors were large and the shell of surrounding bone thin. For this reason, as well as the bone necrosis, supplementary support is required during the healing phase. As a result, we no longer use weak, nonsupportive cancellous bone chips, instead either iliac or fibular strut grafts and/or methylmethocrylate occasionally surrounded by only grafts are inserted. This provides internal support to reduce the danger of postoperative fracture. Ischial weight-bearing braces are now used for extended periods after treatment until sufficient bone consolidation is appreciated. The earliest sign of bone healing has been peripheral sclerosis of the treated area seen on radiograph.

If special care is given to wide skin and subcutaneous tissue retraction, thorough irrigation and meticulous closure, as well as pre- and postoperative antibiotics, the incidence of serious infection should be less than 5 per cent.

Finally, in only one case of 52 was there evidence of disseminated malignancy (possibly a benign lung transplant?), resulting in an incidence of 1.9 per cent of malignant complications. This contrasts strongly to the former Memorial Hospital experience[76] of a 16 per cent fully malignant (lethal) complication rate. It is a distinct possibility that quick and thorough eradication by cryosurgery shortens the course of the disease and the time exposure interval during which a malignancy develops and obviates the need for radiation in many instances. Radiation has also been implicated in malignant transformation of the GCT.

Benign Tumors

Most benign tumors are treated by curettage. If the local destruction is extensive, the bone site may need bone struts or bone plugs in order to help the weight-bearing stability of the bone. However, benign lesions may recur. The worst offenders are usually the aneurysmal bone cyst (ABC) and the simple bone cyst (SBC). Approximately two-thirds of ABC's recurred in a Memorial Hospital series treated by curettage and/or radiation.[84] It is also well known that the SBC, particularly in children under age 10, may recur frequently. Fibrous dysplasia may recur and the latter may yield severe deformities, particularly in the region of the femoral neck, unless the varus deformity is overcome by a valgus overcompensation of the deformed femoral neck. With these recurrent benign diseases, cryosurgery has been, in our experience, a useful adjunct to supplement the usual curettage and bone packing. Indeed, in some situations the healing is prompt after cryosurgery and bone grafting may be unnecessary.

Aneurysmal Bone Cyst

Cure rates are particularly good post-cryosurgery in the treatment of the ABC. The recurrence rate has dropped from 66 per cent to 10 per cent (Fig. 15–14)[84]. In an analysis of the failure group, the obvious result was that very large lesions were not sufficiently frozen to be curative. In our recent cases we have had remarkably good results (unpublished observations, less than 5% recurrence rate).

Aggressive Chondroblastoma

We have also used freezing to cure an aggressive, local recurrent chondroblastoma that had developed 17 apparently benign lung implants. In this case we achieved a 5-year cure without evidence of residual disease. Other patients with similar problems have undergone amputation. We refer you to the reasons why we (Marcove, Mirra, and Huvos) decided against amputation. The main reason was that we believed that the lung "metastases" were not truly malignant but probably lung implants post-curettage (see pp. 226–234 and Figs. 8–86–8–89).[85]

Simple Bone Cyst

The recurrence rate is significant in children under age 10 (30–40%). It is very important to know that many "recurrences" are not recurrences at all but more likely a large residual hole left in the bone post-curettage. A true recurrence of a SBC is characterized by increasing size or destruction, radiologic evidence of bone chip resorption, increasing pain, tenderness, or swelling, and in most cases, refractures. Recurrence is best appreciated on the basis of progressive clinical symptomatology and not simply on a persistent "hole" in the bone. A bone cyst should not be deemed "recurrent" lightly, because if one follows nonsymptomatic operative cases, most do not refracture over the years. In contrast, the vast majority of primary or truly recurrent bone cysts undergo repeated fractures until surgery intervenes. The average number of fractures per patient before the surgeons operate is three.

Cryosurgery has been applied by the author to several cases of SBC with excellent results, but the number of cases is at this time too small to be certain of its residual effect on bone growth because of the bone cyst's proximity to the epiphyseal plate. We place a gelfoam sponge under the epiphyseal plate to minimize possible cryonecrosis. After cryosurgery healing is rapid and vigorous and does not usually require bone graft insertion. The latter, if autogenous, may give more pain than it is worth. At the present time we have not noted clear-cut evidence of epiphyseal plate destruction. On the other hand, Campanacci[84a] has shown a number of cases of SBC that have healed beautifully following the local instillation of steroids. Surgical intervention was not necessary.

If a bone cyst fractures and refractures many times, the patient may develop significant growth deformity, with lack of bone growth, and the head of the humerus may fall into a varus position. As a general rule, if the epiphyseal plate is destroyed at around the age of 10, there will be 1 inch of shortening, and if it occurs at around age 5, there will be 3 inches of shortening.

Fibrous Dysplasia

There are some who say that unless the defective periosteum is removed, the dysplastic process will not be stopped immediately. We have had no experience to confirm that statement. We have to date treated four cases of FD with cryosurgery with excellent results.

In order to treat an impending or resultant "Shepherd's Crook" deformity of the proximal femur we have done the following with great success:

1. Curretted the lesional area.
2. Frozen it.
3. Performed an osteotomy to place the femoral head in an overcorrected valgus position.
4. Placed bone struts (fibular or iliac crest) along the medial border to prevent the head from collapsing in varus.
5. Fixed the neck and head with a nail and plate to maintain the corrected valgus position.

Eosinophilic Granuloma

The younger the patient, the more likely will he have a disease of multiple bones. If the lesion appears solid or packed with cells at surgery, it is much more likely to recur than cystic- or degenerative-looking lesions.

Borderline Enchondroma, Chondrosarcoma, and Unequivocal Grade I to II Chondrosarcoma

Traditionally, adequate treatment of low- to medium-grade chondrosarcoma has consisted of either en-bloc excision or amputation. Chondrosarcomas are notoriously resistant to radiation and even chemotherapy. A number of atypical borderline cartilage "enchondromas" of long and flat bones are treated by curettage. Unfortunately, the bulk of these borderline "enchondromas" are in reality low-grade chondrosarcomas, a number of which have transformed from enchondromas. Biopsy of the enchondromatous areas leads to even more confusion when the tumor recurs in an obviously malignant fashion, usually within 1 to 2 years of curettage.

Once recurrence of chondrosarcoma occurs in an extensively curetted area, it is often hopeless to achieve cure without resorting to amputation. However, when borderline cartilage tumors and definite chondrosarcomas are treated initially by either an adequate en-bloc resection or cryosurgery, the incidence of disastrous recurrence is tremendously reduced. The advantages of cryosurgery, when it is feasible, compared to en-bloc resection, are as follows:

1. Decreased morbidity by saving patient bone stock and articular surfaces and with it, adjacent joint function
2. Irradication of tumors in areas inaccessible to en-bloc resection
3. Improved survival rates and lowered recurrence rates compared to en-bloc resection series. Marcove, *et. al.*,[88] have treated 18 patients with cryosurgery, seven of which were Grade I, and eleven, Grade II. Grade III tumors exhibit highly malignant behavior and metastasize early, particularly those with fibrosarcomatous or osteosarcomatous transformation (see Figs. 8-49–8-51) and require radical procedures.

Our protocol for treatment consists of cryosurgery of the tumor mass by the principles detailed earlier, followed by curettage and appropriate restorative procedures. Soft-tissue masses, when present, were frozen en-bloc with a small layer of normal tissue, usually with the funnel technique. All attempts should be made to include normal bone and soft tissues at the margins of freezing. Occasionally an entire neurovascular bundle that was deemed too close to the tumor to be safely freed was frozen as well.

The patient is then followed by clinical examination and radiographed every 6 to 12 months. Whenever possible, a "second look" procedure should be done within approximately 1 year of surgery to confirm absence of tumor. This should be done even if there is no clinical evidence of disease. Where there were worrisome clinical changes (persistent to increasing pain, poor healing, increasing lysis on radiograph), a repeat biopsy might be done immediately. If tumor is found on the second look, cryosurgery is repeated.

The results have been excellent. All Grade I cases are disease-free following only one cryosurgical procedure. Of the Grade II tumors, five had positive second look procedures. Four of these patients are now disease-free (one metastasized). Two of these five required en-bloc resection to supplement cryosurgery. The follow-up period on these patients ranged from 18 to 104 months (average, 65 months). The 7-year survival rate for these 18 patients is, at this time, 94 per cent. Even more importantly, the number of disease-free patients are also 94 per cent. (One did have metastasis but is still alive with disease.) In control series where one will see a recurrence of Grade I chondrosarcomas, 70 per cent of the recurrences will take place before the fifth year, even though rare cases may not recur until 15 years later.

In one patient who had a tumor of the lumbar region and sacrum, surgical excision would have required hemicorporectomy. Six months after cryosurgery, a second look demonstrated one suspicious area of residual tumor. This area was refrozen. Two years later no residual tumor was seen.

CHEMOTHERAPY

PRINCIPLES. Chemotherapy is being used today on an experimental basis in several large centers for the treatment of soft-tissue and bone sarcomas. It is being employed with increasing frequency in association with local ablative procedures for limb salvage with apparent success, compared to amputation and/or high-dosage radiation alone.[2,42,43,49,50,52]

GOALS. The present goals of chemotherapy are as follows: to slow down the rate of tumor growth and preferably to totally destroy subclinical or clinical metastases; to use as an adjunct with radiation and cryosurgery and/or en-bloc resection for limb salvage procedures; and to shrink or partially or completely necrose the primary tumor.

Application and Principles of Chemo- and Radiotherapy

Osteogenic Sarcoma[55a]

Several large institutions are using various combinations of potent chemotherapeutic agents in association with radiation and local ablative procedures. Most of the reported 1- to 5-year results show a substantial change in projected survivals, even disease-free states, compared to earlier surgical and/or radiation methods alone.[42,43,50,60]

The following sections give a description of the experimental approach and principles of chemotherapy we are at present using at the Memorial Hospital under Dr. Rosen's supervision. We had been using a fifth chemotherapeutic regimen referred to as Trial 5 (T_5), which basically consists of high dose methotrexate with citrovorum rescue plus vincristine; adriamycin, and cytoxan. Every 2 weeks the patients receive one of these three.

History of Chemotherapy Regimen[53,55a]

Initially we noted favorable responses with advanced osteosarcoma to high-dosage methotrexate (HDMTX) and citrovorum factor rescue (CFR). We noted the rapidity in which pain and swelling and tenderness decreased after administration of HDMTX. We also noted the return of the serum alkaline phosphatase (SAP) to normal. However, we also noted that the SAP would rise after 2 to 3 weeks in those patients with the most aggressive disease. Because of this we then began pulsing the HDMTX at 2- to 3-week intervals. These patients then usually eventually developed resistance to the drug. The addition of adriamycin increased the response rate and its duration. We then began alternating adriamycin with HDMTX and CFR giving each drug once a month, each drug being given separately and at 2-week intervals. This regimen produced objective clinical results in 54 per cent of the treated patients. With increased survival came the increased risk of cardiotoxicity to adriamycin cumulative doses. Children on our earlier regimen would accumulate 900 mg./M^2 of adriamycin in 1 year. It was then decided to incorporate cyclophosphamide into the treatment protocol in order to see if it might be useful in helping to control the disease and to aid in the continuation of chemotherapy at 2-week intervals for longer periods of time. We began with a dose of 40 mg./kg. of cyclophosphamide. This dosage was selected because administration of the drug on 1 day would lead to predictable hematologic depression 1 week later and allow us to continue with another drug treatment 2 weeks later. We later added vincristine on the day preceding HDMTX in a theoretically justified attempt to synchronize circulating cells in S—phase at the time of HDMTX administration. We found it useful to see the patient 1 day before HDMTX administration to check the integrity of renal function. This was basically our Trial 5 (T_5) approach.

METHODS. Prior to starting chemotherapy all clinical and pathologic data were reviewed. The patients then underwent evaluation to determine extent of disease; evaluation included stereo chest radiographs or full chest tomography, skeletal survey, bone scan with ^{18}F or ^{99}Tc-diphosphonate, biochemical profile, including serum alkaline phosphatase (SAP), intravenous urogram, and creatinine clearance. All patients received biweekly or monthly chest radiographs. Skeletal survey or bone scans were repeated at 3- to 6-month intervals.

Patients were originally started on chemotherapy after surgical ablation of the tumor. We now find it preferable to begin before surgery and not to operate until the alkaline phosphatase and bone scans revert to normal or near normal for the age. After the start of chemotherapy we test for renal, cardiac, and hematologic function (platelet count, electrocardiogram, hemoglobin, complete blood count). Prior to the administration of adriamycin, an EKG is performed as well as serum glutamic-oxaloacetic transaminase (SGOT) and creatine phosphokinase (CPK). If depression of "T" or "ST" waves is present, the EKG is repeated on subsequent visits until it returns to normal, because persistent EKG changes is an indication for withholding further adriamycin in patients who have had large cumulative doses.

A major toxicity of HDMTX is stomatitis. Severe stomatitis is treated by cleansing the oral mucous membranes with a solution of 3 per cent peroxide and mouth wash. Accompanying oral candidiasis is treated with mycostatin. Oral cellulitis is treated by the appropriate antibiotic to the cultured organism.

Bone marrow depression occurs at about 7 to 12 days after HDMTX and CFR are administered. Depression of WBC below 1500/mm. occurred in 15 per cent of patients. Depression of platelets below 100,000 were seen in 20 per cent of patients. If below 100,000, the patients were often given platelet transfusions, particularly to stem bleeding through the oral mucous membranes.

Adriamycin could produce nausea and vomiting on the day after administration. It would also cause marrow depression and mucosal ulceration on about the tenth day. Cardiotoxicity was carefully guarded against.

Cyclophosphamide, vincristine, and adriamycin are known to cause alopecia. All patients developed temporary alopecia on this regimen.

RESPONSE TO THERAPY.[52] The majority of patients demonstrated objective clinical responses. In one patient chemotherapy shrunk the tumor enough to avoid amputation. One patient had massive shrinkage of pulmonary metastases. At thoracotomy only necrotic tumor was seen.

SUMMARY. The greatest efforts of the treatment team should be directed toward increasing the cure rate in patients with osteosarcoma after the primary tumor has been surgically ablated. The data presented above emphasize the need for a multidisciplinary approach to the treatment of osteosarcoma. The surgical ablation of the primary tumor, utilization of thoracic surgery, chemotherapy to eliminate gross or subclinical lung disease, and the use of subsequent prophylactic chemotherapy may even lead to the salvaging of patients presenting with metastatic disease. However, it is likely that most such patients will eventually become resistant to therapy and will succumb. The latest results (1979) show an almost 75%, 5 year free of disease rate for osteosarcoma treated at Memorial Hospital.[55a]

New Regimen Approach and Other Data from Memorial Hospital, New York City[55a]

We are learning that Cytoxan is more effective if bleomycin and actinomycin D is added. Our Trial 7 (T_7) regimen uses bleomycin, Cytoxan, and actinomycin D in place of Cytoxan alone, as was used in the T_5 regimen.

We are finding the following to be giving us improved results (more massive necrosis of the tumor):

1. In younger children (under age 8), higher doses of methotrexate are necessary for extensive necrosis of local tumor and to prevent lung metastases.
2. We now delay amputation or en-bloc resection until after chemotherapy is started. We evaluate whether alkaline phosphatase is falling below normal, because this gives us a good clinical handle on the degree of tumor necrosis caused by chemotherapy. Also bone scans should revert to normal or near normal; both these improvements should occur within 2 to 3 months.
3. We then proceed to en-bloc resection, if that is feasible. If not, we amputate. If, upon study of the pathologic tissues, we do not find maximum necrosis (90% or better), we will go to higher chemotherapeutic dosages. We are achieving a statistically significant improvement of survival with this T_7 regimen, compared to the T_5 one.

PULMONARY METASTASES. The average time for lung metastases to show up post-amputation is 7.9 months. The average survival after lung metastases appear is 2.9 months. If pulmonary-wedge resections are performed, 30 per cent of patients live 5 years. Half remain disease-free. The contraindications to pulmonary-wedge resection are positive pleural effusion for malignant cells; massive unresectable lung involvement; the discovery at thoracotomy of pleural or intracardiac metastases; and metastases to sites other than lung (usually bone and/or brain). If, in performing the wedge resections, one does not achieve a tumor-free margin, the resection will fail, unless the tumor is 100 per cent necrotic. Pathologic examination should carefully assess margins and degree of tumor necrosis.

SUMMARY. The spread of disease is slower after age 10, but the overall cure rate is about the same, except for upper tibia and fibula lesions, where the cure rate is better. With distal femur lesions, metastases occur just as fast under or over age 10. Patients with a short or longer history of clinical symptoms prior to treatment had the same cure rate statistically.

Ewing Sarcoma

A maximum of 20 per cent of patients with Ewing's sarcoma are cured by amputation alone. Recent reports are showing a tremendous change in the survival rates of patients with Ewing's sarcoma.[20,27,49,52,58,60]

The discussion that follows is from the Memorial Hospital experience of Dr. Rosen,[49] in which the 5-year survival statistics of Ewing's sarcoma patients not presenting with metastatic disease is projected to be 75 per cent.

Background[49]

Initially our group had encouraging results with four drugs, including dactinomycin (actinomycin D), adriamycin, vincristine, and cyclophosphamide (the Ewing's sarcoma T_2 protocol). In 1967 Phillips and Higinbotham reported a superior 5-year survival using megavoltage radiation to the entire involved bone.[46] Many of these patients also received nitrogen mustard, dactinomycin, or Coley's toxin with nitrogen mustard.

MATERIALS AND METHODS. A total of 36 patients were treated. Prior to treatment all data and biopsy material was reviewed. Pretreatment evaluation included chest radiographs, skeletal survey or Tc diphosphonate or fluorine-18 bone scans, a lumbar puncture for tumor cells, urinary vanyl mandelic acid (VMA) and urinary catecholamines (to rule out metastatic neuroblastoma). A distant bone marrow was performed to rule out multifocal or metastatic Ewing's and to rule out lymphoma-leukemia, which may be confused with Ewing's sarcoma.

Treatment consisted of either surgical ablation to the entire involved bone or radiation therapy to the entire involved bone (5000–7000 R).

Radiation therapy to lungs for metastases was given to four patients. Two got whole lung irradiation (1400 R), one received 2100 R for hilar disease, and one, local irradiation for a solitary nodule. Two received radiation to existing bone metastases. Radiation was started concomitantly with the start of T_2 chemotherapy (dactinomycin). Patients having surgical ablation usually begin chemotherapy 2 to 3 weeks following surgery.

The T_2 chemotherapy protocol[55] was revised by deleting one of the two courses of adriamycin after two complete cycles. This was done to reduce cardiomyopathy. The dose of adriamycin was limited to a total cumulative dose at 600 mg./M^2. The dose was limited to 500 mg./M^2 if the patient were to receive incidental irradiation to the heart. Patients received this regimen for a total of eight complete cycles. Chemotherapy was completed in from 8 to 20 months. The interval between doses was 2 weeks. Delays were allowed only for persistent severe mucositis, severe bone marrow depression (WBC less than 2000), or platelets less than 100,000.

Patients received complete blood counts on the days of expected leukopenia or thrombocytopenia and bichemical profiles, monthly chest x-rays, bone survey, bone scans (every 3–6 months) for 3 years. Bone scan was used as an early indication of tumor response or possible recurrence. EKG's were done at appropriate times as described in the preceeding section to monitor cardiotoxicity to adriamycin.

RESULTS. Of the 20 patients who presented without evidence of metastases at 5 years, the actuarial disease-free survival is 75 per cent. Survivors were followed from 31 to 82+ months (median 42 months) from the start of treatment. No patient has relapsed after 36 months. One patient died of cardiac toxicity with no evidence of tumor at autopsy. Of the eight patients who did present with metastases, only one patient appears to be in complete remission following therapy.

Proposed Guidelines to Future Treatment of Ewing's Sarcoma

1. All patients should be individually considered with respect to age, size, expected future growth, size and location of tumor, and probable patient function should they survive the disease.
2. Moderate dose radiation with surgery for the primary tumor is advocated in patients with pelvic disease where excessive pelvic irradiation would cause extreme difficulty of bowel and bladder function and where local recurrence is

high. No patient with a primary ilial or ischial tumor has survived, although two with sacral tumors have been successfully treated with radiation.

3. Young patients with proximal femur lesions where "curative" x-ray therapy might lead to unacceptable hip flexion contracture might do better with moderate-dosage radiation to the total bone following resection of the most tumor-bearing proximal portion. In this instance we advocate preoperative chemotherapy to shrink and control soft-tissue extension. We also propose using an artificial endoprosthesis for the resected bone area.
4. Young patients with lesions about the knee (proximal tibia or distal femur) are initially amputated where the projected length discrepancy between the two knees would be excessive should they survive treatment of irradiation and chemotherapy for primary tumor control. Also they would probably eventually require amputation to ambulate properly anyway. (Unless it is feasible that epiphyseal plates are destroyed on the opposite side projected for an equivalent shortening [Dr. Mirra].
5. Patients with foot lesions where "curative" x-ray therapy would be expected to give poor function with painful gait would function better with surgical treatment to the primary tumor.
6. Chest wall (rib) lesions should be treated with preoperative chemotherapy, wide local excision, and postoperative irradiation (preferably with electron sources to avoid excess irradiation to underlying lung and/or heart).
7. Radiation therapy alone (6000–7000 R) to the entire bone with shrinking fields to spare uninvolved normal soft-tissue structures can be used in nonbulky lesions, including the long bones of the upper extremity and those at the lower extremity where projected leg length discrepancies will not be excessive.

GENERAL PRINCIPLES

Children under age 10 with tumor of the lower extremities would have so much growth inhibition post-therapy and eventual problems with fracturing that great disability is encountered. In these cases amputation and/or bloc resection gives a better quality of survival. However, in such instances we have begun using dactinomycin, adriamycin, vincristine, and cyclophosphamide without irradiation. This is given post-biopsy. At about 2 months post-chemotherapy we give a second look biopsy. If the tumor has decreased in size markedly, shows massive necrosis, and we see reversion to normal bone scans we may elect to perform an en-bloc resection of the involved area using our x-ray data and bone scans to determine the levels of cut. This radical surgery is easier to perform on the Ewing's sarcoma than on the osteosarcoma because the Ewing's soft-tissue component may often shrink completely post-chemotherapy. The en-bloc resection tissues are then thoroughly studied for the degree of necrosis. After en-bloc, 3500 R is given to the remaining entire nonresected bone area. In some cases study of the en-bloc resected tissue may show less than massive necrosis. If not, we advocate using other agents, such as HDMTX with CFR and others. Throw the book at the tumor, if necessary, in an attempt to eradicate all tumor cells. Otherwise the patient will surely not survive.

Other advantages of using chemotherapy followed by en-bloc resection is that the dangers of high-dose radiation effects, such as soft-tissue fibrosis, joint contractures, radiation necrosis, radiation osteitis with fracturing, delayed healing, nonunion and known local recurrence can be avoided. Those effects can be as high as 15 to 20 per cent in the field of high-dosage radiation. In addition, another hazard is radiation sarcoma, which may develop many years later in the survivor group.

One of our patients who had heavy radiation therapy 7 years ago must still use a permanent forearm brace because of repeated fracturing. The quality of survival of another patient with a similar condition treated later is much better. He was first treated by chemotherapy and then partial en-bloc resection of the obvious tumor-bearing area of the radius with insertion of a fibula bone graft. This was followed by a smaller dose (3500 R) of radiation to the remaining radial bone. This has yielded an arm close to normal and well functioning. All other radiation risks are now substantially reduced because of the much lower dosage of radiation being given. The parent of the child who had heavy irradiation, seeing the results of the other type of therapy, asked to have the radius removal and a metal one inserted, but we had to explain to her that surgery through such heavily irradiated area is too dangerous to be risked. We have used this modified approach in at least 10 more patients with similar good results (observations to be published).

Treatment Principles Applicable to Particular Tumors

The following discussion is based upon Marcove's personal experience with over 2,000 personally treated bone tumor cases. The techniques described herein are those that I have found particularly useful.

Metastatic Tumors

Long-stem total hip prostheses are particularly valuable especially with concomitant acetabular disease since the extent of weakened bone due to metastatic disease involvement is often much greater than expected by x-ray analysis alone. If there is acetabular metastatic disease, I advocate curetting the tumor, placing drill holes and placing in the acetabular cup with acrylic. If the tumor can be curetted well, it can be followed up by cryosurgery to destroy residual cells. X-ray therapy, if indicated, can be employed post-operatively to the surgically treated areas.

In tumors that involve the spine, instability is often the most crucial problem, especially if long-term survival is expected. If so, spinal fusion may be helpful before x-ray therapy is given. For example, an intertransverse process fusion can be done and x-ray therapy started 2 to 3 weeks later. The bone grafts usually heal promptly. However, if x-ray is given first, bone healing can be delayed up to 6 months or longer.

In cervical spine disease a posterolateral fusion of Robinson has been found to be very effective. It is much better than anterior fusion because of closer normal apposition to bone at the articular facet area; this means that the bone does not have to creep across intervals of disc at greater distances and an onlay bone graft in the posterolateral mass area can be wired into place and a midline laminectomy, if necssary, can be performed.

METASTATIC RENAL CELL CARCINOMA. This tumor requires special care. It is well known that up to 30 per cent of solitary renal cell carcinomas are curable by amputation if the primary tumor is also removed. With the application of cryosurgery, three out of four cases had a 5-year survival simply by freezing the metastasis *in situ* and thereby salvaging the limb. One case had late metastatic spread after the opposite kidney developed a second renal cell carcinoma. Normally, patients with multiple renal metastases succumb to death quickly. However, one of our cases had a rib and pelvic lesion. The rib lesion was en-bloc resected and the pelvis sacroiliac lesion was frozen. The patient is disease free 8 years later.

Much can be done to palliate patients with metastatic disease by either x-ray, chemotherapy, surgery, cryosurgery, en-bloc resection, and internal fixation devices in addition to the judicious use of acrylic. If there are wide gaps in the bone post-therapy, some form of added metal struts give reinforcement to added acrylic, since it is a particularly brittle substance and may fracture easily.

SPINAL BONE METASTASES. It is useful to perform myelograms prior to therapy in order to see the total extent of the disease, upon which the guidelines to therapy are based. In our experience, radiation therapy alone to these lesions is not nearly as effective as decompression laminectomy, perhaps followed by radiation. Many of the poor results reported in decompression laminectomy procedures appear to be due to the following:

1. Surgical therapy is delayed too long following onset of cord problems or paralysis.
2. The metastases were treated by other methods prior to surgical therapy. It is, therefore, not surprising why surgery has not been very successful under these circumstances.

There certainly is a place for laminectomy in early paralysis, provided that when decompression is to be performed in a dangerous area (e.g., in a region close to upper motor neurones), the patient is in a lateral position and has been given only local anesthesia. This yields much better results because there is less cord transection or crushing due to the maintenance of a protective muscle spasm during the operation. The cause of the irritability of the affected nerves can be readily identified by laminectomy done this way. When discussing this method with Bronson Day, he stated "This is very understandable particularly since all of the early laminectomies were done under local anesthesia." When patients are put under general anesthesia, which releases protective muscle spasm because the patient is turned to be put in place for laminectomy (e.g., face down), irreparable damage may be done by tumor to the cord before laminectomy can even be performed. We have done many cases with much better results as described above.

Prostate

Although prostate cancer may be very common after age 50, once it has metastasized to bone the survival is poor (15%, 5-year survival). Although stilbesterol initially relieves symptoms markedly, it has only a limited impact on overall 5-year survival statistics. It is my belief that these patients should have stilbesterol therapy supplemented by chemotherapeutic agents in maintenance therapy, such as vincristine or colchicine along with cytoxan. We use cytoxan gradually in increasing doses until the white blood count is between 2000 and 3000 cu./mm. The red blood count must be checked every 2 to 3 weeks.

Myeloma

In the management of myeloma most of the symptoms are orthopaedic in nature and an orthopedist should follow the cases closely for spinal instability, impending cord paralysis, which may indicate the need for myelograms and laminectomy and to help plan x-ray therapy ports or to do early fusion where instability can be predicted. Long-bone fractures should be promptly nailed to relieve pain and disability. The maintenance and care of a myeloma patient by a hematologist who does only peripheral bone marrows, neglects dysfunction of the long bones and spinal cord, and treats severe complications poorly that could be handled well by an orthopaedist is ludicrous. On the insistence of Coley and Francis at Memorial Hospital, myeloma patients are managed by a bone oncologist, because most maintenance chemotherapy can also be handled by these experienced people with help from chemotherapists when normal maintenance therapy of cytoxan, vincristine (or colchicine), or Alkeran cannot be further handled. The above medications are simply followed with maintenance of total WBC between 2000 and 3000 cu./mm. The periodic injection of toxic large doses of chemotherapeutic agents rather than the above described maintenance program does not yield as good palliation, in this author's opinion.

Solitary Myeloma and Lymphoma

The usual stated radiosensitivity to myeloma, in Drs. Marcove, Mirra, and Jaffe's opinion (personal communication) appears to be overrated. Therefore, if a patient has localized myeloma a local resection or local cryosurgery should be more curative, at least locally. Proper internal fixation can be done at that time and x-ray therapy can be added postoperatively if the surgeon, radiologist, and pathologist do not believe the tumor has been completely removed. The dismal survival of localized myeloma treated by radiation alone may well be due in some instances to the failure to ever control the tumor in the first place and by subsequent dissemination rather than by necessarily implicating a multifocal disease in every case. Similarly, even a solitary lymphoma and reticulum cell sarcoma, if inadequately locally treated, can become disseminated following inadequate local therapy and may not mean the disease is multifocal in nature and that the chance for survival is poor. This is obvious even in Ewing's sarcoma. Of course, these diseases may be handled by "adequate" radiation therapy because they do not generally show marked radioresistance. However, there are rare lymphoma radioresistant cases. The usefulness of second look biopsies in these diseases has not been established, but, perhaps is indicated especially where a good clinical response, such as soft-tissue mass regression, is not seen.

PATHOLOGISTS NOTE. Perhaps second looks should always be done to rule out viable tumor 3 to 6 months post-radiation. I have seen one case of solitary myeloma show persistent tumor cells for 19 years despite several local doses of radiation. Had cryosurgery or local ablative procedures been performed, the risk of disseminated disease should, upon sound theoretical principles, be reduced.

Osteosarcoma

Where a leg osteosarcoma is too large and a major vessel is involved, an arterial graft may be feasible if care is taken to preserve the long saphenous vein to allow for venous return. If this cannot be done, a distal arteriovenous (AV) shunt should be performed so that the arterial graft will not cause the vein to be thrombosed due to rapid blood flow through an AV shunt. The AV shunt can be closed later.

Where much tumor involves nerves, artery, and perhaps even skin, especially in the femurs where the prognosis is the worst, the whole bone should be removed. However, it is well known that if one can fit a prosthesis on a short upper femur stump, the prosthetic management is facilitated. The comfort of an upper femoral quadrilateral socket is much greater than the pelvic socket necessary for hip joint disarticulation. The energy expended on walking with a high, above-knee stump is much less than hip joint disarticulation (Canadian prosthesis). Therefore, although we remove the entire bone through the hip, longitudinal, posterior, and anterior skin flaps are made, along with salvage of significant lengths of muscles and the neurovascular bundles, as long as the muscles saved are not near the tumor area. The hamstring, adductor, and flexor muscles are sutured through drill holes of the distal shaft of a short Austin-Moore prosthesis (Fig. 15–15). The muscles are then sutured in along with gluteus medius and maximus muscles at normal resting length and in such a balance that the

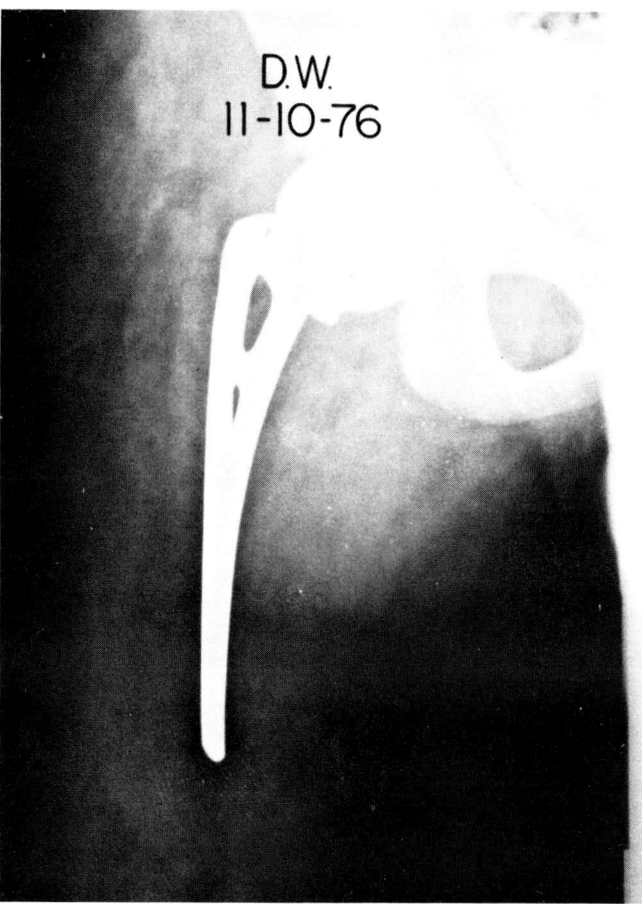

Prosthesis Replacement Post-Amputation for Improved Stump Function

FIG. 15-15. Marcove devised this operation to permit better ambulation in patients with large, unresectable, malignant tumors of the femur. The whole bone has to be removed in these cases. In essence, this is a modified hip joint disarticulation amputation procedure. However, by preserving uninvolved proximal muscle groups and their nerves and by sewing some of them into the prosthesis and modeling the large skin flaps and muscles into a cone shape, the patient can be fitted with a prosthesis and ambulate much better than is possible with the usual hip disarticulation amputation procedures.

prosthetic stumps will be in a functional position. This stump has motion and also serves to fit the quadriceps socket of the above-knee prosthesis and therefore overcomes the problem of whether or not to do a hip joint disarticulation. For, although skip areas up the femur are quite rare (in our experience, less than 2%) they do occur.

Pelvic Malignant Tumors

In selected cases, particularly after regression of tumor post-chemotherapy, bloc excision of various areas of pelvis may be indicated without doing a hemipelvectomy. It should be remembered that a highly malignant sarcoma seen near the sacroiliac joint usually involves the joint and goes through it. Therefore, bloc excision should also remove the alar sacrum. There may be special situations where invasion of this sacrum is obvious and where complete removal of tumor by the above described bloc excision is impossible. But after preliminary shrinkage with chemotherapy, a bloc excision may be possible and any residual tumor in the midline axial skeleton can then be treated by high-dose local radiation therapy. This method is much less dangerous than attempting to treat the original whole tumor with such high-dose radiation therapy.

REFERENCES

En-Bloc Resection, Pulmonary Resections, and Chemotherapy

1. Alexander, J., and Haight, C.: Pulmonary resection for solitary metastatic sarcoma and carcinomas. Surg. Gynecol. and Obstet., *85:* 129, 1947.
2. Beattie, E.J., Jr., Rosen, G., and Martini, N.: The management of pulmonary metastases in children with osteogenic sarcoma with surgical resection combined with chemotherapy. Cancer, *35:* 618, 1975.
3. Benjamin, R.S., Wiernik, P.H., and Bachur, N.R.: Adriamycin. A new effective agent in the therapy of disseminated sarcomas. Med. Pediatr. Oncol., *1:* 63, 1975.
4. Burnel, H.N.: Resection of the shoulder with humeral suspension for sarcoma involving the scapula. J. Bone Joint Surg., *47B:* 300, 1965.
5. Cambell, C.J., Cohen, J., and Enneking, W.F.: New therapies for osteosarcoma. J. Bone Joint Surg., *57A:* 143, 1975.
6. Codman, E.A.: *The Shoulder.* Brooklyn, G. Miller and Co., 1934.
7. Cortes, E.P. *et al.:* Dexorubicin in disseminated osteosarcoma. J.A.M.A., *221:* 1132, 1972.
8. Cortes, E.P., *et. al.:* Amputation and adriamycin in primary osteosarcoma. N. Engl. J. Med., *291:* 998, 1974.
9. Cortes, E.P., *et. al.:* Amputation and adriamycin in primary osteosarcoma. N. Engl. J. Med., *291:* 998, 1974.
10. Dahlin, D.C., and Coventry, M.B.: Osteosarcoma—a Study of 600 cases. J. Bone Joint Surg., *49A:* 101, 1967.
11. Edlich, R.F., *et. al.:* A review of 26 years experiences with pulmonary resection for metastatic cancer. Dis. Chest, *49:* 587, 1966.
12. Francis, K.C., Hutter, R., and Coley, B.: Treatment of Osteogenic Sarcoma. In Treatment of Cancer and Allied Diseases. Pack, G., and Ariels, I.M., eds. Vol. 8, pp. 374–399. New York, Harper & Row, 1964,
13. Francis, K.C., and Worcester, J.N.: Radical resection for tumors of the shoulder with preservation of a functional extremity. J. Bone Joint Surg., *44A:* 1423, 1962.
14. Freidman, M.A., and Carter, S.K.: The therapy of osteogenic sarcoma: current status and thoughts for the future. J. Surg. Oncol., *4:* 482, 1972.
15. Gleidman, M.L., Horowitz, S., and Lewis, F.: Lung resection for metastatic cancer. 29 cases from University of Minesota and a collected review of 264 cases. Surgery, *42:* 521, 1957.
16. Goldenberg, R.R.: Osteogenic sarcoma of the tibia with pulmonary metastasis. Report of a case with 10 year survival. J. Bone Joint Surg., *39A:* 1191, 1957.
17. Goldman, I.D.: The characteristics of the membrane transport of aminoprotein and the naturally occurring folates. Ann. N.Y. Acad. Sci., *186:* 400, 1971.
18. Gravanis, M.B., and Whitesides, T.E., Jr.: The unreliability of prognostic criteria and osteosarcoma. Am. J. Clin. Pathol., *53:* 15, 1970.
19. Higginson, J.F.: A study of excised pulmonary metastatic malignancies. Am. J. Surg., *90:* 241, 1955.
20. Hustu, H.O., Pinkel, D., and Pratt, C.B.: Treatment of clinically localized Ewing's sarcoma with radiotherapy and combination chemotherapy. Cancer, *30:* 1522, 1972.
21. Huvos, A.G., Rosen, G., and Marcove, R.C.: Pathologic aspects of primary osteogenic sarcoma treated by chemotherapy, en-bloc resection and prosthetic bone replacement. A study of 20 patients. Arch. Pathol., *101:* 14, 1977.
22. Jaffe, H.L., and Bodansky, A.: Diagnostic significance of serum alkaline and acid phosphatase in relation to bone disease. Bull. N.Y. Acad. Med., *19:* 831, 1943.
23. Jaffe, N., *et. al.:* Recent advances in the chemotherapry of metastatic osteogenic sarcoma. Cancer, *30:* 1627, 1972.
24. Jaffe, N., *et. al.:* Progress report on high-dose methotrexate in the treatment of metastatic bone tumors. Cancer Chemother. Rep., *58:* 275, 1974.
25. Jaffe, N., *et. al.:* Adjuvant methotrexate and citrovorum factor treatment of osteogenic sarcoma. N. Engl. J. Med., *291:* 994, 1974.
26. Janeck, C.J., and Nelson, C.L.: En-bloc resection of the shoulder girdle, technique and indications. Report of a case. J. Bone Joint Surg., *54A:* 1754, 1972.
27. Johnson, R.E., and Pomeroy, T.C.: Evaluation of therapeutic results in Ewing's sarcoma. Am. J. Roentgenol. Radium Ther. Nucl. Med., *123:* 325, 1971.
28. Lewis, R.J., and Lotz, M.J.: Medullary extension of osteosarcoma. Cancer, *33:* 371, 1974.
29. Lewis, R.J., Marcove, R.C., and Rosen, G.: Ewing's sarcoma: functional effects of radiation therapy. J. Bone Joint Surg., *59:* 325, 1971.
30. Linberg, B.E.: Interscapulo-thoracic resection for malignant tumors of the shoulder joint region. J. Bone Joint Surg., *10:* 344, 1928.
31. Marcove, R.C.: Neoplasms of the shoulder girdle. Orthop. Clin. North Am., *6:* 541, 1975.
32. Marcove, R.C.: New trends in the treatment of osteogenic sarcoma. Orthop. Digest., *3:* 11, 1975.
33. Marcove, R. C.: En-bloc resections for osteosenic sarcoma. Cancer Treatment Report, *62:*225, 1978.

33a. Marcove, R.C., and Huvos, A.G.: Cartilaginous tumors of the ribs. Cancer, *27:* 794, 1971.

34. Marcove, R.C., and Jensen, M.J.: Radical resection for osteogenic sarcoma of fibula with preservation of the limb. Clin. Orthop., *125:* 173, 1977.
35. Marcove, R.C., and Khafagy, M.M.: Total femur and knee replacement using a metallic prosthesis. Clin. Bull., *4:* 69, 1974.
36. Marcove, R.C., and Lewis, M.M.: Prolonged survival

in osteogenic sarcoma with pulmonary metastases. J. Bone Joint Surg., *55A:* 1516, 1973.
37. Marcove, R.C., Lewis, M.M., and Huvos, A.G.: En-bloc upper humeral interscapulo-thoracic resection—the Tikhoff-Linberg procedure. Clin. Orthop., *124:* 219, May 1977.
38. Marcove, R.C., Lewis, M.M., Rosen, G., and Huvos, A.G.: Total femur replacement. Comprehensive Therapy, *3:* 13, 1977.
39. Marcove, R.C., Martini, N., and Rosen, G.: The treatment of pulmonary metastasis in osteogenic sarcoma. Clin. Orthop., *111:* 65, 1975.
40. Marcove, R.C., *et. al.:* Osteogenic sarcoma in childhood. N.Y. State J. Med., *71:* 855, 1971.
41. Morton, D.L., Eilber, F.R., Weisenberger, T.H., Townsend, M., and Mirra, J.M.: Limb salvage using preoperative adriamycin and radiation therapy for extremity soft tissue sarcomas. Aust. N.Z. J. Surg., *48:* 56, 1978.
42. Morton, D.L., *et. al.:* Limb salvage from a multidisciplinary treatment approach for skeletal and soft tissue sarcomas of the extremity. Ann. Surg., *184:* 268, 1976.
43. Morton, D.L., *et. al.:* Adjuvant Chemotherapy in Melanomas and Sarcomas. Adjuvant Therapy of Cancer. Dalman, and Jones, eds. pp. 391–398. Amsterdam, North-Holland Publishing Company, 1977.
44. Pack, G.T., and Baldwin, J.C.: The Tikhoff-Linberg resection of shoulder girdle. Surgery, *38:* 753, 1955.
45. Parrish, F.F.: Allograft replacement of all or part of the end of a long bone following excision of a tumor. Report of 21 cases. J. Bone Joint Surg., *55A:* 1, 1973.
46. Phillips, R.E., and Higinbotham, N.C.: The curability of Ewing's endothelioma of bone in children. J. Pediatr., *70:* 391, 1967.
47. Pratt, B., *et. al.:* Cyclic multiple drug adjuvant chemotherapy for osteosarcoma. Proc. Am. Assoc. Cancer Res., *15:* 19, 1974.
48. Rosen, G.: The development of an adjuvant chemotherapy program for the treatment of osteogenic sarcoma. *In* Frontiers of Radiation Therapy and Oncology. vol. 10, pp. 115–133. Base, S. Karger A., 1975.
49. Rosen, G., *et. al.:* Curability of Ewing's sarcoma and considerations for future therapeutic trials. Cancer, *41:* 888, 1978.
50. Rosen, G., *et. al.:* Chemotherapy, en-bloc resection and prosthetic bone replacement in the treatment of osteogenic sarcoma. Cancer, *37:* 1, 1976.
51. Rosen, G., *et. al.:* High dose methotrexate with citrovorum factor rescue and adriamycin in childhood osteogenic sarcoma. Cancer, *33:* 115, 1974.
52. Rosen, G., *et. al.:* The rational for multiple drug chemotherapy in the treatment of osteogenic sarcoma. Cancer, *35:* 936, 1975.
53. Rosen, G., *et. al.:* Combination chemotherapy and radiation therapy in the treatment of metastatic osteogenic sacoma, Cancer, *35:* 622, 1975.
54. Rosen, G., *et. al.:* Disease free survival in children with Ewing's sarcoma treated with radiation therapy and adjuvant 4 drug sequential chemotherapy. Cancer, *33:* 384, 1974.
55. Rosen, G., *et. al.:* Vincristine, high dose methotrexate with citrovorum factor rescue, cyclophosphamide and adriamycin cyclic therapy following surgery in childhood osteogenic sarcoma. Proc. Am. Assoc. Cancer Res. and Am. Soc. Clin. Oncol., *15:* 172, 1975.
55a. Rosen, G., et. al.: Primary Osteogenic Sarcoma. The rationale for preoperative chemotherapy and delayed surgery. Cancer, *43:* 2163, 1979.
56. Samilson, R.L., Morris, J.M., and Thompson, R.W.: Tumors of the scapula. Clin. or thop., *58:* 105, 1968.
57. Sutow, W.W., and Sullivan, M.P.: Cyclophosphamide therapy in children with Ewing's sarcoma. Cancer Chemother. Rep., *23:* 55, 1962.
58. Sutow, W.W., Sullivan, M.P, and Feinbach, D.J.: Adjuvant chemotherapy in primary treatment of osteogenic sarcoma. Proc. Am. Assoc. Cancer Res. and Am. Soc. Clin. Oncol., *15:* 20, 1974.
59. Tefft, M., *et. al.:* Treatment of rhabdomyosarcoma and Ewing's sarcoma of childhood: acute and late effects on normal tissue following combination chemotherapy with emphasis on the role of irradiation combined with chemotherapy. Cancer, *37:* 1201, 1976.
60. Townsend, C.M., Jr., Eilber, F.R., and Morton, D.L.: Skeletal and soft tissue sarcomas: treatment with adjuvant chemotherapy. J.A.M.A., *236:* 2187, 1976.
61. Wilbur, J.R., *et. al.:* 4 drug therapy and irradiation in primary metastatic osteosarcoma. Proc. Am. Assoc. Cancer Res., *15:* 188, 1974 (Abstr).

Cryosurgery

62. Gage, A.A., Greene, J.C.W., Neiders, M.E., and Emmlings, F.G.: Freezing bone without excision. J.A.M.A., *196:* 770, 1966.
63. Jennings, J.W., Sr.: Production and control of low temperature in cryosurgery. Assoc. Operating Room Nurs., *7:* 1968.
64. Marcove, R.C., Lyden, J.P., and Huvos, A.G.: Giant-cell tumors of bone treated by cryosurgery. An analysis of 25 cases. *In* Latest Developments in Cryosurgery, International Congress Cryosurgery, 1972.
65. Marcove, R.C., Lyden, J.P., Huvos, A.G., and Bullough, P.G.: Giant-cell tumors treated by cryosurgery. An analysis of 25 cases. Proc. Natl. Cancer Conf., *7:* 951, 1973.
66. Marcove, R.C., Lyden, J.P., Huvos, A.G., and Bullough, P.G.: Giant-cell tumor treated by cryosurgery. A report of 25 cases. J. Bone Joint Surg., *55A:* 1633, 1973.
67. Marcove, R.C., Miller, T.R., and Cahan, W.C.: The treatment of primary and metastatic bone tumors by repetitive freezing. Bull. N.Y. Acad. Med., *44:* 532, 1968.
68. Marcove, R.C., and Miller, T.R.: Treatment of primary and metastatic bone tumors by cryosurgery. J.A.M.A., *207:* 1890, 1969.

69. Marcove, R.C., and Miller, T.R.: The treatment of primary and metastatic bone tumors by cryosurgery. S. Clin. N. Amer., *49:*421, 1969.
70. Marcove, R.C., Sadrieh, J., Huvos, A.G., and Grabstald, H.: Cryosurgery in the treatment of solitary or multiple bone metastases from renal cell carcinoma. J. Urol., *108:*540, 1972.
71. Marcove, R.C., Searfoss, R.C., Whitmore, W.F., and Grastald, H.: Cryosurgery in the treatment of bone metastases from renal cell carcinoma. Clin. Orthop., *127:*220, 1977.
72. Marcove, R.C., Weis, L.C., Vagbaiwalls, M.R., Pearson, R., and Huvos, A.G.: Cryosurgery in the treatment of giant-cell tumors of bone. A report of 52 consecutive cases. Cancer, *41:*957, 1978.
73. Rowe, A.W.: Biochemical aspects of cryo-protective agents in freezing and thawing. Cryobiology, *3:*12, 1966.

Giant Cell Tumor

74. Burrows, H.J., Wilson, J.N., and Seales, J.T.: Excision of tumors of humerus and femur, with restoration by internal prostheses. J. Bone Joint Surg., *57B:*148, 1975.
75. Goldenberg, R.R., Campbell, C.J., and Bonfiglio, M.: Giant-cell tumor of bone. An analysis of 218 cases. J. Bone Joint Surg., *52A:*619, 1970.
76. Hutter, R.V., *et. al.:* Benign and malignant giant-cell tumors of bone. Cancer, *15:*653, 1962.
77. Jaffe, H.L.: Giant-cell tumor (osteoclastoma) of bone: Its pathologic delimitation and the inherant clinical implications. Ann. R. Coll. Surg. Engl., *13:*343, 1953.
78. Jaffe, H.L.: *Tumors and Tumorous Conditions of the Bones and Joints.* Philadelphia, Lea & Febiger, 1958.
79. Johnson, E.W., Jr., and Dahlin, D.C.: Treatment of giant-cell tumor of bone. J. Bone Joint Surg., *41A:*895, 1959.
80. Marcove, R.C., Lyden, J.P., Huvos, A.G., and Bullough, P.B.: Giant-cell tumors treated by cryosurgery. Report of 25 cases. J. Bone Joint Surg., *55A:*1633, 1973.
81. Marcove, R.C., Weis, L.D., Vaghaiwalla, M.R., Pearson, R., and Huvos, A.G.: Cryosurgery in the treatment of giant-cell tumors of bone. Cancer, *41:*957, 1978.
82. Mnaymneh, W.A., Dudley, H., and Mnaymneh, L.G.: Giant-cell tumor of bone. An analysis and follow-up study of the 41 cases observed at the Massachusetts General Hospital betweeen 1925 and 1960. J. Bone Joint Surg., *46A:*63, 1964.
83. Parrish, F.F.: Treatment of bone tumors by total excision and replacement with massive autologous and homologous grafts. J. Bone Joint Surg., *48A:*968, 1966.

Benign Tumors

84. Biesecker, J.L., Marcove, R.C., Huvos, A.G., and Mike, V.: Aneurysmal bone cyst. A clinico-pathologic study of 66 cases. Cancer, *26:*615, 1970.

84a. Campanacci, M., De Sessa, L. and Trentani, C.: Scaglietti's method for conservative treatment of simple bone cysts with local injections of methylprednisilone acetate. J. Orthop. and Traumatol.,*3:*27, 1977.

85. Huvos, A.G., Higinbotham, N.L., Marcove, R.C., and O'Leary, P.: Aggressive chondroblastoma. Review of the literature on aggressive behavior and metastases with a report of one new case.
86. Tillman, B.P., Dahlin, D.C., Lipscomb, P.R., and Stewart, J.R.: Aneurysmal bone cyst: an anlysis of 95 cases. Mayo Clin. Proc., *43:*478, 1968.

Borderline Enchondroma, Chondrosarcoma, and Unequivocal Grade I to II Chondrosarcoma

87. Henderson, E.D., and Dahlin, D.C.: Chondrosarcoma of bone—A study of 288 cases. J. Bone Joint Surg., *45A:*1450, 1978.
88. Marcove, R.C., Stovell, P.B., Huvos, A.G., and Bullough, P.G.: The use of cryosurgery in the treatment of low and medium grade chondrosarcoma. Clin. Orthop., *122:*147, 1977.

INDEX

Numerals in *italics* indicate a figure, "t" following a page number indicates a table concerning the subject.